T0342410

Orthopedic Clinical Examination

Michael P. Reiman
PT, DPT, OCS, SCS, ATC, FAAOMPT, CSCS
Duke University Medical Center

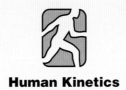

Human Kinetics

Library of Congress Cataloging-in-Publication Data

Orthopedic clinical examination / Michael P. Reiman, editor.
  p. ; cm.
 Includes bibliographical references and index.
 I. Reiman, Michael P., 1965- , editor.
  [DNLM: 1. Musculoskeletal Diseases--diagnosis. 2. Orthopedic Procedures--methods. 3. Physical Examination--methods. WE 141]
   RC925.7
   616.7'075--dc23

                    2015002523

ISBN: 978-1-4504-5994-5 (print)

The web addresses cited in this text were current as of August 2015, unless otherwise noted.

Acquisitions Editors: Madeline Gioja and Joshua J. Stone
Developmental and Managing Editor: Amanda S. Ewing
Copyeditor: Joy Wotherspoon
Proofreader: Red Inc.
Indexer: Susan Danzi Hernandez
Permissions Manager: Dalene Reeder
Senior Graphic Designer: Keri Evans
Cover Designer: Keith Blomberg
Photograph (cover): Digital Vision
Photographs (interior): Neil Bernstein, unless otherwise noted; © Human Kinetics, unless otherwise noted
Photo Asset Manager: Laura Fitch
Visual Production Assistant: Joyce Brumfield
Photo Production Manager: Jason Allen
Art Manager: Kelly Hendren
Associate Art Manager: Alan L. Wilborn
Illustrations: © Human Kinetics, unless otherwise noted
Printer: Walsworth

We thank the Duke University division of physical therapy at Erwin Square Plaza in Durham, North Carolina, for assistance in providing the location for the photo shoot for this book.

The video contents of this product are licensed for educational public performance for viewing by a traditional (live) audience, via closed circuit television, or via computerized local area networks within a single building or geographically unified campus. To request a license to broadcast these contents to a wider audience—for example, throughout a school district or state, or on a television station—please contact your sales representative.

Printed in the United States of America   10   9   8   7   6   5   4   3

The paper in this book was manufactured using responsible forestry methods.

Human Kinetics
1607 N. Market Street
Champaign, IL 61820
USA

United States and International
Website: **US.HumanKinetics.com**
Email: info@hkusa.com
Phone: 1-800-747-4457

Canada
Website: **Canada.HumanKinetics.com**
Email: info@hkcanada.com

                                                                              E6010

This text can be dedicated to no one other than my wife, Kim, and two great kids, Carly and Seth. Not only have you three provided me with the time and availability to undergo this huge endeavor, but you have steadfastly believed in me. I could not have completed a text of this magnitude and quality without your support. I know there were times when this project took precedence over you. Words cannot express how much all of you mean to me, as well as how much I appreciate and love each one of you.

Contents

PART I Review of Anatomy Systems 1

1 Musculoskeletal System 3

Gilbert M. Willett, PT, PhD, OCS, CSCS
Michael P. Reiman, PT, DPT, OCS, SCS, ATC, FAAOMPT, CSCS

2 Nervous System and Pain 25

Michael P. Reiman, PT, DPT, OCS, SCS, ATC, FAAOMPT, CSCS
Adriaan Louw, PT, PhD, CSMT

3 Tissue Injury and Healing 37

Mark F. Reinking, PT, PhD, SCS, ATC
Michael P. Reiman, PT, DPT, OCS, SCS, ATC, FAAOMPT, CSCS

PART II Concepts and Principles of Examination 49

4 Evidence-Based Practice and Client Examination 51

Michael P. Reiman, PT, DPT, OCS, SCS, ATC, FAAOMPT, CSCS

26 Lower Leg, Ankle, and Foot   863

Shefali Christopher, PT, DPT, SCS, LAT, ATC
Michael P. Reiman, PT, DPT, OCS, SCS, ATC, FAAOMPT, CSCS

PART V Examination of Special Populations   943

27 Emergency Sport Examination   945

John DeWitt, PT, DPT, SCS, ATC
Mitch Salsbery, PT, DPT, SCS, CSCS

28 Geriatric Examination   963

Michael Schmidt, PT, DPT, OCS, FAAOMPT
Charles Sheets, PT, OCS, SCS, Dip MDT
Tasala Rufai, PT, DPT, GCS

Foreword

Most books sink like a pebble tossed casually into a pond. Some books have a longer trajectory—a smooth, flat rock skipped a few times across a glassy lake. And then there are books that function like a beacon on a massive coastal rock formation. They guide through the ages—a constant throughout countless academic seasons and storms. Henry Gray's *Anatomy* (1858), William Campbell's *Textbook of Surgical Anatomy* (1911), and Tinsley Harrison's *Principles of Internal Medicine* (1950) are three of those.

Dr. Michael Reiman clearly consulted the lighthouse builder's guide when he conceived of *Orthopedic Clinical Examination*. He embraced rule number one: Massive is good. The book's 29 chapters and more than 1100 pages mean the clinician will find the needed examination for the body part or population in question. The hundreds of photos and 50 videos demonstrate the exams. Detailed and clear tables strip each examination naked; there is no place to hide once Mike and his team has deconstructed, analyzed, and then reconstructed the clinical orthopedic examination.

Orthopedic Clinical Examination will direct current and future generations of clinicians away from the shallow rocks of eminence-based, single special tests that were not rigorously validated. "Special tests are not so special" booms out from many pages. Replacing flawed dogma, the book spotlights tests and test batteries proven in heterogeneous populations of patients who attend for the care of physical therapists, athletic trainers, and primary care doctors.

Because I knew Mike Reiman and his previously published works, I was expecting a comprehensive, quality product about examination. The book I have in my hands is so much more; it's a new keystone for sports physiotherapy, sports medicine, and orthopedics. Mike and his team's ambitious vision emanated from the critical evaluation of previous expert opinion or low-quality research. Profound congratulations for executing that vision.

I am confident that if I see out three or four more decades on earth, *Orthopedic Clinical Examination* will still illuminate the otherwise hidden hazards confronting patients and their clinicians. *Orthopedic Clinical Examination* signals the ideal journey that is accurate, efficient, evidence-based practice.

Karim Khan, MD, PhD, MBA
Professor, The University of British Columbia
Vancouver, Canada
Editor-in-chief, *British Journal of Sports Medicine* **(BJSM)**

Preface

Clinical orthopedic examination is a skill that improves with knowledge and practice. This book provides readers with the knowledge and skills needed to approach the examination process. Each chapter on examination of a specific body part is organized and presented in the same manner. Approaching the examination from a broad to a focused approach (so-called *funnel approach*) and performing specific components of the examination in the same sequence ensures repetition and improved consistency in learning. This book, therefore, is written for the physical therapy, athletic training, and medical student, as well as for any clinician who wants a systematic approach to examination of the orthopedic client. The clinician is encouraged, though, to also use positioning systematically when performing their examination to avoid having the client move excessively, especially if the client is highly irritable symptom wise. Once the clinician has appropriately screened their client for serious pathology, they can use positioning appropriately to assess range-of-motion and muscle performance, for example, in the same position assuming it will not bias the rest of the examination process. The clinician should be well versed in the funnel approach prior to this though.

Due to the complexity of the various types of clients with orthopedic-related pathological presentations, clinicians must examine these clients in a systematic manner. However, with both treatment-based classifications and pathological-based classifications being used in health care fields, the clinician and student are often left wondering which approach to examination is ideal. Additionally, each approach has notable limitations (e.g., not all rotator cuff tears have the same impairments, not all lumbar spines with degenerative disc disease have pain, not all clients appropriately fit a treatment-based classification). The author of this book believes that practicing clinicians should have a good understanding of both approaches because each approach is used by different health care providers. Thus, this book attempts to bridge the gap between treatment-based classifications and pathological-based classifications with the funnel approach to examination. It also presents material at the end of each chapter so that the reader can see common impairments (treatment-based diagnosis) for common pathologies (pathology-based diagnosis).

Currently no other examination book in musculoskeletal medicine has the depth and breadth that this book provides. Many books provide information on anatomy, review of systems, general concepts of the evaluation and examination process, and details of examination for each body region. This book is unique because it covers, in detail, evidence-based and evidence-informed practice diagnostic accuracy values not only for special tests but also for subjective history, observation, diagnostic imaging, and performance-based measures. Books exist that cover these details separately, but none currently has all of this information in one all-inclusive source. In fact, most current books appear to have an over-reliance on the diagnostic accuracy of special tests alone despite multiple studies demonstrating limited clinical utility of these tests. Most books do not include diagnostic accuracy information and figures for diagnostic imaging and performance-based measures. Most texts also do not include diagnostic accuracy information on subjective and other objective findings (besides special tests). Perhaps one of the most impressive components of this text is the dedicated chapter, and emphasis in each chapter in parts III and IV, on triage and differential diagnosis. It is extremely important that the student and practicing clinician have differential diagnostic skills, not only for differential diagnosis of competing joint pain generators but for the ability to screen and diagnose the potential existence of nonmusculoskeletal or serious pathology. No other current text provides all of this information in an easy-to-read, structured format.

The benefits of this book include (1) the organized, systematic approach to body part examination, (2) the details of diagnostic accuracy of not only special tests but also subjective history, observation, diagnostic imaging, and performance-based measures, (3) the quick guide for determining the strength of diagnostic accuracy findings for each of these categories, allowing readers to determine the extent to which they should utilize such findings, (4) its combination of pathology-based and treatment-based diagnoses, (5) the web-based case studies, and (6) web-based videos.

ORGANIZATION

This book provides the reader with a general examination framework to utilize regardless of the body part being examined. The first two parts of this book describe the anatomy of the musculoskeletal system (part I) and the concepts and principles of the examination process (part II). Understanding the content of the musculoskeletal and nervous systems, as well as tissue behavior and healing, is vital for any student or clinician working with clients who have musculoskeletal injuries or dysfunction. Part II details the basic proposed components of the examination sequence. The chapters in parts III (Examination of the Head and Spine) and IV (Examination of the Extremities) provide an organized approach to problem solving, or an examination sequence, that clinicians can apply when evaluating each body area. Screening tests will be used early in the examination sequence, not only to determine the appropriateness of performing an orthopedic examination but also to rule out other potential pain generators and thereby narrow the focus of the examination. Finally, part V covers examination of special populations that require considerations relative to their cohort.

WEB RESOURCE

Perhaps the most unique feature of this text is the web resource, which has case study reviews and interactive questions, videos, and abstract links. For more information on the web resource, see Accessing and Using the Web Resource.

INSTRUCTOR RESOURCES

Instructors have access to a full array of ancillary materials.

- **Image bank.** The image bank contains all of the figures, tables, typeset figures, and technique photos from the book, separated by chapter. These items can be added to lecture slides, student handouts, and so on.
- **Instructor guide.** The instructor guide provides instructors with a sample syllabus and an introduction explaining how to use the instructor and student resources. In addition, chapter-specific files contain chapter outlines and additional resources.
- **Test package.** The test package has more than 400 multiple choice, true or false, fill-in-the-blank, matching, and short answer questions to choose from, based on text material. Instructors can use these questions to customize tests and quizzes.

These ancillaries are available at www.Human Kinetics.com/OrthopedicClinicalExamination.

Accessing and Using the Web Resource

A unique feature of this text is the web resource, which has case study reviews and interactive questions, videos, and abstract links. The web resource is available at www.HumanKinetics.com/Orthopedic ClinicalExamination.

CASE STUDIES

The case studies are based on a logistical flow of what the clinician or student would do next when presented with specific information. These studies present a specific case scenario and a detailed example of what to ask and what options to weigh when making the diagnosis. These cases have an interactive format that allows you to choose various options in a sequenced examination. The goal of the case studies is to help you apply what you have learned in the chapter and implement a systematic, evidence-based, efficient examination sequence. Some of the case studies are supported by videos of the tests used to help make a diagnosis of a specific condition. Within the text, you'll see cross-references to the case studies; here's an example:

Case Studies

Go to www.HumanKinetics.com/OrthopedicClinicalExamination and complete these case studies for chapter 15:

- Case study 1 discusses a 26-year-old female with insidious onset of headaches.
- Case study 2 discusses a 19-year-old male with a facial injury from being hit with a baseball.

VIDEOS

The web resource has 50 videos of many of the special tests, muscle testing, and performance-based measures discussed in the text. These videos allow you to directly visualize the content of the material in the book. These videos are valuable because they provide you with an example of the proper client set-up, positioning of the client and clinician, and the proper performance of the described skill. The determination of positive/negative findings is described for the special tests. Additionally, these videos will serve as resources for you to view whenever you wish. Here are the tests that are demonstrated in the videos:

Chapter 7 Orthopedic Screening and Nervous System Examination

ULNT 1: Median Nerve Bias

Slump Test

Straight Leg Raise (SLR) Test

Chapter 15 Face and Head

Pronator Drift Test

Forearm Rolling Test

Chapter 16 Temporomandibular Joint

Inferior (Caudal) Glide

Lateral Glide

Joint Sounds With Click

Chapter 17 Cervical Spine

Modified Sharp-Purser Test

C1-C2 Rotation: Flexion–Rotation Test (PPIVM)

Prone C0-C1 PAIVM

Prone C1-C2 PAIVM

Prone C2-C3 PAIVM

Spurling's Test

Chapter 18 Thoracic Spine

Thoracic Spine Central PA Mobilization

Cervical Rotation Lateral Flexion Test

Adson's Test

Within the text, you'll see cross-references to the videos; here's an example:

Video 7.5 in the web resource shows a demonstration of this test.

ABSTRACT LINKS

The web resource includes links to hundreds of ICD-10 codes and PubMed abstracts. You can easily access referenced articles including any other aspects of the study you deem worthy of further consideration. Within the text, you'll see cross-references to the abstract links; here's an example:

Abstract Links

Go to www.HumanKinetics.com/OrthopedicClinicalExamination to access abstract links on these issues:

Dix-Hallpike test

Finger tap test

Median nerve upper limb tension test

Pronator drift test

Rinne test

Spurling's test

Weber test

Acknowledgments

There is no way writing a text like this is accomplished alone. I have been blessed with great mentors, colleagues, friends, students, fellow faculty and clinicians, and family members. It is impossible to acknowledge every person who has helped me along the way. There are simply too many great people who have invested in me. It would be remiss to not mention a few, though. Thank you to Human Kinetics for believing in this project. It's impossible for me to thank everyone at Human Kinetics who was instrumental in bringing this book and the ancillaries to fruition. Thank you, Josh Stone, for taking over this project and keeping it moving smoothly. Thank you also for always being a good listener. Thank you, Susi Huls, for the guidance, feedback, and recommendations on the incredible case studies that go along with this book. Thank you, Neil Bernstein and Doug Fink, for the entertainment and your patience during the photo and video shoot. The only way I can think of to thank Amanda Ewing is to say that I simply could not have completed this project without you. To every student I have had the pleasure of interacting with, thank you for continuing to ask for further clarification. Your many thoughtful questions have helped me guide this text into what I hope is a comprehensive yet clearly understandable resource. Most important, I would like to acknowledge my parents, Pat and Marianne Reiman. Again, words cannot express the gratitude I have for the work ethic that you have instilled in me. I am clearly not the most talented writer, teacher, researcher, or clinician, but your example of hard work and words of encouragement have made it possible for this project to come to completion.

I also would like to thank the models from the photo and video shoot for their time and patience in helping to produce outstanding images and video:

Amanda Allen	Matthew McCarty
Anita Aiken	Matthew O'Connell
Erik Carvallio	Carly Reiman
Shefali Christopher	Seth Reiman
Zainab Kothari	Michael Schmidt
Kimberly Kurtz	Greg Wilmoth
Blair Losak	

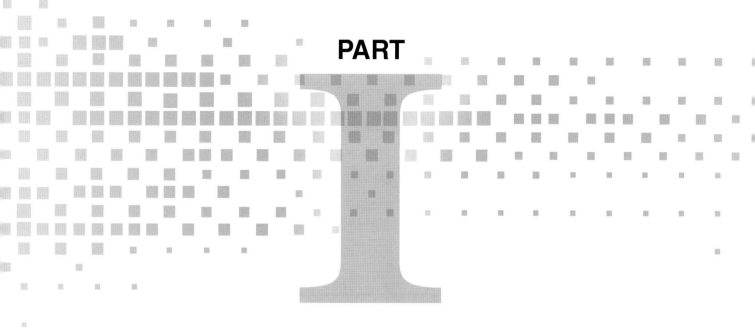

PART

I

Review of Anatomy Systems

Part I of this text reviews the various anatomy systems. It details basic components of the musculoskeletal system and their relation to musculoskeletal injury and examination. It describes the anatomy of the skeletal system, including bone, ligament, tendon, and muscle architecture, as well as joint classifications and various types of joints in the body. Chapter 1 describes differentiation of osteokinematic and arthrokinematic principles and how these concepts relate to the examination of the orthopedic client. It also details soft-tissue structure (e.g., muscle, tendon, nervous system) and function. This part of the text details how injury affects each of these structures and provides guiding principles for the examination of these structures.

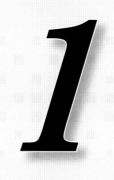

MUSCULOSKELETAL SYSTEM

Gilbert M. Willett, PT, PhD, OCS, CSCS
Michael P. Reiman, PT, DPT, OCS, SCS, ATC, FAAOMPT, CSCS

"In the developed world, musculoskeletal disorders represent the majority of occupational ill-health and work-related illness."[1] With this quote in mind, the overall objective of this chapter is to provide pertinent basic science information about the musculoskeletal system to orthopedic physical therapists. The key elements reviewed in this chapter on the musculoskeletal system are bones, joints, muscle, and related connective tissues.

BONES

Studying skeletal anatomy sometimes gives health professional students and clinicians the wrong impression when it comes to bones. Learning about bones through the use of preserved skeletal models has value, but it can also give the false impression that bone is a rigid, dead structure. In reality, it is dynamic living tissue that serves many purposes and is highly adaptable and capable of remodeling to meet changing needs. Bones provide infrastructure for the human body. They protect essential organs, assist in movement by providing attachment sites for muscles, and store minerals (primarily calcium and phosphorus). They are highly active metabolically, a key factor in maintaining body homeostasis. Bones serve as the second line of defense in preventing acidosis and can adsorb toxins and heavy metals such as lead, minimizing their adverse effects on other tissues.[2] Bones also store fat and produce blood cells in their marrow cavities.

Anatomy and Physiology

Bone is comprised of organic (~40% dry weight) and inorganic materials (~60% dry weight) and a small amount of water.[3] Organic materials include cells and matrix (~90% Type I collagen, as well as proteoglycans, matrix proteins, and cytokines). A variety of cell types can be found in bone, but the primary ones are the three "*O*" cells:[4]

- **Osteoblasts:** These cells form new bone tissue for growth or healing. They produce bone matrix, including the Type I collagen fibers that provide bone with significant strength and flexibility. Osteoblasts develop from mesenchymal stem cells and become osteocytes or line the periphery of bones when they stop forming new bone.

- **Osteocytes:** These cells form a large component of mature bone. Osteocytes have long, branching arms that connect them to neighboring osteocytes. This allows them to exchange minerals and communicate with neighboring cells.

- **Osteoclasts:** These large macrophage-type cells secrete acidic enzymes to break down bone matrix and reabsorb existing bone, thus enabling remodeling of bone.

Inorganic bone components consist of hydroxyapatites (mineral salts), primarily calcium phosphate. These calcium salts are present in the form of tiny crystals, which contribute to bone hardness or rigidity.[5]

Bones have a solid outer shell (cortical, or compact, bone) and a honeycomb inside (known as *cancellous*, *spongy*, or *trabecular bone*). The human skeleton is composed of approximately 80% compact bone and 20% cancellous bone. Cortical bone has an outer periosteal surface and inner endosteal surface. Periosteal surface activity is important for appositional growth and fracture repair. All bone is made up of structural units known as osteons. In cortical bone, an osteon consists of concentric layers (lamellae) of osteocytes and matrix around small blood vessels (haversian canal; figure 1.1). The osteocytes within osteons are interconnected by small channels known as canaliculi. Cortical structure

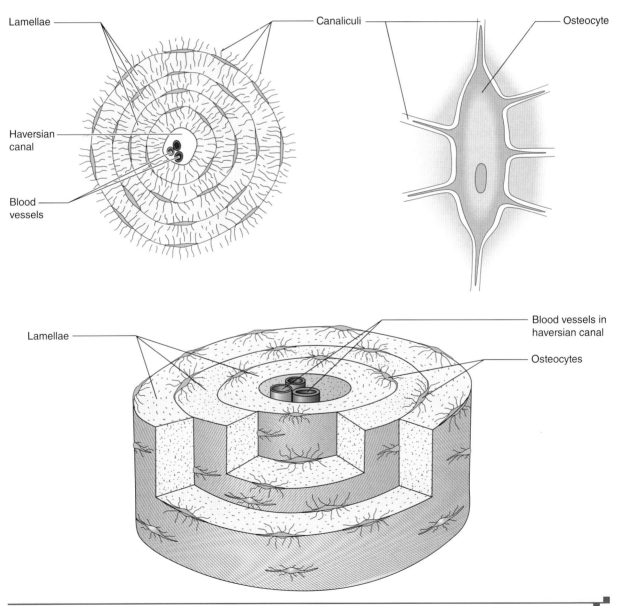

Figure 1.1 Structure of an osteon, including osteocytes and canaliculi.

and microstructure contribute to the mechanical competence of the entire bone. The crystalline component of the structure provides compressive strength and brittleness, while collagen fibrils provide tensile strength and toughness. Cortical bone develops microcracks when stressed in order to dissipate energy during catastrophic loading events. Age-related accumulation of microdamage weakens cortical bone tissue and possibly contributes to increased susceptibility to fracture.[6] Bone formation typically exceeds bone resorption on the periosteal surface, so bones normally increase in diameter with aging.[3]

Cancellous bone (figure 1.2) is made up of a honeycomb network of thin plates (trabeculae) and rods interspersed in the bone marrow compartment. It is found in the ends of long bones near joints, in vertebral bodies, and in flat bones such as the ilium of the pelvis. Cancellous bone is also composed of osteons, called *packets*.[3] Cancellous bone has a higher level of remodeling than cortical bone; however, both engage in the remodeling process.

Mature cortical bone and cancellous bone normally exhibit a lamellar pattern, in which collagen fibrils are laid down in alternating orientations.[3] The mechanism by which osteoblasts lay down collagen fibrils in a lamellar pattern is unknown. Similar to plywood, lamellar bone has great strength resultant from the alternating orientations of collagen fibrils.

This lamellar pattern is absent in woven (immature) bone. In immature bone, the collagen fibrils are laid down in a disorganized manner that makes the bone weaker than lamellar (mature) bone. Woven bone is normally produced during initial formation of primary bone.[3] It may also be seen in association with conditions that result in high bone turnover, such as osteitis fibrosa cystica, Paget's disease, or hyperparathyroidism.

Bone health depends on both nonmechanical and mechanical influences. Nonmechanical factors are broad and encompass individual genetic determinants such as gender, cellular metabolism, and hormone and cytokine production, as well as nutritional components such as calcium and vitamin D. Mechanical factors include loads or stress that influence osteoblast and osteoclast cell activity.[7] Excessive mechanical stress or a prolonged lack of loading can significantly change bone structure. This can result in a variety of musculoskeletal concerns. For example, excessive loading of the lumbar facet joints due to inappropriate postures (exaggerated lordosis) or movements over time can cause hypertrophy of the bony articular processes of the vertebrae. This hypertrophy can create stenosis of the intervertebral foramina and subsequent nerve root impingement. Conversely, lack of loading causes weakening of the bones and increased susceptibility to fracture. The occurrence of these types of fractures in the long bones of the lower limbs of people who depend on wheelchairs for mobility have been well documented.[8] Bones adapt to the physical stresses placed on them through the coordinated action of osteoclasts and osteoblasts.[9] The principle of bone adaptation to stress is known as Wolff's Law. It states that a bone's internal and external architecture change in response to the stresses (or lack thereof) placed on it.[10]

Biomechanical Properties

In order for bones to function normally, they must exhibit a number of mechanical properties. Similar qualities can be found in other infrastructure materials such as wood and steel. Bones have to be able to absorb stress, strain, and shear resultant from the functional demands placed on them. These mechanical properties include anisotropy, viscoelasticity, and loading modes as well as responses due to compression (load-bearing stress) and tension (muscle strain) forces.

Anisotropy is the ability to respond differently to forces applied in different directions. The

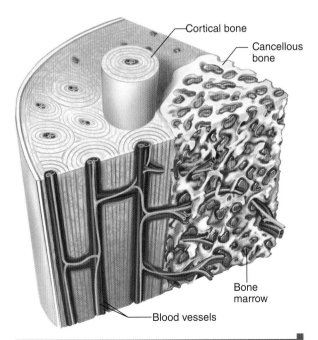

Figure 1.2 Compact cortical bone and spongy cancellous (trabecular) bone.

Cortical bone

Cancellous bone

Bone marrow

Blood vessels

orientation of mineral crystals (rather than the collagen matrix) appears to be the primary determinant of bone anisotropy.[11] These inorganic mineral crystals found in bone also resist compressive forces well. Viscoelasticity is the ability of a material to exhibit both viscous and elastic characteristics when undergoing deformation. Viscous materials (e.g., putty) resist shear flow and strain linearly with time when stress is applied. Elastic materials (e.g., rubber) strain when stretched and quickly return to their original state once the stress is removed. Viscoelastic materials exhibit elements of both of these properties and, as such, exhibit time-dependent strain. This means that the stress depends on not only the strain but also how rapidly the strain occurs. The clinical implications of this are related to bone fracture patterns and subsequent collateral soft-tissue damage. A more rapidly applied load will result in a greater amount of bone fragmentation. The relationships among bone collagen, moisture levels, and mineral levels appear to be the primary influences on bone viscoelasticity.[12] The collagen in bone resists tensile forces well.

Physical therapy clinicians commonly see stress fracture injuries. This type of fracture is a tiny crack that occurs in bones subjected to repetitive stresses (overuse) that eventually accumulate to levels that overwhelm bone's ability to tolerate loading. In these cases, bones fatigue, progressively losing strength or stiffness due to lower level cyclic loading. This fatigue eventually results in failure to tolerate loading. This can happen over time to healthy bones subjected to prolonged stresses or more rapidly to bones weakened by abnormal conditions such as osteoporosis. The accumulation of microdamage impairs the mechanical properties of bone by reducing its elastic properties. Damage accumulates more rapidly in areas of bone under tensile pressures (e.g., muscle insertions), but crack growth (i.e., fracture potential) is greater in areas of bone experiencing compressive forces.[13]

JOINTS

While bones provide infrastructure for the human body, joints allow movement to occur between bones. A joint, or articulation, occurs between two bones. It is comprised of a variety of specialized tissues that enable safe and efficient movement. Joints can be broadly classified into two categories, those with a joint cavity and those without. Because of the clinical emphasis of this text, the primary focus will be on joints with a cavity, also known as diarthrose or synovial joints. They are important components of the musculoskeletal system that enable human body movement. Key anatomical structures, classifications, and important clinical considerations of synovial joints will be addressed. See the section Joint Classifications for a brief review of the other joints found in the human body.

The three distinguishing features of a typical synovial joint are the joint cavity (as previously mentioned), joint capsule, and articular cartilage covering of the bone contact surfaces. In addition, many synovial joints possess unique anatomical specializations, such as ligaments, that allow them to perform optimally. Subsequent sections review these features in greater detail.

Capsule

The joint capsule is vital to the function of synovial joints. It seals the joint space, provides passive stability by controlling or limiting movements, contributes to active (muscular) stability through its proprioceptive nerve endings, and may even help form the contact surfaces of the joint. Its outer layer is composed of a dense fibrous connective tissue that attaches to the bones via specialized attachment zones and forms a sleeve around the joint. Capsules vary in thickness based on the stresses they are subjected to. For example, the hip joint capsule is thicker anteriorly than posteriorly due to the center of gravity passing behind the joint, resulting in a tendency for hyperextension.[14] In some cases, such as the glenohumeral joint, the capsule is locally thickened to form capsular ligaments, and it may also incorporate tendons. If the capsule is injured, it can lead to instability or laxity or can limit movement due to constriction or adhesion to surrounding structures. It is also adversely affected by conditions such as rheumatoid arthritis, osteoarthritis, crystal deposition disorders, bony spur formation, and ankylosing spondylitis.[14] In areas where the capsule connects to bone near the joint, the capsule tissue can become fibrocartilaginous. This change enables it to resist pressures.

The inner layer of the capsule is made up of synovial tissue. It typically consists of loose or fatty areolar tissue on a membrane and a thin layer of tissue only a few cells thick. The synovium produces a fluid with bactericidal properties that nourish and lubricate the avascular cartilage surfaces.[15] Synovial fluid is made up of proteinases, collagenases, hyaluronic acid, and prostaglandins. The viscosity of the fluid changes based on the movement occurring between the joint surfaces. During slow movements, the fluid is more viscous; during fast movements, the fluid becomes less viscous. This adaptation helps to reduce surface friction. Excessive amounts of synovial fluid trapped within a joint (sometimes resultant from joint trauma) may produce swelling, pain, and loss of function.

Cracking or popping of joints is a common occurrence that both clients and clinicians experience. Studies have provided evidence that this phenomenon occurs due to the formation of a cavity within the synovial fluid inside the joint capsule.[16] Unsworth and colleagues demonstrated that traction or stretching of the joint capsule produces a vacuum phenomenon that draws dissolved gas (~80% CO_2) out of the synovial fluid within the joint to form a bubble, which immediately collapses.[16] They theorized that the bubble collapse resulted in an audible pop known as cavitation. Ultrasound and radiographic imaging findings have demonstrated the formation of these bubbles.[17] Interestingly enough, this popping phenomenon has been observed with ultrasound imaging and heard when manually applied traction, such as what would be applied by a clinician to a client, was performed on the metacarpophalangeal joints of a lightly embalmed cadaver. A study using real-time cine magnetic resonance imaging (cine MRI) provided evidence that the sound produced during joint cracking can be attributed to a mechanism known as viscous adhesion or tribonucleation.[18] This occurs when two closely opposed surfaces are separated by a thin film of viscous liquid. Tension between the surfaces resists separation when the surfaces are distracted. When distraction forces overcome the tension adhesion forces, the joint surfaces separate rapidly creating a negative pressure. This negative pressure, combined with the speed with which the surfaces separate, can create a vapor cavity within the synovial fluid. This research offers direct experimental evidence that joint cracking is associated with cavity inception (tribonucleation) rather than collapse of a pre-existing bubble (cavitation).[18]

Cartilage

Cartilage is a strong, flexible connective tissue that covers the end of each bone in a synovial joint. The function of cartilage is to distribute loads, minimize peak stresses on the subchondral bone, and provide a friction-reduced weight-bearing surface. It is remarkably elastic, capable of deforming and regaining its original shape. Cartilage has a low level of metabolic activity and lacks blood vessels, lymphatic vessels, and nerves. Essentially, articular cartilage functions and stands alone. The simple homogeneous appearance of cartilage hides its highly ordered complex structure. This structure appears to remain unchanged unless affected by disease or injury.[19] As with all connective tissues, cartilage is made up of a combination of cells (chondrocytes), collagen fibers, and intercellular matrix material. The collagen fiber components enable shape retention and tensile strength, while the viscous, hydrated matrix absorbs compression forces.

Cartilage exists in three types—hyaline, elastic, and fibrocartilage—and the two most commonly found in joints are hyaline and fibrocartilage. Hyaline cartilage, often called articular cartilage, is the most common type of cartilage found in joints. It covers the ends of long bones where the surfaces articulate and forms the growth plate of long bones during childhood. In order to help joints withstand the compression forces that occur within them, the predominant element in hyaline cartilage is extracellular matrix material. Fibrocartilage forms the intervertebral disks, and it can be found in other locations such as the temporomandibular joint, knee (menisci), and pubic symphysis. Collagen fibers, which help joints maintain shape and withstand tensile forces, are the predominant component of fibrocartilage.

Cartilage is primarily made up of chondrocytes, or cartilage cells, (although fibrocytes have been found on the articular surfaces of some joints such as the temporomandibular joint, or TMJ) and extracellular matrix. Chondrocytes synthesize extracellular matrix components and secrete enzymes that direct cartilage remodeling and regeneration.[20] The biochemical composition of the articular cartilage extracellular matrix determines the biomechanical characteristics of the tissue, such as resilience and elasticity. It has been shown to vary between joints and clients.[21] The extracellular matrix of both hyaline and fibrocartilage consists of water, collagen, proteoglycans, structural glycoproteins, and small amounts of lipid and inorganic components. Water constitutes 60% to 80% of the total weight of hyaline cartilage, slightly less for fibrocartilage.[22]

The organization or structure of hyaline cartilage can be divided into four zones (figure 1.3). The

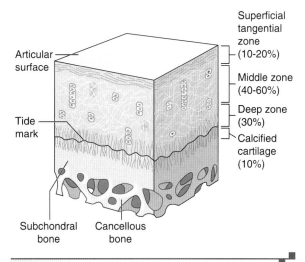

Superficial
tangential
zone
(10-20%)

Middle zone
(40-60%)

Deep zone
(30%)

Calcified
cartilage
(10%)

Articular
surface

Tide
mark

Subchondral
bone

Cancellous
bone

Figure 1.3 Zones of hyaline (articular) cartilage.

collagen organization and amount of proteoglycans in the extracellular matrix vary between zones in order to provide different biomechanical properties. The superficial zone contains the highest collagen content. The collagen fibril orientation is parallel to the joint surface, which suggests that the primary purpose of this zone may be to resist shear stresses. The amount of collagen decreases in each subsequent zone. The middle zone contains random larger collagen fibers and chondrocytes. The deep zone is organized in a compact vertical fashion and is low in water content and rich in proteoglycans. The purpose of this zone is to resist compressive forces. The calcified cartilage zone is where the cartilage transitions to subchondral bone tissue.

Due to the organization of hyaline cartilage and the fact that it is avascular, healing is limited. Chondrocytes may facilitate repair of minor injuries; however, larger lesion repair is restricted because the typical cellular cascade (facilitated by vascular damage in other local tissues) cannot occur. If the cartilage injury is deep enough to involve the vascularized subchondral bone (osteochondral injury), then vascular hemorrhage due to bone damage may enable some repair. This principle is utilized in surgical microfracture and drilling techniques that treat hyaline cartilage defects of the knee joint.

As in the case of bone, articular cartilage has anisotropic qualities that allow it to respond differently to forces applied in varying directions. Cartilage anisotropy occurs under both tension and compression forces. Anisotropy during compression may be essential for normal cartilage function.[23]

Varying collagen fiber alignment and the ratio of collagen to proteoglycan in the extracellular matrix influence the stress tolerances in the different zones of hyaline cartilage.

As a biomaterial, articular cartilage may be considered a porous composite organic solid matrix swollen by water.[24] When cartilage is subjected to a constant load, it exhibits an elastic, rapid deformation response followed by additional slowly occurring deformation over time as fluid flows out of the tissue and into the joint (known as *creep*). Cartilage subjected to constant deformation over time responds with a high initial stress followed by a slowly occurring, progressive decrease in stress. This response is known as *stress relaxation*.[25] Creep and stress relaxation are viscoelastic behaviors of cartilaginous tissues that occur with compression and shearing forces. Flow of interstitial fluid and adaptation responses of the collagen fibers and proteoglycans within the extracellular matrix appear to be responsible for these phenomena. Interstitial fluid flow in and out of the cartilage tissue, promoted by compression and distraction forces, enables the exchange of waste products and nutrition within the cartilage.[24] These dynamic loads can increase or inhibit (if the loads are too frequent or excessive) the biosynthetic activities of the chondrocytes within cartilage.[26]

Cartilage provides a force-bearing surface with low friction and wear. Because of its compliance, it helps distribute the joint surface loads. It is subject to tensile, compression, and shearing forces during functional activities. Studies suggest that particular physical activities alone do not necessarily predispose someone to experience wear and tear of the cartilage (osteoarthrosis). Instead, the way in which the activity is performed, such as a high rate of loading, may be a more important factor for determining whether damage will develop or occur.[27] Clinicians should consider this principle when prescribing training and rehabilitation exercises for improving function while minimizing potential for cartilage injury.

Ligaments

Ligaments are one of the key structures that help stabilize and guide joint movement. They span joints, attach to the bones, and become taut or loose depending on joint position and forces applied. They are a dense connective tissue that is made up of an extracellular matrix of densely packed, crimped bundles of collagen fibers, proteoglycans, elastin, water (~70% of the matrix), and a small numbers of cells (mostly fibrocytes). The collagen fibrils within a ligament fiber contain varying amounts of different types of collagen, elastin, and proteoglycans. Ligaments are often encased in a cellular membrane (epiligament) that is extremely vascular, and contains sensory and proprioceptive nerves. The ligament itself is less vascular, but it does have an organized blood supply and some innervation.[28] Cells in ligaments promote adaptive tissue changes in response to local and systemic factors. Factors that stimulate ligament tissue changes in behavior and responsiveness include loading variations (e.g., due to exercise or immobilization) and changes in hormone level (e.g., menstruation, pregnancy).[28]

The biomechanical properties of ligaments depend on the properties and arrangement of their contents (cells, fibers, matrix) as well as the proportions of those contents. For example, the elastin that is present in small amounts (~5%) of all ligaments forms interdigitated networks among collagen fibrils in order to allow recovery from deformation that occurs with stress. Water and proteoglycans within ligament extracellular matrix provide lubrication and spacing that enable gliding to occur at the collagen fiber matrix.[29] Since ligaments are highly organized fibrous tissues, their mechanical properties are directionally dependent (anisotropic). For example, the human medial collateral ligament has mechanical properties that are 30 times higher for tolerating stress along its longitudinal direction compared to its transverse direction.[30] Ligaments also exhibit viscoelastic behavior and stress or strain responses. During stress, ligaments initially uncrimp (low resistance) as they elongate and then stretch (high resistance) until they reach a point of failure (rupture). During normal activities, ligaments are believed to function at low resistance levels. They also exhibit the viscoelastic qualities of creep and stress relaxation. Hysteresis (energy dissipation) is an additional viscoelastic quality of ligaments. This occurs in response to ligament loading and unloading. Work done during lengthening is greater than work recovered during shortening. The energy that is lost produces heat.

One interesting clinical aspect to consider is the relationship of the viscoelastic properties between ligament and bone. If the loading rate on the bone–ligament complex of a joint is slow, the bone is more likely to fail or break. As the loading rate increases, the bone becomes stronger than the ligament,

and the ligament is more likely to rupture first. At slower loading rates, bony avulsion failures have the greatest probability of occurring. At fast loading rates, ligament tears are to be expected.[31]

Joint Classifications

Joints without a cavity are known as synarthroses. These joints typically allow only small amounts of movement to occur under normal conditions. They are named or classified by how the bones are held together by fibrous or cartilaginous connective tissue. Synarthrodial joints are classified as follows:

1. Fibrous synarthrosis: These joints consist of a tough, fibrous tissue connection between bones. Three types of fibrous synarthroses exist:

- *Sutures.* This is where two bones that are initially separated eventually join together in an interdigitated fashion (suture), and are together by tough fibrous tissue known as Sharpey's fibers. Examples of these joints are found in the skull (cranial sutures). Controversy exists regarding whether any movement occurs between adult cranial bones.

- *Interosseous membrane.* This is a fibrous membrane connection between bones. One example is the interosseous membrane connection between the shafts of the tibia and fibula bones of the leg. Small amounts of movement can occur at these joints. Injuries of these joints (i.e., high ankle sprain) usually occur as a result of extreme forces being placed on the joint. Thus, healing time and rehabilitation needs are significantly increased.

- *Gomphosis.* This is a conical peg-like structure fitting into a socket, surrounded by fibrous-tissue articulation. Examples of these joints are tooth–mandibular or tooth–maxillary articulations. A small amount of tooth movement is allowed by these joints. This is how orthodontic braces can alter tooth alignment and positioning.

2. Synchondroses (amphiarthrosis): These joints consist of a cartilage connection between bones. The intervening cartilage can be hyaline or fibrocartilage, for example, the first sternocostal joint. In this case, hyaline cartilage fills the space between the two bony surfaces. The cartilage connection does allow a small amount of movement to occur between the connected bones.

Joints with a cavity (diarthroses, or synovial joints) can be defined as simple or complex. A simple joint is composed of two bones. A complex joint is composed of three or more bones. In addition, these diarthroses (synovial joints) are named or classified by the shapes of their articulating surfaces or the movement permitted by the shapes of the articulating bone surfaces. The seven joint classifications and their movements are as follows (figure 1.4):

- **Hinge joint (ginglymus):** This is a convex on concave articulation. One example is the humeroulnar joint. Flexion and extension movements occur at these joints.

- **Ellipsoidal joint:** This is a flattened convex ellipsoidal surface on concave articulation. One example is the proximal radiocarpal joint. Flexion and extension and abduction and adduction movements occur at these joints.

- **Saddle joint:** In this convex and concave (saddle-shaped) on a convex and concave articulation, the joint surfaces are oriented at right angles to one another, similar to a rider sitting on a saddle. One example is the carpometacarpal joint. Flexion and extension, abduction and adduction, and circumduction can all occur at these joints.

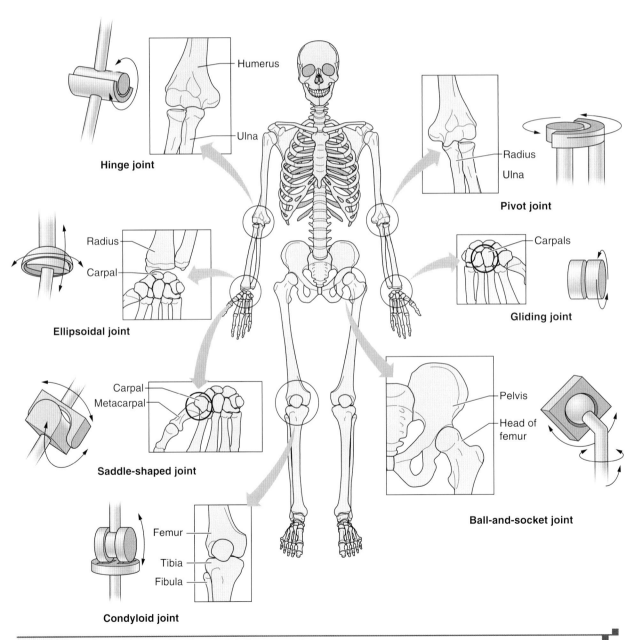

Figure 1.4 Seven joint classifications and their movements.

- **Condyloid joint:** This is an oval-shaped condyle on concave articulation. One example is the tibiofemoral joint. Flexion and extension, abduction and adduction, and a small amount of rotation can occur at these joints.

- **Pivot joint (sellar):** This is a rounded or conical surface on a concave or ring-shaped surface articulation. One example is the proximal radioulnar joint. Spin around a single axis occurs at these joints.

- **Gliding joint (plane):** This is a basically flat surface on flat surface articulation. One example is the intercarpal joints. Sliding movements occur at these joints.

- **Ball-and-socket joint (spheroid):** This is a ball-shaped convex surface on cuplike concave surface articulation. One example is the femoroacetabular joint of the hip. Significant motion in all three planes—flexion and extension, abduction and adduction, and rotation—can occur at these joints.

Anatomical descriptions of joint movements are based on three imaginary planes that intersect the body in anatomical position:

- **Sagittal:** a vertical plane passing longitudinally through the body that divides it into right and left sections.

- **Frontal:** a vertical plane passing longitudinally through the body that divides it into anterior and posterior sections.

- **Transverse:** a horizontal plane passing through the body that divides it into superior and inferior sections.

Three axes exist that are used to describe joint motions in the three planes (figure 1.5). These are perpendicular to the plane in which the motion occurs.

- **Frontal:** perpendicular to the sagittal plane, enables flexion and extension movements.

- **Sagittal:** perpendicular to the frontal plane, enables abduction and adduction movements.

- **Vertical (longitudinal):** perpendicular to the transverse plane, enables medial and lateral rotation movements.

Joint Positions and Movements

Health care professionals who use manual therapy techniques such as joint mobilization and manipulation often use terms such as *loose packed* and *close packed* to describe joint positioning. Loose-packed positioning is typically defined in manual therapy texts as any joint position other than close packed. With loose-packed positioning, the joint surfaces

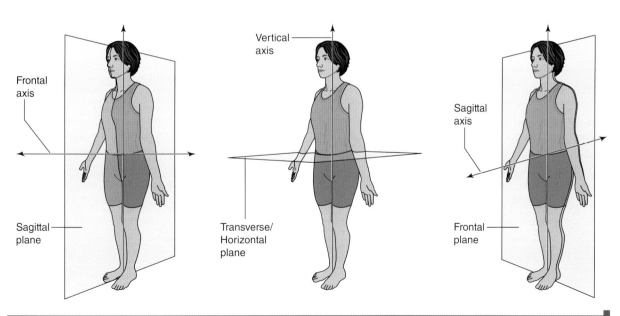

Figure 1.5 The cardinal planes and axes.

are not maximally congruent and surrounding structures (i.e., ligaments, joint capsule) are not maximally taut. Conversely, the term *close packed* is commonly defined as the joint position in which there is maximum contact between the two joint surfaces, and the surrounding structures are maximally taut. A joint that is in a close-packed position should allow minimal translatory motion, thus placing a joint in this position for mobilization is not recommended.

Clearly the definition of close-packed positioning is imperfect in some specific cases, for example, the glenohumeral joint. The glenohumeral close-packed position is commonly described as abduction and lateral (external) rotation. In this position, the anterior capsule is more taut than the posterior capsule, and it is debatable whether the joint surfaces are maximally congruent. However, in spite of the limitations of the definition of close-packed positioning, the concept is useful for understanding and applying manual therapy techniques. It is important to realize there are limitations and exceptions to the concept's definition.

Another joint position definition often used by health care professionals is *resting position*. It is defined as the position of a joint in which the tissues encompassing the joint are under the least amount of stress and in which the joint capsule has its greatest laxity. It may also be termed the *maximal loosely packed position*.[32] Clients often posture or place their joints in this position when swelling is present within the joint in order to minimize discomfort.

Movement at joints is defined in two ways, osteokinematic and arthrokinematic. Osteokinematic motions (also known as physiologic motions) are observable movements of bones in the anatomical planes of motion (flexion and extension, abduction and adduction, medial and lateral rotation). These movements are often quantified by health care professionals using goniometric measurements in order to document client status in terms of joint range of motion. Osteokinematic movements can be passive (performed by a clinician who is moving the limb segment for the client) or active (clients use their own muscles to perform the movement).

Arthrokinematic motions are not readily observable visually or quantifiable by goniometric measurement. They are passive, accessory movements that occur between the two articulating bones at a joint that enable full osteokinematic motion.[33] When someone performs an active osteokinematic movement, these accessory movements occur natu-

rally. They also can be passively assessed by a health care professional who is manually manipulating a client's joint. Grieve described passive assessment of arthrokinematic mobility as any movement mechanically or manually applied to a joint with no voluntary muscular activity by the client.[34] The manual assessment of passive accessory movement available at a joint performed by a clinician is commonly referred to as *joint play assessment*. This assessment is a relatively subjective endeavor.

Arthrokinematic motions include roll, glide (slide), and spin of joint surfaces that occur during physiologic (osteokinematic) movements. Roll is equivalent to a tire rolling on a surface. Glide or slide would be comparable to the tire skidding on a surface. Spin is similar to a figure skater performing a toe spin. In joints, spin involves rotation of one joint surface around a stationary mechanical axis (e.g., radioulnar joint movement during pronation or supination).

A key guideline of joint mobilization commonly used by clinicians is the concave–convex rule. Most joints in the human body are composed of a more convex surface articulating with a concave surface. Kaltenborn proposed that passive joint mobilization techniques in which arthrokinematic glide motion is applied to restore joint mobility should be based on the concave–convex rule.[35] This rule basically states the following:

- If a convex surface is moving on a concave surface, roll and glide occur in opposite directions (figure 1.6*a*).
- If a concave surface is moving on a fixed convex surface, roll and glide occur in the same direction (figure 1.6*b*).

Clinicians who use manual therapy interventions apply this rule to determine which direction they will glide a segment (based on which bone segment they are moving versus stabilizing) to restore normal joint mobility. For example, if a clinician would like to restore knee joint extension range of motion for a client who is lacking full extension, they could choose to glide the tibia in an anterior direction while stabilizing the femur. Recent studies have refuted this rule.[36-39] Based on a review of these studies, Schomacher proposes that the concave–convex rule is a didactic simplification of the lever law during rotatory movements of the joint that does not always follow suit when analyzed in biomechanical research. He states that when considering mobilization glide as an intervention,

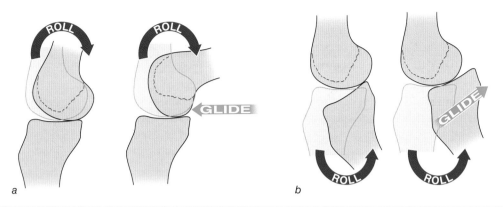

Figure 1.6 *(a)* Convex-on-concave arthrokinematics and *(b)* concave-on-convex arthrokinematics.

it is important not to automatically apply the glide direction normally expected in healthy joints to pathological ones without performing a comprehensive examination first.[40] Restricted gliding may have different causes. Examination findings and subsequent choice of direction of glide for intervention must be determined as part of a thorough clinical reasoning process. An example of this is provided by Johnson and colleagues, who found that posterior glide mobilizations for clients with a diagnosis of glenohumeral joint adhesive capsulitis (frozen shoulder) resulted in greater improvements in lateral rotation range of motion than for those who received anterior glide mobilizations.[39] This result is contrary to the concave–convex rule. Clinicians should consider this information when determining which direction to perform manual glide interventions for restoring joint mobility. The take-home message would be to evaluate thoroughly and choose glide direction based on client response as opposed to blindly following the rule.

SKELETAL MUSCLE AND CONNECTIVE TISSUES

Three classifications of muscles exist in the musculoskeletal system: skeletal (striated or voluntary), smooth (nonstriated or involuntary), and cardiac. Skeletal muscles are named as such because they primarily (but not exclusively) originate and insert on skeletal bones. Approximately 40% of total body weight can be accounted for by skeletal muscle. Skeletal muscles and their associated connective tissues are responsible for both moving and stabilizing the bones and joints of the skeletal system.

They also help distribute loads and absorb shock.[41] This section reviews foundational information concerning these tissues. Skeletal muscles are unable to perform their functions without the nervous system. The nervous system is addressed briefly in this section and in greater detail in chapter 2.

Muscular Anatomy and Physiology

A skeletal muscle (e.g., biceps brachii) can be considered an organ of the muscular system. It is comprised of skeletal muscle tissue, connective tissue, nerve tissue, and vascular tissue. Skeletal muscles have four common characteristics:[42]

- **Contractility:** ability to develop tension in response to a chemical or electrical stimulus. This enables movement of the structures (typically bones) to which the muscles are attached.
- **Excitability:** ability to contract or shorten in response to chemical or electrical stimuli.
- **Elasticity:** ability to stretch.
- **Extensibility:** ability to return to normal resting length.

Grossly, the contractile unit of a muscle that produces movement and force includes the muscle belly and the tendon that attaches the muscle belly to the bone. Contractile muscle tissue has the ability to develop tension in response to chemical, electrical, or mechanical stimuli. Passive tension is provided by noncontractile connective tissue that supports the muscle fiber.[43]

Muscle tissue is comprised of individual, multinucleated cells known as myocytes or myofibers.

These cells are also termed *muscle fibers* in the literature. The fibers (cells) are shaped like long, narrow cylinders and are surrounded by a plasma membrane (known as *sarcolemma*) that encases the cell's numerous nuclei and its cytoplasm (known as sarcoplasm; figure 1.7). Myofibers are typically bundled together. These bundles of fibers are called fasciculi.

Collagen-based connective tissue is a vital component of muscle infrastructure. Sarcolemma is the cell membrane of the muscle fibers. Endomysium is the connective tissue that surrounds the individual muscle fibers and insulates the individual cells from one another. Perimysium ensheathes muscle fasciculi (bundles of myofibers) and epimysium wraps around the entire gross structure of a muscle. Each subsequent layer of muscle connective tissue is tougher and thicker than the previous one. In addition, the epimysium is continuous with the muscle tendon (connective tissue that attaches muscles to their origin and insertion points).[41] The junction where muscle connective tissues merge with the tendon is known as the *myotendinous junction*. This is an area where injuries such as strains often occur.[44] Tendons are addressed in detail later in this section. In summary, skeletal muscles are essentially organized as bundles within bundles, progressing from myofilaments to myofibrils to muscle cells (myocytes or muscle fibers) to fascicles to whole skeletal muscle.

The three primary types of muscle fibers are Type I (slow-twitch), Type IIA (fast-twitch fatigue resistant), and Type IIB (fast-twitch fatigable; table 1.1).[45] Type I slow-twitch muscle fibers generally have low activation thresholds, high aerobic capacity, and low fatigability. Type IIB or fast-twitch muscle fibers on the other hand have high activation thresholds, low aerobic capacity, and high fatigability. Training emphasis for developing Type I muscle fibers should therefore be on high volume (repetition and sets) with low intensity; for Type IIB muscle fiber training, low volume and high intensity. Postural muscles are predominantly Type I muscle fibers because their energy requirements are low but require sustainability. Therefore, program design for these muscle types should emphasize high repetition and sets with minimal resistance. Depending on the muscle and its strength, gravity can often serve as sufficient resistance.

Every skeletal muscle is composed of a combination of the three types of fibers. It is believed that the composition of fiber types is genetically determined. The average person has approximately 50% Type I, 25% Type IIA, and 25% Type IIB fibers in the gastrocnemius muscle.[44] An elite distance runner can have a much higher proportion of Type I fibers, while elite sprinters typically have a much higher proportion of Type IIB fibers.[45] As people age, a greater decrease in the number of Type II fibers generally occurs.

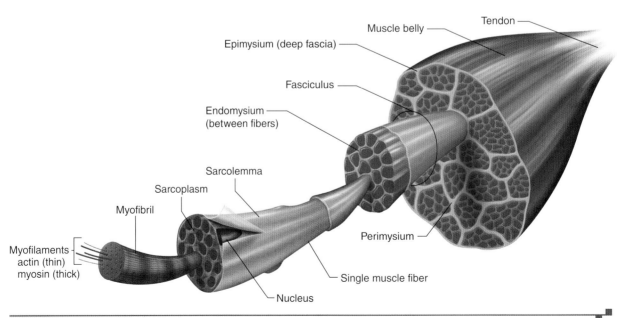

Figure 1.7 Composition of a muscle fiber.

TABLE 1.1   Characteristics of Muscle Fiber Types

	Slow-twitch (Type I)	Fast-twitch fatigue resistant (Type IIA)	Fast-twitch fatigable (Type IIB)
Histochemical fiber profile	Slow oxidative	Fast oxidative glycolytic	Fast glycolytic
Motor units	Small, with low innervation ratio	Medium	Large with high innervation ratio
Twitch response	Slow twitch	Medium	Fast twitch
Order of recruitment	First	Second	Last (usually only when intense effort is required)
Fatigue resistance	High	Reasonably resistant	Low
Recovery after exercise	Rapid	Fairly rapid	Slow
Power output	Low	Moderate to high	High
Aerobic capacity	High	Moderate	Low
Anaerobic capacity	Low	High	High

Stability or postural muscles generally have a higher percentage of Type I, or slow-twitch, muscle fibers. Generally, these muscles have relatively small, slow motor units (small cell bodies, small-diameter axons, and a small number of muscle fibers per motor unit) and are almost continually active during postural activity. Dynamic or mobility muscles, on the other hand, generally respond much faster to a stimulus but also fatigue more rapidly than Type I fibers.

The internal component of a muscle fiber that makes contraction possible is the myofibril. Myofibrils consist of myofilaments (thick and thin filaments) that encompass the length of the cell and lie parallel to each other within the cell sarcoplasm. These filaments are comprised mainly of the proteins actin and myosin. The microstructure of this system appears as a repeating pattern of light and dark striations when viewed microscopically. This is why skeletal muscle is referred to as *striated*. Key terms and definitions for myofilament microstructure follow (figure 1.8).

- **A bands:** dark areas that correspond to the areas where thick filaments are present.
- **I bands:** light areas that contain only thin filaments.
- **Z line:** protein disk within an I band that anchors the thin filaments and connects adjacent myofibrils.
- **H zone:** located in the middle of each A band; this lighter stripe appears corresponding to the region between the thin filaments.
- **M line:** protein fibers that connect neighboring thick filaments.
- **Sarcomere:** the region of the myofibril between two Z lines.

The sarcomere is the basic functional (contractile) component of a myofiber. When contraction occurs, the Z lines move closer together.

While the sarcomere is the basic contractile component of a myofiber, the motor unit is the functional component (see figure 2.1 in chapter 2).

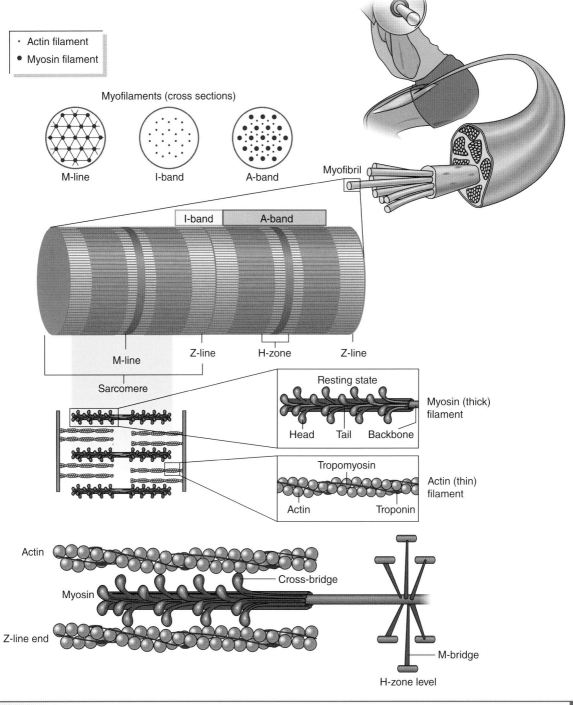

Figure 1.8 Muscle sarcomere.

Motor units are the nervous system connection to the muscle that enables voluntary contraction. Motor neurons (commonly known as *alpha motor neurons*) are nerve cells that connect the central nervous system to the muscle. Muscle fiber contraction occurs by means of excitation and activation of the specific muscle fiber's motor neurons. The nervous system recruits a motor unit by altering the voltage potential across the membrane of the cell body of the alpha motor neuron. This process involves a net summation of competing inhibitory and excitatory inputs.

Alpha motor neuron activation can come from multiple sources, first via recruitment and then by a process of rate coding. Motor units are recruited by the nervous system when the voltage potential across the membrane of the cell body of the alpha motor neuron is altered. Ions flow across the cell membrane and produce an electrical signal, or action potential. The action potential is disseminated down the axon of the alpha motor neuron to the motor end plate at the neuromuscular junction, creating a muscle contraction once the muscle fiber is activated. Increased muscle force is produced when additional muscle fibers are activated.

Individual motor axons from a motor neuron branch out within muscles to synapse on numerous muscle fibers. This wide area of distribution within the muscle ensures that a contraction induced by a motor unit is evenly distributed. This arrangement also reduces the likelihood that injury of one or several alpha motor neurons will significantly alter a muscle's action. An action potential generated by a motor neuron results in a contraction of all of the muscle fibers with which it synapses. A single alpha motor neuron and its associated muscle fibers are the smallest unit of force that can be activated to produce a movement.[46] When an action potential signal is sent from the nervous system, slow-twitch motor units always produce tension first, regardless of whether the intent of the movement is slow or fast.

The fusing of successive summated mechanical twitches in very close proximity of time frame to each other is called *tetanization*. Tetanization represents the greatest force level that is possible for a single muscle fiber.

Sliding Filament Theory

The complex interaction of the chemical, electrical, or mechanical stimuli to produce a muscle contraction has been termed the *sliding filament theory* of muscle contraction.[47] Cross bridging occurs between the myosin and actin myofilaments, with the actin sliding on the myosin chain of myofilaments. This process determines the strength of the muscle contraction.

An electrical stimulus initiates the muscle contraction from the associated motor neurons, causing depolarization of the muscle fiber. Calcium is then released into the cell, where it binds with a regulating protein, troponin. This combination of calcium and troponin causes actin to bind with myosin, initiating the muscle contraction. The muscle will relax once a cessation of the nerve's stimulus causes a reduction in the level of calcium in the muscle.[48] New crossbridges are formed when the stimulation of the muscle fiber occurs at a sufficient level. Crossbridges couple and decouple as myosin and actin interact so that tension can be maintained as the muscle shortens.

During all types of muscular contraction, the myosin and actin filaments remain unchanged in length. During isotonic contractions, the interdigitation between the two sets of filaments changes as the actin filaments slide on the myosin filaments, which results in a change of muscle fiber length. The width of the A bands stays unchanged, while the width of the I bands and H zone vary. As the muscle fibers shorten and the region of the interdigitation increases, the width of the I bands and H zones decrease. In contrast, as the length of the muscle increases and the interdigitation decreases, the width of the I bands and H zones increase (see figure 1.8). The specific sequence of events in muscular contraction is as follows:

1. Action potential is initiated and disseminated down the motor axon.
2. Acetylcholine is released from the axon terminal at the neuromuscular junction.
3. Acetylcholine binds to receptor sites on the motor end plate.
4. Potassium and sodium ions depolarize the muscle membrane.
5. Muscle action potential is disseminated over the membrane surface.
6. Depolarization of T-tubules releases calcium from the lateral sacs of the sarcoplasmic reticulum.
7. Calcium binds to the troponin–tropomyosin complex in actin filaments, releasing the inhibition of actin and myosin binding. The crossbridge between actin and myosin heads is created.
8. Actin combines with myosin adenosine triphosphate (ATP).
9. The energy created produces movement of the crossbridge of myosin and actin.
10. Myosin and actin slide relative to each other.
11. The myosin and actin crossbridge activation continues until the concentration of calcium remains high enough to inhibit the actin of the troponin–tropomyosin system.

12. The crossbridge is broken when stimulation ceases. Calcium moves back into the lateral sacs of the sarcoplasmic reticulum.

Therefore, the sliding filament theory is dependent on the various stimuli. The proper performance of this mechanism of muscle contraction is highly dependent on a properly functioning nervous system.

Muscle Force Production

The total force a muscle is capable of producing is a summation of both its active and passive elements. Contractile elements provide the active force (sliding actin and myosin myofilaments). Noncontractile elements (connective tissues) and the inherent elasticity of the contractile elements contribute to the passive force. The connective tissues that surround the myofilaments (endomysium and perimysium) as well as the myofilaments themselves make up the parallel elastic component of muscles. The muscle tendon that attaches in series with the contractile element and transmits the active contractile force to the bone makes up the series elastic component of muscles. These two elastic components contribute a passive force (tension) in addition to the active contractile force of muscle via energy stored by way of the elastic stretching that occurs in the tissues and the muscle's resultant capacity to return to normal

length when the stretch is released (analogous to stretch and release of a rubber band). Noncontractile tissue force production can occur with either passive stretching or active muscle contraction.

Muscle fiber architecture also influences the muscle's ability to produce contractile force. The two most basic arrangements of muscle fibers are parallel and pennate (fibers aligned at an angle relative to the muscle's force-generating axis; figure 1.9). Rhomboid and biceps brachii muscles are examples of parallel arrangements, and deltoid and rectus femoris muscles are examples of pennate arrangements. Pennate fiber arrangements promote force production while parallel fiber arrangements facilitate shortening. At a given level of fiber tension, a pennate arrangement will result in less force generation compared to a parallel fiber arrangement. However, the pennate arrangement enables more fibers to be packed into a limited space than the parallel arrangement. Thus pennate muscles contain more fibers per unit of muscle volume, which allows them to generate more force than the parallel fiber alignment for muscles of the same size.[49] The amount of force a muscle can generate is also influenced by the velocity of muscle shortening, the length of the muscle at the time it contracts, and the length of time since the muscle last received a stimulus to contract.

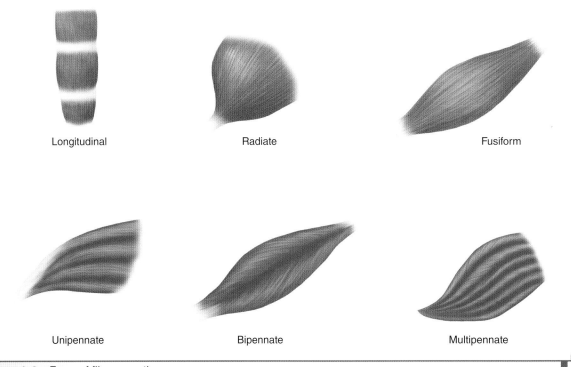

Longitudinal　　Radiate　　Fusiform

Unipennate　　Bipennate　　Multipennate

Figure 1.9 Types of fiber pennation.

A number of different types of muscle contractions exist, all with unique characteristics. For advantages and disadvantages of these different types of contraction, as well as the specific characteristics of each contraction type, see the sidebar. Muscle contractions that result in movement are known as *isotonic*. The basic types of isotonic muscle contraction are concentric, eccentric, and isokinetic. Isometric contractions are not isotonic.

- **Concentric:** A muscle shortens under tension.
- **Eccentric:** A muscle lengthens under tension.
- **Isokinetic:** A muscle lengthens or shortens while a constant velocity is maintained throughout the contraction.
- **Isometric:** A muscle produces tension at a fixed length, but no movement occurs.

Advantages and Disadvantages of Different Types of Muscular Contractions

Note: Concentric and eccentric are components of isotonic and isokinetic contractions. Isokinetic contractions are a unique form of isotonic (both can incorporate eccentric and concentric contractions).

Isotonic

Advantages

- Concentric and eccentric muscle action
- Can improve muscular endurance
- Multiplanar or functional training with free weights
- Can use body weight for resistance
- Can exercise through full ROM
- Inexpensive and readily available with most types of resistive devices
- Can use manual resistance from rehabilitation specialist
- Various components of the training program can be manipulated to maintain workload (reps, sets, weight)

Disadvantages

- Maximally loads muscle at its weakest point in the ROM, especially with elastic tubing
- Muscle only maximally challenged at one point in ROM with free weights and some machines
- Not safe when client has pain during movement
- Potential increased risk of injury at increased speeds of movement
- Difficult to perform at fast functional velocities
- Does not provide reciprocal concentric exercise
- Does not allow for rapid force development
- Unable to spread workload evenly over the entire ROM

Isokinetic

Advantages

- Concentric and eccentric strengthening of same muscle group reciprocally or repeatedly
- Reliable measures with equipment
- Wide range of exercise velocities
- Computer-based visual or auditory cues for feedback

(continued)

Advantages and Disadvantages of Different Types of Muscular Contractions *(continued)*

- Provides maximum resistance throughout ROM
- Safe to perform high- and low-velocity training
- Accommodation for painful arc of motion
- Decreased joint compressive forces at high speed
- Physiological overflow
- Isolated muscle strengthening
- External stabilization

Disadvantages

- Cannot produce angular velocities of many physical activities
- Large and expensive equipment
- Requires assistance and time for set-up
- Cannot use as a home program
- Most units only provide open kinetic chain movement
- Availability of equipment
- Cannot duplicate reciprocal speeds of movement used during most daily and functional activities
- Inconvenience of adjustment of equipment for various joints and ease of various set-ups
- Some artificial parameters until the limb actually moves at the velocity of the dynamometer on the machine

Isometric

Advantages

- Able to be used early in rehabilitation since there is no joint movement
- Angle-specific joint strengthening
- No special equipment needed
- Helps decrease swelling
- Short period of training time
- 20° strengthening overflow throughout ROM

Disadvantages

- Strengthening limited to specific joint angles
- No eccentric work
- Blood pressure concerns with Valsalva maneuver
- Less proprioceptive and kinesthetic training
- No muscle endurance training

Reprinted from J. Loudon, R. Manske, and M. Reiman, 2013, *Clinical mechanics and kinesiology* (Champaign, IL: Human Kinetics), 53-54.

Muscular strength is most commonly measured as the amount of torque a muscle group can generate at a joint. The tension-generating capability of a muscle is related to its cross-sectional area and training state. The amount of force developed in a maximal static action is independent of the fiber type, but it is related to the fiber's cross-sectional diameter. Since Type I fibers tend to have smaller diameters than Type II fibers, a high percentage of Type I fibers is believed to be associated with a smaller muscle diameter and therefore lower force development capabilities.[50] All else being equal, the force a muscle can exert is related to its cross-sectional area rather than its volume.[51] Muscular power is the product of force and velocity. Maximum power occurs at approximately one-third of maximum velocity and at approximately one-third of maximum concentric force. Muscular endurance is the ability of the muscle to exert tension over a period of time. As body temperature elevates, the speeds of nerve and muscle functions increase.

The relationship between muscle fiber length and the force that the fiber can produce at that length is known as the *muscle length–tension relationship*. The distance through which a muscle can lengthen and shorten is determined by the number of sarcomeres in the series. Sarcomere number is not fixed; in adult muscle, this number can increase or decrease.[52] For single muscle fibers and isolated muscle preparations, the greatest force generation is achieved by an active contraction occurring when the fiber is at its normal resting length (neither stretched nor contracted). If the fiber length is increased or decreased beyond resting length, the maximum force it can produce with an active contraction decreases (following the form of a bell-shaped curve known as the *length–tension curve*; figure 1.10).

In a shortened muscle, the overlap of actin and myosin reduces the number of sites available for crossbridge formation. Active insufficiency of a muscle occurs when a muscle is incapable of shortening to the extent required to produce full range of motion at all joints crossed simultaneously.[53]

In a lengthened muscle, the actin filaments are pulled away from the myosin heads so that they cannot create as many crossbridges. Passive insufficiency of a muscle occurs when a two-joint muscle cannot stretch to the extent required for full range of motion in the opposite direction at all joints crossed.[53]

In normal situations (in vivo), the passive elements of a muscle also contribute to force production. For example, a rapid stretch (eccentric contraction) of a muscle increases force during ensuing concentric phase due to the stored energy from the stretch of the passive elastic component. Within the human body, muscle force generation capability increases when the muscle is slightly stretched. Parallel-fiber muscles produce maximum tensions when stretched slightly more than resting length and pennate fiber muscles generate maximum tensions at between 120% and 130% of resting length. This increase in force production is a result of the contribution of the elastic components of muscle (primarily the series elastic component). When a muscle is actively stretched, the series elastic component creates an elastic recoil effect, and the stretch reflex simultaneously initiates the development of tension in the muscle. Thus, a prestretch promotes an additional passive force contribution to muscle shortening. An eccentric contraction followed immediately by a concentric contraction is known as the stretch-shortening cycle. The stretch-shortening cycle starts with an eccentric contraction (typically a small-amplitude stretch at a moderate to fast velocity), and is immediately followed by a concentric contraction. This occurs in muscles during many functional movements such as walking (eccentric stretch of the hip flexor muscles at toe off followed by concentric contraction for swing phase). The benefit of the stretch-shortening cycle is its ability to maximize the work done by the muscle.[54] The increase in muscle length that occurs during the eccentric component of a stretch-shortening cycle is relatively small compared to that which occurs during the controlled lowering of a load. This suggests that the eccentric contractions that occur as part of the stretch-shortening cycle provide greater mechanical efficiency and better energy dissipation than can be achieved with concentric contractions alone.[55] In addition, eccentric contractions can dampen the mechanical effects of impact forces, but they also increase the tissue damage associated with exercise. Evidence suggests that the neural commands controlling eccentric contractions are unique and that this individuality substantially increases the complexity of the strategies that the nervous system must use to control movement.[56]

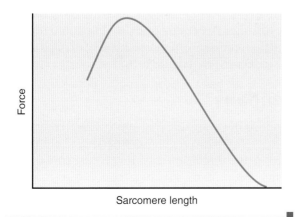

Figure 1.10   Length–tension curve.

The force generated by a muscle is also a function of its velocity. This is known as the *force–velocity relationship*. With concentric muscle contractions, there is an inverse relationship between the concentric force exerted by a muscle and the velocity at which the muscle is capable of shortening. Higher loads will slow the velocity of muscle shortening during concentric contraction. Conversely, the velocity of shortening can be relatively fast when concentric contraction occurs against low loads. The opposite is true with eccentric contractions (figure 1.11).

While concentric contractions provide the propulsive force necessary for such movements as running and jumping, a combination of eccentric and concentric contractions is needed for functional movement.

Muscular power is the product of force and velocity. Maximum power occurs at approximately one-third of maximum velocity and at approximately one-third of maximum concentric force. Muscular endurance is the ability of the muscle to exert tension over a period of time. As body temperature elevates, the speeds of nerve and muscle functions increase. Stronger muscles can produce greater magnitudes of isometric force on the force–velocity curve.

Plyometric strength training activities incorporate the stretch-shortening cycle and are commonly used to enhance athletic performance or functional performance (e.g., for rehabilitation purposes). Eccentric strength training involves the use of resistance that is greater than the person's capacity to generate maximum isometric force. Eccentric and plyometric training are associated with increased muscle soreness due to the potential for heavy eccentric loading of muscles. With both concentric and eccentric strength training, gains in strength over at least the first 12 weeks of training appear to be related to factors such as improved neurological system adaptations of the trained muscle rather than to changes in muscle-tissue characteristics such as an increase in cross-sectional area.[57]

The terms *open* and *closed kinetic chain exercises* are also frequently mentioned in conjunction with rehabilitation programs based on muscle-strengthening exercises. Open kinetic chain exercises are typically defined as non-weight-bearing, with movement occurring at a single joint. With these exercises, the distal segment is allowed to move, and the resistance is usually applied to the distal segment. The knee extension exercise, performed while sitting (moving the knee with resistance applied to the tibia), is an example of an open kinetic chain exercise. Closed kinetic chain exercises are typically defined as load bearing through the shafts of the bones. Movement at multiple joints is required to complete the movement, and the distal segment is usually fixed on a support surface. The resistance may be applied either proximally or distally, or both. An example of a closed kinetic chain exercise would be a squat. Closed kinetic chain exercises have gained popularity over open chain as the exercise of choice for rehabilitation in recent decades. Two common assumptions have apparently led to this popularity. First, closed chain exercises are believed to be safer than open chain exercises because they often place less strain on joint tissues. For example, lower limb closed chain exercises for clients in rehabilitation post anterior cruciate reconstruction place less strain on the ACL graft due to load bearing through the knee joint and cocontraction of the hamstrings. Second, closed chain exercises are believed to be more functional (or more closely reproduce functional movements) than open chain exercises. Therefore, because closed chain exercises are assumed to be safer and promote more normal function, they are often used in place of open chain exercises for rehabilitation.[58]

Tendons

Tendons are comprised of mostly a water–protein matrix and dense regular connective tissue structures (similar to ligaments) that connect muscle to bone. The primary role of a tendon is to transmit muscle-generated force to a bone, which results in movement around a joint. Tendons must also be flexible enough to accommodate movement around

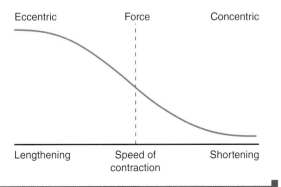

Figure 1.11   Force–velocity curve for eccentric and concentric isotonic contractions.

bone surfaces and to curve under the retinacula that alter the direction of pull. Tendons that function predominantly as force transmitters to bone are termed *positional tendons*. This role requires them to be relatively stiff under loading. Some tendons are also more capable of storing and releasing elastic strain energy based on the composition of their collagen infrastructure (spring-like tendons). This increases efficiency of force production for functions such as gait. One example is the Achilles tendon in the ankle.[59] Tendon collagen architecture is oriented along the lines of stress to optimize function.

While there are slight differences in material and molecular properties between spring-like tendons and positional tendons, there are many similarities in their physiologic composition. The cell type most commonly found in tendons is the tenocyte (fibroblast cells). These spindle-shaped cells are arranged in parallel rows along the lines of stress or muscle loading. They produce collagen and help promote healing after injury. The collagen found in tendons is primarily Type I (makes up ~85% of dry weight of tendons), the most abundant type of collagen in the human body. Tendons also contain some Type III collagen (up to 5% dry weight of tendons). Type III collagen (also known as reticular fibers) provides support and is fibrous in nature, meaning that it contains elastic qualities as well as the typical qualities of collagen. The basic structural unit of collagen is tropocollagen, a long, thin protein produced inside fibroblast cells. Tropocollagen is secreted into the extracellular matrix as procollagen. In addition to collagen, proteoglycans make up approximately 5% of dry weight of tendons. Several key proteoglycans include the following:[60]

- Decorin is the most common proteoglycan in tendon. It regulates collagen-fiber diameter and forms cross-links that enable transfer of loading between collagen fibers.
- Aggrecan holds water and resists compressive forces; therefore, it is commonly found in areas of tendon compression.

Tendons are organized as bundles of bundles, similar to muscle tissue. Their organization is as follows: microfibrils, subfibrils, fibrils, fascicles, and the tendon unit. Tropocollagen forms cross-links to create collagen fibers, which then combine to form microfibrils. Microfibrils bind together to form microscopically visible units, the collagen subfibrils. A group of collagen subfibrils forms a collagen fibril. A group of collagen fibrils forms a fascicle, and

bundles of fascicles make up the tendon. Tendon tissue that inserts into bone undergoes transitions from tendon to fibrocartilage to mineralized fibrocartilage (known as Sharpey's fibers) and finally to bone tissue.[61]

A fine sheath of connective tissue called endotenon envelops each collagen fiber and binds fibers together. A grouping of collagen fibers forms a primary fiber bundle and a group of primary fiber bundles forms a secondary fiber bundle. A group of secondary fiber bundles, in turn, forms a tertiary bundle, and the tertiary bundles make up the tendon. The entire tendon is surrounded by a fine connective tissue sheath called epitenon. Tendons are then surrounded by another connective tissue layer, either a paratenon (e.g., patellar, Achilles tendons) or a synovial sheath (e.g., hand flexor tendons). Paratenon-covered tendons are known for their rich vascular supply (enhances ability to heal), and they are most likely to fail at either the musculotendinous junction or the tendon–bone junction. The paratenon consists of two layers. The deeper layer of the paratenon that connects to the underlying epitenon is known as the mesotenon. The mesotenon conveys vasculature to the underlying muscle tissue. Sheathed tendons are less vascularized and may even contain avascular areas that receive nutrition only by diffusion. This feature allows for smooth gliding of these long tendons but puts them at risk for adhesion development during healing after an injury such as a laceration.

In general, connective tissue is a vital component of nearly every organ. Connective tissue not only functions as a mechanical support for other tissues but also serves as an avenue for communication and transport between tissues. An often overlooked key function of connective tissue is modulation of the healing process. The principal cells involved in immunological defense and injury repair reside within connective tissues.[62]

Similar to other connective tissues described in this chapter (e.g., ligaments and joint capsules), tendons exhibit the biomechanical properties of stress–strain, anisotropy, and viscoelasticity. Their biomechanical properties result from extracellular matrix characteristics. The key constituents of this matrix are collagen, proteoglycans, and water. Similar to ligaments, tendons are highly organized fibrous tissues with mechanical properties that are directionally dependent (anisotropic).[63] Tendons generally contain more collagen and less elastin than ligaments, which makes them better at transmitting the force of muscle contraction to move bones, but somewhat less able to stretch and absorb forces. Tendons typically carry higher stress loads during function than ligaments. Thus, tendon collagen fibers are recruited more quickly than ligament collagen fibers would be when placed under tension. This results in greater stiffness, which enables the bone to transmit force more effectively. Therefore, tendons are less viscoelastic than ligaments. However, they do exhibit viscoelastic behavior with nonlinear elasticity; thus, the rate of force loading on a tendon does influence its mechanical properties. Normal stresses, such as exercise, increase tendon tolerance to loads through remodeling, while disuse or immobilization results in reduction of load tolerance. This has implications for stress progression activities applied during training or injury rehabilitation. Tendon strength (load tolerance) normally increases from birth to maturity and begins to decrease after maturity.[63] Tendons are tolerant to tension forces, but buckle with compression forces. They also demonstrate creep and stress relaxation curves similar to ligaments.

CONCLUSION

Musculoskeletal problems are a growing source of disability, particularly with the increasing population of aging adults. Knowledge of the basic science fundamentals of the musculoskeletal system enables clinicians to build a conceptual model for their orthopedic practice. Ideally, this information will enhance understanding of clinical problems at multiple levels: pathophysiology at the cellular level, gross morphology, and clinical presentation as assessed through history, physical examination, and laboratory findings. Thus, clinicians should improve their ability to address the societal and economic burdens presented by musculoskeletal disorders. Research in the normal biology of musculoskeletal tissues, the diseases and injuries associated with these tissues, and the underlying mechanisms of musculoskeletal tissue regeneration are likely continue to advance and provide additional benefits in the future.

2

NERVOUS SYSTEM AND PAIN

Michael P. Reiman, PT, DPT, OCS, SCS, ATC, FAAOMPT, CSCS
Adriaan Louw, PT, PhD, CSMT

The nervous system is vital to several systems in the body, especially the musculoskeletal system. Therefore, in order to completely and sufficiently examine the musculoskeletal client, the clinician must fully understand the nervous system and know how to examine it. The primary divisions of the nervous system are the central nervous system (CNS) and the peripheral nervous system (PNS). Pain and its neurophysiology is quite complex. This chapter describes various types of pain, the structural divisions of the nervous system, the general function of the nervous system, and the neurophysiology of pain.

STRUCTURAL DIVISIONS OF THE NERVOUS SYSTEM

The two structural divisions of the nervous system are organized into the central nervous system (CNS) and the peripheral nervous system (PNS). The CNS consists of the brain and spinal cord, while the PNS is made up of 43 pairs of nerves arising from the CNS. Of these 43 pairs, the 12 pairs of cranial nerves arise from the base of the brain. The other 31 pairs of spinal nerves originate from the spinal cord.

Central Nervous System

The spinal cord is normally 42 to 45 cm long in adults and has the brain stem and medulla at its upper end. The conus medullaris is the distal end of the spinal cord. In adults, the conus medullaris ends at the L1 or L2 level of the vertebral column.

Three membranes envelop the structures of the CNS: the dura mater, arachnoid, and pia mater. The dura mater is the outermost and strongest of the membranes. The dura forms the dural sac around the spinal cord. It is separated from the bones and ligaments of the vertebral canal by an epidural space, which can become partly calcified or even ossified with age.[1] The pia mater is the deepest of the three layers. It is firmly attached to the outer surface of the spinal cord and nerve roots. The pia mater conveys the blood vessels that supply the spinal cord. It also contains the denticulate ligaments that anchor the spinal cord to the dura mater.[1]

Injury to the CNS is characterized as an upper motor neuron (UMN) lesion. These lesions are located in white columns of the spinal cord and cerebral hemispheres. UMN lesions are characterized by spastic paralysis or paresis, little or no muscle atrophy, hyperreflexive deep tendon reflexes (DTRs) in a nonsegmental distribution, and presence of pathologic signs and reflexes (see the section in chapter 7, Examination of the Physical Health of the Nervous System).

Lower motor neuron (LMN) lesions begin at the alpha motor neuron and include the dorsal and ventral roots, spinal nerve, peripheral nerve, neuromuscular (NM) junction, and muscle-fiber complex. Characteristics of this type of lesions include muscle atrophy and hypotonus, diminished or absent DTR of areas served by a spinal nerve root or a peripheral nerve, and absence of pathologic signs or reflexes.

The differing symptoms between UMN and LMN lesions are the result of injuries to different parts of the nervous system. LMN impairment involves damage to a neurologic structure distal to the anterior horn cell, whereas UMN involves damage to a neurologic structure proximal to the anterior horn cell, namely, the spinal cord or CNS.

Peripheral Nervous System

The peripheral nervous system is composed of the 12 cranial nerves and the 31 spinal nerves. The cranial nerve roots enter and exit the brain stem to provide sensory and motor innervation to the head and muscles of the face. The cranial nerves, their function, and assessment are further discussed in chapter 7 in the section Examination of the Physical Health of the Nervous System.

The spinal nerves are divided topographically into 8 cervical pairs (C1-C8), 12 thoracic pairs (T1-T12), 5 lumbar pairs (L1-L5), 5 sacral pairs (S1-S5), and a coccygeal pair. The posterior (dorsal) and anterior (ventral) roots of the spinal nerves are located within the vertebral canal. The portion of the spinal nerve that occupies the intervertebral foramen, and thus is no longer in the vertebral canal, is referred to as the *peripheral nerve*.

The peripheral nerves are commonly divided into common components: cervical plexus, brachial plexus, lumbar plexus, and sacral plexus. Additionally, nerves in the thoracic region are grouped into either posterior (dorsal) rami or anterior (ventral) rami. For detail on the specific peripheral nerves and their examination, please refer to chapter 7.

Nerve fibers are generally categorized according to function: sensory, motor, or mixed (motor and sensory). Sensory nerves carry afferents (nerves conveying impulses from the periphery to the CNS) from a portion of the skin. They also carry efferents (nerves conveying impulses from the CNS to the periphery). The area of sensory nerve distribution is called a dermatome, and it generally follows the segmental distribution of the underlying nerve distribution.[1]

Motor nerves carry efferents to muscles, and sensory nerves return sensation from muscles, ligaments, and associated tissues. Nerves that innervate muscles also mediate the sensation from the joint that those muscles act on. The law of parsimony, stating that the nervous system activates the fewest muscles or muscle fibers possible to control a joint, exists with muscle recruitment for motor function.

A mixed nerve is the combination of skin, sensory, and motor fibers to one trunk. These nerves would therefore have the characteristics of each of these types of nerves. Therefore, they would provide the functions of each of these nerve types.

As discussed previously, a dermatome is an area of skin supplied by a single nerve. Dermatomes overlap, and pain dermatomes have less overlap than light-touch palpation dermatomes. The degree of dermatome overlap and variability in their description warrants greater investigation and understanding.[2] A myotome is a particular muscle or muscle group innervated by a single nerve root. A sclerotome is an area of bone or fascia supplied by a single nerve root. Assessment of dermatomes and myotomes is also discussed in the examination of the nervous system (chapter 7).

Irrespective of the nerve fiber type, three layers of tissue enclose the peripheral nerves. From outermost to innermost layer, they include the epineurium, perineurium, and endoneurium. The attachment of the epineurium with the surrounding connective tissue is loose so that the nerve trunks are relatively mobile, except where they are tethered by entering vessels or exiting nerve branches.[3]

The four functional parts of the neuron are as follows (figure 2.1):

- **Dendrites** receive information from other nerve cells or the environment.
- **Axons** conduct information to other nerve cells. Axons are often covered by myelin. Myelin is a lipid rich-membrane with a high electrical resistance. It serves to increase the nerve conduction velocity of neural transmissions through the process of salutatory conduction. Along the axon are segments

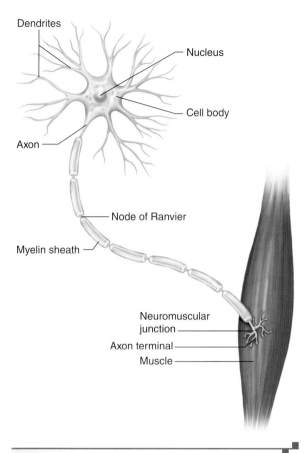

Figure 2.1   The motor unit.

that lack myelin called nodes of Ranvier. The axon extends from the cell body to the muscle, where it divides into either a few or multiple smaller branches.

- **The cell body** contains the nucleus of the cell and performs integrative functions. It is located in the anterior horn of the spinal cord.
- **The axon terminal** is the transmission site for action potentials.

Communication among nerve cells occurs at the synapses. It is here that a chemical is released in the form of a neurotransmitter.

Each muscle contains many motor units, each containing a single motoneuron and its composite muscle fibers. The number of muscle fibers belonging to a motor unit (i.e., the innervation ratio) and the number of motor units within a muscle vary. Activities of relatively low-force contraction have a lower innervation ratio and vice versa.

Motor unit size is determined by the number of muscle fibers that it contains and the size of the motor nerve axon. Fiber number varies from two or three to a few thousand. Muscles performing fine motor control have small-size motor units. These motor units typically have small cell bodies and small-diameter axons. Muscles that are used to produce large forces and large movements typically have a predominance of large-size motor units, large cell bodies, and large diameter axons.

Motor Unit Recruitment

The size principle of motor unit recruitment states that motor units with small cell bodies and few motor fibers are recruited first by the nervous system and then, as force is increased, larger motor units are recruited.[4, 5] Small motor units produce less tension than large motor units and require less energy expenditure, thereby conserving energy. Recruitment strategy is not only based on energy efficiency but also on previous experience, the anticipated magnitude of the required force, and type of muscle action.[5, 6]

Autonomic Nervous System

The autonomic nervous system is the portion of the PNS responsible for innervation of smooth muscle, cardiac muscle, and glands of the body. It primarily functions without our conscious control. The two primary components of the autonomic system include the sympathetic and parasympathetic divisions. In general, these systems function in opposition to each other. The sympathetic division typically functions in actions requiring quick responses, often referred to as *fight or flight*. The sympathetic nervous system is generally located in the thoracolumbar region of the spine and has norepinephrine (except sweat glands) as its principal neurotransmitter. The parasympathetic division functions with actions that do not require immediate action. Some of the primary functions of this division include salivation, lacrimation, urination, food digestion, and defecation. This system is located primarily in the craniosacral region of the spine and has acetylcholine as its principal neurotransmitter.

NEUROMUSCULAR CONTROL

Control of coordinated movements and stability throughout the body requires a properly functioning nervous system. The CNS activates muscles in an integrated fashion to collectively work together to produce the desired motion. The amount of practice required to perform these movements in a properly coordinated fashion should be enough to make changes in the cortical activity of the CNS.[7] The repetition number required to achieve this is quite variable.[7]

Kinesthetic Sense and Proprioception

Proprioception is the sensory abilities required for proper neuromuscular control. Proprioception involves the integration of sensory input concerning static joint position sense, joint movement (kinesthesia), velocity of movement, and force of muscular contraction from the skin, muscles, and joints.[8, 9]

All synovial joints in the body have mechanoreceptors and nociceptors in articular, muscular, and cutaneous structures. Mechanoreceptors are stimulated by mechanical forces (e.g., stretching, relaxation, and compression), and they mediate proprioception. These structures include Pacinian corpuscles, Ruffini endings, the muscle spindle, and Golgi tendon organ–like endings.[10] Table 2.1 provides more discussion on these mechanoreceptors.

Mechanoreceptors appear to protect the joint from injury in three primary ways:

1. They avoid movement of the joint in the pathological range. Extremes of joint motion activate the mechanoreceptors of the ligaments, initiating a spinal reflex with contraction of muscles antagonizing the movement through a ligamentomuscular reflex.[13]

2. They help in balancing the activity between synergistic and antagonistic muscle forces.

3. They appear to generate an image of body position and movement within the central nervous system.

Muscle Spindle

Muscle spindles are fusiform in shape and widely scattered in the fleshy bellies of skeletal muscles.

TABLE 2.1   Types of Mechanoreceptors

Type	Location	Function
Type I: small Ruffini endings	Joint capsule and in ligaments	• Contribute to reflex regulation of postural tone, muscle coordination, and perceptional awareness of joint position • An increase in joint capsule tension, via range of motion, posture, mobilization, or manipulation, increases their frequency of firing[10]
Type II: Pacinian corpuscles	Adipose tissue, cruciate and other ligaments, annulus fibrosus, and fibrous capsule	• Function primarily in sensing joint motion • Regulate motor unit activity of prime movers of the joint • Entirely inactive in immobile joints • Discharge during active or passive motion of a joint, or with applied traction
Type III: large Ruffini endings	In the intrinsic and extrinsic joint ligaments, superficial layers of the capsule, but not in the anterior or posterior longitudinal ligaments	• Detect large amounts of tension • Only become active in the extremes of motion or when strong manual techniques are applied to a joint
Type IV: Nociceptors	Free, noncapsulated nerve endings that form a network of unmyelinated nerve fibers[11, 12]	• Inactive in normal circumstances, but become active with significant mechanical deformation or tension • May also become active in response to direct mechanical or chemical irritation

Each spindle consists of 2 to 10 slender striated muscle fibers that are enclosed within a thin connective tissue capsule and attached at both ends to the epimysium or ordinary striated muscle. These slender muscle fibers, innervated by gamma fibers, are known as *intrafusal fibers.* They are tiny compared with the extrafusal fibers that produce contractile tension within a muscle.[14] Muscle spindles are aligned parallel to the extrafusal fibers. Smaller intrafusal fibers are known as *nuclear chain fibers,* while the larger fibers are designated as *nuclear bag fibers.* The ends of the nuclear chain fibers are attached to the polar parts of the longer nuclear bag fibers (figure 2.2).

The neuromuscular spindle is arranged in parallel to the extrafusal or contractile fibers of the muscle, unlike Golgi tendon organs, which are oriented in series. Therefore, when the tension on the spindle is relaxed, the afferent input from the annulospiral endings ceases, and the muscle relaxes.

The muscle spindle has both sensory and motor components. The purpose of the muscle spindle is to compare the length of the spindle with the length of the muscle that surrounds the spindle.

When a muscle is stretched, the primary sensory fibers of the muscle spindle (Type Ia afferent neurons) respond to both changes in muscle length and velocity by transmitting this activity to the spinal cord in the form of changes in the rate of action potentials. Additionally, secondary sensory fibers (Type II afferent neurons) respond to muscle length changes and transmit this signal to the spinal cord. The Ia afferent signals are transmitted monosynaptically to many alpha motor neurons of the muscle. The activity of the alpha motoneurons is then transmitted via the efferent axons to the extrafusal muscle fiber, which generates force and thereby resists the stretch. The Ia afferent signal is also transmitted polysynaptically through interneurons that inhibit alpha motoneurons of antagonistic muscles, causing them to relax.

Golgi Tendon Organ

Golgi tendon organs (GTOs) are made up of strands of collagen that are connected at one end to the muscle fiber and at the other end to the tendon proper (figure 2.3). Each GTO is innervated by a single afferent Type Ib sensory fiber that branches and terminates as spiral endings around the collagen strands.

When the muscle generates force, the sensory terminals are compressed. This stretching deforms the terminals of the Ib afferent axon. As a result, the Ib axon is depolarized, and it fires nerve impulses

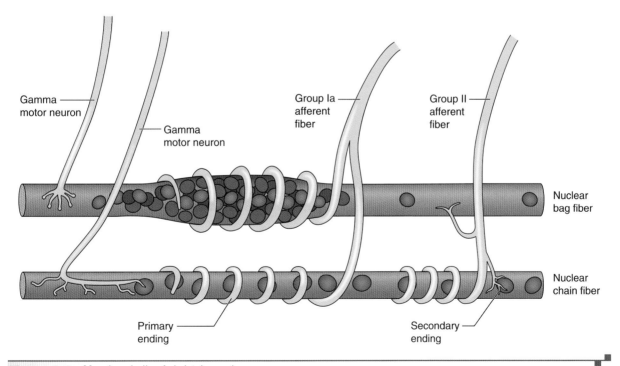

Figure 2.2 Muscle spindle of skeletal muscle.

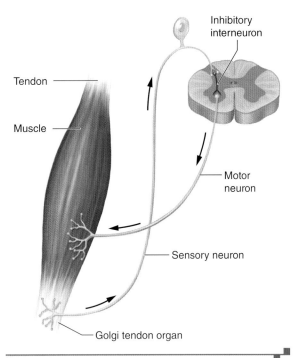

Tendon

Muscle

Inhibitory interneuron

Motor neuron

Sensory neuron

Golgi tendon organ

Figure 2.3 Golgi tendon organ.

that are disseminated to the spinal cord. The action potential frequency signals the force being developed by the 10 to 20 motor units within the muscle. This is representative of whole muscle force.[15]

The Ib sensory feedback generates spinal reflexes and supraspinal responses that control muscle contraction. Ib afferent axons synapse with interneurons within the spinal cord that also project to the cerebellum and cerebral cortex. One of the main spinal reflexes associated with Ib afferent activity is the autogenic inhibition reflex, which helps regulate the force of muscle contractions.

Balance

Balance, or what can be referred to as postural control, involves a complex interaction of integrating sensory input (assessing the body's position and motion in space) and properly executing appropriate muscular responses to control this body position with its own stability limits, as well as within the context of the environment and relative to gravity.[16, 17] Balance requires the proper integration of different body systems (the nervous system and muscular system) and the interaction between these two systems.[17] The nervous system

provides processing of the sensory information of body position and movement in space. This sensory input comes primarily from the visual, vestibular, and somatosensory systems. The musculoskeletal system contributions include postural body alignment, joint integrity, muscle flexibility, muscle performance, and mechanoreceptor sensation. Proper balance requires the integration of the components of each of these systems in unison.

Proper performance of daily tasks requires appropriate static and dynamic balance, as well as the ability to properly react to maintain balance when unexpected external perturbations are placed on the body. These autonomic postural responses include the ankle, the hip, and the stepping strategies.[18] Each of these strategies properly adjusts the body's center of gravity within its own base of support to prevent loss of balance or falling.

- **Ankle strategy:** employed with small perturbations. The muscles around the ankle are used to provide postural stability in the anteroposterior plane. For example, if you are standing on a bus that stops quickly, you would have to lean your whole body forward at the ankles to maintain proper balance.

- **Hip strategy:** employed with larger perturbations. Muscles around the hip and trunk are recruited. For example, if you are standing on a bus that stops quickly, you might lean from your trunk to maintain proper balance.

- **Stepping strategy:** employed if the previous two strategies are not sufficient for maintaining body balance. A step is taken with this strategy. Taking the previous bus example, you would have to step forward with one foot to avoid losing your balance.

Reflexes

A reflex is a subconscious, programmed unit of behavior where a stimulus from a receptor automatically leads to a response from an effector. The two primary types of reflexes are as follows:

- **Muscle stretch reflex.** The muscle stretch reflex is one of the simplest known reflexes. It is dependent on two neurons and one synapse and influenced by cortical and subcortical input, and comes from the stimulation of the GTO and muscle spindle receptors. The quick tap of the reflex hammer on the tendon causes a brief stretch of the tendon and muscle belly, stimulating the intrafusal fiber (muscle spindle) and GTO, which cause the extrafusal fiber to contract. When testing these reflexes, clients should relax and slightly flex the extremity to be tested. The Jendrassik maneuver can be used to enhance a muscle reflex that is difficult to elicit:

- For reflexes in the upper extremity, clients are asked to cross their ankles and try to isometrically abduct their feet.
- For reflexes in the lower extremity, clients are asked to interlock their fingers on each hand and attempt to isometrically pull them apart.

- **Pathologic reflexes.** A number of primitive reflexes are naturally integrated as we develop. Pathologic reflexes occur when a disease process or injury results in loss of the normal suppression by the cerebrum on the segmental level of the brain stem or the spinal cord, resulting in a release of the primitive reflex.[19] The presence of pathologic reflexes is suggestive of CNS (and therefore upper motor neuron) impairment, requiring appropriate referral.

For more details on reflex testing, amplitude, and integrity, as well as examination of the nervous system, see chapter 7 (Orthopedic Screening and Nervous System Examination).

NEUROPHYSIOLOGY OF PAIN

Pain is produced in the brain. This normal experience has many definitions. Pain is based on perception of threat. Threat is an expression of intention to inflict evil, injury, or damage. As it pertains to pain, people may have different threats, based on various factors. For example, in a whiplash study comparing medical doctors' illness and care-seeking behaviors for whiplash associated disorders, compared to people without medical training, a significant difference was observed.[20] Both groups sustained similar injuries; however, the perception of the injury and recovery was seen as a major difference in the ensuing care-seeking behaviors between the groups. Pain is based on perception of threat, since perceptions include the individualistic nature of pain.[21] Clinicians can easily understand this inclusion of perception of threat. Clients exposed to provocative medical terminology proposed to be associated with pain, such as *degenerative disc disease*, *bulging discs*, and *wear and tear* show heightened levels of fear and anxiety.[22] How clients perceive the health of their tissues (correctly or incorrectly) will determine to what extent their brains will produce pain to protect.[21]

Pain is a defense mechanism.[24] Pain, however, is only one of many output systems that are designed to defend. During a pain experience, other biological

Pain Definitions

Pain—An unpleasant sensory and emotional experience associated with actual or potential tissue damage, or described in terms of such damage.

Allodynia—Pain due to a stimulus that does not normally provoke pain.

Hyperalgesia—Increased pain from a stimulus that normally provokes pain.

Hypoalgesia—Diminished pain in response to a normally painful stimulus.

Neuropathic pain—Pain caused by a lesion or disease of the somatosensory nervous system.

Nociception—The neural process of encoding noxious stimuli.

Nociceptive pain—Pain that arises from actual or threatened damage to non-neural tissue; due to the activation of nociceptors.

Central sensitization—Increased responsiveness of nociceptive neurons in the central nervous system to their normal or subthreshold afferent input.

Peripheral sensitization—Increased responsiveness and reduced threshold of nociceptive neurons in the periphery to the stimulation of their receptive fields.

systems engage to protect the body. These become increasingly visibly as pain persists. For example, during a pain experience, motor control, endocrine, immune, language, respiration, posture, energy expenditure, and gastrointestinal function are all altered to deal with the immediate threat. Once the threat (e.g., acute injury) is removed, homeostasis is restored. In persistent pain, these biological defenses become more pronounced. This explains various chronic pain issues such as trigger points, fatigue, widespread sensitivity, and sensitivity to foods.[25, 26]

Tissues contain nociceptors and nociceptive fibers. In the event of an injury or disease, tissues can only tell the brain of danger or nociception. The brain decides to produce pain or not. For example, if an ankle contained pain fibers and a person sprains their ankle crossing a busy street, pain may cause the person to fall down or slow down, endangering their life as speeding traffic heads their way. In this case, pain is not produced by the brain. The person runs out of the way, and when their life is not in danger, their brain produces pain.[26]

Cognitions powerfully affect pain.[25, 27, 28] Various cognitions need consideration; however, two have been heavily implicated in persistent pain states: fear[29-32] and catastrophization.[28, 33]

In most respects, pain has been divided into acute and chronic pain.

- **Acute pain.** Acute pain, by definition, is of sudden onset and expected to last a short time. It can usually be linked clearly to a specific event, injury, or illness (e.g., a muscle strain, severe sunburn, a kidney stone, or pleurisy). People can handle many types of acute pain on their own with over-the-counter medications or a short course of stronger analgesics and rest. The acute pain usually subsides when the underlying cause resolves, such as when a kidney stone or diseased tooth is removed. Acute pain can also be a recurrent problem, with episodes being interspersed with pain-free periods, as in the case of dysmenorrhea, migraine, and sickle-cell disease.

- **Chronic pain.** Chronic pain, by contrast, lasts more than several months (variously defined as 3 to 6 months, but certainly longer than normal healing). Clinically, chronic pain is more challenging to treat due to its inherent complexity. Although improvement may be possible, for many clients, cure is unlikely. Chronic pain can become so debilitating that it affects every aspect of a person's life—the ability to work, go to school, perform common tasks, maintain friendships and family relationships—essentially, it hinders the ability to participate in the fundamental tasks and pleasures of daily living. Chronic pain can be the result of an underlying disease or medical condition, In this case, it may continue or recur after the disease itself has been cured, such as in shingles. It may simply not go away, and flare-ups may occur against a background of persistent pain, as in many instances of low back pain or osteoarthritis. It may also worsen as the disease (such as cancer) progresses.

Pain, Nerves, and Conduction

It could be argued that the gate control theory, more commonly referred to as the *pain gate*, is the predominant mechanism therapists use for understanding pain and developing treatments to modulate a client's pain experience.[34] Since the early 1900s, scientists have focused their attention on various nerve fibers, ultimately leading to a widely accepted classification of nerve fibers based on size and speed of conduction: A, B, and C fibers.[35, 36] These nerve fibers are also typically categorized as being responsible for things such as pain, light touch, or pressure.[35]

- Type A fibers are the thickest and fastest conducting, with a diameter of between 1.5 and 20 microns and a speed of conduction that varies from 4 to 120 m/s, which shows that they have a really fast conduction of impulse. They are myelinated. Examples of type A fibers are skeletomotor fibers and afferent fibers to the skin.

- Type B fibers are medium in size (i.e., they are smaller than type A fibers but larger than type C) and myelinated. They have a diameter of 1.5 to 3.5 microns. Their speed of conduction is 3 to 15 m/s, which shows that they are slower than type A fibers. Examples of type B fibers are preganglionic autonomic efferents.

- Type C fibers are the smallest and thinnest. They are nonmyelinated and have a diameter of 0.1 to 2 microns. Their speed of conduction is 0.5 to 4 m/s, which shows that they have the slowest conduction. Examples of type C fibers are postganglionic autonomic efferents and afferent fibers to skin. Many clinicians are taught that C fibers are pain fibers and are thus responsible, along with A-delta fibers, for conducting pain.

Based on the specialized activity of nerves, Melzack and Wall developed gate control.[34] According to gate control, information is sent to the dorsal horn of the spinal cord, and ultimately to the brain, from various nerve fibers, including thin nociceptive fibers as well as larger diameter fibers dealing with touch, pressure, and vibration. Along the way, the information can be modulated by various interactions, including inhibition by the substantia gelatinosa. Many physical treatments, such as large amplitude passive range of motion, transcutaneous electrical neuromuscular stimulation (TENS), massage, or electrical stimulation, are thought to control pain in part by activating low-threshold, large-diameter, non-nociceptive sensory nerve fibers dealing with touch, pressure, and vibration, which inhibit nociception by closing the gate to nociception at the spinal cord level. Anecdotally, this explains why people rub an injury site or even walk it off, stimulating nerve fibers that in essence override the pain signals.

Although the gate control theory explains many observations regarding pain and modulation, it has various shortcomings, shown by the new, updated research in regard to pain.[27, 37, 38] Gate control cannot account for pain in phantom limb clients or pain in quadriplegics, nor can it account for the complex immune and inflammatory processes that have now been shown to be key components in pain. Furthermore, the pain gate does not take into consideration emotions or descending inhibitory pathways of the brain. Ron Melzack, one of the original authors of the pain gate, has urged clinicians to recognize the shortcomings of the pain gate and embrace the current, more updated view of pain, the brain, and the neuromatrix.[37-40]

Input and Processing Mechanisms in Pain

In an injury or degenerative process, nociceptive fibers send repeated messages to the dorsal horn of the spinal cord. In the spinal cord, repeated stimulation at constant strength of dorsal root afferents (including nociceptive C fibers) can elicit a progressive increase in the number of action potentials generated by motoneurons and interneurons (IN).[41, 42] This process, referred to as *action potential wind-up*, is the consequence of a cumulative membrane depolarization resulting from the temporal summation of slow synaptic potentials. Simply stated, with persistent input from the periphery, changes to the spinal cord second-order neurons, and ultimately brain pathways, leads to a heightened sensitization. With an immediate acute injury, A-delta fibers will send nociception to the spinal cord with the intent to pass the nociceptive message to the brain for action. For example, during a knee injury (medial aspect of the knee), the sensory afferent input will be received into the dorsal horn of the spinal cord (L3) from the affected side (i.e., right side). The nociception from the A-delta fibers chemically activates AMPA receptors (α-amino-3-hydroxy-5-methyl-4-isoxazolepropionic acid receptor) on the second-order neurons via glutamate.[43, 44] Second-order neurons will then relay messages from the spinal cord to the brain.

The nociception is passed on to the brain for interpretation and action. In this acute stage, the pain, although intense, will not usually last. Some of this is due to inhibition via the endogenous mechanisms of the brain, spinal cord, and descending pathways. Descending pathways, usually from the periaqueductal gray (PAG) area produce serotonin, endorphins, opioids, and enkephalins, which inhibit the nociception and ultimately the pain experience.[45] If stimulation of the medial knee persists, then nociceptive fibers will continue firing (in this case, the longer-lasting C fibers).

From the same innervated area on the medial aspect of the knee, A-beta fibers constantly send nociception to the spinal cord for interpretation in the form of light touch. On a daily basis, due to light touch stimulation, this nociception is also passed to the spinal cord, via the L3 dorsal horn, to inform the brain of the light touch. In this case, however, the nociception is blocked at spinal cord level, partly due to actions of the IN. These IN form a connection between other neurons. IN are neither motor nor sensory. In the central nervous system, the term *IN* is used for small, locally projecting neurons, in contrast to larger projection neurons with long-distance connections. Central nervous system IN are typically inhibitory, and they use the neurotransmitter gamma-aminobutyric acid (GABA) or glycine. However, excitatory interneurons using glutamate also exist, as do interneurons releasing neuromodulators like acetylcholine. Following input from A-beta fibers, the interneuron may block the message with a release of GABA. The message ends, and the sensation of light touch from the pants is not registered cortically,[46] so the injured person is not aware of the light touch stimulation around the knee.

With persistent nociception via C fibers, permanent neuroplastic changes are likely to occur. After constant barrage from the C fibers, the IN may die due to high levels of amino acids.[46-49] The end result is a decreased ability to modulate nociception and, ultimately, a pain experience.[43, 44, 46, 50]

Pain, Neuromatrix, and the Brain

The neuromatrix theory was introduced in 1996 by pain scientist Ron Melzack.[40] At the heart of the neuromatrix approach is the brain and, more precisely, an understanding that pain is 100% produced by the brain when it perceives danger and determines that action is required.[27] Traditional pain models such as the pain gate have focused on a rather peripheral view of pain. It seems rather elementary now that the brain must be involved in processing pain. To understand the brain's processing of this nociceptive information and ultimately a pain experience, we need to dispel the belief that a specific pain area exists within the brain, such that when you hit your thumb with a hammer, this area will activate so that you will experience pain.[38] This notion of a single pain area notion was dispelled by observations of clients following cerebral lobotomy and even cerebral hemispherectomy.[51, 52] Multiple studies involving functional brain scanning have now shown that during a painful experience, many different brain areas are active; these areas have now been more comprehensively described.[27, 38, 53, 54] The pain neuromatrix is thus best defined as a collection of brain areas activated during a pain experience.[25] Pain is therefore quite complex, and it involves various areas.

For years, scientists were aware that certain areas of the brain (i.e., anterior cingulate cortex, thalamus, and sensory cortex) were activated during a pain experience. The neuromatrix theory, however, conceptualized that these activated neuronal areas communicate with each other as a network as a means to protect (hence, the names *pain neuromatrix* and *pain neural signature* or *map*). The neuromatrix allows us to update our view of pain, based on this definition of pain by Moseley: "Pain is a multiple system output, activated by an individual's specific pain neuromatrix. The pain neuromatrix is activated when the body tissues are in danger and action is required."[27]

Biological Effects of Pain

Persistent pain, biologically, represents a threat response.[26, 55] The threat response, often assigned to the sympathetic nervous system, is the fight or flight response. The stress response during an immediate threat, however, is significantly more complex, and it involves other bodily systems. During an acute stress response such as acute pain or injury, the body reacts with various systems:

- **Sympathetic nervous system (SNS):** Adrenaline, closely associated with the SNS, is a centrally acting neurotransmitter and a hormone that affects just about all body tissues, but it is best known for regulating heart rate, blood vessel and air passage diameters, and metabolic shifts.[55] The action varies, depending on the tissues and adrenergic receptors; for example, high levels of adrenaline cause smooth muscle relaxation in the airways but cause contraction of the smooth muscle that lines most arterioles. In response to perceived threat, heart rate increases rapidly to pump blood through the body to areas needing blood and oxygen. Adrenaline causes hypervigilance.[56]

- **Muscles:** In an immediate threat response, large muscles able to evade the threat or face the threat are needed. Big, strong leg muscles activate to run away. Arm muscles activate to protect. Smaller muscles are not needed, such as postural muscles or even stabilizing muscles.[57-59] Deactivating these muscles for the immediate threat seems like a good strategy. They should be switched back on when the threat has been removed.

  - **Language:** When startled, expressions include loud, short, sharp, and abrasive words.[60]
  - **Breathing:** With an acute threat, breathing becomes faster and shallower.
  - **Gastrointestinal (GI) system:** Digestion of food is slowed down and even put on hold, allowing for all possible energy and blood flow to be allocated to the immediate, much-needed systems.
  - **Other:** Other responses to stress include blocking desire to reproduce, pain, motivation, and memory.

Once the acute pain experience is dealt with, the stress response dissipates and homeostasis allows the systems to normalize and prepare for the next stress response.[55] This process occurs daily as people are faced with differing stressors. The system, however, is designed to elevate and then calm down; it should not continue to run at elevated levels for prolonged periods. In chronic pain, the stress response is protracted. The stress response is primarily executed by adrenaline initially, followed by cortisol changes in the body.

Adrenaline is a fast-acting neurotransmitter that is likely very effective in the immediate stress response, which should last no longer than several minutes. Cortisol is a more potent and longer-lasting chemical, similar in effect to adrenaline, that is produced to deal with longer-lasting threats.[55] Cortisol is a glucocorticoid steroid hormone produced by the adrenal gland, and is more formally known as hydrocortisone.[55] Its primary function is to increase blood sugar, suppress the immune system, and aid in metabolism of fat, protein, and carbohydrate.[61, 62] The release of cortisol from the adrenal gland is controlled by the hypothalamus. The secretion of corticotropin-releasing hormone (CRH) by the hypothalamus triggers anterior pituitary secretion of adrenocorticotropic hormone (ACTH). ACTH is carried by the cells to the vascular cortex, where it triggers blood secretion.[26, 63, 64]

Cortisol prevents the release of substances in the body that cause inflammation. This is why cortisol is used to treat conditions resulting from overactivity of the B-cell-mediated antibody response, such as inflammatory and rheumatoid diseases and allergies. Cortisol levels are affected by changes in ACTH, depression, psychological stress, and physiological stressors such as illness, surgery, fear, injury, and pain. Cortisol works along with adrenaline to create short-term memories. Long-term exposure to cortisol damages hippocampus cells, limiting learning and altering memory.[65] Cortisol dysregulation increases blood pressure and shuts down the reproductive system, and is associated with weight gain, appetite changes, and obesity.

A more significant effect of cortisol change is its effect on the immune system, specifically pro-inflammatory cytokines. Cytokines are immune molecules that significantly affect tissue healing.[66] During infections, trauma, or injury, cytokines such as interleukin 6 (IL-6) increase 1,000-fold, thus allowing for more ion channels specific to cytokines to open up, potentially resulting in increased sensitivity. This is the process that is seen to occur during a bout of the flu. A major stimulus for the production of cytokines is cortisol. With increased cytokines, there is the further possibility of increased inflammatory processes all over the body, including keeping tissues inflamed.

It is now believed that the complex biological and physiological processes in the nervous system, brain, endocrine system, and immune systems are an integral part of the pain experience. This is often included under the term *neuroscience*. With a prolonged stress response, various long-lasting changes occur:

Sympathetic Nervous System (SNS)

- Adrenal fatigue[67]
- Increased nerve sensitization[68]
- Increased sensitization of the GI system[69-71]
- Development and maintenance of trigger points[72]

Muscle or Motor System

- Postural changes[73]
- Ischemic and fatigued muscles[57]
- Delays in stabilizing muscle contraction[74-76]

Endocrine System

- Fatigue
- Depression
- Memory changes
- Weight gain[77]
- Sleep disturbance

Brain and Central and Peripheral Nervous Systems

- Central sensitization[41, 78]
- Hyperalgesia
- Allodynia

Immune System

- Widespread pain, body part recognition, and inflammation[79-81]

Reproductive System

- Lower sex drive and infertility[82]

Respiration

- Muscle imbalances
- Decreased blood flow and oxygenation of tissues
- Increased pain

Pain is more than just nociception. It involves integrated biological and physiological processes connected with the nervous system, brain, endocrine, immune system, and more. These changes in turn result in various clinical presentations commonly associated with chronic pain.

CONCLUSION

The human nervous system is quite complex. The primary structural divisions of the nervous system include the central (brain and spinal cord) and peripheral nervous systems. Involvement of the CNS results in pathological reflexes and hyperreflexia, while involvement of the PNS results in hyporeflexia. Neuromuscular control is a complex interaction of muscle spindles and Golgi tendon organs. Neurophysiology of pain, also complex in comprehension, has several distinct components with alternative theories on pain processing. Pain is produced in the brain. Pain is complex and involves more than just nociception. Understanding of the mechanisms of the nervous system and pain neurophysiology can assist clinicians in providing the most beneficial examination and subsequent intervention for their clients.

3

TISSUE INJURY AND HEALING

Mark F. Reinking, PT, PhD, SCS, ATC
Michael P. Reiman, PT, DPT, OCS, SCS, ATC, FAAOMPT, CSCS

The human body contains four primary tissue types: connective, epithelial, muscular, and nervous. All organs and organ systems are composed of varying combinations of these tissues, and normal organ and system function is contingent on a healthy state of cells within the four primary tissues. Tissue injury is a direct consequence of injury to cells within the tissue, and it can be caused by many factors, including chemical, mechanical, nutritional, pathogenic, thermal, and radioactive. This chapter focuses on neuromusculoskeletal tissue injury, including calcified and noncalcified connective tissues, muscle, and peripheral nerves. Injury to brain, spinal cord, and epithelial tissues is outside of the scope of this chapter.

Injuries to the noncalcified connective tissues (tendon, ligament, and cartilage), nerve, and muscle are considered soft-tissue injuries. These injuries are classified as either macrotraumatic or microtraumatic.[1] Macrotraumatic injuries, also referred to as acute injuries, involve an imposition of load in excess of tissue tolerance in a single event. Examples of macrotraumatic injuries are fractures, dislocations, lacerations, ligament sprains, muscle strains, and contusions.[1] A client who has experienced a macrotraumatic injury can recall the time, place, and mechanism of the injury.

Microtraumatic injuries, also known as chronic or overuse injuries, are the result of a repetitive overloading of the involved tissue. The forces involved in microtraumatic injuries do not exceed tissue tolerance in a single event; rather, the cumulative, repetitive nature of this loading interferes with the body's normal tissue response and leads to injury. These injuries include tendinitis, tendinosis, tenosynovitis, bursitis, stress fracture, and synovitis. Clients cannot identify a specific time or place a microtraumatic injury occurred; they typically describe it worsening over time.

The mechanical response of tissue to loading can be represented by a stress–strain curve (figure 3.1). In this graphical representation of tissue tolerance, stress is defined as force divided by area, and strain as tissue deformation. As stress is applied to a biologic material, material deformation occurs. Initially, this elastic deformation is temporary. When the load is removed, the material returns to its original state. However, when the stress reaches the yield point on the curve, additional stress causes

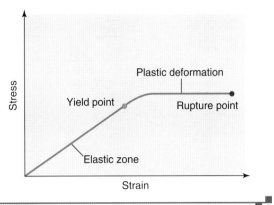

Figure 3.1   Stress–strain curve of skeletal muscle.

Reprinted, by permission, from J. Loudon, R. Manske, and M. Reiman, 2013, *Clinical mechanics and kinesiology* (Champaign, IL: Human Kinetics), 50.

permanent material deformation, or plastic deformation. The ultimate strength of the material is the maximum stress it can accept before complete failure. Most biologic tissues are anisotropic, meaning that they respond to loading differently depending on the type of loading. In this case, the stress–strain curves are likely to look different when comparing, for example, compressive, torsional, and tensile loading. The ability of a tissue to tolerate loading depends on several factors, including the overall health of the tissue, previous tissue injury, age, nutritional status, the magnitude of loading, and the time over which the load is applied.

TISSUE HEALING

When the tolerance of a tissue to loading is exceeded, tissue injury occurs. The body has an intrinsic response to the injury that initiates the tissue healing process. This process is stimulated by damage to blood capillaries within the tissue, releasing plasma and cells (leukocytes, erythrocytes, and platelets) into the region. The presence of these cells in the tissue fluid induces a chemical-signaling process that begins the three-phase process of healing. In most cases of tissue injury, there is progression through the three phases in a predictable manner, resulting in either tissue regeneration (re-creation of the original tissue) or tissue repair (formation of a connective tissue scar). The three phases of healing are the inflammatory phase, the proliferative (or reparative) phase, and the remodeling phase. While these three phases are described in a chronological order, the reality is that the phases are overlapping, with one phase beginning as another phase is ending (figure 3.2). The general duration and characteristics of these phases are summarized in table 3.1.

Inflammatory Phase

The inflammatory phase is stimulated by the extravasation of blood products into the tissue fluid. These products serve as chemoattractants in this tissue environment, stimulating the migration of other cells into the region. Platelets play a critical role in this phase as they aggregate to form a clot and slow the flow of plasma into the tissue fluid. Following a brief time of vasoconstriction limiting blood flow, two chemical cascades occur that cause a rebound vasodilation, bringing necessary healing agents into the injured region. The complement cascade involves activation of multiple proteins present in blood that stimulate mast cells and basophils to release histamine, a powerful vasodilator.[2] The kinin cascade results in the conversion of kallikrein, an inactive enzyme, to bradykinin. This is another powerful chemical agent that facilitates vasodilation and increases capillary permeability.[2] The vasodilation and vessel permeability result in cells such as macrophages and neutrophils invading the region to remove necrotic tissue and potential infectious agents. The consequences of the increased blood flow, fluid movement out of local vessels, and increased cellular activity in the area are the cardinal signs of the inflammatory

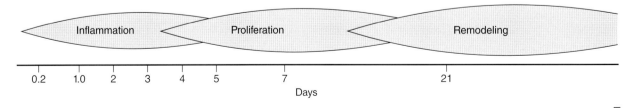

Figure 3.2   Chronology of tissue healing.

Reprinted, by permission, from S.K. Hillman, 2012, *Core concepts in athletic training and therapy* (Champaign, IL: Human Kinetics), 372.

TABLE 3.1 Phases of Healing

Phase	Duration	Characteristics	Goal
Inflammatory	Up to 5 days	At onset of injury, area is warm, red, swollen, and tender.	Stabilize and contain area of injury
Proliferative (reparative)	Up to 21 days	Scar tissue is red and larger than normal because of edema.	Dispose of dead tissue, mobilize fibroblasts, and restore circulation
Remodeling	Up to 1 year or more	Water content of the scar is reduced; vascularity and redness are reduced; scar tissue density increases.	Stabilize and reestablish the area

Reprinted, by permission, from S.K. Hillman, 2012, *Core concepts in athletic training and therapy* (Champaign, IL: Human Kinetics), 373.

process, including swelling, redness, and heat. Pain, another of the cardinal signs of inflammation, is a result of multiple stimuli including direct tissue injury, increased tissue pressure as a result of the fluid accumulation, and pain-stimulating chemicals including bradykinins and histamines.

Growth factors released by the platelets and other cells stimulate the influx of fibroblasts and vascular endothelial cells. These cells begin the process of reconstructing the injured vessels and surrounding tissues. This begins the transition from the inflammatory phase to the proliferative phase. The inflammatory phase is not considered complete until all the remaining necrotic tissue is removed, but the proliferative phase begins before this process of debris removal ends. Typically, the acute inflammatory phase lasts from hours to several days depending on the extent of the tissue damage. However, if adversely affected by poor tissue health, repeated microdamage, inadequate nutrition, infection, ischemia, or other factors, this acute process can develop into a persistent, chronic inflammatory state. Chronic tendinosis (discussed in detail later in this chapter) is a good example of this failed acute inflammatory reaction.

Given the high popularity of nonsteroidal anti-inflammatory drugs (NSAIDs) among the lay population, the term *inflammation* has taken on the connotation of an undesirable condition that should be treated pharmacologically. However, the reality is that the process of inflammation provides the necessary chemical and cellular environment that stimulates the healing process. For this reason, the use of NSAIDs should be discouraged during the acute inflammatory phase given the potential for interference with healing.

Proliferative (Reparative) Phase

The chemotactic migration of fibroblasts and endothelial cells into the injured region marks the initiation of the reparative phase. Microconstruction of new capillary networks, or angiogenesis, begins in the injured region, facilitating the influx of nutrients to facilitate healing. The fibroblast cells, stimulated by growth factors in the region, begin the process of collagen synthesis. Procollagen is synthesized within the fibroblasts and is secreted into the tissue matrix, where it is assembled into fibrils and collagen fibers. In this phase, both Type I and Type III collagen are synthesized, but a greater proportion of Type III collagen is present in fresh wounds. This form of collagen has a lower tensile strength than Type I collagen, so while this initial wound matrix serves as a scaffolding in the injured tissue matrix, it is not yet as strong as the original noninjured tissue. The end result of this fibroblastic process is the development of a collagenaceous scar that has few cells and serves to stabilize the injured tissue matrix.

This proliferative phase of healing can last from days to weeks, again depending on the extent of the original tissue injury. Early in the phase, the tissue may continue to appear swollen and red, since the neovessels being formed tend to leak more than mature vessels and the concentration of vessels is higher than in normal tissue, creating the reddish appearance of the healing region. As the phase progresses, there is a normal degradation of some of the neovessels and maturation of remaining vessels, decreasing the overall perfusion to the area and the amount of tissue fluid in the region. This is recognized visually by the wound becoming less red and taking on a more normal tissue appearance.

Remodeling

The final and longest phase of the healing process is the remodeling phase. During this phase, the scar that was formed in the proliferative phase is either remodeled to a permanent scar (tissue repair) or converted to the original tissue (tissue regeneration). Whether a tissue is repaired or regenerated depends on the tissue type. Bone, for example, is regenerated, whereas muscle is repaired. At the end of the proliferative phase, the tissue is lacking in tensile strength because it has been primarily repaired with a Type III collagenaceous scar.[2] In the case of tissue repair, the Type III collagen is gradually replaced with Type I collagen, increasing the strength of the scar. Specialized fibroblasts referred to as *myofibroblasts* become activated in this phase to assist in contraction of the wound site; these cells contain contractile proteins that allow them to pull the margins of the injured tissues together.

As time passes, the scar tissue is remodeled based on the imposed forces, allowing for normalized function of the injured region. However, in some cases excessive scarring and insufficient remodeling can interfere with function. For example, the condition described as arthrofibrosis occurs when there is periarticular hypertrophic scarring that significantly limits joint motion. This can occur as a result of prolonged joint immobility or infection, and it can also be idiopathic in onset.

In the healing of tendon, ligament, and bone, tissue regeneration occurs during this final phase. As contrasted with tissue repair, there is not the formation of a permanent scar as occurs in muscle or skin; instead, the scar matrix is replaced with the original tissue. The specifics of those processes of healing are described in the following sections on the healing processes of specific tissues.

MUSCLE INJURY

The most common types of muscle injury are strain, contusion, and laceration. A muscle strain is an indirect injury to muscle that is the consequence of excessive lengthening of a muscle combined with an eccentric contraction of the same muscle. An active muscle contraction without stretch or a passive stretch without a muscle contraction is much less likely to induce a muscle strain injury. Muscles that are at risk for strain injury include the two-joint muscles that are subjected to significant lengthening across both joints and muscles with a high proportion of Type II fibers.[3] The preponderance of evidence indicates that muscle strain injuries commonly occur at or near the myotendinous junction.[3-7] The crucial role of the myotendinous junction in force transmission from muscle to tendon may be the primary causative factor in these indirect muscle injuries. To characterize severity, muscle strains have traditionally been classified into three grades:

- **Grade I strain** involves injury to a small number of muscle fibers and causes localized pain with minimal to no loss of muscle performance.
- **Grade II strain** is a tear of a greater number of muscle fibers with associated pain, swelling, diminished muscle performance, primarily linked to pain reproduction with muscle contraction.
- **Grade III strain** is a complete tear across the muscle, resulting in significant pain, loss of anatomic continuity of the muscle, and loss of muscle function.[3-7]

In 2014, Pollock and colleagues[8] proposed a new classification system for muscle injury. Their British Athletic Muscle Injury Classification is based on MRI features of the injury and the anatomic site of the injury. The authors proposed that the specifics of this new system will better direct the clinician in prognosis and treatment of the injury. In this system, muscle injuries are graded from 0 to 4 based on the extent of the MRI signal changes and then are subclassified as a, b, or c depending on whether the injury is in myofascial tissue (a), at the muscle-tendon junction (b), or intratendinous (c). A grade 0 injury has a normal MRI in spite of muscle pain. A grade 1 injury is a small tear (<5 cm), and a grade II injury is a moderate tear between 5 and 15 cm long, or one involving <50% of the tendon cross-section. A grade III injury is an extensive tear (>15 cm), or one involving over 50% of the tendon cross-section. A grade IV injury is a complete muscle or tendon rupture. If this new classification system were widely used, it would provide the clinician with more information about the location and extent of the muscle–tendon injury as compared to the three-stage grading system that is commonly employed at present.

Muscle contusions usually result from a direct blow to the involved muscle. A direct blow to the muscle tissue causes local damage to the muscle with resultant bleeding. The anterior thigh (quadriceps muscle) and the anterior brachium (biceps brachii) are the most common sites for a direct blow muscle injury. A potential adverse effect of a deep muscle contusion is the development of myositis ossificans. This condition is the deposition of bone or cartilage within muscle at the site of a muscle contusion. It is most often associated with contusions involving repeated impact forces to the same muscular region,[9] and it is more common with severe contusions.[5, 9] Muscle laceration, although not common in sport, can occur when there is contact between skin and an environmental hazard (fence, field debris, bleachers) or sports equipment (skate, stick, helmet). The result is a deep cut or gash that disrupts the continuity of the muscle architecture.

Muscle healing is a process of repair, not regeneration as in the healing of bone tissue. Regardless of the mechanism of injury, the healing process occurs in three stages: destruction, repair, and remodeling.[4] In the destruction phase, there is necrosis of the damaged cells followed by formation of a hematoma in the region of the injury. The second phase begins with macrophage-mediated removal of the necrotic tissue and fibroblastic activity producing collagen to begin the formation of a collagen-based scar. In the region of the disrupted myofibers, undifferentiated satellite cells begin a process of differentiation and fuse with the damaged ends of the myofibers. The connective tissue scar within the muscle persists, and the original damaged myofibers are replaced by two fibers that are joined at the scar.[4] In this process of muscle repair, early and excessive stretching of the injured muscle can cause rerupture at the injury site if the scar is not given time to develop and mature. For this reason, early stretching of a muscle strain should be avoided for a few days following injury.[5]

Although not a muscle injury, cramps are a very painful muscle condition that can interfere with daily activities and especially sports participation. These involuntary muscle contractions occur suddenly, and they have been attributed to dehydration, low potassium or low sodium levels, inadequate carbohydrate intake, or very tight muscles. More recent evidence suggests that the mechanism of cramping may involve descending central nervous system influences on Golgi tendon organs and muscle spindles as well as local skeletal muscle factors such as motor unit recruitment and fatigue.[10]

TENDON INJURY

Tendons, which function to transfer contractile forces from muscle to bone, normally consist of tight parallel bundles of primarily Type I collagen fibers organized into fascicles and subfascicles within the tendon. Tendon injury is very common in sport, and it can be classified as macrotraumatic or microtraumatic, with the microtraumatic (or overuse) tendon injury being the more frequent mechanism. Acute macrotraumatic injuries can include rupture, laceration, or contusion. Tendon ruptures, although an acute event, may be the consequence of multiple factors including age, inactivity, repeated microtraumatic injury, prolonged steroid use, or use of fluoroquinolone antibiotics. The spectrum of microtraumatic tendinopathic conditions range from inflammatory conditions (tendinitis or paratenonitis) to chronic degenerative conditions (tendinosis). The following terms are used to describe tendon injuries:

• **Tendinitis:** This traditional view of tendon pathology describes a tendon in which there is an acute inflammatory response to injury or overuse. This condition is characterized by the presence of inflammatory cells (macrophages, neutrophils) as well as hypervascularity, collagen disorganization with fatty infiltration, and fibroblastic proliferation.[11]

• **Tendinosis:** This pathological condition of a tendon is characterized by a chronically degenerative state that is not inflammatory. There is a conspicuous absence of inflammatory cells with the presence of neovascularity, increased proteoglycan content, an increase in Type III collagen, and collagen disorganization. In this chronic state, there is an alteration in the signaling process that differentiates tendon stem cells (TSC) into tenocytes. In tendinosis, the TSC also differentiate into adipocytes, chondrocytes, and osteocytes, resulting in the secretion of fat, bone, and cartilage into the tendinous matrix.[12]

• **Tendon rupture:** This term describes a complete tendon failure, resulting in complete loss of function of that muscle–tendon unit.

• **Tendinopathy:** This term describes a painful tendon without identification of the actual histopathology. It has been recommended as the most appropriate term for clinicians to use in communication with clients because it implies neither an inflammatory nor noninflammatory condition.[13]

- **Paratenonitis (peritendinitis, tenosynovitis, tenovaginitis):** This term refers to a pathologic condition of the outer layer of the tendon sheath. All tendons are enclosed in a connective tissue covering called the epitenon, which contains the vascular, lymphatic, and nerve supplies. In some tendons, the epitenon is surrounded by another connective tissue covering called the paratenon, which is lined by synovial cells. Paratenonitis is inflammatory condition of the paratenon. It is the preferred term to the older terms *peritendinitis, tenosynovitis,* and *tenovaginitis.*[14] De Quervain's syndrome is one example of paratenonitis. Paratenonitis can occur in concert with either tendinosis or tendinitis.

Tendon healing is a regenerative process that is described in three stages: inflammatory, regenerative, and remodeling. The inflammatory stage begins at the time of tendon injury with the migration of erythrocytes, macrophages, and neutrophils to the site of injury. Phagocytosis of necrotic materials occurs, and the leukocytes secrete angiogenic and chemotactic substances that lead to angiogenesis, stimulation of TSC differentiation into tenocytes, and the initiation of collagen production.

During the regenerative (proliferative) phase, Type III collagen, noncollagenous proteins, and proteoglycans are synthesized. The collagen fibers are laid down in a random three-dimensional orientation, forming a scar in the region of tendon injury. Over the course of several weeks, the synthesis of Type III collagen peaks, then begins to slow as there is a gradual shift in the production of Type III to Type I collagen. The focus of the final and longest stage involves the gradual replacement of the Type III scar collagen with Type I collagen and the orientation of the collagen fibrils along lines of strain within the tendon. However, tendon strength is not restored to original levels for a period of up to a full year.[15-18]

The biology of tendon healing as described is best understood in the case of an acute tendon injury with a point-in-time injury to a healthy tendon. In the case of chronic tendon pain as a result of repetitive overuse injury, the process of healing is unlikely to progress through the three stages in a sequential manner. The consequence of the incomplete healing of the tendon from repeated micro-injury is that the tendon likely persists in a state of noninflammatory regeneration or remodeling, where the conversion of Type III to Type I collagen and reorientation of fibers is not completed. Thus, the tendon remains in a state of hypercellularity and neovascularity. The consequence of this is a chronically weakened, painful tendon that is more likely to sustain reinjury. [15]

LIGAMENT INJURY

Ligaments provide joint stability by attaching one bone to another. Ligaments are composed of collagen fiber bundles that are organized in a parallel arrangement, very similar to a tendon. Ligaments can be either intrinsic, a thickening of the joint capsule (e.g., primary hip ligaments: pubofemoral, iliofemoral, and ischiofemoral), or extrinsic, free from the joint capsule (e.g., lateral collateral ligament of the knee). The most common mechanism of a ligament injury is a force causing the associated joint to be moved into an excessive range of motion (ROM), thereby producing excessive lengthening of the ligament. Ligament injuries (sprains) are typically classified in the following manner:

- **Grade I:** involves stretching of the ligament but minimal collagen fiber damage to the ligament. Clinical testing of these injuries reveals little or no increased laxity of the joint.

- **Grade II:** involves stretching of the ligament and tearing of some of the collagen fibers. Clinical testing of these injuries reveals increased joint laxity, but a defined end point (or end-feel).

- **Grade III:** involves maximal stretching of the ligament that results in near or total ligament disruption. Clinical testing of these injuries reveals excessive joint laxity and no firm end-feel.

As in tendon healing, ligament healing has three overlapping stages: reaction, repair and regeneration, and remodeling. The reaction phase occurs in the initial 72 hours post injury, and is an inflammatory-mediated process. As in tendon injury, this stage involves migration of erythrocytes, macrophages, and neutrophils to the site of injury. Phagocytosis of necrotic materials occurs. Through the release of chemotactic substances, additional cells migrate into the region of injury, including fibroblastic cells.

The repair and regeneration phase is marked by high activity of fibroblastic cells, producing a scar matrix of Type III collagen and proteoglycans. Again, as in tendon healing, the initial ligament scar is unorganized tissue that is not yet oriented along the lines of strain imposed on the tendon. Remodeling occurs as the Type III collagen is converted to Type I collagen and as fiber orientation is reorganized along lines of strain. In a healing ligament, the increased collagen content will result in a larger cross-section than that of a normal ligament. In evidence from animal studies, the tensile strength of the healed ligament does not approach the original ligament for periods up to a year.[19-21]

BONE INJURY

The major component of the musculoskeletal system is calcified connective tissue, or bone. Bone serves supportive and protective functions, establishes the lever system that the muscular system acts on to create movement, and provides a reservoir of calcium and phosphorus. Bone is classified as either compact (cortical) or spongy (cancellous), based on the architecture of the mineralization (see chapter 1, figure 1.2). In cortical bone, the functional unit is the osteon, which consists of a central canal with blood supply and nerves that is surrounded by concentric rings, or laminas, of collagen and hydroxyapatite, the calcium-containing mineral in bone. Cancellous bone is composed of a latticework of trabeculae that are arranged along lines of stress. Cortical bone is located in the shafts of long bones, and forms the shell around all bones. Cancellous bone is located within the epiphyses of long bones and in short, flat, and irregular bones.

Bone injuries include fracture and contusion (bruise). Fracture may be a result of direct trauma (like a direct blow from an object or another person) or indirect trauma (such as falling down and twisting the lower leg). Fractures can be either open (compound), where a portion of the fractured bone punctures the skin, or closed. Fracture classifications include transverse, oblique, spiral, or comminuted (figure 3.3). An avulsion fracture is another fracture classification where a piece of bone attached to a tendon or ligament is torn away. These types of fractures are more common in athletes, particularly younger athletes.

Obvious concerns exist with a bone fracture. Besides the immediate concern of fracture stabilization, other concerns associated with fracture include infection, acute compartment syndrome, associated soft-tissue injury, deep venous thrombosis or pulmonary embolism, delayed union or nonunion, and malunion.

Infection of the involved area is more likely to occur with open or compound fractures than with closed fractures due to the break in the skin with open fractures. The clinician should always be cognizant of infection with open fractures and should monitor for signs of infection (e.g., increased skin temperature, redness of the associated skin region, pus-related drainage from the skin, and fever).

Acute compartment syndrome is due to excessive swelling in a muscle compartment related to bleeding from the fracture. These muscle compartments are surrounded by an inelastic fascial sheath. This syndrome commonly occurs in the lower leg region and the flexor compartment of the forearm. This condition causes pain out of proportion to the fracture, pain when the muscles involved are

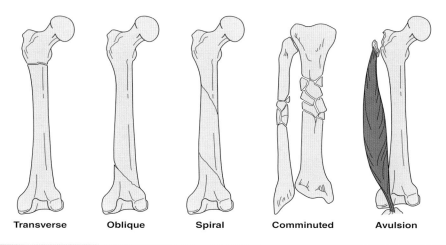

Transverse   Oblique   Spiral   Comminuted   Avulsion

Figure 3.3 Types of fractures.

passively stretched, decreased or lack of pulse in the area, and paresthesia in the involved area. In some cases, this condition may require surgical release of the involved fascial sheath.

Occasionally soft tissues in close proximity to the fracture are also injured. These tissues can be nerves, muscles, ligaments, or vessels. Clinicians must monitor for signs and symptoms associated with involvement of these tissues with both open and closed fractures.

Deep venous thrombosis (DVT) and pulmonary embolism (PE) may occasionally occur after a fracture. This is particularly a concern for fractures in the lower extremities. A DVT is a blood clot in a deep vein. A clot inside a blood vessel is called a thrombosis. DVTs predominantly occur in the lower extremities and may have no symptoms. The nonspecific signs of DVT include pain, swelling, redness, warmness, and engorged superficial veins in the leg. A DVT may go away naturally, but the most serious complication is when a thrombosis dislodges (embolizes) and travels to the lungs to become a life-threatening PE. DVT and PE are grouped together with the term *venous thromboembolism*. Early controlled movement and active muscle contraction (when warranted) can help prevent DVTs and PEs.

Delayed union, or malunion, of a fracture can result in persistent pain and disability that may require surgical correction. Delayed union is a fracture that fails to properly heal after an appropriate amount of time for fracture healing. A malunion of a fracture is a fracture that heals improperly, typically without the correct bony alignment.

Periosteal injury is typically the result of a direct blow to the periosteal region of the bone. This type of bone injury is relatively uncommon. A specific example of a periosteal injury is a *hip pointer*, an injury to the periosteum of the iliac crest caused by a direct blow to this region. Likewise, a direct impact with a blow that is at subfracture threshold may cause bleeding within the bone, or a bone contusion (bruise). These contusions can be subperiosteal, interosseous, or subchondral. More than 80% of anterior cruciate ligament injuries have an associated bone bruise in the lateral compartment of the knee.[22] Some evidence exists that a bone bruise can be a primary source of pain.[23] In the case of subchondral bruising, bone bruising may lead to articular cartilage degeneration.[22]

Bone healing is a regenerative process that can be divided into primary healing and secondary healing. Primary healing occurs following surgical fracture fixation and does not involve formation of a soft cartilaginous callus. In this case, osteoblasts directly deposit mineralized tissue in the fracture site. Most fracture healing, however, is a secondary process that has been described in three phases: inflammatory, reparative, and remodeling.[24] In the inflammatory phase, vasodilation and hyperemia form a local hematoma between the bone ends, which is a result of the migration of inflammatory mediators into the region, including histamines and prostaglandins. As in tendon and ligament injury, phagocytic cells also migrate to the region and initiate the removal of necrotic material. The reparative phase begins as chemical signaling processes cause stem cells to differentiate into osteoblasts, chondroblasts, and fibroblasts. The formation of the callus occurs through both intramembranous and endochondral ossification pathways. Intramembranous ossification occurs in the outer subperiosteal regions of bone and results in direct bone formation without a cartilaginous intermediary. Endochondral ossification involves the formation of a soft cartilaginous callus that is replaced by a bony mineralized callus over time. In the remodeling phase, the calcified callus is gradually replaced by normal bone tissue through the action of osteoclasts and osteoblasts.[25]

The ability of bone to manage imposed loads is affected by the density of the mineral portion of the bone. Assessment of bone density is accomplished through the use of bone densitometers that use X-ray or ultrasound energy to estimate the bone mineral density (BMD). The World Health Organization (WHO) has established a classification system for BMD that is based on the comparison of a person's BMD to the average value for a healthy young woman. Osteoporosis is defined as a BMD that is 2.5 standard deviations or more below the young adult mean (T-score < −2.5). Low bone mass, or osteopenia, is defined as a T-score between −1.0 and −2.5. Low bone mass and degradation of the trabecular microarchitecture (figure 3.4) are major risk factors for fractures of the hip, vertebrae, and distal forearm. Hip and thoracic spine fractures are the most common of osteoporosis-related fractures. Hip fractures have the greatest morbidity and mortality and result in significant loss of function.

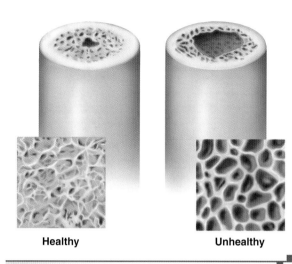

Figure 3.4 Healthy and unhealthy (osteoporosis) bone.

ARTICULAR CARTILAGE INJURY

As mentioned in chapter 1, cartilage is a specialized connective tissue that can be classified as hyaline (articular), elastic, or fibrous (fibrocartilage). Common to all types of cartilage is a proteoglycan matrix with embedded cells (chondrocytes) and collagen. In adults, cartilage is both avascular and aneural, and it relies on diffusion for nutrition and waste disposal. Articular cartilage is the cartilage covering the articular surfaces of the bones, forming a synovial joint typically only a few millimeters thick. Articular cartilage functions to absorb compressive forces and decrease frictional resistance to movement. Damage to the articular cartilage may include partial- or full-thickness defects. Articular cartilage damage is a potentially disabling condition because it can affect the joint's ability to absorb force and allow for movement. Osteoarthritis (OA) is one consequence of prolonged articular cartilage degeneration. Hip and knee OA are the two most common forms of OA. The significant disability and financial burden caused by knee and hip OA are well documented. In 1995, 15% of the United States population had some form of arthritis, and this percentage has been estimated to increase to 19% by 2020.[26] More than 80% of the United States population have radiographically evident OA by age 65, and at least half of these people report symptoms associated with these changes.[26]

Diagnostic imaging techniques such as magnetic resonance imaging (MRI) and magnetic resonance arthrography (MRA), as well as arthroscopy, have been helpful for determining the extent of articular cartilage damage in a joint. The International Cartilage Research Society (ICRS) has developed a classification system for articular cartilage injury.[27] The five grades of injury are described as follows (figure 3.5):

- **Grade 0:** Normal cartilage
- **Grade 1:** Nearly normal cartilage: This cartilage contains soft indentation or surface lesions only.
- **Grade 2:** Abnormal cartilage: Lesions extend from surface to less than half the cartilage depth.
- **Grade 3:** Severely abnormal cartilage: Lesions extend to more than 50% of cartilage depth and may extend into, but not through, the subchondral bone.
- **Grade 4:** Severely abnormal cartilage: Lesions extend through the subchondral bone.

Joint dislocation or subluxation causes a shearing injury to the articular cartilage. Common sites of chondral and osteochondral injuries are the superior articular surface of the talus, the femoral condyles, the patella, and the capitellum of the humerus. These osteochondral injuries may be associated with soft-tissue ligament sprains and muscle strains.

Osteochondritis dissecans (OCD) is a focal lesion of articular cartilage and subchondral bone. The etiology is not well understood, but it involves aseptic necrosis of subchondral bone. Common sites for OCD lesions include the medial femoral condyle, patella, talar dome, and capitellum of the humerus. The ICRS has also developed a grading system for OCD lesions (figure 3.6) based on the stability of the fragment assessed arthroscopically and the continuity with surrounding tissue.[27] OCD I is a stable lesion that is soft but has surface continuity with surrounding tissue. OCD II is also a stable lesion, but it has partial discontinuity. OCD III is a fully discontinuous lesion but is still located in place. OCD IV lesion is a loose fragment within

ICRS Grade 0 - Normal

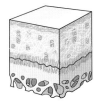

ICRS Grade 1 – Nearly Normal
Superficial lesions. Soft indentation (A) and/or superficial fissures and cracks (B)

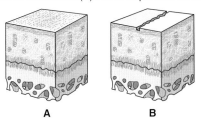

A   B

ICRS Grade 2 – Abnormal
Lesions extending down to <50% of cartilage depth

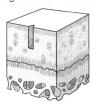

ICRS Grade 3 – Severely Abnormal
Cartilage defects extending down >50% of cartilage depth (A) as well as down to calcified layer (B) and down to but not through the subchondral bone (C). Blisters are included in this Grade (D)

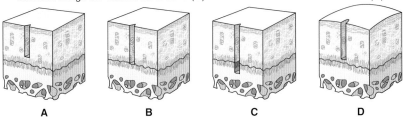

A   B   C   D

ICRS Grade 4 – Severely Abnormal

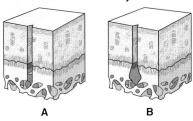

A   B

Figure 3.5   ICRS cartilage injury classification.

Reprinted, by permission, from ICRS Cartilage Injury Evaluation Package, pg. 13. Available: www.cartilage.org/_files/contentmanagement/ICRS_evaluation.pd. By permission of ICRS.

the joint. Surgical treatment is often indicated for OCD, and the specific procedure performed will be based on the grading of the lesion.

Unlike the other tissues discussed in this chapter, adult articular cartilage has a very low metabolic rate and does not have a strong healing response to injury. In fact, a significant healing response to injury does not occur until the defect reaches subchondral bone.[28, 29] In his review of the healing of articular cartilage, O'Driscoll wrote that with articular cartilage damage, cartilage can be "restored, replaced, relieved, or resected."[29] It is significant that intrinsic healing of the cartilage is not among those options. A major challenge of articular cartilage healing is that the healing process replaces hyaline cartilage with fibrocartilage, and the repaired material does not incorporate well into the original cartilage surface.

PERIPHERAL NERVE INJURY

The nervous system is divided into the central nervous system, including the brain and spinal cord, and the peripheral nervous system, including the cranial nerves and spinal nerves. These peripheral nerves include both sensory (afferent) neurons and motor (efferent) neurons. Peripheral nerves include a bundle of axons, where each axon is surrounded by a connective tissue sheath, the endoneurium. Individual axons are clustered together in fascicles and surrounded by another connective tissue sheath, the perineurium. The fascicles of axons are grouped together to form the nerve, which is surrounded by the epineurium. Larger-diameter axons are covered with a material secreted by Schwann cells called myelin, which is composed of proteins, lipids, and water. The presence of myelin increases the conduction speed along the axon. Small-diameter axons, which remain unmyelinated, have slower nerve-conduction velocity.

Peripheral nerves can be damaged by direct trauma (contusion or laceration), indirect trauma by excessive tension or compression, infection, toxic materials, or loss of vascularity. Neurapraxia is the mildest form of injury to a peripheral nerve. It is caused by contusion or compression of a nerve, which leads to segmental demyelination. In this case, nerve conduction is slowed across the region of the axon where myelin has been lost. This condition is temporary because the axon is not disrupted and the loss of myelin is transient. Axonotmesis involves disruption of the axon and interruption of the myelin sheath, but the connective tissue sheaths within the nerve are preserved. Neurotmesis is complete transection of the nerve with loss of continuity of the nerve sheaths. In both of these conditions, there is degeneration of the axon distal to the injury site, referred to as *Wallerian degeneration*. For motor neurons, this leads to denervation of the target muscle.

In the case of segmental demyelination, nerve healing begins with the mitotic division of the remaining Schwann cells. These cells envelop the demyelinated regions of the injured nerve and synthesize myelin to reform the myelin sheath. In the case of axonotmesis or neurotmesis, if the cell body is intact, axonal sprouting can occur from the ends of the damaged axon. If the connective tissue sheath is intact, the axon sprout will grow distally

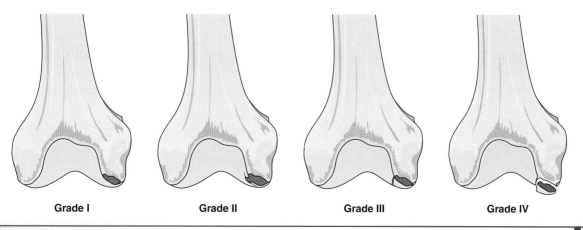

| Grade I | Grade II | Grade III | Grade IV |

Figure 3.6 OCD lesion grading.

and follow the sheath to the target muscle of neural receptor. Once the axon has reestablished its distal connection, the remyelination process is initiated. If there is not a viable sheath (neurotmesis), the axon sprouts will grow without direction, and successful functional reinnervation does not occur.

Injury to a peripheral motor neuron is classified as a lower motor neuron lesion. Classic signs are motor weakness, hypotonicity, diminished deep tendon reflexes, and muscle atrophy. If damage occurs to motor neurons in the brain or spinal cord, the lesion is described as an upper motor neuron lesion. This is characterized by motor weakness, hypertonicity, hyperactive deep-tendon reflexes, and abnormal reflexes such as the Babinski reflex or Hoffmann's sign.

CONCLUSION

Understanding of tissue healing properties is critical to the rehabilitation process. Failure to appreciate and respect the stages of healing by imposing inappropriate rehabilitation strategies could result in disruption of healing tissues and unnecessary delays in healing. As our understanding of the complexities of biologic healing increases, clinicians will be better able to design rehabilitation programs that impose appropriate forces and maximize the tissue environment to facilitate normal healing and progressively return the client to an appropriate level of function.

PART

II

Concepts and Principles of Examination

Part II of this text covers the guiding concepts and principles of the examination process for the orthopedic client. Chapter 4 addresses evidence-based and evidence-informed practice guidelines (e.g., diagnostic accuracy, study quality) and provides a guiding tool for determining the importance of diagnostic accuracy findings. Since there are extensive special tests and studies examining them, refer to this chapter to understand the color coding scheme utilized in this text for an **ideal** versus **good** versus poor finding. Therefore, at a quick glance, greater significance can be placed on **ideal** findings over **good** or poor findings. This chapter also describes in detail how to properly help rule out or rule in the potential presence of pathology and provides the crux of this text, the funnel approach of the examination process. This funnel approach provides the clinician with a systematic, evidence-based examination approach that moves from a broad to narrow focus. Great importance is suggested on the initial components of the examination sequence in this funnel approach because evidence supports significant shifts in post-test probability with the described early components listed here.

Other important components include introduction to client examination (also chapter 4), the client interview and observation of the client in the clinic (chapter 5), and triage and differential diagnosis of potential non-musculoskeletal and other musculoskeletal pathologies (chapter 6). Chapter 7 details the importance and implementation of a proper orthopedic (musculoskeletal) screen and a detailed nervous system examination. Other parts of the funnel approach included in part II are the traditional examination components of range of motion (chapter 8) and muscle performance (chapter 9), as well as special tests (chapter 10), palpation (chapter 11), and physical performance measures (chapter 12). Unlike most other texts, this book highlights gait (chapter 13) and posture (chapter 14) as vital components of the examination sequence. Although they are not delineated specifically as among the eight distinct components of the funnel examination approach, they are included in part II because these discrete examination measures range across the components of the orthopedic client examination (interview, observation, triage, motion tests, muscle performance testing, special tests, palpation, and physical performance measures).

4

EVIDENCE-BASED PRACTICE AND CLIENT EXAMINATION

Michael P. Reiman, PT, DPT, OCS, SCS, ATC, FAAOMPT, CSCS

Examination of the orthopedic client requires a systematic, evidence-informed approach. Understanding the current evidence and integrating the diagnostic accuracy into the examination process affords the clinician the most efficacious use of clinical reasoning when not only interpreting clinical findings but also determining which examination procedures to implement. This chapter describes a thoughtful, clear, and regimented approach to the examination and diagnostic process of the orthopedic client. It illustrates and describes general information on the funnel approach to examination. (See following chapters for additional detail on this examination approach.)

EVIDENCE-BASED PRACTICE AND DIAGNOSTIC ACCURACY

Evidence-based practice (EBP) has been defined as "the conscientious and judicious use of current best evidence in making decisions about the care of individual patients."[1] Central to the concept of EBP is the integration of evidence into the diagnoses and management of clients. Today, there is a strong push toward EBP as the conscientious utilization of the strongest and most recent evidence purported in the literature. Clinical expertise is also vital to the practice of EBP, as stated by Sackett and colleagues:

"Good doctors use both individual clinical exper-tise and the best available external evidence, and neither alone is enough. Without clinical expertise, practice risks becoming tyrannised by evidence, for even excellent external evidence may be inapplica-ble to or inappropriate for an individual patient. With-out current best evidence, practice risks becoming rapidly out of date, to the detriment of patients."[1]

It is possible to have statistical significance with-out having clinical relevance, to have both statistical significance and clinical relevance together, to have clinical relevance without having statistical signifi-cance, or to have neither statistical significance nor clinical relevance. The clinical relevance of research findings is typically not reported in research find-ings, and it has been suggested as paramount to clinical practice.[2] Current best evidence is therefore a balance of the best available evidence supported in the literature and the clinician's sound clinical reasoning. The practicing clinician must rely on the interweaving of these tenets to make the most conscientious, sound decisions when examining and subsequently treating clients.

For these reasons, this text would like the reader to also think in terms of the terminology of evidence-informed practice (EIP). The purpose of EIP is to make clinical decisions with the informa-tion of best evidence. Decisions cannot always be based on evidence alone. This is particularly the case when the evidence supporting or refuting clinical testing is poor. The clinician is referred to the limi-tations of each component of the examination, par-ticularly special testing (as discussed in chapter 10). Many of these tests have less than good ability to assist with differential diagnoses decisions. All com-ponents of the examination, including components not described as standard examination components (e.g., the client's goals, the client's health status), should be used when making clinical diagnosis and treatment decisions.

Diagnostic tests and measures are distinct com-ponents of an EBP model of client examination. A diagnostic test and its results are important tools guiding the clinician to the appropriate diagnosis by revealing the likelihood of whether or not a client has a specific disorder.[3] Diagnostic research should evaluate the validity of the complete diagnostic process and study the evidence of the added value of the different tests used.[4] Not all components of the examination process are equal in their ability to differentiate the presence, absence, or severity of a particular disease or condition present in a client. This likely also depends on the particular pathology. Specific components of the examination process have a stronger diagnostic ability depending on several variables including, but not limited to, the prevalence of the disease, the diagnostic accuracy of the examination component, and the strength of the literature investigating the pathology or examination component.

Prior to discussion of the diagnostic accuracy of various musculoskeletal tests and measures, it is necessary to define terminology central to EBP.

- **Reference standard**—The criterion that best defines the condition of interest.[3] The reference standard should have demonstrated validity that justifies its use as a criterion measurement.[5]
- **Reliability**—The degree of consistency with which an instrument or rater measures a

Critical Clinical Pearls

When making clinical differential diagnoses decisions, keep the following in mind:

- The strengths and weaknesses of the current evidence, as well as other pieces of information (e.g., the client's goals), should help the clinician make informed decisions versus basing the decisions on the evidence alone.
- Each client will have different information affecting their differential diagnosis, such as health status, motivation for improvement, family environment, and so on.
- Each of the above stated variables can have greater influence on the differential diagnosis of a client than actual evidence-based aspects of the examination (e.g., special tests, diagnostic imaging).

particular attribute.[6] Measurements can be affected by random error. In determining the reliability of a measurement, we are determining the proportion of that measurement that is a true representation and the proportion that is the result of measurement error.[7]

- **Validity**—The degree to which a study or test appropriately measures what it intends to measure.[6] Validity attempts to answer the question: Does the test truly measure what it is designed to measure? A test must be reliable to be valid, but a test does not have to be valid to be reliable. Tests that are valid should measure the abilities vital to the sport, occupation, or aspect of activity of daily living.

- **Sensitivity (SN)**—The percentage of people who test positive for a specific disease among a group of people who have the disease. The true positive rate.

- **Specificity (SP)**—The percentage of people who test negative for a specific disease among a group of people who do not have the diagnosis or disorder. The true negative rate.

- **Positive likelihood ratio (+LR)**—The ratio of a positive (+) test result in people with the pathology to a positive test result in people without the pathology. A +LR identifies the strength of a test in determining the presence of a finding, and it is calculated by the following formula: SN / (1 − SP).

- **Negative likelihood ratio (−LR)**—The ratio of a negative (−) test result in people with the pathology to a negative test result in people without the pathology. It is calculated by the following formula: (1 − SN) / SP. The higher the +LR and lower the −LR, the more the posttest probability is altered. Posttest probability can be altered to a minimal degree (+LRs of 1-2, or −LRs of 0.5-1), to a small degree (+LRs of 2-5 and −LRs of 0.2-0.5), to a moderated degree (+LRs of 5-10, −LRs of 0.1-0.2), and to a significant and almost conclusive degree (+LRs greater than 10, −LRs less than 0.1).[3]

- **Positive predictive value (PPV)**—Given a (+) test result, the probability that the client has the condition. Some researchers and clinicians feel that PPV is better than SN since it takes into account the amount of false positives (FP). PPV = TP / (TP + FP), where TP is true positives. Therefore, if the test is (+), the client has X% chance of having the disorder.

- **Negative predictive value (NPV)**—Given a (−) test result, the probability that the client does not have the condition. Again, some believe this is better than SP since it takes into account the number of FNs. Therefore, if the test is (−), the client has X% chance of not having the disorder.

  - SN and SP are properties of the measure, while PPV and NPV are properties of both the test and the population that was tested.

  - Reading the PPV and NPV from the 2 × 2 contingency table is accurate only if the proportion of diseased clients in the sample is representative of the proportion of the diseased people in the population.

- **Overall accuracy**—Proportion of clients who are correctly diagnosed.

Diagnostic accuracy studies compare the results of the test of interest (*index test*) to the best available method for determining disease status (*reference standard* or *gold standard*).[8] Diagnostic components are typically interpreted in terms of SN, SP, +LR, and −LR. Table 4.1 illustrates the manner in which these values are calculated. Tests with high SN will be positive for most people who actually have the problem and, therefore, have a low rate of false negatives. When it is important to not miss a positive case (such as in a fracture), a test with high SN is necessary. This is crucial for screening tests in which positive findings simply indicate the need for more investigation. Therefore, the most meaningful finding with a highly SN test is a negative finding, since it assists the clinician to rule out a disorder with increased confidence. A useful acronym from the Centre for Evidence-Based Medicine is SnNout, meaning a test with high **SN** when **n**egative is used to help rule **out** the condition. The potential for false positives exists with highly sensitive tests. Again, the purpose of these tests is to not miss a positive case. These tests are therefore utilized early in the examination process to screen for the potential of more serious pathology or rule out other potential pain generators.

Tests with high SP will be appropriately negative in clients who do not have the disorder and therefore have a low rate of false positives. Tests with high SP are best for ruling in a disorder. SpPin is the acronym used for these tests. A highly **sp**ecific test

TABLE 4.1   Calculations for Sensitivity (SN) and Specificity (SP)

	FINDINGS FROM GOLD STANDARD	
Findings from index test	**Gold standard positive finding**	**Gold standard negative finding**
Index (clinical) test positive finding	a (true positive)	b (false positive)
Index (clinical) test negative finding	c (false negative)	d (true negative)
	SN = a / (a + c)	SP = d / (d + b)

when **p**ositive is used to help rule **in** the condition. As previously mentioned, this text will use SN for sensitivity and SP for specificity.

In diagnostic studies, values that are within the range of the 95% confidence interval (CI) are considered acceptable. Data presentation is less precise the wider the CI is. The width of the CI is determined by the level of the confidence desired in the study, the variability between and within the clients being investigated, and the sample size.

SN or SP values that qualify as high are usually defined as scores of 95% or greater, especially in a low prevalence setting (few people with the disease).[9] Confidence intervals that are in the 80th percentile, especially the lower 80s, can limit the ability of that measure to rule out or rule in the diagnosis.

Likelihood ratios, both positive and negative, are calculated with the combination of SN and SP. A large +LR can assist the clinician closer to the diagnosis while a small –LR moves the clinician farther away from the diagnosis. Although most of the medical literature is supportive of likelihood ratios over isolated SN and SP, some tests or measures of high SN or SP alone can also provide valuable information. For example, the impressive high SN value with the Canadian C-Spine Rules[10] is extremely helpful to the clinician for ruling out the risk of a

Critical Clinical Pearls

When looking at variously described index tests in this (or any other) text, the clinician should consider the following:

- Tests with high SN and low SP are meaningful because they are helpful to rule out (SnNout) or screen out a potential condition (a good screening tool), but they have the potential for having a high number of false positives (saying a test is positive when it is actually negative). Further use of tests with high SP is required to confirm a diagnosis of the condition when using these tests.

- Tests with high SP and low SN are meaningful because they are helpful to rule in (SpPin) or confirm a potential condition (a good diagnostic tool), but they have the potential for having a high number of false negatives (saying a test is negative when it is actually positive).

- Tests with both high SN and high SP are meaningful because they are helpful to both rule out (screening tool) and rule in (diagnostic tool) a potential condition.

- Screening tools (e.g., Canadian C-Spine Rules for cervical fractures, Ottawa Knee Rules for knee fractures) are designed to have high SN at the expense of low SP. This design is to not miss a fracture when it is there (false negative) versus diagnosing a fracture when it is actually not present (false positive).

- Likelihood ratios and use of disease prevalence are very important variables to consider when looking at index test findings.

cervical spine fracture. The SP of this rule, on the other hand, is not clinically useful at all. Therefore, the clinician can feel comfortable in the fact that this rule will miss very few false negatives. The rule will not likely miss a fracture. On the other hand, the findings will likely lead the clinician to send clients for a radiograph when they actually do not have a fracture (false positive). In this particular instance, it is likely that the clinician (and client) would rather pick up false fractures (false positives) than to miss a fracture that was actually present (false negative).

Although there are no absolute levels of diagnostic accuracy and quality that discriminate studies of higher versus lower clinical applicability, this text suggests some values that the clinician may want to consider when interpreting test findings described. The clinician is reminded however that high SN (or SP) values with poor −LR (or +LR) values are a result of a very low SP (or SN). Screening tests, for example, in this text will be given this consideration. Additionally, the clinician should consider the quality of the study. This text utilizes the Quality Assessment of Diagnostic Accuracy Studies (QUADAS) tool for quality assessment (defined and detailed in the next section of this chapter). The following list is an attempt to quantify the quality of a test or measure described in this text based on the author's previous experience, collaboration with colleagues, and previous report.[11] Colored text is used in the sections of this book that describe findings or test results having diagnostic accuracy (e.g., SN, SP, +LR, −LR). Therefore, the clinician should more strongly consider **good** to **ideal** study findings than findings from studies of lesser quality.

Ruling Out

- **Ideal**: SN of 90 or higher and −LR of 0.20 or lower with tight confidence intervals; QUADAS of ≥10/14
- **Good**: SN of 80 or higher and −LR of 0.50 or lower with tight confidence intervals; QUADAS of ≥9/14

Ruling In

- **Ideal**: SP of 90 or higher and +LR of 5.0 or greater with tight confidence intervals; QUADAS of ≥10/14
- **Good**: SP of 80 or higher, +LR of 4.0 or greater with tight confidence intervals; QUADAS of ≥9/14

With respect to clinical special tests and measures, the clinician should consider many variables. While this is not an exhaustive list, and some of these variables relate to the quality of the study (discussed in the next section), the following are worthy of mention and consideration:

- The clinician should utilize SN tests in the beginning of the examination to rule out potential pathology.
- SP tests, on the other hand, are best utilized later in the examination to rule in or confirm the pathology.
- If a disease process or pathology does not have tests and measures that have high SN or −LR, the pathology should be considered a diagnosis of exclusion. (It will not be able to be ruled out early in the examination process.)
- If a disease process or pathology does not have tests and measures that have high SP or +LR, it will be necessary to screen or rule out other potential pain generator contenders since it is not possible to confirm (or rule in) that particular pathology diagnosis.
- The values of SN, SP, +LR, and −LR must be considered in context: They are simply measuring the metrics of the actual test or measure, not the quality of the study.
- Consider the prevalence and incidence of disease. The Canadian C-Spine Rule (CCSR) for cervical fracture diagnosis, for example, has high SN but poor SP. It has been utilized in emergency department settings with a pretest probability suggestion of 1% to 2%. Therefore, by nature, the prevalence will be very low. That, along with the high SN and low SP, will result in a significant number of FPs. See chapter 10 (Special Tests) for a more detailed explanation of this.
- Consider the clients who were investigated in the study. Are they clients who were likely to have the disease? Were they a cohort of clients likely to have the disease (inflating the SN)?
- Was the examination or measure investigated on clients both likely to have and likely not to have the pathology? If so, the measure is more likely to discriminate those who have and those who do not have the pathology.
- Was the test or measure compared to an appropriate gold standard? Surgery is often such a standard, but not all pathologies (e.g., hamstring injury) require surgery. Therefore the clinical measure is compared to a gold or reference standard with imperfection.

- Along with this, QUADAS scores, although numerical and linear, are not equal. Different biases in a study are not equal and can have different effects on study interpretation.
- The entire examination process must be utilized to increase probability (e.g., subjective history and upper quarter screen [UQS]).
- The goal of the examination process as a unit is to pare down the differential diagnosis with the use of both current best evidence and sound clinical reasoning.
- The clinical special test or measure does not typically define causality. For example, impingement testing in both the shoulder and hip can be attributed to the mechanical abutment of the involved two bones. In the shoulder and hip, impingement has been attributed to both hypomobility and hypermobility factors. Therefore, the special test does not precisely determine the exact mechanism (and therefore the most appropriate intervention) of the bony abutment.

STUDY QUALITY

When searching the evidence for a clinically relevant article on diagnosis, systematic reviews and meta-analysis are the most authoritative types of reports.[12] These types of article are usually less frequent than individual articles, and they are limited in their strength by the studies they include. Systematic reviews and meta-analyses are included in this text when available.

Appraising individual articles is necessary to determine their validity. Simply examining the results and conclusions is not sufficient. The most crucial step in evaluating an article is determining if the methods utilized in the study were free of error and bias.[13-16] If its validity is questionable, the article's results cannot confidently be interpreted.[13]

Quality Assessment of Diagnostic Accuracy Studies (QUADAS)[13] is a tool for measuring the methodological quality of diagnostic accuracy studies in systematic reviews. Inter-rater reliability among separate reviewers has been reported as relatively

Quality Assessment
of Diagnostic Accuracy Studies Scores Tool[13]

Item 1: Was the spectrum of clients representative of those in clinical practice?

Item 2: Were selection criteria clearly described?

Item 3: Is the reference standard likely to classify the target condition correctly?

Item 4: Is the period of time between the reference standard and index test acceptable?

Item 5: Did the whole sample of clients receive verification using the reference standard?

Item 6: Did clients receive the same reference standard regardless of the index test result?

Item 7: Was the reference standard independent of the index test?

Item 8: Was the execution of the index test described in sufficient detail for replication?

Item 9: Was the execution of the reference standard described in sufficient detail for replication?

Item 10: Were the index test results interpreted without knowledge of the reference standard?

Item 11: Was the reference standard interpreted without knowledge of the results of the index test?

Item 12: Were the same clinical criteria available when test results were interpreted as would be in clinical practice?

Item 13: Were uninterpretable/intermediate test results reported?

Item 14: Were withdrawals from the study explained?

Adapted from Whiting et al., 2003.[13]

Critical Clinical Pearls

When looking at the diagnostic accuracy of the various examination components, keep the following in mind:

- SN and SP are characteristics of the actual test (e.g., Lachman's test in the knee). The population does not affect the results.
- Likelihood ratios actually account for those with and without the disease.
- Positive and negative predictive values are influenced by the prevalence of disease in the population that is being tested. If we test in a high prevalence setting, it is more likely that people who test positive truly have that disease than if the test is performed in a population with low prevalence and vice versa.
- Bias in a study (as measured by QUADAS) affects the interpretation of the reported diagnostic values.
- A study with a lot of bias (low QUADAS) score but investigating a special test found to be of strong diagnostic value (high +LR and low –LR) should be interpreted with caution due to study bias. It is unclear if the actual test is a poor test or the study alone is of poor quality.

low, but QUADAS was still suggested as a useful tool for highlighting the strengths and weaknesses of existing diagnostic accuracy studies.[17, 18] It was suggested that clinicians clearly understand the tool prior to its implementation. Clear understanding resulted in notable improvement in reliability among separate reviewers.[18]

The QUADAS tool[13] consists of 14 items, each having a yes, no, or unclear answer option (see the sidebar on page 56). A yes score indicates sufficient information, with bias considered unlikely. A no score indicates sufficient information, but with potential bias from inadequate design or conduct. An unclear score indicates that insufficient information was provided in the article or the methodology was unclear. The total score is the count of all of the criteria that scored yes, which receive a value of 1, whereas no and unclear scores carried a value of 0. The maximum attainable score on the criteria list is 14. Some studies have used a stratification of scoring as high quality and low risk of bias if the QUADAS score was 10 or greater, and low quality and high risk of bias if the study score was less than 10 on the QUADAS.[19-22]

BROAD TO NARROW OR FUNNEL EXAMINATION FOCUS

The entire diagnostic process entails each component described in this text. This examination focus

or sequence will be referred to as *broad to narrow* or the *funnel approach* as advocated by the author and colleagues.[23] The clinician generates a differential diagnosis for each client based on the history (client interview), observation, triage, motion, muscle performance, special tests, palpation, and physical performance measures (figure 4.1). Based on the probability of a particular diagnosis to exist, the findings of each of these components will make shifts in posttest probability based on their diagnostic accuracy (SN, SP, likelihood ratios). Utilizing only one component as the gold standard from which the diagnosis is made is inappropriate clinical practice.

This approach, while comprehensive, is also systematic; it moves from broad to narrow in its approach from the beginning to the end of the examination process. The intent is to start the examination process as comprehensively as possible, including all potential diagnoses. As a result of each systematic step in the examination process, the clinician should narrow down the differential diagnosis list as far as possible. Additionally, the broad-to-narrow approach of the examination is in the sense of moving from less to more isolated examination procedures. For example, in the client interview, the clinician asks broad, open-ended questions that are likely to include multiple potential diagnoses. As the examination continues, the examination process becomes more focused. This is particularly the case after the section for triage or screening and sensitive tests, which is intended to rule out not only the potential for red flags or nonmusculoskeletal disease processes but also

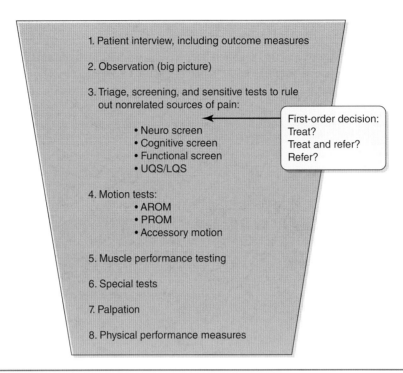

Figure 4.1 Funnel approach of the examination process.
© Michael Reiman

potential pain generators in other joints, as well as other potential diagnoses common to the pain-generating joints.

Observation and triage are also intended to be broad in their focus. Medical systems and neurological screening, in general, assist the clinician in determining the appropriateness of musculoskeletal examination and subsequent intervention. If screening is conclusively negative, the clinician determines that it is appropriate to continue with the rest of the examination process. If screening is not conclusively negative, the clinician is required to make a clinically sound judgment on the appropriateness of immediate referral out to the appropriate medical personnel or on whether an attempt at appropriate intervention will assist in determining the client's status.

Screening tests and upper and lower quarter screens early on in the examination also focus the rest of the examination sequence. Once serious pathology has been screened, the clinician's focus is on determining the pain-generating structure (pain generator). Screening the appropriate upper or lower quarter will narrow the region of examination.

The clinician then systematically works through the rest of the sequences of the examination pro-

cess (motion testing, muscle performance testing, special tests, palpation, and physical performance measures), continuing to screen with increasing focus on validly differentiating among the few remaining diagnoses. Since these diagnoses are similar to each other with respect to nature, severity, and irritability, special tests with high SP are used to minimize confusion with respect to the condition or disorder.[24] Once the clinician has systematically reasoned through the broad-to-narrow-focused examination sequence, they should be able to reasonably determine the client's primary impairments (and thus the treatment-based classification scheme to be used), as well as the most likely pathological presentation of the client. Greater depth of each particular component of the suggested examination process is given in the following sections. For particular details of each component, refer to each respective chapter.

Client Interview

The client interview is likely the initial interaction between the clinician and the client. The clinician has the opportunity to positively or negatively influence the client. Clients described the following factors as indicative of a quality office visit:

thoroughness in routine examinations, spending enough time with them, engaging them, and treating them with courtesy and respect; clinicians did not necessarily interpret these same factors as relevant indicators of a quality visit.[25] Communication and interpersonal skills of the clinician were also deemed as important variables in determining in the minds of the clients how successful clinicians were with an office visit.[26]

Successful communication with the client is dependent on multiple variables including, but not limited to, eye contact with the client, providing clients with the opportunity to describe their current condition without interruption, verbal and nonverbal communication, active listening, time spent with the client, use of facilitative comments, empathy, clarification of the client's statements, and summarizing the client's verbal presentation. Each of these variables is important for a successful interview of the client.

Since the interview is likely the first point of contact with the client, it should also be the time when the clinician starts their differential diagnosis of the client. Properly performing the subjective interview and history of the client allows the clinician to appropriately narrow the focus of potential diagnoses of the client.[27-29] Additionally, the subjective history can be used to determine 76% to 83% of diagnoses with clients.[30, 31]

These variables, aspects of clinical reasoning, components of a standard client interview, and subjective information regarding pain are discussed further in chapter 5.

Outcome measures, more commonly referred to as *self-report measures*, are assessed in the interview. At this point in the examination, the clinician should discuss findings of these outcome measures (if appropriate). Additionally, if clarification is needed with respect to the self-report measure, the client interview is appropriate for this interpretation. These self-report measures are the client's means of subjectively reporting how extensively their pain or dysfunction is affecting them. While these are very focused for each region of the body, the common theme among all of them is the subjective reporting by the client (typically without involvement from the clinician).

Diagnostic imaging can also be interpreted or discussed prior to the appointment or with the client during the interview. Details of outcomes and self-report measures and radiography are presented

in chapter 6 (Triage and Differential Diagnosis) due to their utilization in medical screening.

Observation (Big Picture)

General aspects of observation are discussed in this chapter and referred to throughout the rest of the text. Specific detail regarding observation of posture (chapter 14) and gait (chapter 13) are given later in this text. Essentially, in the observation component of the examination, the clinician is trying to get a broad picture of the client's objective presentation. Nonverbal communication, posture, gait, and transfers are all big-picture assessment components of observation.

Observation of the client requires a systematic approach. Viewing the client from anterior, posterior, and lateral views ensures detail of observation. Limiting errors in observation requires some important variables, including observation from more than one view of the client, multiple observations of the client in the same positions, observation of the client in different positions (e.g., sitting, standing, gait), and determination of eye dominance. Observation of clients takes into account not only how they present in the examination room, but also in the waiting room, their interaction with the secretarial staff (if possible), how they transfer in and out of a chair, how they walk back to the room, how they transfer in the examination room, their gait when they leave, and if possible how they transfer into or out of their vehicle. Viewing the client from more than one view, just like with radiography, will assist the clinician in more completely understanding the client's condition.

Triage and Sensitive Tests

At this point in the examination process, once appropriate data have been gathered, the clinician should determine if it is appropriate to continue with the client's examination or whether high suspicion of red flags or significant medical conditions exist that may contribute to the client's presentation. Interpretation of diagnostic imaging can also assist with differential diagnosis and medical screening relative to whether a primary musculoskeletal component is present in the client's clinical presentation. Details regarding primary imaging modalities, their basic characteristics, and diagnostic accuracy relevant to specific conditions are presented in chapter 6.

Determining Eye Dominance

Most people prefer to use their right eye for viewing. Although the pattern of eye–hand dominance appears related to athletic proficiency for baseball,[32] sighting dominance may not be perfectly correlated with handedness.[33] It has also been suggested that eye dominance may depend on the hand moving toward the target.[33] Regardless, the clinician should have a consistent, reliable intratester method of observation. Determining eye dominance has been suggested multiple ways. One simple option may be for the clinician to make a circle with both hands, focus a stationary object in this circle with both eyes open, and then close one eye at a time while still staring through the hole at the object. The eye that is open in the view where the object remains in the circle is the dominant eye.

Vital sign assessment is a necessity for the clinician examining a client with suspicion of a musculoskeletal condition. Vital signs have diagnostic accuracy applicability and have been shown to be strongly associated with adverse outcomes in triage departments.[34-36] Mandatory assessment of resting blood pressure has been suggested as part of a comprehensive assessment of the client with suspicion of upper cervical instability or cervical artery dysfunction.[37, 38] Careful assessment and reassessment of vital signs should be part of a standard examination and treatment of clients.

Medical screenings include systems review and examination. The client interview should assist the clinician with determining whether medical screening is necessary. Chapter 6 covers medical screening appropriate to the musculoskeletal client in detail. The aim of a screening assessment of the musculoskeletal system (upper and lower quarter screens) is to be sensitive enough to identify the presence of any significant abnormality and to be feasible to perform as part of any general examination. Sensitive tests should be implemented early in the examination as a screening test.[39] Clinicians should use tests of strong screening capability in order to pare down their differential diagnosis of the presenting case.

Performing screening tests and upper and lower quarter screens early on in the examination are especially relevant in vague symptom presentation, multiple-joint referred pain, unexplained atrophy, and unexplained dysfunction connected with gait, balance, or coordination, as well as when the clinician is less confident in where symptoms are being generated from (pain generator). Functional screening can have multiple iterations: Subjective questioning of the client's functional status,

observation of functional tasks, and observation of performance tasks such as stepping up and down a step (observing for strength and quality of motion) are some examples.

At this point in the examination, the clinician must make a clinical decision on the appropriateness of continuing with the examination. The clinician will decide if they should continue with the examination and treatment, cautiously continue with examination or treatment while assessing whether a referral to a more appropriate clinician is necessary, or directly refer the client to a more appropriate clinician.

Motion Tests

Motion testing is comprehensive to include both osteokinematic and arthrokinematic assessment. Comparisons of active range of motion (AROM), resistive range of motion (RROM), and passive range of motion (PROM) assist in determining contractile versus noncontractile tissue involvement. Furthermore, accessory joint play assessment assists in delineating joint involvement. Motion testing is covered in greater detail in chapter 8.

Muscle Performance Testing

Muscle performance is inclusive of muscle strength, power, and endurance. Appropriate suggestions of motor control as a component of this category have also been given and should be warranted. Muscle performance testing, along with motion testing, can also assist with delineating contractile versus noncontractile tissue. This type of testing can help determine the extent of soft-tissue involvement utilizing Cyriax's testing scheme (e.g., strong and painful indicative of minor lesion, weak and pain-less indicative of complete tear or neurological lesion).[40] Chapter 9 also covers other quantitative (e.g., manual muscle testing) and qualitative muscle performance assessments. Global movement assessments, such as a bilateral squat, can serve as screens for the potential of muscle performance, motion, or intra-articular (also assessed with special tests) dysfunction.

Special Tests

Physical examination testing is commonly interpreted as *special tests*. Special tests are extensively published in the literature and various texts. Screening and diagnosis of pathology are far too commonly based heavily on the findings of these tests. Instead, they should be used as one component of a more comprehensive examination process. The approach of this text is to use perspective with regard to these tests. The comprehensive examination process is far superior to over-reliance on special tests alone. Chapter 10 discusses this category of testing.

Palpation

Another component of the examination process that has suffered from overutilization is palpation. Palpation, similar to special tests, has great allure for many clinicians, particularly those wanting to simplify the comprehensive nature of the examination process and those lacking the necessary amount of time for a comprehensive examination approach. Chapter 11 examines palpation and its strengths and weaknesses.

Physical Performance Measures

Physical performance measures (PPMs) are probably the least consistently employed component of the examination sequence. It has been traditionally thought that these measures are most appropriate for only the highest level clients or at the end of a client's treatment (just prior to discharge). Appreciate that, just like other components of the examination sequence, there are levels of PPMs. Depending on the region of the body, there may be very few (and therefore little stratification) or many (and therefore significant stratification) of these measures. Chapter 12 provides greater detail on these measures.

INTEGRATION OF FUNNEL EXAMINATION APPROACH

A systematic approach to using findings (especially those from special tests) reporting SN and SP is suggested in figure 4.2. The use of tests of high SN and low −LR is suggested early in the examination (Triage and Sensitive Tests), with red flags first ruled out. Once it is determined that the client is appropriate for examination or treatment, the clinician continues through additional examination components (e.g., motion tests, muscle performance testing, special tests). Particular emphasis is on motion testing and muscle performance testing to delineate if the client's actual symptoms are reproduced. Additionally, special tests (and possibly imaging) of high SP are helpful to rule in pathology of the determined pain-generating joint(s). Again, caution should be taken when using special tests for diagnosis. Figure 4.2 shows a systematic approach for integrating diagnostic accuracy findings of both high SN (early in the examination—triage and screening) and high SP (later in the examination—special tests—for determination of ruling in pathology). The suggestions for **ideal** and **good** diagnostic accuracy values are again provided here.

THE EXAMINATION CONTINUUM

One primary purpose of this text is to provide a comprehensive approach to examination of each section, as well as to describe the diagnostic capability of the component detailed in each section. Carefully read each component of the examination sequence, decipher the diagnostic capability of each section, and make evidence-informed decisions on the value of each section to increase or decrease the posttest probability that a particular pathology or condition will exist.

A proper examination of a client is a moving target, constantly in motion. In other words, each visit with the client is partly an examination of their status; each pre- and postintervention session performed on the client is an examination. The value of continuous reassessment should be appreciated and respected. Each time the client is seen, some form of reassessment is necessary in order to appreciate the between-session changes in clinical presentation, just as the within-session changes should be

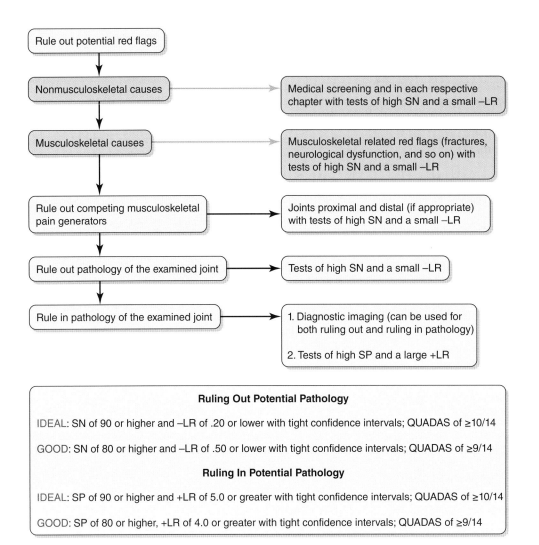

Figure 4.2 Algorithm approach for use of special tests or findings reporting SN and SP. SN = sensitivity; SP = specificity; +LR = positive likelihood ratio; –LR = negative likelihood ratio

© Michael Reiman

appreciated pre and post intervention of a client within a particular session.

The examination of a client should also be recognized as an assessment along a continuum (figure 4.3). Many examination procedures described, including those in this text, are on the *isolated examination* side of the continuum (e.g., ROM, muscle performance, radiology findings, special tests). *Integrated examination* would include measures more applicable to daily tasks, such as sport- and work-related activities (e.g., function). These measures might include administering the physical performance measures section of this text (see chapter 12), as well as simply assessing the client's quality and big-picture quantity assessment of their daily tasks, work tasks, and sports tasks.

While many of these measures are not directly quantifiable in terms of measurement, their quality and tolerance by the client are distinctly important. In fact, it is quite often why the client seeks medical care. Therefore, instead of taking an approach of always proceeding from left to right (from isolated to integrated) on this examination continuum, recognize that it may be necessary to approach the

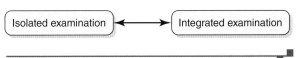

Figure 4.3 The examination continuum.

© Michael Reiman

examination sequence from different locations on this continuum. For example, for someone with broad, diffuse, and nonspecific lower extremity pain, assessment of the client's squatting ability (as with the lower quarter screen) might assist the clinician with determining a potential joint as the true pain generator. The examination then can be performed with the broad-to-narrow approach with that particular joint in mind. This same approach might also work for the athlete with pain with jumping. Assessment from a global perspective (simply watching the athlete jump) may key the clinician into areas of focus for the isolated portion of the examination.

Note that clients likely will move back and forth along this continuum at different points in their rehabilitation process. For example, a client progressing appropriately along post knee injury, but who still has pain with jumping, may require a reassessment where they enter the continuum with a jumping assessment first (toward the integrated side of the continuum). This will help the clinician determine the potential limitation or pain generator from which to then focus the isolated examinations, as described previously.

BASIC PRINCIPLES OF THE EXAMINATION PROCESS

With respect to the examination process, whether it is a systematic approach such as the broad-to-narrow focus described previously or a less regimented process, the clinician must appreciate basic tenets of the examination process. A general outline of these components follows. The clinician should be cognizant of all of these variables when conducting a well-thought-out, systematic examination on a client. The combined utilization of both sound clinical judgment (clinical reasoning) and EBP affords the clinician optimal clinical practice. Greater detail of specific components of the broad-to-narrow examination procedure is given in the following chapters.

Differential Diagnosis

- A primary goal of the exam is to obtain data and rule out or rule in competing diagnoses.
- This goal can be accomplished by selectively provoking the area to implicate it as involved or uninvolved.

Vital Signs

- Essential components of examination include, but are not necessarily limited to, the following (see chapter 6 for more on triage and differential diagnosis):

    Blood pressure

    Heart rate

    Respiration

    Body temperature

    Skin temperature and color

- Monitor client at rest and during activity to assess circulatory system with and without stress.

Bilateral Comparison

- The clinician must always examine the uninvolved side prior to the involved side. This will establish a baseline value from which to relate.
- With this order, the client will be less apprehensive when the involved side is assessed.

Movement Testing Sequence

- Active movements are performed first, then passive movements, then finally resisted isometric movements. This sequence provides the clinician with an idea of what the client believes they can do.
- Painful movements should be performed last to avoid biasing the rest of the examination process.
- If painful movements are tested earlier, the pain that was provoked may influence the rest of the examination. Performing painful movements early in the examination can cause the involved structure to be painful with other movements that are not typically painful, which clouds the examination findings.

Overpressure Application

- Apply overpressure when end-range active movements are negative.
- Gradually apply overpressure with care.
- The intent of overpressure is to more conclusively rule out that structure as a potential pain generator.

Repeat or Sustain Movements if History Indicates

- This is particularly important if the client complains that symptoms are altered by repetitive movements or sustained positions.

Resisted Isometric Movements Performed in a Resting Position

- Stress on the inert tissues is minimal in this position. Symptoms produced in these positions are more likely due to contractile tissue.
- If desired or necessary, isometric testing can be implemented in either shortened or lengthened positions.
  - Shortened (active insufficiency) and lengthened (passive insufficiency) positions are also useful for assessing contractile tissue.
  - Lengthened positions may also be utilized to assess noncontractile structures that stabilize the related joints in that region.

Passive Movements and Ligamentous Testing

- Both the extent of laxity and quality of end-feel of the movement are important.
- End-feels are discussed in greater detail in chapter 8 (Range of Motion Assessment).

Ligamentous Testing

- Repeat testing with increasing stress.
- Start with lighter stress force and increase as per symptoms or response until you are confident in findings.
- As with all forms of testing, use bilateral comparison (noninvolved side tested first) for understanding of force necessary in each particular client.
- Grading of joint instability due to ligamentous dysfunction (sprain) is variable. One proposed grading scheme is outlined in table 4.2.

Muscle Strain Assessment

- Start with light pressure and gradually increase as tolerated and warranted.
- Muscle strains are also graded on a similar scale; see table 4.3.
- As with all testing, bilateral comparison is warranted.

Myotome Testing

- With myotome testing, contractions must be held for 5 seconds since myotome-related weakness can take time to develop.
- Bilateral comparison is warranted.

Potential Exacerbation of Symptoms From Examination

- Warn the client of possible exacerbations in their symptoms due to the examination process itself.
- The client must understand the necessity of provoking their symptoms (i.e., producing their concordant pain to assist with determination of the pain-generating structures) and producing their concordant pain.

Determine Necessity for Referral to a More Appropriate Health Care Provider

- This determination is based on all the information gleaned from the examination and should be based on sound clinical reasoning.
- As always (and as discussed in greater detail in chapter 6), refer the client to a more appropriate health care provider if necessary.

Screening Examination

- Integrate a screening examination early in the examination to determine the appropriateness of the client as a musculoskeletal client.
- Refer to chapters 6 (Triage and Differential Diagnosis) and 7 (Orthopedic Screening and Nervous System Examination) for greater detail regarding this concept.

Examination of Specific Joints

- Use an unchanged systematic approach to the examination that varies only slightly to elaborate certain clues given by the history or by client responses.
- Active movements:
  - Movements are actively performed by the client.
  - Referred to as *physiologic* (or osteokinematic), these movements are ones that the client can obviously perform independently.

TABLE 4.2 Grading of Joint and Ligament Sprains

Sprain or severity	Classification	Translation
Mild	Grade I (1+ instability/1° sprain)	0–5 mm
Moderate	Grade II (2+ instability/2° sprain)	5–10 mm
Severe	Grade III (3+ instability/3° sprain)	10–15 mm
	Grade IV (4+ instability/4° sprain)	15+ mm

mm = millimeters; 1° = 1st degree

TABLE 4.3 Muscle Strain Grading

Strain or severity	Classification	Degree of tissue damage	Clinical findings	Resisted movement interpretation[40]
Normal	Normal	None	Normal appearance	Client tolerates strong resistance with muscle testing and has no pain.
Mild	Grade I (1° strain)	Stretching or tearing of a minimum number of contractile fibers	Client has pain, mild swelling, ecchymosis, corresponding joint stiffness, reflex muscle inhibition, and pain with resistance to muscle testing. Area may have increased temperature to the touch, and there may not be a palpable deformity.	Client tolerates strong resistance but has pain with muscle testing.
Moderate	Grade II (2° strain)	Tearing of a moderate number of contractile fibers	Client has pain, moderate swelling, ecchymosis, corresponding related joint stiffness, reflex muscle inhibition, and pain and weakness with resistance to muscle testing. Area has increased temperature to the touch, and is likely to have a palpable deformity.	Client tolerates minimal resistance (weakness demonstrated) and has pain with muscle testing.
Severe	Grade III (3° strain)	Complete tearing or rupture of all contractile fibers	Client has pain, often significant swelling, ecchymosis, and corresponding related joint stiffness. Area has increased temperature to the touch, and a palpable deformity is present. Reflex muscle inhibition is profound. Client is likely unable to actively move the involved joint. PROM may not be affected, depending on the extent of pain and swelling.	Client tolerates minimal to no resistance (likely unable to move involved joint) and likely has no pain with muscle testing. This may also represent neurological injury.

- Contractile, nervous, and inert tissues are all stressed with active movements.
- Active movements may not be performed with fracture, newly repaired soft tissue, or when active movement is contraindicated.
- Contractile tissue includes muscles, tendons, and their attachment to the bones.
- Nervous tissue includes nerves and associated sheaths.
- Inert tissue includes joint capsules, ligaments, bursa, blood vessels, cartilage, and dura mater.

- On active movements, the clinician should note the following:
  - When and where during each movement the onset of pain occurs
  - Whether the movement increases the intensity and quality of the pain
  - The reaction of the client to pain

- The amount of observable movement or restriction (quantitative assessment)
- The pattern of movement (qualitative assessment)
- The quality and synchrony of movement (qualitative assessment)
- The movement of associated joints (can be both qualitative and quantitative)
- The willingness of the client to move the part
- Any limitation present and its nature

CONCLUSION

This chapter is intended to provide the clinician with a general background and framework of the examination process. Further detail in regard to specific components of the examination are found in the following chapters.

5

CLIENT INTERVIEW AND OBSERVATION

Jonathan Sylvain, PT, DPT, OCS, FAAOMPT
Michael P. Reiman, PT, DPT, OCS, SCS, ATC, FAAOMPT, CSCS

The client interview is the first time in the examination process when there is a direct one-on-one interaction between the clinician and the client. The history is conceivably the most important part of the clinical examination, with the physical examination viewed as complementary and used to confirm hypotheses generated from the history.[1] Purposeful history taking allows the clinician to collect information from clients that can be used as a guide during the physical examination and aid in the identification of the client's concordant sign. The concordant sign is the activity or motion that reproduces the client's pain or chief complaint.[2] During history taking, clinicians often gather information that may reveal the client's concordant sign. In fact, it has been suggested that the subjective history can be used to determine 74% to 90% of diagnoses with clients.[3-6]

The clinician must perform several key functions during this part of the examination, including warmly welcoming the client, alleviating any fear and anxiety they may have with respect to the examination process, and informing the client what the examination process entails. For most clients, this will be the first time they have sufficient time to discuss and interact with a health care provider.[7-9] Additionally, clients relate improved satisfaction with health care providers when the clinician is informative and spends time with them,[10, 11] even when the clinician has less experience than their peers.[10]

EFFECTIVE COMMUNICATION IN THE CLIENT INTERVIEW AND HISTORY

Eliciting a good history and therefore conducting an organized and fruitful client interview and history requires several skills, not the least of which are organizational and communication abilities. Effective communication on the part of the clinician when interviewing a client requires several skills. The clinician must be able to not only ask appropriate questions but also listen to the client, ask follow-up questions based on information the client shares, redirect the line of questioning dependent on this information, and so on.

During consultation, the client must be considered the most valuable source of information. Many clinicians take control during the examination process, not allowing the client to express the reasoning for seeking care. Beckman and colleagues found that in 69% of visits, physicians interrupted client's statements and directed questions toward a specific concern.[12] In another study, physicians redirected clients during their opening statement after a mean of 23.1 seconds. Clients allowed to complete their opening statement required an average of only 6 seconds longer to state their primary concerns.[13] Many clients will not divulge additional relevant information after being interrupted.

The fact that a client interview can be done more or less effectively is demonstrated by the fact that essential diagnostic information can be uncovered from the client interview.[14-17] One's efficiency in communication can be improved through training.[16, 18, 19] It is unlikely that any future technological advances will negate the need and value of compassionate and empathetic two-way communication between clinician and client. The published literature also expresses belief in the essential role of communication: "It has long been recognized that difficulties in the effective delivery of health care can arise from problems in communication between patient and provider rather than from any failing in the technical aspects of medical care. Improvements in provider-patient communication can have beneficial effects on health outcomes."[16] Professional conversation between clients and clinicians shapes diagnosis, initiates therapy, and establishes a caring relationship.[14]

The development and improvement of communication and clinical reasoning skills leads to the clinician "developing an accurate clinical hypothesis, developing an examination and intervention approach to meet the individual's cultural, communication, anatomic, and physiologic needs and abilities, recognizing patient symptoms and signs that necessitate communication with other health care providers, and participating in the decision-making process regarding the selection of appropriate diagnostic testing."[20]

Despite these facts, many health care providers have poor communication skills and perform inadequate client interviews. Many times failure to take a sufficient medical history with proper client communication can lead to mistakes that have clinical and economic consequences.[21-23] In fact, many complaints about health care providers are not about the medical care provided but in regard to poor or insufficient communication.[24] A complex relationship exists between clients' opinions of physician communication and physicians' malpractice history. Clinicians must learn to adapt and tailor their communication styles to each individual client due to variations that exist in clients' intellectual and emotional needs. Clinicians must also develop an understanding of each individual client's desired communication needs.[22]

Communication in primary care physicians is also a significant variable in malpractice claims. Physicians without such claims educated patients on what to expect during their visit, laughed and demonstrated humor, spent more time with patients during routine visits, and sought and facilitated the expression of the patient's opinions, values, and beliefs.[21] For a successful and humanistic encounter at an office visit, the clinician needs to be sure that the client's key concerns have been directly and specifically solicited and addressed. To be effective, the clinician must gain an understanding of the client's perspective on their illness. The whole client must be evaluated because a plethora of conditions may present with manifestations similar to musculoskeletal conditions. Furthermore, client concerns can be wide ranging. Client values, cultures, gender, and preferences need to be taken into consideration.[16]

Clinician skill, rapport, and health-related communication behaviors are key elements of a client interview. Clients are more likely than clinicians to report behaviors demonstrating thoroughness in routine examinations as essential to a quality office visit, such as spending enough time with them, engaging them, and treating them with courtesy and respect.[25] The degree to which these activities are successful depends, in large part, on the communication and interpersonal skills of the clinician.[14]

Certain observable history-taking behaviors are evident between good and poor diagnosticians. Furthermore, these behaviors are evident during the first 3 minutes of the encounter. Behaviors characteristic of good diagnosticians are thoroughness of inquiry about the chief complaint, asking questions in close proximity within a line of reasoning, clarifying or verifying information provided by the client, and summarizing the information at hand. Characteristic behaviors of bad diagnosticians are repeating questions unnecessarily, changing the topic before completing a line of inquiry, inquiring about systems, and inquiring about past history.[26]

A positive working relationship between clinician and client has a positive effect on treatment outcomes, although further research is needed to determine the strength of the relationship.[27] Poor communication, though, can leave clients with an undefined understanding of their diagnosis, prognosis, future management plans, and the therapeutic intent of treatment.[28]

Communicating with a client is a must in order to set up an effective therapeutic alliance. The approach taken is important. Physical therapists tend to apply a paternalistic approach even though clients prefer to share decisions or provide their opinions about treatment options.[29]

The communication relationship with the client encompasses many aspects, including verbal and nonverbal communication, a client-centered interview, the use of empathy, active listening, facilitation, summarization, clarification, and reflection skills. Each of these aspects has specific considerations that the clinician must take into account when engaging in the therapeutic relationship with the client.

Verbal and Nonverbal Communication

Communication is a vital aspect to an effective client encounter.[27, 30, 31] A skilled communicator will listen not only to what is being said but also to what is left unsaid, since communication traditionally incorporates verbal and nonverbal behaviors. Communication is a continuous process that does not stop when verbal communication has.[32] It also involves observing nonverbal body language and noticing any inconsistencies between verbal and nonverbal messages. Nonverbal communication consists of silence, touch, hand gestures, posture, eye contact, facial expressions, and both active and passive listening. The nonverbal component comprises 55% to 97% of communication.[33] Clinicians must be cognizant of nonverbal behaviors. If clients feel they are not being listened to, they may feel that their pain has not been validated, which can lead to feelings of dissatisfaction with their care.[34] Furthermore, research has shown that expert physical therapists focus on verbal and nonverbal communication with clients.[35]

The emotional context of care is especially related to nonverbal communication, and emotion-related communication skills, including sending and receiving nonverbal messages and emotional self-awareness, are critical elements of high-quality care.[36] Effective communication increases client satisfaction and health outcomes.[27, 30, 37]

Verbal behaviors positively associated with health outcomes include empathy, reassurance and support, various client-centered questioning techniques, encounter length, history taking, explanations, both dominant and passive physician styles, positive reinforcement, humor, psychosocial talk, time in health education and information sharing, friendliness, courtesy, orienting the client during examination, and summarization and clarification. Nonverbal behaviors positively associated with outcomes included head nodding, forward lean, direct body orientation, uncrossed legs and arms, arm symmetry, and less mutual gaze.[38]

"By the Way" Syndrome

Clients most often arrive at the clinic with a multitude of questions and concerns. Discussion of each and every issue during a clinical encounter

---

Critical Clinical Pearls

When performing the subjective examination, keep the following in mind:

- The client interview is the most important part of the clinical examination, with the physical exam viewed as complementary and a means of confirming the generated hypothesis.
- Communication, both verbal and nonverbal, is vital to an effective client encounter. Thorough communication increases client satisfaction and health outcomes.
- A clinician's effectiveness in communication can be improved through training and deliberate practice.
- Throughout the consultation, the client must be considered the most valuable source of information.

is often a difficult task. Time constraints and the assumption that clients will begin with their main complaint make it difficult for clinicians to appropriately identify each client's whole agenda.[39] This may lead to a relatively new issue known as *"by the way" syndrome*. It is important for clinicians to attempt to prioritize each client's complaints in an effort to prevent or reduce the frequency of clients waiting to mention issues until the end of their visit. Research has demonstrated that clients raised new problems at the end of the visit in 21% of the cases,[40] and late-arising concerns were more prevalent when physicians did not seek clients' primary concerns during the interview process.[13]

The syndrome occurred in 39% of observed encounters. Its major content was bio-psychosocial (39%), psychosocial (36%), or biomedical (25%), whereas physician responses were mostly biomedical (44%). The physician response was concordant with the client's question in 61% of encounters if the content of the question was psychosocial, 21% if bio-psychosocial, and 78% if biomedical. In 22% of the encounters, clinicians did not give any answer to the client's question, particularly if it was of psychosocial content.[13] Asking about the client's agenda twice or more during the office visit might decrease the appearance of this syndrome.[41] Furthermore, orienting clients to the process of the encounter may inform them when it's most helpful to bring forth concerns, thus encouraging clients to present new problems before the end of the interview.

Clients may comprehend and recall as little as 50% of what health care providers convey during an encounter.[42] Therefore, clinicians must encourage their clients to voice their concerns or need for clarification at any point during encounters. Use of statements such as the following can and will facilitate the exposure of each client's whole agenda: Do you have any questions so far? How does that sound? What else? What other problems would you like to discuss today? What else would you like to accomplish today?

Time Spent With Clients

In visits taking longer than 15 minutes, clients have expressed greater satisfaction about time spent when the clinician discussed test results or findings from the physical examination.[43] Medical providers saved time and reached conclusions faster by asking open-ended questions and listening to their

clients.[44, 45] The clinician should be willing to establish a relationship of active and mutual cooperation with their clients and should make time to do so. Clients must be in a position to freely express their opinions, without hurry or fear. For example, the time spent with clients was found to be the most important ingredient of migraine therapy.[46]

COMMON BARRIERS TO EFFECTIVE COMMUNICATION

As discussed earlier in the chapter, failure to use effective communication skills during a clinical encounter can lead to ineffective care.[21-23] Clinicians should develop an understanding and an awareness of the numerous types of behaviors that can lead to deficiencies during client encounters so that they can avoid them. Common barriers to effective communication include but are not limited to the following:[47, 48]

- Use of medical jargon
- Emotional barriers
- Lack of attention due to disinterest or distractions
- Prejudices and stereotyping
- Differences in beliefs
- Physical or language barriers (e.g., speech, hearing)
- Cultural barriers
- Offering advice before the chief complaint is identified
- Switching the topic

Clinicians should avoid using medical jargon and overcomplicated or unfamiliar terms that may confuse and intimidate the client. Instead, they should emphasize clear, concise, and basic terminology in an effort to appropriately connect with each client. Emotional barriers can be a challenge to overcome. During communication, clinicians must be aware of their own and the client's verbal and nonverbal communication. For example, if the clinician is in a bad mood, their body language may relay to the client that the information being conveyed is bad. Clinicians should not display lack of attention or disinterest and must avoid distractions, since these behaviors will make it difficult for them to develop rapport and trust. Clinicians must be aware of their own preconceived biases and prejudices that can be related to race, gender, age, religion, accent, or previous experiences. They should strive to maintain an open mind to the ideas and opinions of others. Keeping an open mind does not necessarily mean that you have to specifically agree with someone's views, but it does mean that you attempt to develop an understanding. Clinicians must consider physical and language barriers, including but not limited to hearing and vision loss, difficulty reading, and anxiety disorders, which can be barriers to communication.

Clinicians should avoid offering advice, interrupting, or switching the topic with clients before the chief complaint is identified. Often, good listeners are capable of critically evaluating what is being said prior to fully understanding it and listening to what the client is really trying to communicate. Misunderstanding can occur at any time during the communication process. Effective communicators minimize potential misunderstandings and seek client clarification and participation in the communication process to ensure an effective exchange.

Clinicians must conduct a thorough subjective examination that is free of bias. This will lead to an effective secondary physical evaluation that will aid in the development of a hypothesis relating to the client's presentation and the selection of appropriate interventions for providing optimal client outcomes. Communication skills, which involve verbal and nonverbal behaviors, can be taught. Effectiveness in communication can be improved through training. The use of quality communication skills accomplishes the following:

- Aids in more accurately identifying and understanding each client's chief complaint
- Leads to increased client satisfaction with care
- Improves treatment adherence

QUALITIES OF AN EFFECTIVE INTERVIEW

Although the introduction sets the tone of the interview, it is often discounted. The clinician is responsible for orienting the client to the process of the visit. This orientation helps the client set realistic expectations for the visit. An example of an appropriate clinician–client introduction is the following:

"Good morning, my name is _____ and I am going to be your physical therapist. Today we will begin with a discussion of what brings you into the clinic, followed by a physical examination, then we will discuss the findings, and I will leave time for any questions."

Certain components of an interview are paramount for making the client feel comfortable and allowing them to appreciate that this communication process is focused on them. The essential components for effective client–clinician communication are detailed in the following sections.

Setting the Environment

A client-friendly environment that is clean, comfortable, and nonthreatening may help clients to share important personal and private information during the visit. It is the clinician's responsibility to provide an atmosphere that allows for a conducive and productive visit. Therefore, the visit should be performed in an area with minimal noise or distractions and appropriate lighting. The area must be adequately stocked with any items that may be needed.

Open-Ended Questions vs. Closed-Ended Questions

Asking questions is a basic way to gather information during the visit. Clinicians should begin the communication process with the client with an open-ended question and continue using them throughout the interview. Open-ended questions are typically perceived as less threatening, and they allow clients to independently articulate their thoughts and feelings. Here are some examples of open-ended questions:

"What brings you to physical therapy?"

"What can I help you with?"

"I understand that you are experiencing some pain or stiffness. Can you fill me in more?"

"I see from the intake form that you wrote down that your chief complaint is _____. Tell me more about that."

Although the use of open-ended questions can be time consuming and result in gathering unnecessary information compared to closed-ended questions, closed-ended questions fail to gather specific details critical to clinical decision-making[49] because they typically result in inadequate one-word and incomplete replies that impede the discussion.

Eye Contact

Making and maintaining moderate to high levels of eye contact with clients lets them know that the clinician is concentrating on the content of the discussion. Maintenance of eye contact may encourage clients to talk about concerns that they may otherwise keep concealed. Not maintaining eye contact can indicate disinterest, which can keep clients from disclosing additional relevant information.[33]

Note Taking

During clinical visits, clinicians may find it helpful to take notes. Note taking is essential for reflection, but it should not disrupt the interview process. The clinician should stay attentive throughout the interaction. With the implementation of electronic medical records, many clinicians attempt to perform point-of-care charting, which can lead to lack of attentiveness from clinicians. This can make clients feel as if they are not the centerpieces of the visit, which may lead to an ineffective visit.

Facilitation

A facilitative comment by the clinician demonstrates active listening. Active listening is effective in obtaining important clinical information, and it demonstrates that the clinician cares. Here are some examples of active listening responses:

"Can you expand more on that?"

"What do you mean by that statement?"

"So what I hear you saying is . . . ."

"How long has this been going on?"

"How are things going?"

"Uh huh . . . uh huh," "Oh," "All right," "Okay," "I see," or "Hmm . . . ."

Active listening responses appear to serve several functions, including the following:

- Indicate the clinician is attending
- Give the client permission to continue
- Keep the client focused on the story and their chief complaint

There is a difference between listening and passive hearing. Active listening is a communication technique that allows the clinician to concentrate on and comprehend what the client is communicating. Facilitation can be verbal and nonverbal. Staying silent is difficult for many clinicians during the interview process; many interrupt clients at inappropriate times, thus missing important clues and possibly silencing the client and subsequently limiting the information provided.[50]

Ineffective physicians are likely to interrupt the client after only one or two sentences were communicated. Typically, sufficient listening required less than 30 seconds. Often the first minutes were used in rapid dialogue about lab or test results.[12]

Summarizing, Clarifying, and Reflecting

At the completion of the subjective examination it can be helpful to summarize what has been learned during the interaction since it demonstrates to clients that they have been heard. This summary helps to assure that the clinician has developed the correct understanding of the client's views of their problem by pulling together major ideas, facts, and feelings. This also allows the client to incorporate any missed information and clarify where there was any misunderstanding on behalf of the clinician. It gives the clinician an additional opportunity to elicit the client's priorities.

Empathy

Clinicians must remain open minded and must acquire the ability to see things from each client's perspective. This will allow them to understand the problem from the client's perspective and can aid in validating the client's chief complaint. Clinicians must avoid, at all costs, jumping to conclusions and using personal prejudice. All attempts should be made to put the client at ease. As health care clinicians, we must treat clients with empathy and integrity in order to teach, challenge them to promote change in their lives, and aid in their recovery. Here are some ways you can implement empathy within a clinical visit:

- Validate: "I can see how you might think or feel that way."
- Challenge: "Have you thought about this angle or perspective?"
- Promote: "Well, will you try this for me and see what happens?"

STANDARD CLIENT INTERVIEW

During the interview it is a good idea to use a standard form to complete or at least have a standard format of questioning regarding the client's personal and family history. A form or checklist ensures that the clinician utilizes a consistent and thorough approach to cover this information. Prior to the initiation of the interview clients will typically complete a consent to treat form, a pain diagram (figure 5.1), an appropriate outcome measures form, or a medical questionnaire. These forms can aid the clinician during the interview process and subsequent physical examination.

Name: _____ Date: _____

Pain Drawing

Using the symbols given below, mark the area on your body where you feel the described sensations. Include all affected areas.

Aching	Numbness	Pins and Needles	Burning	Stabbing	Other
ΔΔΔ	= = = =	O O O O	X X X X	/ / / /	. . . .

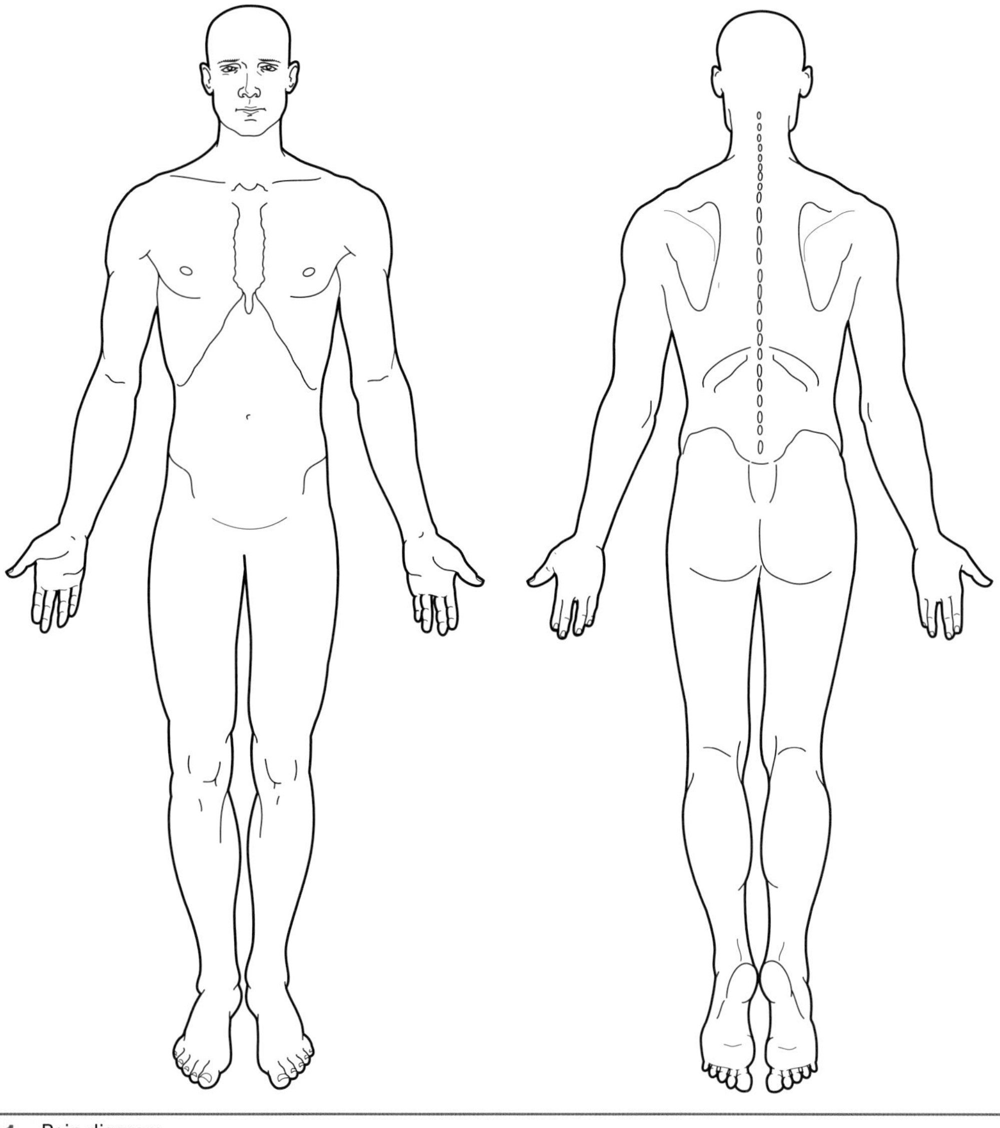

Figure 5.1 Pain diagram.

The client interview must be organized and conducted in a complete and thoughtful manner. The information sought in the interview includes several components (see table 5.1 and chapter 6), and may be ascertained in various sequences, but it must be well planned and organized. The history is principally for triage, during which red flags should be identified and yellow flags assessed.[1] The physical examination is used to confirm suspicions from the history.[1]

Physical Therapy Subjective Interview Process

As previously stated, the client interview is typically the first visit the clinician has with the client. This component of the examination can provide the clinician with a significant amount of information relevant to the probability of the client's presenting diagnosis. Therefore, the objectives of the client

TABLE 5.1 Information to Obtain During a Standard Client Interview

General demographics	Physiological and biographical data: age, gender, height, weight, hand dominance, race or ethnicity, language, education
Social history	Hobbies, social interactions and activities, family or caregiver resources and support, cultural beliefs and values
Employment/school/play	Current and prior employment/school/play, leisure activities, community activities
Living environment	Living environment barriers, devices, equipment
General health status	Perceived and reported function, psychological function, family report
Health habits	Behavioral health risks (e.g., smoking, alcohol abuse), level of physical fitness
Family history	Familial health risks
Medical/surgical history	Involving various systems of the body, involving the area to be treated, related to the area to be treated
Chief complaint about current condition	Reason for being seen, concerns, symptom onset, mechanism of injury, pain location, what aggravates pain, what alleviates pain, previous treatment, previous occurrences
Functional status/activity level	Current and prior status/activity level for activities of daily living (ADLs), work activity, leisure activity
Growth and development	Developmental history, hand dominance
Medications	Medications for current condition, other medications they are taking and the reason they are taking them, possible medication interactions and side effects relevant to the reason they are being seen
Other clinical tests	Laboratory, diagnostic imaging, and other diagnostic tests, review of all available medical records
Review of systems	Gastrointestinal system Urogenital system Cardiovascular system Pulmonary system Musculoskeletal system Neurological system Integumentary system Psychosocial factors

interview primarily include, but are not limited to, the following:

- Identification of red flags
- Classifying the client for treatment or directing clients to the proper health care provider, thereby minimizing and preventing mortality and morbidity
- Hypothesis generation

To perform an effective client interview, clinicians should do the following:

1. Actively listen to each client.
2. Assess verbal and nonverbal communication.
   - Assess tone and delivery of information.
   - Observe nonverbal body language and notice any inconsistencies between verbal and nonverbal messages.
   - Notice silence, touch, hand gestures, posture, eye contact, facial expression, and both active and passive listening.
3. Listen for red flags (for more information, refer to chapter 6).
4. Take the client history.

The client history should be taken in an orderly and systematic sequence. Keep in mind that this process will vary from client to client and visit to visit. Here is how to take a client history.

1. Determine the client's age and gender.

Determining the client's age and gender can assist in assessing for age-related health concerns. For example, growth disorders such as Legg-Perthes and Scheuermann's disease are seen in adolescents and teenagers,[51] whereas degenerative conditions such as osteoarthritis and osteoporosis are more often visited on an older population. Gender can also provide some indication as to predisposition. Typically a combination of gender and age will inform the clinician to particular predispositions. For example, a 60-year-old woman is more likely to have osteoporosis due to hormonal deficiencies from menopause than a 20-year-old woman.

2. Determine the client's activity level.

For each client it is important to ascertain their current and prior employment, leisure activities, and community activities, and if they are a student. This will assist in determining the physicality of their daily activities, thus providing information

about the client's chief complaint that is useful for prognostication purposes. Here are two examples:

- Laborer: may be stronger and less likely to suffer from muscle strain, or may be performing repetitive activities resulting in a muscle strain or injury
- Sedentary individual (i.e., weekend warrior, student, or desk worker): may strain muscles, or may be more susceptible to habitual postural-related strains

3. Determine the mechanism of injury.

Was there any inciting trauma or repetitive activity that led to their chief complaint? Determining the mechanism of injury will assist in determining the cause of the client's symptoms and will elicit a detailed explanation by the client in their own words. It will also allow the clinician to develop an understanding of the longevity of the chief complaint.

Acute

- Symptoms may include sudden and severe pain, swelling, inability to weight bear, tenderness to palpation, difficulty moving joint through full range of motion, weakness, or visible defect in soft tissue or bone.
- Acute condition: usually present for 1 to 10 days.
- It is improper to assume that all acute disorders are irritable.

Subacute/Chronic

- Symptoms may include pain during activity or rest, swelling, tenderness to palpation, difficulty moving joint through full range of motion, or weakness.
- Subacute condition: 10 days to 7 weeks.
- Chronic condition: longer than 7 weeks.
- It is improper to assume that all chronic disorders are nonirritable.

4. Determine the concordant sign or symptom.

This allows the client to describe their chief complaint and aides the clinician in determining the activity or movement associated with the pain.[2, 52] The clinician should try to determine the activities, postures, and positions that initiate concordant symptoms.

5. Determine the nature of the condition.

This is an important aspect that will reveal the severity, irritability, and stage of the client's chief complaint.[2] Determination of the nature of the condition will dictate the aggressiveness of the clinician during the physical examination and subsequent treatment.

Severity is the identification and description by the client of how their problem has affected their daily functioning.

Irritability is the stability of the condition, thus describing how quickly a stable condition degrades to a painful condition. It also allows the clinician insight on whether the pain is constant, periodic, episodic, or occasional, and whether the client is bothered at that very moment. Clients are typically classified as either irritable or nonirritable.

Irritable

- Clients presenting with but not limited to the following:

  Acute trauma/injury

  Fractures

  Acute arthritis

  Acute aggravation of an existing musculo-skeletal condition

- Subjective clues

  Interrupted sleep

  High doses and usage of medications

  Decreased activity levels

  Activity avoidance

- Clinicians should not assume that acute disorders are always irritable.

Nonirritable

- Clients presenting with but not limited to the following:

  Chronic arthritis

  Chronic musculoskeletal conditions that are not typically notably aggravated with daily activities

  Hypomobility status post immobilization due to injury, surgery, or fracture

- Subjective clues

  Report of stiffness

  Intermittent medication use

  Variable activity levels

  Intermittent periods of activity avoidance

Stage is a description of how the client's symptoms or impairments have progressed over time. Thus, have the symptoms become worse, gotten better, or remained the same? Generally, a decrease in symptoms means the condition is improving, whereas an increase or unchanged symptoms can raise concerns.

6. Determine the behavior of the symptoms.

Determining the behavior of the symptoms will aid the clinician in understanding how the symptoms change with time, movement, and activity. The behavior of the symptoms is a snapshot of how the client's chief complaint changes. Is the pain associated with rest? Activity? Certain static postures? Visceral function? Time of day?

- Pain with movement that decreases at rest often indicates a musculoskeletal problem.
- Morning pain that decreases with movement often indicates chronic inflammation and edema, such as with osteoarthritis.[53]
- Pain or aching as the day progresses often indicates increased congestion of a joint.
- Pain at rest and pain at the beginning of movement often implies acute inflammation.
- Pain that is present at rest and during activity may indicate bone pain, or it may be systemic in nature.
- Intractable pain at night may indicate serious pathology.
- Peripheral nerve pain is often reported to increase at night.
- Pain or cramping with prolonged walking that is relieved when seated may indicate lumbar stenosis or vascular issues.[54]
- Facet pain is often relieved by sitting or forward flexion.[55, 56]

7. Determine the location of the symptoms that bother the client.

The clinician should have the client point to the affected area. This allows them to attempt to specify the area of symptoms. In certain instances, if the location of symptoms has changed, it may be useful to have the client point to the site of origin. Also, symptoms may be localized to one area, indicating a specific tissue or joint, for example, the Fortin finger test for sacroiliac joint pain.[57] They may be dispersed about a general area, which may indicate a more severe condition or referral of symptoms.

8. Determine where the pain or symptoms were when the client first had the complaint.

The client will provide specific information about the location of the pain. Some clients will provide a vague description of the pain, while others may be overly descriptive. As clinicians, it is important to discover whether the following have occurred:

- The pain has moved or remained the same.
- There are trigger points, which can give rise to referral pain.
- The pain site or region broadens or moves more distal as lesion worsens, often referred to as *peripheralization*.
- The pain site becomes smaller or more localized as it improves, often referred to as *centralization*.

9. Determine if the client has had the same chief complaint before.

Past treatments and results of these treatments can be helpful with management of the client's chief complaint. This information may also indicate to the clinician which treatments to utilize as well as which to avoid. Also, knowing how long it took to recover and how the current problem is similar or different can provide valuable insight for prognosis of recovery.

10. Determine if the client has exhibited or described fainting, dizziness, and vertigo.

Vertigo and dizziness refer to swaying and spinning sensations. These symptoms can indicate benign conditions or may suggest severe neurological involvement. Therefore, further questioning must occur.

11. Determine if the client has experienced any life or economic stresses.

Life or economic stresses may be affecting the client's condition, recovery, prognosis, and so on. These could include, but are not limited to, the following:

- Divorce
- Marital problems
- Financial problems
- Job insecurity

12. Review and discuss the client's past and present medical history.

Awareness of the client's past medical history provides insight to the following:

- Chronic or serious systemic illnesses that may influence the course of pathology or treatments and necessitate referral to the appropriate medical provider
- Familial history that may be related to the chief complaint, such as tumors, arthritis, heart disease, diabetes, and allergies
- Medications the client takes regularly or has been receiving for treatment of their chief complaint. Clients receiving high doses of

Critical Clinical Pearls

Perform the history in an orderly and systematic sequence, but keep in mind that this process will be different for each client and visit. An effective client interview allows the clinician to do the following:

- Identify red flags that require a referral to an appropriate health care provider, thereby minimizing and preventing mortality and morbidity
- Develop a hypothesis and classify the client for treatment
- Determine the mechanism of injury, concordant sign, nature of the condition, and behavior of the symptoms

steroids for long durations are at increased risk of weakening of soft tissues and osteoporosis. Also, it is important for clinicians to be aware of medications that were taken prior to therapy because some symptoms may be masked due to the medications.

- Diagnostic testing the client has undergone (e.g., diagnostic imaging, blood work, electromyography, nerve conduction studies, electrocardiogram)
- Past and pertinent surgical history

Red Flag Considerations During the Interview Process

A careful subjective examination can aid in uncovering red flags and can provide the examiner with vital information regarding the client's problems. Red flags include the following:[58]

- History of cancer
- Pulsatile abdominal mass
- History of unexplained weight loss
- History of unremitting night pain
- History of fever or chills
- Prolonged corticosteroid use
- Progressive neurologic deficit
- Pathologic changes in bowel and bladder function

Physical therapists should screen for comorbidities, including those considered severe, regardless of the client's anatomical region of symptoms.[59] Signs and symptoms found in the client history and clinical examination may tie a disorder to a serious pathology.[58] Sizer and colleagues recommended categorizing red flags based on the nature and severity of the client's presentation.[58] Furthermore, Grieve outlined three mandatory questions for ruling out red flags for clients presenting with cervical spine pain:[60]

- Any dizziness (vertigo), blackouts, or drop attacks?
- Any history of rheumatoid arthritis (RA) or other inflammatory arthritis, or treatment by systemic steroid?
- Any neurologic symptoms in the arms and legs?

Additional information regarding red flags is presented in chapter 6.

As stated previously, the subjective examination can provide information on disabilities, symptoms, symptom behavior, irritability, and exacerbating, provoking, and relieving factors. The history will also provide information regarding past treatments, and the results of these treatments can provide information about the management of the client and about what treatments may need to be avoided. Additionally, the history will allow the clinician to understand the client's personality and attitude toward their problems and may divulge the client's likelihood to comply with the clinician's instructions.

Access to client demographic and health history prior to the start of the subjective examination is helpful in improving the effectiveness and proficiency of the client interview. In most client settings, a medical record including physician notes and a completed self-patient health history report form can be accessed and viewed before the interview. However, clients are often referred to physical therapy from a variety of sources, and they often present with little diagnostic information. Furthermore, clients may be referred with a nonmedical diagnosis, or in certain parts of the United States (direct access states), they may present without a medical evaluation. If this information is not readily available, contacting the referring physician may be beneficial. If there is limited access to such information due to the practice setting or due to the client taking advantage of direct access, clinician–client interview and communication skills become increasingly more vital.

CLIENT INTERVIEWS RELATIVE TO MUSCULOSKELETAL PAIN

Pain is a complex, multidimensional, and extremely individualized experience.[61, 62] Traditional understandings of pain were that clients' reports of pain were the direct result of physical injury or trauma. Subjective reporting of pain includes characteristics listed in the following sidebar. Current knowledge of pain has uncovered that physical pathology does not always dictate client's pain experiences. Conversely, many clients experience pain with no physical pathology. For example MRI scans routinely exhibit pathology in asymptomatic people,[63, 64] and clients with complaints of chronic low back

Subjective Reporting of Pain

- Onset
  - Traumatic or nontraumatic
  - Immediate or delayed
  - Sudden or insidious
- Location
  - Local or extensive
- Type or quality of pain exhibited
  - Nerve pain: sharp, bright burning, runs in the distribution of that nerve; radiation of pain commonly reported
  - Bone pain: deep, boring, and very localized; limited radiation
  - Vascular pain: diffuse, aching, and poorly localized; may be referred to other areas of the body

- Muscular, ligamentous, bursal pain: usually hard to localize, often indistinguishable, dull, aching, often aggravated by injury, can be referred to other areas
- Severity
  - Pain diagram (figure 5.1)
  - Visual Analogue Scale (figure 5.2)
  - Numeric Pain Rating Scale (figure 5.3)
- Irritability
- Aggravating or alleviating factors
- Constant, continuous, or intermittent

pain can often present with no objective indicators of pathology.[65] Therefore, there must be other factors that contribute to clients' pain perceptions. Contemporary research has demonstrated that cognitive, behavioral, psychological, and social factors play a role in clients' pain perceptions.[66, 67] Increased understanding and awareness will identify clients who require specific pain education and will allow the clinician to provide appropriate reinforcement to clients during the visit in regards to their pain.

Complicating things further is that pain measures are subjective in nature, and the manifestations of

pain vary from client to client and possibly from visit to visit. Difficulty in understanding pain arises due to the fact that there are currently no objective measures for determining the presence and extent of each client's pain. Therefore, the only way we know about our client's pain experience is by how they communicate verbally and nonverbally. Typically clinicians use pain diagrams (see figure 5.1), visual analogue scales (figure 5.2), and numeric pain rating scales (figure 5.3) to subjectively ascertain clients' pain levels. Verbal pain behaviors may include sighing, moaning, groaning, gasping, crying,

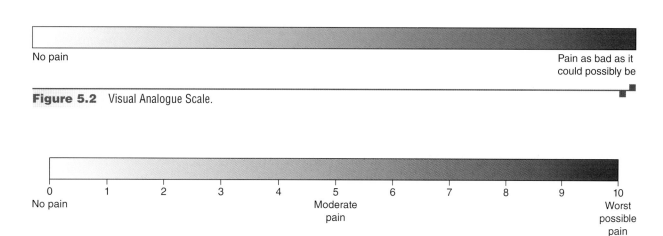

Figure 5.2 Visual Analogue Scale.

Figure 5.3 Numeric Pain Rating Scale.

cursing, whimpering, and using words expressing discomfort (e.g., "ouch," "that hurts") or words of protest (e.g., "stop," "that's enough," "no more"). Nonverbal pain behaviors may consist of facial responses, such as a grimace, frown, wince, eyes closed, eyes wide open with eyebrows raised, looking away in the opposite direction of pain, grin or smile, mouth wide open, or clenched teeth, and body movement, such as bracing of the affected area during movement or rest, limping, restlessness, constant or intermittent shifting of position, massaging the affected area, pacing, withdrawing, clenched fists, rigidity, shaking, or repetitive movement. Assessment of pain behaviors must occur throughout the clinical visit, during movement, and with the client at rest.

Musculoskeletal pain affects between 13.5% and 47% of the general population. Risk factors for musculoskeletal pain include age, gender, smoking, low education, low physical activity, poor social interaction, low family income, depression, anxiety, and sleep disorders, as well as performing manual work and being a recent immigrant, non-Caucasian, and widowed, separated, or divorced.[68]

Musculoskeletal conditions are prevalent, and their influence is extensive. These conditions are a diverse group of disorders with regard to pathophysiology, but they are linked anatomically and by their association with pain and impaired physical function. They encompass a spectrum of conditions, including inflammatory diseases such as rheumatoid arthritis or gout, age-related conditions such as osteoporosis and osteoarthritis, common conditions of unclear etiology such as back pain and fibromyalgia, and those related to activity or injuries such as occupational musculoskeletal disorders, sports injuries, or the consequences of falls and major trauma.[69]

Musculoskeletal conditions are the most common cause of severe long-term pain and physical disability, affecting hundreds of millions of people around the world. They significantly affect the psychosocial status of affected people as well as their families and careers. At any one time, 30% of American adults are affected by joint pain, swelling, or limitation of movement.[70] The prevalence of many of these conditions increases markedly with age, and many are affected by lifestyle factors, such as obesity and lack of physical activity. The increasing number of older people and the changes in lifestyle throughout the world mean that the burden on people and society will increase dramatically.[71] Rheumatoid arthritis,

osteoarthritis, and low back pain are important causes of disability-adjusted life years in both the developed and developing world.[72]

The client interview is vital for developing an understanding of our client's pain. The clinician should attempt to identify the clients' idiosyncratic beliefs, address those beliefs that are inaccurate and potentially maladaptive, and match treatments to clients' biomedical and psychosocial differences.[73]

OUTCOME MEASUREMENTS

Outcome or self-report measures are common methods of having the client assess their pain and function. These measures involve careful evaluation of instrument reliability, responsiveness, and validity. Much work has been dedicated toward the development of these tools. Dedicated self-report functional measures have been created for nearly all body regions or conditions. These measures can be region specific (hip joint), condition specific (osteoarthritis), dimension specific (pain), generic (health profile), or individualized to the client.[74]

Indeed, self-report measures are valuable in defining the client's perspective of their change, but they have been shown to differ substantially from physical performance measures that involve quantification of output, and they are dramatically influenced by changes in pain.[75-82] A reduction in pain after total joint arthroplasty has been associated with clients' self-reported improvements in their functional ability, even though their time to complete performance tasks had doubled.[81] In other words, these clients' perception of their functional ability was inflated in instances of decreased pain.

The relationship between self-reports of pain level and function has frequently been investigated in clients with low back pain (LBP), demonstrating low to moderate levels of association between self-report measures of LBP and physical performance measures (PPMs).[77, 83] Clients systematically and significantly overestimate LBP at preferred and fastest speeds of movement with sit-to-stand tasks. There was also a trend toward underestimating expected pain at slow speeds of movement with the sit-to-stand tasks. An additional concern of self-report measures is that these measures do not always differentiate between whether a specific task is not done or can't be done, and why.[84] Clearly, self-report measures are important, but they should be utilized cautiously. They serve as only one component of the assessment of function.

One commonly used supplemental scale to generic and condition-specific measures is the Patient-Specific Functional Scale (PSFS).[85] The PSFS asks the client to list three activities that are difficult for them to perform as a result of their current condition. The client rates each of these activities on a scale of 0 to 10, with 0 being unable to perform the activity and 10 being able to perform the activity as well as they could prior to the onset of their symptoms.[86] The final PSFS score is the average of the three activity scores. The intraclass correlation coefficient (ICC) test–retest reliability is generally good across multiple pathological conditions.

A commonly used measure for gauging progress in treatment is the Global Rating of Change (GROC) Scale. This is an assessment of the client's self-perceived progress during the course of their treatment. The GROC scale asks the client to rate their progress from a previous point in their care to their current condition. The most frequently used version is a 15-point scale that has points ranging from −7 (a great deal worse) to a +7 (a great deal better). A more recent version, an 11-point scale with a corresponding minimally clinical important difference (MCID) of 2 points, has been suggested.[87]

OBSERVATION

Observation of the client is constant and can be used to gain information on visible defects, functional deficits, and abnormalities of alignment. The clinician should observe each aspect of function while in the presence of the client. Assessment and observation is an ongoing process that begins during the introduction in the waiting area and continues throughout the visit and through the completion of the visit. Generally, the observed deviation should be readily evident. Inspection consists of integumentary inspection, posture, and body symmetry. Skin inspection can provide clues on past and current injuries and postural assessment can lead to clues that contribute to the chief complaint. The clinician must keep in mind that postural asymmetry alone does not necessarily conclude the presence of impairment. A more detailed discussion of what to look for in each body region is discussed in the region-specific chapter sections. A general outline of considerations during the client interview and observation component of the clinical visit is presented in the following sidebar.

Considerations for the Client Interview

1. Assess general body structures
   - Integumentary inspection
     - Atrophy or hypertrophy
     - Edema or effusion
     - Surgical scars: Are there any scars to indicate recent injury or history of injury?
     - Bruising
     - Signs of infection
        A. General symptoms of infection include fatigue, loss of appetite, weight loss, fevers, night sweats, chills, ache, and pains.
        B. Symptoms of wound infection include fever; warm, red, painful, or swollen wound; blood or pus coming from the wound; or a foul odor coming from the wound.
     - Signs of trauma
        A. Ecchymosis
        B. Abrasions
        C. Contusions

(continued)

- Postures: Client postures should be assessed in numerous positions such as sitting, standing, and lying down (refer to chapter 14 for additional detail on posture).
- Somatotype
  - Mesomorph
  - Ectomorph
  - Endomorph
- Fitness level

2. Congenital anomalies
3. Assessment of body alignment
   - Spine
   - Shoulders (scapula, clavicle)
   - Hip
   - Knee
   - Patella
   - Feet
4. Check for asymmetrical stance.
   - Is the client weight bearing symmetrically through bilateral lower extremities? Or is there a weight shift in one direction or a combination of directions?
   - Unloading of an extremity is common due to pain or injury.
5. Any obvious deformity?
6. Are bony contours normal and symmetric?
7. Are soft-tissue contours normal and symmetrical?
8. Are limbs positioned equally and symmetrically?
9. Are color and texture of skin normal?
   - Peripheral nerve lesions can cause loss of skin elasticity, shiny skin, hair loss, skin breakdown, and slow repair of injured skin.
   - Ischemic changes from circulatory problems can cause white, brittle skin, hair loss, and abnormal nails on hands or feet.
10. Is there crepitus, snapping, or abnormal sound in the joints? Is pain present with these sounds?
11. Any heat, swelling, or redness in area being observed?
    - Signs of active inflammatory process or possible infection
12. Psychosocial observations
    - What attitude does the client have toward their condition?
    - Is the client willing to move?
13. Gait
    - Observation of each individual client's gait cycle will begin as clients walk into the clinic and continue during the walk to the treatment room. Observation will reveal whether the client is using an assistive device and, if so, what type of device. Numerous components of gait will be affected by leg length, height, age, and sex. For example, elderly clients may demonstrate decreased cadence, shorter stride and step lengths, longer durations of double-limb support periods, smaller swing-to-support ratios, and a lowered center of gravity from a flexed position. Refer to chapter 13 for a specific discussion of gait. A general assessment of gait will include observation of the following:

- Time variables
  - A. Stance time
  - B. Single-limb time
  - C. Double-limb support time
  - D. Swing time
  - E. Stride time
  - F. Step time
  - G. Cadence
  - H. Speed

- Distance variables
  - A. Stride length
  - B. Step length
  - C. Width of walking base
  - D. Degree of toe out
- Weight acceptance
- Reciprocal arm swing

- Types of observable pathologic gait
  - Antalgic
  - Vaulting
  - Lateral limp
  - Ataxia
  - Trendelenburg
  - High stepping

- Foot drop
- Gluteus medius gait
- Gluteus maximus gait

CLINICAL REASONING

Clinicians routinely visit client presentations with signs and symptoms that do not clearly delineate the specific source of the client's dysfunction. These render clinical reasoning and differential diagnosis as critical decision-making tools. Clinical reasoning provides a bridge between practice and knowledge, and clinically effective care is evidence based and client centered. Clinical evidence should be used to inform clinical expertise, but should not replace it. Expertise aids clinicians in deciding whether the evidence applies to each individual client's situation and, if it does, how it should be used in directing the clinical decision. Evidence-based medicine allows clinicians to apply and present the most efficient interventions for each client.

According to Mattingly and colleagues, a definitive definition of clinical reasoning is challenging because "there is no one-sentence definition that captures the subtlety of how therapists think in the midst of practice."[88] Clinical reasoning cannot be reduced to a definitive definition. However, a proficient definition has been proposed by Jones and colleagues: Clinical reasoning is "the process in which the clinician, interacting with significant others

(patient, caregivers, health care team members), structures meaning, goals, and health management strategies based on clinical data, patient choices, and professional judgment and knowledge."[89]

Currently, there are many proposed models of clinical reasoning. Clinical decision-making models are "routinely viewed along a spectrum; with an assumption of being right on one end and wrong on the other."[90] Modern medical clinical decision-making models explore each client's biological, psychological, and social factors,[91-93] including but not limited to medical comorbidities, illness beliefs, coping strategies, emotional reactions, fear or depression, employment, and economic concerns. This book focuses on diagnostic reasoning, specifically looking at hypothetical deductive decision-making, heuristic decision-making, and a mixed model.

Importance of Clinical Reasoning

The examination process provides the data used in the clinical reasoning process. During this clinical reasoning process, the clinician develops (in a continuous process) multiple competing diagnostic hypotheses. Data that are acquired during the examination process are then used to support or refute the various hypotheses. This process of hypothesis testing guides the format and content of the ongoing examination process until the clinician decides that sufficient information has been obtained to make a diagnostic or management decision.[94]

Decisions will vary from situation to situation and client to client. Many clinicians have difficulty finding the right balance between factors that can affect and influence their decisions.[95, 96] Clinicians must provide current best evidence to clients in an unbiased manner so that the clients can make independent and informed choices on the direction of their treatment. They must remember that "evidence does not make decisions, people do."[95]

Research-enhanced clinical reasoning[95] consists of three interrelated components: clinical and physical circumstances, best research evidence, and client's preferences and actions. Each component must be taken into equal consideration during the reasoning process to allow for an efficacious client visit. Consideration of each component will lead to finding the right treatment for the client, providing it at the right time, and addressing the specific needs and concerns of each particular client.

Clinical reasoning is vital for many reasons, which include but are not limited to the traits in figure 5.4. Each of these traits is a separate and comprehensive component of the clinical reasoning process. Early clinical reasoning models focused on the processes doctors used to arrive at a medical diagnosis.[97, 98] The theories developed within the context of the biomedical model of health were highly focused on a diagnosis and on the implication of physical tissue or impairment as the source of problem. These models limited the client's interaction in the clinical decision-making process. Over the years, a shift toward medicine on the body as a whole and a client-centered process of collaboration has occurred.[99, 100] Influenced by the biopsychosocial model of health, the shift in the clinical reasoning process has transitioned from a procedure occurring only in the clinician's head to one that includes communication between the clinician and client.[92, 93] Clients' preferences and actions can be found within the framework of current clinical reasoning models, and each client must be considered as a whole and not solely from a biomedical standpoint. Clients are informed consumers who expect to participate in the decision-making process. The age of paternalistic clinical practice has passed.

Routinely, clinicians rely on diagnostic clinical reasoning, which is dependent on two processes: the analytic method (hypothetico-deductive reasoning) and the nonanalytic method (pattern recognition). Novice clinicians typically use a hypothetico-deductive reasoning process, compared to more experienced clinicians, who tend to use a combination. Ultimately, the integration of both reasoning processes allows for efficient and accurate clinical decision-making.[101] Most true models are mixed, which eliminates the weaknesses of single models.

Hypothetico-deductive reasoning requires the development of a hypothesis during the clinical evaluation and an acceptance or rejection of the hypothesis during the clinical examination. It is considered a bottom-up approach since it goes from general to specific. Hypothetico-deductive reasoning is very detailed, easy for novice clinicians, and repeatable. But it is slow and arduous, and

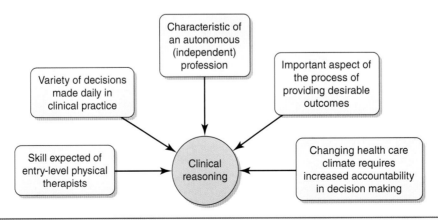

Figure 5.4 Important traits of diagnostic clinical reasoning.

it assumes each assessment is equally beneficial. However, not all diagnoses are definable, most clinical tests are poor, and diagnosis does not dictate treatment. Hypothetico-deductive reasoning does allow for a pathognomonic diagnosis, an on-the-spot decision based on a sign or symptom that is extremely characteristic of a disease.[90]

Heuristic clinical reasoning, or pattern recognition, is considered a top-down approach in which clinicians lump useful findings into coherent groups. It is fast, and it allows experience to assist in decision making, but is also mistake prone and riddled with bias. Pattern recognition should not be interpreted as higher levels of cognition but as a necessary building block in the development of each clinician's clinical reasoning skills.

Research demonstrates that expert clinicians frequently use pattern recognition for clients who present with common dysfunctions and hypothetico-deductive reasoning for complex dysfunctions. Development of expert clinical reasoning is an ongoing process that involves working interpretations and repeated hypothesis generation. Deletion and refinement of clinician-generated interpretations and hypotheses lead to the development of a network of concepts that allows clinicians to develop an understanding of each client's chief complaint.[102, 103]

Although clinicians at all levels of experience use hypothetico-deductive methods of reasoning, experts appear to possess a superior organization of knowledge. Experts often reach a diagnosis based on pure pattern recognition of clinical patterns. With an atypical problem, however, the expert, like the novice, appears to rely more on hypothetico-deductive clinical reasoning. Five categories of hypotheses are proposed for physical therapists using a hypothetico-deductive method of clinical reasoning: (1) source of the symptoms or dysfunction, (2) contributing factors, (3) precautions and contraindications to physical examination and treatment, (4) management, and (5) prognosis.[94]

On a daily basis, clinicians will visit client presentations that vary from well defined to multifactorial and will subsequently treat these clients with simple or complex solutions. During client interaction, components of the clinical examination include (but are not limited to) observation, subjective history, outcome measures, objective examination, and special testing. Each assessment has its own ability to alter the probability of a particular diagnosis.

Expertise in Physical Therapy

Several studies have investigated variables distinguishing master clinicians from novice clinicians. Some traits found in expert orthopedic clinicians include the following:[35]

- Have well-organized knowledge of clinical patterns
- Use metacognition
- Consider the client's understanding, beliefs, and feelings
- Engage in reflection (reflection in action, reflection about action)
- Help shape a client in developing and evolving understanding of problems
- Have the ability to generate a prognosis
- Have the ability to control the environment (ability to focus on the client in a busy environment and to use time efficiently)
- Focus on verbal and nonverbal communication with the client
- Put equal importance on teaching and hands-on care
- Have confidence in predicting effective client outcomes based on knowledge of pathology and experience with healing

Contrary to the deeply engrained beliefs of today's society, research supports the notion that experts in every profession are made, not born. Traditionally, professional expertise has been based on years of experience. Findings by Resnik and Jensen challenge the basic assumption that years of experience are required in order to be classified as an expert.[104] Their research was guided by the grounded theory method, and they performed a retrospective analysis of data. Expertise was defined on the basis of collective client outcomes. Their results revealed that years of experience did not distinguish experts from novice therapists. They found that experts differed in academic and work experience, utilization of colleagues, use of reflection, view of primary role, and pattern of delegation to support staff. "Therapists classified as expert had a patient centered approach to care, characterized by collaborative clinical reasoning and promotion of patient empowerment."[104]

Current research demonstrates that the amount and quality of practice are key factors in the level of expertise people achieve.[105, 106] Specifically, deliberate practice is required. Deliberate practice is "practice that focuses on tasks beyond your current level of competence and comfort."[107] Ericsson and colleagues have discovered that the amount and quality of practice are key factors in the level of expertise people achieve. Deliberate practice entails specific, sustained efforts to do something you can't do well or do at all. Thus, working at what you can't do is what turns you into the expert you are trying to become.

Peak performance reached in the arts and sciences typically occurs in the third and fourth decades of life.[105, 106] Several studies report a consistent relationship between the quality and amount of deliberate practice required to achieve expertise.[108, 109] It is estimated that 10,000 hours of deliberate practice are required. While deliberate practice is fundamental for achieving expertise, mentors are also of vital necessity. They can assist in the following:

- Guide the clinician through deliberate practice
- Help the clinician to learn how to coach themselves
- Engage with metacognition and reflective reasoning
- Provide constructive, even painful, feedback
- Identify aspects of the clinician's performance that will need to be improved at their next skill level

During a clinician's professional career, there may be many pitfalls along the way that can deter the development of expertise:

- Automaticity; plateauing
- Being pushed too fast or too hard by mentors
- Minimal to no practice of history taking, communication, and examination skills

- Inappropriate feedback or lack of meaningful feedback
- Avoidance of engagement in purposeful reflective thinking

Learning From Clinical Reasoning

Learning is the ultimate outcome goal of collaborative clinical reasoning for the clinician and client. To facilitate learning from clinical experiences, reflection must be purposeful, planned, attended to and monitored; clinicians should also set time aside that allows involvement in the processes of metacognition (reflective thinking), discussion with peers and mentors, and incorporation of feedback.[110]

Refinement of clinical reasoning skills with purposeful reflection assists clinicians in identifying each client's clinical presentation and matching it with the most effective treatment[111] while avoiding diagnostic errors.[96] In some instances, it will be necessary for clinicians to view the client's clinical presentation from a different angle. Thus, reflection on action is a critical component during interactions with clients that aids clinicians in developing an accurate diagnosis, resulting in the most effective treatment approach. Collaborative clinical reasoning is fueled by each clinician's knowledge, which is routinely and continuously refined through practice. In order for clinicians to take appropriate action with clients, they must reflect on foundational knowledge, examining, observing, and identifying what is occurring.[94, 103]

Errors during heuristic clinical reasoning are common, and mistakes are often made. Clinicians' cognitive biases can create difficulties during the reasoning process. Developing an understanding and awareness of these biases is important so that

---

Critical Clinical Pearls

The development of clinical expertise requires the following:

- Deliberate practice of skills focusing on areas beyond the clinician's current level of competence
- Effective mentorship and guidance that allows for constructive feedback and assists in identifying aspects of performance that need improvement
- Engagement in purposeful metacognition and reflective reasoning

they can be avoided. Klein describes five noticeable biases that may occur:[112]

1. The representative heuristic: occurs when the clinician approximates something unknown to the closest known thing.

2. The availability heuristic: occurs when the clinician is more inclined to find what they are used to finding or looking for.

3. Confirmatory bias: occurs when the clinician tests until they find confirmation.

4. Illusory correlation: occurs when clinicians create relationships that don't really exist.

5. Overconfidence: overestimating one's knowledge base; considered the most destructive.

CONCLUSION

The client interview is the first time in the examination process where one-on-one interaction between the clinician and client occurs. History taking is reported to be the most important part of the clinical examination, since essential diagnostic information is often revealed. Eliciting a good history requires organizational and communication abilities. Effective communication incorporates verbal and nonverbal behavior. A skilled communicator will recognize a client's vital verbal and nonverbal communication. Clinicians must also develop an understanding of the numerous communication barriers that can lead to deficiencies in order to avoid them.

6

TRIAGE AND DIFFERENTIAL DIAGNOSIS

Michael P. Reiman, PT, DPT, OCS, SCS, ATC, FAAOMPT, CSCS

The color coding for suggestion of **good** and **ideal** diagnostic accuracy values reported in this chapter is without quality scoring (QUADAS), a very important aspect of determination of the clinical utility of such values. Therefore, it is suggested that the reader keep this in mind when interpreting such values.

At the triage and differential diagnosis stage of the examination process, the clinician has accessed any previous medical records (including diagnostic imaging) available to them, had the client fill out the appropriate outcome measures, interviewed the client, and taken a big picture assessment or observation of the client. This is the stage in the examination process where the clinician determines whether to continue with the examination process.

Triage is the process of determining the priority of clients' treatments based on the severity of their condition. The term *triage* originated in World War I when French doctors treated the battlefield wounded at the aid stations behind the front. In the original process, doctors divided wounded soldiers into categories to determine who needed immediate care, who was likely to die, and who was likely to live regardless of what care they received.[1]

The typical approach to screening for medical diagnosis is to review by body systems. This information, a client's signs and symptoms, and the client's medical history are primary components of medical screening and differential diagnosis as defined in the *Guide to Physical Therapist Practice*.[2] The clinician should be cognizant of identifying symptoms overlooked during presentation of the client's chief symptoms.

Screening for nonmusculoskeletal-related pain and dysfunction can often be a complex undertaking. The clinician should be cognizant of appropriate medical screening for each region of the body and should implement it as appropriate. The three key factors that create a need for screening are the following:[3]

1. Side effects of medications
2. Comorbidities
3. Visceral pain mechanisms

While the process of triage in the setting of the battlefield or emergency department has a purpose of ranking survivability and treatment options, the process of triage in the physical therapy examination environment is one of determining whether the clinician will treat the client, treat and then refer the client to another health care provider, or immediately refer the client to a more appropriate health care provider. Essentially this is a process of examining for red flags and signs of serious pathology, determining if the client is appropriate for physical therapy examination and intervention, and so on. If serious pathology has been ruled out and the client is deemed appropriate for physical therapy, the treating clinician will continue with the examination. In some instances, the clinician may deem it appropriate to perform the examination and possibly also begin with a treatment to more clearly elucidate the client's presentation and appropriateness for treatment.

If the medical diagnosis is delayed, or the treating clinician decides to treat and refer, then the correct diagnosis is eventually made when the following occur:[3]

- The client does not get better with physical therapy intervention
- The client gets better, then worse
- Other associated signs and symptoms eventually develop

Numerous examples have been documented of physical therapists using effective multifactorial screening strategies for referred and direct-access clients, leading to timely referrals to physicians. The therapist-initiated client referral to a physician led to subsequent diagnosis of a wide range of conditions and pathological processes.[4]

To assist the clinician in determining appropriateness of therapeutic examination and subsequent intervention, this chapter presents the current evidence on diagnostic accuracy of the various suggested tests and measures. Additionally, this chapter introduces the concept of classifying clients in treatment-based classification (TBC) according to their clinical examination findings. The strengths and weaknesses of the TBC are also addressed.

TRIAGE SCREENING FOR RED AND YELLOW FLAGS

The term *red flags* describes signs and symptoms found in the client history and clinical examination that may tie a disorder to a serious pathology.[5] The term *yellow flags* denotes adverse prognostic indicators. Other colors of flags are also used in triage screening (table 6.1), but this text focuses only on red and yellow flags due to the complexity of discussion required for the other flags.

Red flags denote symptoms or physical findings suggestive of a potentially serious cause for a client's symptoms. They indicate the need for prompt and thorough evaluation on the part of the treating clinician. Additionally, a red flag requires communication with another health care provider, typically a physician. During examination of each client, clinicians should account for red flags that are regional to the area being investigated as well as assess the client as a whole. Commonly described red flags include the following: [3, 5-7]

- Changes in bowel or bladder function
- Changes in muscle tone or range of motion
- Changes in skin or skin lesions

TABLE 6.1 Summary of Flag Color

Flag color	Meaning
Red flag	Serious pathology
Yellow flag	Adverse prognostic indicators (e.g., beliefs, emotional responses, pain behavior)
Blue flags	Perceptions about the relationship between work and health (e.g., feelings of unsupportive work environment)
Black flags	Professional culture, health care policy, and insurance reimbursement environment that the clinician must operate in

- Chest pain with exertion
- Constant excruciating pain
- Constant headache or dizziness
- Fatigue or malaise
- History of cancer
- History of immunosuppression
- History of injection drug use (infection)
- Increased urination with excessive thirst
- Insidious onset of current pain
- Nail bed clubbing
- Nausea and vomiting
- Neurological signs and symptoms
- Night sweats
- No discernible pattern of symptoms
- Pain accompanied by signs or symptoms associated with specific viscera or system
- Pain does not fit the expected mechanical pattern
- Pain that has not improved with therapy treatment
- Pain that has not improved with other conservative treatment
- Pain that improves with treatment, but then gets worse again
- Pain unchanged by movement or rest
- Presence of unusual vital signs
- Rebound tenderness
- Recent infection (within last 6 wk), especially when followed by neurologic symptoms (e.g., Guillain-Barré syndrome), joint pain, or back pain

- Recurrent colds or flu
- Recurrent history of trauma
- Shortness of breath
- Symptoms out of proportion of injury
- Syncope (temporary loss of consciousness)
- Unexplained weight loss (>10% of client's body weight in 10-21 days)
- Unusual menstrual cycle or symptoms

When red flags are noted, clinicians must expeditiously pursue a diagnostic workup. Individual red flags do not necessarily mean the presence of serious pathology; however, the presence of multiple red flags should raise clinical suspicion, and it indicates the need for further investigation. Red flags have not been evaluated comprehensively in any systematic review. The prevalence of systemic or visceral problems masquerading as a neurological or musculoskeletal dysfunction is not fully elucidated. The potential for fairly high false positive rates also exists.[8] In fact, the presence of one red flag by itself has little diagnostic value in the primary care setting.[8]

Yellow flags signal the potential need for more complex management, intensive treatment, or earlier specialist referral. Litigation or the involvement of workman's compensation programs pertaining to the client's pain complaint are also often viewed by the physician as yellow flags. These issues should not, but often do, change the approach to diagnosis and treatment. When yellow flags are present, clinicians need to be vigilant for deviations from the normal course of illness.

The clinician should be cognizant of the fact that previous health care providers may not have

Critical Clinical Pearls

When examining the client, it is important to determine the client's prognosis and potential confounding variables, which may include any of the following:

- Red flags: signs and symptoms suggestive of serious pathology and very poor prognosis in orthopedic clients. In these cases, clients should be referred to appropriate health care clinician.
- Yellow flags: their presence likely suggests poor prognosis, but not serious pathology.
- Blue flags: also can affect prognosis because the client may feel unsupported by employer, which can negatively affect their motivation.
- Black flags: may affect client's prognosis due to limitations with insurance, for example.

appropriately screened the client they are examining. Bishop and colleagues found that <5% of primary care physicians routinely examined for the presence of red flags during an initial screen.[9] The same study demonstrated that 61% of physical therapists screened for the presence of red flags. While this is an improvement compared to primary care physicians, a standard screening process for the presence of red and yellow flags is necessary.

A large majority of the red and yellow flags can be ascertained with the client interview and general observation. Some of them will require hands-on interpretation on part of the clinician. Depending on the presentation and triage staging of the client, the clinician is likely to proceed to physical performance of vital signs and diagnostic imaging findings next in the examination sequence. In those clients with high suspicion of serious pathology, appropriate diagnostic imaging will help clinicians determine the appropriateness of continuing with the examination.

DIAGNOSTIC IMAGING

The use of imaging by clinicians other than physicians is becoming more popular with direct access for physical therapists, increased availability for physical therapists and athletic trainers, and increased education in its clinical utility for the nonphysician. Previous literature suggests that physical therapists have been successfully diagnosing and managing musculoskeletal conditions with direct access and utilization of diagnostic imaging.[10]

Basic competencies regarding physical therapists and imaging are suggested, including being able to do the following:[11]

- Understand the radiographic report and terminology used to describe findings
- Make appropriate referrals for imaging studies based on physical examination and history
- Explain imaging findings to clients and discuss diagnostic imaging with other professionals
- Recognize precautions and contraindications to treatment and modify plans accordingly based on either radiographic report or their own evaluation of the images

Common imaging modalities include radiographs, magnetic resonance imaging (MRI), computed tomography (CT), and ultrasound (US) imaging. The basics of each are discussed in the

following sections. Various other modalities are utilized to assist the clinician with differential diagnosis, including various electrodiagnostic studies. The diagnostic utility of various imaging modalities is listed in table 6.2.

Radiography

Radiography, typically referred to as X-ray, is the traditional initial means of diagnostic imaging for assessment of many injuries. Radiography is the electromagnetic radiation of short wavelengths. The radiograph is considered a shadowgram, since the X-ray passes through the client's body to the film and the radiation reaching the film darkens it. A structure is considered radiodense (relatively white) in the image if it absorbs much of the radiation passing through the tissue. A good example of this is bone tissue. A radiolucent structure is relatively black on the image. A good example of this is fat tissue. Radiodensity, however, is a result of the combined effects of density and thickness.

It is a standard recommendation that at least two images are needed in radiography. These projections should also be at right angles to each other to aid in improving diagnostic ability, as well as improving the dimension of visualization. Several different radiographic views are utilized. An anteroposterior (AP) projection involves the projection of the radiation from the anterior surface of the body to the film located posterior to the client's body. Lateral and oblique views are named according to which surface of the body is located closest to the film. For example, in a right lateral projection, the film receiving the X-ray is located on the right side of the client's body.

Other forms of radiography include myelography, arthrography, stress radiography, and videofluoroscopy. Myelography and arthrography both involve the injection of a contrast medium into the client's body. The radiodensity of the cerebral spinal fluid is increased with a myelogram in order to better outline the thecal sac and nerve roots. In an arthrogram the contrast medium is injected directly into the joint (joint space) to be examined. An arthrogram provides better visualization of joint soft-tissue structures. Stress radiography is a radiograph of a particular joint when it is placed at the extreme of its motion. A common example of this is cervical spine stress radiographs in both flexion and extension to assess for upper cervical spine instability. Videofluoroscopy provides a real-time visualization of a joint's motion and position as it

TABLE 6.2 Diagnostic Imaging for Medically Related Conditions

Pathology	Diagnostic test	Reference standard	SN/SP (%)
MUSCULOSKELETAL RELATED			
Fracture	US	Attending radiologist review of plain film radiographs	**94/92**[12]
Osteoarthritis	MRI	Variable	61/**82**[13]
		Histology	74/76[13]
		Radiographs	61/81[13]
Rheumatoid arthritis	MRI	Variable	20-100/0-100[14]
Osteomyelitis	MRI	Bone biopsy	89 accuracy, +LR 3.8, −**LR 0.14**[15]
	Radiograph		+LR 2.3[15]
	PET	Histology, culture, and 6-month follow-up	**96/91**[16]
	Bone scintigraphy		82/25[16]
	MRI		84/60[16]
CRPS type I	MRI	Criteria specific to diagnostic test for diagnosis of CRPS	35/**91**[17]
	TPBS		79/**88**[17]
	Radiograph		55/76[17]
CARDIOVASCULAR			
Acute coronary syndrome	CTA	American Heart Association for ACS	**95/87**[18]
Obstructive CAD	SPECT	Coronary angiography	88/61[19]
	CMR		89/76[19]
	PET		84/81[19]
CVD due to CAD	CMR	Coronary angiography	**SN 95, NPV 90**[20]
PAD (LE)	MRA	Variable	**92-99.5/64-99**[21]
	CTA		**89-99/83-97**[21]
	US		**80-98/89-99**[21]
DVT	CT	US or venography	96/95[22]
	MRI	Mostly venography	**92/95** (overall)[23]
			SN 94 (proximal LE DVT)[23]
			SN 62 (distal LE DVT)[23]
	US	Venography Formal vascular study	**94/94** (proximal LE DVT)[24]
			64/94 (distal LE DVT)[24]
			89-96/94-99 (proximal LE DVT)[25]
			56-100/**94-100** (UE)[26]
			86/96[27]
	Plethysmography	US or venography	75-91/71-93[28]

(continued)

Table 6.2 *(continued)*

Pathology	Diagnostic test	Reference standard	SN/SP (%)
AAA	US	CT	99/98[29]
	CTA	Surgery	98/95[30]
PULMONARY			
PE	CT	Pulmonary angiogram (or reference test)	53-100/81-100[31]
INTRA-ABDOMINAL/TRUNK			
Thoracic injury	Whole-body CT	Synopsis of hospital charts, subsequent imaging, and interventional procedures	87/99[32]
Abdominal injury	Whole-body CT	Synopsis of hospital charts, subsequent imaging, and interventional procedures	86/98[32] Pooled: **+LR 30/–LR 0.26**[33]
	US	Abdominal CT, laparotomy, or clinical follow-up	79/95[34]
Pelvic injury	Whole-body CT	Synopsis of hospital charts, subsequent imaging and interventional procedures	86/99.8[32]
Acute appendicitis	CT	Surgery	SN 95[35] 96 NPV[35] 94 accuracy[35]
	US	Laparoscopy	94/69[36] 74/39[36]
Injury and hemoperitoneum	US	Abdominal CT scan, laparotomy, or clinical follow-up	79/95[34]
Acute cholecystitis	US	Laparoscopy	100/79[37]
Hepatomegaly	Contrast enhanced CT	H-score cutoffs of 0.92 and 1.08 L/m^2	84/68[38]

SN = sensitivity; SP = specificity; NPV = negative predictive value; US = ultrasonography; CT = computed tomography; CTA = computed tomography angiography; SPECT = single-photon emission computed tomography; CMR = cardiac magnetic resonance; PET = positron emission tomography; ACS = acute coronary syndrome; DVT = deep venous thrombosis; PE = pulmonary embolus; CVD = chronic ventricular dysfunction; CAD = coronary artery disease; PAD = peripheral arterial disease; LE = lower extremity; UE = upper extremity, contrast enhanced; CRPS = complex regional pain syndrome; AAA = abdominal aortic aneurysm

The color coding for suggestion of **good** and **ideal** diagnostic accuracy values reported in this table are without quality scoring (QUADAS), a very important aspect of determination of the clinical utility of such values. Therefore, it is suggested that the reader keep this in mind when interpreting such values.

moves. This has been suggested for midrange joint instability.[39] An additional commonly used means for videofluoroscopy is the placement of intramedullary rods into long appendicular skeleton bones, such as the tibia and femur.

A basic, systematic approach is suggested when evaluating conventional radiographs, the ABCS:

- **A**lignment: This includes the contour, shape, and position of the bone relative to other structures; a fracture or bony exostosis are good examples of alteration in bony alignment.

- **B**one density: Abnormalities include altered bone texture and loss of bone density; altered bone density can be representative of bone sclerosis associated with osteoarthritis or of decreased density associated with osteoporosis and rheumatoid arthritis.

- **C**artilage space: This cannot typically be seen on a radiograph; it is typically represented by a radiolucent area between two articulating bones.

- **S**oft tissue: Dysfunction, such as muscle wasting, intra-articular swelling, and muscle displacement can be utilized to suggest the presence of other dysfunction or disease; improved imaging has provided the clinician with the ability to improve their reading of the potential for soft-tissue dysfunction.

While this sounds simple in its description, radiologists undergo significant amounts of rigorous training to demonstrate competence in radiographic interpretation of images.

Although radiography is utilized for the examination of multiple pathologies, osteoarthritis requires specific mention. Osteoarthritis can affect multiple areas of the body and multiple joints. Definition of osteoarthritis can be multifactorial and can be variable depending on the area of the body or joint. The radiographic definition was originally defined by Kellgren and Lawrence.[40] According to these authors, the following radiological features were considered evidence of osteoarthrosis:[40]

- The formation of osteophytes on the joint margins or, in the case of the knee joint, on the tibial spines

- Periarticular ossicles, found chiefly in relation to the distal and proximal interphalangeal joints

- Narrowing of joint cartilage associated with sclerosis of subchondral bone

- Small pseudocystic areas with sclerotic walls, usually situated in the subchondral bone

- Altered shape of the bone ends, particularly in the head of femur

Magnetic Resonance Imaging

Magnetic resonance imaging (MRI) does not involve ionizing radiation; it produces information via the interaction of tissue with radiofrequency waves in a magnetic field. The image obtained is based on the client's re-emission of absorbed radiofrequencies while in the magnetic field.

Magnetic resonance imaging is ideally suited for evaluating the musculoskeletal system. Since MRI allows for detailed evaluation of both soft and bony tissue without ionizing radiation, it is replacing computed tomography (CT) as the first-line advanced imaging for the client with neck pain. It provides excellent contrast between the spinal cord, intervertebral disks, vertebral bodies, and ligamentous structures and assesses multiple additional aspects of soft-tissue or osseous abnormalities.

Image contrast may be weighted to demonstrate different anatomical structures or pathologies. Each tissue returns to its equilibrium state after excitation by the independent processes of T1 (spin-lattice) and T2 (spin-spin) relaxation. T1 is defined as the relaxation time for the protons to return to this equilibrium net state. T2 is defined as the spin-spin relaxation time, or the relaxation time compared with adjacent protons. Gadolinium is the most common contrast material used in MRI, and it causes significant prolongation of T1 relaxation times. This material is typically used to assess for infection or tumor or to evaluate postoperative clients. MRI has a reported 92% SP in detecting tumor and infection.[41] Table 6.3

TABLE 6.3   Tissue Appearances on T1 and T2 Sequences

	Bright	Dark
T1	Adipose tissue	Air, edema, infection, tumor, inflammation, calcifications
T2	Edema, infection, tumor, inflammation	Air, calcification, fibrous tissue, melanin, protein-rich fluid

Adapted from Laker and Concannon 2011.[42]

lists the basic differences between tissues as seen on T1- and T2-weighted images. Understanding these differences makes accurate MRI interpretation possible.

With the use of MRI, all clients should be screened for the presence of ferromagnetic substances since these are affected by MRI. Pacemakers, hearing aids, spinal cord stimulators, and potentially aneurysm clips and stent materials are common contraindications to MRI. A common caution for closed MRIs is claustrophobia. Improved imaging with open MRIs will assist in avoiding this caution.

Computed Tomography

Computed tomography (CT) is similar to radiography in that it uses X-rays to produce images based on radiodensities. Images displayed by CT are in shades of gray and are in much greater contrast than those with radiography. Imaging characteristics for CT are the same as for a radiograph: Cortical bone is viewed as white, muscle is gray, fat is dark, and air is black. CT is much more similar to image appearance of a radiograph than MRI is. Thus, images with high density, such as bone, will appear bright as they would on radiographs. These same images will appear dark on MRI. MRI is limited in its ability to image cortical bone. MRI clearly displays soft tissue and changes in bone marrow, though, making it ideal for bone tumors, stress fractures, and avascular necrosis.

Computed tomography is excellent for complex osseous abnormalities, instrumented clients, and surgical planning.[42] With advancing technology, submillimeter cuts can be obtained rapidly and compiled to create three-dimensional recreations. Computed tomography myelography combines the detail of CT scanning with the instillation of intrathecal contrast, allowing accurate measurements of central and foraminal canal diameters. The possibility of adverse events and poor pain tolerance is a consideration when determining the use of this imaging modality.

Nuclear Medicine Studies

Nuclear medicine studies have been used as an adjuvant to image lesions that are suspicious for neoplasm or infection within the osseous structures. Radionuclide studies reflect the function of a tissue because it interacts with the specific isotope. The emitted radiation is acquired by a gamma camera and converted into images by the computer's software. As such, the radiation emanates from within the client, and is detected by the imaging device; it is not transmitted through the client from an external source.[42]

Diagnostic Ultrasound

Ultrasound (US) is becoming increasingly popular among various clinicians for the purpose of diagnostic imaging of disease and dysfunction. US creates an image based on ultrasound waves reflected from tissue or tissue interfaces. Differentiation between tissues is based on the amount of US reflected. US images, unlike MRI and CT, are typically viewed in the longitudinal and transverse planes with reference to the viewed structure. The image therefore represents a plane that is continuous

Critical Clinical Pearls

When utilizing diagnostic imaging for client diagnosis, clinicians should consider the following:

- Diagnostic imaging findings suggestive of pathology have been found in several studies and in several body regions of clients who are asymptomatic and without pathology.
- Many times the client's clinical presentation does not match their imaging findings. Therefore, clinicians must treat the client, not the image.
- Diagnostic imaging is one component of the suggested multifaceted funnel examination.
- The various diagnostic imaging modalities have strengths and weaknesses for assessing particular tissue pathology.
- The clinician should be aware of these strengths and weaknesses when choosing the imaging modality.

with the US transducer. US compares favorably in most instances to MRI for soft-tissue diagnosis. In comparison to MRI, it produces greater resolution, requires shorter imaging time, and is of lower cost. Although US can compare favorably to MRI, there are some disadvantages worth mentioning. US has a narrower field of view and limited ability to show intra-articular structures compared to MRI. It is very operator dependent, and structures deep to the bone are not visualized.

VITAL SIGNS

A baseline measurement of vital signs is necessary for measurement of changes over time and, more importantly, the determination of potential disease. Blood pressure (BP), respiratory rate (RR), oxygen saturation (SaO_2), and pulse rate (PR) are basic physiological measures of the cardiovascular and pulmonary systems that should be assessed in a physical therapy examination. Abnormal values at rest will require further assessment prior to initiating any activity requiring significant physical or psychological stress. Additionally, assessment of vital signs can be used to determine whether the client is appropriate for physical therapy at that time or not. Abnormal vital signs may warrant referral to a physician. Specifically in cases such as diabetes mellitus, elevated BP may be associated with elevated blood glucose levels. Consideration of previous medical history, and its relationship with these physiological parameters, is therefore a necessary component of a thorough examination.

Pulse rate, systolic blood pressure (SBP), RR, SaO_2, and the Glasgow Coma Scale (GCS) have been shown to be significantly associated with cardiac arrest within 72 hours among 1,025 critically ill clients in an emergency department. All of these vital signs were also associated with death within 30 days of the cardiac event. These vital signs had high specificity (SP; 99.3 for cardiac arrest and 97.2 for death), but low sensitivity (SN; 11.5 for cardiac arrest and 22.7 for death).[43] Respiratory rate, SBP, and GCS have shown to be strongly associated with adverse outcomes in triage departments as well.[44] In blunt trauma clients with or without TBI, elevated admission SBP was associated with worse delayed outcomes.[45] Thus, these vital signs have diagnostic accuracy value and are of great value when assessing clients for serious pathology.

Assessment of body weight, body mass index (BMI), and height should also be considered. Body mass index can be misleading in the case of the very muscular (and thus potentially very fit) person because it is a measure of body weight compared to height. Therefore, standard guideline definitions of obesity based on BMI should be carefully considered. Body weight is of particular concern with regard to systemic disease when there is a loss of >10% of the client's body weight in 10 to 21 days.[3]

While the previously mentioned parameters are standardly accepted vital signs, sport participation or exercise has been suggested as the fifth vital sign.[46] Sport participation has been associated with a 20% to 40% reduction in all-cause mortality compared with nonparticipation. Clinical studies suggest that playing sports is associated with specific health benefits. Some sports have relatively high injury risk, although neuromuscular training programs can prevent various lower extremity injuries. Exercise has also been suggested as a vital sign, and therefore should be recorded in clients' electronic medical records and routine histories.[46]

Some of the more commonly measured vital signs and their interpretations are listed in the sidebar on pages 98-99. It must be mentioned that the described normal values are general guidelines; some of these have not been universally agreed on.

DIFFERENTIAL DIAGNOSIS AND MEDICAL SCREENING EXAMINATION

Screening has been defined as a method of detecting disease or body dysfunction before someone would normally seek medical care. Medical screening tests are often administered to clients who do not have symptoms, but who may be at high risk for certain adverse health outcomes.[3] Therefore, to more clearly delineate screening of the client with pathology presenting in the musculoskeletal clinic, the terminology *differential diagnosis* or *medical disease screening* is utilized in this text to represent the screening of nonmusculoskeletal-related or neurologic-related pathology as a potential pain generator or contributor to the client's pain that they are being seen for. This type of screening is used to ensure that all possible sources of pathology are assessed; this is especially true if there has been no history of trauma leading to symptoms.

Medical screening covered will include neurological, cardiovascular, pulmonary, intra-abdominal, urological, gastrointestinal, and other

Vital Signs and Their Interpretation

Pulse

Often considered a direct extension of the function of the heart

Location

- Carotid artery: anterior to sternocleidomastoid
- Brachial artery: medial aspect of arm between shoulder and elbow
- Radial artery: at wrist, lateral to flexor carpi radialis tendon
- Ulnar artery: at wrist, between flexor digitorum superficialis and flexor carpi ulnaris tendons
- Femoral artery: femoral triangle; sartorius, adductor longus, and inguinal ligament borders
- Popliteal artery: posterior aspect of knee
- Posterior tibial artery: posterior aspect of medial malleolus
- Dorsalis pedis artery: between first and second metatarsal bones

Interpretation[47]

- Normal for adults is 60-80 beats/min
- Normal for children is 80-100 beats/min
- Rapid and weak = shock, bleeding, diabetic coma, or heat exhaustion
- Rapid and strong = heatstroke, severe fright
- Strong but slow = skull fracture or stroke
- No pulse = cardiac arrest or death

Respiration

- Adult = 12-18 breaths/min[47]
- Children = 20-25 breaths/min
- Shallow = shock
- Gasping or labored = cardiac arrest

Blood Pressure

Systolic: occurs when the heart pumps blood

Diastolic: residual pressure when the heart is between beats

- 15- to 20-year-old males = 115-120/75-80 mmHg
- 15- to 20-year-old females = 105-110/65-75 mmHg
- 15- to 20-year-olds may be excessively high if systolic greater than 135 mmHg
- 15- to 20-year-olds may be excessively low if diastolic is less than 110 mmHg
- Outer ranges of diastolic should not exceed 85 mmHg
- Normal adult 90/60 mmHg to 120/80 mmHg[47] although higher ranges (up to 140/90) have also been suggested as within normal ranges

Temperature

Normal 97.8 to 99.1 °F (36.6–37.3 °C)

Average 98.6 °F (37 °C)[47]

Reflex Testing

An involuntary response following a stimulus

Superficial Reflexes

Caused by a sudden irritation to the skin

Deep Tendon Reflexes

Stimulation of structures under the skin such as tendon and bone

Reflex Grading

See chapter 7.

musculoskeletal conditions. Medical screening is extremely important for the standard examination process of practicing clinicians. Screening out potential nonmusculoskeletal or other musculoskeletal conditions of interest can help the clinician focus their examination on determination of more traditional musculoskeletal pathologies as potential generators of the client's pain or dysfunction.

Neurological

Several neurologically related medical conditions exist that the practicing orthopedic clinician should be cognizant of when performing a screen on clients. Variable clinical presentations, their diagnostic accuracy, and special considerations of the primary neurological pathologies that the orthopedic clinician may encounter are presented here.

Cauda Equina Syndrome

A diagnosis of cauda equina syndrome (CES) must result in a medical referral. For diagnosis of CES, one or more of the following must be present:

- Bladder or bowel dysfunction
- Reduced sensation in saddle area
- Sexual dysfunction
- Possible neurological deficit in the lower limb (motor or sensory loss, reflex change)

No single aspect of CES within the literature achieved unanimity or consensus; however, a majority view indicated that there would be bladder and sensory disturbance. The most commonly cited pathological structure resulting in CES was

identified as the spinal disc.[48] This series shows that saddle sensory deficit has a higher predictive value than other clinical features in diagnosing CES. However, because no symptom or sign has an absolute predictive value in establishing the diagnosis of CES, any client with whom a reasonable suspicion of CES arises must undergo urgent MRI to exclude this diagnosis.[49]

Meningococcal Disease

Five symptoms have clinically useful positive likelihood ratios (+LR) for meningococcal disease:[50]

- Confusion (**+LR = 24.2**)
- Leg pain (**+LR = 7.6**)
- Photophobia (**+LR = 6.5**)
- Rash (**+LR = 5.5**)
- Neck pain or stiffness (**+LR = 5.3**)

The glass test has been suggested by some for differentiating a meningococcal disease–related rash from other rashes. Pressing a solid clear glass against the rash will not make the rash disappear when the rash is due to meningococcal disease. Cold hands and feet had limited diagnostic value (+LR = 2.3), while headache (+LR = 1.0) and pale color (**+LR = 0.3**) did not discriminate meningococcal disease in children. The classic red flag symptoms of neck stiffness, rash, and photophobia are commonly described, but continued investigation regarding their diagnostic accuracy is suggested. These findings, as well as the presence of confusion or leg pain in a child with an unexplained acute febrile illness, suggest the necessity of a detailed assessment to exclude meningococcal disease.[50]

Headache alone is closely associated with severe systolic blood pressure elevation in acute ischemic stroke.[51] Obviously, with several different types of headaches or headache intensities, this must be taken in proper context.

Another variable that must be considered is the client's social environment. For example, freshmen living in dormitories demonstrated an increased risk of meningitis (odds ratio of 3.6) compared with other college students.[52]

Mild Traumatic Brain Injury and Post-Concussion Syndrome

This topic is covered in greater detail in chapter 27 (Emergency Sport Examination), but some information is highlighted here. The Glasgow Coma Scale (GCS) is often utilized to rate mild traumatic brain injury (mTBI). A score of 13 to 15 (normal) is often considered mTBI. Commonly described signs and symptoms for mTBI or post-concussion syndrome of concern for the clinician are a dangerous mechanism onset, headache (typically most common symptom), nausea or vomiting, sensitivity to light and sounds, initial loss of consciousness or dazed expression (GCS of 13-15), deficits in short-term memory, physical evidence of trauma above the clavicles, drug or alcohol intoxication, and seizures.[53-55]

Primary Brain Tumor

Commonly described signs and symptoms for this condition include headache, nausea or vomiting, ataxia, speech deficits, sensory abnormalities, visual changes, altered mental status, and seizures.[56-58] These are commonly described signs and symptoms for other serious pathologies, too. Thus, the clinician should use appropriate clinical reasoning when dealing with clients presenting with such signs or symptoms.

Parkinson's Disease

Tremor as a sign of Parkinson's disease (PD) produced a range of +LRs from 1.3 to 1.5. Clinical features useful in the diagnosis of PD are the following:

- History of the combination of symptoms of rigidity and bradykinesia (**+LR 4.5, −LR 0.12**)
- History of loss of balance (+ LR 1.6–**6.6**, **−LR 0.29–0.35**)
- Symptoms of micrographia (abnormally small, cramped handwriting, or the progression to continually smaller handwriting) (range of + LR 2.8-5.9, range of **−LR 0.30–0.44**)
- History of shuffling gait (range of +LR 3.3–15, range of **−LR 0.32–0.50**).
- Trouble with certain tasks:
  - Turning in bed (+ **LR 13**, −LR 0.56)
  - Opening jars (+ **LR 6.1**, **−LR 0.26**)
  - Rising from a chair (range of +LR 1.9–**5.2**, −LR **0.39**–0.58)

Useful signs include the glabella tap test (**+LR 4.5, −LR 0.13**), difficulty walking heel-to-toe (+LR 2.9, **−LR 0.32**), and rigidity (range of +LR 0.53–2.8, range of **−LR 0.38**–1.6). Therefore, symptoms of tremor, rigidity, bradykinesia, micrographia, shuffling gait, and difficulty with the tasks of turning in bed, opening jars, and rising from a chair should be carefully reviewed in all clients with suspected PD.

The glabella tap and heel-to-toe tests may also be assessed.[59] The glabella tap test or reflex involves a tap on the glabella (space between the eyebrows and above the nose). Normally the client stops blinking after the second or third tap, but clients with PD and certain kinds of cerebral degeneration continue blinking even after many taps. This is a traditional test that has demonstrated limited clinical utility. Most recently, it was found to be of poor clinical utility for PD motor severity.[60] The Simpson-Angus Scale (SAS) was found to be a more valid and reliable measure in evaluating for PD.[61] This scale involves 10 assessments: gait, arm dropping, shoulder shaking, elbow rigidity, wrist rigidity, leg pendulousness, head dropping, tremor, salivation, and the glabella tap.

Myasthenia Gravis

Clients with myasthenia gravis (MG) traditionally complain of weakness in specific muscles, double vision, drooping eyelids, and difficulty chewing and swallowing. The symptoms are typically better after rest and worse with prolonged use of the affected muscles.[62] A history of speech becoming unintelligible during prolonged speaking and the presence of the *peek sign* increase the likelihood of MG (+LR 4.5 and +LR 30, respectively). Their absence does not significantly reduce the likelihood of MG. The identified studies only assessed one other historical feature and sign each (food remaining in the mouth after swallowing and quiver eye movements, respectively), and neither of these significantly changes the likelihood of MG. The ice test is useful when the response is abnormal (summary **+LR 24**), and it diminishes the likelihood of MG when the response is normal (summary **−LR 0.16**). An abnormal sleep test result is useful in confirming the diagnosis (**+LR 53**). The rest and sleep tests make the probability of myasthenia unlikely when results are normal (**−LR 0.52** and **−LR 0.01**, respectively).[62]

The ice pack, rest, and sleep tests for MG all have the same (+) response: complete or almost complete resolution of ptosis or at least a 2 mm increase in palpebral fissure width immediately after the tests. The ice pack test involves placing a latex glove finger filled with crushed ice over the more ptotic eyelid for 2 minutes. The rest test involves placing a glove filled with cotton (placebo) over the more ptotic eyelid while holding the eyes closed for 2 minutes. The sleep test involves leaving the client in a quiet dark room with the eyes closed for 30 minutes.

Weakness of the orbicularis oculi muscle can be indicated by a (+) peek sign. This sign involves the complete closure of bilateral eyelids, followed by involuntary separation of the eyelids within 30 seconds. The sclera begins to then show (i.e., + peek sign). Caution is suggested with utilization of these tests for diagnostic utility.[62, 63]

Cervical Myelopathy

In general, the combination of clinical findings (as opposed to a single finding by itself) is more suggestive of cervical myelopathy (CM). The lack of the presence of at least one clinical finding helped rule out myelopathy (**SN 94, −LR 0.18**), while the presence of three of five (+) findings helped rule in myelopathy (**SP 99, +LR 31**):[64]

- Gait deviation
- (+) Hoffmann's sign
- (+) Inverted supinator sign
- (+) Babinski test
- Age > 45 years

These clinical findings and CM (in general) are discussed in greater detail in chapter 17 (Cervical Spine).

Cardiovascular

Due to the high prevalence of cardiovascular disease, the practicing orthopedic clinician should always be aware of its potential presence. Practicing orthopedic clinicians should be cognizant of several cardiovascular-related medical conditions when performing a screen on their client. Variable clinical presentations, their diagnostic accuracy, and special considerations of the primary cardiovascular pathologies that the orthopedic clinician may encounter are presented here.

Acute Coronary Syndrome

The clinical value for ruling out acute coronary syndrome in clients with chest pain currently relies on different prediction instruments.[65] In a systematic review investigating the clinical utility of such instruments, almost all of the current instruments were found to be investigated in low-biased studies as determined by QUADAS.[66] At the time of this systematic review by Steurer and colleagues, 20 derivation studies had been investigated, 10 of which were validated at least once in 14 validations.[65] The time-insensitive predictive instrument developed by Selker and colleagues[67] (utilizing electrocardiography as a reference standard) found four main risk factors for acute coronary syndrome:

1. Chest pain
2. Shortness of breath
3. Upper abdominal pain or dizziness
4. Age (men > 30 years, women > 40 years)

This predictive instrument demonstrated an SN of 98 or greater, and an SP ranging from 4 to 34 in five different validation studies.[68-72] This rule was deemed the most safe with a false negative rate of 2% or less in most validations, but it was not very efficient. Out of 100 clients with acute chest pain but without acute coronary syndrome, an acute coronary syndrome would be ruled out in only 4 to 34 clients when consistently applying the rule. This has been suggested to yield small limits on its clinical influence and the potential for cost savings.[65]

Another predictive risk score rule has been described:[73]

- Age > 67 years: 1 point
- Insulin-dependent diabetes mellitus: 1 point
- Chest pain: 1 point
- ≥2 chest pain episodes in 24 hours: 1 point
- Prior cardiorespiratory event: 1 point
- ≤1 variable present: **SN 86, SP 50, +LR 1.7, −LR 0.28**

The Marburg Heart Score has also been described as a predictive risk score to assist in ruling out a cardiorespiratory event:[74]

- Age and sex (female ≥65 years, male ≥55 years): 1 point
- Known clinical vascular disease: 1 point
- Client assumes cardiac origin of pain: 1 point
- Pain worse with exercise: 1 point
- Pain not reproducible with palpation: 1 point
- Low risk = 0-2 points, intermediate risk = 3 points, high risk = 4-5 points
- Cutoff value of 3 points: **SN 89**, SP 64, +LR 2.4, **−LR 0.17**

Absence of chest wall tenderness on palpation was the only variable for ruling out myocardial infarction or acute coronary syndrome in a meta-analysis investigating studies with low prevalence of disease. Absence of chest wall tenderness had a pooled SN of 92 for acute myocardial infarction and 94 for acute coronary syndrome. Oppressive pain was less able to rule these conditions out, with a pooled SN of 60 for acute myocardial infarction. Sweating had the highest pooled +LR 2.9, for acute myocardial infarction.[75]

Likelihood ratios of chest pain radiation patterns for myocardial infarction are as follows:[76, 77]

- Into both arms with pain (**+LR 9.7**, −LR 0.64)
- Into right arm with pain (**+LR 7.3**, −LR 0.62)
- Into left arm with pain (+LR 2.2, −LR 0.60)
- Right shoulder pain (+LR 2.2, −LR 0.90)

Other likelihood values worth mentioning are the following:[76, 77]

- Vomiting (+LR 3.5, −LR 0.87)
- Being an ex-smoker (+LR 2.5, −LR 0.85)
- Chest discomfort with indigestion or burning quality (+LR 2.3)
- Sex: male (+LR 1.5, **−LR 0.24**)

Congestive Heart Failure

Many features increased the probability of heart failure, with the best feature for each category being the presence of the following:[78]

- Past history of heart failure (**+LR 5.8**)
- Symptom of paroxysmal nocturnal dyspnea (+LR 2.6)
- Sign of the third heart sound (S3) gallop (**+LR 11**)
- Chest radiograph showing pulmonary venous congestion (**+LR 12.0**)

- Electrocardiogram showing atrial fibrillation (+LR 3.8)

The features that best decreased the probability of heart failure were the lack of the following:[78]

- Absence of past history of heart failure (**−LR 0.45**)
- Symptom of dyspnea on exertion (**−LR 0.48**)
- Rales (−LR 0.51)
- Chest radiograph showing cardiomegaly (**−LR 0.33**)
- Any electrocardiogram abnormality (−LR 0.64)

For dyspneic adult emergency department clients, a directed history, physical examination, chest radiograph, and electrocardiography should be performed. If the suspicion of heart failure remains, obtaining a serum brain natriuretic peptide level may be helpful, especially for excluding heart failure.[78]

Deep Venous Thrombosis

The clinical prediction rule for deep venous thrombosis (DVT) is as follows:[79]

- Active cancer (treatment ongoing or within previous 6 months): 1 point
- Paralysis, paresis, or recent plaster immobilization of the LE: 1 point
- Recently bedridden for 3 days or more, or major surgery within the previous 12 weeks requiring anesthesia: 1 point
- Localized tenderness along the distribution of the deep venous system: 1 point
- Entire leg swelling: 1 point
- Calf swelling at least 3 cm larger than asymptomatic leg (measured 10 cm below tibia tubercle): 1 point
- Pitting edema confined in symptomatic leg: 1 point
- Collateral superficial veins (nonvaricose): 1 point
- Previous DVT: 1 point
- Subtract 2 points if there is an alternative diagnosis at least as likely as a DVT

If score is > 3 = high probability of DVT (53%)

If score is 1-2 = moderate probability of DVT (17%)

If score is 0 = low probability of DVT (5%)

These parameters were useful for ruling in DVT:[80]

- Malignancy (+LR 2.7)
- Previous DVT (+LR 2.3)
- Recent immobilization (+LR 1.98)
- Difference in calf diameter (+LR 1.8)
- Recent surgery (+LR 1.8)

These parameters were useful in ruling out DVT:[80]

- Only absence of calf swelling (−LR 0.67)
- No difference in calf diameter (−LR 0.57)

The Wells clinical score was more valuable than the individual characteristics; it stratified clients into groups with high (**+LR 5.2**), moderate, and low (**−LR 0.25**) probability of DVT. Individual clinical features are of limited value in diagnosing DVT. Overall assessment of clinical probability by using the Wells score is more useful.[80]

Peripheral Arterial Disease

For asymptomatic clients, the most useful clinical findings for diagnosing peripheral arterial disease (PAD) are the presence of claudication (+LR 3.30), femoral bruit (**+LR 4.8**), or any pulse abnormality (+LR 3.1). While none of the clinical examination features help to lower the likelihood of any degree of PAD, the absence of claudication or the presence of normal pulses decreases the likelihood of moderate to severe disease. When considering clients who are symptomatic with leg complaints, the most useful clinical findings are the presence of cool skin (**+LR 5.90**), the presence of at least one bruit (**+LR 5.6**), or any palpable pulse abnormality (**+LR 4.7**). The absence of any bruits (iliac, femoral, or popliteal; **−LR 0.4**) or pulse abnormality (**−LR 0.4**) reduces the likelihood of PAD. Combinations of physical examination findings do not increase the likelihood of PAD beyond that of individual clinical findings.

Clinical examination findings must be used in the context of the pretest probability because they are not independently sufficient for including or excluding a diagnosis of PAD with certainty. The PAD screening score using the handheld Doppler has the greatest diagnostic accuracy.[81]

Abdominal Aortic Aneurysm

Abdominal aortic aneurysm (AAA) should be considered as part of a differential diagnosis in clients who are male, white, over the age of 50 years, have a history of ever smoking, and have a family history of AAA.[82] Screening for AAA with abdominal palpation is suggested. Screening with the use of US imaging has been suggested for men aged 65 to 79 years, although the cost-effectiveness was not clear.[83]

Palpation of the abdominal aorta is done with the client in a supine position with the hips flexed, feet placed flat on table, and abdomen relaxed. The clinician, using their fingertips, first feels deeply for the aortic pulsation, usually found a few centimeters superior to the umbilicus and slightly to the left of midline. The clinician then places an index finger on either side of the pulsating area to confirm that it is the aorta (each systole should move the two fingers apart) and to measure the aortic width. Palpation of the aorta is typically easier in thin clients. The normal aorta is less than 2.5 cm in diameter. If the aorta is larger than this, further investigation with US imaging may be warranted.

- Pooled analysis: SN 39 (AAA of 3.0–3.9 cm), 50 (AAA of 4.0–4.9 cm), and 76 (AAA ≥ 5.0 cm), **+LR 12**, −LR 0.72 (AAA ≥ 3.0 cm), **+LR 16**, −LR 0.51 (AAA ≥ 4.0 cm).[82]
- SN ranged from 33 to 100; SP ranged from 75 to 100 and was not suggested as a screen without US imaging for AAA.[84]

Confidence in the clinical examination is also a variable to consider for posttest diagnosis of AAA. An examination that the clinician considered definite for AAA produced a **+LR of 4.8** and one suggestive of AAA had a +LR of 1.4.[82]

Temporal Arteritis

In a systematic review, the only two historical features that substantially increased the likelihood of temporal arteritis (TA) among clients referred for biopsy were jaw claudication (**+LR 4.2**) and diplopia (+LR 3.4). The absence of any temporal artery abnormality was the only clinical factor that modestly reduced the likelihood of disease (−LR 0.53). Predictive physical findings included temporal artery beading (**+LR 4.6**), prominence of the temporal artery (**+LR 4.3**), and tenderness of the artery (+LR 2.6). Normal erythrocyte sedimentation rate (ESR) values indicated much less likelihood of disease (**−LR for abnormal ESR 0.2**). Therefore, a small number of clinical features are helpful in predicting the likelihood of a positive temporal artery biopsy among clients with a clinical suspicion of disease; the most useful finding is a normal ESR, which makes TA unlikely.[85]

Pulmonary

The only differential diagnosis for pulmonary-related medical conditions discussed with notable diagnostic accuracy is pulmonary embolism. However, the practicing orthopedic clinician should always be cognizant of other potential pulmonary-related medical conditions that may affect the client they are examining.

In a systematic review with meta-analysis, the most useful features (pooled +LR) for ruling in pulmonary embolisms (PE) were syncope (2.4), shock (**4.1**), thrombophlebitis (2.2), current deep venous thrombosis (2.1), leg swelling (2.1), sudden dyspnea (1.8), active cancer (1.7), recent surgery (1.6), hemoptysis (1.6), and leg pain (1.6). The most useful features for ruling out (−LR) PE were the absence of sudden dyspnea (**0.43**), any dyspnea (0.52), and tachypnea (0.56). Many of the analyses involved pooling results that had significant heterogeneity, so the authors recommended that these estimates should be used with caution.[86]

The clinical prediction rule for PE is as follows:[87-89]

- Age 65 years or over: 1 point
- Previous DVT or PE: 3 points
- Surgery or fracture within 1 month: 2 points
- Active malignant condition: 2 points
- Unilateral lower limb pain: 3 points
- Hemoptysis: 2 points
- Heart rate 75-94 beats/min: 3 points
- Heart rate 95 or more beats/min: 5 points
- Pain on deep palpation of lower limb and unilateral edema: 4 points

The clinical pretest probability of PE is as follows:

- 0-3 points is a low, 9% probability of PE
- 4-10 points is an intermediate, 28% probability of PE
- >11 points is a high, 72% probability of PE

With a population prevalence of 24%, this revised Geneva Score had **SN 91**, SP 37.[90]

The Well's Rule for pulmonary embolism is another such probability score:

- Clinically suspected DVT: 3 points
- Alternative diagnosis is less likely than PE: 3 points
- Tachycardia: 1.5 points
- Immobilization (≥3 days) or surgery in previous 4 weeks: 1.5 points

- History of DVT or PE: 1.5 point
- Hemoptysis: 1 point
- Malignancy (with treatment within 6 months) or palliative: 1 point

The clinical probability of PE with the Well's Rule is as follows:[91]

- Score < 2 points is low risk (probability 15% based on pooled data)
- Score 2–6 points is moderate risk (probability 29% based on pooled data)
- Score > 6 points is high risk (probability 59% based on pooled data)

A cutoff of < 2 points: SN **84 (74-89)**, SP 58 (52-65), +LR 2.0, **−LR 0.27**[90]

A cutoff of ≤4 points: SN 60 (49-69), SP 80 (75-84), +LR 3.0, **−LR 0.5**[90]

Intra-Abdominal

Intra-abdominal medically related conditions are a concern to the practicing orthopedic clinician due to their potential pain referral to the spine and hip. Variable clinical presentations, their diagnostic accuracy, and special considerations of the primary intra-abdominal pathologies that the orthopedic clinician may encounter are presented here.

Blunt Intra-Abdominal Injury

The presence of a seat belt sign (contusions and abrasions on the abdomen of a restrained occupant involved in a motor vehicle crash) (**+LR range 5.6-9.9**), rebound tenderness (**+LR 6.5**) (see test description later in the chapter), hypotension (**+LR 5.2**), abdominal distention (+LR 3.8), or guarding (+LR 3.7) suggest an intra-abdominal injury. The absence of abdominal tenderness to palpation does not rule out an intra-abdominal injury (summary −LR 0.61). The presence of intraperitoneal fluid or organ injury on bedside US assessment is more accurate than any history and physical examination findings (adjusted summary +LR 30); conversely, a normal US result decreases the chance of injury detection (**−LR 0.26**).[33] Bedside US has the highest accuracy of all individual findings, but a normal result does not rule out an intra-abdominal injury. Combinations of clinical findings may be most useful for determining whether a client requires further evaluation.[33]

A clinical prediction rule (CPR) has been derived and validated to assist the clinician with ruling out the presence of an intra-abdominal injury after blunt torso trauma.[92] Test performance of the CPR for any intra-abdominal injury (whether treated acutely or strictly monitored only) demonstrated an **SN of 98** in the derivation phase and **96** in the validation phase of the CPR. The SP was 26 in the derivation phase and 30 in the validation phase. +LR and −LR would therefore be 1.4 and **0.13**, respectively.

The CPR for any intra-abdominal injury consisted of the following variables: GCS < 14, costal margin tenderness, abdominal tenderness, femur fracture, hematuria level ≥ 25 red blood cells or high power field, hematocrit level < 30%, and abnormal chest radiograph result (pneumothorax, rib fracture).[92] The practicing physical therapist, athletic trainer, or physician without the ability to determine some of these values should have increased suspicion with the values they can directly assess (e.g., GCS, tenderness of the abdomen or costal margin, and femur fracture assessment with clinical exam).

Appendicitis

An analysis of the most common constellation of signs and symptoms in clients with acute appendicitis consisted of pain and tenderness localized in the right lower quadrant (100% of clients) that exacerbates with movement (98%), feeling unwell (93%), loss of appetite (88%), and rebound tenderness in right lower quadrant (74%).[7] Such signs and symptoms developed relatively quickly (in fewer than 12 hours) in 18% of adult clients and more than half of the clients with a normal body temperature. There did not appear to be any correlation with age, gender, or duration of symptoms in the majority of the clients.[7]

No medical history of physical finding can effectively rule out appendicitis; however, right lower quadrant pain (**+LR 7.3–8.5**), abdominal rigidity (+LR 3.7), and a psoas sign (+LR 2.4) (see test description later in the chapter) all make appendicitis more likely, whereas the absence of right lower quadrant pain (**−LR 0–0.3**) and the presence of previous similar pain make the diagnosis less likely (**−LR 0.3**).[93, 94]

In children with abdominal pain, fever was the single most useful sign associated with appendicitis; a fever increases the likelihood of appendicitis (summary +LR 3.4), and conversely, its absence decreases the chance of appendicitis (**summary −LR −0.32**). In select groups of children, in whom the diagnosis of appendicitis is suspected and evaluation undertaken, rebound tenderness triples the odds of appendicitis (summary +LR 3.0), while its absence reduces the likelihood (**summary −LR 0.28**). Midabdominal pain migrating to the right lower quadrant (+LR range, 1.9–3.1) increases the risk of appendicitis more than right lower quadrant pain itself (summary +LR 1.2). A white blood cell count of < 10,000/MμL decreases the likelihood of appendicitis (summary −LR −0.22), as does an absolute neutrophil count of 6,750/MμL or lower (**−LR −0.06**). Signs and symptoms were found to be most useful in combination, particularly for identifying children who do not require further evaluation or intervention.[95]

In comparison with adults, right lower quadrant abdominal pain, typically identified as a classic symptom of appendicitis, was a much stronger predictor in adults (**+LR 7.3–7.5**) than in children (summary +LR 1.2).[93, 95] Fever, anorexia, nausea, and vomiting were all poor independent predictors of appendicitis in both adults and children. Rebound tenderness and the psoas sign performed similarly in children and adults.[93, 95]

Rebound tenderness (Blumberg's sign) is assessed with palpation at McBurney's point. The supine client is asked to relax as the clinician gently and deeply palpates the right lower quadrant of the abdomen (one-third the distance from the ASIS to the umbilicus). The clinician quickly releases the pressure from this deep palpation. Increased tenderness with the release (rebound technique) over McBurney's point is considered a (+) test for acute appendicitis.

Diagnostic accuracy for tenderness with palpation of this location is as follows:

- **SN 100**, SP 12, +LR 1.1, **−LR 0.0**[96]
- **SN 90**, SP 59, +LR 2.2, **−LR 0.17**[97]

Diagnostic accuracy for rebound tenderness is as follows:

- SN 55, SP 78, +LR 2.5, −LR 0.58[96]
- SN 66, SP 75, +LR 2.6, −LR 0.45[97]

The psoas sign can be elicited in two different client positions. In the supine position, the clinician asks the client to lift the right thigh against the clinician's resistance just proximal to the knee (see chapter 24 Hip). In the side-lying position, the clinician extends the client's top leg at the hip. Increased pain with either maneuver is a (+) sign, and indicates irritation of the psoas muscle by an inflamed appendix (on the right side only, obviously).

Several decision rules have been published for the prediction of a diagnosis of acute appendicitis. The Alvarado model[96] is recommended as the most user-friendly and powerful model for clients presenting to an emergency room with right lower quadrant abdominal pain.[93] The Alvarado clinical decision rule (MANTRELS mnemonic) is as follows:

- **M**igration (pain migrated from epigastric region to right lower quadrant): 1 point
- **A**norexia: 1 point
- **N**ausea and vomiting: 1 point
- **T**enderness in right lower quadrant: 1 point
- **R**ebound pain: 1 point
- **E**levation of temperature: 1 point
- **L**eukocytosis: 1 point
- **S**hift to the left (white blood cell count shifts to the left): 1 point

The maximum total score is 10 points. The rule is considered (+) when a score of ≥7 points is achieved: **SN 81**, SP 74, +LR 3.1, **−LR 0.3** with a score of ≥7.[96]

Acute Cholecystitis

No clinical or laboratory finding had a sufficiently high +LR or low −LR to rule in or rule out the diagnosis of acute cholecystitis without further testing (e.g., right upper quadrant US). Possible exceptions were the Murphy sign (+LR 2.8) and right upper quadrant tenderness (**−LR 0.4**), though the 95% CIs for both included 1.0. Available data on diagnostic confirmation rates at laparotomy and test characteristics of relevant radiological investigations suggest that the diagnostic impression of acute cholecystitis has a **+LR of 25 to 30**. Unfortunately, the available literature does not identify the specific combinations of clinical and laboratory findings that presumably account for this diagnostic success.[98]

Murphy's sign was also found to be a poor screening test (SN 50, −LR 0.5) in another recent study. While it demonstrated much greater clinical utility as a diagnostic test (**SP 98, +LR 25**) there were very large CIs.[37] To perform Murphy's sign, the clinician has the client lie supine and relax. The clinician places one hand ipsilateral to the posterior inferior costal margin and the other hand on the same side in the upper subcostal region anteriorly. As the client draws in a deep breath, the clinician simultaneously palpates the subcostal region deeply.

Pain during inspiration or associated inspiratory arrest is a (+) test.

The physical examination offered limited accuracy when assessing the acute abdomen for acute cholecystitis.[37] It is recommended that clinical gestalt and diagnostic imaging (see table 6.1) be implemented as part of the examination procedure for acute cholecystitis because the existing literature does not support any single finding with strong enough clinical utility to screen or diagnose this pathology.[98]

Hepatomegaly

An increased liver span or volume is suggested to correlate with various liver diseases. Being able to readily palpate a liver edge has some diagnostic ability (+LR 2.0). The probability that the liver edge can be felt below the right costal margin is about 50%. Clients who should be considered for hepatomegaly are those with known or suspected liver disorders, malignancy, and congestive heart failure. Liver US is required to confirm clinical findings.[99]

The liver should be palpated with the client supine and abdomen relaxed. The clinician palpates with the fingers of both hands (hand over hand) over the right upper quadrant of the abdomen in the midclavicular line. The client is asked to take a deep breath (causing the liver to descend toward the fingers) as the clinician palpates deeply in a posterior–superior direction. A (+) test is a readily palpable liver. Diagnostic accuracy of palpation of hepatomegaly is as follows:

- SN 39–42, SP 82–86, +LR 2.2–3.0, −LR 0.68–0.74[100]
- SN 36, SP 83, +LR 2.2, −LR 0.76[101]

Splenomegaly

The prevalence of palpable splenomegaly in an otherwise healthy student population is low, approximating 3%;[102] 12% of normal postpartum women had palpable spleens.[103] Conditions suspicious of splenomegaly include suspected or proven viral illness, malignancy, cirrhosis, suspected portal hypertension, suspected or proven malaria, and connective tissue disorders associated with splenomegaly.[104]

The clinical examination for splenomegaly is more SP than SN, and is best used when ruling in the diagnosis among clients for whom the suspicion is at least 10%. Moreover, the examination should start with Traube's space percussion, followed, if dull, by a supine one-handed palpation. These maneuvers have received more extensive evaluation than other maneuvers, allowing greater confidence in the findings. Middleton's maneuver may work as well.[104]

Percussion of Traube's space requires the client to lie on their right side and the clinician to stand directly behind them. Traube's space (6th rib superiorly, midaxillary line laterally, and costal margin anteriorly) is percussed from lateral to medial margins while client breaths normally. A (+) test is a sound ascertained as uncertain, probably dull, or definitely dull. The diagnostic accuracy of this test is as follows: **+LR 8.2, −LR 0.41** across three studies.[104]

Palpation of the spleen is with the client supine and breathing normally; the clinician stands on the client's right side. The clinician, using their left hand on the posterior aspect of the distal rib cage, lifts the client's rib cage, creating slack in the costal margin region on the right side. The clinician's right hand palpates at the costal margin underneath the ribs to feel the spleen's descent during inspiration. The whole costal margin is palpated. A (+) test is the ability to palpate the enlarged spleen. The diagnostic accuracy of this test is as follows: +LR 2.3, **−LR 0.48** across four studies.[104]

Middleton's maneuver involves the client supine and breathing normally; the clinician stands on the side of the client's left shoulder facing their legs. The clinician curls the fingertips of both hands under the left costal margin and palpates for the spleen while instructing the client to take deep breaths. A palpable spleen is a (+) finding. The diagnostic accuracy of this test is as follows: SN 56, **SP 93, +LR 8.0,** −LR 0.57 (combination of palpation and Middleton maneuver results).[105]

Kidney (Costovertebral Tenderness)

Tenderness over the costovertebral angle posteriorly on the client has traditionally been thought of as a clinical examination for kidney pathology, although the diagnostic accuracy of this maneuver does not appear to have been investigated. To perform this assessment, the client is sitting (or can also be prone). The clinician stands directly behind and to the side of the client, placing a flat hand over the 12th rib at the costovertebral angle. The clinician then raps the back with their hand with a closed fist (using the ulnar border of the fist). A (+) test is subcostal back or flank and lateral abdomen pain.

Urological

Urological-related pathologies are often overlooked as potential contributors to the pain of a client who presents to the traditional orthopedic clinic. Variable clinical presentations, their diagnostic accuracy, and special considerations of the primary urological pathologies that the orthopedic clinician may encounter are presented here.

Four symptoms and one sign significantly increased the probability of urinary tract infections (UTI):

- Dysuria (painful urination) (summary +LR 1.5)
- High frequency of urination (+LR 1.8)
- Hematuria (+LR 2.0)
- Back pain (+LR 1.6)
- Costovertebral angle tenderness (+LR 1.7)

Four symptoms and one sign significantly decreased the probability of UTI:

- Absence of dysuria (**summary −LR 0.5**)
- Absence of back pain (−LR 0.8)
- History of vaginal discharge (**−LR 0.3**)
- History of vaginal irritation (**−LR 0.2**)
- Vaginal discharge on examination (−LR 0.7)

Of all individual diagnostic signs and symptoms, the two most powerful were history of vaginal discharge and history of vaginal irritation, which significantly decreased the likelihood of UTI when present (**−LRs 0.3** and **0.2,** respectively). The combination of signs or symptoms were more powerful (**+LR 24.6** for the combination of dysuria and frequency but no vaginal discharge or irritation) than one sign or symptom by itself.

In women who present with one or more symptoms of UTI, the probability of infection is approximately 50%. Specific combinations of symptoms (e.g., dysuria and frequency without vaginal discharge or irritation) raise the probability of UTI to more than 90%, effectively ruling in the diagnosis based on history alone.[106]

Gastrointestinal

Gastrointestinal contributions to pain in the client presenting to the orthopedic clinician are another often overlooked source requiring proper medical screening. Variable clinical presentations, their diagnostic accuracy, and special considerations of the

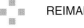

primary gastrointestinal pathologies that the orthopedic clinician may encounter are presented here.

Upper Gastrointestinal Bleed

Among clients who present with a gastrointestinal hemorrhage, an upper gastrointestinal bleed (UGIB) is more likely (incidence 63%) than a lower gastrointestinal bleed (LGIB). Among clients with UGIB, 36% require urgent intervention for severe bleeding.[107] Clients with gastrointestinal bleeding may present with visual evidence of blood loss such as hematemesis (vomiting of blood), hematochezia (bright red blood in stool), melena (black, tarry feces associated with UGIB), or coffee-ground emesis (vomiting). Clients may not always reliably recognize melena as visual evidence of bleeding. A UGIB source should be considered in all clients with evidence of gastrointestinal blood loss.[107]

Demographic and historical features suggestive of UGIB include prior history (**+LR 6.2**), age < 50 years (**+LR 3.5**), and cirrhosis (**+LR 3.1**). Clinical examination features suggestive of UGIB include report of black stool (melena; **+LR 25**) and nasogastric lavage with blood or coffee grounds (**+LR 9.6**). Clients reporting of melenic stool have a **+LR of 5.1 to 5.9**.[107]

Irritable Bowel Syndrome

The community-based prevalence of irritable bowel syndrome (IBS) is estimated to be between 5% and 20% of adults.[108] In clients referred to gastroenterologists for further evaluation, IBS is still likely, with 57% of referred clients diagnosed ultimately with irritable bowel syndrome.[109-111] Lower abdominal discomfort, changes in bowel habit or the nature of the passed stool, flatulence, passage of gas, or a sensation of incomplete rectal emptying all prompt consideration of IBS.[112] Among individual findings, only the presence of looser stools at the onset of abdominal discomfort has an +LR > 2.0. Lower abdominal discomfort has a +LR of 1.3 and a −LR of 0.29. The longer a client experiences symptoms without an alternative diagnosis, the higher the likelihood of IBS.[112]

Other Musculoskeletal Conditions

The majority of this text covers musculoskeletal conditions that are traditionally encountered by the practicing orthopedic clinician. Clinicians do need to be cognizant of other more medically related musculoskeletal-type pathologies. Variable clinical presentations, their diagnostic accuracy, and special considerations of the primary medically related musculoskeletal pathologies that the orthopedic clinician may encounter are presented here.

Septic Arthritis

In a recent review of the literature regarding septic arthritis (SA), the strongest screening variables were a lack of the following: joint pain (**SN 85**), a history of joint swelling (SN 78), and fever (SN 57). In fact, these were the only findings that occurred in more than 50% of clients. Sweats (SN 27) and rigors (SN 19) were of much lower clinical utility.[113]

Osteomyelitis in a Client With Diabetes

Commonly assessed clinical measures for the potential presence of osteomyelitis in a client with diabetes include the presence of a lower extremity ulcer, the area of the ulcer, and a probe-to-bone test. If a bone is exposed in a lower extremity ulcer, it is strongly suggestive of osteomyelitis (**+LR**

Critical Clinical Pearls

When performing a medical screen in an orthopedic (musculoskeletal) client, clinicians should consider the following:

- Typically, musculoskeletal pain is affected by various joint movements.
- Typically, musculoskeletal pain is made worse and better by various components of the examination.
- Lack of change in symptoms in a standard musculoskeletal (orthopedic) examination should alert the clinician to the potential presence of a medically related pathology.

9.2), although the absence of bone exposure is not enough to rule out osteomyelitis (−LR 0.70).

An ulcer area larger than 2 cm² makes osteomyelitis more likely (**+LR 7.2**), while an ulcer area smaller than 2 cm² decreases the likelihood by about half (**−LR 0.48**). Summary results from three studies suggest a positive probe-to-bone test result increases (**+LR 6.4**), while a negative test decreases (**−LR 0.39**) the likelihood of osteomyelitis.

To perform the probe-to-bone test of a foot ulcer, the clinician probes a sterile, blunt stainless steel probe into the wound, assessing for the presence of a rock-hard, gritty structure at the wound base in the absence of any intervening soft tissue. A (+) test is the presence of such a finding. A (−) test result is the inability to probe the base of the wound to the periosteum or bone.

Upper and Lower Quarter Screens

Once nonorthopedic (or nonmusculoskeletal) potential sources of pain are ruled out, the clinician must determine the necessity of an orthopedic screen and detailed examination of the nervous system. Content of this screen and examination are detailed in chapter 7.

TREATMENT-BASED CLASSIFICATION

Traditional and medical model labeling have suggested diagnostic labels for different pathologies. Such medical diagnoses predominantly identify a specific tissue pathology presumed to be the cause of a client's pain and dysfunction. This tissue pathology–based diagnostic labeling follows a pathoanatomic model of disease, where the pain-generating structure is identified. Many clinicians are taught to direct their classification toward this model in terms of, for example, signs and symptoms consistent with labral tear. A primary argument for this approach is that, since physicians use the same approach, clinicians theoretically enhance communication.[114] It has been demonstrated, though, that a specific criterion for each diagnostic label for various dysfunctions is not uniformly defined.[114-116]

More recently, the concept of treatment-based classification was adopted out of the concern that

evidence for efficacious treatment of low back pain (LBP) in the 1990s was elusive.[117] Delitto and colleagues argued that the reason for some treatments failing to demonstrate efficacy in randomized controlled trials was the false assumption that sufferers of LBP are a homogeneous group.[118] The importance of identifying homogeneous subgroups in randomized, controlled trials has been emphasized to avoid problems with sample heterogeneity.[118-122] The process of developing criteria for the identification of homogeneous subgroups within the LBP population is classification. Different potential types of classification schemes might include the following:

- Signs and symptoms: LBP classified according to client presentation of specific signs and symptoms
- Pathoanatomical: LBP classified according to pathology of a lumbar structure
- Psychological: LBP classified according to psychological criteria
- Social: LBP classified according to social criteria

While there are potentially other types of classification schemes than those listed prior, and while each of those listed has relevance, the literature currently supports the classification scheme based on signs and symptoms. Using the classification based on a client's signs and symptoms, and therefore treating clients accordingly, has been termed *treatment-based classification* (TBC). Treatment-based classification is based on the premise that subgroups of clients with LBP can be identified from key history and clinical examination findings.[118] Delitto and colleagues also hypothesized that each subgroup would respond favorably to a specific intervention, but only when applied to a matched subgroup's clinical presentation. Seven different classification groups were originally described in TBC for LBP;[118] however, recent investigations have collapsed the seven classification groups to four: manipulation, specific exercise (flexion, extension, and lateral shift patterns), stabilization, and traction.

The clusters of examination findings and matched interventions used in this TBC approach were principally derived from expert opinion, with little evidence support. Proper classification of clients into the appropriate category has proven reliable.[120, 123-126] Fritz and colleagues [125] and

Brennan and others[127] both provide support for the use of a TBC approach to classification and matched intervention for clients with LBP.

The potential limitations of TBC must be addressed, though. In a recent analysis investigating an algorithmic decision-making model regarding classification, the reliability of proper classification was only moderate (κ −0.52). Additionally, proper classification of those with LBP was a concern. Not all clients met criteria for a subgroup (25.2%).[128]

Therefore, while there are advantages and disadvantages of the various classifications, the approach taken in this text is to list the various commonly described pathologies relevant to each region of the body and, at the end of each pathology outlined, list the TBCs that are most likely to be associated with them. Listing appropriate TBCs is not a suggestion that the TBC method is the best-evidenced approach for classification of clients. In fact, as pointed out previously, this has only received literature support for LBP. It is simply an attempt to help the reader organize their findings from their examination in order to best determine the client's primary impairments and best treat their client.

CONCLUSION

Properly diagnosing a client presenting to the orthopedic clinician's clinic requires triage of the condition, screening for musculoskeletal and non-musculoskeletal serious pathology, and differential diagnosis of potential pathologies. At this point in the examination, the clinician is synthesizing information from the examination to determine if the client is appropriate for continued examination and intervention or referral to a more appropriate medical professional. Utilization of diagnostic accuracy best evidence assists in the determination of proper course of care for the client. Once the client is deemed appropriate for therapeutic intervention, TBC can be of potential benefit for addressing determined impairments.

7

ORTHOPEDIC SCREENING AND NERVOUS SYSTEM EXAMINATION

Michael P. Reiman, PT, DPT, OCS, SCS, ATC, FAAOMPT, CSCS
Adriaan Louw, PT, PhD, CSMT

Once red flags and nonmusculoskeletal contributions to the pain experience have been ruled out, the clinician must determine the contributions to the musculoskeletal pain experience. An efficient way to begin to differentiate the many potential pain referral sources is through the upper and lower quarter screening examination. The components of these screens are detailed in this chapter.

MUSCULOSKELETAL SCREENING

The traditional upper and lower quarter screen consists of testing dermatomes, myotomes, and deep tendon reflexes and possibly includes a cranial nerve and upper motor examination. Typically, a screening exam should be composed of tests with high sensitivity (SN).[1] Since the traditional neurological screen includes tests that are primarily specific (SP) rather than SN,[2] a positive test would help implicate pathology rather than rule it out.

The upper and lower quarter screens are intended to screen for other potentially relevant sources of nociception. These most likely sources are the joints proximal and distal to the pain location. *Referred multijoint pain, vague peripheral pain presentation, uncertainty regarding pain generation, radiating nature of pain, and unexplained gait, balance, coordination, atrophy, or weakness* are all appropriate reasons for employment of the upper or lower quarter screens. Additional reasons to use these screens might include the client's *presenting with an abnormal presentation, suspected psychogenic nociception, and poorly understood mechanism of onset*. It also must be noted that upper and lower quarter screens (at least the entire screen) are not always necessary. The use of these screens must be determined by the client presentation. For example, a client presenting with distinct pain over the acromioclavicular joint and presentation of acromioclavicular joint elevation compared to the other side without referred or unexplained pain would not require the entire upper quarter screen.

Overpressure to the area being examined helps rule out the structure as a potential contribution to the pain experience. When overpressure is applied, it should be done gradually. Overpressure should be applied only if active and passive ROM of the structure are pain free.

Potentially complicating the use of neurological screening measures are wide individual anatomic variations in nerve root innervations and myotome or dermatome descriptions.[1, 2] Symptoms associated with radiculopathies of nerve roots have also been reported to be highly variable and somewhat unpredictable.[3] Despite the limitations, it is generally recommended that reflexes, sensation, and myotomal testing are components of a normal standard of practice examination when indicated. As with all components of the examination, each component is encompassed in the entire examination to make a clinically informed decision regarding the differential diagnosis of the client being seen.

As mentioned, the traditional upper and lower quarter screen consists of testing of dermatomes (figure 7.1), myotomes, and deep tendon reflexes, and possibly examining upper motor (upper and lower quarter) and cranial nerves (upper quarter). The details of these components are listed later in this chapter (see the section Examination of the Physical Health of the Nervous System).

Upper Quarter Screen (UQS)

- Big-picture assessment: general observation for issues that may suggest serious pathology (e.g., significant asymmetry of posture, lack of involved extremity use, bruising or discoloration, swelling, and so on)
- Consciousness, mental status, communication, and cognitive screen (if necessary)
- Cranial nerve examination (if necessary)
- Vital signs
- Motion examination

- Active ROM of cervical spine with or without overpressure: The clinician should be cautious of a (+) Lhermitte's sign of cervical flexion causing a feeling of electrical shock or tingling down the spine. This is thought to signify the possible presence of spinal cord conditions including multiple sclerosis, tumors, or other space-occupying lesions.[4, 5]
    - Full bilateral shoulder flexion with or without overpressure
    - Full bilateral shoulder external rotation (placing bilateral hands behind head) with or without overpressure
    - Full bilateral shoulder internal rotation (reaching behind their back) with or without overpressure
    - Full bilateral elbow or wrist extension with or without overpressure
    - Full bilateral elbow or wrist flexion with or without overpressure
- Myotome examination
    - Resisted cervical rotation or flexion (C1)
    - Resisted cervical extension (C2)
    - Resisted side bending (C3)
    - Resisted shoulder shrug (C4)
    - Resisted shoulder abduction (C5)
    - Resisted elbow flexion and wrist extension (C6)
    - Resisted elbow extension and wrist flexion (C7)
    - Resisted thumb extension or finger adduction (C8)
    - Resisted finger abduction (T1)
- Sensory examination
- Reflex testing
    - Deep tendon reflexes
    - Superficial reflexes (if necessary)
    - Pathological reflexes (if necessary)
- Examination of coordination, balance, and gait (if necessary)

Lower Quarter Screen (LQS)

- Big picture assessment: general observation for issues that may suggest serious pathology

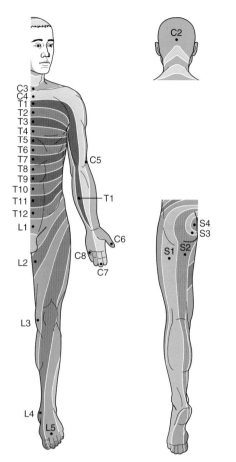

Upper Quarter Screen

C2 Occipital protuberance
C3 Supraclavicular fossa
C4 Acromioclavicular joint
C5 Lateral antecubital fossa
C6 Thumb
C7 Middle finger
C8 Little finger
T1 Medial antecubital fossa
T2 Apex of axilla

Lower Quarter Screen

L1 Upper anterior thigh
L2 Mid anterior thigh
L3 Medial femoral condyle
L4 Medial malleolus
L5 Dorsum 3rd MTP joint
S1 Lateral heel
S2 Popliteal fossa
S3 Ischial tuberosity
S4 Perianal area

Note: Test dermatomes at dots

Figure 7.1 Upper and lower quarter screen dermatome levels.

(e.g., significant asymmetry of posture, lack of involved extremity use, bruising or discoloration, swelling, and so on)

- Consciousness, mental status, communication, and cognitive screen (if necessary)
- Cranial nerve examination (if necessary)
- Vital signs
- Motion examination
  - Active ROM of the spine with or without overpressure
  - Deep squat
  - Full bilateral hip ROM with or without overpressure
  - Full bilateral knee flexion or extension with or without overpressure
  - Full bilateral ankle ROM with or without overpressure
- Myotome examination

  - Single-leg stance (L5-S1 myotome test)
  - Toe walking (S1)
  - Heel walking (L4-L5)
  - Resisted hip flexion (L1-L3)
  - Resisted knee extension (L3-L4) or single leg sit to stand
  - Resisted ankle dorsiflexion (L4-L5)
  - Resisted great toe extension (L5-S1)
- Sensory examination
- Reflex testing
  - Deep tendon reflexes
  - Superficial reflexes (if necessary)
  - Pathological reflexes (if necessary)
- Examination of coordination, balance, and gait (if necessary)

The clinician must always be cognizant of anything that can confound test finding. For example, prior knowledge of lumbar MRI results may introduce bias into the pinprick sensory testing component of the physical examination for lumbar radiculopathy.[6]

If the clinician suspects nervous system involvement, they should determine the extent of nervous system examination necessary. Various components of nervous system examination are appropriate to the practicing orthopedic clinician. These suggested components are listed throughout the rest of this chapter.

EXAMINATION OF THE PHYSICAL HEALTH OF THE NERVOUS SYSTEM

Examination of the nervous system, from an orthopedic standpoint, is comprehensive and variable depending on the client presentation. The clinician should always be cognizant of the potential contribution of nervous system involvement in their client's presentation, especially if there is radiating pain, unexplained pain, or broad, diffuse pain.

General Interview and Observation

As with all orthopedic examinations, the clinician should begin the examination with introduction to the client. Subjective questioning of mechanism of onset, functional limitations, general client observation, and symptom location, severity, and irritability should be implemented. Watching for signs of muscle tone (e.g., hand clawing, muscle fasciculation), muscle wasting, scars, and abnormal movements (e.g., tremor, other uncontrolled movements), as well of any assistive devices the client may present with are all general observations that can assist the clinician during the examination.

Consciousness, Mental Status, Communication, and Cognitive Screen

During the general interview and observation, the clinician can also get an idea of the client's mental status. Asking questions relative to person, place, time, and situation can help the clinician determine if the client is alert and oriented times four (person, place, time, and situation). As the client answers questions, the clinician can also get an appreciation of their language capability, including potential for dysphasia, dysarthria, and dysphonia. Memory can also be assessed with various questioning. The client's personality, emotion, and reasoning should also be appreciated during the subjective interview.

Mini Mental State Examination

The Mini Mental State Examination is an abbreviated mental test that assesses multiple aspects of cognition. The examination requires recall of orientation, recall of registration, language, and the ability to read, calculate numbers, and perform specific tasks.

Glasgow Coma Scale

The Glasgow Coma Scale is a measure of consciousness. In the orthopedic client, this examination is more important in injuries from motor vehicle accidents, concussions, traumatic brain injury, and similar types of injuries. Generally, this scale measures eye, verbal, and motor responses. A score ≥13/15 indicates a mild traumatic injury consistent with concussion. For more information on other measures for determining level of consciousness, potential head injury, and monohemispheric dysfunction, refer to chapter 15 (Face and Head).

Cranial Nerve Examination

Cranial nerves are 12 pairs of peripheral nerves emerging from the brain (first and second pair from the cerebrum and the rest from the brain stem; table 7.1). Clinically, the cranial nerves should be viewed similarly to peripheral nerves in regard to their biological functions of conduction and the need for space, movement, and adequate blood supply.[7] Cranial nerves are especially important in early detection or first contact clinician roles, such as sports medicine and emergency care. For example, cranial nerve testing is increasingly recommended for clinicians examining and treating acute whiplash and concussion clients as a means to screen for any serious brain, brain stem, or vertebral artery injury.

Coordination, Balance, and Gait Examination

Balance and postural control are the most practical and applicable means of testing neuromuscular control, but these domains should be assessed in

TABLE 7.1 Cranial Nerves and Their Examination

Nerve	Afferent (sensory)	Efferent (motor)	Test
I. Olfactory	Smell	—	Identify familiar odors (e.g., coffee)
II. Optic	Sight	—	Test visual fields
III. Oculomotor	—	Voluntary motor: levator of eyelid; superior, medial, and inferior recti Autonomic: smooth muscle of eyeball	Upward, downward, and medial gaze; reaction to light
IV. Trochlear	—	Voluntary motor: superior oblique muscle of eyeball	Downward and lateral gaze
V. Trigeminal (jaw reflex)	Touch, pain: skin of face, mouth, anterior tongue	Voluntary motor: muscles of mastication	Corneal reflex; face sensation; clench teeth and try to open mouth
VI. Abducens	—	Voluntary motor: lateral rectus muscle of eyeball	Lateral gaze
VII. Facial	Taste: anterior tongue	Voluntary motor: facial muscles Autonomic: lacrimal, submandibular, and sublingual glands	Close eyes tight; smile and show teeth; puff cheeks; identify familiar tastes (e.g., sweet and sour)
VIII. Vestibulocochlear (acoustic nerve)	Hearing: ear Balance: ear	— —	Hear watch ticking Hearing tests; balance and coordination tests
IX. Glossopharyngeal	Touch, pain: posterior tongue, pharynx Taste: posterior tongue	Voluntary motor: unimportant muscle of pharynx Autonomic: parotid gland	Gag reflex; ability to swallow
X. Vagus	Touch, pain; pharynx and larynx Taste: tongue, epiglottis	Voluntary motor: muscles of palate, pharynx, and larynx Autonomic: thoracic and abdominal viscera	Gag reflex; ability to swallow Say "Ahhh"
XI. Accessory	—	Voluntary motor: SCM and trapezius muscles	Resisted shoulder shrug
XII. Hypoglossal	—	Voluntary motor: muscles of tongue	Tongue protrusion (if injured deviates toward injured side)

Reprinted, by permission, from J. Loudon, R. Manske, and M. Reiman, 2013, *Clinical mechanics and kinesiology* (Champaign, IL: Human Kinetics), 42.

various means and environments. Various components of balance and postural control exist, and various tests can be implemented for assessment.

• **Anticipatory postural control tests:** observation of client catching something, lifting objects of different weights, and so on. The functional reach test and star excursion balance test are good examples of this type of testing.

• **Dynamic balance tests:** sitting and standing on unstable surfaces are good examples. Comparisons can be made between standing on stable and unstable surfaces. The Romberg test (client standing with bilateral feet together and eyes closed; clinician monitoring for swaying), more advocated as a static balance test, can also be utilized.

- **Reactive postural control tests:** client's responses to a push in a static position. These pushes can be small or large, anticipated versus unanticipated, and so forth.
- **Sensory organization tests:** comparison of balance on stable or unstable surface with respect to eyes open or closed.
- **Vestibular tests:** client's orientation in space relative to vestibular components (e.g., inner ear, balance).
- **Balance during functional activities:** assessing the client's balance and postural control in various environments and tasks that they may encounter.
- **Return-to-sport tests:** These are quite variable depending on the skill domain required to be assessed. Speed, agility, anaerobic power, and so on are various skill domains the clinician may need to assess in clients returning to sport. Various forms of hop testing are suggested as methods of assessing balance, power, and stability. Change-of-direction assessments, such as the T-test, are methods of testing speed, agility, power, and body control that are likely necessary in most sports. Refer to chapter 12 (Physical Performance Measures) for additional detail.
- **Gait:** For more detail, refer to chapter 13. Additionally, for the more neurologically oriented client, the clinician should assess for tremors and tone during gait.

It is beyond the scope of this chapter (and text) to describe all neuromuscular control, muscular performance, or performance tests applicable to various types of clients. For additional detail with respect to this type of testing, refer to chapters 9, 12, 27, and 28, each chapter in parts III and IV, and most notably Reiman and Manske.[8]

Vital Signs

The various vital signs are discussed in detail in chapter 6 (Triage and Differential Diagnosis). Refer to that chapter for the suggested examinations and their components, as well as the diagnostic accuracy of all of these measures.

Conduction

From a therapeutic perspective at least, three primary tests are important in regard to examining the normal functioning of the nervous system:

1. Conduction
2. Movement
3. Palpation

For optimal performance, electrochemical nerve impulses need to travel unhindered from the tissues to the spinal cord (sensory or afferent) and from the spinal cord to the muscles and tissues (motor or efferent). This process is referred to as *conduction*. Traditional conduction includes sensation testing, motor testing, and reflexes.[9, 10]

Reflex, myotome, and sensation testing traditionally compose neurological screening. The diagnostic utility of this type of testing is supported by little evidence. Additionally, the majority of these tests are more specific (SP) than they are sensitive (SN) and thus would serve less well as screening measures.[11-20] Further complicating the use of neurological screening measures are wide individual anatomic variations in nerve root innervations and myotome and dermatome descriptions;[1, 2] symptoms associated with radiculopathies of nerve roots have also been reported to be highly variable and somewhat unpredictable.[3] Despite the limitations of this type of testing, it is generally recommended that reflexes, sensation, and myotomal testing be components of a normal standard of practice examination. As with all components of the examination, each component is encompassed in the entire examination to make a clinically informed decision regarding the differential diagnosis of the client being seen.

Myotome or Motor Function Testing

Conduction is the ability of the efferent system to recruit proper and adequate muscle contraction. Each muscle has specific nerve innervation, and a structured process of assessing the ability of the client to perform an optimal muscle contraction may be used to measure whether the nerve conduction is interrupted. Clinicians are encouraged to memorize and learn the various spinal levels and their respective muscles.

As with sensory testing, the client receives an explanation and demonstration of the impending test. The targeted muscle or muscle group is steadily recruited to a point of maximum contraction and slowly released to avoid injury or sudden strain on the tissues, in effect, following the pattern of a bell-curve buildup, crescendo, and slow release. These break (all-or-nothing) tests establish the integrity of efferent activity of the nervous system. Additionally, clinicians can use scales (refer to chapter 9) to grade the strength of the muscle contraction to further aid in the examination of nerve conduction. Test responses need to be examined in comparison to the uninvolved side or known scales.

Specific myotome testing is described in table 7.2. Weakness of a specific myotome is suggestive

TABLE 7.2 Upper Quarter Myotome Testing

Level	Test	
C1	The clinician keeps the client's head in the mid position. They resist neck flexion or rotation by applying pressure to the chin, rather than to the forehead, and look for any sign of weakness.	
C2	The clinician keeps the client's head in the mid position. They apply force against the back of the head and once again ask the client to resist.	
C3	The clinician applies force against side bending to the left and to the right. They compare the two sides and look for any sign of weakness.	
C4	The clinician stands behind the client with both hands on top of the shoulder blades (supraspinous fossa). (They should not position hands over the upper trap = cranial nerve XI). The clinician asks the client to elevate (shrug) their shoulder blades, then compares left to right sides.	
C5	Abduction of the shoulder	
C6	Elbow flexion and supination and wrist extension	
C7	Elbow extension and pronation and wrist flexion	

(continued)

Table 7.2 *(continued)*

Level	Test	
C8	Flexion of the long finger adductors and thumb extension	
T1	Lumbricales and interossei (finger abduction)	

of that particular nerve root, whereas gross weakness and multisegmental level weakness are more likely suggestive of myelopathy, neuromuscular disease, or peripheral nerve injury.

To perform myotome (muscle strength and power) tests, the client should be in the most comfortable position, but should also be well supported. Important considerations when performing myotome testing include the following (also refer to chapter 4):

- Tests measure strength only. The clinician is not interested at pain at this time, although isometric contraction may cause pain.

- This test is *not* suggested to give a strength scale value. It is just to indicate weakness.

- The clinician should do the following:
  - Watch their own posture when testing
  - Get in good position to test effectively
  - Attempt to *break* the contraction
  - Compare side to side
  - If unsure, test again

Upper Quarter Myotome Testing   Myotome testing (table 7.2) is an essential component of the upper quarter screen. Assessing specific myotome levels can alert the clinician to not only the potential for nervous system involvement but also the potential for other muscle weaknesses that may be related to either that myotome level or the movement that was performed. Detailed testing of other muscles performing the same movement, especially if they are of a different myotome level, can assist with this differential diagnosis.

Lower Quarter Myotome Testing   As with the upper quarter testing, the general considerations described previously apply. Myotome levels are assessed as described in table 7.3.

Sensation Testing

Sensation is tested in various ways. The most commonly described and utilized methods are light touch and pinprick, while other methods include two-point discrimination, vibration, and temperature testing. Generally, dermatome patterns of sensory changes are associated with radiculopathies and multiple level or bilateral patterns of dermatome changes are associated with myelopathies.[4] Sensory testing thus primarily focuses on testing dermatomes and peripheral nerve innervations fields. Clinicians are encouraged to learn these sensory fields, memorize them, and help them guide their physical examinations and clinical reasoning. Due to the overlapping

---

Critical Clinical Pearls

A quick, clinical way to assess sensation may be a combination of the light touch and superficial pain testing methods. In this case, a paper clip is used to test dermatomal fields. It is likely more discreet and time-effective than a light touch test followed by a superficial pain test.

TABLE 7.3 Lower Quarter Myotome Testing

Level	Test	
L1, L2, L3	Hip flexion, with the client sitting and stabilizing themselves with bilateral hands on table. The client lifts the thigh and resists force from the clinician.	
L3, L4	Knee extension is performed a little short of full extension in sitting.	
L4, L5	Dorsiflexion and inversion in sitting. The client performs the combined movements, resisting force from the clinician.	
L5, S1	Big toe extension in sitting	

of the proximal dermatomal fields, the most distal segments of the sensory field should be tested.[9, 10]

To perform sensation testing, the clinician should explain the test to the client. The clinician should ask the client to identify the type of sensation they are experiencing; this could be numbness, pins and needles, pain, or weakness. The client can be seated or standing. The clinician should identify any relevant dermatomes or peripheral nerve innervation fields. It is recommended that clinicians use light touch to measure sensory changes. They should avoid stroking the skin (with either tissue paper or cotton wool) because it stimulates hair follicles, which may affect the findings of the test. Light touch is best performed with a monofilament (i.e., fishing line), dabbing the skin lightly.

Various testing options are available. First, the clinician can ask the client (while their eyes are open) if a tested area feels similar to another, nonaffected body part (i.e., other leg or a point more distal or proximal). The monofilament can be moved in order to develop an outline of the affected area. Next, the clinician asks the client to close their eyes and then spot-checks the affected area, thus stimulating various nonaffected areas and the affected area to establish the extent of the sensory loss.

Once light touch has been established, clinicians can proceed to examine additional sensory tests:

- *Superficial pain.* This sensation is often referred to as *pinprick.* It aims to stimulate A-delta and C-fibers. The clinician presses a sharp pin onto the client's skin and asks the client to report whether the sensation feels sharp or dull or say if they are unsure. The clinician should analyze this response in comparison to an uninvolved body part to establish the sensation to be normal or not.

- *Temperature.* If both light touch and superficial pain sensitivity are normal, a clinician may further test the sensory system using hot and cold sensations. The clinician fills one test tube with the hottest tap water available and another with the coldest water possible. They should ensure the test tubes are dry to avoid evaporation. Then, the clinician applies the test tubes (one at a time) to the affected areas on the client's body and asks the client to differentiate between hot and cold.

- *Proprioception.* Proprioception refers to the ability of the client to correctly identify the

spatial orientation of a body part. In these tests, the clinician gently handles the affected body parts to avoid a lot of pressure, moving them slightly into various positions and then asking the client (whose eyes are closed) to identify the position of the body part. For example, the clinician may move the big toe up and down several times, and then stop the movement with the toe pushed upward and ask the client, "Is the toe up or down?"

- Advanced sensory testing can follow, including two-point discrimination, graphesthesia (ability to use sensory input to identify a number or letter drawn onto the client's hand while visually occluded), and stereognosis (perceiving and understanding the form and nature of objects by the sense of touch).

- These tests are more indicated in advanced pain states, such as complex regional pain syndrome and chronic low back pain.

Clinicians should conduct testing sensation in the upper and lower quarters[9, 10] as follows:

- Use a paint brush or cotton wool to touch the hair.

- Test for pain (sharp) only if necessary.

- May use a pinprick (toothpick or paper clip) since it is more definitive (figure 7.2). Move around the leg, covering the probable affected dermatomes. Map out the area. (Dermatomes

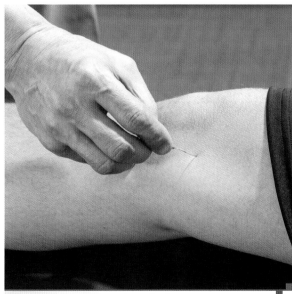

Figure 7.2 L3 dermatome testing.

may vary slightly; what is shown in figure 7.1 is used in this text.)

- Only the end of the dermatome is especially significant.
- The dermatomes overlap proximally, therefore the clinician tests distally.

Reflex Testing

Reflex testing generally involves deep tendon, superficial, and pathological reflex testing. Decreased deep tendon reflexes are suggestive of lower motor neuron dysfunction, most notably of the spinal nerve roots (e.g., radiculopathy), and they are generally considered part of a standard upper or lower quarter screen. Hyperactive reflexes, on the other hand, typically suggest upper motor neuron (UMN) dysfunction.

Reflex testing is a combination of afferent and efferent functions of the nervous system. The term *reflex testing* traditionally refers to muscle-tendinous reflexes. Reflex testing provides a quick stretch (with a tap of a hammer or hand) to a tendon or muscle belly, causing a reflexive contraction of the muscle. Any delay or decreased response to the quick stretch would indicate a nerve conduction issue. A lot of controversy exists as to what constitutes a normal versus an abnormal test. Medical literature uses scales of 1, 1+, and so on, but it has shown a large degree of disagreement among authors.[9, 10] Clinicians should consider a reflex abnormal if it differs from the response from the uninvolved side or other body parts. Based on the contraction, they should qualify the response as either hyperreflexive (increased or exaggerated contraction), hyporeflexive (less of a contraction, more like delay or fatigue), or absent (nonexistent),[21] although other scales are semiquantitatively graded on a scale as described in table 7.4.

Deep Tendon Reflex Testing   Generally, the cervical nerve roots are screened with testing the biceps, brachialis, and triceps tendons, while the lumbar nerve roots are screened with testing the patellar and Achilles tendons (figure 7.3). Some sources also suggest the extensor digitorum brevis, despite the fact that it is often difficult to elicit. The most commonly described deep tendon reflexes and their characteristics are detailed in table 7.5.

Here are some important considerations when performing deep tendon reflex testing:

- Repeat several times for accurate assessment.
- Hold the reflex hammer loosely, but with a firm grip.
- Drop the hammer instead of hitting the area with it.
- If you have difficulty finding a reflex, ask the client to grip their fingers and pull in opposite directions (Jendrassik maneuver).
- Muscle should have slight tension.
- Make the client concentrate on the contraction.
- Positioning the client in prone can assist when assessing the Achilles tendon reflex.[22]
- Determine whether or not you elicit a reflex.
- Compare both sides.
- By comparing side to side, you can decide what is normal for this client.

TABLE 7.4   Reflex Grading

Reflex response	Grade	Definition
Absence of reflex	0	Areflexia
Diminished reflex	1	Hyporeflexia
Average reflex	2	Normal or average
Exaggerated reflex	3	Hyperreflexia
Clonus	4	Spasmodic alteration of muscle contraction or relaxation indicating a nerve irritation

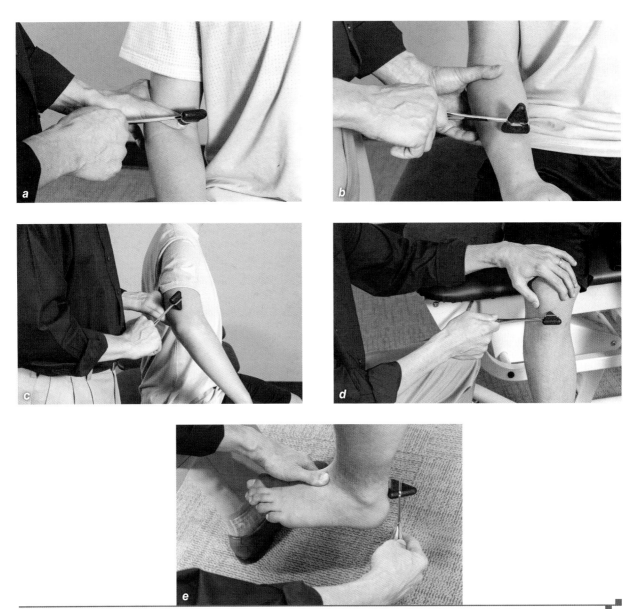

Figure 7.3   Reflex testing for *(a)* biceps, *(b)* brachioradialis, *(c)* triceps, *(d)* patella tendon, and *(e)* Achilles tendon.

Superficial Reflex Testing   Superficial reflexes are motor responses or reflexes elicited by stimulation of the skin. Unlike deep tendon reflexes (monosynaptic reflexes), these reflexes are polysynaptic. They are quite different from muscle stretch reflexes in that the sensory signal must not only reach the spinal cord but also ascend the spinal cord to reach the client's brain. The motor limb then has to descend the spinal cord to reach the motor neurons. This can be abolished by severe lower motor neuron damage or destruction of the sensory pathways from the skin that is stimulated. However, the utility of superficial reflexes is that they are decreased or abolished by conditions that interrupt the pathways between the brain and spinal cord (such as with spinal cord damage). They are graded simply as present or absent, although markedly asymmetrical responses should be considered abnormal as well (table 7.6). Only an absent or reduced superficial reflex has any clinical significance. Clear asymmetry is almost always pathological.

Pathological Reflex Testing   While reflexes and myotome and dermatome testing are suggestive of standard practice, examination for UMN

TABLE 7.5 Common Deep Tendon Reflexes

Reflex	Site of stimulation	Normal response	Segment	SN/SP	Q
Jaw	Mandible	Mouth closes	CN V	NR	NR
Biceps	Biceps tendon (see figure 7.3*a*)	Biceps contraction	**C5**-C6	24/95 14/90	10[13] 9[14]
Brachioradialis	Brachioradialis tendon (see figure 7.3*b*)	Elbow flexion/ FA pronation	C5-**C6**	6/95 17/94	10[13] 9[14]
Triceps	Distal triceps tendon (see figure 7.3*c*)	Elbow extension	**C7**-C8	3/93 14/92	10[13] 9[14]
Patella	Patellar tendon (see figure 7.3*d*)	Knee extension	**L3-L4**	12/96	9[14]
Medial hamstrings	Semimembranosus tendon	Knee flexion	**L5**, S1	NR	NR
Lateral hamstrings	Biceps femoris tendon	Knee flexion	S1-S2	NR	NR
Extensor digitorum brevis	Extensor digitorum brevis tendon	Toe extension	L5, S1	14/91	8[23]
Tibialis posterior	Tibialis posterior tendon	Plantar flexion	L4-L5	NR	NR
Achilles	Achilles tendon (Put tendon on slight stretch with passive dorsiflexion prior to test; see figure 7.3*e*.)	Plantar flexion	**S1**-S2	15/92 85/89	9[14] 6[24]

Q = QUADAS; SN = sensitivity; SP = specificity; CN = cranial nerve; FA = forearm

Bold indicates the primary level.

TABLE 7.6 Superficial Reflexes

Reflex	Description	Normal (or negative) response	Pertinent CNS segment
Upper abdominal	Stroke the skin of abdomen upward toward the midline and above the umbilicus	Umbilicus moves up and toward area being stroked	T7-T9
Lower abdominal	Stroke the skin of abdomen downward toward the midline and below the umbilicus	Umbilicus moves down and toward area being stroked	T11-T12
Cremasteric	Elicited in males by stroking the upper inside of the thigh	Scrotum elevates on the side of inner thigh that is stroked	T12, L1
Anal	Elicited by touching the perianal skin	Contraction of sphincter muscles	S2-S4

testing is likely not needed for all clients. Additional neurologic testing beyond standard practice is suggested when the previous portions of the examination (e.g., interview, observation, and screening) indicate their necessity. Such indications may include, but are not limited to, subjective reports of bilateral extremity involvement, trauma (especially to the spine), gait or balance disturbances, and observation of clonus. Commonly utilized tests for pathological reflex (UMN) testing are listed and described in table 7.7.

Movement

Clinicians interested in examining and treating the physical health of the nervous system require a knowledge of normal nerve movement, or *neu-*rodynamics.[30] One of the main roles of the nervous system is electrochemical communication, described previously in the section on conduction.[10] The nervous system needs to perform these complex signaling processes, while having to deal with movement issues (lengthening, sliding),[30, 31] pressure (tunnels, pinch, surrounding tissues),[9, 10, 30] and blood flow changes (increased and decreased blood flow, blood pressure changes).[9, 10, 30]

Under normal conditions, nerves move quite well.[30-33] Early cadaver studies showed that the nervous system is extremely well designed for handling movement. From a cervical spine neutral position to cervical spine flexion, the spinal cord lengthens approximately 10%,[34] while from cervical spine extension to cervical spine flexion, the cervical cord lengthens approximately 20%.[35]

TABLE 7.7   Pathologic Reflexes (Positive Testing Indicative of UMN Lesion)

Test	Description	(+) Response	SN/SP	QUADAS
Babinski	Stroking the lateral sole of foot in a sweeping motion toward ball of foot	Extension of hallux with or without splaying of other toes	33/**92** 35/77 7/100	10[25] 9[26] 7[27]
Chaddock's	Stroking the lateral side of the foot beneath the lateral malleolus	Same response as above	NA	NA
Oppenheim's	Stroking the anteromedial tibial surface	Same response as above	NA	NA
Clonus	Ankle is taken to end dorsiflexion ROM passively and a quick overpressure into dorsiflexion is applied with pressure to the ankle maintained	>3 involuntary beats will be present	11/96 7/99 13/100	10[25] 7[27, 28]
Hoffmann's (upper extremity)	Flick the terminal phalanx of the index, middle, or ring finger	Reflex flexion of distal phalanx of thumb and of distal phalanx of whichever finger is not flicked (OK sign)	44/75 58/74	10[25] 8[29]

The spinal canal can lengthen approximately 30% from spinal extension to spinal flexion.[36] The peripheral nervous system must be able to accommodate increased movement as well, and research has shown that from a position of wrist and elbow flexion to a position of wrist and elbow extension, the median nerve must adapt to a nerve bed that is almost 20% longer.[37]

Neurodynamic tests, therefore, are tests to examine the ability of the client's nervous system to accommodate to movement. The tests furthermore examine physiologically whether the nervous system has adequate blood, as well as the system's sensitivity and ability to handle movement and compression and pressure changes. These tests can be performed actively or passively, although passively ensures end ROM assessment if that is necessary.

Active Neurodynamics

In the past, tests were almost always performed as passive; that is, they were led by clinicians. With increased understanding of pain, nerve sensitivity, and client care, it is recommended where possible that clients perform the active neurodynamic test before the passive version. The client can control the amount of pain or sensitivity they able or willing to go into. If no issues are identified during the active tests, the more elaborate, time-consuming physical tests, especially upper limb tests, may not be needed. Remember that the nervous system is very susceptible to anxiety[38] and catastrophization.[39]

Passive Neurodynamics

Passive neurodynamic tests follow the active tests if needed. The clinician should explain the test to the client and avoid provocative terminology.[40] They should be gentle and should slowly and carefully engage barriers to movement. A good clinician can feel barriers before a client expresses a symptom (e.g., pain). They should not always look for pain. Many clients will develop tightness or resistance before pain. Due to the complexities of pain, clinicians should be careful in analyzing the symptoms.

Neurodynamic tests assess the mechanical movement of the nervous system tissues as well as their level of sensitivity to mechanical stress or compression.[9, 41] A very important consideration would be how to analyze the finding of a neurodynamic test. If a client extends their arm out to the side and they develop a pull, ache, or even pain in the wrist, what causes it? It can be a nerve, likely median, but it can also be from a joint, tendon, or the skin.[10, 30, 31] A helpful way to determine if the nervous system is a likely cause of the symptoms is structural differentiation. Structural differentiation is the process whereby an evoked response is altered with the adding or subtracting of a remote body part. The fact that the nervous system is continuous would imply, for example, that if wrist extension causes pain and neck side flexion increases or decreases the evoked response, the chance of it being neurogenic in nature increases. No muscles connect the wrist to the neck; no joint connects the neck to the wrist.

What is a positive test? Only 20% of clients may actually report their pain during neurodynamic testing.[42] Given the complexities of the nervous system (blood supply, immune responses, muscle spindles), clients may actually report a variety of muscle symptoms including tightness, pulling, and stretching or neurological symptoms such as pins and needles, numbness, or burning. Clinicians may compare left and right and normal data from research. They should utilize structural differentiation to further enhance examination and add subjective examination clues.[43] The ultimate question as to a positive test is if the examination finding should be addressed to help increase the client's function.

Upper Limb Neurodynamic Tests

The upper limb neurodynamic test (ULNT) neurodynamically tests the brachial plexus; through having the client perform selective movements, the clinician can differentiate between the three major nerves supplying the upper extremity:[9, 10]

- Median nerve
- Ulnar nerve
- Radial nerve

Four neurodynamic tests (passive assessment) are discussed in the upper limb:

- ULNT 1 Median nerve dominant using shoulder abduction
- ULNT 2a Median nerve dominant using shoulder depression and external rotation
- ULNT 2b Radial nerve dominant using shoulder depression and internal rotation
- ULNT 3 Ulnar nerve dominant using shoulder abduction and elbow flexion

Unless subjective examination directs otherwise, the clinician may wish to first screen upper limb neurodynamics with active screens.[10] The active neurodynamics allow the clinician to determine the client's willingness to move and their level of irritability.

Active neurodynamic screens are a quick client self-assessment that determines the potential irritability the client may have with neurodynamic testing (figure 7.4a-c). The tests are active movements as detailed in the actual passive tests that follow.

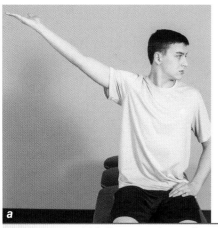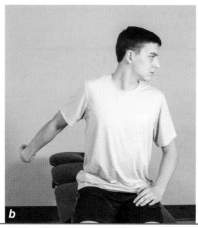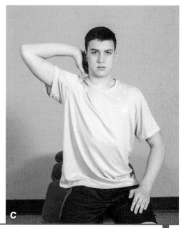

Figure 7.4   *(a)* Active screen for median nerve bias, *(b)* active screen for radial nerve bias, and *(c)* active screen for ulnar nerve bias.

ULNT 1: MEDIAN NERVE BIAS

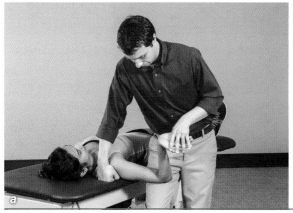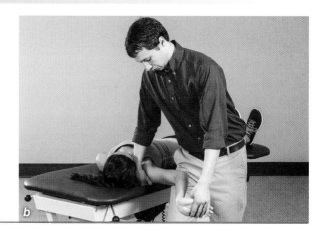

Figure 7.5

Client Position	Lying supine, with the side to be assessed close to the edge of the table. If possible, *do not* use a pillow.
Clinician Position	Standing in stride, facing the client. One hand controlling the client's shoulder and the other controlling the hand, including the fingertips and thumb *(a)*.
Movement	The clinician places the fist of their arm (the one closest to the client) on the table above the client's shoulder to keep it from elevating during abduction. The clinician abducts the client's arm to the point of resistance by using their thigh to walk the arm up into the abduction position *(b)*. With the client's elbow still flexed, the clinician supinates the client's forearm and extends the wrist and fingers, including the thumb. The clinician then externally rotates the shoulder. Next, they extend the client's elbow. By strictly maintaining the earlier components, the clinician may add neck side bend-

 Video 7.5 **in the web resource shows a demonstration of this test.**

ing toward or away from the tested side. They should take care not to rotate the client's head—this is pure side bending. The important part of neurodynamic tests is to maintain load from the beginning of the test to the completion of the test. Furthermore, clinicians should be sure to *identify* and *interpret* symptoms and symptom changes from one step to another. They must inquire about any symptoms as they add components of the ULNTs.

Assessment   A (+) test is defined by the following criteria:

- Reproduction of client's symptoms
- Side-to-side differences (reproduces concordant pain on involved side and nonconcordant symptoms on noninvolved side)
- Affected by a distant component: contralateral neck side bending increases symptoms or ipsilateral side bending decreases symptoms.

Statistics   **SN 97 (90-100)**, SP 22 (12-33), +LR 1.3, **−LR 0.12**, QUADAS 10, in a study of 82 clients suspected to have cervical radiculopathy or carpal tunnel syndrome (mean age 45 ± 12 years, 41 women, duration of symptoms NR), using a reference standard of electromyography and nerve conduction study.[13]

Notes
- Elbow extension can also be a good comparative sign, but cervical side bending is typically suggested.
- Indications: symptoms in the arm, head, neck, and thoracic spine; any neurological symptoms that imply impaired nervous tissue.
- Biomechanics: Shoulder abduction stresses the C5, C6, and C7 nerve roots.

ULNT 2A: MEDIAN NERVE (USING SHOULDER DEPRESSION AND EXTERNAL ROTATION)

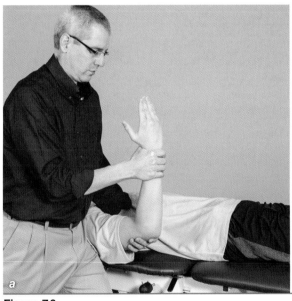 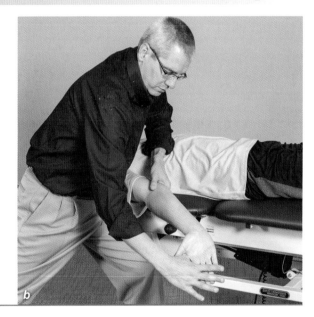

Figure 7.6

Client Position   Lying across the table, in a slightly diagonal orientation, with the scapula of the side to be tested at the edge of the table

Clinician Position   Standing at the head of the table

Movement   The clinician holds the client's right wrist with their right hand and the client's elbow with their left hand *(a)*. This position allows minimal hand change, thus allowing a smoother and better-controlled movement. The clinician's thigh rests against the client's shoulder. Using the thigh, the clinician carefully prevents abduction of the client's shoulder. This positioning allows the clinician to closely watch the client's face for nonverbal cues. The clinician carefully externally

(continued)

ULNT 2a: Median Nerve (Using Shoulder Depression and External Rotation) *(continued)*

rotates the client's whole arm, and then carefully slides their fingers down the client's fingers and extends the client's fingers and wrist *(b)*. They should carefully abduct the client's arm until they locate symptoms or resistance. Releasing the shoulder depression will help them differentiate neural tissue sensitization. If needed, clinicians can add or subtract neck side bending.

Assessment   A (+) test is defined by the following criteria:

- Reproduction of client's symptoms.

- Side-to-side differences (reproduces concordant pain on involved side and nonconcordant symptoms on noninvolved side).

- Affected by a distant component: Contralateral neck side bending increases symptoms or ipsilateral side bending decreases symptoms; additionally release of shoulder depression eliminates symptoms.

Statistics   NR

ULNT 2B: RADIAL NERVE

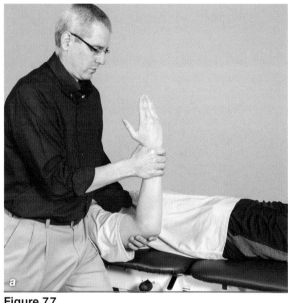 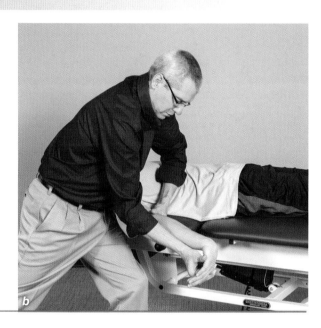

Figure 7.7

Client Position   Lying across the table, in a slightly diagonally orientation, with the scapula of the side to be tested at the edge of the table

Clinician Position   Standing at the head of the table

Movement   Clinician holds the client's right wrist with their right hand and the client's elbow with their left hand *(a)*. This position allows minimal hand change, thus allowing for smoother and better-controlled movement. The clinician's thigh rests against the client's shoulder. Using the thigh, the clinician carefully prevents abduction of the client's shoulder. This positioning allows the clinician to closely watch the client's face for nonverbal cues. By reaching under the client's arm, the clinician internally rotates it. This is the *key factor* of this test. Inevitably the client's forearm will go into pronation. The clinician should use their left hand to keep the client's elbow from flexing *(b)*. They should carefully abduct the client's arm until they locate symptoms or resistance. Taking off the shoulder depression will help the clinician differentiate neural tissue. Additionally, they can choose neck movements.

Assessment   A (+) test is defined by the following criteria:

- Reproduction of client's symptoms.

- Side-to-side differences (reproduces concordant pain on involved side and nonconcordant symptoms on noninvolved side).

- Affected by a distant component: Contralateral neck side bending increases symptoms or ipsilateral side bending decreases symptoms; additionally release of shoulder depression eliminates symptoms.

Statistics   SN 64 (45-83), SP 30 (17-42), +LR 0.9, –LR 1.2, QUADAS 10, in a study of 82 clients with carpal tunnel syndrome (mean age 45 ± 12 years, 41 women, mean duration of symptoms 183 days), and using electrophysiological examination as a reference standard[44]

ULNT 3: ULNAR NERVE

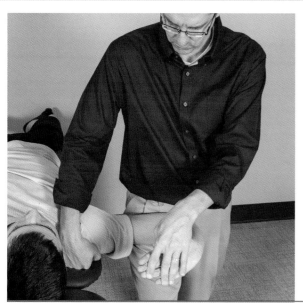 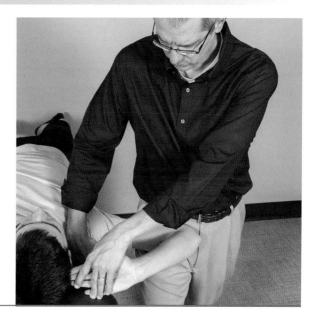

Figure 7.8

Client Position   Lying supine, with the side to be assessed close to the edge of the table. If possible, *do not* use a pillow.

Clinician Position   Stride-standing position

Movement   The clinician places the fist of their arm (the one closest to the client) on the table above the client's shoulder to keep it from elevating during abduction. They extend the client's wrist and fingers, pronate the client's forearm, flex the client's elbow, and externally rotate the client's whole upper arm. They should place the client's elbow against their ASIS or thigh and then carefully move the client's arm into abduction. Cervical side bending away from and toward the side being tested (and symptoms) may add or release neural load.

Assessment   A (+) test is defined by the following criteria:

- Reproduction of client's symptoms.
- Side-to-side differences (reproduces concordant pain on involved side and nonconcordant symptoms on noninvolved side).
- Affected by a distant component: Contralateral neck side bending increases symptoms or ipsilateral side bending decreases symptoms.

Notes   Any neurological symptoms arising from the C8 and T1 nerve roots would indicate using the ULNT 3. Disorders such as golfer's elbow may also indicate the use of the ULNT 3. Any neurological symptoms provoked by movements above the head may indicate the use of the test.

Lower Limb Neurodynamic Tests

As with upper limb tension testing, clinicians should assess neurodynamic dysfunction in the lower extremity in a systematic and defined manner, as described previously. The tests for the lower extremity primarily consist of the straight leg raise (SLR) test and the femoral nerve test. The slump test is commonly described in this category as well, although it might also be argued as an overall system neurodynamic assessment. It is suggested that the slump test is a completely different test than the SLR test.[9, 10] The slump test is best indicated in chronic conditions, suspected canal problems, and functional positions.[9, 10] The dura is tightest at T6. Additionally, the C6, L4, and posterior knee have been described as normal tension points, where the nervous system is normally most tight.[9, 10] Therefore, it is normal for clients to feel a stretch or slight burn in this region.

SLUMP TEST

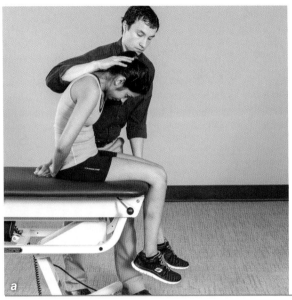 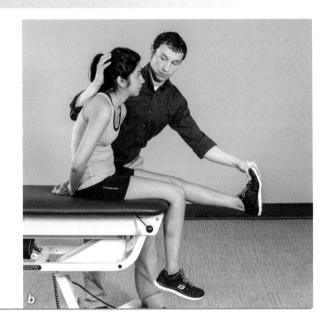

Figure 7.9

As with all neurodynamic tests, the slump test should be performed gently and gradually. As with the other neurodynamic techniques, clinicians should conduct testing in a step-by-step manner and monitor symptoms after each of the following systematic steps:

 Video 7.9 **in the web resource shows a demonstration of this test.**

Client Position	Sitting on table with the thighs well supported and the back of their knees against edge of the table; hands placed behind their back
Clinician Position	Sitting on the table or standing next to the client's affected side

Movement   The clinician asks the client to slump. They then assess for symptoms by gently placing their elbow on the thoracic spine (applying no pressure), and then gently putting two fingers on the client's head (again, no pressure). The clinician asks the client to gently flex the cervical spine, and then assesses for any symptoms *(a)*. The clinician asks the client to actively extend the good leg first until they feel any resistance, and then assesses for any symptoms. Next, the clinician asks the client to extend the symptomatic side. The clinician may need to passively extend the client's knee to full extension in order to rule out symptoms. They should assess for symptoms and compare to the other side. When the point of resistance is reached, the clinician should ask the client to gently extend their head and then notice whether any changes in the leg and back symptoms occur *(b)*. They can add dorsiflexion to increase tension. The clinician should check signs and symptoms at each stage of the test. They can also perform the whole test passively for the client to get a better feel for the resistance. The following order of implementation of movement can help structural differentiation of symptom provocation:

- Spine symptoms are more likely provoked with the following movement sequence: slump, neck flexion, knee extension.

- Leg symptoms are more likely provoked with the following movement sequence: dorsiflexion, knee extension, slump, neck flexion.

In a normal young person, extension of the knee and dorsiflexion may be decreased by 15° to 20° due to muscle shortening.

Assessment   A (+) test is defined by the following criteria:

- Reproduction of client's concordant pain.

- Symptoms are different from those on the other side (reproduces concordant pain on involved side and nonconcordant symptoms on noninvolved side).

- Symptoms are affected by a distant component movement (typically it is best to use head movement as the distant component).

Statistics - **SN 83 (NR)**, SP 55 (NR), +LR 1.8, **−LR 0.32**, QUADAS 11, in a study of 105 clients with suspicion of discogenic pathology (mean age 42.7 ± 9.8 years, 36 women, 72% of cases' mean duration was greater than 3 months), using CT or MRI as a reference standard[19]

- SN 84 (NR), SP 83 (NR), +LR 4.9, −LR 0.19, QUADAS 7, in a study of 75 clients with clinical suspicion of disc herniation (mean age of 38-40 years in symptom and control groups, 20 women, symptom duration of less than 12 weeks), using MRI as a reference standard[45]

STRAIGHT LEG RAISE (SLR) TEST

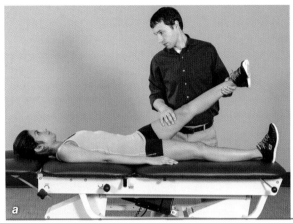 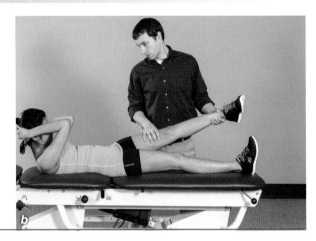

Figure 7.10

As with all neurodynamic tests, the SLR test should be performed gently and gradually. As with the other neurodynamic techniques, clinicians should perform testing step by step and monitor symptoms after each of the following systematic steps:[9, 10, 30]

 Video 7.10 **in the web resource shows a demonstration of this test.**

Client Position	Supine, with bilateral legs relaxed and leg to be assessed close to edge of table
Clinician Position	Standing next to client's leg to be assessed, directly facing client
Movement	The clinician should perform the test on the good leg first for the client's comfort and understanding of testing. Whether using a pillow or not (not using a pillow is preferred), the clinician should be sure to keep the position constant for reassessments. The clinician comfortably grasps the client's leg above the malleolus with one hand and places their other hand above the client's knee to maintain knee extension. Next, they comfortably raise the client's leg straight up. The traditional test has been described with slight hip adduction and internal rotation *(a)*.[9] The clinician feels for any resistance and compares side to side. They can accomplish further sensitization with foot dorsiflexion and internal rotation.
Assessment	A (+) test requires all three of the following criteria to be present: • Reproduction of client's concordant pain. • Symptoms are different than those on the other side (reproduces concordant pain on involved side and nonconcordant symptoms on noninvolved side). • Symptoms are affected by a distant component movement (head movement) *(b)* or bias with the foot and ankle as suggested by many other sources.
Statistics	• Pooled analysis: **SN 92 (87-95)**, SP 28 (18-40), +LR 2.9, **–LR 0.29** in a systematic review of 16 studies with surgery as a reference standard.[46] • Pooled analysis: **SN 91 (82-94)**, SP 26 (16-38), +LR 2.7, **–LR 0.35** in a systematic review of 17 diagnostic studies with surgery only as a reference standard.[47] • **SN 97 (NR)**, SP 57 (NR), +LR 2.2, **–LR 0.05**, QUADAS 10, in a study of 274 clients with pain radiating into leg (mean age 46 ± 12 years, 135 women, median duration of symptoms 19 days), using MRI as a reference standard.[48] • SN 89 (NR), SP 14 (NR), +LR 1.0, –LR 0.78, QUADAS 7, in a study of 55 clients with unilateral sciatica (mean age and gender NR), using surgery as a reference standard.[49]

- SN 98 (NR), SP 44 (NR), +LR 1.8, –LR 0.05, QUADAS 7, in a study of 100 clients with lumbar disc protrusions (and 36 control clients with LBP and sciatica, but normal myelogram and no surgery; mean age and gender NR), using surgery as a reference standard.[18]
- SN 52 (NR), SP 89 (NR) +LR 4.7, –LR 0.54, QUADAS 7, in a study of 75 clients with clinical suspicion of disc herniation (mean age of 38-40 years in symptom and control groups, 20 women, symptom duration of less than 12 weeks), using MRI as a reference standard.[45]
- Agreement between SLR and Slump test (κ = 0.64) in a study of 45 clients with unilateral leg pain (mean age 46 ± 11 years, 23 women, mean duration of symptoms was 5.6 ± 5.7 months).[43]
- Women were 7.5 times more likely and men were 23 times more likely to test (+) for SLR test when in personal injury program than in workmen's compensation.[50]
- The SLR test is generally considered an assessment of the L5, S1, and S2 nerve roots as they are completely stretched at 70° per findings in a cadaver study.[51] The clinician must consider client variability with respect to this finding.

Special Considerations Multiple biases of the SLR test exist for various distal lower extremity nerves:[9]
- Sural nerve: hip flexion, knee extension, ankle dorsiflexion, and foot inversion
- Tibial nerve: hip flexion, knee extension, ankle dorsiflexion, foot eversion, and toes extended
- Common peroneal nerve: hip flexion and internal rotation

Lasègue's test is similar in that the client reports pain below the knee, which increases with neck flexion and decreases as head returns to neutral. The bowstring test is a variation of this test. The clinician (after performing a SLR test), keeps the client's thigh in the same position and passively flexes the client's knee 20°, reducing symptoms. The clinician then applies pressure to the popliteal region with a thumb or finger to re-establish the painful radicular symptoms. No diagnostic accuracy values have been reported for this test.[52]

WELL LEG RAISE TEST (CROSSED STRAIGHT LEG RAISE)

Essentially, the client and clinician positions and the movement are the same as for the SLR test, except that raising the noninvolved side elicits symptoms down the involved side.

Assessment A (+) test requires all three of the following criteria to be present:
- Reproduction of client's concordant pain.
- Symptoms are different than the other side (reproduces concordant pain on involved side and nonconcordant symptoms on noninvolved side).
- Symptoms are affected by a distant component movement (typically it is best to use head movement as the distant component).

Statistics
- Pooled analysis: SN 28 (22-35), **SP 90 (85-94)**, +LR 2.8, –LR 0.36 in a systematic review of 16 studies with surgery as a reference standard[46]
- SN 24 (NR), SP 100 (NR), QUADAS 7, in a study of 55 clients using unilateral sciatica and surgery as a reference standard[49]
- SN 43 (NR), SP 97 (NR), +LR 14.3, –LR 0.59, QUADAS 7, in a study of 100 clients with lumbar disc protrusions (and 36 control clients with LBP and sciatica, but normal myelogram and no surgery; mean age and gender not reported), using surgery as a reference standard[18]

Critical Clinical Pearls

When performing neural tension and discogenic symptom tests (e.g., SLR, well leg SLR, slump), the clinician should keep the following in mind:

- Progress slowly with testing, especially if the client has a high degree of symptom irritability.
- Sequentially perform the step-by-step movements.
- Maintain each previous position or movement when performing the next movement.
- Always perform the examination on the uninvolved side first.

FLIP SIGN (SITTING SLR)

The flip test is a sitting version of the SLR test.

Client Position	Sitting on table with legs off to one side, maintaining upright posture
Clinician Position	Sitting directly to the side of the client
Movement	The clinician places the open palm of one hand against the client's distal thigh, depressing it against the table, and places the other hand under the heel cord so that the client's heel rests in the palm. Next, the clinician gradually extends the affected limb at the knee.
Assessment	With genuine sciatic tension, no resistance or complaints are noted until approximately 45° of knee extension is reached, but continuance of elevation past that point (toward full knee extension) is attended with an acute reversal of the lumbar lordosis. The client may have a tendency to fall backward, flipping back onto their arms as the name of the drill suggests. The most reliable response is not a flip but rather the demonstration of pain on extension of the knee. The term *sitting SLR test* is therefore recommended as a more accurate name.[53]
Statistics	• 67 clients with sciatica and MRI scans confirming disc protrusion and nerve root compression were examined.[53]

- 33% had no pain.
- 39% had pain on full extension of knee +/– leaning back with hands in braced position.
- 28% had pain and resisted full extension of knee +/– leaning back with hands in braced position.

• SN of supine SLR was 67, compared with SN of 41 of the seated SLR test (P = 0.003) on 71 consecutive clients referred to neurologic surgery clinic, and using MRI as a reference standard.[54]

PRONE KNEE-BEND (PKB) TEST

Both versions of the prone knee-bend test measure L1, L2, L3, and L4 tension. As with all neurodynamic testing, the clinician should be sure that the findings are relevant to the client's complaint. Neurodynamic testing of the femoral nerve can be performed with the following technique:[9, 10]

Client Position	Prone, with head turned to side to be assessed
Clinician Position	Standing on side of leg to be assessed, directly facing client
Movement	The clinician grasps the client's leg just above the malleolus and stabilizes their pelvis with the other hand on the posterior superior iliac spine. The clinician passively flexes the knee of the leg to be assessed until symptoms are produced. Once symptoms are produced, sensitizing movements can include ankle plantar flexion or dorsiflexion, or head movements. Knee flexion restricted between 0° and 90° could test several structures: femoral nerve, psoas, rectus femoris, the fascia, and so on.
Assessment	A (+) test is reproduction of concordant symptoms on the involved side and not present on the noninvolved side.

FEMORAL NERVE TENSION IN SIDE LYING TEST

Another version of L1-L4 neurodynamic testing is the femoral nerve tension in side lying test (also known as the prone knee bending in side lying test). This version may be preferred as it is difficult to bias with head movement in the previously stated version. The femoral nerve tension in side lying test involves the following sequence of movements:

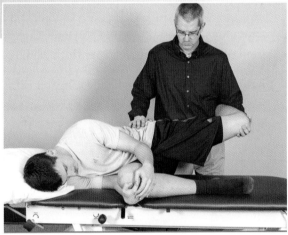

Figure 7.11

Client Position	Side lying, with symptomatic side facing the ceiling
Clinician Position	Standing directly behind the client
Movement	The client flexes the bottom leg, holding it at the knee, and slumps the upper body with neck flexion. The clinician stabilizes the client's pelvis and flexes the knee of the top leg to 90°. The clinician gently extends the hip until resistance is felt. While keeping the leg at the point of discomfort, the clinician asks the client to extend their cervical spine. If possible, this can be performed passively. Adding cervical spine flexion or extension creates a very powerful structural differentiation, with extension decreasing and flexion increasing symptoms in clients with neural tension. Any alteration of thigh or groin symptoms with neck movements would implicate the nervous system.
Assessment	A (+) response for these tests should include all of the following: • Reproduction of client's concordant pain. • Symptoms are different than the other side (reproduces concordant pain on the involved side and nonconcordant symptoms on the noninvolved side). • Symptoms are affected by a distant component movement (typically it is best to use head movement as the distant component).

Palpation

Palpation has been highlighted in physical medicine, especially regarding its poor inter- and intrarelater reliability. More precisely, palpation has shown poor reliability in spine assessments for hypo- and hypermobility. There is better reliability in palpating the area and provoking pain or not. Nerve palpation has gained increased attention by showing increased reliability in mechanosensitivity, SN, and SP.[43, 55-60]

Nerve palpation is important for relearning nerve anatomy and pathways of nerves. It has been shown to help with diagnosis and could help with treatment (e.g., neural massage for the more superficial nerves). Nerves change their shape and amount of connective tissue based on function. Areas with more connective tissue are less sensitive. More sensitive nerves are found around the large-spanning elbow and knee. Nerves are round compared to tendons. They slide around and may give typical neurogenic responses. Nerves are sensitive and vulnerable in tunnels, where they branch off; over hard bony areas, they are fixed.[10] The following are suggested sites for nerve palpation.[10]

Median Nerve

The median nerve is most easily palpated (primarily for symptom reproduction) in the upper arm. The clinician places the client's arm in approximately 80° of shoulder abduction. They then palpate the midline axilla to biceps tendon (figure 7.12). The clinician can also indirectly palpate the median nerve in the carpal tunnel.

Ulnar Nerve

The ulnar nerve can also be palpated in the upper arm. The clinician should palpate the inferior aspect of the upper extremity, in line with axilla and cubital tunnel, placing the arm again in slight abduction (figure 7.13). The ulnar nerve can also be palpated in the cubital tunnel. This nerve can also be more sensitive to touch once it exits the cubital tunnel and branches. The clinician can also palpate the Guyon canal lateral to the pisiform bone and medial to the hook of the hamate, assessing for symptom reproduction.

Radial Nerve

The radial nerve is not easily palpable, but clinicians can palpate at the radial spiral groove, the arcade of Frohse (supinator arch), the anterior lateral aspect of forearm, and where the nerve crosses the anatomical snuffbox, assessing for symptom reproduction.

Saphenous Nerve

Clinicians can find the saphenous nerve at the adductor canal (Hunter's canal), palpating the medial tibial plateau of the knee (figure 7.14). As with all nerve palpation, symptom reproduction is the primary finding.

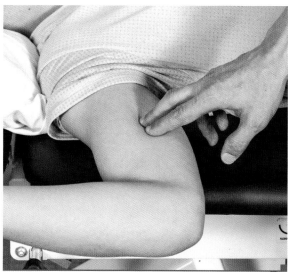

Figure 7.12 Palpation of the median nerve in the upper arm.

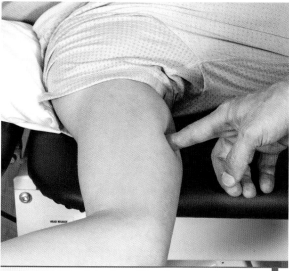

Figure 7.13 Palpation of the ulnar nerve in upper arm.

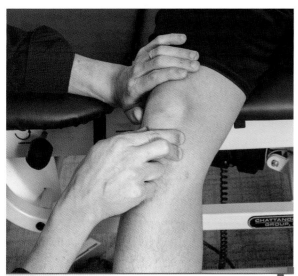

Figure 7.14   Palpation of saphenous nerve at medial tibial plateau.

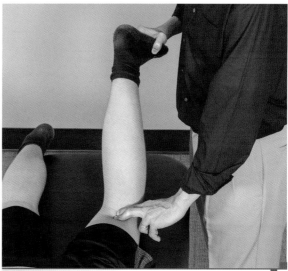

Figure 7.15   Palpation of tibial nerve in the popliteal space.

Lateral Femoral Cutaneous Nerve

The lateral femoral cutaneous nerve is implicated in conditions such as meralgia paresthetica. Clinicians should palpate it slightly anterior and lateral of the anterior superior iliac spine of the pelvis, looking for symptom reproduction.

Sciatic Nerve

The sciatic nerve is palpated along the medial one-third of the buttock. Clinicians will perform an indirect palpation due to the depth of this nerve in the buttock, assessing for symptom reproduction. For additional detail on palpation of the sciatic nerve, refer to chapter 19 (Lumbar Spine).

Tibial Nerve

The tibial nerve is palpated in the midline of the posterior knee (popliteal space). Clinicians can use hip and knee flexion, as well as ankle dorsiflexion and plantar flexion, to assist with palpation for symptom reproduction (figure 7.15). Additionally, they can palpate the tibial nerve along the posterior tarsal tunnel (posterior to medial malleolus). Again, symptom reproduction is primary finding.

Common Peroneal Nerve: Knee

The common peroneal nerve can be palpated posterior to the superior tibiofibular joint (figure 7.16). Nerve movement can be felt with ankle movements.

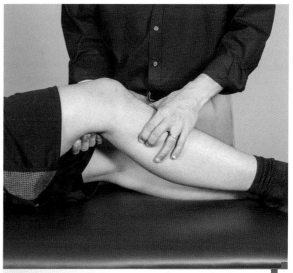

Figure 7.16   Common peroneal nerve palpation at the superior tibiofemoral joint.

Deep Peroneal Nerve

The deep peroneal nerve can be palpated for symptom reproduction just lateral to the extensor hallucis longus tendon (figure 7.17). Clinicians should palpate at the distal aspect of this tendon, just prior to the metatarsal phalangeal joint and then just lateral for the nerve.

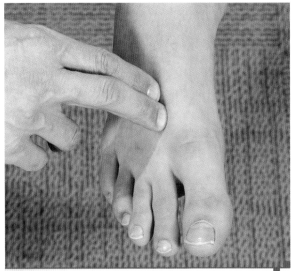

Figure 7.17 Deep peroneal nerve palpation, lateral to the extensor hallucis tendon.

Sural Nerve

Clinicians should palpate the sural nerve between the Achilles tendon and lateral ankle. They should try to palpate just off the Achilles and then move to the lateral calcaneus, assessing for symptom reproduction.

PERIPHERAL NERVE EXAMINATION

As detailed previously, the examination of the nervous system is comprehensive and complex. The clinician should be concerned not only with the detail of the nervous system examination as described prior, but with the peripheral nervous system as well. As mentioned, the findings of the upper and lower quarter screen may suggest the necessity for differentially diagnosing myotome versus peripheral nerve involvement. Details of the peripheral nerves, their segmental levels, origins, and sensory or motor contributions are presented in table 7.8 (Peripheral Nerves of the Upper Extremity) and table 7.9 (Peripheral Nerves of the Lower Extremity).

- Cervical plexus: C1-4
- Brachial plexus: C5-T1
- Lumbar plexus: L1-4 (T12)
- Sacral plexus: L5-S4
- Sacrococcygeal plexus: S5-Co1

TABLE 7.8 Peripheral Nerves of the Upper Extremity

Peripheral nerve	Origin	Sensory	Motor
CERVICAL PLEXUS (C1-C4) SENSORY BRANCHES			
Small occipital nerve (C2, C3)	Cervical plexus	Skin of lateral occipital portion of scalp, over mastoid process	—
Great auricular (C2, C3)	Arises from anterior rami of C2 and C3 and emerges from behind SCM before ascending on it to cross over parotid gland	Ear and face over ascending ramus of mandible	—
Cervical cutaneous (C2, C3)	Cervical plexus	Skin over anterior portion of neck	—
Supraclavicular (C3, C4)	Cervical plexus	Skin over clavicle and upper deltoid and pectoral regions, as low as 3rd rib	—

Peripheral nerve	Origin	Sensory	Motor
CERVICAL PLEXUS (C1-C4) MUSCULAR BRANCH			
Phrenic nerve (C3-C5)	From cervical plexus over scalene anterior and between subclavian artery and vein to enter thorax behind SC joint, then descends to diaphragm	Pericardium, diaphragm, and part of costal and mediastinal pleurae	Diaphragm
BRACHIAL PLEXUS (C5-T1; C4, T2 OCCASIONALLY DESCRIBED)			
Dorsal scapular (C5)	Shares C5 root with long thoracic nerve	Shoulder and subaxillary region	Rhomboid major and minor, levator scapulae
Long thoracic nerve (C5-C7)	Ventral rami of C5-C7 roots	—	Sole innervation of serratus anterior
Nerve to subclavius (C5-C6)	Upper trunk of brachial plexus	—	Subclavius
Suprascapular (C5-C6)	Anterior division of upper trunk	2/3 shoulder capsule, glenohumeral and AC joints	Supraspinatus, infraspinatus
Lateral pectoral (C5-C7)	Lateral cord	—	Pectoralis major
Medial pectoral (C8-T1)	Medial cord	—	Pectoralis major, pectoralis minor
Upper subscapular (C5-C6)	Posterior cord	—	Subscapularis
Thoracodorsal (middle subscapular; C6-C8)	Posterior cord	—	Latissimus dorsi
Lower subscapular (C5-C6)	Posterior cord	—	Subscapularis, teres major
Medial antebrachial cutaneous (C8-T1)	Medial cord	Medial surface of forearm	—
Medial brachial cutaneous (C8-T1)	Medial cord	Medial surface of arm	—
Musculocutaneous (C4-C6)	Terminal branch of lateral cord	Anterolateral aspect of forearm (palmar surface)	Coracobrachialis, biceps brachii, brachialis
Axillary (C5-C6)	Last nerve off posterior cord	Lateral shoulder (sergeant's patch)	Deltoid, teres minor
Radial (C6-C8, T1)	Direct continuation of the posterior cord	Posterior aspect of arm, antebrachial region of forearm, dorsal surface of forearm, dorsal aspect of radial 1/2 of hand, posterior aspect of first interosseous space	Triceps, anconeus, and upper portion of the extensor–supinator group of forearm muscles; posterior interosseous innervates all extensor muscles of wrist except extensor carpi radialis brevis and longus

(continued)

Table 7.8 *(continued)*

Peripheral nerve	Origin	Sensory	Motor
Median (C5-T1)	Combination of inferior branch of lateral cord and superior branch of medial cord	Skin of palmar aspect of thumb and lateral 2 1/2 fingers as well as distal ends of same fingers	Pronator teres, pronator quadratus, palmaris longus, flexor carpi radialis, flexor digitorum superficialis, radial portion of flexor digitorum profundus, flexor pollicis longus, abductor pollicis brevis, opponens pollicis, superficial head of flexor pollicis brevis, 1st and 2nd lumbricales
Ulnar (C8, T1)	Inferior branch of medial cord	Dorsal and palmar aspects of ulnar border of hand, including 5th finger and ulnar border of 4th finger	Median 1/2 of flexor digitorum profundus, flexor carpi ulnaris, palmaris brevis, abductor digiti quinti, opponens digiti quinti, flexor digiti quinti, deep head of flexor pollicis brevis, adductor pollicis, dorsal and palmar interossei, ulnar lumbricales

TABLE 7.9 Peripheral Nerves of the Lower Extremity

Peripheral nerve	Origin	Sensory	Motor
Iliohypogastric (T12, L1)	Lumbar plexus	—	—
Ilioinguinal (L1)	Lumbar plexus	Area along the inguinal ligament	—
Genitofemoral (L1-L2)	Lumbar plexus	Middle upper part of anterior thigh below inguinal ligament, skin of scrotum or labia	Cremasteric muscle, quadratus lumborum, psoas muscle
Femoral (L2-L4)	Lumbar plexus	Lower 2/3 of medial thigh to foot Above knee (anterior cutaneous nerve) Knee and medial shin to foot (saphenous nerve)	Sartorius, pectineus, and quadriceps muscle group (rectus femoris, vastus medialis, vastus lateralis, vastus intermedius, articularis genu)
Obturator (L2-L4)	Lumbar plexus	Groin and inner thigh to medial knee	Obturator externus, adductor brevis, adductor magnus, adductor longus, gracilis

Peripheral nerve	Origin	Sensory	Motor
Lateral femoral cutaneous (L1-L3)	Lumbar plexus	Anterolateral thigh, most notably proximal 1/3	Only sensory
Superior gluteal (L4-S1)	Sacral plexus	Posterior sacral portion of buttock	Gluteus medius and minimus, tensor fascia lata, hip joint
Inferior gluteal (L5, S1, S2)	Sacral plexus	Posterior sacral portion of buttock	Gluteus maximus
Sciatic (L4, L5, S1-S3)	Lumbosacral plexus	—	Short head of biceps femoris, semitendinosus, semimembranosus, long head of biceps femoris, adductor magnus
Tibial (L4, L5, S1-S3)	Sacral plexus/sciatic nerve	Calcaneus region	Gastrocnemius, popliteus, plantaris, soleus, tibialis posterior, flexor digitorum longus, flexor hallucis longus
Common fibular (peroneal; L4, L5, S1, S2)	Sciatic nerve	Popliteal space, superior and inferior articular branches to the knee joint and the lateral sural cutaneous nerve	Branches into superficial and deep peroneal nerve branches
Superficial fibular (peroneal)	One of two primary branches of common fibular nerve	Anterior surface foot and distal 2/3 of anterior distal lower extremity	Peroneus (fibularis) longus, peroneus brevis
Deep fibular (peroneal)	One of two primary branches of common fibular nerve	Anterior surface distal foot and web spaces between 1st and 2nd toes	Tibialis anterior, extensor digitorum longus, extensor hallucis longus, peroneus tertius, extensor digitorum brevis
Sural	Common fibular and tibial nerves	Distal lateral 1/3 of lower leg and lateral border of foot	Sensory
Medial plantar	Tibial nerve	Plantar surface of foot, medial region	Flexor digitorum brevis, abductor hallucis, flexor hallucis brevis, first lumbricale, lateral lumbricales, dorsal interossei
Lateral plantar	Tibial nerve	Plantar surface of foot, lateral region	Quadratus plantae, abductor digiti quinti, flexor digiti quinti, opponens digiti quinti, plantar interossei, adductor hallucis (transverse and oblique), dorsal interossei

CONCLUSION

Screening the orthopedic client is necessary when the client has vague multijoint pain, unexplained signs or symptoms, or uncertainty regarding pain generation. The orthopedic client screen for both the upper and lower quarter examines not only the joint and contractile tissue, but also the inert, non-contractile tissues. A major noncontractile tissue assessed during the upper and lower quarter screen is the nervous system. This chapter details the upper and lower quarter screens, as well as particularly important aspects of a more comprehensive neurological system examination.

RANGE OF MOTION ASSESSMENT

Michael P. Reiman, PT, DPT, OCS, SCS, ATC, FAAOMPT, CSCS

Range of motion (ROM) is an essential assessment for the clinician in terms of determining impairments that the client may present with. Mobility assessment can be global in nature (e.g., looking at someone squat down to pick something off the floor) or isolated in nature (e.g., goniometric measurement of a specific joint motion). The assessment of ROM therefore can be relatively qualitative or quantitative. For the purposes of general ROM screening, qualitative may be more appropriate, but for purposes of documentation and determination of progress with intervention, quantitative is more appropriate. It must be mentioned though that qualitative assessment is essential as well. Full ROM performed poorly is not a goal in the rehabilitation setting.

This chapter details components of ROM assessment. For basic aspects of these concepts and figures detailing them, see chapter 1. The reason for mentioning and detailing some of these concepts here again is to provide additional context relative to ROM.

RANGE OF MOTION AND FLEXIBILITY

Joint motion is classically viewed as the amount of joint ROM. Essentially it is a combination of osteokinematic and arthrokinematic motion. ROM can be active (AROM: the client performs independently), active-assistive (AAROM: the client requires some assistance to perform), and passive (PROM: the clinician passively performs the requisite motion without assistance from the client). Flexibility, on the other hand is determined by the extent of tissue extensibility of the periarticular and connective tissues that cross the joint. Several types of tissue can determine a joint's ability to move: the muscle itself, tendons, ligaments, connective tissue, bone, adipose tissue, skin, and neural tissue. The motion available at a joint is typically a combination of joint osteokinematic and arthrokinematic motion, as well as soft-tissue flexibility. The details of each of these components are outlined in this chapter.

Joint Motion

Motion in a joint can be considered from two different perspectives. The proximal segment of the joint can rotate around the relatively fixed distal segment. More commonly, the distal segment can rotate around the relatively fixed proximal segment. As mentioned in chapter 1, joint motion is a component of both osteokinematic and arthrokinematic movement.

Osteokinematics

Osteokinematic motion is also referred to as physiologic motion. These motions occur as movement of a bone on the other bone in the joint in the anatomical planes of motion (sagittal, frontal, and transverse). These motions are quantified with ROM measurements with a goniometer (AROM, AAROM, and PROM), as discussed later in this chapter. The axis of rotation for osteokinematic motions is oriented perpendicular to the plane in which the rotation occurs.[1]

Arthrokinematics

Arthrokinematic motion is commonly described as joint-related mechanical movement (roll, slide, and spin motion) at the joint level (figure 8.1).[2, 3] Roll is when one portion of the joint surface rolls on the other, like a car tire rolling down the road. An example is the femoral condyles rolling over the tibia (via the menisci) with knee flexion and extension. As a bone segment rolls, new equidistant points on the rolling surface come into contact with new equidistant points on the opposing surface. Spin occurs as an object rotates about a fixed axis, similar to a top spinning on a tabletop or a car tire spinning when the car is stuck in the snow and the driver is pressing on the gas pedal, yet the car is not moving. An anatomical example of joint spin occurs at the superior radioulnar joint with pronation and supination. Glide, or slide, is when one articulating surface translates relative to another, similar to

car tires sliding on the ice after the driver has just slammed on the brakes. An example of gliding is the relative concave tibia gliding along the femoral condyles with knee flexion and extension. During glide, the same point on the gliding bone comes into contact with new points on the opposing surface. The gliding accessory component is the basis of most joint mobilization techniques.

This motion is involuntary, and has been described as the joint play available at a joint. This accessory joint play has been described as involuntary movement present in all synovial joints.[4] Kaltenborn describes joint play as short, straight-lined passive bone movement.[2] Essentially, accessory joint play is involuntary articular joint movement (arthrokinematic movement) necessary for the client to achieve full osteokinematic movement. For the initial description of osteokinematic and arthrokinematic motion, see chapter 1.

Joint Mobility of the Spine

Osteokinematic and arthrokinematic motion are traditionally described and considered for the appendicular skeleton (extremities). Assessment of both of these types of motion is also important and necessary for the spine. Passive physiological movement of the spine along the anatomical planes of motion is referred to as *passive physiological intervertebral motion* (PPIVM), while joint-related mechanical movement (roll, slide, and spin motions) at the joint level in the spine is referred to as *passive articular (or accessory) intervertebral motion* (PAIVM).

PPIVMs have been rated on a 5-point ordinal scale, with 0 and 1 indicating hypomobility, normal anchored at 2, and 3 and 4 indicating hypermobility. Pain response can also be used, although its diagnostic utility is unknown.[5]

Restricted mobility in the spine with PAIVMs is typically determined subjectively, which should always be cautioned due to its nature of individual interpretation. Ratings of mobility limitations along with reproduction of client's concordant pain have

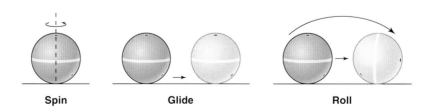

Figure 8.1 Arthrokinematic motions.

Reprinted, by permission, from J. Loudon, R. Manske, and M. Reiman, 2013, *Clinical mechanics and kinesiology* (Champaign, IL: Human Kinetics), 6.

much greater diagnostic accuracy, especially in the cervical spine.[6, 7]

The concave–convex theory of arthrokinematic motion was initially described by MacConaill.[8] The construct of this theory is that the joint surface geometry determines the accessory movement pattern during physiological movement.[9] The rule states that when a concave surface moves on a convex surface, roll and glide occur in the same direction. When a convex surface moves on a concave surface, roll and glide occur in the opposite direction. Refer to figure 1.6 for an illustration demonstrating this concept.

Close-Packed Position

In a close-packed position, the joint surfaces have the following characteristics:

- Maximally congruent
- Maximally compressed
- Joint capsule and ligaments are maximally tense
- Maximal stability of a joint
- Little to no distraction; therefore, further movement is possible
- Intracapsular space and volume are minimal

Loose-Packed Position

The loose-packed position of a joint encompasses all other positions of a joint other than the close-packed position. Therefore, the resting position of a joint is loose packed.

Resting Position

The resting position of a joint is that in which the joint surfaces have the following characteristics:

- Least joint congruency
- Least joint compression
- Capsule and ligament are maximally relaxed
- Minimal stability of a joint
- Maximal distraction, and greatest movement is available
- Intracapsular space and volume are maximal

End-Feel

End-feel is defined as the extreme of each passive movement of the joint that transmits a specific sensation in the clinician's hands.[10, 11] It is a sensation that the clinician feels at the end of the joint play or PROM. End-feel classification descriptions are as follows:[11]

- **Bone to bone**—The end-feel of the joint is hard, as when a bone engages another bone.
- **Springy block**—May suggest internal derangement, but may also represent a capsular or ligamentous end-feel.
- **Abrupt check**—An unexpected restriction imposed by a muscular spasm.
- **Soft-tissue approximation**—A normal end-feel where the joint can be pushed no farther secondary to engagement to another body part.
- **Empty**—No end-feel is felt since the movement is too painful and the examiner is unable to push the joint to its end range.

From these original descriptions, end-feel classifications have been adopted to include normal and abnormal by several sources, both in written literature[12, 13] and anecdotally:

Critical Clinical Pearls

Close-packed, loose-packed, and resting positions are commonly described joint positions.

- Close-packed is the joint position where the joint is the most taut and limited in movement.
- Loose-packed is every other position of the joint besides the close-packed position.
- Resting position is the joint position where the joint is the least taut and has the greatest amount of movement.
- Resting position is a position in loose-packed.
- Close-packed and resting positions are opposite from each other.

Normal end-feels

- **Hard (bone to bone)**—An abrupt, hard stop to movement when one bone contacts another bone (e.g., elbow extension: the olecranon contacts the olecranon fossa).

- **Soft (soft-tissue approximation)**—When two body surfaces come together a soft compression of tissue is felt (e.g., elbow flexion: the forearm and upper arm soft tissue approximates).

- **Firm (soft tissue stretch)**—A firm or spongy sensation that has some give when a muscle is stretched (e.g., passive ankle dorsiflexion performed with the knee extended is stopped due to tension in the gastrocnemius muscle).

- **Capsular stretch**—A hard arrest to movement with some give when the joint capsule or ligaments are stretched (e.g., stretching leather sensation with passive shoulder external rotation).

Abnormal (pathological) end-feels

- **Hard (bone to bone)**—An abrupt stop to movement, bone-to-bone contact, or bony grating sensation; when rough articular surfaces move past one another (e.g., a joint that contains loose bodies, degenerative joint disease, dislocation, or fracture).

- **Soft**—A boggy sensation that indicates the presence of synovitis or soft-tissue edema (e.g., an acutely inflamed knee joint with effusion, unable to fully extend).

- **Firm**—A springy sensation or a hard arrest to movement with some give, indicating muscular, capsular, or ligamentous shortening (e.g., adhesive capsulitis).

- **Springy block**—A rebound is seen or felt with this motion; suggestive of internal derangement in the joint (e.g., a meniscus tear blocking full joint ROM).

- **Empty**—Any end-feel that cannot be ascertained due to pain; the client requests the movement be stopped; indicates pathology (e.g., abscess, neoplasm, acute bursitis or joint inflammation, fracture).

- **Spasm**—A hard sudden stop to passive movement that is often accompanied by pain (e.g., indicative of acute or subacute arthritis, severe active lesion, or fracture). If pain is absent, a spasm end-feel may indicate a lesion of the central nervous system with resultant increased muscular tone.

Capsular Pattern

A capsular pattern of restriction is a limitation of pain and movement in a joint-specific range of motion. These characteristic patterns of restriction are based on empirical or anecdotal findings that have since come under significant scrutiny.[14-16] A capsular pattern suggests that a specific ratio of limited motions means that the capsule is a primary component of restriction for the client's ROM. For example, the capsular pattern in the glenohumeral joint has external rotation as the most limited motion, followed by abduction, and then internal rotation. Therefore, the greatest percentage of ROM restriction is with external rotation greater than abduction greater than internal rotation. A noncapsular pattern of restriction is a limitation in a joint in any pattern other than capsular. It may indicate the presence of a joint derangement, a restriction of one portion of the capsule only, or an extra-articular lesion obstructing joint ROM.[10]

The close-packed, loose-packed, and resting positions for each joint are presented in their respective chapters. Additionally, the described normal values for ROM, end-feel, and theoretical capsular patterns for these joints are also presented in the respective tables for each joint.

Irritability (Reactivity)

Irritability, or reactivity, is a term used to define stability of a present condition. In other words, irritability represents how quickly a stable condition degenerates in the presence of pain-causing inputs. Clients who exhibit irritable symptoms may respond poorly to an aggressive examination and treatment approach. The irritability of the client will dictate the comprehensiveness of the examination and intervention. Different degrees of irritability will have different characteristics, and should be treated accordingly. Here are the degrees of irritability:

- **High degree:** Clients typically have pain before the restriction is determined by the clinician.

- **Moderate degree:** Clients typically have pain at the restriction determined by the clinician.

- **Low reactivity:** Clients typically have no pain at the restriction determined by the clinician.

Joint Mobility

Full and pain-free ROM suggests normalcy for that movement, although it is important to remember that normal ROM is not synonymous with normal motion. Normal motion implies that the control of the ROM is also present. Control of the motion is a factor of muscle flexibility, joint stability, and central neurophysiologic mechanisms. Altered ROM (either increased or decreased from normal) can result in the presence of dysfunction either directly at the site of alteration or in a corresponding area that has to compensate for this alteration.

- **Joint hypomobility.** A joint that is hypomobile moves less than what is considered normal for the joint on the other extremity or other side of the spine. Here are the characteristics of a single hypomobile joint:

    - Loss of osteokinematic motion at the involved joint
    - Loss of arthrokinematic or accessory motion at the involved joint
    - Increased pain at end range
    - Abnormalities of the surrounding soft tissue (e.g., muscle spasm, guarding)
    - Restricted mobility of surrounding tissue

These tissue changes have been shown to result in an increase in intra-articular pressure during movement.[17]

- **Joint hypermobility.** Hypermobility is a joint that has what is considered increased motion as compared to the joint on the other extremity or the other side of the spine. Hypermobility has been defined as a laxity associated with symptoms manifested by the client's inability to control the joint during movement, especially at end range.[18] Here are the characteristics of a single hypermobile joint:

    - Increased osteokinematic motion of the involved joint
    - Increased arthrokinematic or accessory motion at the involved joint
    - Pain and muscle stiffness produced with prolonged positioning
    - Pain and muscle stiffness likely relieved somewhat by movement out of the prolonged positioning
    - Ligamentous tenderness in the accessible ligaments
    - Joint predisposed to joint locking

A client presenting with either hypomobility or hypermobility may not necessarily have pathology in that joint. Ideally, the clinician is looking for reproduction of their concordant pain with assessment of the specific joint.[19, 20]

The client may have hypo- or hypermobility on both sides of the extremities or spine. The clinician must always consider the overall tissue mobility when assessing the client's mobility status. The client with hypermobility may simply have generalized joint hypermobility (GJH) versus instability (a pathological condition manifesting as pain due to excessive joint play). Generalized joint hypermobility is a condition in which most of an individual's synovial joints move beyond the normal limits, with the age, gender, and ethnic background of the client taken into account.[21] Because of differing definitions and case identifications, the prevalence of GJH in published reports varies from 5% to 43% in adults[22, 23] and 2% to 55% in children.[24] Generalized joint hypermobility has a higher incidence in girls than boys[25, 26] and in those of African or Asian descent when compared with their Caucasian counterparts.[26, 27] Generalized joint hypermobility is also a recognized feature of many heritable disorders of connective tissue, such as Ehlers-Danlos syndrome,

Critical Clinical Pearls

Joint motion consists of osteokinematic and arthrokinematic motion.

- Arthrokinematic motion (i.e., roll, glide, and spin of one joint surface on the other) is required for proper osteokinematic motion.
- Dysfunctional arthrokinematic motion (limited) will result in limited osteokinematic motion.
- Dysfunctional arthrokinematic and osteokinematic motion can present as either joint hypomobility or joint hypermobility.

osteogenesis imperfecta, and Marfan syndrome.[28] Many of these disorders are associated with symptoms of chronic fatigue and widespread musculoskeletal pain, which may result from the GJH.[28]

Generalized joint hypermobility is diagnosed through a set of major and minor criteria—a combination of symptoms and objective findings—that include arthralgia, back pain, spondylosis, spondylolysis and spondylolisthesis, joint dislocation or subluxation, soft-tissue rheumatism, marfanoid habitus, abnormal skin, eye signs, varicose veins, hernia, or uterine or rectal prolapse.[26] Other specific tests and clinical criteria have been developed (table 8.1). These tests are clinically applicable and easy to administer, and they have demonstrated good to excellent reliability.[26, 29, 30]

TABLE 8.1 Hypermobility Objective Measures

Hypermobility objective measure	Description	Cutoff indicating hypermobility
Modified 9-point Beighton scale[31-34]	1 point for each side that meets each criterion • Passive 5th finger MCP dorsiflexion/hyperextension > 90° • Passive apposition of thumb to forearm in wrist flexion • Hyperextension of elbows > 10° • Hyperextension of knees > 10° • Flex spine so palms flat on floor from standing with knees fully extended	≥3[34] ≥4[31-33] ≥5[35]
Modified 5-point Carter & Wilkinson[36]	1 point for each side that meets each criterion • Passive 5th finger MCP dorsiflexion/hyperextension > 90° • Passive apposition of thumb to forearm in wrist flexion • Hyperextension of elbow > 5° • Hyperextension of knee > 5° • Flex spine so palms flat on floor from standing with knees fully extended	≥2[36]
Modified 10-point Carter & Wilkinson[37]	1 point for each side that meets each criterion • Passive hyperextension of fingers to parallel with forearm • Passive thumb to forearm flexor aspect • Elbow hyperextension > 10° • Knee hyperextension > 10° • Dorsiflexion of ankle > 30°	≥5[37]

Hypermobility objective measure	Description	Cutoff indicating hypermobility
Brighton criteria	Major criteria • Beighton score of ≥4/9 (either currently or historically) • Arthralgia for >3 months in 4 or more joints Minor criteria • Beighton score of 1, 2, or 3/9 • Arthralgia in 1 to 3 joints; back pain; or spondylosis, spondylolysis /spondylolisthesis • Dislocation or subluxation in >1 joint, or in 1 joint on >one occasion • ≥3 soft-tissue lesions • Marfanoid habitus • Skin striae, hyperextensibility, thin skin • Eye signs: drooping eyelids, myopia, or antimongoloid slant • Varicose veins, hernia, or uterine-rectal prolapses	2 major criteria or 1 major and 2 minor criteria 4 minor criteria 2 minor criteria or findings in 1st degree relatives
8-point Wynne & Davies[38]	1 point for each side that meets each criterion • Thumb to volar aspect of forearm • 5th MCP hypertension > 90° • Elbow hyperextension • Knee hyperextension	≥5[38]

MCP = metacarpal phalangeal joint

A simple five-part questionnaire has demonstrated good statistical properties in diagnosing GJH.[39] Overall the questionnaire correctly identified 84% of all cases and controls. This simple and reproducible questionnaire for detecting GJH could be of particular use as an adjunct in the clinical assessment of chronic, diffuse pain syndromes where hypermobility is often missed yet is potentially treatable.[39]

While dislocations, subluxations, and sprains are commonly reported in people with GJH,[40] reports in the current literature are inconclusive as to whether the risk of lower-limb joint injury during sport is greater in hypermobile participants compared with their nonhypermobile peers. Conflicting evidence of the relationship between hypermobility and joint injuries has been reported among ballet dancers[33, 41] and gridiron players.[42]

Although a couple of systematic reviews have also been unable to definitively determine any difference in the risk of lower-limb joint injury sustained by hypermobile sporting participants,[43, 44] others have found that GJH was associated with knee joint injury.[45, 46] The knee injuries were especially common among players participating in contact sports. GJH was not associated with ankle injury or overall with lower-limb joint injuries. The authors did express caution interpreting these results because they may have been obscured by the differences between studies in methods of measurement and by the inclusion of a wide range of sports.[45, 46]

The average age at onset of symptoms for GJH was 6.2 years old.[40] The major presenting complaint was arthralgia in 74%, abnormal gait in 10%, apparent joint deformity in 10%, and back pain in 6%. Of these children, 12% had "clicky" hips at birth and 4% had actual congenital dislocatable hip. A history of recurrent joint sprains was seen in 20% and actual subluxation or dislocation of joints in 10%. Some experienced difficulties at school: 40% had experienced problems with handwriting tasks, 41% had missed significant periods of schooling because of symptoms, and 48% had major limitations of school-based physical education activities. Outside of school, 67% had limitations with other physical activities and 43% described a history of easy bruising. Examination revealed that 94% scored ≥4/9 on the Beighton scale, with knees (92%), elbows (87%), wrists (82%), hand metacarpophalangeal joints (79%), and ankles (75%) being most frequently involved.[40]

The clinician should also be cognizant of nonjoint-related symptoms in these clients. Less than 20% of the same cohort of children had urinary tract infections, as well as speech and learning difficulties. The degree of relationship between GJH and these other symptoms is undetermined.[40]

Clinicians are urged to utilize the different objective measures for GJH as part of their examination. These objective measures could help the clinician differentiate diagnoses related to hypermobility and hypomobility of a particular body area.

Flexibility

Flexibility can be defined as the ability to move joints fluidly through complete ranges of motion without injury.[47] While flexibility is probably not regarded as a major parameter for assessment in human performance, it is integral to dynamic human movement and pain-free function. Prolonged low-load stretching in animals has been shown to increase muscle length and hypertrophy,[48, 49] as well as permanently lengthen connective tissue. Similar results have been achieved in human subjects with osteoarthritic hips[50] and joint contractures.[51] Evidence of similar effects in healthy shortened muscles has yet to be obtained.[52]

Optimal body alignment and proper agonistic–antagonistic muscle relationships have been advocated by many experts.[53-55] Functionally shortened muscles have the capability of reciprocally inhibiting their antagonistic counterpart.[53-55] This can lead to increased potential for future injury and less-than-optimal function. The terms *upper crossed syndrome* and *lower crossed syndrome*[53] have been used to refer to such imbalances. Specific muscles have

been shown to have a predisposition for tightness (e.g., pectoralis major and minor, upper trapezius, suboccipital muscles, hip adductors and flexors, and erector spinae) and thereby to inhibit their antagonistic muscle groups (e.g., lower trapezius, gluteal muscles, deep neck flexors, and rectus abdominis). The clients display typical postures[53] as a result of muscle imbalance between antagonistic muscle groups. The clinician should assess for these muscle imbalances by testing both muscle strength and muscle length, but the clinician should be cognizant of abnormal posture in clients without symptoms. As with all components of the examination process, determination of pathology requires comprehensive findings suggestive of such pathology. Isolated findings may simply be incidental findings and should be supported with other findings in the examination for determination of their true relevance in the client's dysfunction.

GONIOMETRY

Osteokinematic ROM is measured in degrees of rotation with a measuring device called a goniometer. Goniometry, then, is the measurement of the available osteokinematic (physiological) ROM at a joint, whether it is AROM, AAROM, or PROM. Goniometry may be used to determine both a precise joint position and the total amount of motion available at that joint. During an examination when AROM deficits or dysfunctions are confirmed by corresponding PROM deficits, the next step is to quantify those limitations of motion. This quantitative analysis of motion is completed by the use of a goniometer and is measured in degrees of motion.

The intent of this section is not to provide a comprehensive summary of the studies examining reliability and validity of goniometry. The goniometric reliability and validity are affected by the procedure implemented. Each respective chapter describes the reliability and validity of goniometric assessment of that particular region of the body. In general, this assessment method does demonstrate adequate reliability and validity.[12] For specific details on reliability and validity, refer to the chapters in this text on individual regions of the body and especially to Norkin and White[12] for greater detail on these values and specific details on goniometry.

ROM varies among clients and is influenced by variables such as age, gender, and generalized joint mobility. Several studies have demonstrated that older adult groups typically have less ROM of the extremities and the spine than younger adult groups. These age-related changes are typically joint and motion specific and may affect men and women differently. Gender does appear to be a variable affecting ROM. Women have been shown to have more ROM across the age ranges in multiple different joints.[56-58]

The instrument chosen to assess joint ROM depends on the degree of accuracy required in the measurement and the time and resources available to the clinician. Radiographs, motion analysis systems, photographs, electrogoniometer, flexometer, or plumb line may give objective, valid, and reliable measures of ROM, but they are not always practical in the clinical setting. The instruments used for clinical measures are dependent on the motion being measured, and the instrument's accuracy, availability, cost, ease of use, and size. The universal goniometer is the instrument most commonly used to measure joint position and motion in the clinical setting. The majority of measurement techniques discussed in this book describe the use of this tool. Other commonly clinically applicable tools include the bubble inclinometer and the cloth tape measure.

Universal goniometers are usually made of plastic or metal, and they typically have a scale from 0° to 360° (plastic) or from 0° to 180° (metal). The body of the universal goniometer is the central component, and its center is typically the axis of the goniometer (which is thus placed over the axis of the joint to be measured). The stationary arm is a structural part of the body of the goniometer that cannot be moved independently from the body. It is typically placed over the bone of the joint (or body part of the segment) that is not moving with the measurement (e.g., the humerus when measuring elbow flexion). The moving arm is attached to the center of the goniometer, and is free to move on the body. It is typically placed over the bone or body part that is moved (either actively or passively) to measure the joint motion (e.g., the forearm when measuring elbow flexion). The length of the stationary and moveable arms, as well as the size of the body, depends on the type of goniometer. For example, smaller goniometers are necessary for measuring toe and finger ROM. In fact, specific types of goniometers are often necessary for these body parts.

The basic technique of goniometry is dependent on multiple variables, including the body part, type of goniometer used, position of the client, and so on.

The technique outlined here is general in nature, and it should be modified dependent on the previously described variables.

1. Select a universal goniometer.
2. Differentiate between the movable and stationary arms.
3. Find the line in the middle of the movable arm and follow it back to the number scale on the body of the goniometer.
4. Properly align the client accordingly.
5. The axis of the goniometer should be placed appropriately over the axis of the joint to be assessed with respect to the fact that many joints may make the axis move slightly.
6. The stationary arm should be aligned over the portion of the joint (or segment) that is relatively stationary or not moving, with the midline of that arm along the midline of the segment.
7. The movable arm should be aligned over the portion of the joint (or segment) that will be moved, with the midline of that arm along the midline of the segment.
8. The client is instructed on the testing method.
   - If it is an AROM measurement, the clinician demonstrates the motion and then asks the client to perform the same motion.
   - If it is a PROM measurement, the clinician demonstrates the motion and then guides the client's body through that motion for the measurement.
9. At the end of the available ROM, the clinician takes the measurement and records it as appropriate.
10. Repeated measurements of the motion may be necessary in some cases.

Various scales of measurement are utilized in goniometry. The 0° to 180° notation system or neutral zero method for the extremities utilizes 0° for flexion–extension and abduction–adduction when the body is in anatomical position. The term *hyperextension*, for example, in this system would describe a greater than normal extension ROM. The 180° to 0° notation system defines anatomical position as 180°. A ROM begins at 180° and proceeds in an arc toward 0°. The 360° notation system also defines anatomical position as 180°.

QUALITATIVE ASSESSMENT OF MOTION

Motion of a particular body segment or movement can also be assessed qualitatively. Some of these assessments can also be done quantitatively. For example, motion analysis systems can assess for both qualitative and quantitative quality of movement, with complex and expensive testing methods typically reserved for motion analysis labs in universities or research facilities. Less complex assessments can include assessing the client with daily task movements or specifically designed motion screen assessments (Functional Movement Screen, Y-Balance Test, and so on). It is strongly recommended that clinicians utilize such measures as components of their assessment methods because these integrated movements are likely the limitations that their clients are encountering. Chapter 12, Physical Performance Measures, lists some of the more commonly used assessments in this category.

CONCLUSION

The assessment of ROM includes both quantitative and qualitative aspects. The more traditional form is quantitative. Traditional goniometry is an example of a method for quantitative assessment. Goniometry is a standard method of assessment of ROM that can be utilized to measure current status, progress, and changes over time. Range of motion in a joint is measured with goniometry and is generally an osteokinematic assessment, although normal arthrokinematic motion is necessary for completing full osteokinematic motion.

9

MUSCLE PERFORMANCE AND NEUROMUSCULAR CONTROL

Michael P. Reiman, PT, DPT, OCS, SCS, ATC, FAAOMPT, CSCS

Descriptions of muscle performance typically include the terms *strength*, *power*, and *endurance*. Performance by a muscle, depending on its called-on action or requirements, may include one or all three of these components. This chapter outlines these components as well as the factors affecting them. It also discusses means of clinically measuring muscle performance.

COMPONENTS OF MUSCLE PERFORMANCE

The primary components of muscle performance include strength, power, and endurance. Each

of these components of muscle performance has distinct characteristics, which are outlined in the following sections.

Strength

Strength is the ability of the muscle to exert a maximal force or torque at a specified or determined velocity. Strength can be measured in terms of force, torque, or work.[1] Functional strength relates to the ability of the neuromuscular system to produce, reduce, or control forces that are either contemplated or imposed during functional activities in a smooth, coordinated fashion.[2, 3] The effect of strength on function depends on both absolute and relative strength. *Absolute strength* is the most force a muscle can generate, or the maximum amount of weight a person can lift once (one-repetition max, or 1RM) irrespective of body weight. *Relative strength* is absolute strength divided by the person's body weight. Therefore, if a client can bench press 200 lbs (91 kg) and they weigh 150 lbs (68 kg), their relative strength is 1.33.

Using relative strength is a means of equalizing strength relative to the person's size. Larger people typically have much greater absolute strength than smaller people, but their relative strength may be much more equal. For example, a 300 lb (136 kg) person who squats 350 lbs (159 kg; relative strength of 1.17) and a 150 lb person who squats 175 lbs (79 kg; 1.17) will have the same relative strength.

Power

Power is the rate of work, or amount of work per unit time. Muscular power is the amount of work produced by a muscle per unit time (force × distance / time).[2, 3] Therefore, since velocity is equal to distance over time, power is equal to force × velocity. The rate of force production is an essential element in the production of power. The greatest power is produced by exerting the most force in the shortest amount of time. Power can be improved by either increasing strength or by reducing the amount of time required to produce force.

To develop optimal levels of speed strength (starting, explosive, and reactive), clients must train with heavy loads (85–100%) and light loads (30%) at high speeds. In order to recruit and synchronize as many motor units as possible, clients should lift heavy loads (85–100% of 1RM) as quickly as they can. Training by lifting relatively light loads of approximately 30% of maximum weight at high speeds is superior to plyometric training and traditional weight training (80–90% of 1RM) in developing dynamic athletic performance.[4] A more recent synthesis of the literature demonstrated that lighter loads (typically <50% 1RM) were most effective for upper body multi-joint athletic power, while loads of 45% to 70% 1RM were most effective for lower body multi-joint power.[5] Therefore, a foundation of strength is necessary for power development, but higher speed of the movement with lighter loads is typically shown to be most effective for power training (especially in the upper extremities).

Power is necessary not only for sport-related activity, but for daily activity as well. Activities such as tripping and avoiding falling or jumping quickly out of the way of a vehicle to avoid getting hit are activities that require power. Both speed of movement and adequate strength are necessary for successfully performing these activities.

Endurance

Endurance refers to the ability to perform low-intensity, repetitive, or sustained activities over a prolonged period of time without fatigue.[6] Endurance can be further broken down into local muscle endurance and general endurance. General endurance is often referred to as cardiorespiratory endurance. Local muscle endurance, however, refers to the ability of a muscle to contract repeatedly against a load (resistance), generate and sustain tension, and resist fatigue over an extended period of time.[6] Activities requiring cardiorespiratory endurance also require muscular endurance, although tasks requiring muscular endurance do not always require cardiorespiratory endurance.

Local muscle endurance deficits require the clinician to train the client with high volume and low intensity to replicate the proper function of these muscles. Cardiorespiratory endurance can be similarly accomplished with large muscle group movements. Movements that replicate functional

---

Critical Clinical Pearls

The components of muscular performance are the following:

- Strength
- Power
- Endurance

All of these components have distinct characteristics and should be assessed and trained accordingly.

tasks and activities should be of particular importance to the client with orthopedic dysfunction.

FACTORS AFFECTING MUSCLE PERFORMANCE

Typically, muscle performance (and hence client function) is dependent on a combination of strength, power, and endurance. Since each of these components of muscle performance has unique characteristics, different factors can affect them. These factors follow. For greater detail on these variables, please refer to chapter 1.

- **Neural control and adaptation.** Muscle strength generally increases when more motor units are involved in the contraction, the motor units are greater in size, or the rate of firing is faster. Much of the improvement in strength evidenced in the first few weeks of resistance training is attributable to neural adaptations such as efficiency of movement and skill acquisition of learning the movement.

- **Muscle fiber arrangement.** The angle of pennation is the angle created between the fiber direction and the line of pull. Fusiform and longitudinal muscle fibers, where the muscle fibers lie parallel to the long axis of the muscle, have little or no angle of pennation, while other arrangements of muscle fibers demonstrate some degree of pennation. Muscle fibers can contract to about 60% of their resting length, and the force is in the same direction as the muscle fiber. Most human muscles have pennation angles that range from 0° to 30°.[7] Only a portion of the force of pennate muscles goes toward producing motion of a bony lever. The more oblique an angle of pennation, the less force the muscle fibers are able to exert. Pennation of the muscle fibers appears to enhance force during high-speed concentric muscle action, particularly at ROM extremes, but may reduce force capability for eccentric, isometric, or low-speed muscle actions.[7, 8] This potential decrease in force is offset because pennate muscles usually have larger a physiological cross-sectional area (PCSA). The PCSA is the sum total cross-sectional area of all muscle fibers within the muscle. Assuming full activation, the maximal force potential of a muscle is proportional to the sum of the cross-sectional area of all its fibers.

- **Muscle length.** A muscle can generate the most force at resting length and less force when in an elongated or a shortened state (refer to the discussion on active and passive insufficiency later under the item Muscle Length–Tension Relationship on this list). The shape of the total muscle length–tension curve can vary considerably, however, between muscles of different structure and function.[9] Refer to chapter 1 for greater detail on muscle length.

- **Joint angle.** Changes in strength throughout the joint ROM affect force capability. The amount of torque exerted about a given joint varies throughout the joint's ROM because of the relationship between force and muscle length, as well as the geometric arrangement of muscles, tendons, and joint structures. The joint angle is likely related to the muscle length, length of the lever arm acting on a muscle, and so forth. All these variables require careful consideration on the part of the clinician when planning a treatment or assessment.

- **Muscle fiber type.** The different muscle fiber types (Type I, Type IIa, and Type IIb), along with their specific primary characteristics, are detailed in chapter 1. Generally, Type I fibers are predisposed for endurance or duration activities, while Type IIb are predisposed for explosive, anaerobic activities. Some muscles, such as the rotator cuff, paraspinals, and gluteus medius require high volume training or endurance due to their endurance requirements with activities. Exercise prescription therefore should account for this and should be adapted to address such issues.

- **Muscle fiber diameter.** The amount of force developed in a maximal static action is independent of the fiber type but is related to the fiber's cross-sectional diameter. Since Type I fibers tend to have smaller diameters than Type II fibers, a high percentage of Type I fibers is believed to be associated with a smaller muscle diameter and therefore lower force-development capabilities. All else being equal, the force a muscle can exert is related to its cross-sectional area rather than its volume.[10]

- **Muscle force–velocity relationship.** The rate of muscle change, whether the muscle is lengthening or shortening, substantially affects the force a muscle can develop when it contracts. As the speed of a muscle's shortening increases, the force it is capable of producing decreases. During a lengthening (or eccentric) muscle contraction, the force production differs from a shortening (or concentric) contraction.[11]

- **Muscle length–tension relationship.** A muscle's force-production capability is related to its length. The relationship between the length of a muscle and its force capability is referred to as the length–tension curve (see chapter 1). Maximum force is produced near a muscle's normal resting length. An example worthy of consideration for the practicing orthopedic clinician is the use of resistive tubing or bands. These bands increase in tension (and therefore resistance) the more they are stretched. Performing an exercise where the muscle is actively insufficient (maximal cross bridging of actin and myosin and muscle shortening) or passively insufficient (least amount of actin and myosin cross bridging or maximal muscle lengthening) against maximal resistance of the tubing is not appropriate exercise prescription and therefore is not suggested.

• **Specificity of required activity.** Specifically training a muscle or group of muscles to achieve the wanted goals (e.g., strength, power, endurance, stabilization) is of paramount importance. It is beyond the scope of this chapter to cover this issue in detail, and the reader is advised to consult elsewhere.[3] General parameters are discussed here. Training or testing the different parameters of muscle performance (strength, power, and endurance) requires different program designs (table 9.1). Strength training typically involves a load of 80% to 100% of the maximum amount of weight a person can lift in one repetition (1RM), with approximately one to six repetitions. Power training, as previously mentioned, requires a foundation of strength. The primary component of power training after strength is established is velocity of movement. Therefore, since velocity is inversely proportional to the amount of load lifted, the load will have to be relatively lighter to accomplish the necessary velocity. Endurance training can involve many methods (e.g., circuit training), but the common theme is high repetitions with lighter loads. The relative work-to-rest ratio for endurance training is the lowest among the three parameters of muscle performance.

• **Age.** Muscle performance is thought to increase in a client until about 30 years of age; then, as the client ages, there are noted decreases in muscle performance.[12-15] Along with these decreases in muscle performance, there are decreases in muscle size and a decrease in the number of muscle fibers.

• **Gender.** Gender is a variable to consider that affects muscle performance. Men are generally stronger than women in absolute strength.[16, 17]

TABLE 9.1 Comparison of Training Characteristics for Developing Muscle Performance

	Strength	Power	Strength and endurance	Endurance
Load (% of 1RM)	80–100%	Strength/force (70–100%) Velocity (30–45%) or up to 10% body weight	50–70%	Circuit training (40–60%)
Repetitions	Very low to low 1-6	1-5 (strength) 5-10 (power)	12-25	Moderate to high (15-30+)
Sets	3-5	4-6	2-3	2-5
Rest period	3-6 min	2-6 min	30-60 s	45-90 s (1:1 work–rest ratio)
Speed of performance	Slow to medium (speed of effort is as fast as possible)	Fast/explosive	Slow to medium	Medium
Primary energy source	Phosphagen Anaerobic glycolysis	Phosphagen	Anaerobic glycolysis/aerobic	Aerobic

---

Critical Clinical Pearls

Several variables affect muscular performance. Each of these variables can have unique influence on muscular performance. Clinicians should consider and account for these variables when assessing and prescribing exercise for their orthopedic clients.

CLINICAL MEASURES OF MUSCLE PERFORMANCE

Measuring muscle performance can include both objective measurements (quantitative) and measurements of function or combinations of subjective and objective measures (some qualitative). Measurement of strength specifically can be accomplished by various means.

Quantitative Assessment

Quantitative measures of muscle performance include anthropometry and different methods of assessing the strength, power, and endurance capability of a muscle or muscle group. These include manual muscle testing, handheld dynamometry, and isotonic and isokinetic testing.

Anthropometry

Anthropometry is the science of measuring the size, weight, and proportions of the human body. Limb circumference has been used to approximate muscle size. Limb circumference is generally measured with a tape measure and is often assumed to correlate with muscle power and strength, with greater circumference and muscle bulk indicating greater strength. Several studies suggest that limb girth correlation with strength is misleading. Cooper and colleagues[18] evaluated the relationship between thigh circumference and muscle strength and power as measured by isokinetic dynamometry and found no correlation between the torques produced at the knee by the knee extensors and flexors and thigh circumference measures at three levels. In addition, Hortobagyi and colleagues[19] also found that individual differences in muscle strength correlate poorly with segmental girth measurements.

Manual Muscle Testing

Manual muscle testing (MMT) is used to test the strength of individual muscles or muscle groups.

Muscles with a common action or actions can be tested either as a group or individually. It can be difficult to isolate muscles individually. Additionally, muscles typically work in synergistic patterns functionally. Thus muscle group or action testing is typically described in muscle testing texts.

MMT is performed by applying manual resistance to a limb or body part. This resistance is typically applied at a point in the limb's ROM where the muscle being tested is most efficient. A muscle that is fully shortened (active insufficiency) or fully lengthened (passive insufficiency) will be weaker than a muscle in mid ROM. There is considerable difference in the amount of force that various muscles can hold against. The application of resistance throughout the arc of motion (make, or active resistance, testing) in addition to resistance applied at only one point in the available ROM (break testing) can help determine the true strength of the muscle.[20] The client must be positioned to isolate the muscle to be tested in either situation, and the effect of gravity must be considered with testing for muscle grade.

Muscle strength is typically graded on a numeric scale of 0 to 5, although various grading schemes have been described (table 9.2). All the grades above 1 may be scored as the number alone or with a score of the number with a + or − to delineate slightly stronger (+) or weaker (−) than the respective number grade. A break test should be used when testing the strength of muscles with a grade higher than fair (3/5).[20] This is performed by applying pressure to the tested segment, in addition to gravity, to determine the maximal effort the client can exert. The clinician gradually applies more pressure until the effort by the client is overcome.[20] When a muscle can move a body part only against gravity, its strength is graded as 3/5. When testing weak muscles with less than 3/5 strength, a position that minimizes gravity and that generally involves moving the body part in the horizontal plane is best to use.

The MMT scale is easy to apply, but it is important to realize that these scores are relative. A score of 4 does not indicate that a muscle is twice as strong

TABLE 9.2 Manual Muscle Testing Grading Definitions and Scoring

Grading definition	Qualitative score	Various described numerical scores			Groupings
Complete full ROM or maintain end testing ROM against maximal resistance	Normal	5	10	100%	All positions of full ROM with some degree of resistance
Gives or yields to an extent at end testing ROM with maximal resistance	Good	4	8	80%	
Moves through full ROM and holds end testing ROM against mild resistance	Fair (+)	3 (+)			
Moves through full ROM against gravity but additional resistance causes the muscle to give	Fair	3	6	60%	All positions of some amount of ROM against gravity but no resistance
*Moves through >half ROM against gravity without resistance	Fair (−)				
*Moves through <half ROM against gravity without resistance	Poor (+)	2 (+)			
Muscles complete full ROM in a gravity-minimized position (horizontal plane most typically)	Poor	2	4	40%	All positions of some amount of ROM in a gravity-minimized position
*Muscles complete partial ROM in gravity-minimized position (horizontal plane most typically)	Poor (−)	2 (−)			
Contractile activity of the muscles is detected either visually or with palpation, although joint movement does not occur as a result of this muscle activity.	Trace	1	2	20%	Either contractile or noncontractile muscle activity
No muscle activity to palpation or visualization	0	0	0	0%	

* = less commonly described grades

as one with a score of 2. Furthermore, validity of high scores may be limited by the strength of the clinician performing the test. Additionally, MMT has been shown to be less capable of detecting strength deficits in stronger muscles than in weaker muscles.[21] MMT is the fastest and most efficient means of assessing muscle strength in the clinical setting, and it provides information not obtained by other procedures.[20]

Handheld Dynamometry

Handheld dynamometers can be used to test the strength of individual muscles or muscle groups. This small device fits in the clinician's hand and is placed at precise locations on a client's limb in an effort to assess the force generated by various muscles or groups of muscles. Handheld dynamometers are inexpensive, convenient, and lightweight; they require minimal setup time and training and can be used in a wide variety of settings.[22] Handheld dynamometers overcome some of the limitations of MMT, particularly the subjectivity and nonlinearity of grading muscle force production. They also have good to very good reliability. These devices therefore are popular and well accepted in clinical practice.[23-26] However, as with MMT, consistent locations and client positions must be used for accurate and reliable results.

Isotonic Testing

Isotonic testing involves lifting a fixed mass against gravity. This testing can be performed using weight machines or free weights. Many isotonic strength-testing protocols exist, including the 1RM and the 10RM. A 10RM is the maximum amount of weight the client can lift and lower 10 times. The 10RM test was first developed by DeLorme and Wilkins.[27] Isotonic testing of all types has been criticized because it is limited by the *sticking point*, or the weakest point, in the ROM; therefore, it measures only the maximum strength at this point.[28] The more recent literature calls this type of strength testing *dynamic testing* because it involves both a concentric (muscle shortening) and eccentric (muscle lengthening) contraction.[29] A great benefit of this type of testing is that it can easily be used to replicate a client's functional requirements. Activities of daily living such as stepping up onto a step and sitting down in a chair can serve as both assessments and training modules in the rehabilitation of a client when appropriate.

Isokinetic Testing

Isokinetic strength testing measures force production during fixed-velocity movement with an accommodating resistance.[30, 31] The tests are performed using an electrically powered device that maintains a chosen velocity of movement while maximizing the resistance throughout the ROM. Many isokinetic strength-testing devices are available. All have components for testing movement of different joints, and some are able to assess open and closed kinetic chain movements. Isokinetic devices can be programmed for velocities from 1° to 500° per second. There are many advantages to this type of testing, including the provision of objective data, isolated joint strength assessment, and so on. There are also several disadvantages to this type of testing, including (but not limited to) the fact that this type of testing is very expensive and that the machinery requires a lot of space. Isokinetic testing can provide information about subtle changes in strength that may not be detectable by MMT.[30, 32] For example, such testing revealed that some postsurgical knee arthroscopy clients had strength deficits of as much as 31% despite testing 5/5 for strength with MMT.[32] An additional limitation of isokinetic testing is that it does not isolate specific muscles but rather measures combined strength for moving in a single plane such as knee flexion or extension.

Qualitative Assessment

Qualitative measures of muscle performance primarily include assessment of the client's quality of movement. Assessing movement quality in all three planes of movement requires monitoring for compensations in each plane. Some assessments of qualitative movement can also be measured quantitatively with complex biomechanical analysis that is not common in the traditional physical therapy clinic. Other qualitative measures of muscle performance could include various subjective questionnaires that clients fill out regarding their functional capabilities. It is beyond the scope of this text to cover complex biomechanical motion analysis system assessment. Refer to the chapters on specific body parts and regions for additional details on subjective questionnaires and muscle performance assessment.

Some of the more common qualitative assessments of muscle performance for the practicing clinician include the relationship in movement between the scapula and humerus (scapulohumeral rhythm), gait dysfunctions (e.g., Trendelenburg gait, gluteus maximus gait), going into valgus (or medial collapse) with a single-leg squat, and so on.

Muscle Integrity and Damage

Resistance muscle testing can also be utilized to differentially diagnose the type of tissue involvement in the presenting pathology or dysfunction. Interpretation of resistive movement can prove a valuable resource in differentiating what type of structural tissue is involved.[33] Pain with a muscle contraction generally indicates an injury to the muscle or a capsular structure.[33] Combining findings from the isometric, passive joint motion, and joint distraction and compression tests can assist the clinician with determining the type of tissue at fault (table 9.3). If they can isolate and then apply tension to a structure, clinicians can then determine the integrity of that structure.[33]

Pain with muscle testing may indicate a muscle or joint injury. Pain occurring consistently with resistance, irrespective of the muscle's length, likely indicates a muscle tear. Weakness with muscle testing is also differentiated according to the position of the muscle. Muscle weakness throughout the ROM is more likely representative of pathological weakness versus weakness only at certain positions (positional weakness). Strength testing interpretation according to Cyriax[33] is described as follows:

- A strong resistance provided on the part of the client that is also painless is indicative of normal contractile tissue.
- A strong resistance provided on the part of the client that is also painful is indicative of a minor tear of the contractile tissue (grade I injury).
- A weak resistance provided on the part of the client that is also painful is indicative of a major tear of the contractile tissue (grade II injury). Additionally, others suggest that this representation may also be indicative of a tumor or of minor muscle damage and inflammation induced by (for example) eccentric exercise.[34]

TABLE 9.3   Differential Diagnostic Characteristics of Inert Versus Neural Versus Contractile Tissue Involvement in Clients' Presentation

Diagnostic characteristic	Inert	Neural	Contractile
Pain with testing?	Most likely, but tension in joint swelling may limit testing to pain-free ROM	Most likely	Definitely yes
Type of pain	Dull (more chronic nature) to sharp (acute) depending on acuteness of injury	Burning	Dull and aching; client likely to cramp with testing
Paresthesia with testing?	Not likely	Most likely	Not likely
Dermatomal distribution?	Not likely	Most likely	Not likely
Peripheral nerve distribution (sensory)?	Not likely	Most likely if peripheral nerve involvement	Not likely
End-feel noted with testing	Firm tension/boggy	Most likely a stretch or binding/increasing tension feel	Muscle spasm

- A weak resistance (or none, including the inability to move the involved joint) provided on the part of the client that is also painless is indicative of a complete rupture (grade III) of neurologic involvement.

Pain that occurs on the release of the contraction (but not during the resistance testing) is thought to be of articular nature due to the joint glides occurring once the tension is released. To comprehensively assess muscle integrity, a combination of resistance and length of the muscle must be assessed. A few considerations are worthy of mention:

- Pain that occurs with resistance, along with pain noted when the muscle is maximally stretched passively, indicates muscle impairment.
- Resistance testing of the muscle at a fully lengthened position places it in passive insufficiency (chapter 1); therefore minimal force is likely required. This position also tightens the inert components of the muscle (and likely the corresponding region of the joint) and tests for muscle tears at the tenoperiosteal region of the muscle.
- Resistance testing of the muscle at midrange position tests the overall power of the muscle. This is the position where the muscle is likely the strongest due to myosin and actin overlap (chapter 1).

- Resistance testing of the muscle at a fully shortened position is used for determination of the presence of palsies. The muscle is in active sufficiency. Therefore, the muscle is biomechanically in its weakest position.
- Active and passive insufficiency of the muscle being tested must be taken into consideration. The muscle naturally will be weaker in these positions than in midrange.

Muscle strain injuries usually involve muscle failure at the junction between the muscle and the tendon.[35, 36] After this, localized bleeding, swelling, redness, and pain typically result from the inflammatory process. Various grading scales are used to describe muscle strains. Grade I is often described as a minor strain with minimal muscle tearing, grade II is a moderate strain, and grade III is a complete tear of the muscle (refer to chapter 3 for additional detail).

CONCLUSION

Muscle performance testing has many components as well as many methods of assessment. Both qualitative and quantitative assessment methods should be employed by the clinician ascertaining the client's function. The particular method of muscle performance assessment chosen should be individualized based on the particular relevant aspects of the client being assessed.

10

SPECIAL TESTS

Michael P. Reiman, PT, DPT, OCS, SCS, ATC, FAAOMPT, CSCS

This chapter addresses clinical special tests and their applicability in clinical practice. All of the tests described in this text, for the most part, do not require special equipment and have been described as being performed on typical clients presenting with suspected conditions. Refer to chapter 4 (Evidence-Based Practice and Client Examination) for background information relevant to this chapter (diagnostic accuracy, reference standard, study quality, and so on). Chapter 4 should be read in detail prior to reading this chapter.

Physical examination testing is commonly interpreted as *special tests*. Special tests are extensively published in the literature and various texts. Screening and diagnosis of pathology is frequently based heavily on interpretation of these testing methods for determining the origin of the client's complaints or the pain-generating structure.

Although some of the studies investigating special tests may reflect everyday clinical practice, the complete diagnostic process encompasses all components discussed in this text. Tests used for diagnostic purposes cannot be deemed simply good or bad; rather the test may provide important information for certain clients under certain conditions but not for others. The majority of special tests are deficient as stand-alone tests for determining the specific pathology.[1-12] Screening and diagnosis of pathology is far too commonly based heavily on the findings of these tests. Instead, they should be used as simply one component of a more comprehensive examination process (the entire funnel paradigm).

Diagnostic research should evaluate the validity of the complete diagnostic process and study the evidence of the added value of the different tests used.[13] The entire diagnostic process entails each component described in this text, not simply special testing alone. One must remember that evidence does not make decisions, people do. The clinician should rely on the use of all eight components of the examination process set forth in this text (client interview, observation, triage or screening, mobility, muscle performance, special tests, palpation, and physical performance measures) as well as clinical reasoning and the client's values and characteristics to make the most informed clinical decision when examining a client. Relying on only one of the eight (or even a couple of the eight) examination components is not sensible clinical practice. Additionally, "clinical evidence should be used to inform but not to replace clinical expertise."[14] Good clinicians use both clinical expertise and the best available evidence, and neither alone. In fact, the clinician must consider that even excellent external evidence may be inapplicable to or inappropriate for an individual client.[15]

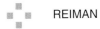

Critical Clinical Pearls

The clinician should use a comprehensive approach to examination of the orthopedic client that includes the following:

- All eight components of the examination funnel approach
- Appropriate clinical reasoning
- Both their clinical expertise and the best available current evidence
- The client's values and characteristics

Using several, or at least more than one, tests and measures can improve the probability that a client is correctly diagnosed with a specific condition. A trend is to include a cluster of tests to more accurately predict a positive or negative result. Clinical prediction rules are tools used by clinicians to determine the likelihood that a client is presenting with a given disorder, based on a number of variables that have been shown to have predictive validity in revealing clients most likely to have specific disorders.[16] These clusters and clinical prediction rules use multiple tests as a group, rather than a single test or multiple tests used in isolation. This grouping of tests is intended to improve their predictive ability. Using these clusters of tests as a single entity is advocated for predicting the possibility of a positive or negative result from clinical testing. But again, even this grouping of tests is one component of a more comprehensive process, as outlined in this text.

EXAMINATION PROCEDURE

Special test performance, like many components of the examination process, should be systematic and purposeful. Simply performing special tests for the purpose of conclusive diagnosis or screening is not advocated. Again, they are one component of a more comprehensive examination approach.

- **Preparation.** As with all components of the examination process, the client should be properly prepared for the examination. The clinician must explain the examination process, including reasons for its use, necessity of relaxation, and potential sensations that the client may perceive. The area to be examined must be properly exposed and prepared prior to special test performance. As with all types of testing, the clinician must first examine the noninvolved (or region closely associated) side (if appropriate) for several reasons (comparison to normal, understanding of expectations on part of the client). Observational assessment of the client in general, as well as of the involved region, should be utilized prior to palpation of the area. Observing the client in general can give the clinician an appreciation of the client's current level of irritability, while observation of the area may also alert the clinician to any observable features diverging from the normal.

- **Testing implementation.** As with all types of examination testing, the clinician should have a systematic approach to implementation. Once the client is prepared, the test should be implemented as described in the literature. Client position, clinician position, and movement of the test are described in each of the chapters in parts III and IV. The clinician should pay particular attention to stabilization, hand placement, movement, and so on to properly perform the testing.

- **Testing interpretation.** Interpretation of the test requires comprehension of a (+) versus (−) response. A (+) test for each test described in parts III and IV is given after description of test implementation. In addition to consideration of SN, SP, +LR, −LR, and QUADAS values, the clinician should consider the other information described for each test. In particular, the prevalence of the disease, the demographics of the study population, the reference standards utilized in the study, and whether or not there were independent and blind comparisons are particular concerns of study quality and interpretation. For each of the tests described, the confidence intervals (CIs) are reported for both SN and SP when reported by the authors or calculable by the data from the study. This allows the reader to appreciate the degree of variability in the SN and SP findings. Wide CIs suggest caution with interpretation due to their significant variability.

DIAGNOSTIC APPLICATION OF SPECIAL TESTS

As mentioned in chapter 4, highly SN (and low –LR) tests are suggested to be performed in the triage section of the examination (e.g., early in the examination process) not only to help rule out the potential for more serious pathology but also to assist with limiting the competing differential diagnoses. Highly specific (SP) (and high +LR) tests, on the other hand, should be utilized later in the examination process (advocated after muscle performance testing and prior to palpation in this text). The ideal and suggested format is a combination of highly SN (and low –LR) tests early in the exam and highly SP (and high +LR) tests later in the exam.

An example using the Canadian C-Spine Rule (CCSR)[17] is provided to demonstrate a suggested implementation. In this study of 8,924 alert and stable clients presenting to the emergency room with blunt trauma to the head or neck, stable vital signs, and a Glasgow Coma Scale of 15, the CCSR was applied to all 8,924 clients. Figure 10.1 is the final 2×2 diagnostic accuracy table once all testing was completed.

Once the CCSR is completed, the clinician knows only that there are 5,192 total positive results. At this point in the examination process, it is unclear which are TPs and which are FPs. With an SN of 100% (due to 0 FN), the clinician can be assured that there were no missed fractures. Due to the nature of tests with high SN, though, it is possible for several FPs to exist.

The 5,192 total positive results post CCSR then underwent radiography (a highly SP test with SP ranging from 93-99 depending on the study). The use of such a highly SP test after use of a highly SN test (as previously suggested here) resulted in the discrimination of TP (151) versus FP (5,041). Most of the total positives after the application of the CCSR were FP, hence the low PPV and overall prevalence of fractures (1.7%) in this study. Again, the nature of a test with high SN is to capture all potential positives (TP + FP, hence capturing some that actually do not have a fracture) with the examination and to minimize the number of FN (in this case, to not miss a fracture).

A very simplistic explanation of using tests with high SN first then highly SP tests later in the exam is the following example. Suppose there is a piece of land with two fishing ponds, but only the first pond has fish in it. The two owners want to keep the largest fish in just the first pond and put the smaller fish in the second pond. They take a net that spans the width of the first pond and has holes in it that are small enough that no fish will escape. They stand on both sides of the pond and sweep the length of the pond, essentially capturing all the pond's fish in the net (as well as most other moveable contents). They take these fish and put them in the second pond. They then take a net with holes large enough to let the smaller fish escape yet capture the large fish and sweep the second

	(+) radiograph	(−) radiograph	Total (+)
CCSR (+)	TP 151	FP 5041	5192 (+)
CCSR (−)	FN 0	TN 3732	3732 (−)
	151 fx's	10,773 ≠ fx	8924

SN = 151 / (151 + 0) = 100%   PPV = 39%
SP = 3732 / (5041 + 3732) = 35%   NPV = 100%
(+) LR = 1.5   Prevalence = 151 / 8924 × 100 = 1.7%
(−) LR = 0

Figure 10.1 2×2 contingency table for cervical fracture using CCSR. CCSR = Canadian C-Spine Rule; TP = true positives; FP = false positives; FN = false negatives; TN = true negatives; SN = sensitivity; SP = specificity; +LR = positive likelihood ratio; −LR = negative likelihood ratio; PPV = positive predictive value; NPV = negative predictive value

pond. This process captures only the largest fish. The owners then take the largest fish captured with the second net and place them back in the first pond. In this example the first net is like an SN test, capturing all potential targets (as well as other targets, or FPs) and minimizing missing any of them (no FNs). The second net is similar to an SP test, only capturing the particular target.

As mentioned in chapter 4, PPV and NPV are properties of both the test and the population being tested (prevalence affects outcome). Reading the PPV and NPV directly from a table is accurate only if the proportion of diseased clients in the sample is representative of the proportion of diseased people in the population. In each chapter in parts III and IV, the sample of clients investigated for each special test is listed. These tests are typically performed on a

select client cohort, affecting their PPV and NPV. The CCSR example described earlier is such an example. The clients undergoing testing were a particular set of clients, not a random sample of clients. The clients in this sample had a high suspicion of having the pathology in the first place.

As mentioned previously, the CCSR is strongly weighted to SN and poor SP (see figure 10.1). Application of this information can be applied with use of pretest probability and the use of a Fagan's nomogram. Assuming a pretest probability of 1% for a fracture, the use of the CCSR versus the example of subjective reporting of prolonged corticosteroid use provides significantly different results (figures 10.2 and 10.3). With a +LR of 1.5 and a −LR of 0, the posttest probability of a fracture existing is only ~1.3% (red arrow), but the posttest probability of a fracture *not existing*

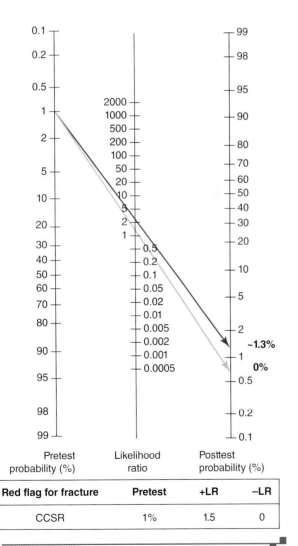

Red flag for fracture	Pretest	+LR	−LR
CCSR	1%	1.5	0

Figure 10.2 Fagan's nomogram calculation posttest probability of fracture based on CCSR.

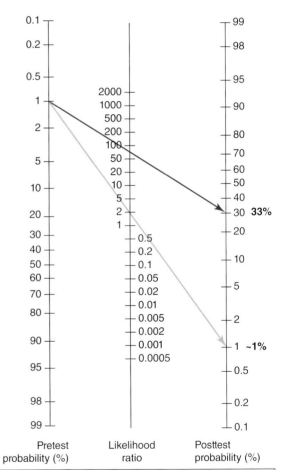

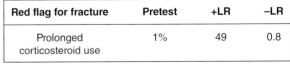

Red flag for fracture	Pretest	+LR	−LR
Prolonged corticosteroid use	1%	49	0.8

Figure 10.3 Fagan's nomogram calculation posttest probability of fracture based on prolonged corticosteroid use.

Critical Clinical Pearls

- Tests of very high SN and a low –LR are useful in situations where the clinician is screening the client for red flag conditions, such as fractures.
- The very low –LR, for example 0 in the case of the CCSR, essentially helps rule out the potential for missing a fracture due to 0 FNs.
- Hence, these tests are intended to cast a broad net that captures all potential target clients.
- Tests with poor SP and +LR are not intended to diagnose such conditions and thus have many FPs.

is 0% (green arrow). Again, the CCSR is poorly designed for predicting the presence of a fracture, but extremely well designed for predicting the *absence* of a fracture. The prolonged corticosteroid use, on the other hand, provides a different interpretation. With a +LR of 49 and a –LR of 0.8, the posttest probability of a fracture existing is 33% and the posttest probability of a fracture not existing is ~1%. The presence of a potential fracture's existence improved after testing when prolonged corticosteroid use was used as the testing metric, while the posttest probability of the absence of a fracture existing significantly improved when the CCSR was utilized. Again, separate tests must be used in different parts of the exam (SN tests early and SP tests later to confirm diagnosis).

CONCLUSION

Special tests are suggested as distinct components of a more comprehensive examination. Clinicians should utilize each of the eight primary components outlined in this text as individually important components of the exam process that, when combined with each of the other components, clinical reasoning, and client values and characteristics, affords them the greatest ability to determine the presence or absence of a particular dysfunction or pathology. Reliance on any one component of the examination process is not best evidence practice.

11

PALPATION

B. James Massey, PT, DPT, OCS, FAAOMPT

Palpation is the use of a clinician's sense of touch to clarify and quantify specific parameters of a client's tissue status through direct physical contact. It is a tool that physically links the clinician to the client in the context of addressing a complaint. As with many physical examination techniques, palpation requires procedural skill and an understanding of related evidence for optimal clinical utility. Though authors of clinical guidelines and textbooks commonly include palpation for the purposes of diagnosis, clinicians must respect both the limitations of palpation for diagnostic purposes and the indications of palpation for impairment qualification. Cyriax writes that palpation should be used "more to define, than find."[1]

Palpation is a prime example of a physical examination component that is strengthened by the three pillars of evidence-based practice: clinical expertise, scientific evidence, and client perspective. Clinical experience may provide multiple opportunities for comparison that allow a clinician to discriminate a perceived sensation when palpating a target structure as well as improve procedural efficacy over time. Application of the best available evidence will allow clinicians to identify limitations in their ability to integrate palpation findings throughout the clinical reasoning process. The client's perspective is essential to consider with palpation for the purposes of establishing an appropriate rapport and identifying areas of need for client education. Appropriate application of technique and interpretation of findings may aid a clinician throughout the process of determining a working diagnosis, prognosis, and therapeutic intervention plan.

PALPATION PROCEDURE

Palpation is performed with the clinician's skilled and purposeful application of external force to a client's body tissue during diagnostic and treatment procedures. Several cognitive and physical processes for the client and the clinician contribute to the manner in which this act affects the provision of health services. A multitude of variables may affect a clinician's ability to appropriately execute the procedure and assess the implications of the results. To fully appreciate the art and science of palpation, clinicians must critically analyze the process of palpation as a whole.

Preparation

First, the client is prepared for palpation. A verbal description of the procedure should be provided to the client to ensure that they are informed of the process and potential outcomes. An explanation of possible immediate outcomes (e.g., provocation, perceived pressure sensation) should include instruction that the client convey a description of the perceived sensation to the clinician. The client's description should include the parameters of location, quality, quantity, and relation to primary or secondary complaints. Clinicians should explain their expectation that clients differentiate between symptoms that are or are not associated with a specific complaint of interest. This qualification will improve the clinician's ability to determine the relevancy of a finding to diagnosis and intervention planning. Additionally, employing a constructive and collaborative manner, the clinician should inform the client of the option to discontinue this component of the examination, should they choose to do so. Provision of this option may provide a sense of control for the client during a relatively passive procedure, as well as facilitate a caring rapport.

The clinician must assist clients to assume a comfortable position that allows access to the structures that are targeted for palpation. Prioritizing the client's comfort may contribute to satisfaction and rapport, but it is also practical. Positioning a client such that minimal energy is required to maintain the position promotes relaxation of muscle tissue, allowing the clinician to observe the quality of tissue deep to the muscle structures. Actively contracted muscle tissue, whether volitional or nonvolitional, does not allow the tissue deformation that is necessary to access structures deeper than the contractile tissues. Also, if a client is positioned such that a tissue structure would not be expected to provoke a response (symptom or sign) under nonpathologic conditions, the clinician can identify abnormalities and compare clinical observations to the client's overall presentation. This concept is discussed further in the section Palpation Components of the Musculoskeletal Examination.

The area that is to be palpated should be exposed in a way that allows the clinician to visually identify anatomical location while respecting the client's dignity. Visual inspection during palpation is required to improve accuracy of the procedure, identify abnormalities, prevent wound contamination, and observe for physical responses to palpation. Additionally, in regard to both clinical efficiency and risk management, maintaining visual contact may help clinicians avoid palpating anatomical structures that are not pertinent to the examination.

The clinician's positioning also may affect the procedure and the interpretation of findings. Clinicians must find a position that allows them to apply the appropriate force to a targeted area and to perceive findings. They should minimize reach away from their body, diminishing complexity of a maneuver and gross force production. When applying force to the client's tissues, extreme joint positions of the clinician's upper extremities should be avoided to improve comfort, safety, and accuracy. Application of excessive force during palpation may result in a false provocation of an adverse response, while insufficient force may result in a failure to identify a sign or symptom. Additionally, inappropriate force may limit a clinician's ability to perceive variation in physical parameters of a palpated area, which is discussed further in the following section.

Locating and Defining the Target Structures

The clinician must be able to identify anatomic structures that they palpate for findings to contribute to the clinical reasoning process. They may utilize a number of strategies for navigating the body during palpation, including recall of anatomic knowledge, adjusting location in relation to other known anatomic structures, assessing tissue for an expected capacity to deform from palpation force, and assessing the shape and size of a suspected structure. When palpating a structure, the clinician should search for observable boundaries of a tissue to appreciate size and shape. This may be facilitated by mobilizing the finger in a direction perpendicular to the perceived or expected orientation of the tissue fibers.

Additionally, a clinician may assess the physical response of a tissue to a particular type of mechanical loading, thereby identifying a structure from the expected function. For example, a clinician may provide isometric resistance to identify a specific muscle (based on the muscle's action). They may then follow along the muscle to the insertion or origin tendons and follow along the tendons to the insertion point on bone. The muscle is identified by an easily observable change in tissue quality with activation, and inert structures are identified in relation to the muscle tissue. Further navigation of the body may be made when certain structures are identified in this manner, such as location of the scaphoid for tenderness testing in comparison to the anatomical snuffbox created by the thumb's extensor and abductor tendons.

Application of Force

Following appropriate preparation, the clinician may initiate the palpation examination. The clinician applies force to a targeted tissue, typically the epidermis, and that force is transmitted through other body tissues. The differentiation of tissues may be described as a process of perceiving variations in the relative densities of various tissues. For manual palpation tests to be valid, a standardized finger pressure needs to be applied.[2] After this force locally stimulates sensory receptors in the clinician's fingertips, the sensory input is transmitted through the peripheral nervous system via axonal potentiation. After passing through the dorsal column tracts of the spinal cord and the ventroposterior nuclei of the thalamus, the input is received by the primary sensory cortex. Different regions of the brain contribute to interpretation of the stimulus and response.

Initially, physical parameters of the force application that may affect the stimulus of sensory receptors include mass of the clinician's and client's (targeted and intermediary) tissues, velocity of the clinician's hands, contact area, and direction relative to the orientation of the tissue structure (subject to the type of mechanical loading imposed by the force and the type of sensory receptor). Sensory stimuli may be altered for the client by local sensitization that results from trauma-induced inflammation and innervation of pathologic and nonpathologic tissues. Local density of the activated sensory receptor has been proposed to correlate with sensitivity to mechanical stimulus, though there may not be a similar relationship between pain sensation and local nociceptor density.[3] Central neurologic factors that may affect stimulus interpretation include somatosensory cortex mapping parameters and central sensitization.

Once force is applied, the clinician observes the response to mechanical stimulus through visual inspection and subjective report. Findings from visual inspection may include facial expression, withdrawal of a palpated structure, local or regional muscle activity, tissue deformation, and skin discoloration. The subjective response may include verbal description of the perceived sensation or other audible interjection (such as "ouch"), and often requires clarification by the clinician. The client may require further prompting to express symptom location, nature, quantity, and relation (in regard to primary or secondary complaints).

Assessment

A clinician must assess the relationship of observations to variable factors of the palpation procedure and other examination findings, as well as the relative value of findings for the episode of care (working diagnosis, prognosis, and therapeutic intervention plan).

• **Palpation procedure.** Determine the significance of a finding, given the relationships between symptom location and established anatomic pain referral patterns, physical findings and limitations in the research properties of palpation, the gross quantity of force elicited and the physical properties of a structure, tissue mass and physical observations, and subjective reaction and physical parameters of force application (if the response is a reasonable reaction to the action).

• **Other examination findings.** Given the findings from the preceding examination components, the clinician must determine the implications of palpation findings on the working diagnosis or therapeutic intervention plan. Because a clinical hypothesis (e.g., working diagnosis, expected response to intervention) has been defined prior to palpation, the clinician must determine if the findings support, refute, or modify the clinical hypothesis, or perhaps not affect it. A clinician may improve this skill by applying principles of clinical expertise, scientific evidence, and client perspective.

• **Relative value of findings.** The clinician must determine the relative value of palpation findings in regard to diagnosis and therapeutic intervention. The diagnostic process is described as the generation of a preliminary diagnosis hypothesis, progressive modification and refinement of the hypothesis, and verification of a hypothesis and plan for further action.[4] The first step, hypothesis generation, should have been performed prior to palpation. During the process of hypothesis generation, the clinician has defined a hypothetical framework that is based on demographic probabilities, recognized a clinical pattern from the subjective examination and preceding physical examination components, and considered the seriousness of the suspected health condition. Palpation is typically performed during the second and third steps of the diagnostic process. During the modification and refinement of a hypothesis, palpation findings provide grounds to identify the need for further data, provide context for interpreting subsequent and preceding examination components, and add or remove other diagnoses. A clinician may incorporate palpation findings for the confirmation or elimination of a diagnosis when verifying a diagnosis, based on clinical patterns developed from experience and research literature. Additionally, the clinician should continue to integrate pertinent findings from palpation during ongoing assessment throughout the episode of care, noting changes in status in relation to expected change in status.

PALPATION COMPONENTS OF THE MUSCULOSKELETAL EXAMINATION

Palpation procedures are performed to obtain data that are pertinent to a client's clinical presentation. The physical requirements of a procedure vary based on the type of data a clinician intends to collect. During the physical examination, clinicians may use palpation to appreciate provocation of concordant symptoms, temperature, sensation, edema, tissue quality, muscle activation, and mechanical abnormalities. Because the relative value of specific data varies among clinical presentations, the clinician should identify the need for specific palpation components for each client.

Local Tenderness and the Working Diagnosis

Frequently throughout orthopedic literature, local tenderness to palpation is included as a component of diagnostic criteria for musculoskeletal injuries. Clinical diagnoses are further discussed in respective chapters on various body regions. Refer to table 11.1 for examples of musculoskeletal health conditions that have been reported to include focal tenderness as a criterion of diagnosis.

Clinicians must be cautious when determining the relationship between symptom provocation during palpation and a client's primary or secondary complaints, though the link is commonly utilized for localization of a lesion related to the client's primary complaint. Cyriax suggests that "the least reliable way to diagnose in soft tissue lesions is to palpate immediately for tenderness in the area outlined by the client."[1] Many factors may skew the ability of both the client and clinician to appropriately utilize symptomatology throughout the processes of diagnosis and therapeutic intervention.

Local provocation may be useful for implicating a pain generator when referred pain of the client's concordant sign occurs.[25] Errors of reasoning may be attributable to the client's description of a painful stimulus or the clinician's interpretation of the client's reaction to a stimulus. Often, local discomfort may be mistaken for provocation of symptoms related to a client's complaint due to poor communication. Because a client likely lacks understanding of the clinician's goal with palpation, the clinician carries the responsibility of administering an effective examination. If pain is verbalized during palpation, asking the client, "Is this the same pain that caused you to come for treatment, or is this different?" may aid in establishing a relationship between symptoms and complaints. Palpation of the contralateral structure (if applicable) may aid in discriminating between concordant symptoms and unrelated tenderness. Incorrectly establishing a relationship between a working diagnosis and a

---

Critical Clinical Pearls

When planning palpation for refinement of a diagnostic hypothesis, clinicians should do the following:

- Reflect: Clinicians should isolate the parameters of the information they may gain from palpation (e.g., severity of guarding, presence or absence of tenderness, severity of tenderness) and determine how these parameters will affect their working diagnosis.
- Consider innervation and sensory distribution of tissues that have suspected involvement.
- Identify the manner in which other examination findings may affect utility of palpation findings (e.g., excessive superficial tissue of a client may limit a clinician's ability to isolate structures deep to that tissue, and findings may have limitations for hypothesis modification).

TABLE 11.1   Focal Tenderness as a Criterion for Diagnosis of a Musculoskeletal Lesion

Body region	Health condition
Head and face[5]	Temporomandibular joint dysfunction
Thoracic spine and ribs[6, 7]	Costochondritis, slipping rib syndrome
Lumbosacral spine[8]	Sacral stress fracture
Shoulder and upper arm[2, 9-11]	Glenoid labrum lesion, AC joint pathology, internal impingement, partial ruptures of biceps tendon or tendinitis, humeral periostitis (humeral shin splints), humeral stress fracture, subacromial impingement
Elbow, wrist, and hand[11]	MCL injury, snapping triceps syndrome, ulnar neuropathy, radiocapitellar joint pathology (fractures, arthrosis, a symptomatic posterolateral synovial plica, or radial bursa), LCL injury, lateral epicondylopathy, radial tunnel syndrome, olecranon stress fracture or olecranon apophysitis, olecranon bursitis, gout
Hip[12-14]	Athletic pubalgia, osteitis pubis, piriformis syndrome, injuries of gluteus minimus and medius, femoral neck/head stress fracture
Knee and thigh[15-17]	Knee meniscus lesion, acute hamstring injury
Ankle, foot, and lower leg[18-23]	Ankle impingement syndromes (anterolateral, anteromedial, posteromedial, posterior), plantar fasciopathy, Achilles tendinopathy, ankle syndesmosis injury, Haglund's deformity, stress fractures of the calcaneus
Other[24]	Pediatric physeal ankle fracture

AC = acromioclavicular; MCL = medial (tibial) collateral ligament; LCL = lateral (fibular) collateral ligament

tender area that is unrelated may lead to misdiagnosis and inappropriate intervention.

In addition, other cognitive factors that may affect one's response to a perceived sensation (or anticipated sensation) include fear of pain, fear of movement (kinesophobia), anxiety of pain, rumination, magnification, sense of helplessness, or misrepresentation due to secondary gain. Though a client's reaction to a stimulus may be perceived as unwarranted or excessive by a clinician, it is important to acknowledge the multitude of nonmalicious contributors or causes to a reaction. Each clinician must respect their own scope of practice and clinical expertise when assessing a painful response and must integrate findings throughout the clinical reasoning process based on sound logic.

Appropriate interpretation of symptoms during palpation is essential to the provision of safe and effective health services. To improve the reliability of provocation from the palpation examination, the clinician may use a score of 0 to 3, with each rating sequentially corresponding to "no tenderness," "mild tenderness," "moderate tenderness," or "severe tenderness."[2, 26, 27] This score should be recorded for each anatomical location based on the client's response and feedback during the palpation.

Trigger Points

The trigger point is defined as "the presence of discrete focal tenderness located in a palpable taut band of skeletal muscle, which produces both referred regional pain (zone of reference) and a local twitch response."[28] Trigger points are classified as *active* or *latent*. Active trigger points are described as those that are associated with local and referred pain in a specific distribution, whereas latent trigger points are asymptomatic.[29] Trigger points may be related to the negative effects of sustained low-level contractions or dynamic repetitive contractions.[30] Continued activity causes a cascade of oxygen and glucose depletion, increased anaerobic glycolytic function of oxygen-deprived musculature, excessive lactic acid production, and stasis of that lactic acid.[30] Additionally, peripheral sensitization may contribute to local tenderness.

The diagnosis of a trigger point is primarily based on findings from palpation; diagnostic criteria include a palpable band, local and referred tenderness, and a local twitch response.[28, 30] Palpation procedures that have been described for trigger-point identification include flat, pincer, and deep palpation.[31] The process of flat palpation involves the slow translation of fingertips over a suspected muscle, such that "the skin is pushed to one side, and the finger is drawn across the muscle fibers."[31] Similarly, snapping palpation has been described as like the "plucking of a violin. . . used to identify the specific trigger point."[31] Pincer palpation involves approximating the muscle tissue between the first and second digits in a "rolling manner while attempting to locate a taut band."[31] Deep palpation is used for provocation testing of deeper muscle tissues.

Few quality research studies have investigated diagnostic criteria for trigger points. Authors of literature reviews have generally reported observations of poor reliability for the diagnosis of trigger points.[29, 32] From a review of clinical studies, Lucas and colleagues reported a higher reliability for subjective criterion (tenderness [κ range, 0.22–1.0] and pain reproduction κ range [0.57–1.00]), as opposed to objective criterion (taut band κ range, −0.08–0.75; local twitch response κ range −0.05–0.57).[29] Similarly, Myburgh and colleagues reported that they observed reproducible findings including local tenderness of the trapezius (κ range, 0.15–0.62), pain referral of the gluteus medius (κ range, 0.298–0.487), and pain referral of the quadratus lumborum (κ range, 0.36–0.501).[32] It is also notable that only two studies were found to be of sufficient quality.

Temperature

The clinician should palpate the surface temperature of an anatomical area because abnormalities may indicate changes in vascular function. This is typically examined by gently palpating the tissue, typically the epidermis, with the pads of the fingers or dorsum of the hand to appreciate a gross temperature. This gross finding may be compared with an expected normal temperature, or with other areas of the client's body that are not suspected to contribute to the pathophysiologic process. Greater, or warm, temperatures may indicate a local or regional inflammatory response, global or local infection, thrombosis, hematoma, hyperthermia, or increased activity levels. Lesser, or cool, temperatures may indicate peripheral vascular disease, obstruction or laceration of proximal vascular structures, hypothermia, hypovolemic shock, and other systemic illness. Though findings of greater or lesser temperatures than normal may be related to a number of pathophysiologic processes, considering the context of a client's complaint may aid causative reasoning.

Many clinical presentations may indicate surface temperature examination, though certain presentations may increase the relative value of abnormal findings in an orthopedic clinical setting based on the need to identify serious health conditions. Identification of surface temperature abnormalities during physical examination should be prioritized in the context of postoperative management, examination of clients with greater relative risk for thrombosis, following acute musculoskeletal injury, and examination of clients with subjective or objective findings that indicate a serious health condition.

Sensation

Testing of sensory function is typically performed during the neurologic screening or neurologic examination components of a physical examination, though abnormalities of sensation that are identified during the palpation examination should be noted and further investigated as appropriate. If not specifically examined during the neurologic examination, light-touch or deep-pressure sensory impairments may be observed with palpation. If new sensory impairments become apparent, the clinician must reassess the need for further neurologic testing.

Edema

If a clinician observes signs and symptoms consistent with edema (e.g., swelling) based on visual inspection or anthropometric measurements (e.g., circumference measurements, volumetric displacement), they should palpate the structures to observe the quality of the tissues. Swelling may be observed locally at an involved structure or at the area surrounding the structure, or regionally due to disruptions of fluid uptake by the circulatory system.

Graded forces should be applied to the area to observe the quality of the edema. First, the area should be palpated gently to assess for gross density of the fluid and pain provocation. Because acute inflammation due to local musculoskeletal injury may sensitize the surrounding tissue,[33, 34] a clinician may defer further palpation if symptoms are provoked. The clinician should note whether reports of pain are concordant or nonconcordant. If tolerated by the client, the clinician may apply a more sustained pressure (approximately 3-5 s) through the fingers with enough force to deform the tissue. The edema is considered *pitting* if an imprint is visually observed after removing the finger and *nonpitting* if the form of the tissue immediately returns. If peripheral pitting edema has not been medically assessed and managed, action should be taken to ensure that the client is assessed and managed by the appropriate medical provider due to the seriousness of potential origins or contributors. Peripheral pitting edema may be related to systemic illness, vascular obstruction (e.g., thrombosis, tumor), infection, or pregnancy.[35-37] The clarification of swelling as peripheral pitting edema or local response to a musculoskeletal lesion may aid in differentiation of the client's diagnosis and identification of serious health conditions.

Tissue Quality

Tissue quality may be described as the state of a client's tissue, given the expected physical properties of the tissue in nonpathologic conditions. The tissue's expected physical properties vary by tissue type, though a clinician may assess the state as a function of the relative resistance they encounter with the application of force. Greater resistance to force may indicate a more dense structure (such as bone), while lesser resistance may indicate less dense tissues (such as adipose tissue). Abnormalities in the gross quantity of force required for deformation of the tissue may indicate an altered state for a particular tissue. For example, one would expect muscle tissue to be more pliable than bone tissue and less pliable than any superficial adipose tissue. One would also expect muscle tissue to be less firm than the bone tissue to which it attaches, though more firm than adipose tissue. A clinician may assess for abnormality by comparing a structure to a noninvolved contralateral structure (if applicable) or to findings from previous client encounters.

Muscle Activity

The function of a muscle is to move or stabilize the structures to which it attaches. This is performed by active contraction of the muscle tissue, thereby placing a tensile load on tissue such that the distance between the attachment sites increases or decreases in a controlled manner. When activated, the muscle tissue has increased fullness due to the shortening of contractile units. During palpation, clinicians may observe this gradual increase in fullness, as well as decreased pliability and increased difficulty with tissue deformation.

For examination purposes, the clinician locates the target tissue and applies pressure to the muscle belly with the fingertips or palmer surface of the fingers (pending the size of the muscle). The clinician may cue the client to perform a volitional contraction by asking them to activate the muscle or to complete the action of the muscle. If no activation is observed, the clinician may attempt facilitation strategies to promote activation. Facilitation strategies may include gently tapping of the muscle belly with the fingertips, assisting with motion for the muscle's action to diminish resistance, providing resistance that opposes the muscle's action, or asking the client to simulate a daily activity that will likely result in activation of the muscle. The clinician should observe for substitution strategies that the client may rely on to decrease muscular demands.

Though the functions of the muscle to be examined should be based on the client's presentation, the clinician may test ability to activate, strength, endurance, power, and timing of activation during functional activity performance. Inability to regulate force production may indicate upper motor neuron dysfunction.[38] If the clinician suspects a central neurologic origin of abnormalities, they should refer the client for further neurologic assessment and management as appropriate. Diminished activation may be a sign of neurologic dysfunction or muscle function impairments.[38] Additionally, researchers have described the inhibition of a muscle or group of muscles due to a painful stimulus.[39-41]

Arthrogenic muscle inhibition (AMI) has been described as "continued reflex inhibition of musculature surrounding a joint following injury or joint effusion."[40] Muscle performance impairments related to AMI have been reported to contribute to secondary impairments that are related to functional compensation strategies.[41] Compensation strategies may cause damage to joint structures by resulting in abnormal joint loading during activity performance. Rice and McNair described that quadriceps inhibition following ACL injury "may impair dynamic knee stability, physical function, and quality of life, increase the risk of re-injury to the knee joint, and contribute to the development and progression of osteoarthritis (OA)."[41] AMI has also been described in regard to shoulder and neck pain related to scapular muscle inhibition and hip joint effusion related to gluteus maximus inhibition.[39, 40] Clinicians should consider employing palpation for targeted muscle activation to test for impairments that are reported to be common for specific client populations.

When palpating muscle tissue, the resting activity level of the structure should be noted. If the client were positioned such that a targeted muscle is able to be in a relaxed state, the clinician would expect the muscle tissue to be pliable, but firm. An increase in the resting activity level of a muscle may be related to a protective response to painful stimuli (known as *guarding*), neurologic dysfunction, anxiety or fear, or volitional contraction. Resting activation may be addressed with verbal cueing to relax and reassure the client, though the clinician should note the resting activity if no change is observed. Further examination should be performed to differentiate the factors contributing to abnormal findings, though the clinician may not be able to determine a specific origin.

Palpation by the clinician, or by the client following proper instruction, may be utilized as a biofeedback tool for muscle activation when related impairments are identified. The procedure for palpating the muscle tissue does not differ from that performed during examination, though immediate feedback is provided for the purpose of training motor performance. In the context of orthopedic clinical practice, this technique has been described as an intervention strategy to address impaired motor function for a variety of clinical presentations.

Among clients with low back pain (LBP), motor performance impairments of lumbar paraspinal (multifidus) and abdominal musculature (transversus abdominis) have been commonly reported in regard to activation quality and quantity.[42] Researchers have included palpation for lumbar multifidus (LM) and transversus abdominis (TrA) activation as a testing method or during coordination training for purposes of biofeedback.[43-45] Though examination and intervention techniques for palpating activation of the LM and TrA are commonly taught in entry-level programs and utilized in clinical environments, empirical evidence that investigates the research properties (reliability, validity, efficacy measures) of such methods is limited, and their utilization is cautioned.

Palpation for Mechanical Abnormalities of a Joint

Palpation for indicators of mechanical dysfunction within a joint is often described as a component of the orthopedic physical examination. Certain commonly used techniques vary by professional discipline, though many techniques are universal in the orthopedic examination. The techniques take many forms, including the following.

Crepitus or Clicks and Pops

Crepitus occurs during joint movement, and is defined as a "crackling or rattling sound made by a part of the body."[46] The origin of clicking and popping joint sounds has been the subject of debate in many clinical settings, though explanations are typically mechanical in nature. Joint noises have been described as a common clinical observation and diagnostic criterion for a number of musculoskeletal diagnoses, including the following: osteoarthritis of the knee,[47, 48] osteoarthritis of the hip,[49] osteoarthritis of the shoulder,[50] posterior tibial tendon dysfunction,[51] loose bodies and osteochondral lesions within a joint,[11, 52, 53] de Quervain's disease,[54] rotator cuff tears,[55] patellofemoral pain syndrome,[56] and temporomandibular joint dysfunction.[57]

Specific Response to a Special Test

Many special tests not only require palpation for preparation and positioning but also utilize palpation findings for administration of the test. This component may vary by the purpose and body region of the test. Joint instability tests often require palpation of a joint line or bony landmark to observe or quantify movement, such as tests for upper cervical ligament stability[58, 59] and varus and valgus stress testing of the elbow and knee.[60, 61] Palpation may be utilized to aid in assessment of suspected contractile unit disruption, as with the rent test for rotator cuff tears[62] or the biceps crease index and the hook test for distal biceps tendon tears.[63] Palpation may also be used to identify a mechanical dysfunction that results with predetermined joint forces, such as with McMurray's test for knee meniscus lesions[16, 61, 64] and the scaphoid shift test for scaphoid instability.[65] Several tests for sacroiliac joint (SIJ) dysfunction involve palpating for symmetry of bony pelvic landmarks and changes to symmetry with positional change, though there is a paucity of diagnostic literature that demonstrates sufficient research properties for clinical application.[60] Many tests for thoracic outlet syndrome involve palpation of the radial pulse to observe for change; such tests include Adson's test, the hyperabduction test, and Wright's test.[60] Palpation for provocation is discussed in the earlier section Provocation of Concordant Symptoms, though it is notable that many special tests describe focal tenderness at a specific location as a positive test.

ABDOMINAL PALPATION

During subjective and physical examinations, a clinician who provides health care services in an orthopedic setting may observe symptoms or signs that are suggestive of a nonmusculoskeletal origin. There is significant overlap of pain referral patterns among of the musculoskeletal system (especially the trunk and proximal joints of the extremities) and the digestive system, cardiopulmonary systems, circulatory system, and urogenital system. Autonomous health care providers in this setting must utilize the most effective strategies for identifying findings that are suggestive of nonmusculoskeletal origin, determining a safe and appropriate plan of action for the client, and facilitating referral for further assessment as appropriate.

In the *Description of Specialty Practice for Orthopedic Physical Therapy*, authors report the distribution of client encounters for board-certified specialists by body region.[66] From this data, one may observe that the majority of clients receive services for complaints that may overlap in pain referral patterns with other body systems. Encounter distributions, by body regions that may refer symptoms in similar patterns as the digestive and urogenital systems, are as follows: cervical spine (15%), thoracic spine (5%), lumbar spine (20%), pelvic girdle and abdomen (5%), shoulder girdle (15%), and hip (5%). Health care providers who provide services in orthopedic settings must be able to provide an appropriate abdominal screening examination to aid in identification of digestive and urogenital system health conditions.

Following visual inspection for abnormalities (e.g., distention, contour abnormalities), the clinician should position a stethoscope over the four abdominal quadrants and the midline to auscultate peristaltic sounds.[67] Though the location of an examination technique varies by location of the organ that is being assessed, the components of the abdominal examination include palpation (for direct tenderness, rebound tenderness, gross size abnormalities, and inflammation), percussion, and auscultation of bowel sounds. Instruction for the abdominal screening examination is limited, since the topic is beyond the scope of this chapter. Additional detail of technique and diagnostic accuracy is given in chapter 6 (Triage and Differential Diagnosis).

PULSE PALPATION

Vascular structures may be palpated to assess for pulse or vascular distention. Pulses are typically palpated in the context of assessment for occlusion, dissection, and cardiovascular function. Pulse is a function of the force of ejection from the left ventricle to the aorta, as well as elasticity of vascular structures. Pulse is described as a diagnostic component for certain clinical presentations, as well as a vital sign to be observed and monitored. Pulses are typically assessed in regard to presence (present or absent), regularity (regular or irregular), rate (beats per minute), rhythm, or quality (strong, weak, thready). Certain regular irregularities are commonly associated with specific clinical presentations and may be further classified. Body position (relative to gravity) at the time of pulse examination should be planned and noted.

Peripheral pulse palpation is performed in anatomic locations that are specific to commonly assessed arteries. Pressure is applied as the minimal force necessary to sense pulsation. Here are some commonly assessed peripheral pulses:

• **Common carotid artery:** Palpated at the anterior border of the sternocleidomastoid muscle, lateral to the thyroid, this pulse is typically easy to palpate. When palpating for the carotid pulse, a clinician should always be cautious to avoid occluding the vessel or provoking a vasovagal response.

• **Brachial artery:** The clinician palpates the medial aspect of the upper arm, deep to the biceps brachii muscle, approximately two-thirds of the distance from the axilla to the elbow. The brachial artery is commonly palpated for infants.

• **Radial artery:** This anatomic location is most commonly used during the vital signs assessment. The clinician palpates on the anterior surface of the distal lateral forearm, just medial to the lateral border of the radius.

- **Femoral artery:** Typically palpated with the client in a supine position, the clinician palpates for this pulse midway from the pubic tubercles and the anterior superior iliac spine (ASIS), just distal to the inguinal ligament. The femoral pulse is commonly palpated during clinical examination of the abdomen.

- **Popliteal artery:** The clinician palpates the popliteal space on the posterior aspect of the knee. This is performed with the client in a position of slight knee flexion.

- **Posterior tibial artery:** The clinician palpates slightly distal and inferior to the posterior aspect of the tibia's medial malleolus.

- **Dorsalis pedis artery:** On the dorsal foot, the clinician palpates between the tendon of the extensor hallucis longus muscle and tendon of the extensor digitorum longus that extends to the second toe. Though palpation of this pulse is a common component of clinical examinations involving the lower extremities, an absent pulse may commonly lead to a false positive for occlusion. Researchers have reported incidence of an absent pulse on clinical examination from 4% to 12%. Anatomic studies have been performed to investigate incidence rates of an absent artery, and researchers have reported values ranging from 1.5% to 14.2%.[68] The clinician should consider that a client's absent dorsalis pedis pulse may not be an indicator of pathology.

When observed in an extremity, an absent or weak pulse may indicate thrombosis (due to vessel occlusion) or dissection of a vascular structure. Thrombosis and infection are serious potential complications to surgical interventions; palpation of surface temperature (of the tissue surrounding the incision) and pulse (pending the type of procedure) should be standard examination procedures.

Pulse rate may be assessed as a vital sign (rate and rhythm) and monitored for response to a stimulus (such as exertion, positional change relative to gravity, or drugs). Normative values of rate are reported as 55 to 100 beats per minute for adults, though they may be slower for athletes or faster for children and infants.[67] Heart rates that are lower than normative values are considered bradycardias, whereas heart rates higher than normative values are tachycardias. When monitoring response to a stimulus, a baseline measurement should be taken at rest. The rate should be compared to the baseline measurement and assessed for normal response to a known stimulus. For example, a client's pulse rate follows a known pattern in response to exercise. Variation from the normal pattern may indicate an adverse response that is related to cardiopulmonary disease. Abnormal pulse rates could be observed when examining clients who have a number of health conditions related to the cardiovascular and pulmonary systems.

BONY LANDMARK PALPATION

Typically, landmarks are identified with palpation for the purposes of anatomical navigation and structural assessment. Because the rigidity of bone make it a distinguishable and unique body tissue, certain known prominences demonstrate excellent clinical utility as beacons by which to locate or compare other structures of established spatial relation. In regard to body mapping, this technique is described to facilitate other clinical testing procedures. Examples of this may include location of the femoral artery in relation to the pubic tubercles and ASIS to examine femoral pulse, the gluteus medius tendon in relation to the greater trochanter of the femur and the iliac crest for tenderness testing, or the ASIS and the patella to measure hip abduction range of motion.

Structural assessment may be performed in many contexts. In regard to symmetry assessment, clinicians compare relative positions of landmarks with a contralateral counterpart. Palpation of the spine should be utilized to assess for asymmetry from side to side as well as assessment of interspinous space between corresponding levels. Side-to-side asymmetry of the spinous processes from one level to the next may indicate the presence of a rotational dysfunction.[69] Palpation of interspace between corresponding spinous processes can give an appreciation for the vertical height between corresponding vertebral levels. If two spinous processes have very little to no space between them, the clinician should suspect decreased size of the intervertebral disc or increased lumbar lordosis (which would approximate the spinous processes). Observation and palpation from the side would give an appreciation for the extent of lumbar lordosis. Localized tenderness over the facet joints without other root tension signs or neurologic signs may indicate facet joint pain.[70]

Prior to observing and palpating a client for asymmetry or dysfunction, the clinician should determine which eye is their dominant eye. In order to assess eye dominance, the clinician can make a circle with both hands and place and look through the circle at a nonmoving object (such as a clock on the wall) with both eyes open. From this same point of view, the clinician then closes one eye at a time and looks through the same circle. Whichever eye is open when the nonmoving object appears in the circle is the dominant eye.

JOINT MOTION

Palpation for the purpose of clarifying or quantifying joint motion is typically performed in the context of manual therapy assessment or intervention. Joint motion palpation techniques are highly controversial. A primary challenge for determining the value of findings from palpation of joint motion is the significant variation of practice among clinicians who commonly use such assessment techniques. This controversy demonstrates the importance of considering the current body of evidence throughout the provision of client services.

Joint mobility testing is most commonly described as testing for passive accessory motion or passive physiologic motion. Passive accessory motions are tested by reproducing the accessory motion of a targeted joint (roll, spin, or glide), and then qualifying and quantifying this motion. When joint motion is interpreted to be excessive in comparison to normal expected motion, it is considered a hypermobility. Joint motion that is less than normal expected motion is considered a hypomobility.

Specific to mobility testing of the spine, passive accessory intervertebral motion (PAIVM) testing is commonly used to describe procedures in which the clinician applies force on a bony landmark of the vertebra to appreciate the gross amount of motion. Passive physiologic intervertebral motion (PPIVM) tests are typically performed such that an osteokinematic motion is reproduced. The clinician palpates a specified anatomic structure, typically the spinous process, and notes the proportion of motion relative to the adjacent segments. Research properties for joint mobility testing procedures are discussed further in the respective body region chapters.

CONCLUSION

Robert E. Kravetz writes that "the healing properties of touch, a simple form of client communication, are often overlooked and underutilized in our everyday practice."[71] Human contact physically links the clinician to their clients, establishing an attentive and caring rapport. To their clients, the clinician who integrates effective palpation skills into diagnostic and therapeutic procedures represents the caregiver who is present and focused on the client's complaint. Though many clinical presentations include tenderness as a diagnostic criterion, the utility of palpation spans beyond traditional provocation testing. Palpation is a tool that may be used to coordinate muscular activation during functional activity training, appreciate mechanical properties of joint structures, or improve efficacy of other physical examination components. Touch is a ritual that conveys the focused and skilled effort of an invested health care provider.

Critical Clinical Pearls

When testing joint mobility, clinicians should do the following:

- Ensure security of the stabilized segment (typically the proximal segment) to aid in limiting osteokinematic motion such that arthrokinematic motion may be isolated
- Identify the orientation of the joint's articular surfaces to plan the direction and location of force applied to the mobilized segment
- Increase contact area with the stabilizing and mobilizing segments to improve the client's ability to relax musculature that surrounds the joint of interest
- Place the pad of a finger on the joint line to aid in palpation of joint motion

12

PHYSICAL PERFORMANCE MEASURES

Robert J. Butler, PT, DPT, PhD

Function is measured in a number of different ways, including through the use of impairment measures, self-report measures, and physical performance measures (PPMs). Each of these measures has unique contributions and dedicated limitations to the measurement of function. Physical performance measures, or what have also been termed *performance-based measures* or *functional testing*, attempt to assess the person as a whole versus their specific components (muscle performance, range of motion) or specific impairments (decreased joint play, special testing). While many of these local, isolated measures have demonstrated causal relationships for postinjury assessment, they often simply test and measure just one parameter of function. The clinician must consider how impairments, client perceptions, and biopsychosocial measures affect performance on PPMs. Additional concerns with PPMs are that they have been poorly investigated with respect to diagnostic accuracy of injury prediction, and their correlation to other measures of impairment and disability (e.g., muscle performance, joint mobility, and proprioception) are mostly unclear. The clinical utility of PPMs is traditionally thought to exist as a measure for return to sport or potential injury prediction, or for those clients with very high levels of function post injury. Other measures are addressed in their respective areas of this book. For greater detail on all of the PPMs, refer to the work of Reiman and Manske.[1]

OVERVIEW OF TESTING HIERARCHY

Physical performance measures have a natural progression associated with requiring the client's body to control increasing load and momentum (table 12.1). The entry point from which these tests should start is with a simple assessment or screening of single body-weight motor control that examines the constructs of fundamental motor control and balance competency. Once competency and physiologic symmetry have been established with a given body-weight task, it is appropriate to then examine competency and symmetry of higher-level movement constructs that require motor control under higher levels of load, incorporate momentum, and require maintenance for longer durations of time. The end of the continuum of testing should incorporate agility, aerobic capacity, and sport-specific testing to optimize functional return and athlete durability when returning to sport. The majority of this literature has been focused on performance in the lower extremity; as a result, this initial section focuses on lower extremity PPM with an additional section in the end targeted on upper extremity PPM and general core stabilization tests.

SINGLE BODY-WEIGHT PHYSICAL PERFORMANCE MEASURES

Physical performance measure tests of a single body weight aim to identify competency of movement with the client's own body weight alone as resistance. Poor performance on these tests is often associated with deficient and painful movement on PPMs that require greater motor control demands. These tests can be divided into two sections: fundamental motor competency and balance competency. This section covers three fundamental motor competency measures and two balance measures.

Functional Movement Screen

The Functional Movement Screen (FMS) is a set of seven tests aimed at screening for movement competency and pain-free motion of a client using their own body weight as resistance.[2, 3] The seven tests of the FMS are the deep squat, hurdle step, in-line lunge, shoulder mobility, active straight-leg raise, trunk stability push-up, and rotary stability. Each test is scored from 0 to 3, with 0 being painful

TABLE 12.1 Proposed Levels for the Progression of the Functional Assessment

Levels for the assessment of function	Screens, assessments, and tests
Single body weight: fundamental motor competency	Functional movement screen Selective functional movement assessment Lateral step-down
Single body weight: balance competency	Single-leg stance Star excursion balance test/lower quarter Y balance test
>Single body-weight load	Vertical jump testing Single-leg anterior hopping Drop vertical jump test
>Single body-weight load + momentum	Triple hop/triple crossover hop Triple hop for time
Agility	Pro agility shuttle (5-10-5) Timed triangle Illinois agility test
Endurance and aerobic capacity	300 yd (274 m) shuttle Lower extremity functional test Multistage fitness test
Upper extremity	Closed kinetic chain upper extremity stability test Upper quarter Y balance test One-arm hop test Seated shot-put throw
General core stabilization	Prone bridge and plank Lateral flexor endurance and side bridge

and 3 meeting the criteria to successfully complete the full range of motion of the test without pain. Scores of 1 and 2 suggest some level of nonpainful compensation that does not meet the criteria for completion of the test, with a score of 1 indicating a greater limitation than a score of a 2. Five of the FMS tests have a bilateral component and should be scored independently. In addition to the movement-based tests, three clearing tests examine end-range pain that is not tested during the FMS: the impingement test, prone press-up, and quadruped flexion clearing test. When analyzing a client's FMS, the clinician should understand the number of painful tests, the number of asymmetries present, the number of scores of 1, and the composite score (sum of the scores across the seven tests). Additionally, clinicians can examine each individual test to determine whether the client is ready to progress or if they need to regress or maybe potentially to lateralize their training in order to attain the movement competency goals. Current research on the FMS suggests that scores on the FMS can be reliable between raters and across days.[3-5] Poor performance or asymmetry on the test has been associated with an elevated risk for musculoskeletal injuries in some populations.[6-8]

Selective Functional Movement Assessment

The Selective Functional Movement Assessment (SFMA) is a way to look at basic motor control competency that may be associated with the limitations in the functional tasks looked at under the client's own body weight.[1] This movement appraisal can serve as an intermediary step between functional limitations and isolated range of motion and muscle testing. The SFMA is utilized to assess movement competency with a more focused appraisal of spinal motion and with the expectation of identifying similar pain associated with the client's primary complaint. The SFMA examines seven basic motor control patterns: cervical mobility, shoulder mobility, multisegmental flexion, multisegmental extension, multisegmental rotation, single-leg stance, and deep squat. The movements have specific standards that need to be met to determine whether the movement is adequate (functional) or deficient (dysfunctional). During the testing, clinicians should also monitor pain at the joint of primary concern and note whether any secondary pain is developed. Scoring of the test has initially been reported to be reliable but dependent on experience in using the SFMA.[9]

Lateral Step-Down Test

The lateral step-down (LSD) test assesses frontal plane competency during a unilateral squat from a standardized height.[10] The focus of the test is to examine what secondary plane deviations and balance strategies are required for completing the maneuver. The LSD sums the number of compensations that occur in order to complete the lateral step-down activity. The test is completed off a standard 8 in. (20 cm) step with the hands placed on the hips. The criteria that are scored are use of arm strategy, trunk lean, pelvic motion in the secondary planes, medial knee deviation (second toe and medial border of the foot as landmarks), and ability to perform the test without touching down with the nontested limb. Fewer than two total errors should occur during the test in order to exhibit competency of performance. This test serves as a good indicator of potential lower extremity compensations when a greater level of load is placed on an isolated lower extremity.[11, 12]

Critical Clinical Pearls

When performing the Functional Movement Screen, clinicians should keep the following in mind:

- Clients should complete the test without warming up.
- When identifying the score on the FMS, clinicians should use the checklist to ensure that all criteria were met to achieve a 3 and mark down which limited part of the movement led to a score that was not a 3.
- Clinicians should factor in performance on the FMS to the overall exercise programming (i.e., clients shouldn't squat with additional weight if their body weight alone is causing a deficit [i.e., a 1 on the FMS deep squat]) and break down patterns to identify whether limitations are due to motor control or joint mobility limitations.

Single-Leg Stance (SLS) Test

Single-leg stance test serves as a basic test of a fundamental static balance strategy.[13] To complete the standardized single-leg stance test, a client should stand up straight with their feet together. The client then lifts one thigh so that it is parallel with the ground and the knee is bent to 90°. To exhibit fundamental static balance competency, a cutoff point of 10 seconds is expected in order to progress to higher level dynamic balance tasks; however, it should be of note that the 10 second threshold is below what would be considered normal for most age groups. Average performance in adult populations is about 30 seconds per side.[13] The client should complete this test while standing independently on each leg. Insight into fundamental static balance competency can also be accomplished by completing this test with the client's eyes closed (eyes closed after the leg is in the air) while using the same time cutoff point for successful SLS. If a client cannot complete the fundamental SLS test with eyes open, there is minimal need for further balance testing, however it can be beneficial to test SLS with eyes closed to understand how removing the sensory input affects SLS.

Star Excursion Balance Test

The Star Excursion Balance Test (SEBT) protocol was originally developed as a way to assess dynamic balance across eight independent reach directions (figure 12.1).[14] Performance of the test requires the client to maintain unilateral stance while reaching with the contralateral limb in a variety of directions. A recent review of the literature by Gribble and colleagues recommended a reduction in number of reach directions from eight to three (anterior, posteromedial, and posterolateral) to improve the efficiency of the testing process.[15] The standardized SEBT protocol requires the client to keep their hands on their hips while reaching in the different directions and their heel in contact with the floor. When the client reaches the furthest distance they can reach, they lightly touch their foot down. The client practices each reach direction four times before the clinician collects the three performance trials in order to minimize the learning effect associated with the test. Performance on the test is measured by calculating normalized reach distances and average normalized (leg length measured from ASIS to medial malleolus) reach distances (composite scores), as well as reach asymmetry scores (in cm) for each independent direction. A derivation of the SEBT is the Y balance test (YBT) developed by Plisky and colleagues.[16] The Y balance test protocol is performed with a standardized test kit to allow for increased efficiency with set-up. The primary difference between the traditional SEBT and YBT protocol is that for the YBT protocol, the client does not need to keep their hands on their hips or their heel on the ground during the test. Performance on SEBT and YBT has been reported to be reliable across raters and days.[14] Poor performance or reach asymmetry on the SEBT or YBT has been associated with increased risk for musculoskeletal injury in athletic populations.[17-19]

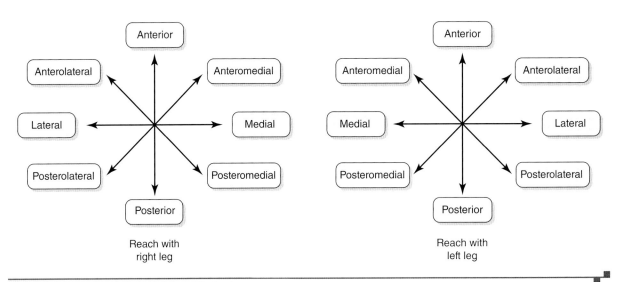

Figure 12.1 Star Excursion Balance Test set-up.

Reprinted, by permission, from M. Reiman and R. Manske, 2009, *Functional testing in human performance* (Champaign, IL; Human Kinetics), 109.

SINGLE BODY-WEIGHT LOADING

After examining basic movement and balance competency under a single body weight, the client should be tested under conditions of higher level loading. This incremental increase in performance demands allows for proper targeting of intervention strategies and environments that promote improvement of movement abilities under tasks with a greater demand.

Vertical Jump Testing

The double-leg vertical jump is a test that examines concentric lower extremity power.[20] This test can be used as an indicator to examine overall lower extremity performance for jumping competency. The double-leg vertical jump can be assessed using a vertimax testing apparatus or a foot switch device. (The foot switch device measures on and off for contact time, which can serve as an indirect measure of jump height.) To conduct the test, the clinician has the client start in a bilateral stance and then jump as high as possible off of both legs and land while keeping their balance. Countermovement of the lower extremity and natural upper extremity movement are expected and allowable in order to maximize the performance on the task. In order to be considered a complete trial, the client must statically hold the bilateral landing for 2 seconds prior to taking a step. The bilateral task can serve as a marker for lower extremity function; however, the task should also be performed unilaterally since unilateral deficits can be masked during bilateral tasks.[21]

The single-leg vertical jump (SLVJ) is a test that examines concentric unilateral power.[22] Deficits in tasks of this nature are often observed following injury.[20] The SLVJ should be completed for symmetry and competency before testing higher level demands on the lower extremity (such as shear forces and momentum). The client's side-to-side values for height and flight time should be within 10% before higher-level or multiple direction landing abilities are examined. Clinicians should also consider total height in examining basic competency in lower extremity power. Performance on these measures has previously been established to be reliable, and poor performance has previously been reported as an indicator for future anterior knee pain.[23-25]

Single-Leg Anterior Hop

Single-leg anterior hopping (SLAH) can be divided into a number of phases to examine normative values and establish symmetry comparisons to assess lower extremity function.[26] SLAH examines lower extremity power and stability and adds the demand for controlling anteroposterior force components in addition to the vertical forces tested in the SLVJ. To clarify the differences in jumping and hopping, a jump is a two-leg movement and a hop is a jump off of a single leg.[26-28] The countermovement and upper extremity movement contributions are considered standard and acceptable for the performance of the test. Similarly, in this protocol it is expected that all landings are held for 2 seconds in order to be counted.[27]

SLAH protocol should be completed by utilizing a series of maximal unilateral broad hops: one-leg hopping to two-leg landing, one-leg hopping to opposite-leg landing, and one-leg hopping to same-leg landing.[27-28] The first iteration of the test that should occur is the one-foot hop to two-foot landing in order to provide additional stability during the eccentric landing. Values (distance traveled) for the opposite side hopping should be within 5% of the one- or two-leg hopping values. However, values for the same-side single-leg broad hop should be between 10% and 15% of the opposite-side single-leg broad hop. Performance on these tests has been established to be reliable across testing periods and to provide an indicator of lower extremity function.[26, 27]

Drop Vertical Jump Test

The drop vertical jump test is utilized to screen for movement deficits with a level of loading during a jump landing.[29] The test is conducted with a standard stool or step that is 31 cm in height and a video camera that is placed perpendicular to the stool to assess the change in the frontal plane position of the knee from standing to peak medial position. To conduct the test, the clinician has the client stand on top of the stool with their feet shoulder-width apart. At this point in time the clinician starts the video recording and asks the client to drop directly down to the floor and perform a maximal vertical jump with a similar motion as that of grabbing a basketball rebound. The clinician stops the video and then tracks and records the change in the horizontal distance of the knee from initial contact to peak medial motion, as seen in the video.

Critical Clinical Pearls

When performing the drop vertical jump test, keep the following in mind:

- Make sure your camera positions are perpendicular to the frontal plane of the performance to minimize perspective error.
- If analyzing the sagittal plane as well, keep the focal center of the camera perpendicular to the landing area.
- When addressing deficient areas that can be contributing to deficits on the DVJ, assess proximal as well as distal factors.

Average motion on this measure is 4.15 cm (95% CI: 3.74–4.55 cm). Research on measures similar to this has suggested it to be associated with an increased risk of ACL injury in some studies.[30] In addition, a number of studies have examined the ability to modify this mechanical deficit through plyometric training programs.[31]

SINGLE BODY-WEIGHT LOADING AND MOMENTUM

After establishing the performance of the client on tests of elevated load, the clinician can increase the demands on the task by utilizing tests that include not only elevated load but also momentum. The control of momentum requires faster timing and control of joint mechanics, which is integral to the examination of clients in the rehabilitation setting in order to determine readiness for return to sport.

Triple Hop and Triple Crossover Hop

The next iteration of the single-leg broad-hop protocol involves the triple-hop sequence.[32, 33] The triple-hop sequence is carried out using the triple hop and triple crossover hop. The guidelines regarding lower extremity countermovement and upper extremity movement are similar to the single-leg anterior-hop protocol. The triple-hop protocol consists of how far a client can hop over a total of three consecutive hops (figure 12.2*a*). The final landing for this series of hops should be held for 2 seconds

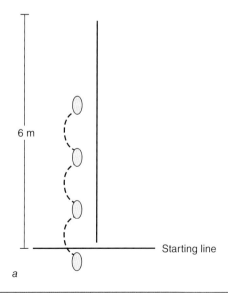
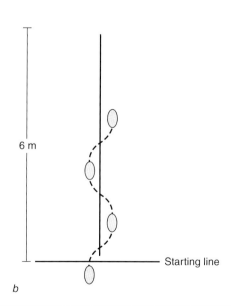

Figure 12.2 *(a)* Triple hop and *(b)* triple crossover hop.

in order to assess momentum control of the task. The results of this test should optimally be three times the single-leg hopping distance of the ipsilateral single-leg broad jump. The triple crossover hop adds a medial–lateral performance aspect to the test. For the triple crossover hop, the clinician places a taped line 6 in. (15 cm) wide along the jumping path. Performance of this test requires the client to jump laterally, then medially, and then one last time laterally over the line in order to complete the test (figure 12.2b). If the client does not clear the 6 in. tape or does not hold the final landing, then the trial is not counted. Performance of this test should be within 10% of the linear triple hop. These measures have previously been established as being reliable measures that correlate with subjective measures of function.[26, 27, 32, 33]

Six-Meter Hop for Time

The 6 m hop for time is a test of combined power and agility. The test set-up consists of a 6 m distance marked off (figure 12.3) and requires a stop watch.[32] When the clinician gives the verbal direction to begin the activity, the client jumps on a single leg as fast as possible to complete the 6 m distance. The clinician starts the timer when giving the verbal command and stops it when the client crosses the 6 m line. This test is completed independently for

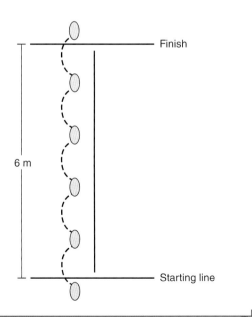

Figure 12.3 Six-meter timed hop.

Reprinted, by permission, from M. Reiman and R. Manske, 2009, *Functional testing in human performance* (Champaign, IL; Human Kinetics), 154.

each side, and symmetry of performance should be within 5%. Previous research on this measure has found it to be a reliable and relevant measure in assessing unilateral function in athletes.[22, 33]

AGILITY

Agility is the next level of performance that needs to be examined along the continuum of client function. Agility assessments need to examine performance in multiple directions of motion during a relatively short burst of activity.

Pro Agility 5-10-5

The pro agility 5-10-5 test (figure 12.4) examines fundamental agility performance over a short distance.[33] To conduct the test, the clinician should set up three cones in a line, 5 yards (4.6 m) apart. The client starts at the central cone with their body parallel to the line of cones. When the clinician gives a verbal command, the client runs to the left and then back past the center cone to the cone on the right, and then returns as fast as possible past the center cone. The clinician starts the timer when giving the verbal command and stops it once the client passes the center cone for the final time. Previous research has suggested that there should not be asymmetries in performance in clients following the test even if the client exhibits asymmetries on isolated single-leg landing tasks.[29]

Timed Triangle

The timed triangle is an agility test that incorporates angular cutting (figure 12.5). The test is completed with a series of six cones (inner and outer set of three cones). The base of the set of cones is placed 10 yards (~10 m) apart from each other. The top of the triangle should be placed 26 ft (8 m) perpendicular to the midpoint of the base of the triangle. An additional set of cones should be placed 1 yard (~1 m) outside each corner cone in order to create a normalized turning radius for each corner. Additional cones can be placed 1 yard around the perimeter to control the performance environment. The test starts with the client standing at the middle of the base of the triangle. Following a verbal command, the client should run around the triangle three times, staying within the

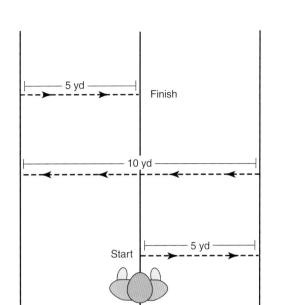

Figure 12.4 Pro Agility 5-10-5.

Reprinted, by permission, from M. Reiman and R. Manse, 2009, *Functional testing in human performance* (Champaign, IL; Human Kinetics), 193.

controlled performance environment. The test should be conducted running in both clockwise and counterclockwise directions in different trials. The client should complete the direction for each trial two times, and the clinician should average the trials. Performance in both directions should be within 10% of each other.

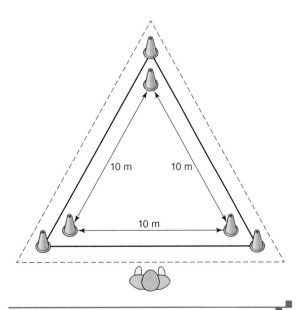

Figure 12.5 Timed triangle test.

Illinois Agility Test

The Illinois Agility Test (figure 12.6) incorporates linear speed along with cutting in a 10 m × 5 m space.[34] The clinician should set up four cones at the corner of the space. Along the midline of the space, the clinician places a series of four cones spaced 3.3 m apart. The client starts the drill at a bottom left cone facing the testing set-up so that all cones are in front of and to the right of them. To begin the task, the client runs forward to the 10 m line, and then turns and runs back to the starting line and rounds the bottom cone. Next the client weaves in and out of the cones along the midline of the space. When reaching the last cone, the client turns around and weaves back through the cones. After finishing this task, the client runs down to the far 10 m line again before returning back to the starting line. Excellent performance of the test is <15.2 seconds for males and <17.0 seconds for females.[1]

AEROBIC CAPACITY

Long-term aerobic capacity is important to examine in all clients due to the correlation of this construct to

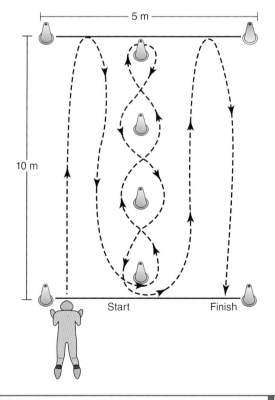

Figure 12.6 Illinois agility test.

Reprinted, by permission, from M. Reiman and R. Manske, 2009, *Functional testing in human performance* (Champaign, IL; Human Kinetics), 199.

client durability. In assessing aerobic capacity, the clinician should test this construct in multiple durations and with tests that include repeated attempts in order to examine the fitness capacity of the client.

300-Yard Shuttle Run

The 300-yard (274 m) shuttle run (figure 12.7) provides a linear indicator of anaerobic endurance.[1, 36] The test is set up with two markers 50 yards (45 m) apart from each other. The client starts at one of the markers and runs to the other one as fast as they can. The client touches the other marker and then returns to the other marker as fast as possible. The client covers this distance a total of six times, completing 300 yards. The aim of this test is to complete it in <60 seconds. Repetitive tests can also be done with 2-minute rest periods interspersed to examine the effect of exertion on multiple test performance.

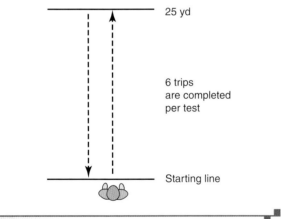

25 yd

6 trips are completed per test

Starting line

Figure 12.7 300-yard shuttle run.

Reprinted, by permission, from M. Reiman and R. Manske, 2009, *Functional testing in human performance* (Champaign, IL; Human Kinetics), 264.

Lower Extremity Functional Test

The lower extremity functional test (LEFT; figure 12.8) is a longer duration test of agility and aerobic capacity.[35, 37] The test is set up using four cones that are placed 30 ft (9 m) apart in the anteroposterior direction and 10 ft (3 m) apart in the mediolateral direction. The mediolateral cones are set up at the midpoint of the anteroposterior distance. Performance of the LEFT consists of forward runs, backward runs, side shuffle, carioca, figure-eight runs, 45° cuts, and 90° cuts completed two times. The clinician records the total time needed for the client to complete the testing protocol. Clinical recommendations for performance on the LEFT is <100 seconds for males and <120 seconds for females.[38] This measure has been found to be reliable across days.[39]

Multistage Fitness Test

The multistage fitness test (also known as the 20 m shuttle, the yo-yo, and the beep test) is a common test that estimates aerobic power and $\dot{V}O_2max$.[40, 41] To set up the test, the clinician places two cones 20 m apart.[40] The clinician uses a standard audio track to monitor the timing of the runs between the two cones. The audio track beeps when the client is supposed to be in contact with a cone. The distance between beeps becomes shorter and shorter to require an increase in client speed. Once the client is not present at a cone for two beeps in a row, the clinician stops the test. The clinician records performance on the test as the number of levels and number of shuttles that the client completed before the beep that ended the test. This test can take up to 23 minutes to complete. As a result of

Critical Clinical Pearls

When examining performance on the 300-yard shuttle, consider the following:

- It can be very helpful to track the splits of each shuttle to examine maintenance or decrements in time during the whole performance.
- It can be helpful to have the client run a flat-out 300-yard sprint on a track to factor in the stop-and-go cutting effect on the limitations of performance.
- Use a heart rate monitor to identify heart rate recovery during the 2-minute rest period to factor in the general conditioning aspect of the performance.

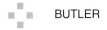

1. Forward sprint (A-C-A)
2. Retro sprint (A-C-A)
3. Side shuffle right – face in (A-D-C-B-A)
4. Side shuffle left – face in (A-B-C-D-A)
5. Cariocas right – face in (A-D-C-B-A)
6. Cariocas left – face in (A-B-C-D-A)
7. Figure 8s right (A-D-C-B-A)
8. Figure 8s left (A-B-C-D-A)
9. 45° cuts right – plant outside foot (A-D-C-B-A)
10. 45° cuts left – plant outside foot (A-B-C-D-A)
11. 90° cuts right – plant outside foot (A-D-B-A)
12. 90° cuts left – plant outside foot (A-B-D-A)
13. Crossover 90° cuts right – plant inside foot (A-D-B-A)
14. Crossover 90° cuts left – plant inside foot (A-B-D-A)
15. Forward sprint (A-C-A)
16. Retro sprint (A-C-A)

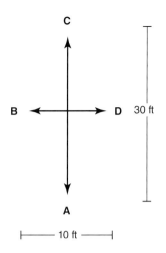

Figure 12.8 Lower extremity functional test.

Reprinted, by permission, from M. Reiman and R. Manske, 2009, *Functional testing in human performance* (Champaign, IL; Human Kinetics), 265.

this, the test serves as an indicator of higher-level aerobic capacity. Performance standards are age and sport specific.[42] Performance on the test can also be utilized to provide an estimate of $\dot{V}O_2$max based on established equations.[41]

UPPER EXTREMITY

Limited research has been conducted on functional assessment of the upper quarter. However, a series of progressive tests have been described in order to obtain an understanding of the limits of performance in the upper quarter as it relates to stability, motor control, and power. These tests can provide insight as to when limitations begin to be observed along the continuum of upper quarter function.

Closed Kinetic Chain Upper Extremity Stability Test

The closed kinetic chain upper extremity stability test (CKCUEST; figure 12.9) examines closed chain upper extremity stability, strength, and endurance. The clinician sets up the test by placing two pieces of tape 3 ft (1 m) apart from each other in parallel.[44] The client then assumes a push-up position within the boundary created by the tape. The client then is given 15 seconds to tap their hands as many times as possible from line to line, reaching across the body with the hand. The clinician records the number of touches performed to assess performance of this measure. The test can be modified in order to make comparisons between left and right stabilizing arms.

In this case, the client would reach in a single direction for 15 seconds and then complete the task in the opposite direction. Performance on this should be in the range of 18 to 28 taps using the bilateral tapping protocol.[44, 45] The test has been found to provide reliable measures in client populations as well as in uninjured groups.[46]

Upper Quarter Y Balance Test

The upper quarter Y balance test (YBT-UQ) examines end-range stability of the upper quadrant while maintaining core stability (figure 12.10). The test is completed using the standard Y balance test kit.[47] The client positions their body perpendicular to the front rail of the test kit and assumes the top of the push-up position, placing the hand on the side of their body closest to the stance platform on top of the stance platform, with the fingers together and the thumb next to the starting line. To conduct the test, the clinician has the client use the hand resting on the front rail to move the reach indicator in the medial (with respect to the stance limb), inferolateral, and superolateral directions, without resting the reach hand on the ground. The goals for performance on the test are to have physiologic symmetry between limbs (<4 cm for medial reach, <6 cm for posteromedial and posterolateral reach). In addition to symmetry, an average reach across all reach directions normalized to limb length, measured from C7 to tip of longest finger with the arm abducted 90°, is calculated and examined for both right and left limbs to examine overall competency (composite score) on the test. This value

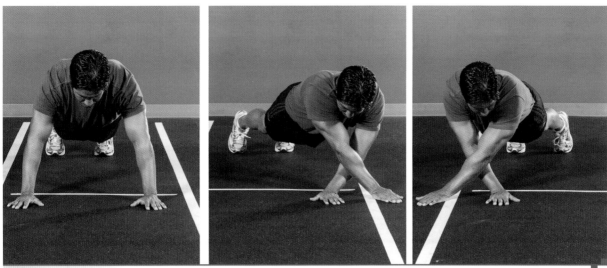

Figure 12.9 Closed kinetic chain upper extremity stability test.

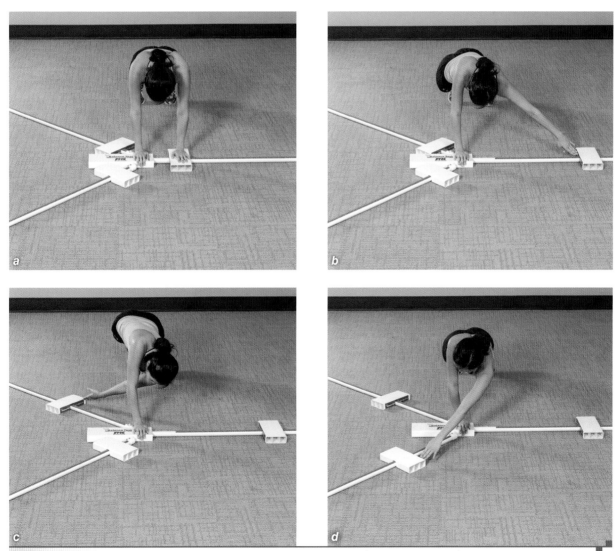

Figure 12.10 Upper quarter Y balance test: *(a)* starting position YBT-UQ, *(b)* medial YBT-UQ reach, *(c)* inferolateral YBT-UQ reach, and *(d)* superolateral YBT-UQ reach.

should be >85% limb length.[22, 45, 47] Overall performance should be considered as being a product of combined shoulder and core stabilization based on research by Westrick and colleagues.[45]

One-Arm Hop Test

The one-arm hop test is a higher-level test of arm strength and power as well as core stability. The test is completed by having the client assume the plank position of a one-arm push-up.[48] For this set-up position, the client should have a flat back and place the feet shoulder-width apart. Directly next to the client's hand a step (10.2 cm) is placed that serves as the elevated surface to which the client needs to hop. On hearing the verbal command to complete the exercise, the client needs to hop up to the elevated surface and down to the starting position five times. The time it takes to complete the activity is recorded and scored for both left and right sides. In male collegiate athletes, these values have been observed to be within the 6-second range, and no differences have been found between dominant and nondominant sides.[48]

Seated Shot-Put Throw

The seated shot-put throw (figure 12.11) is a test that isolates upper extremity strength and power.

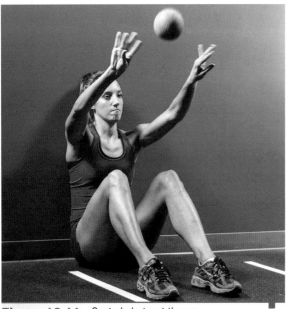

Figure 12.11 Seated shot-put throw.

A 10 lb (4.5 kg) ball is standardized to use.[49] To complete the task, the client should sit with their back against a wall and their knees bent to 90°. The client should then clutch the ball with both hands and push it forward from the center of their chest. Several practice trials are allotted to accommodate to the test before completing three performance trials. The average of the three trials should be used for analysis. Previous work on this test has correlated performance on the test to bench press power; however, the strength of the relationship is lowered when accounting for body mass.[50]

GENERAL CORE STABILIZATION

Basic core stabilization is a prerequisite for efficient peripheral movement. Historically core stabilization has been assessed in a high threshold position to identify the isometric limitations of the core. Information received from these testing postures can drive effective training strategies aimed at normalizing core function.

Prone Bridge

The prone bridge or plank (figure 12.12) is a test to examine high threshold isometric stabilization of the trunk and core musculature.[1, 35, 51] In order to complete the task, the client positions themselves in prone while being propped up on their elbows. When instructed, the client lifts their pelvis off the ground in a straight line between the ankles and shoulders. The client should hold this position until they are unable to maintain it due to fatigue or pain. Normative values for this have been observed to differ between males (92.9 ± 29.3) and females (51.2 ± 19.9) as well. Performance on the test is affected by the onset of pain and history of back pain.[51]

Endurance of Lateral Flexors

The lateral trunk flexor endurance test or side plank (figure 12.13) is the frontal plane complement to the prone bridge, and assesses high-threshold isometric stabilization bilaterally.[1, 52, 53] On command, the client lifts their hips up off the surface so that

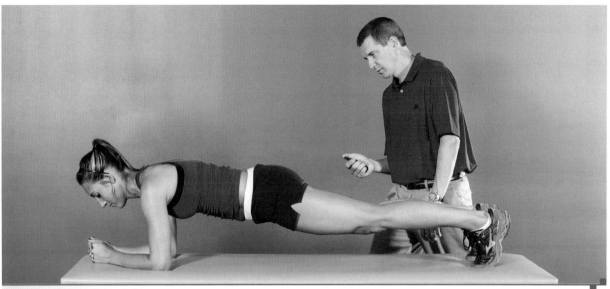

Figure 12.12 Prone bridge.

their pelvis is in line with their feet, knees, and head. The client should hold this test position as long as possible until unable due to fatigue or pain. The goal of the test is to hold the position for 30 seconds on each side. The test is scored on a 1 to 5 scale, with a 1 representing the client being unable to lift their hip off the table and scaled to a 5 where the client is able to hold the position for 20 to 30 seconds. If a client is unable to lift their hips off the ground in this position, the test is modified to be completed with the knees bent, which decreases the difficulty of the test.

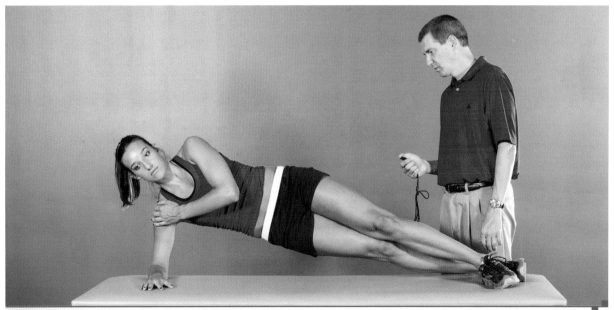

Figure 12.13 Lateral trunk flexor endurance test.

CONCLUSION

Implementation of PPMs for postinjury assessment should be a criterion-based progression with consideration for personal and biopsychosocial concerns. The PPM may be unable to accurately portray the client's true physiological ability due to psychological or other nonphysical variables. For example, it was demonstrated that clients with higher fear-avoidance beliefs were less able to perform more difficult trunk endurance testing post lumbar microdiscectomy than their colleagues with lower fear-avoidance beliefs.[9] In such a case, simply measuring the PPM would not accurately portray the client's dysfunction. As proposed by Reiman and Manske, the examination of a client is along a continuum.[54] This continuum includes impairment-based measures (decreased strength and range of motion), self-reported outcome measures, and PPMs. The combination of all of these testing approaches measures the concept of a client's function. Assessment of a client's function should be criterion-based (lower level assessments must be successfully completed prior to higher levels of assessment).

GAIT

Janice K. Loudon, PT, PhD, SCS, ATC

Select portions of this chapter are reprinted, by permission, from J. Loudon, R. Manske, and M. Reiman, 2013, *Clinical mechanics and kinesiology* (Champaign, IL: Human Kinetics), chapters 17 and 18.

Human locomotion is a repeated series of synchronous movements that involves multiple joint segments of the human body. This movement requires fully functioning musculoskeletal, neuromuscular, and cardiorespiratory systems. A keen observer can detect problems with any of the systems based on deviations in a client's gait. As thus, a gait assessment should be one component of every orthopedic examination. This chapter focuses primarily on the musculoskeletal system's contribution to walking and running gait. Normal walking and running kinematics and kinetics are discussed first, followed by common faults found in each locomotion mode. The breakdown of each gait phase will help the clinician understand and identify gait faults.

WALKING GAIT

In general, walking gait is a sequential, semipredictable, and efficient mode of locomotion.[1] The body's ability to control vertical and horizontal displacement allows for efficient forward motion. This efficient motor pattern is based on six determinants:

1. Pelvic rotation in the transverse plane: On the swing side, the pelvis moves anteriorly to advance the limb forward.

2. Lateral pelvic tilt: On the swing side, the pelvis drops approximately 1 in. (2.5 cm).

3. Lateral shift: The body shifts approximately 1 to 2 in. (2.5–5 cm) toward the stance limb.

4. Knee flexion: The knee flexes up to 45° during preswing.

5. Ankle dorsiflexion: The ankle dorsiflexes during the late phase of midstance as the body progresses forward.

6. Heel rise: During the last portion of stance, the heel raises during preswing.

A disturbance in any one of these determinants results in gait deviations that can be grossly observed and in an increase in energy expenditure.[2]

Walking Gait Sequence

A full gait cycle is the sequential completion of a single limb's stance phase and swing phase. Further, it can be described as the period between right initial contact and right initial contact (or left initial contact and left initial contact), or stride length. Step length is the distance between right foot contact and left foot contact. The stance (stride) phase is when the reference foot is on the ground; it is made up of five subphases: initial contact, loading response, midstance, terminal stance, and preswing. The swing phase is when the reference foot is off the ground; it includes the initial swing, midswing, and terminal swing. These phases are taken from the Rancho Los Amigos (RLA) terminology.[3] A comparison of traditional gait sequence terminology with Rancho Los Amigos terminology is included in figure 13.1. Traditional terminology refers to points in time, whereas the RLA terminology refers to lengths of time. The next section looks at the individual phases of gait.

With normal walking speed (1 m/s), the stride phase makes up 60% to 62% of the whole gait cycle. Single support occurs when only one foot is on the ground and occurs during the middle portion of the stance phase. Double support occurs when both feet are on the ground and at the beginning and end of the stance. Figure 13.1 displays each phase of the gait sequence.

Initial contact is defined as the point when the foot contacts the ground. In normal gait, this contact is made by the heel. However, in gait sequences like those of people with cerebral palsy, initial contact may be with the mid- or forefoot. Initial contact is the shortest phase of the stance phase.

Loading response is the phase from initial contact until the contralateral leg leaves the ground. During loading response, weight is rapidly transferred onto the outstretched limb, and the limb is decelerating. This along with initial contact is the first period of double-limb support, since the contralateral limb is on the ground. The initial contact phase and the loading response phase together make up 10% of the gait cycle.

Midstance is the period when the contralateral extremity lifts off the ground and continues to a position in which the body has progressed over and ahead of the supporting extremity. Midstance

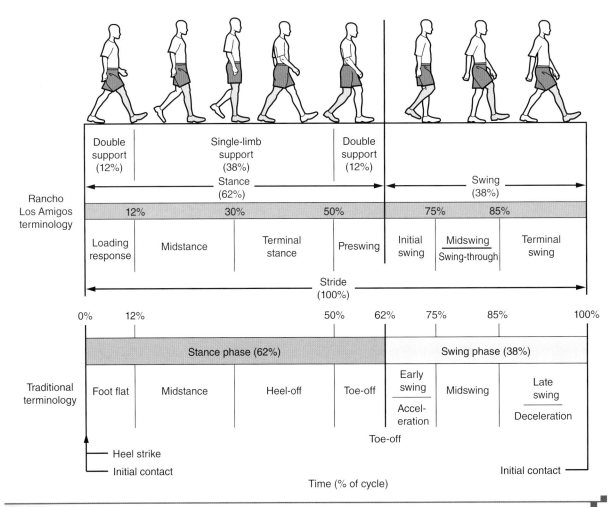

Figure 13.1 Ranch Los Amigos and traditional terminology for the walking gait cycle.

Reprinted, by permission, from J. Loudon, R. Manske, and M. Reiman, 2013, *Clinical mechanics and kinesiology* (Champaign, IL: Human Kinetics), 356.

makes up 20% of the gait cycle and is a period of single-limb support.

Terminal stance occurs from midstance to a point just before initial contact of the contralateral extremity. In normal gait, the heel is leaving the ground as progression over the stance limb continues. The body moves ahead of the limb, and weight is transferred onto the forefoot. Terminal stance lasts for 20% of gait cycle, and is the second period of single-limb support.

Preswing is the final phase of stride and takes place from just after heel-off to toe-off. A rapid unloading of the limb occurs as weight is transferred to the contralateral limb. Preswing is the second period of double-limb support and makes up 10% of the gait cycle. Preswing occurs during loading response on the opposite side.

The swing phase is when the foot is not on the ground. It consists of initial swing, midswing, and terminal (late) swing. Swing phase is 38% to 40% of the total gait cycle. These three phases are equally divided with regard to time. Initial swing is the acceleration phase and is described as the time the foot leaves the ground until maximal knee flexion in swing. During this phase, the thigh begins to advance as the foot lifts off the floor. Midswing begins after initial swing and continues until the airborne tibia is in a vertical position. The thigh continues to advance as the knee begins to extend and the foot clears the ground. Terminal (late) swing is the deceleration phase. The knee is extending as the limb prepares to contact the ground.

Walking Gait Kinematics

The kinematics during walking gait are complex.[4] Table 13.1 lists the primary joints, joint positions, external moments, and muscle movement for each phase of the gait cycle. This section focuses on joint positions. The head, arms, and trunk (sometimes referred to as HAT) are usually considered in literature as a rigid unit and are not discussed here.

TABLE 13.1   Lower Extremity Kinematics During Gait Phase

	Anatomical position	Muscles	External moment
SUBTALAR JOINT			
IC	Inverted (2°)	Tibialis posterior (eccentric)	ND
LR	Pronated (5°)	Tibialis posterior (eccentric)	ND
MS	Moving into supination	Tibialis posterior (concentric)	ND
TS	Supinated (max)	Peroneals (eccentric)	ND
PS	MTP dorsiflexed (70°)	Peroneals (eccentric)	ND
S	Supinated	Peroneals (concentric)	NA
ANKLE JOINT			
IC	Dorsiflexed	Pretibials (eccentric)	Plantar flexion
LR	Plantar flexed	Pretibials, soleus (eccentric)	Plantar flexion
MS	Early: neutral; late: dorsiflexed	Soleus (eccentric)	Dorsiflexion
TS	Dorsiflexed (10°)	Soleus (eccentric)	Dorsiflexion
PS	Plantar flexed (20°)	Plantar flexors (concentric)	Dorsiflexion
S	Plantar flexed, neutral	Pretibials (concentric, isometric)	NA
KNEE JOINT AND TIBIA			
IC	Extended, externally rotated	Quadriceps and hamstrings (co-contraction)	Extension
LR	Flexed (15°), internally rotating	Quadriceps (eccentric)	Flexion
MS	Neutral	Early: quadriceps (concentric); popliteus, gastrocnemius	Neutral
TS	Extended (0°), externally rotating	Hamstrings (eccentric), gastrocnemius (concentric) for knee flexion	Extension

(continued)

Table 13.1 *(continued)*

	Anatomical position	**Muscles**	**External moment**
PS	Flexed (45°), externally rotated	Popliteus (concentric), rectus femoris (eccentric)	Flexion
S	Flexed, late; extension (65°)	Early: hamstrings (concentric); late: hamstrings and quadriceps to stabilize knee in extension	NA
HIP JOINT			
IC	Flexed (35°), slight adduction and external rotation	Hip extensors (eccentric)	Flexion
LR	Flexed, internally rotating	Gluteus maximus, hamstrings (concentric), gluteus medius (eccentric) in frontal plane	Flexion
MS	Early: neutral, internal rotation→ external rotation, abduction	Iliopsoas (eccentric), gluteus medius (isometric)	Neutral
TS	Extended, externally rotated	Tensor fasciae latae (eccentric)	Extension to neutral
PS	Neutral	Rectus femoris (concentric), adductors (eccentric)	Neutral to flexion
S	Early; neutral, flexed, adduction	Psoas (concentric), adductors (eccentric), hamstrings (eccentric)	NA

IC = initial contact; LR = loading response; MS = midstance; TS = terminal stance; PS = preswing; ND = not described; NA = not applicable

Reprinted, by permission, from J. Loudon, R. Manske, and M. Reiman, 2013, *Clinical mechanics and kinesiology* (Champaign, IL: Human Kinetics), 358.

Subtalar Joint

At initial contact, in normal gait, the contact is made on the lateral side of the heel and the subtalar joint (STJ) is minimally supinated. From initial contact through loading response, the STJ pronates. At the midpoint of midstance, the foot begins to resupinate to get the foot ready for push-off. During terminal stance and preswing, the great toe moves into maximal extension, creating the windlass effect, a passive lifting of the arch due to the plantar fascia.

Talocrural Joint

The talocrural joint range of motion is between 5° of plantar flexion and 5° of dorsiflexion at heel strike. The remainder of the foot slowly lowers to the floor as the gait cycle progresses. During loading response and early midstance, the talocrural joint is in relative plantar flexion because the stance leg is in front of the body. As the body progresses over the fixed foot, the talocrural joint moves into relative dorsiflexion (midstance) until the heel leaves the ground, readying it for push-off. Maximal dorsiflexion (10° or greater) is required at terminal stance. If dorsiflexion is lacking, substitutions such as STJ pronation or early heel rise will occur. During swing, the talocrural joint returns to dorsiflexion to clear the ground and to get ready for initial contact.

Knee Joint

During initial contact, the tibia is externally rotating due to the distal influence (STJ supination) and the opposite limb swing. In the sagittal plane, the knee joint remains relatively straight during this phase. As the STJ pronates and the tibia internally rotates during loading response and the beginning of midstance, the knee moves into slight flexion to help with shock absorption. At preswing, the knee passively flexes to 45° as the heel lifts off the ground. During initial swing, the knee maximally flexes to 60° to allow the foot to clear the ground. Knee flexion is one of the determinants of gait and is needed to minimize vertical translation and conserve energy.

Hip Joint and Pelvis

The hip joint has key motion in all three planes during the gait cycle. In the sagittal plane, the hip joint is in flexion (25–35°) at initial contact, and then moves into extension as the body progresses over the fixed foot. The hip reaches maximal extension during terminal stance (15–25°) and then begins to move back into flexion during preswing through the swing phase. The pelvis is anteriorly rotated until midstance, where it moves posterior 8° to 10°.

In the frontal plane, the hip moves in relation to the action of the pelvis. The pelvis is level at initial contact and the hip is in neutral abduction. During loading response, the pelvis rises on the stance side (4°) and slightly drops on the swing side. The hip is in adduction. In the transverse plane, the femur mirrors the action of the tibia. After the foot contacts the ground, the primary motion is internal rotation until the opposite heel strike.

Walking Gait Kinetics

Human locomotion has been described as a series of controlled falls and catches.[3] The falls are a result of gravitational forces, pulling the body toward the center of the Earth. The muscles of the lower extremity are responsible for controlling these gravitational forces. In addition, three rockers (heel, ankle, and metatarsal heads) add to the gravitational control and momentum conservation during stance. These rockers describe the anatomical pivot points during crucial phases of the gait cycle. The first rocker is the heel rocker. It occurs from initial contact to loading response and is the period when the foot is decelerating towards the ground. During the first rocker, the joints are absorbing impact and the muscles are working eccentrically. The second rocker, ankle rocker, is defined from foot flat to midstance and is characterized by the control of the ground reaction force as the foot remains flat and the tibia translates anterior. The third rocker occurs during terminal stance and preswing as plantar flexion arrests the tibia and the fulcrum pivots to the metatarsal heads.

Foot and Ankle

The primary extrinsic muscles working at the STJ during gait are the anterior tibialis and posterior tibialis. These muscles work eccentrically to decelerate pronation.[5] Toward the end of the stance phase, the foot invertors work concentrically to lock the foot into supination. The peroneal muscles work eccentrically to fine-tune the supination. The pretibial muscles (anterior tibialis, extensor digitorum, and extensor hallucis longus) are active during the first rocker, working eccentrically to control foot slap. As the ground reaction force (GRF) passes through the heel, an external plantar flexion moment is created. During the second rocker, the soleus is working eccentrically to control the anterior displacement of the tibia. This is also a period of force absorption. The third rocker is a period of acceleration, and the plantar flexors are working concentrically. Deceleration of the first two rockers must be counterbalanced by the third rocker. The pretibial muscles work concentrically in swing to hold the foot in dorsiflexion to prevent foot drag.

Knee Joint

At initial contact the muscle activity around the knee is variable.[6] The quadriceps and hamstring co-contract to help stabilize the knee joint. During the loading response, the GRF creates an external flexion moment, and the quadriceps work eccentrically to absorb energy and counteract the external moment. Midstance is characterized by minimal to no muscle activity as the ligaments around the knee and the external extensor moment help to stabilize the joint. The external moment changes to flexion during terminal stance and the rectus femoris becomes active to eccentrically control knee flexion. During swing, the knee motion is passive, so little muscle activity is necessary; the rectus femoris may work to limit knee flexion.

Hip Joint

During the first rocker, the hip extensors work eccentrically to control hip flexion. As the hip is extending in second rocker, the gluteal muscles work concentrically to accelerate the body forward. As swing begins, the hip drives forward into flexion with contraction of the hip flexors, primarily the

---

Critical Clinical Pearls

During normal walking gait, three rockers occur that aide in gravitational control and momentum conservation:

- 1st rocker: a *heel rocker* that occurs from initial contact to loading response
- 2nd rocker: also termed the *ankle rocker*, occurs from foot flat to midstance
- 3rd rocker (*forefoot rocker*): occurs during terminal stance and preswing

iliopsoas muscle. Late in midstance, hip extension is passive and is limited by the iliofemoral ligament. The hip continues to extend into the third rocker, where it reaches maximal extension.

The stance side gluteus medius is the primary muscle that controls hip and pelvic motion. The same muscle group will concentrically raise the pelvis on the swing side to help with foot clearance during late swing. The adductor magus works on a fixed front limb to cause internal rotation. Terminal stance is characterized by external rotation of the femur as the adductor magnus now works eccentrically to stabilize the pelvis.

Ground Reaction Force

Newton's third law states that for every action there is an equal and opposite reaction. In terms of gait, the equal and opposite reaction that occurs when the foot is on the ground is the ground reaction force (GRF). The ground reaction force can be resolved into three vector forces: vertical, anteroposterior, and medial–lateral forces. Figure 13.2 displays the vertical GRF. The vertical ground reaction force averages 110% to 140% of the body weight (BW) with normal walking. The anteroposterior GRF is 20% and the medial–lateral is 5% BW.

Center of Pressure

The center of pressure (COP) is the cumulative forces in a given area at an instance in time. The path of the COP for walking is displayed in figure 13.3. At initial contact of the heel, the COP is located just lateral to the midheel. It progresses along the lateral midfoot, which corresponds to the midstance of gait. At terminal stance and heel-off, the COP is located under the medial forefoot. Center of pressure can be used to determine the amount of forces distributed on an area, especially when it is excessive. For example, a client with diabetic peripheral neuropathy may develop sores on the feet and be unaware of the incidence. The COP pathway would help the clinician determine if the insulting forces can be minimized with the use of an orthotic or change in footwear.

Joint Moments

Moments, or torques, are placed on the joints as a result of the GRF. These external moments vary depending on the phase of gait. The external moments are counterbalanced by muscle contraction, which creates an internal moment. Figure 13.4 depicts the external moments at the foot, knee, and hip at each phase of the stance phase. At initial contact, the external moment at the ankle is posterior, which is in the plantar flexion direction. If unopposed by muscle action, the ankle would plantar flex because of the external moment. However, during this phase of gait, the pretibial muscles are active to control the plantar flexion external moment so that the foot lowers slowly to the ground. At the knee and hip, the external moment is anterior to the joint axes. At the knee this creates an external extension moment and at

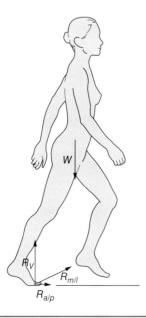

Figure 13.2   Ground reaction forces: one vertical (R_v) and two horizontal ($R_{a/p}$; $R_{m/l}$).

Reprinted, by permission, from J. Watkins, 2010, *Structure and function of the musculoskeletal system*, 2nd ed. (Champaign, IL: Human Kinetics), 302.

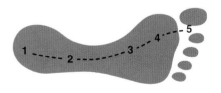

Key

1 = Initial contact (heel strike)

2 = Loading response (foot flat)

3 = Midstance

4 = Terminal stance (heel-off)

5 = Preswing (toe-off)

Figure 13.3   Center of pressure during the gait cycle.

Reprinted, by permission, from P. Houglum, 2010, *Therapeutic exercise for musculoskeletal injuries*, 3rd ed. (Champaign, IL; Human Kinetics), 359.

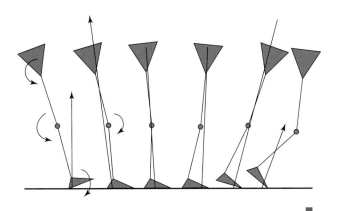

Figure 13.4 External moments about the hip, knee, and ankle during walking gait.

Reprinted, by permission, from J. Loudon, R. Manske, and M. Reiman, 2013, *Clinical mechanics and kinesiology* (Champaign, IL: Human Kinetics), 363.

the hip an external flexion moment. Again, the muscle activity at these joints will counteract the external moment. The last column in table 13.1 lists the external moment at the hip, knee, and ankle for the stance phase of gait. An imbalance between internal and external moments will disrupt the normal gait cycle.

Gait Parameters

In quantifying gait, the clinician can measure both distance and temporal measurements. The following sections list common gait parameters and average values.

Distance Variables

Step and stride length are routinely measured in a gait analysis, and they are relatively easy to record.[7] Right step length is the longitudinal distance from left to right initial contact (figure 13.5). Left step length is the distance from right to left initial contact. The average step length in an adult is 64 to 74 cm.[8] Stride length is equivalent to initial contact to initial contact of the same limb. In adults the average stride length is 1.33 to 1.63 m (average = 1.41 m), with men on the higher end of the range and women on the lower end of the range.[3] Stride length should equate to the sum of right and left step lengths. This distance is less in women, in elderly people, and in people with musculoskeletal and neurological deficiency.[9]

Step width is the distance between feet. Normally it is 5 to 10 cm (2–4 in.). A wider step width may be indicative of poor balance. Step angle is the amount of toe-out in the foot. Normally this angle is 4 to 8° (average = 7°).

Temporal Variables

Temporal variables describe time values such as how fast someone walks. Gait velocity on average is 1.23 to 1.37 m/s (3 mph; 5 kmph) for adults.[10] Gait velocity (speed) = step length × cadence, in units of distance / time. Step rate or cadence is the number of steps per time and equates to just less than 2 steps/s or 111 to 117 steps/min. On average, the rate for women is usually 6 to 9 steps/min higher than for men. Additionally, the time spent in stance (stance time), swing (swing time), double support, and single support can be calculated. Reported values for distance and temporal parameters are as follows:

Stride length (m)	1.33 ± 0.09 to 1.63 ± 0.11
Step length (m)	0.70 ± 0.01 to 0.81 ± 0.05
Step width (cm)	0.61 ± 0.22 to 9.0 ± 3.5
Foot angle (°)	5.1 ± 5.7 to 6.8 ± 5.6
Gait speed (m/s)	0.82 to 1.60 ± 0.16
Cadence (steps/min)	100 to 131
Stance time (s)	0.63 ± 0.07 to 0.67 ± 0.04
Swing time (s)	0.39 ± 0.02 to 0.40 ± 0.04

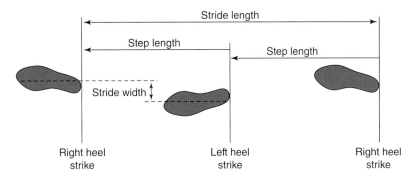

Figure 13.5 Distance variables in stride length, step length, and stride width.

Reprinted, by permission, from P. Houglum, 2010, *Therapeutic exercise for musculoskeletal injuries,* 3rd ed. (Champaign, IL: Human Kinetics), 353.

Walking Gait Disturbances and Mechanical Faults

As previously stated, walking gait is a very efficient mode of locomotion. Conservation of energy is achieved by minimizing the center of gravity displacement in both in the vertical and horizontal planes. Earlier, six anatomical determinants were identified as being important for the conservation of energy. In addition, five attributes of gait are important for maximizing gait efficiency. These attributes are stability in stance, foot clearance in swing, prepositioning of the foot for initial contact, adequate step length, and energy conservation. Deviations in one or more of the attributes are common in pathological or abnormal gait patterns. An example of a deficiency in stance stability is abnormal foot position such that weight distribution and balance are poor. A child with cerebral palsy who has an equinus (plantar flexed club foot) deformity will be unable to bear weight on a flat foot, compromising the base of support. This is one reason many people with cerebral palsy use an assistive device. Other deficiencies in the attributes of gait are found in table 13.2.

Another way to look at the phases of gait so that gait deviations can be described is to use the functional phases of gait.[3] The three phases are labeled weight acceptance, single-limb support, and swing-limb advance. Weight acceptance includes initial contact and loading response. The single-limb support includes midstance and terminal stance, when only one limb is in contact with the ground. Swing-limb advance includes the last phase of stance, preswing, and the entire swing phase. Table 13.3 breaks down the functional phases of gait and the possible gait deviations that can occur at the major joints.

Classic Abnormal Walking Gait Patterns

Many gait abnormalities are identified by the pathological cause of the gait rather than the joint or muscle impairment.[11] Listed here are common abnormal gait patterns. However, the clinician should understand that generalizing a gait pattern is not ideal. Descriptive terms such as the ones listed in table 13.3 are preferable.

Antalgic (Painful) Gait

An antalgic gait occurs as a result of pain in one or both lower extremities. The stance phase of the affected limb will be shorter relative to the opposite side. Because of pain, less time is spent on the involved side. The shortened stance time is a result of a shorter step length. Because of this shortened time, the swing phase of the uninvolved side will also be shorter. In addition, walking velocity and cadence will be decreased.

Arthrogenic Gait

An arthrogenic gait is a result of stiffness in one or more joints of the lower extremity. This gait is characterized by a forward lean, decreased hip and knee range of motion, and a relatively longer limb on the stiff side. Gait deviations could include vaulting or circumduction of the reference limb. The clinician may notice an increase in plantar flexion on the opposite side to counter the relatively long leg.

Ataxic Gait

An ataxic gait is common in people with cerebellar problems. This gait deviation is a result of poor balance. The client will walk with a broad base of support and hands held out to the side to improve stability.

TABLE 13.2 Attributes of Gait

Attribute	Attribute deficiency
Stability in stance	Abnormal foot position; poor balance
Foot clearance in swing	Loss of knee motion; inadequate dorsiflexion
Prepositioning for initial contact	Inadequate foot position; landing on toes
Adequate step length	Inadequate knee extension; unstable foot; inadequate push-off
Energy conservation	Bouncy gait that increases the center of gravity excursion; uncoordinated movement between the hip, knee, ankle

Reprinted, by permission, from J. Loudon, R. Manske, and M. Reiman, 2013, *Clinical mechanics and kinesiology* (Champaign, IL: Human Kinetics), 365.

TABLE 13.3   Gait Deviations During the Functional Phases of the Gait Cycle

Joint	Deviation (impairment) and possible cause
WEIGHT ACCEPTANCE	
Trunk	Backward lean: to decrease demand on hip extensors (gluteus maximus)
	Forward lean: due to increased hip flexion (joint contracture or muscle weakness)
	Lateral lean: right or left weak hip abductors
Pelvis	Contralateral drops: weak hip abductors on reference limb
	Ipsilateral drops: compensation for shortened limb
Hip	Excessive flexion: hip flexion contracture, excessive knee flexion
	Limited flexion: weakness of hip flexors, decreased hip flexion
Knee	Excessive flexion: knee pain, weak quadriceps, short leg on opposite side
	Hyperextension: decreased dorsiflexion, weak quadriceps
	Extension thrust: intention to increase limb stability
Ankle	Forefoot contact: heel pain, excessive knee flexion, plantar flexion contracture
	Foot flat contact: dorsiflexion contracture, weak dorsiflexors
	Foot slap: weak dorsiflexors
Toes	Up: compensation for weak tibialis anterior
SINGLE-LIMB SUPPORT	
Trunk	Backward lean: to decrease demand on hip extensors (gluteus maximus)
	Forward lean: due to increased hip flexion (joint contracture or muscle weakness)
	Lateral lean: right or left weak hip abductors
Pelvis	Contralateral drops: weak hip abductors on reference limb
	Ipsilateral drops: compensation for shortened limb
	Anterior pelvic tilt: hip flexion contracture
Hip	Limited flexion: weakness of hip flexors, decreased hip flexion
	Internal rotation: weak external rotators, femoral anteversion
	External rotation: retroversion, limited dorsiflexion
	Abduction: reference limb longer
	Adduction: secondary to contralateral pelvic drop
Knee	Excessive flexion: knee pain, weak quadriceps, short leg on opposite side
	Hyperextension: decreased dorsiflexion, weak quadriceps
	Extension thrust: intention to increase limb stability
	Wobbles: impaired proprioception
	Varus: joint instability, body deformity
	Valgus: lateral trunk lean, joint instability, bony deformity
Ankle	Excessive plantar flexion: weak quadriceps, impaired proprioception, ankle pain
	Early heel-off: tight dorsiflexors
	Increased pronation: subtalar joint deformity
Toes	Up: compensation for weak tibialis anterior
SWING-LIMB ADVANCE	
Trunk	Backward lean: to decrease demand on hip extensors (gluteus maximus)
	Forward lean: due to increased hip flexion (joint contracture or muscle weakness)
	Lateral lean: right or left weak hip abductors
Pelvis	Hikes: to clear swing limb
	Ipsilateral drops: weak hip abductors on contralateral side

(continued)

Table 13.3   *(continued)*

Joint	Deviation (impairment) and possible cause
	SWING-LIMB ADVANCE
Hip	Limited flexion: weakness of hip flexors, decreased hip flexion, hip pain
Knee	Limited flexion: excess hip flexion, knee pain
	Excess flexion: knee contracture, weak quadriceps
Ankle	Excessive plantar flexion: weak quadriceps, impaired proprioception, ankle pain
	Drag: secondary to limited hip flexion, knee flexion, or excess plantar flexion
	Contralateral vaulting: compensation for limited flexion of swing or long swing limb
Toes	Inadequate extension: limited joint motion, forefoot pain, no heel-off
	Clawed or hammered: imbalance of long toe extensors and intrinsics, weak plantar flexion

Reprinted, by permission, from J. Loudon, R. Manske, and M. Reiman, 2013, *Clinical mechanics and kinesiology* (Champaign, IL: Human Kinetics), 366.

Contracture Gait

In a contracture gait, the client has limited motion at one or more joints of the lower extremity. If the contracture is at the hip in flexion, the client will present with increased lumbar lordosis and knee flexion. Besides these compensations, the client may walk with a flexed trunk because the hip flexors do not allow a full upright posture. If the contracture is with knee flexion, the client will present with increased ankle dorsiflexion on the uninvolved side and early heel rise on the involved side. A plantar flexion contracture at the ankle will create knee hyperextension and forward bending of the trunk.

Gluteus Maximus Gait

This gait is characterized by weakness in the gluteus maximus, which results in a backward lurch position to compensate for the lack of control of hip extension. This gait is sometimes referred to as a *myopathic gait*.

Gluteus Medius (Trendelenburg) Gait

This gait deviation occurs in the frontal plane, and is characterized by hip abductor muscle weakness on the stance side. The primary role of the gluteus medius is to stabilize the pelvis in the frontal plane. When weakness exists in this muscle, excessive hip drop occurs on the opposite side (swing side). In some cases this occurs bilaterally, and the client will walk with a wobbling gait. Possible causes of this gait pattern are hip arthritis, congenital hip dislocation, or coxa vara. Limiting the gluteus medius activation will reduce the compression across the hip joint, thereby lessening the pain.

Hemiplegic

This gait occurs after a cerebral vascular accident when one side of the body has been affected by paralysis. This gait pattern is also referred to as a *spastic gait*. The client will shuffle on the involved side. Many times the upper extremity is held in a tonic position of shoulder adduction, elbow flexion, and wrist flexion, and the fingers are held in a grasping position.

Parkinsonian Gait

As the name implies, this gait is found in people with Parkinson's disease. The gait is characterized by reduced stride length and short, rapid shuffling

Critical Clinical Pearls

Several differences exist between running gait and walking gait. Some differences found in running are the following:

- A double float phase, where both feet are off the ground
- Decreased cycle time (0.7 seconds versus 1 second with walking)
- Higher vertical ground reaction force (2-5 × body weight)
- Narrower base of support

steps with a slightly increased walking base. In addition, people with this gait pattern will hold their arms out to the side without swinging. They may demonstrate an increased gait velocity once in stride, but then are unable to stop suddenly.

Scissors Gait

The scissors gait is characterized by hip adduction and forceful thrusting of the limb forward with limb advancement. This gait is common in people with spastic paralysis of the lower extremity. It is also referred to as a diplegic gait.

Steppage (Drop Foot) Gait

The steppage gait occurs in people with weak dorsiflexors or peripheral neuropathy. This type of gait is characterized by exaggerated hip and knee flexion in order to lift the foot high enough to clear it from the ground.

RUNNING GAIT

The running cycle is comparable to the walking cycle in that each consists of a stance phase and swing phase. However, a couple of major differences are that during the stance phase of running there is no double support and during the swing phase there is a point when both feet are off the ground, called *double float*. Also, the running cycle is quicker, lasting approximately seven-tenths of a second, whereas the walking cycle takes on the average 1 second. One further difference is the magnitude of the ground reaction force which can be as high as 5 × body weight during running compared to 1.5 × body weight with walking.

Running requires better balance than walking because there is no double support phase, and the base of support is narrower with running. Running also requires more strength of the lower extremity

to decelerate the greater ground reaction forces. Additionally, if you look at the range of motions required for walking and running, you will notice that running requires more motion at the ankle and knee. The knee flexion and ankle dorsiflexion is required for attenuating impact forces. The narrower base of support creates more adduction of the limb.

Running Sequence

The running gait sequence includes the stance and swing phases. The stance phase (also referred to as the *support phase*) is defined as the period in the gait cycle when the foot is on the ground, and it takes up 38% to 45% of the total running cycle. Three purposes for the stance phase are to establish contact with the supporting surface, provide a stable base so the opposite extremity can move through its swing phase, and advance the body forward over a fixed foot. The running cycle stance phase consists of foot strike (initial contact), midsupport (midstance), and take-off. Figure 13.6 displays the running cycle. Table 13.4 breaks down the running mechanics into the different phases and presents the joint motions and working muscles for each phase.

Foot strike, or initial contact, is defined as the point when the foot makes the first touch with the ground. At this point, the loading forces are controlled eccentrically. Runners may contact the ground with the heel, the midfoot, or the forefoot. More than 70% of long distance runners use a heel strike running gait.[12] Recent conversation has emphasized the use of minimal to no footwear to promote a midfoot strike.[13] A midfoot strike may help to minimize braking forces and hip and knee joint forces.[14] However, to date, there is no evidence that a midfoot or forefoot strike pattern minimizes injury in the long distance runner. In fact, forefoot striking has been associated with greater force through the ankle and Achilles tendon.[15]

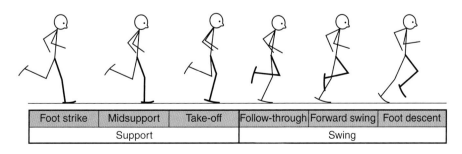

Foot strike	Midsupport	Take-off	Follow-through	Forward swing	Foot descent
Support			Swing		

Figure 13.6 Running gait cycle.

Reprinted, by permission, from J. Watkins, 2010, *Structure and function of the musculoskeletal system*, 2nd ed. (Champaign, IL: Human Kinetics), 30.

TABLE 13.4 **Running Gait**

		Hip	**Knee**	**Foot**
Foot strike	Joint motion	20–50° flexion	15–20° flexion	5–10° dorsiflexion for rearfoot strikers
	Muscle activity	Eccentric: gluteus maximus, gluteus medius, tensor fasciae latae, hamstrings Concentric: adductors	Concentric: hamstrings, gastrocnemius, popliteus Quadriceps contraction	Eccentric: tibialis anterior, toe extensors
Midsupport	Joint motion	30° flexion	20–40° flexion	20° dorsiflexion
	Muscle activity	Eccentric: gluteus medius and tensor fasciae latae to control pelvis Eccentric: gluteus maximus, hamstrings to control limb in flexion	Eccentric: quadriceps to control knee flexion	Eccentric: gastroc-soleus complex, tibialis posterior
Take-off	Joint motion	10° extension	0° flexion	25° plantar flexion
	Muscle activity	Concentric: hamstrings, gluteus maximus, gluteus medius Eccentric: trunk musculature	Eccentric: quadriceps	Concentric: gastroc-soleus complex, peroneals, toe flexors Eccentric: toe extensors
Follow-through	Joint motion	5° extension	20–125° flexion	10° plantar flexion
	Muscle activity	Eccentric: adductors to control pelvis, hip flexors to control hip extension, internal rotation of limb	Concentric: medial hamstrings	Concentric: gastrocnemius
Forward swing	Joint motion	10–60° flexion	125° flexion	10° plantar flexion
	Muscle activity	Concentric: iliopsoas, rectus femoris, tensor fasciae latae	Hamstrings and quadriceps contraction	Eccentric: pretibial muscles to control ankle
Foot descent	Joint motion	40° flexion	40–20° flexion	10° dorsiflexion
	Muscle activity	Concentric: gluteus maximus and hamstrings decelerate flexing thigh, gluteus medius, tensor fasciae latae	Eccentric: hamstrings	Concentric: pretibial muscles

Reprinted, by permission, from J. Loudon, R. Manske, and M. Reiman, 2013, *Clinical mechanics and kinesiology* (Champaign, IL: Human Kinetics), 371.

When the foot is flat on the ground, midsupport begins. From initial contact to midsupport, the body is absorbing the ground reaction forces; this is the braking phase. The ankle and knee are at their maximum flexion angle, and the subtalar joint is pronating as the foot adapts to the ground. The lower limb is primarily working eccentrically to break the forward momentum of the body.

Once the runner's body moves anterior to the stance leg, the propulsion phase begins until the foot leaves the ground (take-off). The concentric contraction of the lower limb muscles along with stored potential energy in the tendons help propel the body forward. The arms provide some upward lift, promote efficient movement and balance, and

help reduce rotation forces through the body. It is during the stance phase that the greatest risk of injury arises, since forces are acting on the body and muscles are active to control these forces, and joints are being loaded.

The swing phase (sometimes referred to as the *recovery phase*) is when the foot is off the ground; it makes up about 55% to 62% of the total running cycle. The purpose of the swing phase is to return the limb to a position that is ready for foot contact. Additionally, during this phase, the swinging limb adds momentum to the body, thereby increasing efficiency. The swing phase includes follow-through (initial swing), forward swing (midswing), and foot descent (terminal swing). Follow-through is characterized as the end of backward momentum of the leg, where the knee reaches maximal flexion (60°). The limb begins to drive forward as forward swing begins. As the limb prepares for foot contact, foot descent begins. It is during the swing phase that the period of double float, when neither foot is on the ground, happens. Double float occurs at the beginning and end of the swing phase.

Running Kinematics

This section describes motion of the lower and upper extremities during running. More range of motion is required of the shoulder, elbow, hip, knee, ankle, and foot during running as compared to walking.

Initial Contact to Midsupport

During running, motion at the hip occurs primarily in the sagittal plane. At foot contact, the hip is flexed to approximately 45° and immediately begins to move toward extension, reaching around 20° of flexion by midsupport. Hip flexion helps with absorption of impact forces during this initial ground contact. Motion in the frontal and transverse planes is much less than what is found in the sagittal plane. The hip adducts relative to the pelvis at foot contact. Similar to lateral pelvic tilt, this is a shock-absorbing mechanism. The amount of hip adduction is approximately 6°. Hip motion in the transverse plane during running is similar to walking gait; the hip is in slight external rotation and then moves into internal rotation up until midsupport.[16]

At contact, the knee should be flexed around 20°. Knee flexion continues to approximately 40° during midsupport. The ankle is dorsiflexed and reaches 20° during midsupport.

At initial contact, the subtalar joint is inverted (supinated) as the foot hits the ground. The ankle is dorsiflexed, around 10° for rearfoot strikers; the knee is flexed to 15° to 20°, and the hip is flexed between 20° and 50°. As the running gait continues, the talus plantar flexes, adducts, and inverts on the stabilized calcaneus to produce subtalar pronation. An adducted position of the talus (pronation) increases tibial internal rotation because of the congruity of the articulations at the talocrural joint.

Midsupport to Take-Off

From midsupport to toe-off, the hip joint moves from 20° of flexion to 5° of extension. This change in motion helps to propel the runner's body for-ward. From midsupport to toe-off, the hip progressively abducts and should be in a position of abduction by the time the foot leaves the ground. The hip then returns to a more neutral position at toe-off.[17] During take-off, the knee extends and then begins to flex again once the foot leaves the ground. By toe-off, the ankle is plantar flexed to around 25° and the knee extends to 0°. The hip continues to move to 10° of extension.

Swing Phase

As the limb moves into the swing phase, the hip continues to extend to approximately 20°. At the same time, the pelvis is moving from a position of posterior tilt to anterior tilt. Inadequate anterior tilt or rotation of the pelvis during late stance phase may cause the runner to excessively extend the femur; this may increase tensile stresses to the iliofemoral ligament and anterior joint capsule.[18] The hip then changes directions and moves into flexion as it initiates forward swing. The hip reaches maximal flexion (65°) during this portion of swing. As the foot readies itself for ground contact, the hip moves from 65° of flexion to 40° of flexion. The return of the hip into extension helps to reduce the horizontal velocity of the foot prior to contact and possibly minimize the ground reaction force.[18]

During swing, the hip abducts (8°) but returns to adduction just prior to foot contact. Motion at the hip will mirror the motion of the pelvis in this plane, and this combined motion is thought to help minimize shoulder and head movement.[19] Increased femoral adduction has been linked to various injuries in the knee and hip joints.[20] A variation in hip position has been reported in swing (internally rotated versus neutral), although it would seem that a neutral hip would be more advantageous than excessive internal rotation.

Peak knee flexion occurs during forward swing, reaching close to 125° in elite runners. The extreme flexion serves to shorten the lever arm of the limb to improve swing acceleration. During swing, the ankle moves from a position of plantar flexion to dorsiflexion as the foot descends to the ground.

The main function of the upper body and arm action is to provide balance and assist with drive.[21] In the transverse plane, the arms and trunk move to oppose the forward drive of the legs. The arms are held relaxed with the elbow angle at 90° or less. The hands should remain relaxed. The normal arm action during distance running involves shoulder extension to pull the elbow straight back; then, as the arm comes forward, the hand will move slightly across the body. Excessive arm crossover will cause excessive trunk rotation.

Running Kinetics

The forces on the lower extremity with running are measured using vertical ground reaction forces (VGRF). Running research has shown that the force increases as the running speed increases, and it is in the range of 2 to 3.5 times body weight.[22] In visualizing the VGRF, as in walking, there appear to be two peaks. Impact peak is not as dramatic as with walking, and is dependent on location of foot strike (e.g., rearfoot striker versus a forefoot striker; figure 13.7). The increase in VGRF that occurs from transitioning from walking to jogging is a function of the change in center-of-gravity velocity.[23] It has been reported that increasing step or stride rate will decrease joint forces.

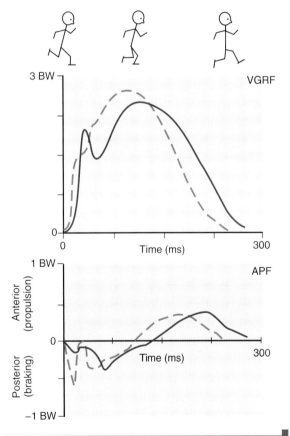

Figure 13.7 Ground reaction force–time curves (vertical and horizontal components) for a heel striker (solid line) and forefoot striker (dashed line). BW = body weight; VGRF = vertical ground reaction force; APF = anteroposterior ground reaction force.

Reprinted, by permission, from P.M. McGinnis, 2015, *Biomechanics of sport and exercise*, 2nd ed. (Champaign, IL: Human Kinetics), 352.

Braking Phase

Braking phase is another way to describe the initial phase of stance during running. The braking phase occurs from initial contact to foot flat. This phase represents a period of deceleration. The muscles are working eccentrically to control joint motion and gravity. The motion of the foot, ankle, and knee is coordinated to absorb the vertical landing forces on the body. During the initial phase of stance, the body is absorbing the ground reaction forces. The lower limb is primarily working eccentrically to control the forward momentum of the body. At the hip, the primary muscles working are the quadriceps, hip extensors, hip abductors, and hamstrings. The hip joint extensor, the gluteus maximus, generates power during this phase to pull the body forward by actively extending the hip after swing.[24] In the frontal plane, the gluteus medius is working to control or slow frontal plane lateral pelvic tilt. The hamstring is active before foot strike and demonstrates continued EMG activity into the propulsion phase. Its initial activity is responsible for slowing the rapidly extending knee in preparation for contact.

During the braking phase, the eccentric strength in the calf and quadriceps muscles is required to control the knee and ankle joints; otherwise the knee and ankle would collapse or rotate inward. In fact, the quadriceps and calf muscles are active prior to initial contact, and most of their activity occurs between initial contact (IC) and midstance (MS) to help control the braking forces.

Propulsion Phase

Once the runner's body moves anterior to the stance leg, the propulsion phase begins; it lasts until the foot leaves the ground. More specifically, the propulsion phase occurs from flat foot to toe-off. This phase represents a period of powerful concentric contraction. During the propulsion phase, the ankle and knee motion are the opposite of the motion in the braking phase.

The concentric contraction of the lower limb muscles, along with stored potential energy in the tendons, helps to propel the body forward. Here, the ankle, knee, and hip combine in a triple extension movement to provide propulsion upward and forward.[25] The calf, quadriceps, hamstring, and gluteal activity during the propulsion phase is less than during the braking phase, because the propulsion energy comes mainly from the recoil of elastic energy stored during the first half of stance. The gastrocnemius generates the primary propulsion during the propulsive phase.[26] In addition, the hip flexors are dominant in the propulsion phase. This activity continues through the first half of swing. This muscle group initially is decelerating hip extension but then becomes the primary force generation for forward swing. The gluteus medius contracts concentrically to abduct the hip and provide hip lift.[27]

The calf, quadriceps, hamstring, and gluteal activity during the propulsion phase is less than during the braking phase because the propulsion energy comes mainly from the recoil of elastic energy stored during the first half of stance.

Swing Phase

During the swing phase of running, the hip flexors work concentrically to bring the swing limb forward to ready it for impact. The gluteus maximus works eccentrically to control this motion.[28] The hip abductors and external rotators are working eccentrically to control motion in the frontal and transverse planes. The gluteus medius muscles (abductors) are of primary importance in providing lateral stability. Their contraction prior to and during the braking phase prevents the hip from dropping down too far to the swing-leg side. The muscles will be acting eccentrically, or even isometrically, to prevent this movement.

Running Injuries

Running is a common mode of exercise for millions of people. Unfortunately, accompanying this activity is a high incidence of injury. According to a systematic review by Van Gent and colleagues,[29] the incidence may be as high as 80%. These injuries are commonly due to repetitive tissue loading over many cycles.[30] The most common running injuries are patellofemoral pain syndrome, iliotibial band syndrome, plantar fasciitis, tibial stress fracture, and Achilles tendinopathy. A summary of common running injuries and possible contributing factors can be found in table 13.5. Potential causes of running injuries can be classified as nonmodifiable and modifiable.

Nonmodifiable Factors

Nonmodifiable factors are related to anatomical structure, age, and sex. Running involves repetitive impact, and each runner has a limit to the amount of stress their tissue can tolerate before breakdown. Even a slight biomechanical abnormality could induce injury.[31] Several theories implicate struc-

ture and function as causative factors for running injuries. Differences in foot structure are associated with common overuse injuries.[32] Tong and Kong[33] found that the strength of this relationship is low. Theoretically, a flexible foot allows for more shock absorption than does a rigid foot. However, excessive or prolonged pronation has been attributed to faulty alignment (patellofemoral pain syndrome) and excessive muscle activity (shin splints).[34] When the foot is at maximal pronation, the tibia should be at maximal internal rotation, and the knee should be flexed. This position occurs during midsupport. Past this point, the knee begins to extend; however, in some runners, the STJ is still in pronation, and this will cause excessive torsion in the system, especially at the knee.[35, 36] The runner with excessive eversion may also display excessive internal rotation of the tibia, which can also influence knee and hip mechanics.[37] A runner with a rigid foot is unable to dissipate the ground forces through foot mobility, so this stress is passed on to the tibia and up the leg. These runners are more prone to stress fractures in the tibia, lateral ankle sprains, and iliotibial band syndrome.[32]

Recently, attention has been focused on the hip and pelvis as causative factors for a variety of common running injuries. The alignment of the femur and tibia is important for alignment of structures such as the patella. Increased motion of the hip or pelvis in the frontal and transverse planes has been associated with patellofemoral pain syndrome,[27, 38] iliotibial band syndrome,[20] and tibial stress fractures.[39]

Modifiable Factors

Modifiable factors are those factors that can be changed, such as the environment, technique, or training. Specifically, the research suggests that the biggest predictors of injury are total volume of running and sudden changes in volume or intensity of running.[40]

Running terrain can be a factor that contributes to injury. Running surface directly affects the magnitude of the ground reaction forces. Asphalt and concrete are associated with higher forces as compared with a grass surface. An advantage of a harder surface is that better traction occurs between the surface and the runner's shoe or foot. A trade-off with grass, dirt, and sand is less force but less traction and more joint range of motion than is needed in the lower extremity. A person with an unstable ankle may prefer the harder surface to minimize the chance of injury or reinjury.

TABLE 13.5 Common Running Injuries

Running injury	Contributing factors	Movement error	Treatment strategy
Anterior knee pain	Laterally tilted patella Weak quadriceps Tight lateral structures Excessive hip IR Rearfoot pronation Weak core	Increased hip adduction and IR Knee valgus Inactive foot and ankle in propulsion	Quadriceps strengthening Hip and core strengthening Running retraining Patellar taping
Iliotibial band syndrome	Adducted gait Ilium anteriorly rotated Weak hip abductors and external rotators Functional leg-length discrepancy Genu varum Limited great toe extension	Excessive femoral rotation Overstriding	Strengthening hip external rotators Soft-tissue massage Superior tibiofibular joint mobilization Cross-training
Exercise-related leg pain	More common in women Higher BMI Leg-length discrepancy Training error	Increased tibial shock Overstriding Increased heel strike	Retraining for softer landing ST joint mobilization and manipulation Calf stretching Hip strengthening Taping Orthotics
Achilles tendinopathy	Facilitated segment L5-S1 Heel-height change in shoes Training or surface errors (hills) Joint mechanics; anterior talus, plantar flexed cuboid	Overstriding Forefoot strike Excessive vertical displacement Abnormal pronation Propulsive whip Poor ankle rocker	Heel lift Slow return to running Core stability Dural stretching Taping Orthotics Strengthening anterior tibialis, soleus, FHL Eccentric heel raises
Plantar fasciitis	Hallux limitus Forefoot varus Subtalar varus Abnormal pronation Tight calf Improper footwear Tight hamstrings	Strike control Soft strike Active heel-rise retraining Excessive hip IR Dynamic valgus at knee	Arch taping Orthotics Night splint ST joint mobilization and manipulation Calf stretching FHL strengthening
Proximal hamstring strain	Hamstring dominant pattern over gluteal muscles vs. hamstrings Neural restriction Proximal adhesions Eccentric overload Pelvic malalignment SI hypo- or hypermobility L5 radiculopathy	Overstriding Unilateral strike variance	Eccentric hamstring loading Slump stretching Gluteal strengthening Core stability Hip ROM Soft-tissue massage Kinesiology tape

IR = internal rotation; ST = subtalar; FHL = flexor hallucis longus; BMI = body mass index

One possible cause of many running injuries is overstriding. This is a common fault in novice runners. Overstriding contributes to excessive braking forces. The correct movement patterns of the hip, knee, and ankle combined with correct activation and strength of the major leg muscles will help control braking forces during running, resulting in a more efficient action using tendon elastic energy and minimizing landing forces. Since running speed is equal to stride length multiplied by stride frequency, one way to improve running rate is to increase stride frequency, or cadence. Recommended cadence for long-distance runners is 160 to 180 steps/min.

Rapid increases in training pace or volume are common training errors. Although it has not been validated, applying the 10% rule to a running program can be used as a guide. The runner should not increase pace or volume more than 10% per week. It is also recommended to increase these factors one at a time. If pace is increased, then mileage should be restricted for a period of time. Also, the long run for a week should not exceed 30% of the total weekly running mileage. In addition, adequate rest between training sessions is important to allow remodeling of the tissues. A rest period of 48 to 72 hours is recommended between successive training sessions. Cross-training can be used to supplement this relative rest period.

BIOMECHANICAL ANALYSIS OF WALKING AND RUNNING

Biomechanical analysis of walking or running involves measurement of kinematic or kinetic data. These measurements require some sort of instrumentation, which may be as simple as a yard stick or as sophisticated as a three-dimensional motion analysis system. Measurement techniques are constantly evolving as technology improves. This section focuses on instrumentation that is commonly used in the clinic.

Kinematic Evaluation

Kinematic evaluation involves observing limb or joint position, displacement, velocity, and acceleration. These measures will help the clinician decide if the client's motion falls within normal limits or if a deviation is present. Identification of gait deviations during walking or running provides information that may help the clinician determine the cause of a client's complaint. Additionally, it will help determine the course of treatment. Identifying gait deviations is a learned skill and requires a trained eye. When it comes to running, it is almost impossible to identify faults without visually slowing the motion. A great way to do this is with some type of video capture system. The current technology allows us to easily and objectively analyze gait for baseline and progression. Additionally, it gives the client immediate feedback and can be replayed repeatedly to modify faulty movement patterns with walking or running.

Basic equipment needed for video gait analysis includes a camera, tripod, motion capture software, and playback device. The type of movement (walking or running) and the requirements of the analysis largely determine the camera and analysis system of choice. Standard video provides 60 samples per second, which are perfectly adequate for walking. Capturing running will require a digital video capture system that has a higher sampling rate. For both qualitative and quantitative analysis, however, a consideration often of greater importance than camera speed is the clarity of the captured images. It is the camera's shutter speed that allows user control of the exposure time, or length of time that the shutter is open when each picture in the video record is taken. The faster the movement being analyzed, the shorter the duration of the exposure time required to prevent blurring of the image captured.

For two-dimensional analyses, one camera is adequate. Video observation should be viewed from the anterior, posterior, and lateral views. Therefore, the camera will need to be positioned in these three different positions. To prevent angle distortion, the camera should be placed so it is as close to perpendicular to the plane of the subject as possible. Some sort of reflective marker placed on the subject is helpful for identification of joint centers. Typically, these markers are placed on the ASIS, PSIS, greater trochanters, lateral knee, and lateral malleoli.

For research purposes, a detailed quantitative study of walking or running kinematics will require six to eight video cameras and a playback unit with higher rates of picture capture. The equipment used is much more sophisticated and expensive for running compared to walking. Much of today's biomechanical analysis software is capable of providing graphical outputs displaying kinematic and kinetic quantities of interest within minutes after a motion has been digitally captured by the cameras.

Once the video is captured, the clinician should develop a standard strategy for examination. Examples of a walking analysis and running analysis form are included in figures 13.8 and 13.9. To analyze the gait pattern, several computer software programs are available (at cost or free) that allow digitization of joint motion. The clinician would freeze-frame the point of interest from the video clip and then determine joint angles with the software tools. Angles of interest may include calcaneal eversion in the posterior view, frontal plane projection angle in the anterior view, and peak knee flexion angle during midsupport. Ideal angle values are found in table 13.6.

Gait Mats

Gait mats are systems that provide information on temporal and spatial measures during walking gait. The mat consists of a long mat or strip of carpet that serves as a walkway. Embedded within the carpeted mat are foot switches that are triggered to close by pressure when a subject walks over them. The switches are connected to a computer that computes temporal and spatial gait parameters such as step length, stride length, and gait speed.

Accelerometers

An accelerometer is a transducer used for the direct measurement of acceleration. These devices can be very light and small in size. The accelerometer is attached as rigidly as possible to the body segment or other object of interest, with electrical output channeled to a recording device. Three-dimensional accelerometers that incorporate multiple linear accelerometers are commercially available for monitoring acceleration during nonlinear movements. Accelerometers may be used to determine the acceleration rate of the limb. Milner and colleagues used accelerometers to determine tibial shock values.[41] These researchers found that female runners with a history of tibial stress fracture exhibited higher

tibial shock and impact loading as compared to a control group.[41]

Kinetic Evaluation

Measurement of forces and muscle activity (kinetics) are more difficult to obtain than kinematic variables; therefore, force and muscle activity are not frequently measured in the clinic. Tools for measuring kinetic variables in biomechanics include force platforms and electromyography (EMG).

Force Platform

Force platforms or force plates are instruments that measure the ground reaction force. Ground reaction forces are measured as vertical, forward and back, and side to side. Previous discussions of GRF are found in the kinetic sections for walking and running. The force plate surface is rectangular. This surface can vary in size, but 40 cm by 60 cm is common. The plate is placed into the floor so that it is flush with the walking surface. This placement minimizes a change in gait sequence due to an uneven surface. The force plate typically houses a strain gauge or piezoelectric set-up. For large quick forces such as those produced with running, a piezoelectric force plate is required. In a complete biomechanics lab, the force plate is synchronized with the kinematic video devices so that the video data can be synchronized with the force data.

EMG

Electromyography measures the electrical activity of a contracting muscle via surface electrodes placed on the skin over a superficial muscle or via indwelling electrodes that are implanted within the muscle. In gait, EMG is useful in determining the timing of muscles. For example, a runner who tends to adduct their limb past the midline during stance may benefit from biofeedback using an EMG electrode placed on the posterior gluteal muscles. The runner could then watch the EMG activity of those muscles and elicit gluteal muscle firing during stance.

Subject: _____

Observer: _____

Overall Inspection (Observe from front, back, and side)

Yes

❏   Shoes off

❏   Asymmetry of limb movement: _____

❏   Asymmetry of step length, stride length, foot angle: _____

Foot and Ankle

❏   Excessive drop of MLA? When: _____

❏   Lack of MLA drop? When: _____

❏   More than two toes showing from behind = _____ and is the same left to right.

Knee

❏   Is genu valgum present? When: _____

❏   Is genu varum present? When: _____

❏   Is genu recurvatum present? When: _____

❏   Full extension not achieved at initial contact.

Hip

❏   Excessive adduction during stance?

❏   Excessive femoral IR during stance?

❏   Lack of hip flexion during initial contact.

❏   Is a Trendelenburg gait present?

❏   Lack of hip extension during terminal stance/preswing.

❏   Does the hip circumduct during swing?

Trunk and UE

❏   Is excessive flexion, side bending, or extension observed? _____

❏   Arm swing is not symmetrical: _____

❏   Arm swing is not reciprocal with the LE: _____

❏   Arm swing crosses the body? _____

❏   Other observations: _____

Figure 13.8   Walking gait analysis form.

Name _____ Tape # _____ Date _____

Footwear _____ Orthotics_____

Treadmill speed: _____ Incline: _____ Cadence: _____

Rear

❑   Lateral head motion _____

❑   Center of mass _____

❑   Thoracic rotation _____

❑   Scapular position _____

❑   Lumbar sidebending _____

❑   Lateral pelvic tilt _____

❑   Pelvic transverse rot _____

❑   Pronation/supination _____

❑   Foot crosses midline (increased hip adduction) _____

❑   Increased foot pivot _____

Side

❑   Trunk (lean) _____

❑   Shoulder/elbow position (90°) _____

❑   Tight hands _____

❑   Proper hip extension (15–20°) _____

❑   Low knees (decreased hip flexion) _____

❑   Overstriding _____

❑   Asymmetrical leg swing _____

❑   Increased foot slap _____

❑   MTP extension _____

Front

❑   Head position _____

❑   Center of mass (increased vertical) _____

❑   Shoulders (level) _____

❑   Arms cross midline _____

❑   Trunk lean _____

❑   Excessive hip rotation (increase femoral rotation) _____

❑   Knee alignment (varus/valgus) _____

❑   Tibial rotation _____

❑   Heel strike: heel _____ mid _____ forefoot _____

❑   Outward toeing _____

Figure 13.9   Running gait analysis form.

TABLE 13.6   Video Analysis: Assessment of Joint Angles

View	Joint	Ideal angle
Anterior	Knee valgus angle	Less than 7°
	Hip adduction during stance	5–7°
	Trunk angle with vertical plane	Minimal
Posterior	Calcaneal eversion angle	Less than 8°
	Contralateral pelvic drop	Less than 7°
Lateral	Knee flexion at initial contact	15–20°
	Peak knee flexion (stance)	40°
	Hip flexion at peak knee flexion	20°
	Hip extension (late stance)	10–15°
	Shoulder motion	25° flexion; 10° extension
	Elbow position	90°

CONCLUSION

Analysis of walking and running gait requires an understanding of the kinematics and kinetics that occur during each gait phase. This chapter presents a detailed description of walking and running gait. Specific ranges of motion and muscle actions are presented for the lower extremity for both gaits. In addition, musculoskeletal faults are detailed in table format for easy access.

14

POSTURE

Michael P. Reiman, PT, DPT, OCS, SCS, ATC, FAAOMPT, CSCS

Posture of the human body, regardless of the position, can have a significant effect on a client's examination and treatment progress. Specific postural deficits can be correlated with specific pathological dysfunctions. Clients with an excessive forward head and bilaterally rounded shoulders have been shown to have higher incidence of upper quarter dysfunctions, while those with excessive genu valgus in the frontal plane have demonstrated a higher frequency of lower extremity pathology and dysfunction. However, it should also be mentioned that abnormal posture is common in people without pathology. Therefore, the clinician assessing normal posture and hence the potential for postural dysfunction should be keenly aware of the potential deficiencies with postural assessment. As has been elucidated throughout this text, landmark palpation and interpretation also have notable limitations. Refer to chapter 11 (Palpation) as a reminder of the means for minimizing the potential for error with these assessments.

BODY TYPE

Prior to assessing the client's posture, the clinician should perform an assessment of their body type. The client's body type can be a significant factor relative to their posture. The term used to describe a client's body type is *somatotype*. Somatotype is a combination of bone structure, bone density, and musculature. All of these variables are genetically encoded. Three primary somatotype classifications have been described: endomorph, mesomorph, and ectomorph (figure 14.1).

The client with an *endomorph* body type has a heavy or fat body build. These body types are typically described as more round in appearance and soft. These clients are more likely to have a large waist and short limbs, and the proximal portion of their arms and legs will be disproportionately larger than the distal portion of the same limb. Due to this asymmetrical distribution of body mass, these clients may likely present with postural dysfunctions of increased lumbar lordosis (to offset the increased abdominal mass), bilaterally rounded shoulders (due to the proximal trunk and arm body mass), as well as a general appearance of slouched posture. *Mesomorphs* have a muscular, athletic body build. While these clients may have a high body mass index (BMI) similar to endomorphic clients, their body mass is larger in muscular content and therefore much more favorable than that of the endomorphic client. Mesomorph clients also likely have strong bones (due to the positive stress on their bones) and a generally good posture. A client with an *ectomorph* body type is one with a very thin build and much less muscle mass than the client with a mesomorph body type. These clients are suggested

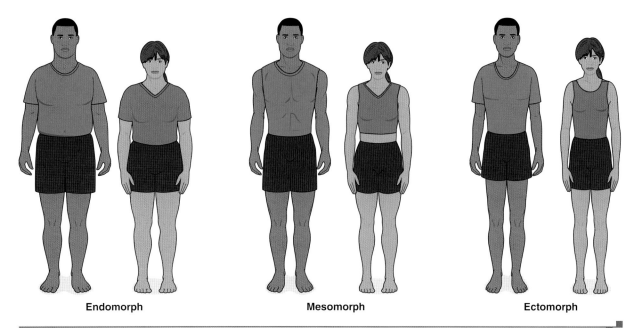

| Endomorph | Mesomorph | Ectomorph |

Figure 14.1 Somatotypes.

Reprinted, by permission, from NSCA, 2008, Age- and sex-related differences and their implications for resistance exercise, Avery D. Faigenbaum. In *Essentials of strength training and conditioning*, 3rd ed., edited by T.R. Baechle and R.W. Earl (Champaign, IL: Human Kinetics), 145.

to be at future risk for osteoporosis with aging since they have less progressive positive stress on their skeletal structure and they tend to have increased kyphotic posture.

When assessing a client's body type, the clinician should be cognizant of the likelihood that the client will likely have a combination of two of these body types. Many clients are not strictly one body type versus the other.

OPTIMAL STANDING POSTURE

Posture, whether it is optimal or dysfunctional, can be assessed in any position the client can assume. Again, it is worthy of mention that optimal or normal posture can be quite variable for different clients. Posture should always be viewed from two different viewpoints whenever possible. Since posture is typically most frequently assessed in the standing position, the two views would be either anterior or posterior for one perspective and a lateral view for the second one.

Body segments are aligned vertically, and the line of gravity will pass through or run very close to all joint axes. Slight deviations from the optimal posture are to be expected because of individual variations in body structure. Traditional assessment of optimal posture is with plumb line measures. In this instance, a plumb line is dropped from the ceiling; passing through the external auditory meatus or center of ear, it can be used to represent the line of gravity. In normal standing posture, the center of mass is directly anterior to the second sacral vertebra in most instances. At each joint in the body there is an external moment (due to gravity) acting

Critical Clinical Pearls

Various body types have different postural characteristics:

- Endomorph body type is generally described as a body build that is heavy or stout.
- Mesomorph body type is generally described as a body build that is muscular and athletic.
- Ectomorph body type is generally described as a body build that is skinny or thin.

on that joint, while an internal moment (due to contractile and noncontractile tissue) acts to resist this external moment. Table 14.1 lists the major joints of the body, the external moments acting on them, and the internal moments (passive and active opposing forces) resisting these external moments.

Therefore, with normal standing posture, muscle activity throughout the body should be minimal. The farther the line of gravity is away from the center of the joint, the greater the muscle activity on the antagonistic muscle group will be to oppose the gravitational moment. The muscles with the greatest electrical activity in normal, quiet stance are soleus to maintain upright posture, iliopsoas to counteract posterior moment at hip joint, gluteus medius and tensor fascia latae to control lateral pelvic tilt, and erector spinae muscle group to counteract anterior moment at the trunk.

Anteroposterior View

The plumb line, when dropped from the ceiling, should bisect the body into equal sides (left and right) when viewed both anteriorly (figure 14.2) and posteriorly (figure 14.3). Alignment in this view is as such (from cranial to caudal):

- Head and neck straight (no rotation or side bending)
- Equal distance between ears and sides of head
- Equal distance between eyes
- Plumb line bisects the midline of occiput through spinous process of vertebrae and directly through gluteal cleft
- Spine straight without lateral curvature
- Equal paraspinal muscle size
- Nose, chin, suprasternal notch, sternum, and umbilicus are bisected into equal halves
- Equal height of shoulders (dominant shoulder may be lower)
- Medial border of scapulae equidistant from spine
- Inferior angle of scapulae equal
- Rib cage symmetrical
- Elbows with equal carrying angles
- Iliac crest equal height
- ASIS and PSIS equal height
- Greater trochanters equal height
- Gluteal folds equal height

TABLE 14.1 Major Joints and Gravitational Moments

Joints	Line of gravity	Gravitational moment	Passive opposing forces	Active opposing forces
Atlantooccipital	Anterior	Flexion	Ligamentum nuchae, tectorial membrane	Posterior neck muscles
Cervical	Posterior	Extension	Anterior longitudinal ligament	Deep cervical flexors
Thoracic	Anterior	Flexion	Posterior longitudinal ligament, ligamentum flavum, supraspinous ligament	Thoracic extensors (paraspinal muscles)
Lumbar	Posterior	Extension	Anterior longitudinal ligament	Abdominals, hip flexors
Sacroiliac joint	Anterior	Flexion	Sacrotuberous ligament, sacrospinous ligament, long dorsal ligament, interosseous ligament	Hip extensors, lumbar extensors
Hip joint	Posterior	Extension	Iliofemoral ligament	Iliopsoas
Knee joint	Anterior	Extension	Posterior joint capsule, posterior cruciate ligament	Hamstrings
Ankle joint	Anterior	Dorsiflexion	Posterior tibiofibular ligament	Soleus

Reprinted, by permission, from J. Loudon, R. Manske, and M. Reiman, 2013, *Clinical mechanics and kinesiology* (Champaign, IL: Human Kinetics), 341.

- Equal hamstring muscle size
- Equal distance between knee joints
- Patellae facing forward and equal height
- Popliteal fossa equal height
- Equal calf muscle size
- Achilles tendon and calcaneus in neutral alignment
- Equal distance between ankle joints and medial malleoli
- Longitudinal arch of foot not excessively high or flat
- Toes in natural alignment
- Feet toed out 5° to 18°

In both the anterior and posterior views, the ears, shoulders, iliac crests, fibular heads, and lateral malleoli should be level (in the same plane). In throwing athletes, or with people who are dominant on one arm, it is common for the dominant shoulder to be lower (or more caudal) than the nondominant arm. This is referred to as the *handiness pattern*.[1]

Bilateral arms should be equidistant from the trunk, with an equal carrying angle (5–15°). Bilateral palms should face toward the body with thumbs facing anterior. The posterior view should demonstrate bilateral scapulae equidistant from the spine and level to each other in the superior–inferior direction. The scapulae normally rest 2 to 3 in.

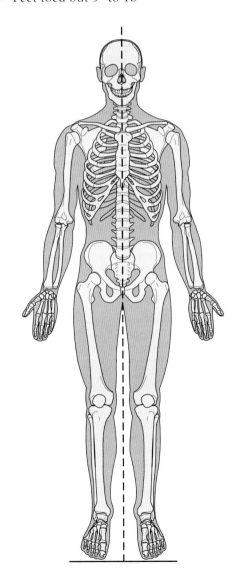

Figure 14.2 Ideal posture, anterior view. In this and subsequent similar figures, the dashed line represents a plumb line.

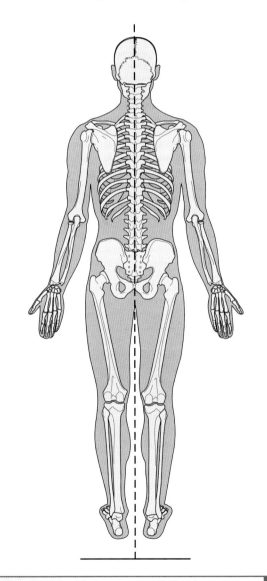

Figure 14.3 Ideal posture, posterior view.

(5–8 cm) from the spine and at the level of between the second and seventh thoracic vertebral levels.

The spinous processes throughout the spine should be in line vertically with each other without any noticeable curvature in the frontal plane (scoliosis). Bilateral iliac crests should be level. The rib cage and trunk should be symmetrical on each side without appearance of a lateral shift or deviation of the trunk in the frontal plane. Posteriorly, the gluteal fold should be vertical and the bilateral gluteal masses should be symmetrical. There should be a slight genu valgus at bilateral knees with the patellae facing directly forward. Posteriorly, the popliteal creases should be level and horizontal. The feet should be abducted slightly (5–18°), but remain symmetrical. Posteriorly, the Achilles tendons should be relatively vertical and symmetrical to each other.

Lateral View

Lateral view assessment of posture must be done from both the right and left sides of the client. As with the anterior and posterior view assessments, clinicians should start the assessment by viewing from cranial to caudal. With a lateral view, the plumb line ideally should line up accordingly (figure 14.4):[1]

- Through the external auditory meatus
- Through the odontoid process
- Through the bodies (to slightly posterior) of the cervical vertebrae
- Through the acromioclavicular joint of the shoulder
- Slightly anterior to the thoracic kyphosis
- Slightly posterior to the lumbar lordosis
- Through the greater trochanter of the femur, slightly posterior to the center of the hip joint
- Slightly anterior to the center of the knee joint and posterior to the patella
- Slightly anterior to the lateral malleolus, through the calcaneocuboid joint of the ankle

OTHER POSTURE POSITIONS

The orthopedic clinician should consider observing a client's sitting and lying down positions and trans-

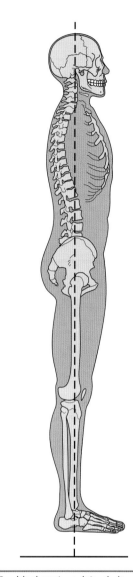

Figure 14.4 Ideal posture, lateral view.

fer activities as additional postural assessments. This is particularly important because a static measure of standing posture can be of limited clinical utility when the client complains of pain or dysfunction when they are performing dynamic tasks.

Sitting posture is of particular importance for the client with an occupation or leisure activity that mostly involves sitting. As with standing posture, the ideal sitting posture is characterized by minimal muscle activity. In the ideal posture, the spine is erect, the shoulders are aligned directly over the hips, the hips are flexed to 90°, and the feet are completely supported on a stable surface.[2] Sitting without proper spine support results in a significant increase in muscle activity to maintain an upright posture.[3]

Assessment of sitting posture, as with standing posture, should be done from anterior, posterior, and lateral views. Some specific considerations for meeting ideal sitting posture at a computer work station include the following:

- Head vertical with computer screen (or primary view at client's station) at eye level

- Shoulders relaxed and level (not rounded)

- Elbows at 90°

- Wrists in neutral to slight extension and supported

- Trunk upright with back support

- Hips and knees at 90°

- Feet completely supported

A back support in a chair that is too high will promote lumbar flexion, while a support that is too low will not provide enough stability to the spine. A chair without arm rests or one that causes the client to support their wrists on their typing surface will promote shoulder muscle activity to prevent the arms from dangling. A seat of the chair that is too low will promote overall flexed posture, while a seat that is too high may cause the client's feet to be unsupported and increase the pressure on the client's posterior thighs.

Sitting posture does not significantly increase intradiscal pressure in the spine compared to standing;[4] in fact, at least one study has suggested that intradiscal pressure is less in sitting than standing.[5] Generally speaking, trunk-forward flexion, a rounded trunk when lifting weight, and trunk flexion with rotation are the most stressful movements to the intervertebral discs of the spine.[5, 6]

Some important considerations from these studies include the facts that increased muscle activity acting on the spine in these sitting or trunk-flexed postures increases intradiscal pressure and that clients should constantly change position to promote nutrition to the disc.[4, 5]

Lying posture is important to assess due to the amount of time a client will spend sleeping. It is generally suggested that the clinician assess the client in their normal resting or sleeping posture. Generally speaking, the client's spine, head, and pelvis should be in a relatively normal, neutral position whether they are in a side-lying or supine position. Obviously, the client may assume multiple adapted positions. The principal factor when assessing lying posture is to attempt to avoid positions that will place undue stress on the client's body (and provoke pain), such as too many pillows in side-lying or supine positions promoting excessive head side bending (side-lying) or excessive head flexion (supine). Excessive trunk side bending should also be avoided. Pillow positioning can assist with these potential poor postures. For the client with complaints of pain due to excessive hip adduction in side-lying position, the use of pillows between their knees may be an option for avoiding such positions. Additionally, a pillow under the hips or between the knees when side lying can improve alignment and relieve stress on the spine.[1]

Transfer postures should be noted because these activities are often those that clients complain most of experiencing pain with. For the client with low back pain (for example), clinicians should observe how they perform sit to stand, supine to sit, getting in and out of a car, lifting, and so on, since these activities require a lot of trunk motion and muscle activity. Often teaching the client how to use their legs with sit-to-stand movements and lifting, and so on can make a significant improvement in their pain and dysfunction.

The clinician should also assess for symmetry of movement with transfer activities. Symmetry of movement can minimize the muscle activity requirement and, hence, the demands placed on the person to successfully complete such tasks.

ABNORMAL POSTURES

Posture that is abnormal is quite difficult to quantify due to the variable client presentations, both with and without pain, dysfunction, or pathology. As with all components of the comprehensive examination, the clinician is reminded to carefully ascertain the relevance of perceived abnormal. If the client demonstrates abnormal posture, the clinician should try to categorize such posture accordingly in order to properly address the appropriate dysfunction. Categorization of dysfunctional posture previously described in the literature ranges from simply stating the abnormal position (e.g., forward head) to describing syndromes (e.g., upper and lower crossed syndrome).

Crossed syndrome is the concept of neuromuscular imbalances between groups of muscles resulting in poor posture, loss of mobility, and an increase in joint loads.[7] According to this theory, certain muscle groups tend to be either tight (tonic muscles) or weak (phasic muscles). Muscles prone to tightness are generally readily activated with any movement, creating abnormal movement patterns. Janda describes two crossed syndromes: lower and upper crossed syndrome.

Lower crossed syndrome (figure 14.5) is characterized by tightness of the thoracolumbar extensors on the posterior side that crosses with tightness of the iliopsoas and rectus femoris on the anterior side. Antagonistic muscle weaknesses would include the deep abdominal muscles anteriorly and the gluteus maximus and medius posteriorly.

Upper crossed syndrome is characterized by tightness of the deep neck flexors, upper trapezius, and levator scapulae on the posterior side crossed with tightness of the pectoralis major and minor on the anterior side. Corresponding antagonistic muscle group weaknesses include the deep neck flexors anteriorly and the middle and lower trapezius posteriorly. This pattern of muscle imbalance between the tight and weak muscles creates joint dysfunction, specifically at the atlantooccipital joint, C4-5, cervicothoracic junction, glenohumeral joint, and T4-5.[2]

Addressing these dysfunctions requires consistent client education, strengthening of the weak muscle groups, and stretching of the tight muscle groups. Strengthening of the weak antagonists is particularly beneficial for maintaining the corrected posture.[2]

General postural dysfunctions related to muscle imbalances are commonly seen by the orthopedic clinician (table 14.2). Forward head posture with occiput extension is a very common postural defect. These clients may present with suboccipital muscle tightness and deep neck flexor weakness (upper crossed syndrome). Clients with this postural dysfunction are prone to posture-related headaches and cervicogenic headaches. Cervicogenic headaches are as a result of upper cervical spine dysfunction that, in some instances, can be related to postural imbalances.

A common postural dysfunction that is also present with clients with a forward head posture is bilaterally rounded and internally rotated shoulders. Tight muscles in these clients would likely include the latissimus dorsi and pectoral muscles. Tight pectoral muscles are also common contributors to increased thoracic kyphosis, which is correctable with verbal and tactile cueing (versus a static dysfunction that is not correctable with these cues).

Tight hip flexors are common contributors to postural dysfunction of increased lumbar lordosis and limited hip flexion with such tasks as gait. Weak hip abductors can contribute to postural dysfunction statically and dynamically (especially with gait, running, and jumping) to increased genu valgus at the knee. Weak hip external rotators can contribute to increased femoral internal rotation, a common

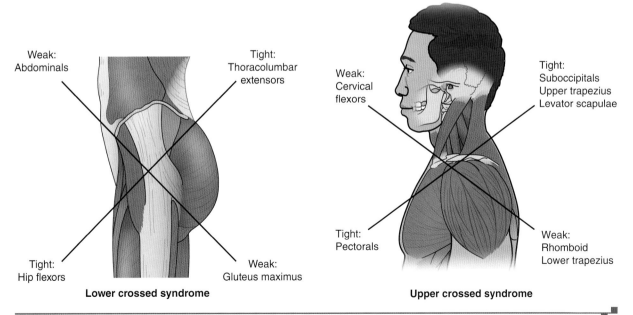

Figure 14.5 Lower and upper crossed syndrome.

TABLE 14.2 Muscle Imbalances as a Result of Postural Defects

Postural defect	Muscles that are short	Muscles that are long (may be weak)
Forward head position Atlantooccipital extended to allow person to keep eyes level from lower cervical flexion Lower cervical spine flexion TMJ clenched Scapulae abducted and elevated Humeral internal rotation	Levator scapulae Sternocleidomastoid Scalenes Suboccipital muscles Upper trapezius Pectoralis major and minor Serratus anterior Latissimus dorsi Subscapularis	Hyoid muscles Deep neck flexors (e.g., longus colli and capitis) Lower cervical and thoracic erector spinae Middle and lower trapezius Rhomboids
Anterior tilt of scapulae	Pectoralis minor Biceps	Lower trapezius Middle trapezius Serratus anterior
Scapular downward rotation	Rhomboids Levator scapulae Latissimus dorsi Pectoralis minor Supraspinatus	Upper trapezius Serratus anterior Lower trapezius
Scapular abduction	Serratus anterior Pectoralis major Pectoralis minor Shoulder external rotators	Middle trapezius Lower trapezius Rhomboids
Humeral medial rotation	Pectoralis major Latissimus dorsi Shoulder internal rotators	Shoulder external rotators
Humeral anterior glide	Shoulder external rotators Pectoralis major	Shoulder internal rotators
Thoracic kyphosis	Pectoralis major Pectoralis minor Internal obliques	Thoracic spine extensors Middle trapezius Lower trapezius Rhomboids
Flat thoracic spine	Thoracic erector spinae Scapular retractors	Scapular protractors Anterior intercostal muscles
Lordotic (flexible spine) Pelvis: anterior Lumbar: flexion Hip: flexion	Lumbar extensors Hip flexors	Abdominals Hip extensors
Flat back (stiff spine) Pelvis: posterior Lumbar: flexion Hip: extension	Abdominals Hip extensors	Lumbar extensor muscles Hip flexor muscles

Postural defect	Muscles that are short	Muscles that are long (may be weak)
Swayback Pelvis: posterior Lumbar: flexion Hip: extension Thoracic spine relatively posterior in relation to lumbar spine	Upper abdominals Hip extensors	Lower abdominals Hip flexors Lower lumbar extensors
Handiness pattern Shoulder girdle low on dominant side Iliac crest high on dominate side	Ipsilateral trunk muscles	Contralateral trunk muscles Ipsilateral shoulder girdle muscles
Scoliosis	Muscles on concave side Hip adductors Foot supinators on short side	Muscles on convex side Hip abductors Foot pronators on long side
Femoral anteversion	Hip internal rotators	Hip external rotators
Femoral retroversion	Hip external rotators	Hip internal rotators
Genu valgum	Hip internal rotators Hip adductors	Gluteus medius
Genu varum	Hip adductors	Iliotibial band
Genu recurvatum	Quadriceps	Hamstrings

Reprinted, by permission, from J. Loudon, R. Manske, and M. Reiman, 2013, *Clinical mechanics and kinesiology* (Champaign, IL: Human Kinetics), 343.

component of which has been described as lower extremity medial collapse (increased hip adduction and medial rotation beyond normal ranges with dynamic tasks).

Pes planus (flat foot posture) is a common postural dysfunction that can either be static due to structural abnormalities or dynamic due to lack of muscular control either proximally at the hip or more locally at the foot (posterior tibialis muscle performance dysfunction, for example).

Different general posture presentations can also be commonly found in clients (figure 14.6). Kypholordotic posture presentation is one of excessive kyphosis in the thoracic spine and corresponding excessive lordosis in the lumbar spine. A flat back posture is one in which the lumbar spine has less than normal lordosis or a flattened lumbar spine. Swayback posture presentation is one of a relatively flattened lumbar spine and a corresponding posterior sway of the thoracic spine relative to the vertical plumb line.

Postural dysfunction results from either structural or functional faults. Structural faults result from either congenital or developmental anomalies, disease, or trauma.[1, 8, 9] Such structural faults include excessive thoracic kyphosis due to Scheuermann's

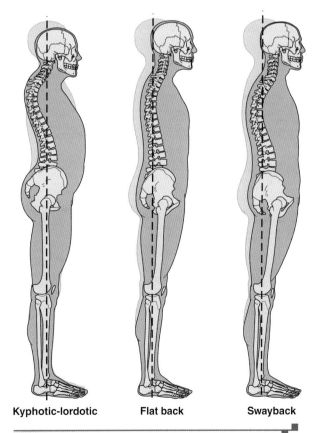

Kyphotic-lordotic   **Flat back**   **Swayback**

Figure 14.6 General posture presentations.

Critical Clinical Pearls

Different postural dysfunctions have different clinical presentations:

- With each presentation, a particular muscle group is shortened, while the agonist of this muscle group is lengthened.
- Muscles that are both shortened and lengthened from their normal length are suggested to be weak.
- Clinicians should always assess the muscle strength and performance to determine the actual muscle performance of a muscle group that is suspected to be either short or lengthened.
- Many clients, both with and without pathology, function just fine with muscles that are deemed to be shorter or lengthened more than what is normal.

disease (figure 14.7), scoliosis, and congenital leg length discrepancy. Structural faults often require bracing, specific exercise prescription, and occasionally surgical correction (if necessary). Functional faults are those that typically result from poor posture habits.[1, 8, 9] Upper and lower crossed syndromes are common examples of functional faults.

Scoliosis is a postural dysfunction that involves both the frontal and transverse planes. It is named for the shape of the presentation of the spine. A C-curve is a single curve and an S-curve is a double curve. The curve is named for the side of the convexity and the region where the curve is located (figure 14.8). Figure 14.8*b* demonstrates a right thoracic scoliosis, with the convexity (apex) of the curve on the right side in the thoracic spine region. A right thoracic, left lumbar curve is demonstrated in figure 14.8*e*.

In scoliosis the spine will side bend and rotate in contralateral directions. In a right thoracic spine C-curve, for example, the thoracic spine is left side bent but right rotated. Since it is right rotated, the rib cage on the right side is prominent posteriorly. This posterior prominence of the rib cage is called a *rib hump*. The rib hump may not be seen readily in a normal upright standing posture, but with trunk forward flexion (Adam's test) it can be more clearly seen (figure 14.9). Scoliosis and its assessment are described in greater detail in chapters 18 (Thoracic Spine) and 29 (Pediatric Examination).

Radiographic measurement of scoliosis is described as the Cobb angle. This angle, developed by orthopedic surgeon John Robert Cobb, was originally utilized to measure coronal plane deformity on anteroposterior plane radiographs in the classification of scoliosis. It has subsequently been adapted to classify sagittal plane deformity, especially in clients with thoracolumbar spine fractures. The Cobb angle is an angle measured radiographically that is commonly accepted by the Scoliosis Research Society as the gold standard measurement for scoliosis, although a 2° to 7° measurement error potential does exist.[10] To measure the Cobb angle, do the following (figure 14.10):

1. Locate the most tilted vertebra at the top of the curve and draw a parallel line to the superior vertebral end plate.
2. Locate the most tilted vertebra at the bottom of the curve and draw a parallel line to the inferior vertebral end plate.
3. Erect intersecting perpendicular lines from the two parallel lines.
4. The angle formed between the two parallel lines is the Cobb angle.

For vertebral fractures, the Cobb angle is the angle formed between a line drawn parallel to the superior end plate of the vertebra one level above the fracture

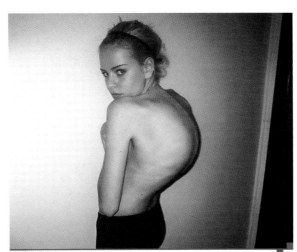

Figure 14.7 Scheuermann's disease.

emily tropea/Fairfax Media

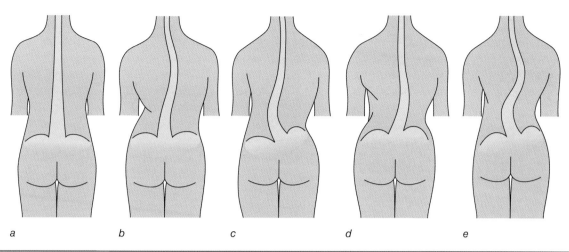

Figure 14.8 Forms of scoliosis: *(a)* normal orientation of the vertebral column, *(b)* right thoracic scoliosis, *(c)* left lumbar scoliosis, *(d)* right thoracolumbar scoliosis, and *(e)* bilateral scoliosis (right thoracic and left lumbar).

Reprinted, by permission, from J. Watkins, 2010, *Structure and function of the musculoskeletal system,* 2nd ed. (Champaign, IL: Human Kinetics), 150.

and a line drawn parallel to the inferior end plate of the vertebra one level below the fracture. The Cobb angle is the preferred method of measuring posttraumatic kyphosis in a recent meta-analysis of traumatic spine fracture classification.[11]

DYNAMIC POSTURE

Traditional examination of posture primarily encapsulates static assessment. While examination of these postures is important for the orthopedic client, it is worthy of mention that static postural abnormality does not always equate to pain, dysfunction, or poor health.[12] More dynamic postural dysfunctions have been suggested as more relevant to pathology.[13-17] Therefore, clinicians should examine the client during movements, particularly those the client encounters in daily and work-related activities. For the athlete, this would also include movements done during their sporting activities. Of particular importance in the dynamic postural

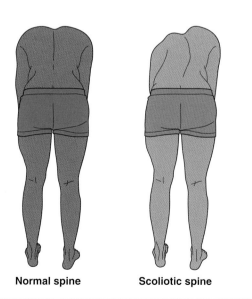

Normal spine   **Scoliotic spine**

Figure 14.9 Normal spine versus scoliotic spine in trunk flexion (Adam's test) positions. See figure 14.8 for normal versus scoliotic spine in upright positions.

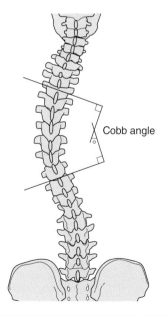

Cobb angle

Figure 14.10 Cobb angle measurement.

assessment is observing and examining the client during movements that reproduce the client's pain. These movements are also especially helpful to use as a retest measure to determine whether the therapeutic intervention was beneficial.

PALPATION ASSESSMENT OF THORACIC POSTURE

Beyond observation, postural assessment of the spine, particularly the thoracic spine, can be assisted with palpation (figure 14.11). This is a general

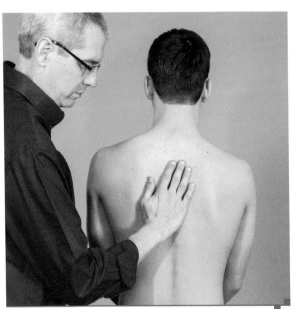

Figure 14.11   Palpation of thoracic posture.

light palpation assessment method that can be followed up with more detailed joint mobility assessments (as described in chapter 18, Thoracic Spine) if necessary. The clinician will assess for postural curvature, symmetry of the rib cage from side to side and cranial to caudal, as well as skin and soft-tissue mobility. Clinicians should stand directly behind the client and use a relaxed, open-hand purchase as they slide their hand up and down, as well as side to side along the length of the spine. Clinicians can also have the client sit in an upright, normal posture position to assess for differences in the previously mentioned characteristics in the normal position versus client's natural position.

CONCLUSION

Body posture is a distinct observation skill that clinicians should always integrate into their clinical examination of the orthopedic client. Posture examination requires an understanding of commonly described accepted normal standards. It is important to appreciate that various postural presentations are present in clients with and without pain, dysfunction, or pathology. The clinician should be cognizant of such information and be careful to determine the relevance of the client's so-called abnormal posture.

III

Examination
of the Head and Spine

Part III details examination of the head and spine, covering the face and head (chapter 15), temporomandibular joint (chapter 16), cervical spine (chapter 17), thoracic spine (chapter 18), lumbar spine (chapter 19), and the sacroiliac joint and pelvic girdle (chapter 20). It highlights the importance of screening for serious pathology, such as consciousness and head injury (face and head), cervical artery dysfunction and cervical instability (cervical spine), vertebral compression fractures (thoracic spine), as well as cauda equine syndrome (lumbar spine). It also provides the latest evidence to afford the clinician the best ability to properly rule out or rule in these pathologies. It also covers other less serious pathologies in great detail with the latest supporting evidence.

In part III, the clinician is introduced specifically to the application of the funnel examination approach. At the end of each chapter in parts III and IV, in a section titled Common Orthopedic Conditions, each of the eight components of the funnel examination, as well as the supporting evidence (or lack thereof) for each component, is described in detail respective to the body part highlighted in that chapter. This section also provides ICD-9 and ICD-10 coding for each of the pathologies outlined. The listed ICD codes should be particularly helpful to the clinician with the recent conversion to ICD-10. At the end of each pathology, suggested treatment-based classifications are available that will help guide appropriate interventions. Great detailed evidence with a color code scheme is also provided here so that the clinician, once again, can quickly discern if the evidence supporting the testing measures is **ideal** versus **good** versus less than good.

15

FACE AND HEAD

Michael P. Reiman, PT, DPT, OCS, SCS, ATC, FAAOMPT, CSCS

Examination detail regarding the face and head is typically less extensively described than are most other areas of the body in musculoskeletal medicine. The region's close relationship to the temporomandibular joint (chapter 16) and cervical spine (chapter 17) often lead to grouping these sections as one entire unit. Although these sections are described in independent chapters in this text, clinicians should consider the close and interdependent relationship among these regions.

The face and head, while not commonly encountered pathology for the orthopedic clinician, is an area worthy of individual consideration. This chapter covers the funnel approach examination sequence for the face and head, describing current best evidence as well as clinical suggestions appropriate for this area.

CLINICALLY APPLIED ANATOMY

The facial skeleton is composed of the mandible (lower jaw), maxilla (upper jaw), nasal bones, and the palatine, lacrimal, zygomatic, and ethmoid bones. The facial skull has several cavities for the nose (nasal), eyes (orbital), and mouth (oral; figure 15.1). Several

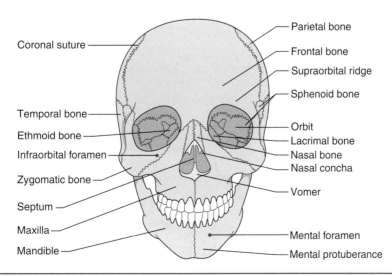

Coronal suture
Parietal bone
Frontal bone
Supraorbital ridge
Sphenoid bone
Temporal bone
Ethmoid bone
Infraorbital foramen
Zygomatic bone
Orbit
Lacrimal bone
Nasal bone
Nasal concha
Septum
Vomer
Maxilla
Mandible
Mental foramen
Mental protuberance

Figure 15.1 Anatomy of the skull.

small openings also allow nerves and blood vessels to penetrate the bony structures of the skull.

The 12 cranial nerves are the primary control for the muscles of the face and head. These nerves, and their function, are listed in chapter 7 (see the section Cranial Nerve Examination). Assessment of these nerves, and their function, is essential to the client with a face and head musculoskeletal injury.

The eyelid is the skin protective covering over the external portion of the eye. It protects the eye from foreign bodies, distributes tears over the surface of the eye, and limits the amount of light entering the eye. The eye itself is composed of the sclera, cornea, and iris, as well as the lens

and retina (figure 15.2). The sclera is the dense white portion of the eye. The cornea separates the watery fluid of the anterior chamber of the eye from the external environment. The iris is a circular, contractile muscular disc that controls the amount of light entering the eye. It also contains pigmented cells that give the eye its color. The lens is a crystalline structure directly behind the iris that permits images from various distances to be focused on the retina. The retina is the primary sensory structure of the eye. It transforms light impulses into electrical impulses, which are then transmitted to the brain by the optic nerve and are registered as the object seen.

The outer ear is composed of cartilage covered with skin. The middle ear (figure 15.3), composed of the tympanic membrane (eardrum), malleus (hammer), incus (anvil), and stapes (stirrup), sends vibration to the cochlea when sound is encountered. The cochlea, part of the inner ear, transmits the sound waves to the vestibulo-cochlear nerve (cranial nerve VIII), which then transmits the electrical impulses to the brain for interpretation of the sound. The other part of the inner ear, the semicircular canals, plays a significant role in balance maintenance.

The outer nose is also cartilage covered with skin. The nose is divided into two chambers by a septum (figure 15.4). These chambers are lined with a mucous membrane containing hairs that collect debris from inspired air. These air-filled spaces are named for the facial bones in which they are located:

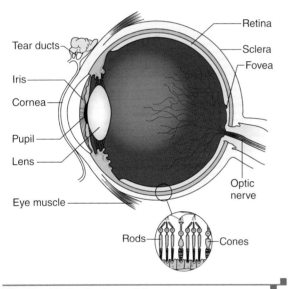

Figure 15.2 Anatomy of the eye.

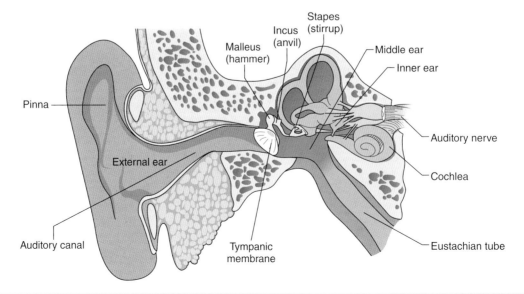

Figure 15.3 Anatomy of the ear.

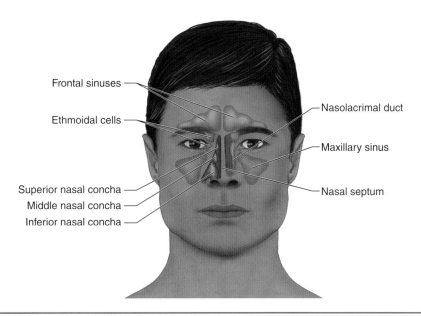

Figure 15.4 Anatomy of the nose and sinuses.

- **Maxillary sinuses:** the largest of the paranasal sinuses, located under the eyes in the maxillary bone.
- **Frontal sinuses:** located superior to the eyes in the frontal bone.
- **Ethmoidal sinuses:** formed by several discrete air cells within the ethmoid bone between the nose and the eyes.
- **Sphenoidal sinuses:** located in the sphenoid bone.

CLIENT INTERVIEW

The interview is typically the first encounter the clinician will have with the client. As discussed in chapter 5 (Client Interview and Observation), this component of the examination can provide the clinician with a significant amount of information relevant to the probability of the client's presenting diagnosis. For purposes of this text, the interview is described relative to each body part or section, but generally includes subjective reports by the client, as well as findings from their outcome measures. Additionally included in this section is radiographic imaging. While clinicians should consider avoiding biasing their examinations by interpreting findings of radiographic imaging prior to seeing clients (in most cases without concerns for red flags and major medical-related issues), this point in the examination is most likely where clinicians will encounter radiographic imaging. Additionally, in some instances, clinicians must interpret radiographic imaging early in the examination to rule out serious pathology prior to continuing with other components of the examination sequence.

Subjective

As with all injured clients, the mechanism of injury should be one of the first questions the clinician asks the client with a face and head injury. A mechanism of direct impact to the head or indirect impact from a fall should alert the clinician to the possibility of the potential for traumatic brain injury (TBI). The term *mild TBI* (MTBI) is now used in place of *concussion* in the nomenclature according to the Centers for Disease Control and Prevention (CDC) and the World Health Organization (WHO). Traumatic brain injury is a clinical diagnosis of neurological dysfunction following head trauma, typically presenting with acute symptoms of some degree of cognitive impairment. The American Academy of Neurology (AAN) defines MTBI as a biomechanically induced brain injury resulting in neurologic dysfunction.[1] MTBI results in a constellation of physical, cognitive, emotional, or sleep-related symptoms and may or may not involve a loss of consciousness (LOC). Duration of symptoms is highly variable, and symptoms may last from several minutes to days, weeks, months, or even longer in some cases.[2]

Clinicians have a greater awareness of potential short- and long-term sequelae of athletes who suffer brain injuries, such as increased propensity for reinjury, cognitive slowing, early onset Alzheimer's, second impact syndrome, and chronic traumatic encephalopathy.[2-8] Greater detail with respect to concussion is given in chapter 27 (Emergency Sport Examination). The clinician should ascertain the client's level of alertness. Alertness and orientation to person, place, time, and situation is often described as normal and "alert and oriented × 4." The Glasgow Coma Scale (GCS; described later in this chapter) is a necessary tool for determining the potential for brain injury, especially on the acutely injured client.

Assuming there are no major considerations for significant potential of brain injury, the clinician should determine the location and extent of the client's pain. Pain drawings, pain scales, and descriptions of type of pain should all be employed to determine the significance of the pain presentation.

The client should be questioned as to the potential presence of paresthesia, abnormal sensation, or lack of sensation. Questions regarding loss of smell, vision, taste, hearing, and balance issues would alert the clinician to the potential for specific cranial nerve involvement. Aggravating and alleviating factors should be determined. Is the pain position dependent? Answers to these types of questions can determine the significance of the client's pain presentation, as well as the potential necessity for outside referral and concern for red flag issues (see chapter 6, Triage and Differential Diagnosis).

Headaches can be a common presentation for the client with face and head pain. Headaches are quite complex and require a careful questioning and examination. Headaches without a particular pattern or ones progressively worsening without any form of relief should always be considered for potential non-musculoskeletal causes until proven otherwise. See the section Common Orthopedic Conditions of the Face and Head later in this chapter for more detail on headache presentation.

Dizziness is also a concern. Again, the clinician should always be careful with questioning and exam-ination of these types of clients. Further detail on diz-ziness is also presented in the later section Common Orthopedic Conditions of the Face and Head.

The severity of the client's injury can be suggested by all of the variables discussed previously, as well as by ability to solve simple mathematical problems, normal speech, vision, and the level of the client's irritability, concentration, and memory. Clients who present concerns in any of these areas should be further investigated.

Speech problems can be quite complex. *Dysarthria* is a defect in articulation, enunciation, or rhythm of speech. It is often characterized by slurring, slowness of speech, and indistinct speech. *Dysphonia* is a disorder of vocalization characterized by the abnormal production of sounds from the larynx. The primary complaint with dysphonia is hoarseness. *Dysphasia* is the inability to use and understand spoken and written words as a result of disorders involving cortical centers of speech in the cerebral hemisphere.

Concerns related to vision, hearing, and smell should also be determined. Each of these issues could be related to the client's current condition or they could be preexisting. Careful subjective questioning should be able to determine this distinction. These potential dysfunctions should also be considered potentially significant for more serious pathology, including (but not limited to) cranial nerve dysfunction, Horner's syndrome, and non-musculoskeletal red flag concerns.

Outcome Measures

Refer to chapters 16 (Temporomandibular Joint) and 17 (Cervical Spine) for appropriate measures.

Diagnostic Imaging

Severe trauma to the face is a strong indication for radiological investigation. In the client with maxil-lofacial trauma, the radiological exploration should answer two major questions: (1) Do the fractures

---

Critical Clinical Pearls

Differentiation of the most common orthopedic-related speech disorders:
- Dysarthria: defect in articulation, enunciation, or rhythm of speech
- Dysphonia: abnormal production of sound (e.g., hoarseness)
- Dysphasia: deficiency in the generation of speech and sometimes also in its comprehension

involve areas that may alter the physiologic function of the sinuses, mouth, nasal vault, or orbit? (2) Will the fracture result in any cosmetically detectable abnormality? The goal of the radiological work-up is to define the number and exact location of the fractures, to determine if there is any depression, elevation, or distraction of the fracture fragments, and to assess concomitant soft-tissue complications. Conventional plain radiography and computed tomography (CT) scans are the traditional diagnostic tools for maxillofacial injuries, with CT being the long-term gold standard.[9, 10] Each of these modalities has limitations, as pointed out in the following respective sections.

The role of imaging is to detect fractures, describe their morphology and topography, and evaluate adjacent soft-tissue damage. CT is the imaging method of choice for an accurate diagnosis and depiction of the complex anatomic structures of the maxillofacial region (table 15.1). Magnetic resonance imaging (MRI), on the other hand, plays a limited role, mainly in the assessment of lesions of orbital soft tissues.[11] CT and MRI are well-established imaging modalities for examining the facial nerve as well as the course of the facial nerve itself. MRI has a superior soft-tissue contrast to CT that enables imaging of the facial nerve itself. Therefore, the normal facial nerve and pathologic changes of the facial nerve are readily visualized from the brain stem to the parotid gland.[12]

Radiographs

A disadvantage of this imaging modality for maxillofacial injuries is that the superimposition of images of overlying structures sometimes makes definite radiological interpretation difficult.[9, 13] An additional disadvantage is that real-time visualization is impracticable without digital technology; thus, only one hard-copy image of two-dimensional plane films is available for evaluation.[14]

Magnetic Resonance Imaging

MRI is mainly beneficial for soft-tissue and nerve-lesion involvement. Generally, it also has limited application in facial and head bone pathology.

Computed Tomography

Disadvantages of CT include high cost and high radiation exposure. In addition, with clients who have metallic implants, there can be blurring of the image due to artifacts generated by the metal.[14]

TABLE 15.1 Diagnostic Accuracy of Imaging Modalities for the Face and Head

Pathology	Diagnostic test	Gold standard	SN/SP
Head and neck injuries	Whole-body CT	Synopsis of hospital charts, subsequent imaging and interventional procedures	85/99[15]
Facial injuries	Whole-body CT	Synopsis of hospital charts, subsequent imaging and interventional procedures	80/99[15]
Zygomatic arch fracture	US	Plain radiograph and CT	100/100[16]
		Variable	>90/>90[14]
Infraorbital margin fracture	US	Plain radiograph and CT	90/100[16]
Orbital fracture		Variable	56-100/85-100[14]
Frontozygomatic suture separation	US	Plain radiograph and CT	25/100[16]
Nasal bone fracture	US	CT	95/100[17]
		Variable	90-100/98-100[14]
			84/75[18]
	Radiographs	Clinical examinations	50-64/58-72[18]
Mandibular fracture	US	Variable	66-100/52-100[14]

US = ultrasonography; CT = computed tomography

The color coding for suggestion of **good** and **ideal** diagnostic accuracy values reported in this table are without quality scoring (QUADAS), a very important aspect of determination of the clinical utility of such values. Therefore, it is suggested that the reader keep this in mind when interpreting such values.

Ultrasonography

Recently, multiple studies have investigated the diagnostic accuracy of ultrasonography (US) as an imaging modality for maxillofacial injuries. A fair amount of evidence justifies the use of diagnostic US in maxillofacial fractures, especially fractures involving the nasal bone, orbital walls, anterior maxillary wall, and zygomatic complex. The SN and SP of US have been reported to be generally comparable with CT.[14]

Review of Systems

Refer to chapter 6 (Triage and Differential Diagnosis) for details on review of systems relevant to the face and head.

OBSERVATION

To properly observe the face and head, the clinician should view them from the front, back, and both sides. Particular attention should focus on position and shape of the eyes, mouth, nose, ears, and teeth. Clinicians should also look for deformity, imbalance or asymmetry, swelling, atrophy, drooping at rest and with facial expressions (e.g., Bell's palsy), and lacerations. They should examine facial bone features for symmetry and distortion, as well as the general head and face posture. Is the client holding their head and face in a relatively neutral position? If they are not, where is the asymmetry presenting from (e.g., cervical spine, facial distortion from injury)? General appearance of facial expression is often an indicator of the client's overall feeling. For example, clients in acute distress are not likely to smile or exhibit a positive facial expression. If the client appears confused, the clinician should have heightened awareness of the potential for more sinister issues.

When viewing from the front, the clinician should also pay particular attention to the appearance of the client's eyes. Eye asymmetry can be a concern for vestibular, cranial nerve, and other pathological concerns that the clinician should be cognizant of. Eye tracking, nystagmus, and other movement asymmetries should also be assessed to alert the clinician of potential serious pathological concerns. Although assumed, it is worthy of mention that significant asymmetries, discolorations, altered eye activity, impaired function, pain, and lacerations, bruises, and swelling should be considered significant concerns for potential referral

to a physician until proven otherwise. Pupil size and symmetry should be assessed. Dilation unilaterally may be the result of a sympathetic nerve response following blow to the face or head and intracranial hemorrhage, and it should be taken seriously.[19]

Asymmetry of other facial features, particularly bony or cartilage structures, may indicate trauma and the potential for fracture. Missing, cracked, or chipped teeth should also alert the clinician for the potential of traumatic injury. Discoloration in the area is another concern. For example, Battle's sign, shown by blue and purple discoloration of the skin in the mastoid area (postauricular area), has been suggested to indicate the potential for temporal bone or basilar skull fracture. Battle's sign was shown to have a positive predictive value (PPV) of 66% for intracranial lesions in an emergency service for clients with a Glasgow Coma Scale of 13 to 15.[20] Other clinical signs of basilar skull fracture include otorrhea (discharge of cerebrospinal fluid from nose or ear) or rhinorrhea (excessive discharge from nose), hemotympanum (presence of blood in tympanic cavity of middle ear), laceration of the external auditory canal, and periorbital ecchymosis with tarsal plate sparing (raccoon eyes). These signs may take several hours to develop.[21] Raccoon eyes has been associated with anterior skull base fractures in more than 70% of cases.[22]

TRIAGE AND SCREENING

Triage and screening is a necessary component of the examination process that should be done prior to continuing with the examination. Ruling out serious pathology is paramount at this stage. (Refer to chapter 6, Triage and Differential Diagnosis, as well as chapter 17, Cervical Spine, for cervical spine related red flags.) Pain generation from other related (or close-proximity) structures also helps the clinician more accurately determine the necessity of continuing with the other examination components to identify the actual source of the client's pain. Additionally, implementing strong screening tests (tests of high SN and low –LR) at this point in the examination is suggested for narrowing down the competing diagnoses of the respective body region (predominantly cervical spine, in this case) when this is applicable.

Ruling Out Serious Face and Head Pathology

If the clinician encounters a client in an acute injury situation, especially with the possibility of trauma as a mechanism, there are additional triage concerns. Besides those discussed here, the clinician is reminded of chapter 6 (Triage and Differential Diagnosis), chapter 17 (Cervical Spine), and the description of observable findings (e.g., Battle's sign and raccoon eyes) just previously mentioned.

Glasgow Coma Scale

The Glasgow Coma Scale (table 15.2) is an important tool for assessment regarding the conscious or unconscious client's level of consciousness. Decorticate (arms, wrists, and fingers flexed, upper limbs adducted, and legs extended, internally rotated, and plantar flexed) and decerebrate (extension, adduction, and hyperpronation of arms, along with same response in legs as with decorticate) posturing are abnormal responses that require immediate referral to physician.

With any client who has sustained facial trauma, a thorough history and comprehensive physical examination centering on the head and neck

TABLE 15.2 Glasgow Coma Scale

	Score
EYE OPENING	
Spontaneous	4
To speech	3
To pain	2
No response	1
BEST MOTOR RESPONSE	
Follows motor commands	6
Localizes	5
Withdraws	4
Abnormal flexion	3
Extensor response	2
No response	1
VERBAL RESPONSE	
Oriented	5
Confused conversations	4
Inappropriate words	3
Incomprehensible sounds	2
No response	1

Scoring: minimum score = 3; maximum score = 15. Greater levels of consciousness represented by higher scores. Mild disability (13-15); moderate disability (9-12). Clients with scores of 3-8 are usually said to be in a coma (severe disability, vegetative state score is <3).

region as well as proper radiological assessment are essential.[23] Determination of the necessity for radiographic imaging is an inexact science, but some observable measures have been investigated that may assist in this determination.

All of the following signs have ideal ability to help **rule in** nasal fracture; none were helpful for ruling out nasal fracture:[24]

- Epistaxis (SP 98, +LR 14.0)
- Presence of inflammation in the area (SP 92, +LR 7.0)
- An acute septal injury (SP 100, +LR Inf)

All of the following signs have good ability to help **rule in** nasal fracture; none were helpful for ruling out nasal fracture:[24]

- Airway obstruction present (SP 96, +LR 4.8)
- Lateral deviation of nose present (SP 96, +LR 4.5)

All of the following signs have less than good ability to help rule in nasal fracture; all have poor ability to help rule out nasal fracture:[24]

- Irregular nasal dorsum present (SP 92, +LR 3.6)
- Nasal wound present (SP 70, +LR 1.5)

Ottawa Subarachnoid Hemorrhage Rule

The majority of the preceding measures, therefore, are unimpressive in their ability to rule out fractures and are not overwhelmingly helpful for ruling in fractures and intracranial damage. The Ottawa Subarachnoid Hemorrhage Rule has been investigated for the ability to rule out the presence of a subarachnoid hemorrhage in a client presenting with acute headache. This clinical decision rule is a tool the clinician can utilize to rule out the possibility of a subarachnoid hemorrhage existing in the client older than 15 years who presents with an acute headache (maximum intensity within 1 hour).[25]

Investigation for subarachnoid hemorrhage should be undertaken if ≥ 1 of these high-risk variables is present:

- Age ≥ 40 years
- Neck pain or stiffness
- Witnessed loss of consciousness
- Headache onset during exertion: **SN 99 (94-100)**, SP 28 (26-30), +LR 1.4, **−LR 0.04**[25]

- Thunderclap headache (instantly peaking pain)
- Limited neck flexion on examination: **SN 100 (97-100)**, SP 15 (14-17), +LR 1.2, **−LR 0.0**[25]

This rule is not for new neurologic deficits, previous aneurysms, subarachnoid hemorrhage, brain tumors, or history of recurrent headaches (≥ 3 episodes over the course of ≥ 6 months).

Canadian Computed Tomography Head Rule

As discussed in chapter 17 (Cervical Spine), determination of whether or not imaging is necessary and the extent of imaging are not clearly elucidated. The Canadian CT Head Rule (similar to the Canadian C-Spine Rule discussed in chapter 17) is a decision rule that attempts to limit false negative findings. The Canadian CT Rule is required only for clients with minor head injuries with any of the following findings:

High risk (for neurological intervention)

- GCS score < 15 at 2 hours after injury
- Suspected open or depressed skull fracture
- Any sign of basal skull fracture (hemotympanum, raccoon eyes, cerebrospinal fluid otorrhea or rhinorrhea, Battle's sign)
- Vomiting ≥ 2 episodes
- Age ≥ 65 years

Medium risk (for brain injury on CT)

- Amnesia before impact > 30 min
- Dangerous mechanism (pedestrian struck by motor vehicle, occupant ejected from motor vehicle, fall from height >3 ft [1 m] or five stairs)

- High or medium risk criteria: **SN 99-100** for neurosurgical intervention cases and **SN 80-100** for any intracranial injury, SP 39-51 in a systematic review and economic evaluation.[26]
- High risk criteria: **SN 99-100**, SP 48-77 for injury requiring neurosurgical intervention in a systematic review of 19 studies, 4 of which included CCHR high risk.[27]

The rule is not applicable if any of the following apply:

- Non-trauma causes
- GCS < 13
- Age < 16 years
- Coumadin or bleeding disorder
- Obvious open-skull fracture

Regarding pediatric clients, three high-quality clinical decision rules (CDRs) have been identified: CATCH (Canadian Assessment of Tomography for Childhood Head Injury), CHALICE (Children's Head Injury Algorithm for the Prediction of Important Clinical Events), and PECARN (Pediatric Emergency Care Applied Research Network). Currently none has been proven superior to the other, and it is suggested that their validity and cost-effectiveness requires further study.[28, 29]

Ruling Out Pain Generation From Other Related Structures

Suspicion of cervical instability or cervical artery dysfunction should be addressed as discussed in the cervical spine chapter (chapter 17) prior to proceeding with the examination. The upper quarter screen will determine cervical spine range of motion (ROM) and the potential for the cervical spine as a

---

Critical Clinical Pearls

Various clinical decision rules have been described for clients presenting with acute facial or head trauma:

- Glasgow Coma Scale: utilization for the determination of the consciousness level of the client
- Ottawa Subarachnoid Hemorrhage Rule: utilized in clients who present with an acute headache to rule out potential subarachnoid hemorrhage
- Canadian Computed Tomography Head Rule: utilized to determine if radiographic imaging is necessary in clients with minor head injuries
- CATCH, CHALICE, and PECARN: all utilized in pediatric clients with head injury

pain generator to the client's complaints of face and head pain. Additionally, pain generation due to radiculopathy can be reasonably screened (or ruled out) as described here:

- Radiculopathy or discogenic-related pathology: ruled out with a combination of Spurling's test and the upper limb neurodynamic test (median nerve bias)
- Spurling's test: **SN 93 (77-99), SP 95 (76-100), +LR 19.6, –LR 0.07,** QUADAS 9[30]
- Median nerve upper limb neurodynamic test: **SN 97 (90-100),** SP 22 (12-33), +LR 1.3, **–LR 0.12,** QUADAS 10[31]
- Arm squeeze test (described for cervical nerve root compression): SN 95 (85-99), SP 96 (87-99), +LR 24, –LR 0.05, QUADAS 8[32]

Additionally, as with any joint, clearing active range of motion (AROM) with and without overpressure is necessary. AROM of all motions as per the upper quarter screen described in chapter 7 should be implemented. In order to fully clear the cervical spine, full AROM (with overpressure if pain-free) must be present.

MOTION TESTS

Because there are no articular joints for the face and head (besides the craniomandibular complex,

which is covered in chapter 16), no motion assessments (i.e., AROM, passive range of motion [PROM], accessory motions, flexibility) are required.

MUSCLE PERFORMANCE TESTING

Refer to chapters 16 (Temporomandibular Joint) and 17 (Cervical Spine) for information on muscle performance testing specific to the face and head.

SPECIAL TESTS

As mentioned in chapter 10 (Special Tests), in many cases the clinician is overly dependent on the performance and interpretation of special test findings with respect to differential diagnosis of the client's presenting pain. Utilization of special tests for ruling in (or diagnosing) a particular pathology should occur at this point in the examination process. It is also hoped that the clinician has a much clearer picture of the client's presentation prior to this point in the examination and will therefore depend minimally on special test findings with respect to diagnosis of the client's pain.

Index of Special Tests

Vestibular Dysfunction

Dix-Hallpike Test

Monohemispheric Dysfunction: Tumor

Finger Tap Test
Pronator Drift Test
Finger Rolling Test
Forearm Rolling Test
CPR for Unilateral Cerebral Lesions

Examination of the Ear

Weber Test (hearing loss)
Schwabach Test (hearing loss)
Rinne Test

Case Studies

Go to www.HumanKinetics.com/OrthopedicClinicalExamination and complete these case studies for chapter 15:

- Case study 1 discusses a 26-year-old female with insidious onset of headaches.
- Case study 2 discusses a 19-year-old male with a facial injury from being hit with a baseball.

Abstract Links

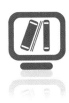

Go to www.HumanKinetics.com/OrthopedicClinicalExamination to access abstract links on these issues:

Dix-Hallpike test	Rinne test
Finger tap test	Spurling's test
Median nerve upper limb tension test	Weber test
Pronator drift test	

VESTIBULAR DYSFUNCTION

DIX-HALLPIKE TEST

Client Position	Typically long sitting with legs extended on table (or sitting with legs off end of table if necessary)
Clinician Position	Standing directly behind client
Movement	The clinician rotates the client's head approximately 45° *(a)*, and quickly passively lowers the client to supine with head in rotation and 20° extension (off end of table) position *(b)*. The clinician observes the client's eyes for about 45 seconds for nystagmus.
Assessment	If rotational nystagmus occurs, test is (+) for benign paroxysmal positional vertigo (BPPV). The fast phase of the nystagmus is toward the affected ear. The fast phase is defined by the rotation of the top eye, either clockwise or counterclockwise.
Statistics	• Published estimates of SN ranged from 48 to 88; estimates of SP were lacking.[33]
	• SN 79 (65-94), SP 75 (33-100), +LR 3.2, –LR 0.28, in a critical review of literature for diagnosis of BPPV.[33]
	• Side-lying performance of Dix-Hall-pike: **SN 90 (79-100)**, SP 75 (33-100), +LR 3.6, **–LR 0.14**[33]

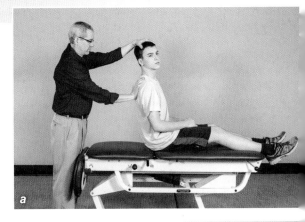

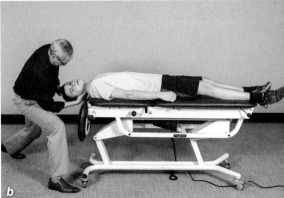

Figure 15.5

MONOHEMISPHERIC DYSFUNCTION: TUMOR

FINGER TAP TEST

Client Position	Sitting or standing
Clinician Position	Standing, monitoring client
Movement	The clinician asks the client to tap the index finger of one hand to the interphalangeal joint of the thumb on the other hand as many times as possible in 10 seconds. The clinician makes a side-to-side comparison in repetitions.
Assessment	A (+) test is a difference of ≥5 repetitions between sides.
Statistics	SN 73 (not reported, or NR), **SP 88 (NR)**, **+LR 5.9**, –LR 0.31, QUADAS 9, in a study of 170 clients with a suspected abnormality in the nervous system (mean age 54.6 years, male–female ratio of 1.5:1, mean duration of symptoms NR) and computed tomography as a reference standard.[34]

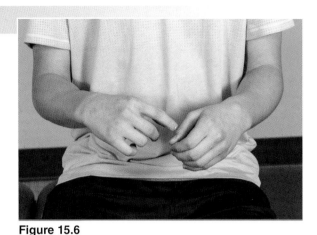

Figure 15.6

PRONATOR DRIFT TEST

Video 15.7 **in the web resource shows a demonstration of this test.**

Client Position	Sitting or standing
Clinician Position	Standing, monitoring client
Movement	The client flexes bilateral shoulders to 90° with full elbow extension and supination *(a)*. The clinician asks the client to close their eyes and maintain that position for up to 2 minutes.
Assessment	A (+) test is a gradual drift of the involved-side forearm into pronation *(b)*.
Statistics	• **SN 92 (NR), SP 90 (NR), +LR 9.2, –LR 0.09**, QUADAS 9, in a study of 170 clients with a suspected abnormality in the nervous system (mean age 54.6 years, male–female ratio of 1.5:1, mean duration of symptoms NR) and computed tomography as a reference standard.[34]
	• SN 22 (12-36), SP 100 (83-100), +LR Inf, –LR 0.88, QUADAS 8, in a study of 46 clients with a single cerebral hemisphere lesion (age range 21-83 years, 18 women, mean duration of symptoms NR) and CT as a reference standard.[35]

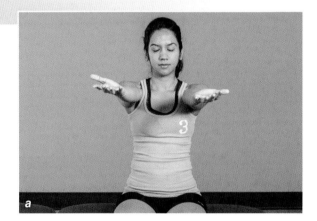

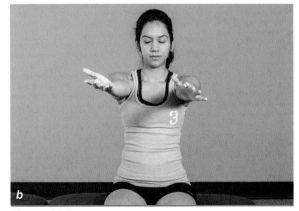

Figure 15.7

FINGER ROLLING TEST

Client Position	Sitting or standing
Clinician Position	Standing, monitoring client
Movement	The clinician asks the client to roll bilateral fingers around each other in a symmetrical pattern.
Assessment	A (+) test is one finger orbiting around the other, with the involved finger moving less.

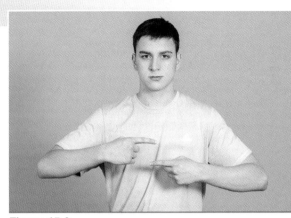

Figure 15.8

Statistics
- SN 41 (NR), **SP 93 (NR)**, +LR 5.9, –LR 0.63, QUADAS 9, in a study of 170 clients with a suspected abnormality in the nervous system (mean age 54.6 years, male–female ratio of 1.5:1, mean duration of symptoms NR) and CT as a reference standard.[34]

- SN 33 (21-47), SP 100 (83-100), +LR Inf, –LR 0.77, QUADAS 8, in a study of 46 clients with a single cerebral hemisphere lesion (age range 21-83 years, 18 women, mean duration of symptoms NR) and CT as a reference standard.[35]

FOREARM ROLLING TEST

Video 15.9 **in the web resource shows a demonstration of this test.**

Client Position	Sitting or standing
Clinician Position	Standing, monitoring client
Movement	The clinician asks the client to roll bilateral forearms around each other in a symmetrical pattern.
Assessment	A (+) test is one forearm orbiting around the other, with the involved arm moving less.

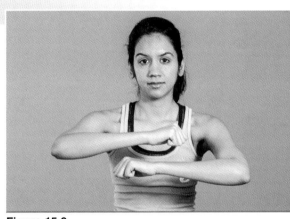

Figure 15.9

Statistics
- SN 46 (NR), **SP 98 (NR)**, +LR 18.2, –LR 0.56, QUADAS 9, in a study of 170 clients with a suspected abnormality in the nervous system (mean age 54.6 years, male–female ratio of 1.5:1, mean duration of symptoms NR) and computed tomography as a reference standard.[34]

- SN 24 (14-38), SP 100 (83-100), +LR Inf, –LR 0.76, QUADAS 8, in a study of 46 clients with a single cerebral hemisphere lesion (age range 21-83 years, 18 women, mean duration of symptoms NR) and CT as a reference standard.[35]

CPR FOR UNILATERAL CEREBRAL LESIONS

Combination of three maneuvers:

- Pronator drift
- Finger tap
- Deep tendon reflexes

Statistics
- (+) = all 3 (+); (−) = >1 (−): SN 75 (NR), **SP 98 (NR)**, **+LR 30.2**, −LR 0.25
- (+) = >1 (+); (−) = all 3 (−): **SN 98 (NR)**, SP 86 (NR), +LR 7.3, **−LR 0.03**, QUADAS 9, in a study of 170 clients with a suspected abnormality in the nervous system (mean age 54.6 years, male–female ratio of 1.5:1, mean duration of symptoms NR) and computed tomography as a reference standard.[34]

EXAMINATION OF THE EAR

WEBER TEST (HEARING LOSS)

Client Position	Sitting, relaxed
Clinician Position	Standing behind or to the side of client
Movement	The clinician places a vibrating tuning fork on the center of the client's forehead.
Assessment	A normal response is the sound being heard in the center without lateralization to either side. A (+) response for conductive hearing loss is the sound being heard on the side of conductive loss. A (+) response for sensorimotor loss is the sound being heard better on the unaffected side.
Statistics	+LR 1.6–1.7, −LR 0.70–0.76, making it an inaccurate screening and poor diagnostic test for hearing loss[36]

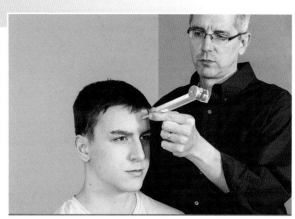

Figure 15.10

SCHWABACH TEST (HEARING LOSS)

Client Position	Sitting in a relaxed position
Clinician Position	Standing or sitting by the client
Movement	The clinician alternately places the vibrating tuning fork against the client's affected mastoid process until the client can't hear a sound (timing the duration) and then against their own non-affected mastoid process until the clinician can no longer hear a sound (again timing the duration).
Assessment	A (+) test is not hearing the sound for equal amounts of time.
Statistics	NR

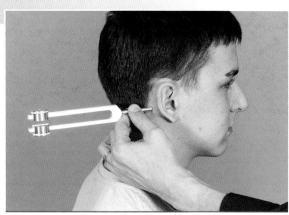

Figure 15.11

RINNE TEST

Client Position	Sitting in a relaxed position
Clinician Position	Standing by the client
Movement	The clinician places the vibrating tuning fork against the client's mastoid bone *(a)*. The clinician times the length of time the client can hear the sound. The clinician then quickly positions a still-vibrating tine 1 to 2 cm from the auditory canal *(b)* and asks the client to again indicate when they can no longer hear the sound. The clinician then compares the number of seconds the sound was heard by bone conduction and by air conduction.
Assessment	An air-conducted sound should be heard for twice as long as bone-conducted sound.
Statistics	SN 73 (NR)[37]

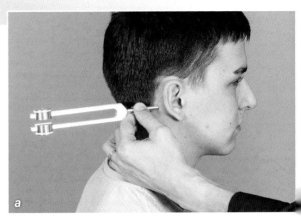

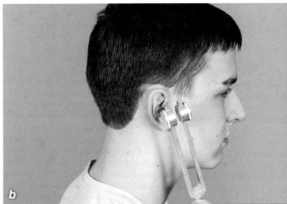

Figure 15.12

PALPATION

Palpation of the face and head (as with all regions of the body) should be systematic. As with observation, clinicians should pay particular attention to the appearance or palpation of swelling, asymmetry, and the appearance of discoloration, possibly indicating serious pathology. Directly facing the client, the clinician should palpate for symmetry and normal contour of the frontal bone, nasal bone, maxilla, and mandible. To assess for clicking, as described in chapter 11, the clinician can palpate bilateral temporomandibular joints with and without the client's opening their mouth.

If the clinician has experience performing this technique, they can also assess the temporomandibular joint with the client's mouth open. Observation and palpation (if necessary) of the client's teeth may alert the clinician of the possibility for referral to a dentist for loose, cracked, or chipped teeth.

Palpation of the client's sinuses could also be clinically important. The frontal sinuses are located above the eyebrows on the distal aspect of the frontal bone and the maxillary sinuses are located just below the eyes. Palpation in this area creating pain or pressure should be further investigated if significant.

The clinician can palpate the top of the skull and hair for normal appearance and feel, making note of any asymmetry from side to side, swelling, and so on. Facing the back of the client's head, the clinician can palpate the cervical spine as noted in chapter 17, as well as the external occipital protuberance, mastoid processes, bilateral ears, and posterior skull, again making note of any asymmetry from side to side and swelling.

PHYSICAL PERFORMANCE MEASURES

No specific physical performance measures (PPMs) are available for the face and head. Refer to chapter 17 (Cervical Spine) for relevant PPMs.

COMMON ORTHOPEDIC CONDITIONS OF THE FACE AND HEAD

While it is impossible to distinctly describe various pathological presentations of the face and head, there are evidence-based findings supportive of particular pathologies of this region of the body. Therefore, the intent of this section of the chapter is to present current evidence-supported findings suggestive of face and head pathologies. As previously described in chapter 4 (Evidence-Based Practice and Client Examination), though, not all examination findings are absolutely supported with clinical evidence, and the clinician should also rely on clinical experience and input from the client when performing differential diagnosis of a client's presentation of pain and dysfunction.

Monohemispheric Dysfunction: Tumor

ICD-9: 191; 225

ICD-10: D33.2 (benign neoplasm of brain, unspecified)

I. Client Interview

Subjective History

- Complaints of facial drooping, difficulty with blinking, closing the eye, smiling, and other motor activities of the face
- May complain of headache, light-headedness, blurred vision, or lethargy[35]

II. Observation

- Inability to perform simple math calculation has less than good ability to help rule in (SP 95, +LR 3.4) monohemispheric dysfunction (MD).[35]
- Difficulty with right–left discrimination (SP 100, +LR Inf), reading (SP 100, +LR Inf), and writing (SP 100, +LR Inf) all have less than good ability to help rule in MD.[35]
- A visual field defect (SP 95, +LR 4.4), facial weakness (SP 95, +LR 3.4), and optokinetic nystagmus (SP 100, +LR Inf) all have less than good ability to help rule in MD.[35]

III. Triage and Screening

- All non-musculoskeletal causes, as well as causes from related joints, should be ruled out.
- History is used for triage, during which red flags should be identified and yellow flags assessed.[38]
- An alert, asymptomatic client without distracting injury or neurological deficit who is able to complete a functional ROM examination may be safely cleared from cervical spine immobilization without radiographic evaluation (SN 98).[39]
- Ruling out traumatic skull fracture:
  - Battle's sign: When present, it had a PPV of 66% for intracranial lesions in an emergency service for clients with a Glasgow Coma Scale of 13-15.[20]
  - Raccoon eyes: When present, this was associated with anterior skull base fractures in more than 70% of cases.[22]
- Canadian CT Head Rule: when (−) among high or medium risk criteria or high risk criteria alone, this rule has ideal ability to help **rule out** (SN 99-100) neurosurgical intervention cases and good to ideal ability to help **rule out** (SN 80-100) any intracranial injury.[26]
- Ottawa Subarachnoid Hemorrhage Rule: When (−), this rule has ideal ability to help **rule out** (SN 99-100, −LR 0.04) subarachnoid hemorrhage in an acutely appearing client coming to the emergency room with a headache.[25]
- Canadian C-Spine Rule: This demonstrated better diagnostic accuracy (SN range 90-100) than either the NEXUS criteria (SN range 83-100)[40] or physician clinical judgment alone (SN 92)[41] and, therefore, an improved ability to help **rule out** an actual fracture.
- Alar ligament testing:
  - Significant variability in diagnostic accuracy (SN 69-100, −LR 0.29–0.31; SP 72-96, +LR 18-Inf) with

improved ability to help **rule in** versus **rule out** alar ligament insufficiency with less complex testing.[42]

- Better ability to help **rule in** (SP 96-100, +LR 18-Inf) versus **rule out** (SN 72, −LR 0.30) alar ligament insufficiency with more complex testing.[42]

- Sharp-Purser test: demonstrates stronger ability to help **rule in** (SP 96, +LR 17.3) than rule out (SN 69, −LR 0.32) transverse ligament insufficiency.[43]

- More complex transverse ligament testing is also better able to help **rule in** (SP 99, +LR 65) than rule out (SN 65, −LR 0.35) transverse ligament insufficiency.[42]

- Cervical rotation is helpful for **ruling in** (SP 100, +LR 83.3) potential vertebrobasilar ischemia.[44]

- Combined cervical extension and rotation is helpful for **ruling in** (SP 98, +LR 4.2) potential upper cervical neurovascular compromise.[45]

- Radiculopathy or discogenic-related pathology: ruled out with a combination of Spurling's test and upper limb tension test (median nerve bias).

  - Spurling's test: **SN 93 (77-99)**, **SP 95 (76-100)**, **+LR 19.6**, **−LR 0.07**, QUADAS 9[30]

  - Median nerve upper limb tension test: **SN 97 (90-100)**, SP 22 (12-33), +LR 1.3, **−LR 0.12**, QUADAS 10[31]

IV. Motion Tests

- Client has limited motion of facial muscles on involved side.

V. Muscle Performance Testing

- Facial weakness described in observation.

VI. Special Tests

- Finger tap (SP 88, +LR 5.9), pronator drift (SP 90, +LR 9.2), finger rolling (SP 93, +LR 5.9), and forearm rolling (SP 98, +LR 18.2) have **good** ability to help rule in MD.[34]

- Having pronator drift, finger tap, and deep tendon reflexes all (+) has **good** ability to help rule in (SP 98, +LR 30.2) MD.

- Having pronator drift, finger tap, and deep tendon reflexes all (−) has **good** ability to help rule out (SN 98, −LR 0.03) MD.

VII. Palpation

- Client may have decreased sensation and possibly hypersensitivity in facial nerve innervation region.

VIII. Physical Performance Measures

- None appropriate

POTENTIAL TREATMENT-BASED CLASSIFICATIONS

- Referral to physician

Headaches

Headache is a commonly described pathology. The International Headache Society (IHS)[46, 47] has, using the International Headache Classification, grouped headaches into either primary or secondary headaches.[48] Primary headaches include migraines, tension-type headache (TTH), cluster headache and other trigeminal autonomic cephalalgias, and other primary headaches (primary stabbing headache, primary cough headache, primary exertional headache, primary headache associated with sexual activity, hypnic headache, primary thunderclap headache, hemicrania continua, and new daily persistent headache [NDPH]). Secondary headaches likely occur in forms that the client has had previously, but they are now worsening. These headaches are generally more difficult to classify. These have been classified by the IHS as headaches attributed to any of the following:[48]

- Trauma or injury to the head or neck

- Cranial or cervical vascular disorder

- Nonvascular intracranial disorder

- Substance or its withdrawal

- Infection

- Disorder of homoeostasis

- Headache or facial pain attributed to disorder of the cranium, neck, eyes, ears, nose, sinuses, teeth, mouth or other facial or cervical structure

- Psychiatric disorder

Migraine Headache

ICD-9: 346.0

ICD-10: G43.109 (migraine with aura); G43.009 (migraine without aura)

Migraine headaches have been further subclassified into migraines without aura, migraine with aura, childhood periodic syndromes that are commonly precursors of migraine, retinal migraine, complications of migraine, probable migraine, and episodic syndromes that may be associated with migraine (recurrent gastrointestinal disturbance, benign paroxysmal vertigo, and benign paroxysmal torticollis).[47]

I. Client Interview

Subjective History[47, 49, 50]

- Migraine with an aura is characterized by focal neurological symptoms preceded or accompanied by a headache. Some clients also experience a premonitory phase hours or days prior to the headache. Premonitory and resolution symptoms include hyperactivity, hypoactivity, particular food cravings, depression, and repetitive yawning.

- Migraine without aura headache attacks typically last 4 to 72 hours.[47]

- Migraine without an aura is often aggravated by avoidance of routine physical activity.[47]

- Migraine with aura typically spreads over ≥5 minutes, and each individual aura symptom lasts 5 to 60 minutes.[47]

- The presence of photophobia with a headache helps **rule in** (+LR 5.8) a migraine-type headache.[51]

- Predictors suggesting migraine headache using the mnemonic POUNDing are present (Pulsating, duration of 4-72 hOurs, headache is Unilateral, Nausea is associated with headache, and the headache is Disabling). If four of the five criteria are met, the +LR for definite or possible migraine is 24 (95% confidence interval [CI], 1.5–388); if three are met, the +LR is 3.5 (1.3–9.2), and if two or fewer are met, the +LR is 0.41 (0.32–0.52).[51]

- Migraine is more likely in women 20 to 40 years of age.

- Pain is more likely unilateral versus bilateral.

Outcome Measures[47, 49, 50]

- The Migraine Screen Questionnaire (MS-Q) asks the client five yes or no questions regarding headaches or migraine episodes without headaches that they may have experienced in their lifetime:

  - Do you have frequent or intense headaches?

  - Do your headaches usually last more than 4 hours?

  - Do you usually suffer from nausea when you have a headache?

  - Does light or noise bother you when you have a headache?

  - Does headache limit any of your physical or intellectual activities?

A cutting point indicating suspicion of migraine was established at ≥4 points, while a <4 score indicated no suspicion of migraine.[52]

- The MS-Q is better able to help **rule in** (SP 97, +LR 27.3) than **rule out** (SN 82, −LR 0.19) migraine headaches.[53]

II. Observation[47, 49, 50]

- Migraine with brainstem aura can have dysarthria, vertigo, ataxia, decreased level of consciousness, or diplopia.[47]

- Migraine aura–triggered seizure: a seizure triggered by migraine with aura.[47]

- Benign paroxysmal torticollis: recurrent episodes of head tilt, perhaps with slight rotation, that remit spontaneously. Typically occurs in infants and small children, with onset in the first year.[47]

  - Other potential signs: pallor, irritability, malaise, vomiting, or ataxia.

  - Neurological examination is normal between attacks.[47]

III. Triage and Screening

- All non-musculoskeletal causes, as well as causes from related joints, should be ruled out.

- History is used for triage, during which red flags should be identified and yellow flags assessed.[38]

- An alert, asymptomatic client without distracting injury or neurological deficit who is able to complete a functional ROM examination may be safely cleared from cervical spine immobilization without radiographic evaluation (SN 98).[39]
- Ruling out traumatic skull fracture:
  - Battle's sign: When present, it had a PPV of 66% for intracranial lesions in an emergency service for clients with a Glasgow Coma Scale of 13 to 15.[20]
  - Raccoon eyes: When present, it was associated with anterior skull base fractures in more than 70% of cases.[22]
- Canadian CT Head Rule: when (−) among high or medium risk criteria or high risk criteria alone, it has ideal ability to help **rule out** (SN 99-100) neurosurgical intervention cases and good to ideal ability to help **rule out** (SN 80-100) any intracranial injury.[26]
- Ottawa Subarachnoid Hemorrhage Rule: when (−), it has ideal ability to help **rule out** (SN 99-100, −LR 0.04) subarachnoid hemorrhage in an acutely appearing client coming to the emergency room with a headache.[25]
- Canadian C-Spine Rule: demonstrated better diagnostic accuracy (SN range 90-100) than either the NEXUS criteria (SN range 83-100)[40] or physician clinical judgment alone (SN 92)[41] and, therefore, an improved ability to help **rule out** an actual fracture.
- Alar ligament testing:
  - Significant variability in diagnostic accuracy (SN 69-100, −LR 0.29–0.31; SP 72-96, +LR 18-Inf) with improved ability to help **rule in** versus **rule out** alar ligament insufficiency with less complex testing.[42]
  - Better ability to help **rule in** (SP 96-100, +LR 18-Inf) versus **rule out** (SN 72, −LR 0.30) alar ligament insufficiency with more complex testing.[42]
- Sharp-Purser test: demonstrates stronger ability to help **rule in** (SP 96, +LR 17.3) than rule out (SN 69, −LR 0.32) transverse ligament insufficiency.[43]

- More complex transverse ligament testing is also better able to help **rule in** (SP 99, +LR 65) than rule out (SN 65, −LR 0.35) transverse ligament insufficiency.[42]
- Cervical rotation is helpful for **ruling in** (SP 100, +LR 83.3) potential vertebrobasilar ischemia.[44]
- Combined cervical extension and rotation is helpful for **ruling in** (SP 98, +LR 4.2) potential upper cervical neurovascular compromise.[45]
- Radiculopathy or discogenic-related pathology: ruled out with a combination of Spurling's test and upper limb tension test (median nerve bias).
  - Spurling's test: **SN 93 (77-99), SP 95 (76-100), +LR 19.6, −LR 0.07,** QUADAS 9[30]
  - Median nerve upper limb tension test: **SN 97 (90-100),** SP 22 (12-33), **+LR 1.3, −LR 0.12,** QUADAS 10[31]

IV. Motion Tests

- Typically there are not any particular motion restrictions due to this type of headache.
- Painful or limited restrictions may exist (joint arthropathy found at C0 through C3 levels, with restrictions of C1-C2 being the most common),[54-58] although there is no evidence of these restrictions in migraine HAs.[59]
- A 10° or greater ROM loss with the cervical flexion–rotation test suggests C1-C2 involvement in cervicogenic-related headaches. This test is better at helping to **rule in** (SP 100) versus **ruling out** (SN 86) cervicogenic headache attributable to a C1-C2 dysfunction.[58]

V. Muscle Performance Testing

- Hemiplegic migraine: migraine with aura including motor weakness[47]

VI. Special Tests

- Typically there are not any particular special tests for this type of headache.
- Dizziness and unsteadiness can cause joint reposition errors in cervical spine.[60]

VII. Palpation

- Tenderness can be association with palpation with migraine, but it is less likely due to this type of headache.

VIII. Physical Performance Measures

- Cranial cervical flexor endurance test (if appropriate)

POTENTIAL TREATMENT-BASED CLASSIFICATIONS

- Headache
- Pain most likely
- Exercise and conditioning as a long-term resolution

Tension-Type Headache

ICD-9: 307.81; 339.1

ICD-10: G44.2 (tension-type headache)

Tension-type headache (TTH) is very common, and has a lifetime prevalence of 30% to 78% in the general population.[47] This type of headache, as by its name, has a primary component of muscle-related tension involvement. This type of headache has been divided into episodic and chronic subtypes. The exact mechanisms of TTH are unknown.

I. Client Interview

Subjective History[47, 49, 50]

- More likely has bilateral presentation with complaints of pressing or tightening quality
- Pain often described as dull and throbbing, and is likely variable in duration
- Does not appear to be gender or age specific
- Increased stressful activity a likely predisposing factor
- May be associated with elevated blood pressure and increased activity

II. Observation[47, 49, 50]

- Client may appear acutely distressed, with pain posturing and guarded patterns of movement.
- Forward head and rounded shoulders may be likely present.

III. Triage and Screening

- All non-musculoskeletal causes, as well as causes from related joints, should be ruled out.

- History is used for triage, during which red flags should be identified and yellow flags assessed.[38]
- An alert, asymptomatic client without distracting injury or neurological deficit who is able to complete a functional ROM examination may be safely cleared from cervical spine immobilization without radiographic evaluation (SN 98).[39]
- Ruling out traumatic skull fracture:
  - Battle's sign: When present, it had a PPV of 66% for intracranial lesions in an emergency service for clients with a Glasgow Coma Scale of 13 to 15.[20]
  - Raccoon eyes: When present, it was associated with anterior skull base fractures in more than 70% of cases.[22]
- Canadian CT Head Rule: When (−) among high or medium risk criteria or high risk criteria alone, this rule has ideal ability to help **rule out** (SN 99-100) neurosurgical intervention cases and good to ideal ability to help **rule out** (SN 80-100) any intracranial injury.[26]
- Ottawa Subarachnoid Hemorrhage Rule: When (−), it has ideal ability to help **rule out** (SN 99-100, −LR 0.04) subarachnoid hemorrhage in an acutely appearing client coming to the emergency room with a headache.[25]
- Canadian C-Spine Rule: It demonstrated better diagnostic accuracy (SN range 90-100) than either the NEXUS criteria (SN range 83-100)[40] or physician clinical judgment alone (SN 92)[41] and, therefore, an improved ability to **rule out** an actual fracture.
- Alar ligament testing:
  - Significant variability in diagnostic accuracy (SN 69-100, −LR 0.29–0.31; SP 72-96, +LR 18-Inf) with improved ability to help **rule in** versus **rule out** alar ligament insufficiency with less complex testing.[42]
  - Better ability to help **rule in** (SP 96-100, +LR 18-Inf) versus **rule out**

(SN 72, −LR 0.30) alar ligament insufficiency with more complex testing.[42]

- Sharp-Purser test demonstrates stronger ability to help **rule in** (SP 96, +LR 17.3) than rule out (SN 69, −LR 0.32) transverse ligament insufficiency.[43]

- More complex transverse ligament testing is also better able to help **rule in** (SP 99, +LR 65) than rule out (SN 65, −LR 0.35) transverse ligament insufficiency.[42]

- Cervical rotation is helpful for **ruling in** (SP 100, +LR 83.3) potential vertebrobasilar ischemia.[44]

- Combined cervical extension and rotation is helpful for **ruling in** (SP 98, +LR 4.2) potential upper cervical neurovascular compromise.[45]

- Radiculopathy and discogenic-related pathology: ruled out with a combination of Spurling's test and upper limb tension test (median nerve bias).

  - Spurling's test: **SN 93 (77-99)**, **SP 95 (76-100)**, **+LR 19.6**, **−LR 0.07**, QUADAS 9[30]

  - Median nerve upper limb tension test: **SN 97 (90-100)**, SP 22 (12-33), +LR 1.3, **−LR 0.12**, QUADAS 10[31]

IV. Motion Tests

- Clients are not likely to have any particular motion restrictions particular to this type of headache.

- A 10° or greater ROM loss with the cervical flexion–rotation test suggests C1-C2 involvement in cervicogenic-related headaches. This test is better at helping to **rule in** (SP 100) versus **ruling out** (SN 86) cervicogenic headache attributable to a C1-C2 dysfunction.[58]

V. Muscle Performance Testing

- Clients are not likely to have any particular motion restrictions specific to this type of headache.

- If client has forward head and rounded shoulders posture, they likely will have deep neck flexor and scapula retractor weakness.

VI. Special Tests

- Dizziness and unsteadiness can cause joint reposition errors in cervical spine.[60]

VII. Palpation

- Pericranial tenderness is often present.[47]

VIII. Physical Performance Measures

- Cranial cervical flexor endurance test (if appropriate)

POTENTIAL TREATMENT-BASED CLASSIFICATIONS

- Headache
- Pain most likely
- Exercise and conditioning as a long-term resolution

Trigeminal Autonomic Cephalgia: Cluster Headache

ICD-9: 339.00; 339.01; 339.02

ICD-10: G44.0 (other headaches)

Trigeminal autonomic cephalgias, especially cluster-type headaches, do not have an aura. These headaches tend to be more chronic in nature.

I. Client Interview

Subjective History[47, 49, 50]

- Often described as attacks of severe, strictly unilateral pain that is orbital, supraorbital, temporal, or in any combination of these sites, lasting 15 to 180 minutes and occurring from once every other day to eight times per day.

- Several signs or symptoms ipsilateral to the headache may be present:
  - Nasal congestion
  - Eyelid edema
  - Forehead and facial sweating
  - Sensation of fullness in the ear
  - Miosis or ptosis

II. Observation[47, 49, 50]

- Observe for signs discussed in the interview section (ptosis, forehead, and facial sweating)

III. Triage and Screening

- All non-musculoskeletal causes, as well as causes from related joints, should be ruled out.

- History is used for triage, during which red flags should be identified and yellow flags assessed.[38]

- An alert, asymptomatic client without distracting injury or neurological deficit who is able to complete a functional ROM examination may be safely cleared from cervical spine immobilization without radiographic evaluation (SN 98).[39]

- Ruling out traumatic skull fracture:
  - Battle's sign: When present, it had a positive predictive value of 66% for intracranial lesions in an emergency service for clients with a Glasgow Coma Scale of 13 to 15.[20]
  - Raccoon eyes: When present, it was associated with anterior skull base fractures in more than 70% of cases.[22]

- Canadian CT Head Rule: When (−) among high or medium risk criteria or high risk criteria alone, it has ideal ability to help **rule out** (SN 99-100) neurosurgical intervention cases and good to ideal ability to help **rule out** (SN 80-100) any intracranial injury.[26]

- Ottawa Subarachnoid Hemorrhage Rule: When (−), it has ideal ability to help **rule out** (SN 99-100, −LR 0.04) subarachnoid hemorrhage in an acutely appearing client coming to the emergency room with a headache.[25]

- Canadian C-Spine Rule: It demonstrated better diagnostic accuracy (SN range 90-100) than either the NEXUS criteria (SN range 83-100)[40] or physician clinical judgment alone (SN 92)[41] and, therefore, an improved ability to **rule out** an actual fracture.

- Alar ligament testing:
  - Significant variability in diagnostic accuracy (SN 69-100, −LR 0.29–0.31; SP 72-96, +LR 18-Inf) with improved ability to help **rule in** versus **rule out** alar ligament insufficiency with less complex testing.[42]
  - Better ability to help **rule in** (SP 96-100, +LR 18-Inf) versus **rule out** (SN 72, −LR 0.30) alar ligament insufficiency with more complex testing.[42]

- Sharp-Purser test: It demonstrates stronger ability to help **rule in** (SP 96, +LR 17.3) than rule out (SN 69, −LR 0.32) transverse ligament insufficiency.[43]

- More complex transverse ligament testing is also better able to help **rule in** (SP 99, +LR 65) than rule out (SN 65, −LR 0.35) transverse ligament insufficiency.[42]

- Cervical rotation is helpful for **ruling in** (SP 100, +LR 83.3) potential vertebrobasilar ischemia.[44]

- Combined cervical extension and rotation is helpful for **ruling in** (SP 98, +LR 4.2) potential upper cervical neurovascular compromise.[45]

- Radiculopathy and discogenic-related pathology: ruled out with a combination of Spurling's test and upper limb tension test (median nerve bias).
  - Spurling's test: **SN 93 (77-99)**, **SP 95 (76-100)**, **+LR 19.6**, **−LR 0.07**, QUADAS 9[30]
  - Median nerve upper limb tension test: **SN 97 (90-100)**, SP 22 (12-33), +LR 1.3, **−LR 0.12**, QUADAS 10[31]

IV. Motion Tests

- A 10° or greater ROM loss with the cervical flexion–rotation test suggests C1-C2 involvement in cervicogenic-related headaches. This test is better at helping to **rule in** (SP 100) versus **ruling out** (SN 86) cervicogenic headache attributable to a C1-C2 dysfunction.[58]

V. Muscle Performance Testing

- Assess for deep neck flexor and scapula retractor weakness

VI. Special Tests

- Dizziness and unsteadiness can cause joint reposition errors in cervical spine.[60]

VII. Palpation

- Suboccipital and cranial muscles may have secondary tenderness.

VIII. Physical Performance Measures

- Cranial cervical flexor endurance test (if appropriate)

POTENTIAL TREATMENT-BASED CLASSIFICATIONS

- Headache
- Pain most likely
- Exercise and conditioning as a long-term resolution

Cervicogenic Headaches or Cervicocranial Syndrome

ICD-9: 339.0 (other headache syndromes); 784.0 (headache)

ICD-10: G44 (other headache syndromes); R51 (headache)

Refer to Chapter 17, Cervical Spine.

Facial and Skull Fractures

ICD-9:

- Facial fracture (802)
- Skull fracture (800.0; 804.9)

ICD-10:

- Facial fracture (S02.92XS)
- Skull fracture (S02.1)

Differential Diagnosis of Most Common Headache Types

Type	Gender and age	Symptom area	Frequency/ Duration	Aggravating factors	Associated symptoms
Cervicogenic	Any age, more likely in females	Unilateral; does not change sides; frontal, orbital	Episodic or chronic; 2-3x week; may last hours to days	Sustained postures, neck movements, with or without trauma	Neck pain or stiffness, a 10^0 or greater ROM loss with the cervical flexion-rotation test suggest C1-C2 involvement in cervicogenic related headache; photophobia are not common
Migraine	More likely in females, 20-40 years of age	More likely unilateral	Without aura: typically lasts 4-72 hours With aura: typically spreads over ≥ 5 minutes, and each individual aura symptom lasts 5-60 minutes	Physical exertion; certain foods; environmental stresses	Aura; photophobia; POUNDing (Pulsating, duration of 4-72 hOurs, headache is Unilateral, Nausea is associated with headache, and the headache is Disabling)
Tension	Not gender or age specific	More likely bilateral	Episodic or chronic; may last hour to days (variable in duration)	Emotional stress; muscle tension; not often related to trauma; often related to elevated blood pressure and increased activity	Cervical muscle tightness/ tension; cervical joint related dysfunction possible; photophobia and nausea/ vomiting are not common
Cluster	Any age, probably more likely in females	Unilateral, orbital, supraorbital and/or temporal	Last 15-180 minutes and occurring from once every other day to 8 times/day	Symptoms are often severe	Nasal congestion, eyelid edema, forehead and facial sweating, sensation of fullness in the ear, miosis or ptosis

I. Client Interview

Subjective History

- Nasal fractures are either the most or second most (mandible) common bone injury of the face, and third most frequent of all body fractures.[24, 61]

- 40% of facial trauma injuries include fractures of the nasal bone.[62]

- Motor vehicle accidents and interpersonal violence are the main causes of nasal and general fractures.[61]

- Motorcycle accidents are the most common mechanism for mandibular fractures, as well as for the presence of more than one facial bone fracture.[63]

- Motorcycle accidents are also the only significant risk factor for maxillary fractures.[63]

- Fractures of the zygomatic and nasal bones are mainly associated with activities involving animals (riding and stock farming) and sports.[63]

- Sports with high speed and high impact, especially without facial guard protection, result in more facial bone fractures than low-speed and low-impact sports.[64]

- Alcohol consumption is often a contributing factor to facial fractures.[61]

- Male–female ratio of nasal fractures is 4:1[61]

- Incidence of facial fractures tends to increase with age.[63]

- Prevalence of carotid artery injury in clients with basilar skull trauma is 2%.[65]

Diagnostic Imaging

- Refer to table 15.1 for details regarding particular fractures, imaging, and their particular diagnostic accuracy values.

II. Observation

- All of the following signs have ideal ability to help **rule in** nasal fracture; none were helpful for ruling out nasal fracture:[24]
  - Epistaxis (SP 98, +LR 14.0)
  - Presence of inflammation in the area (SP 92, +LR 7.0)
  - An acute septal injury (SP 100, +LR Inf)

- All of the following signs have good ability to help **rule in** nasal fracture, none were helpful for ruling out nasal fracture:[24]
  - Airway obstruction present (SP 96, +LR 4.8)
  - Lateral deviation of nose present (SP 96, +LR 4.5)

- All of the following signs have a less than good ability to help rule in, and poor ability to help rule out nasal fracture:[24]
  - Irregular nasal dorsum present (SP 92, +LR 3.6)
  - Nasal wound present (SP 70, +LR 1.5)

III. Triage and Screening

- All non-musculoskeletal causes, as well as causes from related joints, should be ruled out.

- History is used for triage, during which red flags should be identified and yellow flags assessed.[38]

- An alert, asymptomatic client without distracting injury or neurological deficit who is able to complete a functional ROM examination may be safely cleared from cervical spine immobilization without radiographic evaluation (SN 98).[39]

- Ruling out traumatic skull fracture:
  - Battle's sign: When present, it had a PPV of 66% for intracranial lesions in an emergency service for clients with a Glasgow Coma Scale of 13 to 15.[20]
  - Raccoon eyes: When present, it was associated with anterior skull base fractures in more than 70% of cases.[22]

- Canadian CT Head Rule: When (−) among high or medium risk criteria or high risk criteria alone, it has ideal ability to help **rule out** (SN 99-100) neurosurgical intervention cases and good to ideal ability to help **rule out** (SN 80-100) any intracranial injury.[26]

- Ottawa Subarachnoid Hemorrhage Rule: When (−), it has ideal ability to help **rule out** (SN 99-100, −LR 0.04) subarachnoid hemorrhage in an acutely appearing client coming to the emergency room with a headache.[25]

- Canadian C-Spine Rule: It demonstrated better diagnostic accuracy (SN range 90-100) than either the NEXUS criteria (SN range 83-100)[40] or physician clinical judgment alone (SN 92)[41] and, therefore, an improved ability to help **rule out** an actual fracture.

- Alar ligament testing:
  - Significant variability in diagnostic accuracy (SN 69-100, −LR 0.29–0.31; SP 72-96, +LR 18-Inf) with improved ability to help **rule in** versus **rule out** alar ligament insufficiency with less complex testing.[42]
  - Better ability to help **rule in** (SP 96-100, +LR 18-Inf) versus **rule out** (SN 72, −LR 0.30) alar ligament insufficiency with more complex testing.[42]

- Sharp-Purser test: It demonstrates stronger ability to help **rule in** (SP 96, +LR 17.3) than rule out (SN 69, −LR 0.32) transverse ligament insufficiency.[43]

- More complex transverse ligament testing is also better able to help **rule in** (SP 99, +LR 65) than rule out (SN 65, −LR 0.35) transverse ligament insufficiency.[42]

- Cervical rotation is helpful for **ruling in** (SP 100, +LR 83.3) potential vertebrobasilar ischemia.[44]

- Combined cervical extension and rotation is helpful for **ruling in** (SP 98, +LR 4.2) potential upper cervical neurovascular compromise.[45]

- Radiculopathy or discogenic-related pathology: ruled out with a combination of Spurling's test and upper limb tension test (median nerve bias).

- Spurling's test: **SN 93 (77-99)**, **SP 95 (76-100)**, **+LR 19.6**, **−LR 0.07**, QUADAS 9[30]

- Median nerve upper limb tension test: **SN 97 (90-100)**, SP 22 (12-33), +LR 1.3, **−LR 0.12**, QUADAS 10[31]

IV. Motion Tests

- Any movement relative to the fracture should be suspected to be painful, limited, and guarded.

V. Muscle Performance Testing

- Any movement or strength assessment relative to the fracture should be suspected to be painful, limited, and guarded.

VI. Special Tests

- For ruling out traumatic fractures, head, and cervical spine injuries, see prior section Triage and Screening.

- Dizziness and unsteadiness can cause joint reposition errors in cervical spine.[60]

VII. Palpation

- It is suspected that the region relative to the fracture will be painful and likely swollen.

VIII. Physical Performance Measures

- Not appropriate acutely

POTENTIAL TREATMENT-BASED CLASSIFICATIONS

- Pain and stabilization most likely

- Exercise and conditioning as a long-term resolution

Dizziness

ICD-9: 780.4

ICD-10: H81.9 (unspecified disorder of vestibular system)

Dizziness compromises a variety of symptoms:[66]

- *Light-headedness or presyncope.* This is a sensation of impending loss of consciousness due to a momentary decrease in cerebral blood flow. It often occurs when standing up from supine too quickly.

- *Disequilibrium.* This imbalance or unsteadiness is experienced while standing or walking. It is caused by various factors including diminished vision, loss of vestibular function, defects in proprioception, and motor dysfunction from the central or peripheral nervous system.
- *Oscillopsia.* This is the subjective illusion of visual motion. While vertigo occurs with the eyes open or closed, oscillopsia only occurs when the eyes are open. Clients with bilateral loss of vestibulo-ocular reflex (VOR) frequently experience oscillopsia during head movements.
- *Vertigo.* The illusion of movements of oneself or the environment is due to an imbalance of tonic neural activity in the vestibular-cortical pathway. It is commonly exacerbated by head movements and accompanied by nausea and vomiting. Clients usually report rotational vertigo, although they occasionally describe a sensation of linear displacement or tilt.

Cervicogenic dizziness tends to be a controversial diagnosis because there are no diagnostic tests to confirm that it is the cause of the dizziness. Cervicogenic dizziness is a diagnosis that is provided to people who have neck injury or pain as well as dizziness and in whom other causes of dizziness have been ruled out.

I. Client Interview

Subjective History

- See prior information for respective complaints per condition.

II. Observation

- Ocular tilt reaction (OTR) refers to the trio of head tilt, ocular torsion, and skew deviation. Skew deviation is in reference to one eye focusing or appearing to be lower than the other. The head tilt is typically toward the lower eye as well.

III. Triage and Screening

- All non-musculoskeletal causes, as well as causes from related joints, should be ruled out.
- History is used for triage, during which red flags should be identified and yellow flags assessed.[38]
- An alert, asymptomatic client without distracting injury or neurological deficit who is able to complete a functional ROM examination may be safely cleared from cervical spine immobilization without radiographic evaluation (SN 98).[39]
- Ruling out traumatic skull fracture:
  - Battle's sign: When present, it had a positive predictive value of 66% for intracranial lesions in an emergency service for clients with a Glasgow Coma Scale of 13 to 15.[20]
  - Raccoon eyes: When present, it was associated with anterior skull base fractures in more than 70% of cases.[22]
- Canadian CT Head Rule: When (−) among high or medium risk criteria or high risk criteria alone, it has ideal ability to help **rule out** (SN 99-100) neurosurgical intervention cases and good to ideal ability to help **rule out** (SN 80-100) any intracranial injury.[26]
- Ottawa Subarachnoid Hemorrhage Rule: When (−), it has ideal ability to help **rule out** (SN 99-100, −LR 0.04) subarachnoid hemorrhage in an acutely appearing client coming to the emergency room with a headache.[25]
- Canadian C-Spine Rule: It demonstrated better diagnostic accuracy (SN range 90-100) than either the NEXUS criteria (SN range 83-100)[40] or physician clinical judgment alone (SN 92)[41] and, therefore, an improved ability to help **rule out** an actual fracture.
- Alar ligament testing:
  - Significant variability in diagnostic accuracy (SN 69-100, −LR 0.29–0.31; SP 72-96, +LR 18-Inf) with improved ability to help **rule in** versus **rule out** alar ligament insufficiency with less complex testing.[42]
  - Better ability to help **rule in** (SP 96-100, +LR 18-Inf) versus **rule out** (SN 72, −LR 0.30) alar ligament insufficiency with more complex testing.[42]
- Sharp-Purser test demonstrates stronger ability to help **rule in** (SP 96, +LR 17.3) than rule out (SN 69, −LR

0.32) transverse ligament insufficiency.[43]

- More complex transverse ligament testing is also better able to help **rule in** (SP 99, +LR 65) than rule out (SN 65, −LR 0.35) transverse ligament insufficiency.[42]

- Cervical rotation is helpful for **ruling in** (SP 100, +LR 83.3) potential vertebrobasilar ischemia.[44]

- Combined cervical extension and rotation is helpful for **ruling in** (SP 98, +LR 4.2) potential upper cervical neurovascular compromise.[45]

- Radiculopathy or discogenic-related pathology can be ruled out with a combination of Spurling's test and upper limb tension test (median nerve bias).

  - Spurling's test: **SN 93 (77-99)**, **SP 95 (76-100)**, **+LR 19.6**, **−LR 0.07**, QUADAS 9[30]

  - Median nerve upper limb tension test: **SN 97 (90-100)**, SP 22 (12-33), +LR 1.3, **−LR 0.12**, QUADAS 10[31]

IV. Motion Tests

- Cervicogenic dizziness is postulated to have an upper cervical motion restriction. The clinician should perform a comprehensive motion assessment in cases of such suspicion.

V. Muscle Performance Testing

- Suboccipital and cranial muscles may have secondary tenderness.

VI. Special Tests

- The Dix-Hallpike maneuver has a less than good ability to help rule out (when negative; SN 79, −LR 0.28) and help rule in (when positive; SP 75, +LR 3.2) BPPV.[33]

- Dizziness and unsteadiness can cause joint reposition errors in cervical spine.[60]

VII. Palpation

- Suboccipital and cranial muscles may have secondary tenderness.

VIII. Physical Performance Measures

- Cranial cervical flexor endurance test (if appropriate)

POTENTIAL TREATMENT-BASED CLASSIFICATIONS

- Pain and stabilization most likely

- Exercise and conditioning as a long-term resolution

Bell's Palsy

ICD-9: 351.0

ICD-10: G51.0 (Bell's palsy)

Bell's palsy is an acute unilateral facial nerve paresis or paralysis with onset in less than 72 hours that does not have an identifiable cause. It is a rapid unilateral facial nerve paresis or paralysis, and is the most common diagnosis associated with facial nerve weakness or paralysis. It leads to the partial or complete inability to voluntarily move facial muscles on the affected side of the face. Bell's palsy is more common in pregnant women, people 15 to 45 years of age and those with diabetes, upper respiratory ailments, or compromised immune systems. Clinicians should assess the client using history and physical examination to exclude identifiable causes of facial paresis or paralysis in clients presenting with acute-onset unilateral facial paresis or paralysis. Routine diagnostic imaging and laboratory testing are not recommended for this diagnosis unless other, more serious pathologies are suspected.

I. Client Interview

Subjective History

- Complaints of facial drooping, difficulty with blinking, closing the eye, and smiling

- May have neurological symptoms of facial paresthesia and tingling

- Can complain of headache or neck pain, memory problems, balance problems, and ipsilateral paresthesia and weakness

II. Observation

- Likely to present with facial drooping on involved side and inability to smile or frown on ipsilateral side

- Likely to have difficulty with closing eye on that side (may have complaints of dry eyes and so forth)

III. Triage and Screening

- All non-musculoskeletal causes, as well as causes from related joints, should be ruled out.

- History is used for triage, during which red flags should be identified and yellow flags assessed.[38]

- An alert, asymptomatic client without distracting injury or neurological deficit who is able to complete a functional ROM examination may be safely cleared from cervical spine immobilization without radiographic evaluation (SN 98).[39]

- Ruling out traumatic skull fracture:
  - Battle's sign: When present, it had a PPV of 66% for intracranial lesions in an emergency service for clients with a Glasgow Coma Scale of 13 to 15.[20]
  - Raccoon eyes: When present, it was associated with anterior skull base fractures in more than 70% of cases.[22]

- Canadian CT Head Rule: When (−) among high or medium risk criteria or high risk criteria alone, it has ideal ability to help **rule out** (SN 99-100) neurosurgical intervention cases and good to ideal ability to help **rule out** (SN 80-100) any intracranial injury.[26]

- Ottawa Subarachnoid Hemorrhage Rule: When (−), it has ideal ability to help **rule out** (SN 99-100, −LR 0.04) subarachnoid hemorrhage in an acutely appearing client coming to the emergency room with a headache.[25]

- Canadian C-Spine Rule: It demonstrated better diagnostic accuracy (SN range 90-100) than either the NEXUS criteria (SN range 83-100)[40] or physician clinical judgment alone (SN 92)[41] and, therefore, an improved ability to help **rule out** an actual fracture.

- Alar ligament testing:
  - Significant variability in diagnostic accuracy (SN 69-100, −LR 0.29-0.31; SP 72-96, +LR 18-Inf) with improved ability to help **rule in** versus **rule out** alar ligament insufficiency with less complex testing.[42]
  - Better ability to help **rule in** (SP 96-100, +LR 18-Inf) versus **rule out** (SN 72, −LR 0.30) alar ligament insufficiency with more complex testing.[42]

- Sharp-Purser test: It demonstrates stronger ability to help **rule in** (SP 96, +LR 17.3) than rule out (SN 69, 0.32) transverse ligament insufficiency.[43]

- More complex transverse ligament testing is also better able to help **rule in** (SP 99, +LR 65) than rule out (SN 65, −LR 0.35) transverse ligament insufficiency.[42]

- Cervical rotation is helpful for **ruling in** (SP 100, +LR 83.3) potential vertebrobasilar ischemia.[44]

- Combined cervical extension and rotation is helpful for **ruling in** (SP 98, +LR 4.2) potential upper cervical neurovascular compromise.[45]

- Radiculopathy and discogenic-related pathology can be ruled out with a combination of Spurling's test and upper limb tension test (median nerve bias).
  - Spurling's test: **SN 93 (77-99)**, **SP 95 (76-100)**, **+LR 19.6**, **−LR 0.07**, QUADAS 9[30]
  - Median nerve upper limb tension test: **SN 97 (90-100)**, SP 22 (12-33), +LR 1.3, **−LR 0.12**, QUADAS 10[31]

IV. Motion Tests

- The client has limited motion of facial muscles on involved side.

V. Muscle Performance Testing

- The client has limited strength of facial muscles on involved side.

- The client may have ipsilateral upper extremity weakness.

- The clinician should assess for deep neck flexor and scapula retractor weakness.

VI. Special Tests

- There are no particular special tests for this pathology.

VII. Palpation

- Clients are likely to complain of decreased sensation and possibly hypersensitivity in facial nerve innervation region.

VIII. Physical Performance Measures

- Cranial cervical flexor endurance test (if appropriate)

POTENTIAL TREATMENT-BASED CLASSIFICATIONS

- Pain most likely initially
- Exercise and conditioning long-term

CONCLUSION

Examination of the face and head can be a complex undertaking. Integration of best evidence as described in this chapter, as well as the systematic examination approach, is suggested to minimize further complicating the differential diagnosis of this region of the body. A systematic, evidence-based funnel approach suggests to the practicing clinician the importance of all components of the examination process. Additionally, it suggests that the clinician focus on ruling out or screening for potential competing pathologies early in the examination process and attempting to rule in or diagnose particular pathologies later in the examination process. Utilization of a systematic screening process early in the examination *funnels* or narrows down potential competing diagnoses that can then be more likely ruled in with more SP findings or testing.

16

TEMPOROMANDIBULAR JOINT

Michael P. Reiman, PT, DPT, OCS, SCS, ATC, FAAOMPT, CSCS

The temporomandibular system consists of the temporomandibular joint (TMJ) and the associated neuromuscular system. A temporomandibular disorder (TMD) can result from a defect of one or both. The prevalence of TMD can be difficult to determine because many studies utilize different diagnostic qualifications and investigative designs. Prevalence estimates range from 5% to 60%.[1] Symptoms may be unilateral or bilateral and can involve the face, head, or jaw.[2] The collection of conditions affecting the TMJ and masticatory muscles, the so-called TMD, can be classified according to the Research Diagnostic Criteria for Temporomandibular Disorders. Of the three subgroups—muscle disorders (group I), disc displacements (group II), and arthralgia, arthritis, and arthrosis (group III)—the muscle disorders are most frequently seen in community sample studies; group II and group III diagnoses are less prevalent.[3] Additional detail regarding this classification scheme is given at the end of the chapter (Common Orthopedic Conditions of the Temporomandibular Joint).

A TMD is clinically characterized by pain in the temporomandibular region or in the muscles of mas-

tication, pain radiating behind the eyes, pain in the face, shoulder, neck, or the back, headaches, ear ache or tinnitus, jaw clicking, locking or deviation, limited jaw opening, clenching or grinding of the teeth, dizziness, and sensitivity of the teeth lacking oral disease.[4] Symptoms of TMD can often resemble other medical conditions. Orofacial pain, on the other hand, is commonly described to include chronic headache, neck pain, TMD, and atypical facial pain, among other related conditions. TMDs rarely have an isolated cause, and studies have shown that numerous factors are typically involved. Therefore, the client interview can be complicated by the multidimensional nature of TMD's clinical presentation.

CLINICALLY APPLIED ANATOMY

The craniomandibular complex consists of the cranial articulation at the temporal bone on each side of the head in front of the ear and the two condyles of the mandible. Each joint is referred to as the TMJ. The craniomandibular complex allows for functional movement of the jaw during chewing (mastication), speech, and various facial expressions. The TMJ is one of the most frequently moved joints in the body, and its design reflects its variety of functional demands. The function of the TMJs is also closely related to that of the cervical spine, and it can be influenced by postural adaptations. Posture dysfunctions of the cervical spine can have a significant influence on the TMJ.

The TMJ includes the temporal bone and mandible. The mandible is essentially suspended from the temporal bones on either side of the skull by ligaments. The mandible is a U-shaped bone with condyles on each end (figure 16.1). The body of

the mandible is relatively horizontal; it receives the lower teeth at the alveolar process at the upper margin of the body. Notable markings on the interior of the body of the mandible are the digastric fossa, site of the attachment of digastric muscles on the inferoanterior aspect of the anterior portion of the body, and the mylohyoid line, the area of attachment of the flat mylohyoid muscle on the interior surface of the body of the mandible.[5] The ramus is the more vertical component of the mandible. At the superior end of the ramus are two projections, the coronoid process and the mandibular condyle. The coronoid process is the anterior bony projection that provides attachment for the temporalis and the masseter muscles. The most superior portion of the coronoid process rests deep in the zygomatic arch, and its anterior aspect can be palpated posterior to the third molars high in the intraoral cavity. The mandibular notch is the area between the coronoid process and the mandibular neck. The mandibular condyle articulates with the disc (figure 16.2) and together with the disc and the temporal bone forms the TMJ, the unilateral component of the craniomandibular complex. The TMJ articulation is reinforced (as are all synovial joints) with a joint capsule and ligamentous support (figure 16.3).

At the lateral aspect of the temporal bone is the mandibular fossa. The mandibular fossa receives the mandibular condyle, but only a portion of the fossa is suitable for the loading and weight bearing required for proper functioning of the TMJ. The most superior bony portion of the mandibular fossa forms the roof of the TMJ.

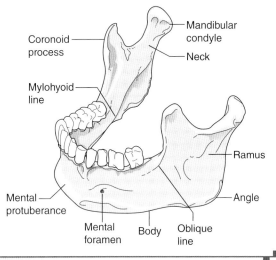

Figure 16.1 TMJ anatomy.

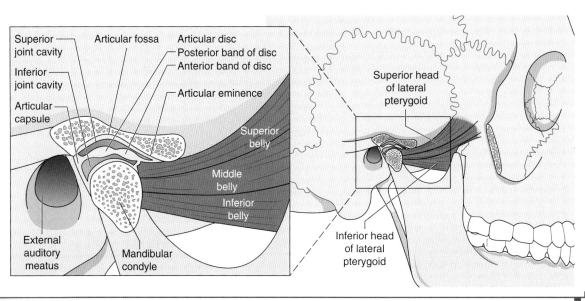

Figure 16.2 Anatomy of the TMJ joint.

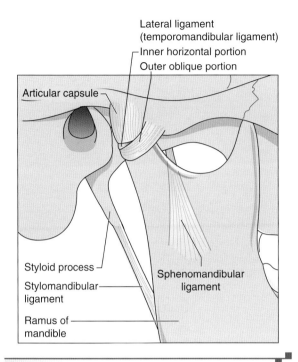

Lateral ligament
(temporomandibular ligament)
Inner horizontal portion
Outer oblique portion

Articular capsule

Styloid process

Stylomandibular
ligament

Ramus of
mandible

Sphenomandibular
ligament

Figure 16.3   Ligaments of the TMJ.

The cartilaginous covering of the temporal bone in the TMJ is fibrocartilage rather than the hyaline cartilage typically associated with synovial joints. Compared with hyaline cartilage, fibrocartilage allows for increased tolerance of repetitive or high loads as well as improved ability to repair damage sustained during micro- or macrotrauma. Activities that contribute to microtrauma of the TMJ include fingernail biting, lip chewing, gum chewing, tooth grinding (bruxism), and jaw clenching. These activities repetitively load the joint and over time can produce a sequence of degenerative changes to the joint such as joint laxity, disc dysfunction, and changes to the articular cartilage.

The articular eminence is the downward-sloping anterior border of the fossa. The fibrocartilage lining the trabecular bone of the articular eminence is thick, especially at the middle third of the eminence, and is well suited for repetitive and high-force loading. There is no bony block on the anterior eminence that might prevent the mandibular condyle from translating forward off of the eminence. Infrequently, in hypermobile joints, the mandibular condyle may dislocate anteriorly and lodge anterior to the articular eminence. This occurs most often with excessive opening of the mouth during yawning.[6]

Other bones related to the TMJ complex include the styloid process, a thin bony projection from the tympanic plate that provides attachment for ligaments and muscles. The zygomatic process is the squamous portion of the temporalis bone that articulates with the zygomatic bone to form the arch of the cheek bone. The maxillae on each side fuse to form the hard palate of the mouth and the maxillary arch that receives the upper teeth.

Each TMJ is divided into an upper joint space and a lower joint space by the articular disc. Each joint space has a separate joint capsule with its own synovial lining. The lower joint is formed by the mandibular condyle and the inferior surface of the articular disc. This joint functions as a ginglymus (or hinge) joint, with the primary movement of rotation. The articular eminence of the temporal bone and the superior surface of the articular disc form the upper joint of the temporomandibular complex. The upper joint is classified as an amphiarthrodial joint or a plane joint; translation between the disc and the articular eminence is the primary movement available.

The movements available at the TMJ (figure 16.4) are mouth opening (mandibular depression) and closing (mandibular elevation), mandibular protrusion and retrusion, and mandibular lateral excursion (or deviation). Mandibular depression and elevation are sagittal plane movements involving mandibular condyle anterior rotation in the lower joint and translation in the upper joint. Mandibular protrusion and retrusion involves bilateral condylar translation in the upper joint; anterior for protrusion and posterior for retrusion. Lateral excursion involves contralateral condyle protrusion (anterior translation in upper joint) and ipsilateral condyle spinning.

CLIENT INTERVIEW

Pain is often the primary complaint and therefore the reason for the client with TMD to seek intervention. Since pain is an arbitrary construct, determining a clear relationship between a client's pain and the relevant dysfunction that they present with is not always discernible. In fact, a systematic review found no clear evidence for a relationship between clinical and MRI diagnoses and findings. Several studies in this systematic review reported a relationship between clinical pain and an internal derangement diagnosed with MRI, but the calculated odds ratio (OR) for this relationship was generally low (1.54–2.04). ORs for the relationship between pain and disc displacement without reduction (4.82) or

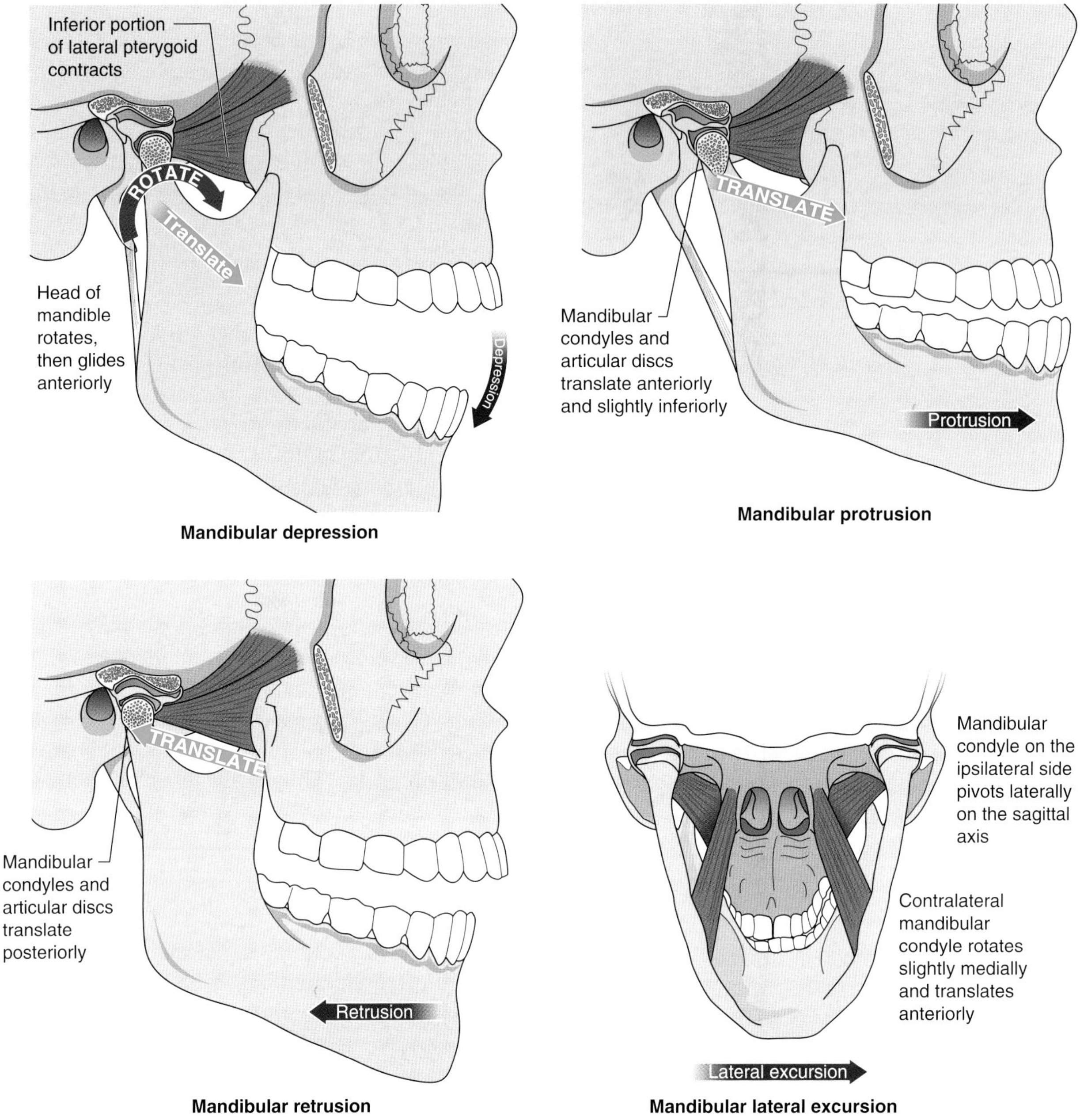

Inferior portion
of lateral pterygoid
contracts

ROTATE

Translate

Head of
mandible
rotates,
then glides
anteriorly

Depression

Mandibular depression

TRANSLATE

Mandibular
condyles and
articular discs
translate anteriorly
and slightly inferiorly

Protrusion

Mandibular protrusion

TRANSLATE

Mandibular
condyles and
articular discs
translate
posteriorly

Retrusion

Mandibular retrusion

Mandibular
condyle on the
ipsilateral side
pivots laterally
on the sagittal
axis

Contralateral
mandibular
condyle rotates
slightly medially
and translates
anteriorly

Lateral excursion

Mandibular lateral excursion

Figure 16.4   TMJ movements.

between crepitation and disc displacement without reduction (3.71) were higher.[7] This is reflective of the diagnostic accuracy values of the special testing for TMD, which is discussed later in this chapter. While clinicians should consider avoiding biasing their examinations by interpreting findings of radiographic imaging prior to seeing clients (in most cases without concerns for red flags and major medical-related issues), this point in the examination is most likely where clinicians will encounter radiographic imaging. Additionally, in some instances, clinicians must interpret radiographic imaging early in the examination to rule out serious pathology prior to continuing with other components of the examination sequence.

Subjective

As with all clients presenting for examination, the clinician must clarify if trauma had any involvement in the client's clinical presentation. Motor vehicle and other related accidents have been known to cause TMD. Additionally, trauma due to dental management, opening the jaw very wide, and eating have also been reported as possible contributors to TMD.[8] Undergoing traditional orthodontic treatment has not been shown to increase the prevalence of TMD.[9] The clinician must also consider the possibility of previous head and neck trauma contributing to TMD. Mandible condyle fracture[10] and, to a lesser degree, whiplash[11, 12] have demonstrated the possibility of contributing to TMD.

Pain present in the TMD client occurs typically with opening and closing the mouth. Pain with opening the mouth fully is suggested as an extra-articular problem, while pain associated with biting firm objects is an intra-articular problem.[13] Limited opening of the mouth can be due to anterior disc displacement. If the client has pain with biting or chewing objects, it should be clarified whether chewing is painful on both sides of the mouth or just on one side. Chewing on one side of the mouth is often the result of malocclusion.[13] Pain on the side opposite of the side of chewing may concern the clinician with respect to an intra-articular problem as well. Compression on the chewing side will likely cause tensile stretch loads on the contralateral side. Additionally, soft-tissue extra-articular structures must also be considered in this case. Careful palpation and resistive testing will assist in this differential diagnosis.[14-17] The clinician must also consider the possibility of issues with the client's teeth and therefore the necessity for referral to a dentist.

Regarding pain, as is typical of a comprehensive orthopedic examination, the severity or intensity, level of irritability, nature, and stage of the client's pain and presentation must be clearly delineated. Along with this, the specific location of their concordant versus discordant pain must be elucidated. Due to the interdependent relationship of orofacial pain, delineation between other relevant potential pathology (e.g., headaches, cervical spine pathology, non-musculoskeletal pain) is necessary. Aggravating and easing factors for the client's pain should also be asked. Finding a characteristic pain pattern, the location of pain, and aggravating or easing factors are very helpful for determining not only the potential for musculoskeletal-related pain versus non-musculoskeletal pain but the potential pain generator as well. Also, as part of a standard comprehensive examination, inquiry into the possible presence of paresthesia, abnormal sensation, or lack of sensation must be determined. Cranial nerve assessment may or may not be a significant component of the client with orofacial pain.

The client may also complain of clicking, catching, or crepitus with chewing.[14-17] Clicking is the result of abnormal motion of the disc and the mandible. Clicking early in the motion of opening the mouth suggests a more recent condition, and it is more likely that the disc is not displaced anteriorly very much in front of the mandibular condyle. A click later in the opening of the mouth suggests a more chronic problem, with the potential for further anterior disc displacement. With disc displacement (subluxation) or dislocation, the later the click with opening and the earlier the click with closing, the more suggestive it is that the disc displacement is further anterior. A click noted with both opening and closing of the mouth is described as a *reciprocal click*. It is typically believed that the later the click happens (further the mouth is opened) with opening and the sooner it happens (more open the jaw is at the time of the click) with closing, the greater the anterior displacement of the disc. The late click therefore happens with close to end range of opening, and the early click happens with the beginning of closing the mouth in this example.

Sleeping posture and sleeping habits should be discussed with the client during the interview. Pain with sleeping directly on the painful side may be an indicator of pain with compression to the joint, while pain with sleeping on the contralateral side may be an indicator of pain with distraction or tension on the joint. Bruxism, or nonfunctional grinding and clenching of the teeth, typically occurs during sleep, but may also occur with early awakening. Typically, symptoms associated with bruxism are severe with awakening; over time, they can cause damage to the TMJs.[18] The client should also be questioned regarding the combination of symptoms of pain and stiffness present when they awaken. As with other joints, this may be suggestive of intra-articular damage. In fact, a history of stiffness on waking with pain on function that disappears as the day goes on suggests osteoarthritis.[13]

Any history of headaches or current complaints must be ascertained. Due to the classification of orofacial pain including both TMD and various forms of headaches, the client with one of these conditions very well could present with the other. Additionally, the International Headache Society Classification Scheme includes TMD as part of its schema.

Stressful life events have been more frequently reported in a group of TMD clients than in a non-affected control group.[19] These clients exclusively presented with muscle-related symptoms.[20] Anxiety,[21] depression, somatoform disorders, and personality disorders[22] have been suggested to be more frequent in groups of TMD clients compared to controls. In a study by Kinney and colleagues,[23] 40% of TMD clients qualified for at least one personality disorder, with obsessive compulsive disorder being the most common.

Gender and age are also variables for the clinician to consider for the client with TMD. Women are more aware of the symptoms and as a result outnumber men in many studies regarding prevalence of these disorders.[24] In another study, persistent TMD was associated with female gender, older age, psychological distress, widespread body pain, and taking medication.[25]

Outcome Measures

Outcome measures for TMD should include relevant outcome measures for related areas, namely the cervical spine. Refer to chapter 17 for additional detail in this regard.

There is significant discrepancy between authorities over the precise clinical features, and hence the diagnostic criteria, for TMD.[2] The terminology used to describe this symptom group is quite variable. At least four pain classifications are used for description of orofacial pain, each with their strengths and weaknesses. The Research Diagnostic Criteria for Temporomandibular Disorder (RDC/TMD) is a dual-axis system that utilizes physical examination, as well as a self-report 31-item questionnaire. The strength of this instrument has been described as its ability to grade and measure both physical and psychological components of the client's pain.[26] A distinct disadvantage of this tool is that the physical examination component of it was designed to be performed by specialists, maxillofacial surgeons. Therefore, its clinical applicability to others is unknown.

Since there is the suggestion of psychiatric diagnosis and TMD,[21-23] the clinician may want to utilize relevant measures as part of their clinical examination and re-examination. The major Research Diagnostic Criteria for Temporomandibular Disorders Axis II measures demonstrated psychometric properties suitable for comprehensive assessment and management of TMD clients. The Depression instrument's normal versus moderate to severe cutoff point was good at identifying current-year depression and dysthymia (SN 87%, SP 53%). Nonspecific Physical Symptoms did not have high utility for detecting psychiatric disorders (SN 86%, SP 31%).[27]

As with all areas, re-examination of the client should include relevant outcome measures and assessment of progress. Again, two relevant clinical measures for this include the Global Rating of Change (GROC) and the Patient-Specific Functional Scale (PSFS).

Diagnostic Imaging

A suggested reference standard (gold standard) for diagnosis of TMD according to the RDC/TMD classification scheme is a comprehensive history and examination, as well as imaging that includes a panoramic radiograph, bilateral TMJ, magnetic resonance imaging (MRI), and bilateral TMJ computed tomography (CT; table 16.1).[28] The comprehensive extent of diagnostic imaging suggested may not be necessary, appropriate, or clinically available in many instances outside of research studies designed specifically for diagnostic accuracy of these tools.

Radiographs

Plain radiographs are often the first choice of imaging modality for TMD. The more common views include anteroposterior (AP), lateral transcranial, transpharyngeal, and transorbital. Panoramic radiography is also commonly implemented on a fairly routine basis, especially by dentists. The AP view is a good image for condylar shape and contour. The lateral view allows the clinician to also view the position of the condylar heads with the mouth open and closed, the extent of condylar movement with mouth opening, and the relationship of the TMJ to the other bony structures of the head and cervical spine. Panoramic radiography provides information about the teeth and other areas of the mandible; however, the relationship between the condyle and glenoid fossa is not seen in this film.

Tomography is a good method for depicting osseous or bony changes with arthrosis in TMJ. The major disadvantage of tomography is the lack of visualization of the soft tissue of TMJ, which is also a problem with plain film radiography.

Arthrography involves small amounts of iodinated contrast injected under fluoroscopy. If the disc is perforated, contrast flows into both the superior and inferior joint recesses. However, the arthrographic needle can inadvertently puncture the meniscus and cause iatrogenic filling of both joint spaces.

Magnetic Resonance Imaging

Magnetic resonance imaging is most frequently used for differentiation of soft-tissue-structure

TABLE 16.1   Diagnostic Accuracy of Various Imaging Modalities for the TMJ

Pathology	Diagnostic test	Gold standard	SN/SP
Disc displacement with reduction	US	MRI	Pooled analysis: 79/91[29] 76/82[30]
	MRI	Cryosections of cadaver	90/100[31]
Disc displacement without reduction	US	MRI	Pooled analysis: 76/82[29] 79/91[30]
Disc displacement (general)	US	Variable	13-100/62-100[32]
Anterior disc displacement	Arthrography	Variable	90/80[33]
	CT		66/68[33]
	MRI		86/63[33]
Joint effusion	US	Variable	71-84/74-100[32]
Bone marrow changes	MRI	Biopsy during surgery	78/84[34]
Condylar erosion	US	Variable	70-94/20-100[32]
Condylar osseous changes (cadaver skulls)	MDCT	Observation of skull	25-50/86-87[35]
	CBCT		23-40/83-90[35]

US = ultrasonography; MRI = magnetic resonance imaging; CT = computed tomography; MDCT = multidetector computed tomography; CBCT = cone beam computed tomography

The color coding for suggestion of **good** and **ideal** diagnostic accuracy values reported in this table are without quality scoring (QUADAS), a very important aspect of determination of the clinical utility of such values. Therefore, it is suggested that the reader keep this in mind when interpreting such values.

involvement, including the visualization of disc displacements, but also for the study of bone mineral density of the condyle. Cytokines play an important role in TMJ pathology. For example, IL-1beta, which has been associated with TMJ pain, hyperalgesia, and anterior bite opening, is mostly absent in the synovial fluid of healthy joints.[3]

Computed Tomography

As with other areas of the body, CT is advantageous over MRI and is typically superior to radiography in the imaging of bony structures. CT involves ionizing radiation. It can be used to diagnose internal derangement issues of the TMJ since the disc has a slightly higher density than the surrounding muscle and soft tissue.

Ultrasound

Diagnostic US imaging is becoming more popular and favorable for assessment in the TMJ. As with other areas of the body, US imaging is cheaper than MRI or CT scans. Again, a potential disadvantage for the use of US in orthopedic assessment is that the reliability of this imaging modality depends on the operator.

Review of Systems

Refer to chapter 6 (Triage and Differential Diagnosis) for detail on review of systems relevant to the temporomandibular joint.

OBSERVATION

Observation of the client with craniomandibular dysfunction starts with general overall posture. Poor posture, such as forward head and bilaterally rounded shoulders (e.g., upper crossed syndrome), has long been suggested to contribute to TMD. The clinician should also observe for overall facial appearance. Does the client appear to be in acute distress due to pain? Head posture out of alignment in any of the three planes of movement should also be assessed. Specific to the TMJ, does the client's jaw rest in midline with the rest of their face?

General appearance of the face (as with the head and face observation) must account for any asymmetry, scars, discoloration, swelling, and so on. Any observable feature out of the normal should be investigated in greater detail with subjective questioning, as well as physical examination. Clenching of the jaw, typically observable with increased temporalis or masseter muscle activity, should be noted if present. While jaw clenching may provoke acute muscle tenderness, it has not been proven to be analogous to myogenous TMD.[36]

Increased muscle activity can be noted in other ways with these clients. Stressful life events can be frequent in TMD clients.[20] These clients will have muscle-related symptoms,[19] and they are therefore likely to present with protective posturing and muscle guarding that can be observed.

A normal fit of the upper and lower teeth is when the upper teeth are slightly forward of the lower teeth. Missing teeth or inappropriate pressure on the joints can contribute to TMD. Malocclusion, a misalignment of teeth or incorrect relation between the teeth of the two dental arches, has various presentations. It is often referred to as irregular bite, crossbite, or overbite. Malocclusion may be seen as crooked, crowded, or protruding teeth. It will often affect the client's appearance, speech, and ability to eat. Malocclusion is discussed in detail in the section Common Orthopedic Conditions of the Temporomandibular Joint at the end of this chapter (also see figure 16.19). Bruxism, or grinding of upper and lower teeth, is most common during sleep, although a subjective report can have observable features. Continued grinding of teeth may present as wearing of the teeth, especially noticeable anteriorly. The correlation between anterior teeth wear and TMD is not strong, however.[36]

During the interview the clinician can also observe for the client's ability to naturally converse with them. While difficulty with speech is typically a significant concern for conditions such as dysarthria, dysphasia, and dysphonia, it may also indicate musculoskeletal dysfunction of the TMJ. Inability or unwillingness to open the mouth fully may be an indicator of the potential for disc displacement, muscle spasm, and other musculoskeletal-related conditions. As always, though, limitations in speech must be clearly differentially diagnosed as musculoskeletal- or non-musculoskeletal related.

Generalized joint hypermobility (GJH) has long been believed to contribute to TMD. While GJH may contribute to TMD,[37] including in children,[38] the exact relationship between GJH and TMD remains unclear and requires more stringent investigation.[39]

TRIAGE AND SCREENING

Triage and screening is a necessary component of the examination process that should be done prior to continuing with the examination. Ruling out serious pathology is paramount at this stage of the examination. (Refer to chapter 6, Triage and Differential Diagnosis, as well as chapter 17, Cervical Spine, for cervical spine related red flags.) Pain generation from other related (or close-proximity) structures also helps the clinician more accurately determine the necessity of continuing with the other examination components to identify the actual source of the client's pain. Additionally, implementing strong screening tests (tests of high SN and low −LR) at this point in the examination is suggested for narrowing down the competing diagnoses of the respective body region (predominantly cervical spine, in this case) when this is applicable.

The clinician should also address any suspicion of cervical instability or cervical artery dysfunction, as discussed in the cervical spine chapter (chapter 17), prior to proceeding with the examination. The upper quarter screen will determine cervical spine ROM and the potential for the cervical spine as a pain generator to the client's complaints of shoulder pain. Additionally, assessment of pain generation due to radiculopathy can be accomplished primarily with the Spurling's test and the median nerve upper limb neurodynamic test (tests of high SN and low −LR):

- Spurling's test: **SN 93 (77-99)**, **SP 95 (76-100)**, **+LR 19.6**, **−LR 0.07**, QUADAS 9[40]
- Median nerve upper limb neurodynamic test: **SN 97 (90-100)**, SP 22 (12-33), +LR 1.3, **−LR 0.12**, QUADAS 10[41]

Additionally, as with any joint, clearing AROM with or without overpressure is necessary. In order to fully clear the cervical spine, full AROM (with overpressure if pain-free) must be present. In order to fully clear the temporomandibular joint, full AROM (with overpressure if pain-free) must be present. Detail in this regard is described in the following section.

The diagnostic accuracy of SN tests is variable and is mostly limited with respect to clinical utility. Refer to the sections Special Tests and Common Orthopedic Conditions of the Temporomandibular Joint later in this chapter for specific details of tests.

MOTION TESTS

Measurement of motion at the TMJ is unique due to the nature of the joint. Many of the measure-

TABLE 16.2   TMJ Arthrology

Joint	Close-packed position	Resting position	Capsular pattern	ROM norms	End-feel
TMJ	Full occlusion	Teeth separated by 2-3 mm	Restriction in inferior glide	40-55 mm opening 3-6 mm protrusion 3-4 mm retrusion 10-12 mm lateral excursion	• Soft-tissue stretch for opening • Bony during full occlusion of teeth • Firm for protrusion and retrusion • Capsular for lateral excursion

TMJ = temporomandibular joint; mm = millimeters

ments are for distance (millimeters of movement). As with all joints, ROM norm values, end-feel, capsular pattern, and closed- and open-packed positions are listed in table 16.2. Additionally, refer to figure 16.4 regarding arthrokinematics of the TMJ.

The potential for both hypo- and hypermobility exist in the TMJ, similar to other joints with joint capsules. While it has commonly been believed that generalized joint hypermobility is associated with TMD, it is still not clear whether this association exists.[39]

Passive and Active ROMs

Goniometry of the TMJ is typically most appropriate with a ruler or measure stick versus with a goniometer. The clinician should wear a glove when performing these assessments. Consideration of the type of gloves worn is suggested due to latex allergies and so on in some clients.

MANDIBLE DEPRESSION (OPENING OF MOUTH)

See figure 16.13b for active range of motion (AROM) and figure 16.14 for passive range of motion (PROM).

Client Position	Sitting in upright posture, cervical spine in neutral
Clinician Position	Standing directly to the side of the client
Movement	The clinician stabilizes the posterior aspect of the client's occiput with one hand (if necessary) and purchases the mandible with the other (positioning it between the thumb and index finger) (for PROM). The clinician passively pulls the mandible inferiorly until they perceive a firm end-feel (due to stretching of the joint). They measure the distance between the upper and lower central incisor teeth with a ruler. These motions can be performed actively by the client without assistance from the clinician. Active range of motion should be performed prior to PROM to determine the client's willingness to move. Additionally, palpation of the joint can be performed during AROM.
Assessment	Clinician assesses for amount of ROM, end-feel, quality of the movement, client response, potential difference between AROM and PROM, and so on.

MANDIBLE PROTRUSION

See figure 16.15 for AROM.

Client Position	Sitting in upright posture, cervical spine in neutral
Clinician Position	Standing directly to the side of the client
Movement	The clinician stabilizes the posterior aspect of the client's occiput with one hand (if necessary) and purchases the mandible with the other (positioning it between the thumb and index

(continued)

Mandible Protrusion *(continued)*

finger) (for PROM). The client may assist the movement by pushing the chin anteriorly as far as possible until a firm end-feel (due to stretching of the joint) is perceived. The clinician measures the distance between the upper and lower central incisor teeth with a ruler. These motions can be performed similarly actively by the client without assistance from the clinician. Active range of motion should be performed prior to PROM to determine the client's willingness to move.

Assessment Clinician assesses for amount of ROM, end-feel, quality of the movement, client response, potential difference between AROM and PROM, and so on.

MANDIBLE LATERAL DEVIATION

See figure 16.16 for AROM.

Client Position Sitting in upright posture, cervical spine in neutral

Clinician Position Standing directly to the side of the client

Movement The clinician stabilizes the posterior aspect of client's occiput with one hand (if necessary) and purchases the mandible with the other (positioning it between the thumb and index finger) (for PROM) and then moves the mandible to the side until they perceive a firm end-feel (due to stretching of the joint). The clinician measures the distance between the most lateral points of the upper and lower cuspid (or first bicuspid) teeth with a ruler. This motion can be performed similarly actively by the client without assistance from the clinician. Active range of motion should be performed in the sitting position and done prior to PROM to determine the client's willingness to move.

Assessment Clinician assesses for amount of ROM, end-feel, quality of the movement, client response, potential difference between AROM and PROM, and so on.

Passive Accessories

As with all passive accessory testing, clinicians must take care with respect to client comfort and potential for reproduction of concordant pain. The clinician should wear a glove when performing these assessments. Consideration of the type of gloves worn is suggested due to latex allergies and so on in some clients.

INFERIOR (CAUDAL) GLIDE

 Video 16.5 **in the web resource shows a demonstration of this test.**

Client Position Supine

Clinician Position Standing or sitting at the client's head facing the client

Stabilization The rest of the client's body on the table serves as a stabilizing force, and the clinician's cranial hand and chest stabilize the client's cranium as well.

Movement and Direction of Force The clinician places their caudal or distal thumb on the superior aspect of the client's posterior teeth and their fingers along the client's lateral mandible. The clinician, purchasing primarily with their thumb, transmits the distraction force directly caudal or inferior; force involves low-velocity oscillations or sustained stretch.

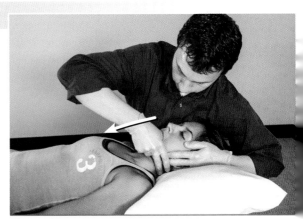

Figure 16.5

Assessment   Assessment is done for joint play/passive accessory motion, client response, and end-feel. Reproduction of concordant pain suggests dysfunction. Impaired joint mobility or end-feel may also suggest dysfunction if concordant pain is also reproduced.

ANTERIOR GLIDE

Client Position	Supine
Clinician Position	Standing or sitting at the client's head facing the client
Stabilization	The rest of the client's body on the table serves as a stabilizing force, and the clinician's cranial hand and chest stabilize the client's cranium as well.
Movement and Direction of Force	The clinician places their caudal or distal thumb on the superior aspect of the client's posterior teeth and their fingers along the client's lateral mandible. The clinician, purchasing primarily with their thumb, provides a slight initial caudal force prior to a subsequent anteriorly directed force. Force involves low-velocity oscillations or sustained stretch.

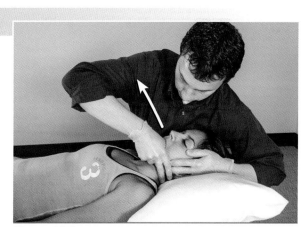

Figure 16.6

Assessment   Assessment is done for joint play/passive accessory motion, client response, and end-feel. Reproduction of concordant pain suggests dysfunction. Impaired joint mobility or end-feel may also suggest dysfunction if concordant pain is also reproduced.

MEDIAL GLIDE

Client Position	Supine
Clinician Position	Standing or sitting at the client's head facing the client
Stabilization	The rest of the client's body on the table serves as a stabilizing force, and the clinician's cranial hand and chest stabilize the client's cranium as well.
Movement and Direction of Force	The clinician, using their caudal or distal thumb, purchases the superior aspect of the client's posterior teeth and their second and third fingers of same hand on the lateral aspect of client's mandible, stabilizing the cranium. The clinician imparts distraction inferiorly followed by medial direction

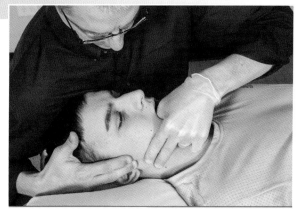

Figure 16.7

primarily through the second and third fingers extra-orally (clinician can use finger over finger placement if needed), stabilizing the client's cranium with the hand and chest. Force involves low-velocity oscillations or sustained stretch.

Assessment   Assessment is done for joint play/passive accessory motion, client response, and end-feel. Reproduction of concordant pain suggests dysfunction. Impaired joint mobility or end-feel may also suggest dysfunction if concordant pain is also reproduced.

LATERAL GLIDE

 Video 16.8 **in the web resource shows a demonstration of this test.**

Client Position	Supine
Clinician Position	Standing or sitting at the client's head facing the client
Stabilization	The rest of the client's body on the table serves as a stabilizing force, and the clinician's cranial hand and chest stabilize the client's cranium as well.
Movement and Direction of Force	The clinician, using their caudal or distal thumb, purchases the medial aspect of the client's mandible and their second and third fingers of same hand on the lateral aspect of the client's mandible, stabilizing the cranium. They impart distraction inferiorly, followed by a glide in the lateral direction, primarily via their thumb (on medial aspect of condyle), providing stabilization with their cranial hand. Force involves low-velocity oscillations or sustained stretch.
Assessment	Assessment is done for joint play/passive accessory motion, client response, and end-feel. Reproduction of concordant pain suggests dysfunction. Impaired joint mobility or end-feel may also suggest dysfunction if concordant pain is also reproduced.

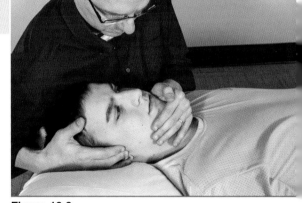

Figure 16.8

MEDIAL OR LATERAL GLIDE (EXTRA-ORAL)

Client Position	Supine
Clinician Position	Standing or sitting at the client's head facing the client
Stabilization	The rest of the client's body on the table serves as a stabilizing force, and the clinician's cranial hand and chest stabilize the client's cranium as well.
Movement and Direction of Force	The clinician purchases the client's lateral mandible with their thenar eminence, stabilizing the client's cranium. The clinician then imparts a medially directed force (or relative lateral force is applied on contralateral TMJ) with the thenar eminence, continuing to stabilize the cranium. Force involves low-velocity oscillations or sustained stretch.
Assessment	Assessment is done for joint play/passive accessory motion, client response, and end-feel. Reproduction of concordant pain suggests dysfunction. Impaired joint mobility or end-feel may also suggest dysfunction if concordant pain is also reproduced.

Figure 16.9

Critical Clinical Pearls

When performing joint play testing for the TMJ, clinicians should keep the following in mind:

- The part of the joint below the disc (inferior joint cavity or caudal disc articulation with the mandibular condyle) primarily has a rolling motion.
- This rolling motion is typically the initial movement of TMJ joint arthrokinematics.
- The part of the joint above the disc (superior joint cavity or cranial disc articulation with the articular eminence) primarily has a gliding motion.
- This gliding motion is typically the latter portion of TMJ joint arthrokinematics.
- Protrusion and retrusion predominantly involve a gliding motion.

Flexibility

Refer to chapter 17 (Cervical Spine) for flexibility assessments appropriate for the temporomandibular joint.

MUSCLE PERFORMANCE TESTING

Muscle performance testing of the craniomandibular complex, as in most regions of the body, is difficult to clinically isolate. Rather, it is a movement-based examination not specific to a particular muscle. Hence, a more function-based assessment is used instead of isolated muscle testing. This importance is ADL appropriate due to the daily tasks of eating, chewing, talking, and so forth. The following are manual muscle tests of the TMJ.

MANDIBLE DEPRESSION (JAW OPENING)

Client Position	Seated with bilateral knees flexed over edge of table
Clinician Position	Standing directly to the side of the client
Movement and Assessment	The clinician stabilizes the client's head with one hand and provides resistance with the other hand in a superior direction, then attempts to close the client's jaw.
Grading	• Functional: Client completes the available ROM and holds against strong resistance.
	• Weak functional: Client is able to open mouth two or three finger widths and to take some resistance.
	• Nonfunctional: Minimal motion occurs.
	• 0: No voluntary mandible depression occurs.
Primary Muscles	Lateral pterygoid
	Digastric
Secondary Muscles	Mylohyoid and geniohyoid muscles
Primary Nerves	Nerve to lateral pterygoid
	Nerve to digastric

MANDIBLE ELEVATION (JAW CLOSING)

Client Position	Seated with bilateral knees flexed over edge of table
Clinician Position	Standing directly to the side of the client
Movement and Assessment	The clinician stabilizes the client's head with one hand and provides resistance in an inferior direction with the other hand, and then attempts to open the client's jaw.
Grading	• Functional: Client closes jaw tightly.
	• Weak functional: Client closes jaw, but clinician can open mouth with less than maximal resistance.
	• Nonfunctional: Client closes mouth but tolerates no resistance.
	• 0: Client cannot completely close mouth.
Primary Muscles	Masseter
	Temporalis
	Medial pterygoid
Primary Nerves	Masseteric nerve
	Nerve to medial pterygoid

MANDIBLE LATERAL DEVIATION

Client Position	Seated with bilateral knees flexed over edge of table
Clinician Position	Standing directly in front of the client
Movement and Assessment	The clinician stabilizes the contralateral side of the client's head with one hand, while providing resistance in a lateral direction with the other hand to move the client's jaw toward the midline.
Grading	• Functional: Client completes available ROM and holds against strong resistance.
	• Weak functional: Motion is decreased and resistance is minimal.
	• Nonfunctional: Minimal motion occurs and no resistance is tolerated.
	• 0: No motion occurs.
Primary Muscles	Lateral pterygoid
	Medial pterygoid
Primary Nerves	Nerve to lateral pterygoid
	Nerve to medial pterygoid

MANDIBLE PROTRUSION

Client Position	Seated with bilateral knees flexed over edge of table
Clinician Position	Standing directly in front of the client
Movement and Assessment	The clinician stabilizes the back of the client's head with one hand and provides resistance with the other hand in a posterior direction horizontally.
Grading	• Functional: The client completes available ROM and holds against strong resistance.
	• Weak functional: Motion is decreased where there is no discernible gap between upper and lower teeth; tolerates only slight resistance.
	• Non-functional: Minimal motion occurs and no resistance is tolerated.
	• 0: No motion occurs.
Primary Muscles	Lateral pterygoid
	Medial pterygoid
Primary Nerves	Nerve to lateral pterygoid
	Nerve to medial pterygoid

SPECIAL TESTS

As mentioned in chapter 10 (Special Tests), in many cases the clinician is overly dependent on the performance and interpretation of special test findings with respect to differential diagnosis of the client's presenting pain. Utilization of special tests for ruling in (or helping to diagnose) a particular pathology should occur at this point in the examination process. It is also hoped that the clinician has a much clearer picture of the client's presentation prior to this point in the examination and will therefore depend minimally on special test findings with respect to diagnosis of the client's pain.

Clinical special testing for TMD is currently limited. Some of the limitations in the current literature include the quality of the studies, as well as the subclassification of the clients. As discussed later in the section Common Orthopedic Conditions of the Temporomandibular Joint, the classification of TMD suffers from limited diagnostic accuracy as well. Therefore, due to a lack of clear findings indicating compelling evidence for or against a diagnosis of TMD with these tests, as well as the low quality of many of the studies, the data are suggested to be insufficient for supporting or rejecting these tests.[42] Clustered testing appears to be of greater benefit than isolated testing.[43]

Index of Special Tests

Audible Joint Sounds

Crepitation	Joint Sounds With Click	Reciprocal Click

Pain

Pain With Posterolateral TMJ Palpation	Pain in TMJ With Mouth Opening

Mouth Movements

Limited Active Mouth Opening	Limited Protrusive Movement	Deviation of Mouth During Opening
Limited Passive Mouth Opening	Restricted Lateral Condylar Translation	Cluster Testing

Case Studies

Go to www.HumanKinetics.com/OrthopedicClinicalExamination and complete these case studies for chapter 16:

- Case study 1 discusses a 49-year-old female with face and jaw pain, especially with chewing.
- Case study 2 discusses a 67-year-old male with jaw pain and grinding of the jaw with movement.

Abstract Links

Go to www.HumanKinetics.com/OrthopedicClinicalExamination to access abstract links on these issues:

Crepitation   Reciprocal click

Joint sounds with clicks   Restricted lateral condylar translation

AUDIBLE JOINT SOUNDS

CREPITATION

Client Position	Seated with mouth relaxed
Clinician Position	Standing to the side to be tested
Movement	The clinician places the stethoscope over TMJ and instructs the client to open their mouth *(a)*, deviate it laterally *(b)*, and bite down *(c)*.
Assessment	A (+) test is crepitus sounds noted during the movements.

Statistics

- Disc displacement with reduction (DD-R): SN 2 (not reported, or NR), SP 91 (NR), +LR 0.21, −LR 1.08, QUADAS 9, in a study of 273 clients with various characteristics of TMD (mean age 33.2 years, 221 women, mean duration of symptoms NR), and using MRI as a reference standard[44]

- DD-R: SN 11 (NR), SP 64 (NR), +LR 0.29, −LR 1.39, QUADAS 7, in a study of 40 clients with TMJ complaints (mean age 32.6 years, 27 women, mean duration of symptoms NR), and using MRI as a reference standard[17]

- Disc displacement with no reduction: (DD-NR): SN 16 (NR), **SP 97 (NR)**, **+LR 5.3**, −LR 0.86, QUADAS 9, in a study of 273 clients with various characteristics of TMD (mean age 33.2 years, 221 women, mean duration of symptoms NR), and using MRI as a reference standard[44]

- DD-NR: SN 71 (NR), SP 89 (NR), +LR 6.4, −LR 0.33, QUADAS 7, in a study of 40 clients with TMJ complaints (mean age 32.6 years, 27 women, mean duration of symptoms NR), and using MRI as a reference standard[17]

- Osteoarthritis (OA): SN 45 (NR), SP 86 (NR), +LR 3.2, −LR 0.64, QUADAS 7, in a study of 200 clients, using arthroscopy as a reference standard[45]

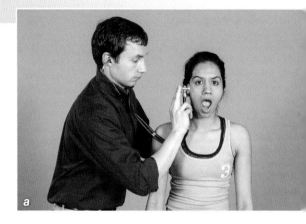

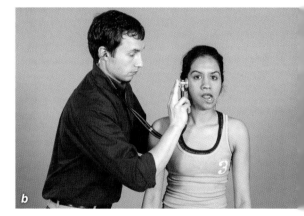

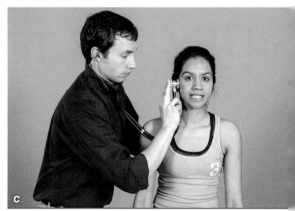

Figure 16.10

JOINT SOUNDS WITH CLICK

Video 16.11 in the web resource shows a demonstration of this test.

Client Position	Seated with mouth relaxed
Clinician Position	Standing to the side to be tested
Movement	The clinician places the stethoscope over the TMJ and instructs the client to open their mouth *(a)*, deviate it laterally *(b)*, and bite down *(c)*.
Assessment	A (+) test is clicking sounds noted during the movements.
Statistics	
Palpation of Click	• DD-R: SN 46 (35-56), SP 66 (58-73), +LR 1.3, −LR 0.82, QUADAS 12, in a study of 194 clients with TMD (mean age 55.3 years, 153 women, symptom duration NR), and using MRI as a reference standard[14]
	• DD-NR: SN 49 (40-58), SP 66 (58-73), +LR 1.4, −LR 0.77, QUADAS 12, in a study of 194 clients with TMD (mean age 55.3 years, 153 women, symptom duration NR), and using MRI as a reference standard[14]
Auscultation of Click	• DD-R: SN 89 (75-97), SP 20 (7-41), +LR 1.1, −LR 0.53, QUADAS 7, in a study of 40 clients with TMJ complaints (mean age 32.6 years, 27 women, mean duration of symptoms NR), and using MRI as a reference standard[17]
	• DD-NR: SN 29 (10-56), SP 20 (7-41), +LR 0.37, −LR 3.5, QUADAS 7, in a study of 40 clients with TMJ complaints (mean age 32.6 years, 27 women, mean duration of symptoms NR), and using MRI as a reference standard[17]

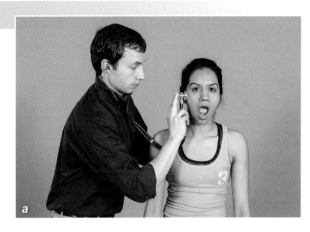

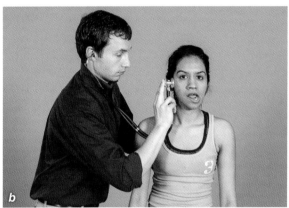

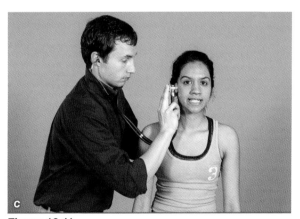

Figure 16.11

RECIPROCAL CLICK

Client Position	Seated with mouth relaxed
Clinician Position	Standing to the side to be tested
Movement	Clinician palpates the client's lateral TMJs bilaterally as they open their mouth fully *(a)* and then close their mouth to normal resting position *(b)*.
Assessment	Clicking noted with both opening and closing of the mouth is a (+) test.
Statistics	• DD-R: SN 76 (NR), SP 95 (NR), +LR 15.2, –LR 0.25, QUADAS 8, in a study of 70 clients (90 temporomandibular joints) with various related pathology (mean age, gender, and duration of symptoms NR), and using MRI as a reference standard[16]
	• DD-NR: SN 4 (NR), SP 52 (NR), +LR 0.08, –LR 1.85, QUADAS 8, in a study of 70 clients (90 temporomandibular joints) with various related pathology (mean age, gender, and duration of symptoms NR), and using MRI as a reference standard[16]

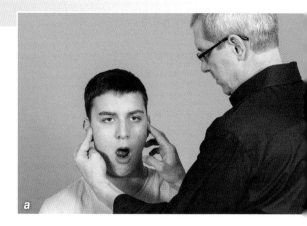

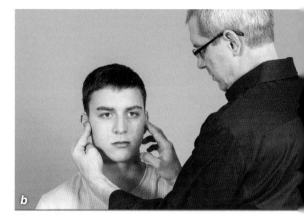

Figure 16.12

PAIN

PAIN WITH POSTEROLATERAL TMJ PALPATION

Client Position	Seated with mouth relaxed
Clinician Position	Standing directly in front or to the side of the client next to the TMJ to be tested
Movement	The clinician palpates the client's temporalis and masseter muscles with the client's mouth clenched *(a)* and the submandibular muscles with the mouth open. The clinician then palpates the client's TMJ externally *(b)*, both laterally and posteriorly.

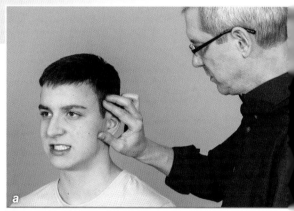

Figure 16.13

Assessment	A (+) test is concordant pain during testing.
Statistics	• DD-R: SN 100 (91-100), SP 20 (7-41), +LR 1.3, –LR 0, QUADAS 7, in a study of 40 clients with TMJ complaints (mean age 32.6 years, 27 women, mean duration of symptoms NR), and using MRI as a reference standard[17]
	• DD-NR: SN 66 (NR), SP 67 (NR), +LR 2.0, –LR 0.51, QUADAS 8, in a study of 70 clients (90 temporomandibular joints) with various related pathology (mean age, gender, and duration of symptoms NR), and using MRI as a reference standard[16]

Effusion SN 84-85, SP 62-69, +LR 2.3-2.7, –LR 0.24, QUADAS 12, in a study of 194 clients with TMD (mean age 55.3 years, 153 women, symptom duration NR), and using MRI as a reference standard[14]

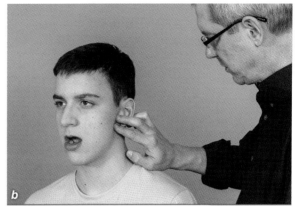

Figure 16.13

PAIN IN TMJ WITH MOUTH OPENING

Client Position	Seated with mouth relaxed
Clinician Position	Standing at the side to be tested
Movement	The clinician instructs the client to open their mouth as far as they can.
Assessment	A (+) test is a reduction in full mouth opening.
Statistics	• DD-R: SN 17 (NR), SP 70 (NR), +LR 0.56, –LR 1.19, QUADAS 9, in a study of 273 clients with various characteristics of TMD (mean age 33.2 years, 221 women, mean duration of symptoms NR), and using MRI as a reference standard[44]
	• DD-R: SN 44 (NR), SP 31 (NR), +LR 0.64, –LR 1.81, QUADAS 8, in a study of 70 clients (90 temporomandibular joints) with various related pathology (mean age, gender, and duration of symptoms NR), and using MRI as a reference standard[16]
	• DD-NR: SN 74 (NR), SP 57 (NR), +LR 1.72, –LR 0.46, QUADAS 8, in a study of 70 clients (90 temporomandibular joints with various related pathology), and using MRI as a reference standard[16]
	• DD-NR: SN 59 (NR), SP 88 (NR), +LR 4.9, –LR 0.47, QUADAS 9, in a study of 273 clients with various characteristics of TMD (mean age 33.2 years, 221 women, mean duration of symptoms NR), and using MRI as a reference standard[44]

MOUTH MOVEMENTS

LIMITED ACTIVE MOUTH OPENING

Client Position	Seated with mouth in resting position
Clinician Position	Standing directly in front of client monitoring for movement
Movement	The client opens their mouth as far as possible.
Assessment	A (+) test is limited mouth opening.
Statistics	• DD-R: SN 5 (NR), SP 70 (NR), +LR 0.18, –LR 1.36, QUADAS 9, in a study of 273 clients with various characteristics of TMD (mean age 33.2 years, 221 women, mean duration of symptoms NR), and using MRI as a reference standard[44]
	• DD-NR: SN 43 (NR), SP 84 (NR), +LR 2.6, –LR 0.68, QUADAS 9, in a study of 273 clients with various characteristics of TMD (mean age 33.2 years, 221 women, mean duration of symptoms NR), and using MRI as a reference standard[44]

(continued)

Limited Active Mouth Opening *(continued)*

- DD-R: SN 11 (NR), SP 59 (NR), +LR 0.26, –LR 1.50, QUADAS 7, in a study of 40 clients with TMJ complaints (mean age 32.6 years, 27 women, mean duration of symptoms NR), and using MRI as a reference standard[17]
- DD-NR: SN 77 (NR), SP 87 (NR), +LR 6.1, –LR 0.27, QUADAS 7, in a study of 40 clients with TMJ complaints (mean age 32.6 years, 27 women, mean duration of symptoms NR), and using MRI as a reference standard[17]

LIMITED PASSIVE MOUTH OPENING

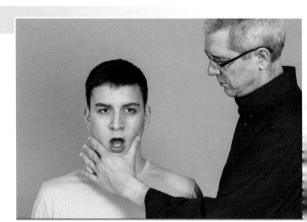

Figure 16.14

Client Position	Seated with mouth in resting position
Clinician Position	Standing directly in front of client monitoring for movement
Movement	The clinician passively opens the client's mouth as far as possible.
Assessment	A (+) test is limited mouth opening.
Statistics	• DD-R: SN 29 (NR), SP 29 (NR), +LR 0.41, –LR 2.4, QUADAS 8, in a study of 70 clients (90 temporomandibular joints) with various related pathology (mean age, gender, and duration of symptoms NR), and using MRI as a reference standard[16]

- DD-NR: SN 76 (NR), SP 69 (NR), +LR 2.5, –LR 0.35, QUADAS 8, in a study of 70 clients (90 temporomandibular joints) with various related pathology (mean age, gender, and duration of symptoms NR), and using MRI as a reference standard[16]

LIMITED PROTRUSIVE MOVEMENT

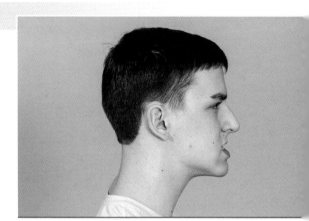

Figure 16.15

Client Position	Sitting with mouth in resting position
Clinician Position	Standing directly in front of client monitoring for movement
Movement	The client protrudes their mandible as far as possible.
Assessment	A (+) test is limited in full protrusion.
Statistics	• Adhesions: SN 90 (NR), SP 40 (NR), +LR 1.5, –LR 0.25, QUADAS 7, in a study of 200 clients using arthroscopy as a reference standard[45]
	• DD-R: SN 29 (NR), SP 38 (NR), +LR 0.47, –LR 1.87, QUADAS 8, in a study of 70 clients (90 temporomandibular joints) with various related pathology (mean age, gender, and duration of symptoms NR), and using MRI as a reference standard[16]

- DD-NR: SN 62 (NR), SP 64 (NR), +LR 1.7, –LR 0.59, QUADAS 8, in a study of 70 clients (90 temporomandibular joints) with various related pathology (mean age, gender, and duration of symptoms NR), and using MRI as a reference standard[16]

RESTRICTED LATERAL CONDYLAR TRANSLATION

Client Position	Sitting with mouth in resting position
Clinician Position	Standing directly in front of client monitoring for movement
Movement	The client laterally deviates their mandible from one side to the other.
Assessment	A (+) test is restricted or reduced movement of one side of mandible compared to the other.

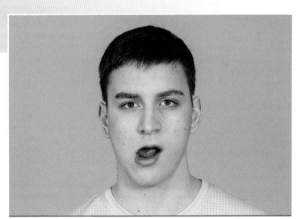

Figure 16.16

Statistics
- DD-R: SN 15 (NR), SP 34 (NR), +LR 0.22, –LR 2.5, QUADAS 8, in a study of 70 clients (90 temporomandibular joints) with various related pathology (mean age, gender, and duration of symptoms NR), and using MRI as a reference standard[16]

- DD-R: SN 66 (NR), SP 76 (NR), +LR 2.8, –LR 0.45, QUADAS 8, in a study of 70 clients (90 temporomandibular joints) with various related pathology (mean age, duration, and symptoms NR), and using MRI as a reference standard[16]

- DD-R: SN 11 (NR), SP 56 (NR), +LR 0.24, –LR 1.59, QUADAS 9, in a study of 273 clients with various characteristics of TMD (mean age 33.2 years, 221 women, mean duration of symptoms NR), and using MRI as a reference standard[44]

- DD-NR: SN 78 (NR), SP 83 (NR), +LR 4.4, –LR 0.27, QUADAS 9, in a study of 273 clients with various characteristics of TMD (mean age 33.2 years, 221 women, mean duration of symptoms NR), and using MRI as a reference standard[44]

- DD-NR: SN 69 (NR), SP 81 (NR), +LR 3.6, –LR 0.4, QUADAS 10, in a study of 137 consecutive clients with TMD (mean age 33.0 ± 15.4 years, 124 women, mean duration of symptoms NR) and 23 volunteers (mean age 19.6 ± 0.5 years, 20 women, and mean duration of symptoms NR), and using MRI as a reference standard[46]

DEVIATION OF MOUTH DURING OPENING

Client Position	Seated with mouth relaxed
Clinician Position	Standing to the side to be tested
Movement	The client is instructed to open their mouth as far as it will go. At this position, they are asked to deviate their mandible laterally in each direction.
Assessment	A (+) finding is any deviation from midline during opening or asymmetry in lateral deviation once the mouth is fully open (limited deviation to one side indicates it has already deviated some with normal opening).

Figure 16.17

Statistics
- DD-R with correction: SN 44 (NR), SP 83 (NR), +LR 2.6, –LR 0.67, QUADAS 8, in a study of 70 clients (90 temporomandibular joints) with various related pathology (mean age, gender, and duration of symptoms NR), and using MRI as a reference standard[16]

(continued)

Deviation of Mouth During Opening *(continued)*

- DD-R without correction: SN 18 (NR), SP 41 (NR), +LR 0.30, −LR 2.0, QUADAS 8, in a study of 70 clients (90 temporomandibular joints) with various related pathology (mean age, gender, and duration of symptoms NR), and using MRI as a reference standard[16]

- DD-NR with correction: SN 14 (NR), SP 57 (NR), +LR 0.33, −LR 1.5, QUADAS 8, in a study of 70 clients (90 temporomandibular joints) with various related pathology (mean age, gender, and duration of symptoms NR), and using MRI as a reference standard[16]

- DD-NR without correction: SN 66 (NR), SP 83 (NR), +LR 3.9, −LR 0.41, QUADAS 8, in a study of 70 clients (90 temporomandibular joints) with various related pathology (mean age, gender, and duration of symptoms NR), and using MRI as a reference standard[16]

- DD-R: SN 92 (NR), SP 31 (NR), +LR 1.3, −LR 0.25, QUADAS 7, in a study of 40 clients with TMJ complaints (mean age 32.6 years, 27 women, mean duration of symptoms NR), and using MRI as a reference standard[17]

- DD-NR: SN 35 (NR), SP 8 (NR), +LR 0.38, −LR 8.19, QUADAS 7, in a study of 40 clients with TMJ complaints (mean age 32.6 years, 27 women, mean duration of symptoms NR), and using MRI as a reference standard[17]

Critical Clinical Pearls

When examining limited joint motion at the TMJ, keep the following in mind:

- Capsular restriction will likely result in deviation toward the involved side.

- Restricted motion that occurs near normal opening (minimal opening limitation) is more likely a translation arthrokinematic restriction.

- Restricted motion that occurs near early opening (very limited opening) is more likely a rolling arthrokinematic restriction.

- Regarding a double click, the later in opening the initial click occurs and the earlier the second click occurs, the more anteriorly displaced the disc is likely to be.

CLUSTER TESTING

Pain in TMJ on palpation, function, and opening, with MRI as a reference standard for DD-NR

Pooled analysis: SN 68 (59-76), SP 68 (59-76), +LR 2.1, −LR 0.47, across two studies (n = 172 clients)[43]

Cluster (ROM, muscle–joint palpation, and joint sounds) with MRI as a reference standard for DD-R

Pooled analysis: SN 67 (60-74), SP 79 (74-83), +LR 3.0, −LR 0.42 across two studies (n = 282 clients)[43]

Cluster (ROM, muscle–joint palpation, and joint sounds) with MRI as a reference standard for DD-NR

Pooled analysis: SN 54 (47-61), SP 87 (83-90), +LR 4.1, −LR 0.66, across two studies (n = 282 clients)[43]

PALPATION

An association between the extent of tenderness and TMD has been shown (e.g., the greater the tenderness over the TMJ, the more severe the TMD).[47] Additionally, clients with localized or generalized muscle tenderness had more TMJ clicking than those without muscle tenderness.[47] The client with suspected TMD requires palpation examination of relevant cervical spine and head and face structures. Refer to chapter 17 (Cervical Spine) and chapter 15 (Face and Head) for additional detail on relevant structures of palpation. Specific to the TMJ, gentle and cautious palpation of the muscles of mastication can be necessary for many clients. These structures should be palpated for tenderness, structure, and normalcy. The primarily accessible and relevant musculature includes the masseter and temporalis bilaterally (figure 16.18 and 16.13*a*).

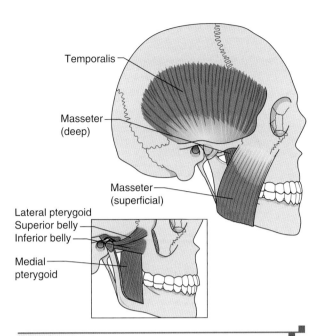

Figure 16.18 Masseter and temporalis muscles.

The TMJ joint itself should be palpated (see figure 16.13*b*). The easiest way to palpate the proximal mandible condyle or joint is posteriorly (this is typically easiest with palpation with a finger in each of the client's ears) or just anterior to the ears. The joint should also be palpated laterally in the same location. With palpation, the clinician can also assess for potential clicking or popping in the joint, as well as the amount and quality of condylar movement.

PHYSICAL PERFORMANCE MEASURES

No specific physical performance measures (PPMs) are available for the temporomandibular joint. The reader can refer to chapter 17 (Cervical Spine) for relevant PPMs for the temporomandibular joint.

COMMON ORTHOPEDIC CONDITIONS OF THE TEMPOROMANDIBULAR JOINT

While it is impossible to distinctly describe various pathological presentations of the temporoman-

dibular joint, there are evidence-based findings supportive of particular pathologies of this region of the body. Therefore, the intent of this section of the chapter is to present current evidence-supported findings suggestive of temporomandibular pathologies. As previously described in chapter 4 (Evidence-Based Practice and Client Examination), though, not all examination findings are absolutely supported with clinical evidence, and the clinician should also rely on clinical experience and input from the client when performing differential diagnosis of a client's presentation of pain and dysfunction.

There is significant discrepancy between authorities over the precise clinical features, and hence the diagnostic criteria, for TMD.[2] The terminology used to describe this symptom group is quite variable. The American Academy of Orofacial Pain (AAOP) classification utilizes broad categorization, including myogenous TMD, sometimes called TMD secondary to myofascial pain and dysfunction, and arthrogenous TMD, that is, TMD secondary to true articular disease. Myogenous TMD is more common. In its pure form, it lacks apparent destructive changes of the TMJ on radiograph and can be caused by multiple etiologies such as bruxism and other dentition-related aspects as well as stress and anxiety.[48]

Three other pain classifications are used for the orofacial region: the International Association for the Study of Pain classification system, the International Headache Society classification system, and the Research Diagnostic Criteria for Temporomandibular Disorder (RDC/TMD). The RDC/TMD Axis I diagnostic examination procedure employs a set of standardized clinical and questionnaire items. This procedure allows for assignment of TMD clients to any of three diagnostic groups that include eight subdiagnoses:[26]

- Group I: muscle disorders—(Ia) myofascial pain; (Ib) myofascial pain with limited opening
- Group II: disc displacements—(IIa) disc displacement with reduction; (IIb) disc displacement without reduction with limited opening; (IIc) disc displacement without reduction without limited opening
- Group III: arthralgia, arthritis, and arthrosis—(IIIa) arthralgia; (IIIb) osteoarthritis; (IIIc) osteoarthrosis

RDC/TMD nomenclature, especially that of group III, is not universally employed. Of the three subgroups, it was found that the muscle disorders were most frequently seen in community sample studies.[3]

Of particular concern to the practicing clinician is the diagnostic accuracy of this classification system. This dual-axis system proved to be finer to other instruments since it can be used to grade and measure both physical and psychological components.[26] However, revision of the current diagnostic algorithm is warranted due to only the myofascial pain's being without differentiation between normal and limited opening (targets set at SN ≥ 70, S ≥ 95).[28] Of additional concern is the applicability of this tool, which was designed to be implemented by maxillofacial surgeons. Therefore, its clinical applicability would seem limited. The 31-item questionnaire is a self-report measure.

Group I Muscle Disorders: (Ia) Myofascial Pain and (Ib) Myofascial Pain With Limited Opening

Myogenous Classification (AAOP)

ICD-9: 729.1 (myalgia and myositis, unspecified); 524.60 (temporomandibular joint disorders, unspecified)

ICD-10: M60.9 (myositis, unspecified); M26.60 (temporomandibular joint disorders, unspecified)

Diagnostic accuracy of the RDC/TMD Axis I diagnosis (group I):

- Group Ia: SN 65, **SP 92**, **+LR 8.1**, −LR 0.38, QUADAS 10, in a study of 614 clients with suspected various TMD (age range 18-70, duration of symptoms ranged from 0-72 months) and RDC/TMD Axis I diagnostic examination procedure utilizing a set of standardized clinical and questionnaire items[26] as a reference standard.[28]

- Group Ib: **SN 79**, **SP 92**, **+LR 9.9**, **−LR 0.23**, QUADAS 10, in a study of 614 clients with suspected various TMD (age range 18-70, duration of symptoms ranged from 0-72 months) and RDC/TMD Axis I diagnostic examination procedure utilizing a set of standardized clinical and questionnaire items[26] as a reference standard.[28]

- Combined: **SN 87, SP 98, +LR 43.5, −LR 0.13,** QUADAS 10, in a study of 614 clients with suspected various TMD (age range 18-70, duration of symptoms ranged from 0-72 months) and RDC/TMD Axis I diagnostic examination procedure utilizing a set of standardized clinical and questionnaire items[26] as a reference standard.[28]

I. Client Interview

Subjective History

- Pain localized over one or more of the masticatory muscles (usually masseter or temporalis).

- Fatigue with chewing.

- May have limited mandibular function secondary to pain.

- With myofascial pain, clients may have associated symptoms: tinnitus, vertigo, toothache, tension-type headaches.

- With myofascial pain, clients may have referral of pain.

Outcome Measures

- The Research Diagnostic Criteria for Temporomandibular Disorders instruments are better at **ruling out** (SN 86-87, −LR 0.25–0.45) than ruling in (SP 31-53) biobehavioral presentation.[27]

- Visual Analogue Scale (VAS), Numerical Scale (NS), Behavior Rating Scale (BRS), and Verbal Scale (VS) have been advocated in TMD clients.[2]

- Global Rating of Change (GROC) and Patient-Specific Functional Scale (PSFS) are recommended for assessment of intervention.

Diagnostic Imaging

- This category of TMD is much less likely to have (+) diagnostic imaging findings.[2, 49]

- Age, gender, and coarse crepitus, but no pain-related variables, were associated with increased risk of degenerative findings in TMJ tomograms.[50]

- Maximal opening < 40 mm for mandibular depression was associated with a posterior condyle-to-articular tubercle relation on opening in TMJ tomograms.[50]

- Refer to table 16.1 for various diagnostic accuracies regarding imaging and various pathologies (too numerous to mention here).

II. Observation

- Monitor for upper crossed syndrome and general poor posture.

III. Triage and Screening

- All non-musculoskeletal causes, as well as causes from related joints, should be ruled out.
- Rule out discogenic-related pathology:
  - Spurling's test: **SN 93**, **SP 95**, **+LR 19.6**, **−LR 0.07**, QUADAS 9.[40]
  - Median nerve upper limb tension test: **SN 97**, SP 22, +LR 1.3, **−LR 0.12**, QUADAS 10.[41]

IV. Motion Tests

- Sometimes clients will have limited AROM of mouth opening (mandibular depression) dependent on muscles involved (mandible depressors, protruders, elevators).
- Decreased mandibular ROM is likely with this classification of TMD.[49]

V. Muscle Performance Testing

- Pain in the TMJ during resistive movements provides no benefit for ruling in or ruling out TMD.[15]

VI. Special Tests

- Almost all described special tests are relative to DD-R and DD-NR. The clinician should understand that myogenous pain contribution to TMD can coexist with disc displacement and should clinically reason the appropriateness of special tests as described.
- Pain in TMJ on palpation, function, and opening, with MRI as a reference standard for DD-NR, may be appropriate for the myogenous category due to each of the listed restrictions having a myogenous component. Unfortunately, this cluster of testing has very limited ability (with pooled analysis) to help rule out (SN 68, −LR 0.47) or rule in (SP 68, +LR 2.1) TMD.[43]

VII. Palpation

- Involved masticatory muscles are likely tender to palpation (again, most likely are masseter and temporalis).
- Despite traditional descriptions of its clinical utility, palpation of the lateral pterygoid muscle lacks evidence support, and has been suggested to be discontinued.[51]
- It is nearly impossible to palpate the inferior portion of the lateral pterygoid anatomically.[52]
- Care must be taken when judging findings of palpation of lateral pterygoid due to findings of palpation of this structure not reaching acceptable values of SN 80 and SP 77 in the myofascial pain diagnosis.[53]
- Clients with localized or generalized muscle tenderness had more TMJ clicking than those without muscle tenderness.[47]
- Jaw clenching may provoke acute muscle tenderness, but it has not been proven to be analogous to myogenous TMD.[36]

VIII. Physical Performance Measures

- See chapter 17 (Cervical Spine).

POTENTIAL TREATMENT-BASED CLASSIFICATIONS

- Pain, mobility, exercise, and conditioning are most likely.

Group II Disc Displacements: (IIa) Disc Displacement With Reduction, (IIb) Disc Displacement Without Reduction With Limited Opening, and (IIc) Disc Displacement Without Reduction Without Limited Opening

Arthrogenous Classification (AAOP)

ICD-9: 524.6 (temporomandibular joint disorders, unspecified)

ICD-10: K07.6 (temporomandibular joint disorders), M26.6 (temporomandibular joint disorder, unspecified)

Diagnostic accuracy of the RDC/TMD Axis I diagnosis (group II):

- SN 3-38, SP 88-99, +LR 0.25–38, −LR 1.1–0.62, QUADAS 10, in a study of 614 clients with suspected various TMD (age range 18-70, duration of symptoms ranged from 0-72 months) and RDC/TMD Axis I diagnostic examination procedure utilizing a set of standardized clinical and questionnaire items[26] as a reference standard.[28]

I. Client Interview

Subjective History

- Headache, TMJ sounds, and pain in the face or neck.[54]
- More likely to have history of trauma, history of jaw lock, TMD complaints with activities including seeing dentist, and so on.[49, 54]
- Early morning pain and stiffness likely; often improved with mandibular activity (if capsular restriction is predominant).[49]
- Pain and fear or apprehension noted with mandible depression, especially with disc displacement that has history of not reducing pain or causing significant pain.[49]

Outcome Measures

- The Research Diagnostic Criteria for Temporomandibular Disorders instruments are better at helping to **rule out** (SN 86-87, −LR 0.25–0.45) than ruling in (SP 31-53) biobehavioral presentation.[27]
- Visual Analogue Scale (VAS), Numerical Scale (NS), Behavior Rating Scale (BRS), and Verbal Scale (VS) have been advocated in TMD clients.[2]
- Global Rating of Change (GROC) and Patient-Specific Functional Scale (PSFS) are recommended for assessment of intervention.

Diagnostic Imaging

- Age, gender, and coarse crepitus, but no pain-related variables, were associated with increased risk of degenerative findings in TMJ tomograms.[50]
- Maximal opening < 40 mm for mandibular depression was associated with a posterior condyle-to-articular tubercle relation on opening in TMJ tomograms.[50]
- US (**SP 82-91**)[29, 30] and MRI (**SP 100**)[31] serve better to help rule in than rule out disc displacement; disc displacement with reduction is slightly more diagnostic than without reduction.
- Refer to table 16.1 for various diagnostic accuracies regarding imaging and various pathologies (too numerous to mention here).

II. Observation

- Look for deviation and deflection with mandible depression and elevation.[49, 50, 54, 55]
- The relationship between GJH and TMD remains unclear.[39]

III. Triage and Screening

- All non-musculoskeletal causes, as well as causes from related joints, should be ruled out.
- Rule out discogenic-related pathology:
  - Spurling's test: **SN 93**, **SP 95**, **+LR 19.6**, **−LR 0.07**, QUADAS 9[40]
  - Median nerve upper limb tension test: **SN 97**, SP 22, +LR 1.3, **−LR 0.12**, QUADAS 10[41]

IV. Motion Tests

- Decreased mandibular ROM is present with this classification of TMD.[49]
- Look for limited active mandibular opening, lateral deviation (typically to involved side most notably), and protrusion (deviation to involved side) with capsular restriction or disc displacement anteriorly on that side.[49]

V. Muscle Performance Testing

- Pain in the TMJ during resistive movements provides no benefit to rule in or rule out TMD.[15]

VI. Special Tests

- Deviation (+LR 6.4) and crepitation (+LR 5.9) as single tests and crepitation, deflection, pain, and limited mouth opening as a cluster of tests are the most valuable for helping to **rule in** DD-NR (+LR 6.4), while the test cluster click, deviation, and pain helps **rule out** DD-R (−LR 0.09).[43]

- No single test or cluster of tests was conclusive and of significant value for ruling in DD-R.[43]

- Pain in TMJ on palpation, function, and opening, with MRI as a reference standard for DD-NR, may have some limited ability to help **rule in** (SP 87, +LR 4.1) TMD.[43]

VII. Palpation

- Observe for tenderness of muscles in the jaw or head and sounds on condylar movement. Women had a higher prevalence of these signs.[54]

- The greater the tenderness over the TMJ, the more severe the TMD.[47]

- Clients with localized or generalized muscle tenderness had more TMJ clicking than those without muscle tenderness.[47]

- Despite traditional descriptions of its clinical utility, palpation of the lateral pterygoid muscle lacks evidence support and has been suggested to be discontinued.[51]

- It is nearly impossible to palpate the inferior portion of the lateral pterygoid anatomically.[52]

VIII. Physical Performance Measures

- See chapter 17 (Cervical Spine).

POTENTIAL TREATMENT-BASED CLASSIFICATIONS

- Pain, mobility, exercise, and conditioning are most likely.

Group III Arthralgia, Arthritis, and Arthrosis: (IIIa) Arthralgia, (IIIb) Osteoarthritis, and (IIIc) Osteoarthrosis

Arthrogenous Classification (AAOP): Inflammatory Disorders (Capsulitis/Arthritis)

ICD-9: 524.69 (other specified temporomandibular joint disorders)

ICD-10: M26.69 (other specified disorders of temporomandibular joint)

Diagnostic accuracy of the RDC/TMD Axis I diagnosis (group III):

- Group IIIa: SN 53, SP 86, +LR 3.8, −LR 0.55, QUADAS 10, in a study of 614 clients with suspected various TMD (age range 18-70, duration of symptoms ranged from 0-72 months) and RDC/TMD Axis I diagnostic examination procedure utilizing a set of standardized clinical and questionnaire items[26] as a reference standard.[28]

- Group IIIb/IIIc: SN 15, **SP 98-99**, **+LR 7.5–15**, −LR 0.87, QUADAS 10, in a study of 614 clients with suspected various TMD (age range 18-70, duration of symptoms ranged from 0-72 months) and RDC/TMD Axis I diagnostic examination procedure utilizing a set of standardized clinical and questionnaire items[26] as a reference standard.[28]

I. Client Interview

Subjective History

- Pain in TMJ or in front of ear.
- Pain exacerbated by jaw function.
- May have limited mandibular function secondary to pain.
- Early morning pain and stiffness likely; often improved with mandibular activity (if capsular).[49]
- These conditions are frequent in TMD due to the cyclical nature of TMD. Clients have chronic pain, learn to adapt, then experience an exacerbation of symptoms.[56]
- Pain can be present in clients with both DD-R and DD-NR, despite the fact that these conditions are traditionally chronic in nature. The acute pain experienced by the client is most likely due to capsulitis or synovitis.[56]

Outcome Measures

- The Research Diagnostic Criteria for Temporomandibular Disorders instruments are better at helping to **rule out** (SN 86–87%, −LR 0.25–0.45) than ruling in (SP 31–53%) biobehavioral presentation.[27]
- Visual Analogue Scale (VAS), Numerical Scale (NS), Behavior Rating Scale (BRS), and Verbal Scale (VS) have been advocated in TMD clients.[2]

- Global Rating of Change (GROC) and Patient-Specific Functional Scale (PSFS) are recommended for assessment of intervention.

Diagnostic Imaging

- US (SP 74-100) is better able to help **rule in** than rule out joint effusion.[32]
- MRI (SP 84) is slightly better able to help **rule in** than rule out bone marrow changes.[34]
- CBCT (SP 83-90) and MDCT (SP 86-87) are better able to help **rule in** than rule out condylar osseous changes.[35]
- Age, gender, and coarse crepitus, but no pain-related variables, were associated with increased risk of degenerative findings in TMJ tomograms.[50]
- Maximal opening < 40 mm for mandibular depression was associated with a posterior condyle-to-articular tubercle relation on opening in TMJ tomograms.[50]
- Refer to table 16.1 for additional detail on various diagnostic accuracies regarding imaging and various pathologies (too numerous to mention here).

II. Observation

- Clients may have limited mouth opening or deviation with mouth opening.
- Monitor for upper crossed syndrome and general poor posture.
- Capsular restriction will have lateral jaw deviation with mandible depression (as described in the Motion Tests section that follows).

III. Triage and Screening

- All non-musculoskeletal causes, as well as causes from related joints, should be ruled out.
- Rule out discogenic-related pathology:
  - Spurling's test: **SN 93**, **SP 95**, **+LR 19.6**, **−LR 0.07**, QUADAS 9[40]
  - Median nerve upper limb tension test: **SN 97**, SP 22, +LR 1.3, **−LR 0.12**, QUADAS 10[41]

IV. Motion Tests

- Pain becomes worse with clenching or biting down on involved side.[49]
- Decreased mandibular ROM is present with this classification of TMD.[49]
- Clients have limited active mandibular opening, lateral deviation (typically to involved side most notably), and protrusion (deviation to involved side) with capsular restriction on that side.[49]
- Crepitus, grinding, or clicking may be noted, especially with arthrosis or arthritis.[49]

V. Muscle Performance Testing

- Pain in the TMJ during resistive movements provides no benefit for ruling in or ruling out TMD.[15]

VI. Special Tests

- Almost all described special tests are relative to DD-R and DD-NR. The clinician should understand that the contribution of pain from arthralgia, arthrosis, or arthritis to TMD can coexist with disc displacement and should clinically reason the appropriateness of special tests as described.
- ROM limitation, muscle-joint pain, and joint sounds with MRI reference standard for DD-NR may be most appropriate for this category. Unfortunately, this cluster of testing has limited ability (with pooled analysis) to help rule out (SN 68, −LR 0.47) or rule in (SP 68, +LR 2.1) TMD.[43]
- Pain in TMJ on palpation, function, and opening, with MRI as a reference standard for DD-NR, may be appropriate for this category. Unfortunately, this cluster of testing has limited ability (with pooled analysis) to help rule out (SN 54, −LR 0.66) TMD, with some ability to help **rule in** (SP 87, +LR 4.1) TMD.[43]

VII. Palpation

- Tenderness to palpation over joint and corresponding musculature can be present.
- The greater the tenderness over the TMJ, the more severe the TMD.[47]
- Clients with localized or generalized muscle tenderness had more TMJ clicking than those without muscle tenderness.[47]

- Despite traditional descriptions of its clinical utility, palpation of the lateral pterygoid muscle lacks evidence support, and has been suggested to be discontinued.[51]
- It is nearly impossible to palpate the inferior portion of the lateral pterygoid anatomically.[52]

VIII. Physical Performance Measures

- See chapter 17 (Cervical Spine).

POTENTIAL TREATMENT-BASED CLASSIFICATIONS

- Pain, mobility, exercise, and conditioning are most likely.

Differential Diagnosis of Temporomandibular Disorders

In general, the current diagnostic accuracy of the various tests for TMD make it difficult for clinicians to discriminate the various pathologies.

Muscle Disorders

- Myofascial pain: Clients often have tinnitus, toothache, and tension-type headaches; pain is often localized to masticatory muscles, but clients may have referral of pain.
- Myofascial pain with limited opening: same as preceding list but with limited ability to open mouth.

Disc Displacements

- Disc displacement with reduction
- Disc displacement without reduction with limited opening
- Disc displacement without reduction without limited opening
  - All with likely history of trauma, pain, apprehension with opening, especially those clients without disc reduction
  - Cluster testing helpful for ruling in disc displacement without reduction
  - No tests significant for ruling in disc displacement with reduction

Arthralgia, Arthritis, Arthrosis

- Arthralgia
- Osteoarthritis
- Osteoarthrosis
  - Pain is often exacerbated with jaw function for all categories.
  - Clients with all conditions are likely to have limited mandibular function and stiffness, especially in morning.
  - Typically these conditions are chronic in nature.

Bruxism ▪ ▪ ▪ ▪ ▪ ▪ ▪ ▪ ▪ ▪ ▪ ▪ ▪ ▪ ▪ ▪

ICD-9: 327.53 (sleep-related bruxism)

ICD-10: G47.63 (sleep-related bruxism)

Bruxism is clenching of the teeth, causing them to grind during sleep or on early awakening. Clients are often unaware that they clench and grind their teeth. Bruxism can occur during both the day and night, although sleep-related bruxism is often the bigger problem because it is harder to control. The cause of bruxism is not completely agreed on, but daily stress may be the trigger. Some clients probably clench their teeth and never have symptoms. Whether or not bruxism causes pain and other problems may involve a complicated mix of factors: the amount of stress the client is encountering, how long and tightly they clench their teeth, whether or not their teeth are misaligned, posture, the client's ability to relax, diet, and sleeping habits. Symptoms often can include any of the following: anxiety; stress or tension; depression;

earache; eating disorders; headache; tooth sensitivity to hot, cold, or sweetness; insomnia; and sore or painful jaw. The client with bruxism will likely have a combination of these signs and symptoms.

Malocclusion

ICD-9: 524.4 (malocclusion, unspecified)

ICD-10: M26.4 (malocclusion, unspecified)

Malocclusion, a misalignment of teeth or incorrect relation between the teeth of the two dental arches, is often referred to as irregular bite, crossbite, or overbite. Malocclusion may be seen as crooked, crowded, or protruding teeth, and it can have profound effects on speech, eating, and overall sense of well-being due to appearance. The most common types of malocclusion are the following:

- Upper protrusion: The upper front teeth are more anterior than the lower front teeth. This is commonly referred to as *buck teeth*. A small lower jaw, pacifier use, and thumb-sucking have all been postulated as potential contributors to this condition.

- Crowded teeth: Too little room for teeth can cause crowding, which can prevent permanent teeth from coming in properly or at all (impaction).

- Overbite: The upper front teeth overlap too far down on the lower front teeth.

- Open bite: The upper and lower front teeth do not overlap.

- Overjet: The upper front teeth angle out horizontally.

- Underbite: The lower front teeth are farther forward than the upper front teeth.

- Crossbite: Any or all of the upper front teeth fit into the wrong side of the lower teeth (medial or lateral horizontal movement from neutral).

A commonly described classification system for malocclusion is normal occlusion, class I occlusion, class II malocclusion, and class III malocclusion (figure 16.19). Normal occlusion is the generally accepted normal presentation of upper and lower teeth relationship. In class I malocclusion, although the upper and lower molars are properly positioned, the teeth crowd together or have too much space. Crossbites, rotations, and overlapping can also occur in severe cases. In class II malocclusion, the

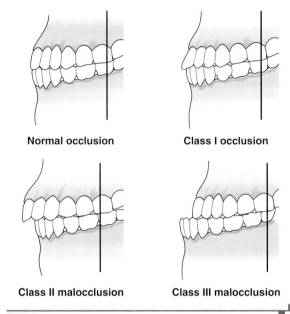

Figure 16.19 Malocclusion classifications.

lower molars fit with the upper molars, but they are positioned toward the throat, drawing the mandible posterior (retrognathia). This is commonly referred to as an overbite. In a class III malocclusion, the lower molars are far forward of the upper molars, creating a jutting jaw (prognathia) and a crossbite with the upper teeth. This is commonly referred to as an underbite.

An association between molar loss and pain, clicking, and progression to locking in these clients has been suggested, but it does not demonstrate a strong correlation.[55]

CONCLUSION

The TMJ and craniomandibular complex is becoming increasingly more recognized as a potential pain-generating complex for the client with pain in the upper quarter, neck, face or head. As with most other body parts, accurately differentially diagnosing the potential pathologies requires a systematic, evidence-based funnel approach. The vast majority of special tests for the TMJ demonstrate limited diagnostic accuracy. Therefore, as with all body regions, clinicians should use the entire examination sequence and all of its components when examining this body region.

17

CERVICAL SPINE

Michael P. Reiman, PT, DPT, OCS, SCS, ATC, FAAOMPT, CSCS

Neck pain and corresponding disability is a common dysfunction. Twenty-five percent of clients receiving outpatient physical therapy have neck pain.[1] Neck pain prevalence in those over the age of 25 years is 20.6%, behind only low back and shoulder pain.[2] Neck pain is second only to low back pain (LBP) in annual workers' compensation costs in the United States.[3] At any given point in time, 10% to 20% of the general population reports neck problems,[4-7] with 54% of those people having experienced pain within the last 6 months.[8] The prevalence of neck pain increases as one ages. Additionally, it is most common in women around the fifth decade of life.[7, 9, 10]

As high as 37% of those with neck pain will develop chronic neck pain for at least 6 months.[6, 7] Similar to the clients with chronic LBP, the longer these clients are off work, the less likely they will be to return to previous work levels. Age > 40 years, a long history of neck pain, bicycling as a regular activity, loss of strength in the hands, worrisome attitude, poor quality of life, and less vitality have been demonstrated to be predisposing factors for the development of chronic neck pain.[11] Obviously, avoiding progression to chronicity is key to successful recovery for these clients.

CLINICALLY APPLIED ANATOMY

The cervical spine allows for more motion than any other region of the spine. Thirty-seven joints make up the cervical spine. The cervical spine consists of seven vertebrae, and it has been divided into four anatomical units: the atlas, the axis, the C2-C3 junction, and the rest of the cervical vertebrae (figure 17.1).[12] The third through seventh vertebrae

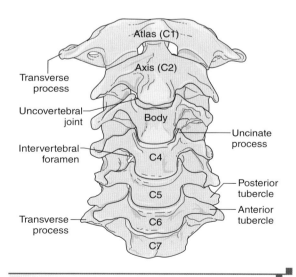

Figure 17.1 Anterior view of cervical spine.

287

follow a typical morphology with minor variations. These lower cervical vertebrae are often described as a functional unit.

The craniovertebral junction is a collective term that refers to the occiput, atlas, axis, and supporting ligaments. This region of the spine is designed for a large amount of movement. The lower five cervical vertebrae have load-bearing, stability, and mobility functions. These vertebrae are common in their characteristic osteology and function. The vertebral body, as well as its superior and inferior end plates, typically has a greater transverse diameter than anteroposterior diameter and height.

Due to the presence of the uncinate processes along the posterolateral edges, the superior surface of the body of a lower cervical vertebra is concave in the frontal plane, while the superior surfaces slope forward and downward in the sagittal plane. The inferior surface of the vertebra is concave with an anterior lip that projects anteroinferiorly toward the anterior superior edge of the vertebra below.[13]

The transverse processes of the cervical spine have a groove for the spinal nerves exiting the spinal cord. Two parts of each transverse process have been described, an anterior and posterior tubercle (figure 17.2). The transverse processes have several muscle attachments, while the spinous process primarily has ligamentous attachments.

The spinous processes extend inferiorly and are typically short and slender. These spinous processes are bifid at their tip. Their length decreases slightly from C2 to C3, remains constant from C3 to C5, and significantly lengthens at C7 (figure 17.3).[14]

Each vertebra has a superior and inferior articular facet that articulates with the vertebra either above or below. Each articular facet is teardrop shaped with the superior facet facing superior and posterior, while the inferior facet faces inferior and anterior. The average horizontal angle of the joint planes of the middle cervical segments is approximately 45° between the transverse and horizontal planes. Upper cervical levels are closer to 35° and lower levels approximate 65°, although clinically the joint planes are thought of as passing at an angle, that if extended, would pass through the client's nose.

The primary joint articulations in the cervical spine are the atlantooccipital joint, atlantoaxial joint, intervertebral joints, and the facet joints. The atlantooccipital joint (C0-1) is primarily involved in cervical nodding motion, while the atlantoaxial (C1-2) joint functions predominantly with rotation.

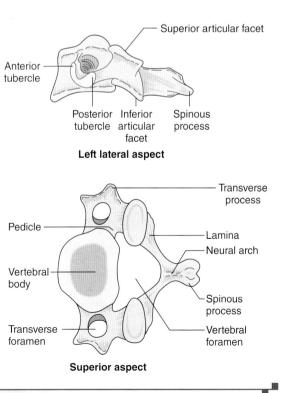

Figure 17.2 Typical cervical vertebra.

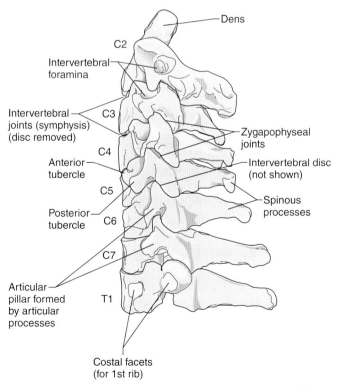

Figure 17.3 Lateral view of cervical spine.

The facet joints in the cervical spine perform flexion, extension, side bending, and rotation.

CLIENT INTERVIEW

The interview is typically the first encounter the clinician has with the client. As previously discussed in chapter 5 (Client Interview and Observation), this component of the examination can provide the clinician with a significant amount of information relevant to the probability of the client's presenting diagnosis. For purposes of this text, the interview is described relative to each body part or section, but generally includes subjective reports by the client, as well as findings from their outcome measures. Additionally included in this section is radiographic imaging. While clinicians should avoid biasing their examination by interpreting findings of radiographic imaging prior to seeing the client (in most cases without concerns for red flags and major medical-related issues), this point in the examination is most likely where clinicians will encounter radiographic imaging. Additionally, in some instances, clinicians must interpret radiographic imaging early in the examination to rule out serious pathology prior to continuing with other components of the examination sequence.

Subjective

As with all regions of the body, the subjective examination for the client with neck pain should be deliberate and focused. Determining pain location can be very helpful in differentiating the potential pain generator. Since pain generated at the cervical spine can produce upper extremity radicular pain, careful differential diagnosis is necessary. Inquiring as to location of pain, movements that aggravate pain, mechanism of onset, symptom duration, and relieving factors can help the clinician determine if the presenting upper extremity pain is due to cervical spine causes or otherwise.

Cervical discogenic pain typically causes pain in a dermatomal pattern. Irritation of the nerve or nerve root may not necessarily present with a specific dermatomal pattern. An additional consideration is the possible presentation of Cloward areas. Cloward, using provocative discography of the cervical discs, demonstrated that disc injuries in the cervical spine can refer pain to the tho-

racic spine, especially along the medial scapular border. For example, it was discovered that the C3-4 disc referred pain to the cervicothoracic junction and ipsilateral upper trapezius, the C4-5 disc referred to the superior-medial border of the scapula, the C5-6 disc referred to the midscapular level, and the C6-7 disc referred to the lower scapular level. All of the these referral zones were to the ipsilateral side of the medial scapular border.[15] More recent findings not only support the findings of Cloward but also demonstrate the value of pain drawings on the part of the client.[16, 17]

The pain location can be helpful in determining the pain generator. While the location of pain presentation for clients with radiculopathy can be variable, clients are most likely to have pain above the elbow (SP 93) and typically in the cervical spine region.[18] Pain isolated to a specific area of the cervical spine has been more commonly described for clients with mechanical neck pain and cervicogenic-related headaches.[11]

Pain referral from the facet joint is dependent on the level of dysfunction (figure 17.4). While there are discrepancies among sources, typically pain in the occipital region was referred from C2-3 and C3, while pain in the upper posterolateral cervical region was referred from C0-1, C1-2, and C2-3. Pain in the upper posterior cervical region was referred from C2-3, C3-4, and C3; that in the middle posterior cervical region from C3-4, C4-5, and C4; and that in the lower posterior cervical region from C4-5, C5-6, C4, and C5. In addition, pain in the suprascapular region was referred from C4-5, C5-6, and C4; that in the superior angle of the scapula from C6-7, C6, and C7; and that in the midscapular region from C7-T1 and C7.[19]

Upper cervical spine pain location has been more common in cervicogenic-related headaches,[20-24] although the clinician should be cognizant of the potential for cervical spine instability.[11] Additionally, concern for arterial damage should be heightened with a reasonable mechanism and broad, vague pain distribution (figure 17.5).

Specific questions of concern for serious pathology or red flag concerns are listed later in this chapter (see the section Triage and Screening) as well as in chapter 6. Regarding the mechanism of injury, Grieve[25] suggests three mandatory questions that, when positive, should heighten the clinician's concern for serious pathology:

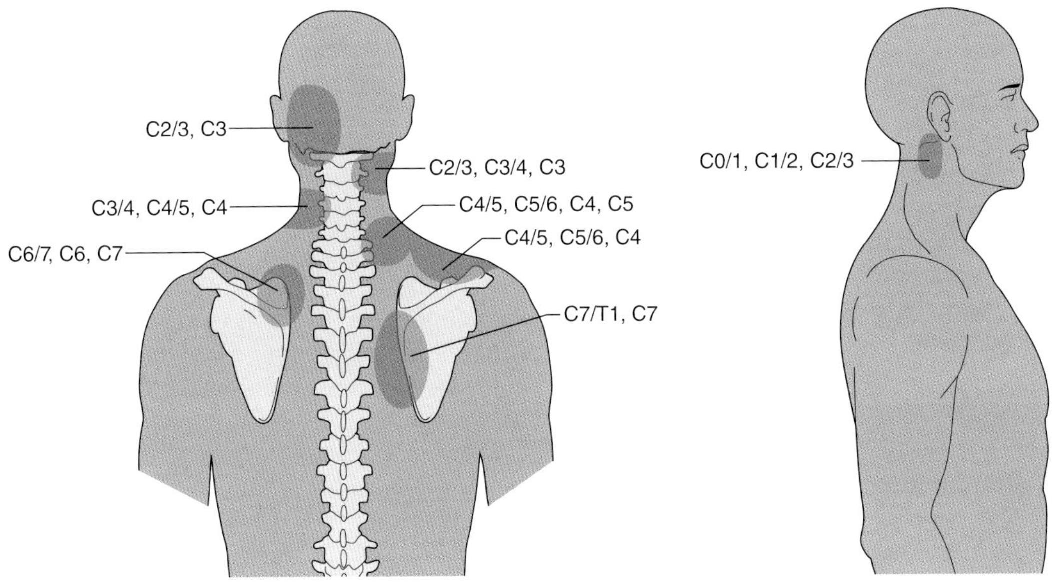

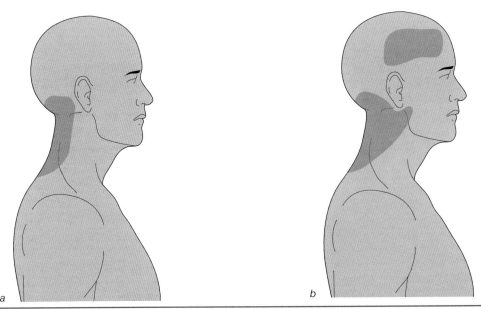

C2/3, C3

C2/3, C3/4, C3

C3/4, C4/5, C4

C4/5, C5/6, C4, C5

C6/7, C6, C7

C4/5, C5/6, C4

C7/T1, C7

C0/1, C1/2, C2/3

Figure 17.4 Main referred pain distributions for the cervical spine.

1. Any dizziness (vertigo), blackouts, or drop attacks?
2. Any history of rheumatoid arthritis (RA) or other inflammatory arthritis or treatment by systemic steroid?
3. Any neurological symptoms in arms and legs?

Understanding the answers to these particular questions can assist the clinician in determining the extent of the follow-up examination. In fact, these questions could determine whether the client can appropriately continue with the examination or needs referral to another health care provider or further testing. With deliberate questioning the clinician can also ascertain whether or not the client has sensory or muscle deficits. This understanding again would assist with prioritization of the continued examination.

a

b

Figure 17.5 Typical pain distribution relating to *(a)* vertebral artery dissection and *(b)* internal carotid artery dissection.

The mechanism of onset is of significant importance. As is discussed in the section Triage and Screening, specific traumatic mechanisms should alert the clinician to the possibility of the potential for serious pathology, red flags, or the need for additional diagnostic imaging.[26, 27] Questions regarding motor vehicle accidents or high-level trauma should be detailed to the extent of fully understanding the mechanism. High-grade lesions to the alar ligament, transverse ligament, and the posterior atlantooccipital membrane were most common in those clients with a head rotated posture versus facing ahead posture.[28] Elongation-induced vertebral artery injuries were also found in head rotated postures versus nonrotated postures.[29] Severe injuries to the transverse ligament and the posterior atlantooccipital membrane were more common in front than in rear-end collisions.[28]

If the risk of serious pathology is deemed low and the clinician reasons continuing the examination is prudent, the severity, irritability, nature, and stage of the client's pain should be delineated. Understanding the extent of these variables will help the clinician determine not only the pain generator but also the extent of disability and seriousness of the client's current condition. The severity and irritability of the client's condition could determine the acuity of the condition as well as the extent of the condition. Typically, but not always, more chronic conditions are less severe and irritable. Asking about the client's tolerance of daily tasks can be a good determiner of severity and irritability. Notable increases in pain level with minimal daily activity should alert clinicians to the fact that they may not be able to complete the full examination in one visit due to a probable high degree of irritability. A pain level that is consistently high (7/10 or greater) has been suggested to be a determining factor for classification in the pain control treatment-based classification category.[30]

Looking for a collection of similar subjective findings is helpful for the clinician. Clients with cervical radiculopathy, for example, have described the following: having a loss of feeling (SP 92), their most bothersome location of symptoms is in the neck (SP 90) and in the arm above the elbow (SP 93), with greater pain there than in the shoulder or scapula or below the elbow (SP 83 for both). While the collection of these findings together strengthens the case for cervical radiculopathy, none of the subjective history from this study showed the ability to rule out cervical radiculopathy if they were not present.[18]

Description of the nature of the pain, as well as aggravating or relieving factors, is helpful in determining not only the potential pain generator, but also the possibility that the pain is not mechanical in nature. Pain with Valsalva maneuver, for example, helps rule in (SP 94, +LR 3.7) the possibility of cervical radiculopathy.[18] More seriously, pain that is constant and unrelieved by rest or positioning has long been suggested as a risk for being potentially nonmusculoskeletal in nature. Pain of this presentation should be treated as such until proven otherwise.

Inquiring about specific job and leisure activities that are aggravating and relieving can be valuable information in determining the client's clinical presentation. Limited mobility and concordant pain serve both screening (SN 100) and diagnostic (SP 100) capability for the client with pain related to mechanical facet joints.[31] Unilateral upper cervical region pain that is accompanied with limited cervical spine rotation at C1-2 is more diagnostic (SP 100) than screening (SN 86),[24] while chronic neck pain associated with abnormal cervical spine motion is characteristic of whiplash-associated disorder (WAD).[32] Finally, decreased cervical rotation is characteristic of cervical radiculopathy[18] and is expected in stenosis.

The client's age can assist in determining the potential pathology or pain generator. Older age is suggested and has been predictive of certain pathologies, including cervical stenosis and myelopathy.[33] Meanwhile clients with mechanically related neck pain are more likely to be younger than 50 years of age.[11]

Headaches (HAs) are a common complaint. The International Headache Society suggests four primary types of HAs: migraine, tension-type, cluster and other trigeminal autonomic cephalalgias, and other primary HAs.[34] It has been reported that 14% to 18% of HAs are cervicogenic in nature with upper cervical spine pain presentation. The orthopedic or sports clinician will very likely encounter clients with cervicogenic-related HAs. More detail regarding the differentiation between the types of HAs is listed in the back of the chapter (see the section Common Orthopedic Conditions of the Cervical Spine) under the diagnosis cervicogenic HA. In short, cervicogenic HAs typically have a mechanical nature to them but do not have an aura, and they are aggravated by neck movement and palpation of the upper cervical spine.[34]

Some other questions of importance to ask the client include their current health status, any family history that may be relevant to their current condition, their normal job and leisure activities (even if

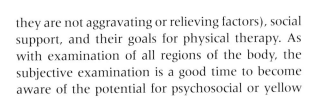

they are not aggravating or relieving factors), social support, and their goals for physical therapy. As with examination of all regions of the body, the subjective examination is a good time to become aware of the potential for psychosocial or yellow flag issues.

Outcome Measures

Reliable and valid self-report questionnaires are useful in assessing pain, function, disability, and psychosocial status in clients with neck pain.[35] In fact, consistent evidence shows that client self-assessment questionnaires may have utility in routine clinical practice and research by characterizing clients' clinical presentation and subjective functional effect of neck pain and course over time.[35] The clinician should always be cognizant of the client's interpretation of their symptoms, or how pain affects their daily life, as well as the potential for psychosocial issues that may affect prognosis. Outcome measures are a good tool for assessing these constructs.

The Neck Disability Index (NDI) is one of the more common outcome measures utilized for the client with cervical dysfunction. It is available in multiple languages as well. The NDI contains 10 items: 7 related to activities of daily living, 2 related to pain, and 1 related to concentration. Each item is scored from 0 to 5, and the total score is expressed as a percentage, with higher scores corresponding to greater disability.[36] Despite the fact that it has been described as a one-dimensional measure, the NDI has demonstrated that it is strongly correlated (>0.70) to a number of similar indices and is moderately related to both physical and mental aspects of general health.[37] Additionally, the NDI has been shown to possess adequate SN.[38, 39] The minimum detectable change (MDC) for the NDI is around 5/50 for uncomplicated neck pain and up to 10/50 for cervical radiculopathy.[37] The minimal clinical important difference (MCID) for clients with mechanical neck pain is 9.5 points or 19%.[40] Others have suggested a MDC of 10.2 and 7.5 on the MCID.[41] Therefore, it likely is pathology dependent when interpreting the level of clinically important change.[37]

The Patient-Specific Functional Scale (PSFS) has been shown to be a reliable tool for cervical spine clients. The intraclass correlation coefficient (ICC) valued for clients with cervical radiculopathy was 0.82. The MDC in the same population was 2.1 points with an MCID of 2.0.[42] While there are other reported measures for the cervical spine, the NDI demonstrates the strongest clinical utility. A recent practice guideline gave the NDI a strong recommendation.[11]

The Global Rating of Change (GROC) is a favorable scale for demonstration of client progression with treatment. As with all regions of the body, an 11-point GROC scale with a corresponding minimal clinically important difference (MCID) of 2 points is suggested.[43]

Diagnostic Imaging

As with other regions of the body, diagnostic imaging can be very beneficial in providing detailed information for the clinician regarding assessment of the client (table 17.1). However, as with other areas of the body, this information can be either misleading or irrelevant. Imaging studies often report findings that might have little to do with neck pain:[44]

- No evidence exists that the degree of cervical lordosis or kyphosis can accurately identify cervical muscle spasm or distinguish clients with whiplash-associated disorder (WAD) from those without WAD.

- No evidence exists that magnetic resonance imaging (MRI) accurately detects specific trauma-related findings in the cervical spine in the absence of fracture or major ligamentous disruption.

- Degenerative changes observed in MRI are common in asymptomatic subjects and increase with age. These are not well correlated with neck pain.

- The validity of high-intensity signal MRI findings in the upper cervical spine ligaments to identify acute whiplash injury has not been demonstrated.

- No evidence exists that common degenerative changes on cervical spine MRI are the cause of pain in clients with clinically suspected cervicogenic headache.

Radiographs

Plain radiography of the cervical spine has certain advantages over more advanced imaging techniques. Imaging is inexpensive, quick, and easy to perform, and exposes the client to significantly less radiation than computed tomography (CT) scans. However, radiographs are insensitive to many dis-

TABLE 17.1   Diagnostic Accuracy of Various Imaging Modalities for the Cervical Spine

Pathology	Diagnostic test	Gold standard	SN/SP (95%CI)
CAD/ vertebrobasilar circulation	CTA	Clinical follow-up until day 90 including MRA and DSA	100/90[45]
	US		38.5/100[45]
	CT	Variable	Pooled analysis: 79/97[46]
	TCD	DSA	87/80[47]
Acute unstable cervical spine injury following blunt trauma	CT	Variable	>99.9/> 99.9[48]
Cervical spine injuries	Plain radiograph	Variable	Pooled analysis: SN 52/SP not calculated due to gold standard variability[49]
	Plain radiographs: standard views of the cervical spine (lateral, anteroposterior, open-mouth odontoid, and submental views)	Radiographic interpretations	81/93[50]
	Adding oblique views to the above standard views		76(69-83)/90(87-93)[50]
	CT	Variable	Pooled analysis: SN 98/SP not calculated due to gold standard variability[49]
	CCHR	Variable	99-100/48-77[51]
WAD	MRI	Clinical findings and interobserver reliability	33/73[52]

CI = confidence interval; CAD = cervical artery dysfunction; CT = computed tomography; CTA = computed tomography angiography; DSA = digital subtraction angiography; US = ultrasound imaging; MRA = magnetic resonance arthroscopy; CCHR = Canadian Computed Tomography Head Rule; DSA = digital subtraction angiography; TCD = transcranial Doppler ultrasound; WAD = whiplash-associated disorder

The color coding for suggestion of good and ideal diagnostic accuracy values reported in this table are without quality scoring (QUADAS), a very important aspect of determination of the clinical utility of such values. Therefore, it is suggested that the reader keep this in mind when interpreting such values.

orders of the cervical spine, and these disorders may require adjuvant advanced imaging confirmation. In clients without a history of trauma, plain radiographs are often ordered for the workup of neck pain or radicular upper extremity pain. However, in those with nonspecific neck pain, plain radiographs are unlikely to be helpful in the diagnosis.[53] The history should alert the clinician regarding when further workup and imaging will be necessary.

Red flags initially described for acute low back pain can be used in the assessment of clients with neck pain. These red flags include age of onset less than 20 years or greater than 55 years, constitutional symptoms, history of cancer, immunosuppression, and drug abuse.[54] Evaluation may include laboratory work as well as plain radiographs. Early

disease may be missed, and normal results of radiographs should not preclude further workup.[55] In spite of the high prevalence of a single red flag (80% in those presenting with low back pain to a family physician), only 1% to 3% of those were of serious pathology.[56]

Plain radiographs and advanced imaging may also be obtained for clients with chronic neck pain who have failed a trial of conservative care or for clients with neurologic signs of radiculopathy.[54] The American College of Radiology has developed a set of criteria for the appropriate use of imaging in clients with chronic neck pain.[57] Plain radiographs may not need to be obtained if further imaging with either CT or magnetic resonance imaging (MRI) is pursued. In these cases, a plain radiograph is unlikely to add diagnostic value or alter the management plan.[55]

Routine anteroposterior (AP) and lateral views may show loss of vertebral disc space height, facet arthropathy, spondylolisthesis, malalignment, fracture, and congenital osseous abnormalities. Oblique views are often ordered to evaluate the foramen, but this is highly dependent on client positioning. The findings are more conclusive with CT and MRI. Flexion–extension views may be added to evaluate for instability, particularly if a spondylolisthesis is found on lateral views.[55] Greater than 3.5 mm of translational displacement or 20° of angular motion during these views is significant and suggests instability.[14] Flexion–extension views may be indicated in cases with high suspicion of instability, such as significant injury, history of prior fusion, rheumatoid arthritis, and Down syndrome. The open-mouth odontoid view is needed if there is a history of trauma or in the presence of disorders that affect the atlantooccipital junction.[55] Indications for more advanced imaging include any concern for infection or malignancy, such as constitutional symptoms, immunocompromise, or history of cancer. Neurologic impairment on examination should prompt more advanced imaging.[54]

The CCSR (Canadian C-Spine Rule)[26] and National Emergency X-Radiography Utilization Study (NEXUS)[27] are clinical decision rules that the clinician can use to determine the necessity of radiographs for their client. These rules were designed for utilization on the acutely injured client. Both in comparison studies and individually, the CCSR has outperformed the NEXUS (table 17.2). In a recent systematic review, based on studies with modest methodological quality and one direct comparison, the CCSR was found to have stronger diagnostic accuracy than the NEXUS criteria.[58]

The NEXUS criteria were developed to stratify clients into low- and higher-risk groups for those with blunt trauma. Clients meeting the following criteria have a low probability of injury and do not require further imaging:[27]

- No midline cervical tenderness
- No altered level of consciousness or intoxication
- No abnormal neurologic findings
- No painful distracting injuries

Clients meeting all of the NEXUS criteria are classified as low risk and may be cleared on the basis of history and physical examination alone. Higher-risk clients require imaging before receiving clearance.[27]

Alternatively, the Canadian C-Spine Rules may be followed to determine which among the awake and alert trauma clients require further imaging.[26] The Canadian C-Spine Rules are as follows (for alert [GCS = 15] and stable trauma clients where cervical spine injury is a concern):[26]

Step 1: Any high-risk factor that mandates radiography?

- Age ≥ 65 years, or
- Dangerous mechanism, or
- Paresthesia in extremities

TABLE 17.2 Canadian C-Spine Rules and NEXUS Diagnostic Accuracy

Diagnostic test	Gold standard	SN/SP
CCSR	Systematic review	90-100/1-77[58]
CCSR	Cross-validation	100/42.5[26] (alert and stable trauma clients; original study)
CCSR	C-spine radiography	100/37.7[69] (paramedics out of hospital)
CCSR Physician clinical judgment without use of CCSR	C-spine radiography	100/44[59] 92/54[59]
NEXUS	Systematic review	83-100/2-46[58]
NEXUS	Variable	92.7/37.8[70]

CCSR = Canadian C-Spine Rule, NEXUS = National Emergency X-Radiography Utilization Study

Step 2: Any low-risk factor that allows safe assessment of range-of-motion?

- Simple rear-end motor vehicle crash, or
- Able to sit in the emergency department, or
- Able to ambulate, or
- Delayed-onset neck pain, or
- Absence of midline tenderness

Step 3: Ability to rotate neck 45° to the right and left?

- Clients who meet *any* criteria in step 1 require radiographs.

Clients not meeting any criteria in step 1 proceed to step 2.

Clients who do not meet criteria in step 2 require radiographs.

Clients who are unable to perform step 3 require radiographs.

Clients who are able to perform all 3 steps and rotate neck 45° to the right and left do not require radiographs.

In a recent systematic review, the Canadian C-Spine Rule's SN ranged from 90 to 100 and the SP ranged from 1 to 77. For the NEXUS, SN ranged from 83 to 100 and the SP ranged from 2 to 46. One study directly compared the accuracy of these two rules using the same cohort and found that the Canadian C-spine Rule had better accuracy. For both rules, a negative test was more informative for reducing the probability of a clinically important cervical spine injury. The Canadian C-Spine Rule demonstrated better diagnostic accuracy than the NEXUS criteria; specifically, it produced fewer false negatives and hence had an improved SN and decreased risk of missing an actual fracture.[58] The Canadian C-Spine Rule was found superior to unstructured physician clinical judgment as well. In a study comparing physician judgment with and without the use of this rule, the SN with the use of the rule was 100, while the SN without the use of the Canadian C-Spine rule was only 92.[59]

A recent meta-analysis determined that an alert, asymptomatic client without distracting injury or neurological deficit who is able to complete a functional ROM examination may be safely cleared from cervical spine immobilization without radiographic evaluation (SN 98).[60] The clinician is cautioned, though, since an SN of less than 100 requires a few false-negative interpretations (and therefore missing an actual fracture).

In regard to what specific views of radiographs are required, generally AP, lateral, and open-mouth odontoid views are obtained. A swimmer's view may be added if the lateral view fails to adequately visualize the C7-T1 junction. The open-mouth odontoid view requires the client to be awake and cooperative, which may not be possible in obtunded or unconscious clients. This view may also be difficult to obtain in the young pediatric population, and it is not suggested for clients younger than 5 years.[61] Pediatric clients are at an increased risk of higher cervical injuries than adults, and any question of injury to the upper cervical spine in this client population should be evaluated with a CT scan.[62] Flexion and extension views may also be obtained in alert clients to assess for ligamentous injury, although it has been advocated that they are inferior to MRI for this purpose.[63] Lateral view radiographs have shown that providing an evaluation of the dynamic lateral instability of the atlantoaxial joint can be useful for early diagnosis of atlantoaxial lesions in RA.[64]

A growing body of evidence suggests that CT images should replace all plain radiographs in the setting of blunt trauma because of the low SN of radiographs for identifying clinically significant injury.[65, 66] Any client with whom adequate views cannot be obtained should undergo more advanced imaging.[66] Modern CT alone has been suggested sufficient for detecting unstable cervical spine injuries in trauma clients. Adjuvant imaging is unnecessary when the CT scan is negative for acute injury.[48] Less certain is whether CT should replace plain radiography as the initial screening test for less injured clients who are at low risk for cervical spine injury but still require radiographic imaging.[49] More recent findings suggest the improved ability to rapidly exclude injury provides further evidence that CT should replace radiography for the initial evaluation of blunt cervical spine injury in clients at any risk for injury.[66]

Magnetic Resonance Imaging

Since MRI allows for detailed evaluation of both soft and bony tissue without ionizing radiation, it is often replacing CT as the first-line advanced imaging for the client with neck pain. It provides excellent contrast between the spinal cord, intervertebral discs, vertebral bodies, and ligamentous structures and assesses multiple additional aspects of soft tissue or osseous abnormalities. Reliability of readings on MRI for cervical spine pathologies such as radiculopathy is considerable. Interobserver reliability of MRI evaluation in clients with cervical radiculopathy was substantial for root compression, with or without clinical information. Agreement on the cause of the compression (i.e., herniated disc or spondylotic foraminal stenosis) was lower, though.[67] Magnetic resonance imaging is suggested for the confirmation of correlative compressive lesions (disc herniation and spondylosis) in cervical spine clients who have failed a course of conservative therapy and who may be candidates for interventional or surgical treatment, with a grade B recommendation.[68]

MR imaging findings significantly associated with whiplash injuries were occult fracture (P < 0.01), bone marrow contusion of the vertebral body (P = 0.01), muscle strain (P < 0.01) or tear (P < 0.01), and the presence of perimuscular fluid (P < 0.01). While 10 findings thought to be specific for whiplash trauma were significantly (P < 0.01) more frequent in clients (507 observations), they were also regularly found in healthy control subjects (237 observations). MRI at 1.5 T reveals only limited evidence of specific changes to the cervical spine and the surrounding tissues in clients with acute symptomatic whiplash injury compared with healthy control subjects.[52]

Computed Tomography

As mentioned previously, a recent meta-analysis demonstrated that CT alone is capable of ruling out cervical spine instability in trauma clients.[48] To what extent it serves as the first line of imaging in less traumatically injured clients is apparently still debated.

Computed tomography myelography combines the detail of CT scanning with the instillation of intrathecal contrast, allowing accurate measurements of central and foraminal canal diameters. Adverse events associated with myelography are reported to be 4.9% with a cervical approach and 3.4% with a lumbar approach. Client tolerance is relatively low, and pain after the procedure is common.[71] Although CT myelography is considered the criterion standard for advanced imaging of the spine, and correlation with surgical findings in radiculopathy is as high as 90%, the possibility of complications and radiation exposure to the client lend support to the suggestion that MRI be the considered first-line study for ambulatory neck pain clients requiring advanced imaging.[55]

A grade B recommendation states that CT myelography is suggested for the evaluation of clients with clinical symptoms or signs that are discordant with MRI findings (e.g., foraminal compression that may not be identified on MRI). Computed tomography myelography is also suggested in clients who have a contraindication to MRI.[68]

Catheter angiography has been the gold standard for the diagnosis of vertebral artery injuries (VAIs); however, new 16-slice computed tomography angiography seems to have sensitivity and specificity close to that of catheter angiography.[72] The clinician should, as always, be cognizant of the imaging modality's strengths and weaknesses when interpreting imaging findings.

Nuclear Medicine Studies

In the cervical spine, nuclear medicine studies have been used as an adjuvant to image lesions that are suspicious for neoplasm or infection within the osseous structures. Single-photon emission CT (SPECT) is the most common type of nuclear medicine study of the spine. Although abnormal findings on SPECT scans have shown strong correlation with MRI findings for pathologies such as cervical spondylosis and facet joint pain, the radiation exposure and cost should be kept in mind with this procedure.[55]

Ultrasound

The utility of ultrasound or ultrasonography (US) as a diagnostic tool is significantly limited in the cervical spine due to its inability to image through bone into the central canal or intervertebral foramen. Ultrasonography does have the advantage of not using ionizing radiation, and it may reduce cost. The main disadvantage of US in the cervical spine compared to other real-time imaging such as fluoroscopy is the inability to reliably assess for cervical radicular arteries. Assessing these arteries is imperative for avoiding catastrophic outcomes with epidural steroid injections.

Nerve Root Blocks

Selective nerve root block with specific dosing and technique protocols may be considered in the evaluation of clients with cervical radiculopathy and compressive lesions identified at multiple levels on MRI or CT myelography to discern the symptomatic levels. Selective nerve root block may also be considered to confirm a symptomatic level in clients with discordant clinical symptoms and MRI or CT myelography findings. All of the above were grade C recommendation by Bono and colleagues.[68]

Electromyography

Bono and colleagues found that the evidence was insufficient to make a recommendation for or against the use of electromyography for clients in whom the diagnosis of cervical radiculopathy was unclear after clinical examination and MRI.[68]

Others

No evidence supports using cervical provocative discography, anesthetic facet, or medial branch blocks in evaluating neck pain.[35] The use of more advanced imaging appears favorable to these modalities.

Review of Systems

Refer to chapter 6 (Triage and Differential Diagnosis) for details on review of systems relevant to the cervical spine.

OBSERVATION

Cervical spine posture is often described in radiography reports. These reports describe the degree, or lack thereof, of lordosis in the client's neck. While this information is often used to describe to the client the relevance of their posture to pathology, interpreting these findings requires caution. As mentioned previously, there is no evidence that the degree of cervical lordosis or kyphosis can accurately identify cervical muscle spasm or distinguish clients with WAD from those without WAD.[44]

Clients with torticollis will adapt a characteristic pattern of postural compensation regardless of the type or cause of the torticollis. The typical compensated head posture for the client with torticollis is ipsilateral side bending and contralateral rotation of the head.

As with all regions of the body, side-to-side and front-to-back asymmetry should be assessed. Upper crossed syndrome is commonly described in clients demonstrating tight suboccipital and pectoral muscles along with weak deep neck flexor and scapula retractor muscles, giving the appearance of a forward head and bilaterally rounded shoulders. More detail on this presentation is given in chapter 14 (Posture).

A side-to-side asymmetry of upper trapezius vertical height should include the differential diagnosis of handedness and the potential for an elevated or cervical rib. Typically, handedness will demonstrate increased muscle mass on the ipsilateral side, which may give the appearance of increased vertical height of the corresponding upper trapezius muscle, although the dominant shoulder girdle in athletes is commonly lower in appearance than the nondominant shoulder.

An elevated first rib should correlate with a specific mechanism, as well as the potential for a (+) cervical rotation lateral flexion test (see chapter 18, Thoracic Spine). Cervical ribs (a rib coming off of C7 versus T1 and typically without a bony articulation anteriorly to the manubrium) are rare with the overall prevalence of 0.74%, with a higher rate in women compared with men (1.09% and 0.42%, respectively). The presence of elongated C7 transverse processes (transverse apophysomegaly) was also noted in these clients, with an overall prevalence of 2.21%. They were also more common in women (3.43%) than in men (1.13%).[73]

Clients with Down syndrome often adopt an abnormal head posture, particularly in cases of incomitant strabismus (disorder in which the eyes don't look in exactly the same direction at the same time), nystagmus (rhythmic, oscillating motions of the eyes), or both.[74, 75] While the specific abnormal posture can vary, the most likely presentation is leaning the head toward the involved side.[75] Other postural deviations that the clinician should monitor for are those due to vestibular migraine,[76] dizzying headache,[77] glaucoma,[78] and mouth breathing.[79] For example, the client with vestibular or dizziness-related complaints will more likely avoid turning their head, and the mouth-breathing client is likely to have a forward head posture.

TRIAGE AND SCREENING

Triage and screening is a necessary component of the examination process that should be done prior to continuing with the examination. Ruling out serious pathology (refer to chapter 6, Triage and Differential Diagnosis) and pain generation from other related (or close-proximity) structures helps the clinician more accurately determine the necessity of continuing with the other examination components to identify the actual source of the client's pain. Additionally, implementing strong screening tests (tests of high SN and low –LR) at this point in the examination is suggested for narrowing down the competing diagnoses of the respective body region (thoracic spine and shoulder in this case) when this is applicable.

Ruling Out Serious Pathology and Red Flags

Signs and symptoms found in the client history and clinical examination may tie a disorder to a serious pathology.[80] Commonly described red flags in the cervical spine are cervical myelopathy, ischemic stroke, meningitis, mild traumatic brain injury (mTBI), primary brain tumor, fracture, cervical artery dysfunction (CAD), cervical myelopathy, inflammatory or systemic disease, complete nerve injuries of the cervical spine and shoulder region, Pancoast tumor of the superior sulcus of the lung, and inflammatory or systemic disease. The Pancoast tumor will present with nagging pain in the shoulder and scapular border, with potential progression into the upper extremity (primarily ulnar nerve distribution) and nonmusculoskeletal presentation.

Cervical myelopathy is an upper motor neuron disease due to pressure on the spinal cord (central nervous system). Therefore, clinical presentation for the client with myelopathy will typically have hyperreflexia, bilateral symptoms, unsteady gait, presence of pathological reflexes, bowel and bladder disturbances, multisegmental weakness or sensory changes (or both), and potential muscle wasting of the hand intrinsic muscles, although these traditional measures are more diagnostic than screening and are currently investigated in limited strength studies.[81]

Ischemic stroke often presents with a sudden onset of a severe headache. In fact, a severe headache itself is closely associated with severe systolic blood pressure elevation in acute ischemic stroke.[82] Additionally, the client may have a history of hypertension, concurrent elevated blood pressure, trunk and extremity weakness, and altered mental state. Other potential signs or symptoms could include vertigo, vomiting, and aphasia.[82, 83]

Meningitis often presents with a headache. Other common symptoms include seizures and sleepiness. The clinician should monitor for gastrointestinal signs of vomiting and symptoms of nausea. Other common findings include fever, photophobia, confusion, and a positive slump test (see chapter 7).[84, 85] Confusion (**+LR 24**), leg pain (**+LR 7.6**), photophobia (**+LR 6.5**), rash (**+LR 5.5**), and neck pain or stiffness (**+LR 5.3**) were found to be the most clinically useful symptoms of meningococcal disease, while headaches (**+LR 1.0**) were not discriminatory for the disease.[86] Freshmen who lived in dormitories had an elevated risk of meningococ-

cal disease (odds ratio of 3.6) compared with other college students.[85]

Mild traumatic brain injury (mTBI) or *post-concussion syndrome* is still a very complex entity that is not completely understood. Refer to chapters 15 (Face and Head) and 27 (Emergency Sport Examination) for additional detail on this syndrome. Common characteristics of this syndrome include the following:[87, 88]

- Dangerous injury mechanism
- Headache
- Nausea or vomiting
- Sensitivity to light and sounds
- Loss of consciousness, appearing dazed; an initial Glasgow Coma Scale of 13 to 15 (refer to chapter 7, Orthopedic Screening and Nervous System Examination)
- Deficits in short-term memory
- Physical evidence of trauma above the clavicles
- Drug or alcohol intoxication
- Seizures

Commonly described signs or symptoms of a *primary brain tumor* include headache, gastrointestinal signs of vomiting and symptoms of nausea, ataxia, speech deficits, sensory abnormalities, visual changes, altered mental status, and seizures.[89-91] Since these are signs or symptoms characteristic of various other cervical spine–related pathologies, including previously mentioned red flags, it behooves the clinician to critically discern their presence and relevance.

While there is considerable concern for the clinician to rule out the potential for red flags, they must also consider prevalence of such conditions existing. Individual red flags do not necessarily mean the presence of serious pathology; however, the presence of multiple red flags should raise clinical suspicion, and indicates the need for further investigation. Red flags have not been evaluated comprehensively in any systematic review; however, the incidence of spinal tumors is very low. In the academic and private practice setting, this reached 0.7% and 0.1%, respectively, of the populations examined[92] and for those with complaints related to low back pain presenting to a family physician,[56] suggesting that the chance of missing serious pathology, especially in the private practice setting, is exceptionally low. Radiographs do not and should not compensate for an inadequate assessment as a result of, for example, time constraints.

Clearance of Cervical Spine Injury

The potential for serious cervical spine pathology must be ruled out prior to proceeding with the examination. The Neck Pain Task Force recommends that people seeking care for neck pain should be triaged into four groups:[44]

- Grade I: Neck pain with no signs of major pathology and no or little interference with daily activities
- Grade II: Neck pain with no signs of major pathology, but interference with daily activities
- Grade III: Neck pain with neurologic signs of nerve compression
- Grade IV: Neck pain with signs of major pathology

In the emergency room after blunt trauma to the neck, triage should be based on the NEXUS criteria or (currently more preferably) the Canadian C-spine Rule (see table 17.2). Those with a high risk of fracture should be further investigated with plain radiographs or CT scan (refer to previous Radiographs section for detail). In ambulatory primary care, triage based on history and physical examination alone, including screening for red flags and conducting neurologic examination for signs of radiculopathy, has been suggested.[44]

The International Federation of Orthopaedic Manipulative Physical Therapists (IFOMPT) has produced a consensus document on cervical spine clearance prior to initiation of manual therapy intervention. As pointed out in this document, clinicians should consider several variables when attempting to clear the cervical spine for continued assessment or intervention (figure 17.6).[93]

The subjective history of the client is used to make an informed decision on the probability of the existence of serious pathology and contraindications to treatment. Red flags discussed previously and in chapter 6 should alert the clinician

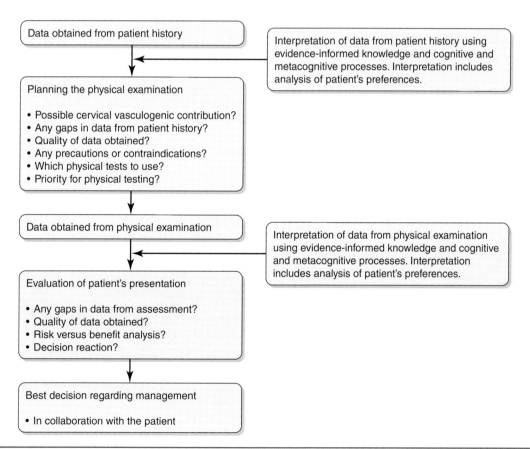

Figure 17.6 Flowchart of clinical reasoning regarding clearance of the cervical spine.

to the possibility of serious pathology. Also, a side-impact collision in a motor vehicle accident (MVA)[94] and one with the client turning their head[29] were shown to be more likely to cause vertebral artery elongation.

As outlined in figure 17.6, the physical examination for cervical spine clearance (if to be undertaken) must be planned carefully. The clinician must consider the risks of such testing, specifically if there are any precautions or contraindications. Risk factors for physical examination testing should also be assessed. A Delphi study identified the following risk factors being associated with the potential for ligamentous or bony compromise of the upper cervical spine:[95]

- History of trauma (e.g., whiplash, MVA)
- Throat infection
- Congenital collagenous compromise (e.g., syndromes such as Down and Ehlers-Danlos)
- Inflammatory arthritides (e.g., rheumatoid arthritis, ankylosing spondylitis)
- Recent neck, head, or dental surgery

Risk factors for cervical artery dysfunction (CAD), internal carotid, or vertebrobasilar arterial pathology that can be assessed during the history are the following:[96, 97]

- Past history of trauma to the cervical spine or cervical vessels
- History of migraine-type headaches (odds ratio 3.6)[98]
- Hypertension
- Hyperlipidemia or hypercholesterolemia
- Cardiac disease, vascular disease, previous cerebrovascular accident or transient ischemic attack
- Diabetes mellitus
- Long-term use of steroids
- History of smoking
- Recent infection (odds ratio 1.6)[98]
- Anticoagulant therapy
- Being immediately postpartum
- Absence of plausible mechanical explanation for symptoms
- Trivial head or neck trauma (odds ratio 3.8;[98] odds ratio 23[99])

Additionally, major and minor risk factors have been previously delineated:[100-102]

Major Risk Factors

- Hypertension (BP > 140/90)
- Hypercholesterolemia
- Hyperlipidemia
- Diabetes
- Family history of MI, angina, TIA, stroke, PVD
- Smoking
- BMI > 30
- Repeated or recent injury (including repeated manipulations)
- Upper cervical instability

Minor Risk Factors

- Estrogen-based contraceptive
- Hormone replacement therapy
- Infection (systemic)
- Poor diet
- RA or other connective tissue syndrome
- Blood-clotting disorder
- Fibromuscular dysplasia
- Hypermobility
- Erectile dysfunction
- BMI 25-29

The authors of the IFOMPT framework suggest a risk–benefit strategy when determining the action to be undertaken with the client with suspicion of potential CAD.[103] The authors suggest that a high number or severe nature of risk factors have a low predicted benefit of testing or utilization of manual therapy, and therefore clinicians should avoid treatment, while a low number or low nature of risk factors suggests that clinicians should employ treatment or assessment with care and continual monitoring for change and new symptoms.[93, 103]

Cervical Stability Testing

Cervical spine stability testing is warranted in any client suspected to have potentially serious pathology in the cervical spine. Likely mechanisms, similar to the Canadian C-Spine Rule, include traumatic episodes. If the client complains of signs or symptoms suggestive of CAD, it is advised that the clinician must implement the Canadian C-Spine rule followed by cervical stability testing before assessing for CAD. Additional signs and symptoms suggestive of the need for cervical stability testing include occipital numbness and tingling, severe limitation in active range of motion (AROM) of the cervical spine in at least one plane of motion, and signs or symptoms suggestive of cervical myelopathy.

As alluded to previously, the clinician should be cognizant of the fact that clients with rheumatoid arthritis[64, 104] and Down syndrome[105, 106] have a higher predilection toward upper cervical spine instability than most other clients. The clinician should also consider several other variables including (but not limited to) the mechanism and the extent of the expected trauma. For example, an abnormal alar ligament was the most commonly injured ligament or membrane in subjects with WAD.[28]

Careful monitoring of the client's presentation throughout the examination is of paramount importance for the client with the suspicion of CAD or upper cervical instability. Loss of balance, gait disturbance, guarded posturing, and anxiety are but a few of the observations that should alert the clinician to the potential for these serious conditions.

Several tests for cervical stability are described in the literature. Some have stronger diagnostic accuracy and clinical utility than others. Additionally, some are more technically difficult to perform. In the following techniques, the more technically difficult tests will be delineated as such. Decision on which tests to utilize for the client requires sound clinical reasoning throughout the entire examination process.

ALAR LIGAMENT TESTING

Client Position   Sitting in upright posture

Clinician Position   Standing to the side of the client

Movement   The clinician palpates the client's spinous process (SpP) of C2 with one hand (left as shown), and then passively side bends the client's head minimally with the other hand (right as shown). With side bending to the right, the SpP should immediately kick to the left—here, the clinician is primarily testing the left alar ligament. They should perform the opposite procedure for the right side. They can also perform this drill in supine, using their thumb or finger on the side of the SpP of C2 opposite to the direction the client's head is bent in. A variation of this test involves palpation of the C1 transverse process to assess for movement between C1 and C2.[107]

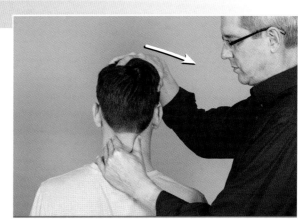

Figure 17.7

Assessment   The test is considered (+) if the SpP does not immediately move to the contralateral side of the side bending motion.

Statistics   • SN 69 to 100, SP 72 to 96, +LR 18-Inf, –LR 0.29–0.31, QUADAS 7, in a study of 122 clients (92 with and 30 without a diagnosis of whiplash-associated disorder, type 2; mean age 20.3 years for controls, 42.6 for symptomatic clients; 78 total were female; mean duration of symptoms 5.7 years), and using a reference standard of MRI[107]

   • Reliability: 0.69–0.71 κ)[107]

Note   The diagnostic accuracy values reported previously are for the variation of this test as reported by Kaale and colleagues.[107]

ALAR LIGAMENT STRESS TEST

! **This is a more technically difficult test.**

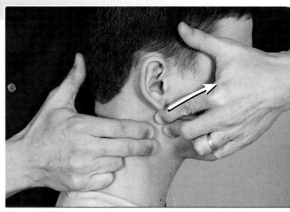

Figure 17.8

Client Position	Sitting with bilateral upper extremities relaxed at side
Clinician Position	Standing close to the client, with their trunk stabilizing the client's trunk
Movement	The clinician places both hands on the same side of the client's cervicooccipital junction. With their caudal hand (right as shown), they stabilize the client's C2 by pressing their second and third fingers against the lateral aspect of C2, pulling this part backward (posterior). The test of the ligament is performed by an upward pull into rotation with two fingers on the cranial hand (left as shown), placing their third finger under the lateral mass of atlas (C1) and their second finger under the mastoid process. The clinician performs the test with different angles of cervical rotation to locate the exact test position that gives the maximal movement between C1 and C2.
Assessment	The test of the alar ligaments assesses the quality of rotation between the occiput, atlas, and axis. Insufficiency of the ligament gives a hypermobile function in this area. A (+) test is excessive movement between C1 and C2 and/or reproduction of concordant pain (myelopathic symptoms).

Reliability
- Right: (κ) coefficient: 0.71 (0.58–0.83)[107]
- Left: (κ) coefficient: 0.69 (0.57–0.82)[107]

Statistics
- Right: SN 69 (56-81), SP 100, +LR Inf, –LR 0.31
- Left: SN 72 (60-84), SP 96 (91-100), +LR 18, –LR 0.30, QUADAS 7, in a study of 122 clients (92 with and 30 without a diagnosis of whiplash-associated disorder, type 2; mean age 20.3 years for controls, 42.6 for symptomatic clients; 78 women; mean duration of symptoms 5.7 years), and using a reference standard of MRI[107]

Notes
- The clinician should take care to maintain the client's head in neutral (avoid side bending away) by using their trunk.
- The clinician should use the pads of their fingers versus their fingertips for client comfort with this test.
- This test requires significant clinician skill to perform.

TRANSVERSE LIGAMENT STRESS TEST

Client Position	Supine with upper extremities relaxed at sides
Clinician Position	Sitting at client's head
Movement	The clinician places their deltopectoral groove on the client's forehead. With the mobilizing hand (right as shown), the clinician lifts the client's occiput and C1 together cranially as they use their other hand (left as shown) to monitor the SpP of C2.

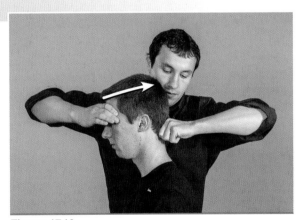

Figure 17.9

Assessment	A (+) test is reproduction of symptoms (myelopathic type, etc.), and/or if the SpP of C2 does not lift off the index finger. These symptoms could include soft end-feel, muscle spasm, dizziness, nausea, nystagmus, a lump sensation in the throat, or paresthesia of the lip, face, or limb.
Statistics	NR (not reported)
Note	The clinician should make sure to not lift their hand or the index finger of the hand palpating (and therefore assessing) the SP of C2 to avoid the possibility of a false (–) test result.

MODIFIED SHARP-PURSER TEST

 Video 17.10 **in the web resource shows a demonstration of this test.**

 Use extreme caution with this test.

Figure 17.10

Client Position	Sitting with neck semiflexed (20–30°), bilateral upper extremities relaxed at their side
Clinician Position	Standing up close to the client with their trunk stabilizing the client's trunk
Movement	The clinician places one hand (right as shown) on the client's forehead, and uses their other hand (left as shown) to pinch grip the spinous process of C2. Applying posterior pressure through the client's forehead (with right hand as shown), the clinician posteriorly translates the occiput and atlas.
Assessment	Firm end-feel is desired for a (–) test result. Reproduction of myelopathic symptoms during forward flexion, decrease in symptoms during the anterior-to-posterior movement, or a sliding motion of the head posteriorly in relation to the axis indicates a (+) test for atlantoaxial instability. Sliding may also be accompanied by a clunk (the approximation of the dens and posterior region of the anterior ring of the atlas).
Statistics	• SN 69 (50-84), SP 96 (89-99), +LR 17.25, –LR 0.32, (subluxation > 4 mm), QUADAS 8, in 123 clients with rheumatoid arthritis (gender, age, and duration of symptoms NR), using a criterion reference of radiographic imaging[108]

(continued)

Modified Sharp-Purser Test (continued)

- Modified κ (agreement): 0.29–0.67 in a study of 11 children with Down syndrome, utilizing four clinicians and a reference standard of flexion radiographs (subluxation > 5 mm)[109]

Notes
- If (+), the clinician should put a cervical collar on the client and send them to a physician or the emergency department.
- If the client starts in full cervical flexion, the unique feature of this test is that the stress component is intended to relieve symptoms rather than aggravate them.
- It is worthy of mention that all clients in this study had rheumatoid arthritis.

TRANSVERSE LIGAMENT

 This is a more technically difficult test that requires significant clinician skill to perform.

Client Position	Sitting with bilateral upper extremities relaxed
Clinician Position	Standing close to the client with their trunk stabilizing the client's trunk

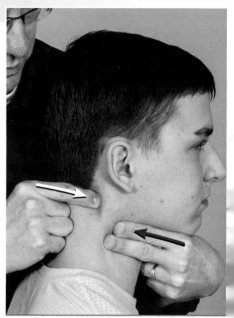

Figure 17.11

Movement The clinician stabilizes the client's C2 with a frontal grip (caudal hand, left in this case), pressing their thumb against the frontal part of the left lateral process (not seen), while pressing their second and third fingers against the right lateral process. This finger grip must not give the client a feeling of strangling. The clinician performs the test movement by pressing their thumb against the posterior part of the left lateral mass of the atlas while holding their second finger against the lateral mass on the client's C1 (atlas) on the opposite side (cranial hand, right in this case). At the same time, the clinician presses these fingers firmly against the inferior part of the client's occiput.

The flexed fingers (3-5) support the grip from below. The clinician presses C1 forward (occiput follows the movement of atlas) and C2 backwards, testing the translation of the dens (axis) in the space from the transverse ligament to the posterior part of C1. The clinician performs the test from a neutral position between C1 and C2, and through several steps of increasing flexion.

Assessment A (+) test is excessive translation of the atlas or reproduction of concordant pain (myelopathic symptoms). The test of the transverse ligament assesses the anterior/posterior translation of the atlas against the axis.

Reliability (κ) coefficient: 0.69 (0.55–0.83)[107]

Statistics SN 65 (51-79), SP 99 (96-100), +LR 65, –LR 0.35, QUADAS 7, in a study of 122 clients (92 with and 30 without a diagnosis of whiplash-associated disorder, type 2; mean age 20.3 years for controls and 42.6 for symptomatic clients; 78 women; mean duration of symptoms 5.7 years) and using a reference standard of MRI.[107]

TECTORIAL MEMBRANE

> **!** **This is a more technically difficult test that requires significant clinician skill to perform.**

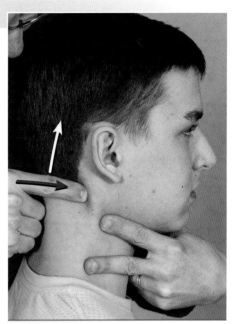

Figure 17.12

Client Position	Sitting with bilateral upper extremities relaxed
Clinician Position	Standing up close to the client with their trunk stabilizing the client's trunk
Movement	The clinician places the posterior hand (left as shown) that performs the passive test movement in the client's suboccipital region. The clinician forms their first and second fingers into a semicircle and presses them against the lower part of the client's occiput, supporting them from below with flexed fingers 3, 4, and 5. C1 is following the anteriorf and cranial movement of the occiput. The clinician stabilizes the client's C2 with a frontal grip from finger 2 on the anterior hand (left as shown). The test movement goes forward (anterior), combined with a traction force (posterior hand). The clinician performs this test with different angles of flexion and degrees of traction.
Assessment	A (+) test result is given by an excessive translation between occiput-C1 and C2 and/or reproduction of concordant pain (myelopathic symptoms). The test of the tectorial membrane assesses the degree of ventral horizontal translation between the bones in the atlantooccipital axis (C0-C1-C2).
Reliability	(κ) coefficient: 0.93 (0.83–1.03)[107]
Statistics	SN 94 (82-106), SP 99 (97-101), +LR 94, –LR 0.06, QUADAS 7, in a study of 122 clients (92 with and 30 without a diagnosis of whiplash-associated disorder, type 2; mean age 20.3 years for controls and 42.6 for symptomatic clients; 78 total were female; mean duration of symptoms 5.7 years), using a reference standard of MRI.[107]

POSTERIOR ATLANTOOCCIPITAL MEMBRANE TEST

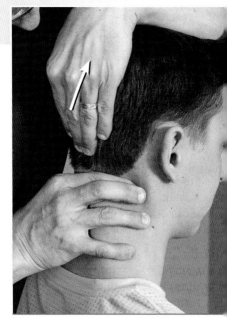

Figure 17.13

! This is a more technically difficult test that requires significant clinician skill to perform.

Client Position	Sitting with bilateral upper extremities relaxed
Clinician Position	Standing up close to the client with their trunk stabilizing the client's trunk
Movement	The clinician places both hands in the client's suboccipital region. The caudal (right as shown) hand stabilizes the client's C1 by a downward pressure with the thumb and fingers placed on the lateral mass of atlas. The clinician forms a grip with their cranial (left as shown) hand, directing the fingers downward. The clinician performs this test by pulling with the cranial hand in the opposite direction of the downward pressure performed by the caudal hand. They repeat this pulling repeated several times through different angles of flexion.
Assessment	The test of the posterior atlantooccipital membrane assesses the stability in the posterior part of the neck between the occiput and atlas. A (+) test is excessive translation and/or reproduction of concordant pain (myelopathic symptoms).
Reliability	(κ) coefficient: 0.97[107]
Statistics	SN 96 (87-104), SP 100, +LR Inf, –LR 0.04, QUADAS 7, in a study of 122 clients (92 with and 30 without a diagnosis of whiplash-associated disorder, type 2; mean age 20.3 years for controls and 42.6 for symptomatic clients; 78 total were female; mean duration of symptoms 5.7 years), using a reference standard of MRI.[107]

TEST FOR A JEFFERSON FRACTURE

Client Position	Supine with arms relaxed at sides
Clinician Position	Standing at head of table
Movement	The clinician palpates both transverse processes (TP) of C1. The mobilizing hand (right as shown) utilizes a pincer grip on the TP of C1, while the stabilizing hand (left as shown) blocks the other TP of C1 in a manner most comfortable to the client. While blocking one side of C1, the clinician compresses the other side.
Assessment	A normal or (–) test results in a hard nonyielding end-feel. Excessive movement or reproduction of the client's symptoms suggests the potential for disruption in the ring of the atlas.
Statistics	NR

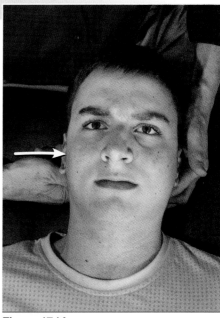

Figure 17.14

Cervical Artery Dysfunction Testing

Cervical artery dysfunction is a multifactorial disease, requiring a multifactorial assessment. Testing for CAD represents assessment of both posterior and anterior circulation in the neck. Vertebrobasilar insufficiency (VBI) testing has been the traditional testing but accounts only for testing of the vertebrobasilar artery complex (posterior circulation). More recent terminology utilizes CAD to account for the anterior circulation (internal carotid) as well.

When this type of testing is performed, the Canadian C-Spine Rules and NEXUS followed by cervical stability testing should have already been implemented. The potential correlation between upper cervical instability and CAD does exist. In a recent study, approximately 0.5% of all trauma clients were reported to have vertebral artery insufficiency (VAI), and 70% of all traumatic VAIs had an associated cervical spine fracture. Cervical spine translation injuries and transverse foramen fractures are most commonly cited as having a significant association with VAIs. The incidence of neurologic deficits secondary to VAI ranges from 0% to 24%.[72]

CAD testing is controversial and has been suggested to lack precision in diagnostic accuracy. Some anecdotal evidence, as well as evidence-based research, suggests that despite various guidelines advocating specific screening procedures for this type of testing, support for their ability to accurately identify clients at risk is lacking.[60] Additionally, CAD may be present in clients with subjective reports of vertigo and visual disturbances that are reproduced with CAD physical examination procedures.[110]

All of these findings underlie the importance of clinical reasoning during the subjective examination. In a case study design utilizing manipulative physiotherapists, the therapist's hypothesis generation in relation to CAD was mainly based on the subjective examination; no new pathoanatomic hypotheses were generated in the physical examination. The major indicators of CAD involvement were dizziness, particularly if associated with other symptoms (visual disturbances, history of trauma, and headache) and if exacerbated by cervical spine movements. Therapists demonstrated a lack of confidence in functional positional testing.[111]

It is proposed that vascular red flag presentations mimic neuromusculoskeletal cervicocranial syndromes. This reasoning presupposes that some clients who have poor clinical outcomes, or a serious adverse response to treatment, may be those who actually present with undiagnosed vascular pathology.[101] In the most recent systematic review on this topic, it was not possible to draw firm conclusions about the diagnostic accuracy of premanipulative tests.[112] Despite a thorough screening prior to treatment, there is still an element of risk. Clinicians should avoid sustained end-of-range rotation and quick-thrust rotational manipulations until there is a stronger evidence base for clinical practice.[113]

It is worth mentioning that selected manual therapy intervention techniques have been investigated for their effect on blood flow to the brain. In healthy adults, the positions of cervical spine neutral, rotation, rotation distraction (similar to a Cyriax manipulation), C1-C2 rotation (similar to a Maitland or osteopathic manipulation), and distraction were investigated. Blood flow to the brain did not appear to be compromised by these positions. In fact, it was determined that (in healthy adults) positions using end-range neck rotation and distraction do not appear to be more hazardous to cerebral circulation than more segmentally localized techniques.[114] Therefore, due to the complex nature of CAD, various testing modalities have been described. Their purpose, evidence, and limitations and advantages are listed in table 17.3.

Cervical Rotation Statistics

SN 57 (NR), **SP 100 (NR)**, +LR 83.3, −LR 0.44, QUADAS 9, in a study of 46 clients with vertebrobasilar ischemia and 40 control clients examined during head rotation using transcranial Doppler ultrasonography as a reference standard.[115]

Combined Cervical Extension and Rotation Statistics

- SN 21 (NR), SP 100 (NR), +LR 6.3, −LR 0.81, QUADAS 6, in 27 asymptomatic clients (mean age 62 years, 6 women) and 23 students (mean age 21 years, none were female) with transcranial Doppler measurement of blood flow as a reference standard.[116]

- SN 9 (NR), SP 98 (NR), +LR 4.2, −LR 0.93, QUADAS 7, in 1,108 clients (mean age, sex, and duration of symptoms not detailed) examined for potential neurovascular compromise and using duplex ultrasonography as a reference standard.[117]

The clinician should also be cognizant of ruling out the potential for vestibular dysfunction. One test with lower risk is the dizziness test. This test attempts to differentiate dizziness due to vestibulocochlear dysfunction versus CAD. The head is

TABLE 17.3 Functional Positional Testing for Cervical Artery Dysfunction

Test	Purpose	Evidence	Limitation and advantages
Cervical rotation	Affects flow in contralateral vertebral artery. Limited effect on internal carotid artery.	Poor SN, variable SP. Blood flow studies support effect on vertebral artery flow.	Only assesses posterior circulation. Interpret with caution.
Cervical extension	Affects flow in internal carotid arteries. Limited effect on vertebral arteries.	No specific diagnostic utility evidence available. Blood flow studies; internal carotid artery flow.	Primarily assesses anterior circulation.
Blood pressure	Measure of cardiovascular health.	Correlates to cervical arterial atherosclerotic pathology.	Reliability dependent on clinician. Continuous, not categorical, measure.
Cranial nerves	Identifies nerve dysfunction resulting from ischemia	No specific diagnostic utility evidence available.	Reliability dependent on experience.
Eye exam	Assists in diagnosis of possible neural deficit related to internal carotid artery.	No specific diagnostic utility evidence available.	May be early warning of serious underlying pathology.

Data from Kerry and Taylor 2006; Kerry and Taylor 2009; Cook and Hegedus 2008.[100-102]

passively rotated in one direction and symptoms are assessed. If dizziness is noted, it is not clear whether these symptoms are due to vestibulocochlear or CAD. If the head is held stationary, and the client is asked to actively rotate their body (producing rotation of the head in the same direction as the first part of this test), and dizziness is again noted, it is suggested that the dizziness is due to CAD. Vestibulocochlear dysfunction is produced by movement of the head (positioning of the head), while CAD is produced by the position of the head relative to the trunk (whether the head is moved on the trunk or vice versa).

A test with implied higher risk is the Dix-Hallpike test for benign paroxysmal positional vertigo (BPPV). Clients with BPPV report repeated episodes of vertigo with changes in head position.

Physical examination for these clients requires that each of the following criteria be fulfilled:[118]

- Vertigo associated with nystagmus is provoked by the Dix-Hallpike test.
- There is a latency period between the completion of the Dix-Hallpike test and the onset of vertigo and nystagmus.
- The provoked vertigo and nystagmus increase and then resolve within a time period of 60 seconds from onset of nystagmus.

The estimated diagnostic accuracy of the Dix-Hallpike test is as follows:

- SN 79 (65-94), SP 75 (33-100), +LR 3.2, −LR 0.28 with a criterion reference diagnosis by neurologists and otolaryngologists across various studies.[119]

Critical Clinical Pearls

When assessing the potential existence for CAD, keep the following in mind:

- A comprehensive, detailed examination is necessary.
- CAD testing is ongoing as soon as the clinician first interacts with the client and incorporates multiple aspects of the funnel examination (e.g., interview, observation, and screening).
- Client involvement in the decision-making process is required and suggested by the International Federation of Orthopaedic Manipulative Physical Therapists.[93]
- Utilization of the CCSR and NEXUS may be a necessary component, but clinicians must realize that the diagnostic accuracy of these tools for ruling out cervical spine fractures is relative for acutely injured clients presenting in the emergency room.
- Clinicians should monitor for risk factors associated with the potential for ligamentous or bony compromise of the upper cervical spine.[95]
- Clinicians should monitor for risk factors for CAD that can be assessed during the history.[96, 97]
- Clinicians should monitor for other traditionally suggested subjective complaints (e.g., dysphagia, dysarthria, diplopia, double vision, nausea, numbness) and objective signs (e.g., ataxia, nystagmus).
- Clearance of potential upper cervical instability is necessary prior to CAD testing.
- Some of the suggested stability tests of the upper cervical spine are complex. The clinician should become proficient in these tests before implementing them.
- CAD testing is controversial and has been suggested to lack precision in diagnostic accuracy. Support for testing ability to accurately identify clients at risk has been suggested to be insufficient.[60]
- Some literature also suggests that many clinicians demonstrate a lack of confidence in functional positional testing.[111]
- Current best evidence suggests the utilization of the suggested flowchart of clinical reasoning regarding clearance of the cervical spine by the International Federation of Orthopaedic Manipulative Physical Therapists[93] as listed earlier in this chapter.

Ruling Out Pain Generation From Nonorganic or Psychological-Related Sources

Nonorganic symptoms and signs have been described in the medical literature dating back to the early part of the 20th century, and they were initially felt to be an indication of malingering. As medical research advanced, however, it became apparent that these symptoms and signs were more closely correlated with psychological distress and abnormal illness behavior rather than malingering.[120] Waddell's signs have been long-held testing methods to assess for nonorganic signs contributing to pain (see chapter 19, Lumbar Spine). Sobel and colleagues[120] have developed a standardized set of eight physical examination signs (some of Waddell's lumbar spine signs extrapolated to the cervical spine and three additional signs that they developed). These signs were standardized and proven reliable.[120]

1. **Tenderness**
   - *Superficial.* Clinician palpates the cervical spine region, comprised of the posterior aspect of the cervical and upper thoracic spine. A (+) test is if the client complains of pain with light touch or light pinching of the skin.
   - *Nonanatomic.* The areas of the cervical, thoracic, lumbar, and brachial regions are deeply palpated. If the client also had concomitant low back pain, then pain on deep palpation of the low back was discounted and the region of the arm was added to the criteria.

2. **Simulation:** When a simulation test is performed, the client is under the assumption that the painful area is being tested when, in reality, it is not. A test is considered (+) if the client reports pain with the physical exam maneuver.
   - *Rotation of head, shoulder, and trunk in the sitting position.* With the client sitting on the examination table facing the clinician, the clinician rotates the client's trunk to the right and left using the client's shoulders. The clinician must take care to observe that the head is rotating in the same plane as the shoulders.
   - *Rotation of the head, shoulder, trunk, and pelvis while standing.* Similar to the sitting test, the clinician rotates the client's shoulders, trunk, and pelvis to the right and left as one unit. Care must be taken to observe that the head is rotating in the same plane as the shoulders, trunk, and pelvis. A (+) test is if the client complains of neck pain with rotation.

3. **Range of motion:** To test for cervical rotation, the clinician asks the seated client to rotate their head as far as possible to the right and then left. A (+) test is when rotation is less than 50% of normal in each direction. This test was devised based on the fact that the majority of cervical rotation occurs in the upper cervical spine, and the majority of cervical spine lesions are in the mid to lower cervical spine.

4. **Regional disturbance:** For motor or sensory changes to be classified under this category, the deficit has to fall out of what is considered normal neuroanatomy. For example, a client who reports loss of sensation involving half of the body or an entire upper extremity would be considered to fall into this category as long as multiple nerve root or peripheral nerve injury has been ruled out. Care must be taken to rule out multiple nerve root or peripheral nerve injuries before considering that either or both of the regional disturbance subcategories are positive.
   - *Sensory loss.* For this test to be considered (+), the client must report diminished sensation to either light touch or pinprick in a pattern that does not correspond to a specific dermatome of a nerve root or peripheral nerve. Frequently, clients will report loss of sensation of the entire upper extremity or below the elbow.
   - *Motor loss.* On formal manual muscle testing, weakness is detected in a nonanatomic pattern. The hallmark of this test is giveaway weakness. In addition, a test would also be considered (+) if, on observation, the client demonstrates normal muscle strength, but exhibits weakness on formal testing. For example, the client uses their elbow extensors to get up onto the examination table but is then noted to have less than antigravity strength on manual muscle testing of the elbow extensors.

5. **Overreaction:** In this study, this category was considered (+) if the clinician felt that the client was overreacting during the examination. Examples of overreaction were reported to include rubbing the affected area for more than 3 seconds, grimacing due to pain, and

sighing. For the clinician, this is a very subjective category. Therefore, clinicians must take care not to let their own emotional feelings about the client interfere with the assessment of whether or not the client is overreacting to the examination. In addition, the clinician must take into account that there can be a considerable degree of cultural variation in the response to painful maneuvers.

Ruling Out Pain Generation From Other Related Structures: Thoracic Spine

The thoracic spine can be a pain generator for pain in the cervical spine. Serious pathology, such as fracture in the thoracic spine, is of primary concern.

Thoracic Spine Fractures

- Closed-fist percussion sign: **SN 88 (75-95), SP 90 (73-98), +LR 8.8, −LR 0.14,** QUADAS 10[121]

- Supine sign: **SN 81 (67-91), SP 93 (83-99), +LR 11.6, −LR 0.20,** QUADAS 10[121]

Additionally, as with any joint, clearing AROM with or without overpressure is necessary. AROM of all motions as per the lower quarter screen described in chapter 7 should be implemented. In order to fully clear the thoracic spine, full AROM (with overpressure if pain-free) must be present.

Sensitive Tests for the Cervical Spine

Radiculopathy and discogenic-related pathology can be ruled out with a combination of Spurling's test and the upper limb neurodynamic test (median nerve bias) (tests of high SN and low −LR):

- Spurling's test: **SN 93 (77-99), SP 95 (76-100), +LR 19.6, −LR 0.07,** QUADAS 9[122]

- Median nerve upper limb neurodynamic test: **SN 97 (90-100),** SP 22 (12-33), +LR 1.3, **−LR 0.12,** QUADAS 10[18]

- Arm squeeze test (described for cervical nerve root compression): SN 95 (85-99), SP 96 (87-99), +LR 24, −LR 0.05, QUADAS 8[123]

Additionally, as with any joint, clearing AROM with or without overpressure is necessary. In order to fully clear the cervical spine, full AROM (with overpressure if pain-free) must be present. Detail in this regard is described in the following section.

MOTION TESTS

The cervical spine has a relatively unique complex biomechanical and anatomical nature. As with all regions of the body in orthopedic medicine, it is necessary to understand the reliability of motion assessment. The various cervical spine joints, their positions, end-feel, and ROM norm values are listed in table 17.4.

TABLE 17.4   Cervical Spine Arthrology

Joint	Close-packed position	Resting position	Capsular pattern	ROM norms	End-feel
OA joint	Not described	Not described	Extension and side bending equally limited. Rotation and flexion are not affected.	Combined flexion and extension reported to range from 14–35°; side bending reported to range from 2–11°; axial rotation reported to range from about 0–7°.	Firm for all motions
C1-C2	Not described	Not described	Restriction with rotation	Flexion–extension is approximately 10°; rotation is approximately 40°.	Firm for all motions
C3-C7 (typical cervical spine) facet joint	Full extension	Midway between flexion and extension	Side bending and rotation are equally limited; extension is more limited than flexion.	Flexion: 50° Extension: 60° Right side bending: 45° Left side bending: 45° Right rotation: 80° Left rotation: 80°	Firm for all motions

Assessment of cervical spine ROM is reliable across various clients and measurement devices.[124-126] The ICC values ranged from 0.45 to 0.79 with the use of a bubble inclinometer for clients with and without neck pain.[127] Client estimates of reduced neck ROM are not accurate compared to clinician measurement.[35]

Soft-tissue lesions may affect neck motion as reflected by active range of motion (AROM). Among clients with WAD, increasing severity of lesions to the alar ligaments was associated with a decrease in maximal flexion and rotation. A similar pattern was seen for lesions to the transverse ligament. An abnormally posterior atlantooccipital membrane was associated with shorter range of left rotation. No significant association was found in relation to lesions to the tectorial membrane, but very few clients had such lesions. Since lesions to different structures seem to affect the same movement, AROM alone is not a sufficient indicator for soft-tissue lesions to specific structures in the upper cervical spine.[128] Clients with other pathologies have also been shown to have limitations in ROM. Mean cervical spine ROM was reduced in clients with cervicogenic headache.[129]

Elderly clients have been shown to have decreased ROM in all planes compared to their younger counterparts, for both men and women.[130, 131] The elderly group also had a wider variation of cervical ROM values as compared to the younger group. Women were found to have greater ROM in all cohort age groups.[130]

Passive and Active ROMs

Active ROM of the cervical spine can be generally assessed with observation and previous components of the examination. The clinician can get an idea of the client's AROM with the client interview and observation. The client unwilling or unable to move their head comfortably should be suspected of having limited AROM, and possibly spinal instability, until proven otherwise.

In the cervical and lumbar spine, it may be particularly beneficial to also perform combined motions. These are often referred to as *quadrant positions*. Therefore, if the single-plane movements were unremarkable for reproduction of the client's pain, the clinician may want to also implement these combined motions to further test these regions of the spine. Posterior quadrants would involve the motions of extension, side bending, and rotation to the same side, while anterior quadrants would involve the combined active motions of flexion, side bending, and rotation to the same side. Additionally, these measures provide the clinician with a nice big-picture assessment of the client's functional status, degree of irritability, and willingness to move.

CERVICAL FLEXION

Client Position	Sitting with arms relaxed
Clinician Position	Standing directly to the side of the client
Goniometer Alignment	The clinician positions the fulcrum over the external auditory meatus, places the proximal arm either perpendicular or parallel to the table, and aligns the distal arm with the base of the nose.
Movement	The clinician places one hand on the back of the client's head and the other hand on the client's chin. The clinician passively pulls the client's chin down toward their chest to end range flexion (normal end-feel is firm). This motion can be performed similarly actively by the client (without assistance from the clinician). Active range of motion should be performed prior to passive range of motion (PROM) to determine the client's willingness to move.
Assessment	Clinician assesses for amount of ROM, end-feel, quality of the movement, client response, potential difference between AROM and PROM, and so on.

CERVICAL EXTENSION

Client Position	Sitting with arms relaxed
Clinician Position	Standing directly to the side of the client
Goniometer Alignment	The clinician positions the fulcrum over the client's external auditory meatus, places the proximal arm either perpendicular or parallel to the table, and aligns the distal arm with the base of the nose.
Movement	The clinician places one hand on the back of the client's head and the other hand on their chin. The clinician passively lifts the client's chin up away from their chest to end range extension (normal end-feel is firm). This motion can be performed similarly actively by the client (without assistance from the clinician). Active range of motion should be performed prior to PROM to determine the client's willingness to move.
Assessment	Clinician assesses for amount of ROM, end-feel, quality of the movement, client response, potential difference between AROM and PROM, and so on.

CERVICAL ROTATION

Client Position	Sitting with arms relaxed
Clinician Position	Standing directly behind the client
Goniometer Alignment	The clinician positions the fulcrum over the center of the cranial aspect of the client's head and aligns the proximal arm parallel to the bilateral acromion processes and the distal arm with the tip of the client's nose.
Movement	The clinician places both hands on the sides of the client's face and passively rotates their head to the side to be assessed to end range rotation (normal end-feel is firm). This motion can be performed similarly actively by the client (without assistance from the clinician). Active range of motion should be performed prior to PROM to determine the client's willingness to move.
Assessment	Clinician assesses for amount of ROM, end-feel, quality of the movement, client response, potential difference between AROM and PROM, and so on.

CERVICAL SIDE BENDING

Client Position	Sitting with arms relaxed
Clinician Position	Standing directly behind the client
Goniometer Alignment	The clinician positions the fulcrum over the spinous process of the client's C7 and aligns the proximal arm with the spinous processes of the thoracic spine and the distal arm with the midline of the head.
Movement	The clinician stabilizes the contralateral shoulder with one hand and places the other hand on top of the client's head. Stabilizing the shoulder, the clinician passively pulls the client's head toward the opposite shoulder to end range side bending (normal end-feel is firm). This motion can be performed similarly actively by the client (without assistance from the clinician). Active range of motion should be performed prior to PROM to determine the client's willingness to move.
Assessment	Clinician assesses for amount of ROM, end-feel, quality of the movement, client response, potential difference between AROM and PROM, and so on.

Passive Accessories

Passive accessory (articular) intervertebral motion (PAIVM) is a term commonly used to describe accessory joint play in the spine, while *passive physiological intervertebral motion* (PPIVM) is a term commonly used to describe passive ROM of the spine. Depending on the method of assessment, these terms (and therefore techniques) sometimes can be difficult to differentiate. Attempts will be made in the spinal sections to differentiate between these techniques and terms, but the reader is reminded of this difficulty in distinction.

Once all joint play assessments are complete, the clinician should be able to discern which facet joint is restricted (assuming there is facet joint dysfunction). For the C0-C1 joint, restricted posterior gliding of the occipital condyle is found with C0-C1 flexion and contralateral side bend. Restricted anterior gliding of the condyle is found with extension and the ipsilateral side bend. Assessment of the C1-C2 joint is predominantly with rotation, as described. The inability of a facet joint to go down and back (or posterior and inferior) in the typical spine would be found with extension, contralateral side glide, and ipsilateral rotation. The inability of a facet joint to go up and forward would be found with flexion, ipsilateral side glide, and contralateral rotation.

C0-C1 (ATLANTOOCCIPITAL) JOINT: SEGMENTAL MOBILITY TESTING

C0-C1 FLEXION AND EXTENSION (PPIVM)

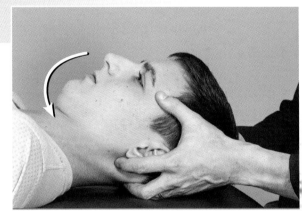

Figure 17.15

Client Position	Supine with head at top of table
Clinician Position	Standing at head of table facing client
Movement	The clinician palpates the transverse processes of C1 with their index fingers if possible. The clinician flexes and extends the client's head at the upper cervical spine only. The axis for this motion is through the ears.
Assessment	Assessment is done for joint motion, client response, and end-feel. Reproduction of concordant pain suggests dysfunction. Impaired joint mobility or end-feel may also suggest dysfunction if concordant pain is also reproduced.

- OA (C0-C1) joint flexion assesses for the ability of that joint to posteriorly glide. A restriction (lack of joint play or restricted end-feel) reveals either bilateral or unilateral limited posterior glide.
- OA (C0-C1) joint extension assesses for the ability of that joint to anteriorly glide. A restriction (lack of joint play or restricted end-feel) reveals either bilateral or unilateral limited anterior glide.

Notes
- The amount of movement is small (14–35°) and difficult to assess because the mid-cervical spine kicks into motion easily.
- If restricted motion is noted, a side bending assessment is suggested to determine the side of involvement.

C0-C1 SIDE BENDING (PPIVM)

Client Position   Supine with head at top of table

Clinician Position   Standing at head of table facing client

Movement   The clinician palpates the transverse processes of the client's C1 with their index fingers. The clinician side bends the head only with the 3rd through 5th fingers of bilateral hands via the mastoid process. The axis of movement is through the nose—no deflection should be seen; otherwise movement is taking place in the mid-cervical spine. During the assessment of right side bending (as shown here), the right transverse process should become more prominent as the right C0 moves medial, inferior, and anterior (MIA).

Assessment   Assessment is done for joint motion, client response, and end-feel. Restricted joint mobility or end-feel and/or reproduction of concordant pain suggest potential dysfunction.

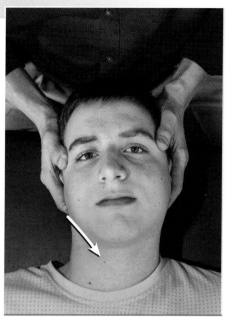

Figure 17.16

- Side bending: The ipsilateral condyle moves MIA and the contralateral condyle moves lateral, posterior, and superior (LPS). Right side bending example: right side OA joint moves MIA, left OA joint moves LPS.

- Restricted right side bending: Either restricted right MIA or left LPS movement occurs.

- Restricted MIA movement will be noted with ipsilateral side bending and anterior glide (described previously). In above example, right side bending and anterior glide restriction would indicate right OA joint anterior glide restricted.

- Restricted LPS movement will be noted with contralateral side bending and posterior glide (described previously). In above example, right side bending and posterior glide restriction would indicate left OA joint posterior glide restricted.

C1-C2 (ATLANTOAXIAL) JOINT

ACTIVE MOTION SCREEN

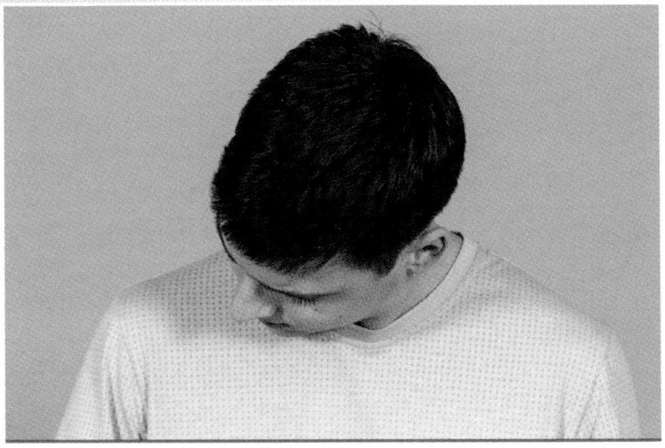

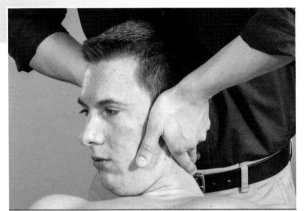

Client Position	Sitting in upright posture with neutral spine and scapulae retracted
Clinician Position	Monitoring posture and symmetry of movement from side to side
Movement	The clinician has the client flex the cervical spine maximally to reduce the contribution of the lower segments. The clinician asks the client to fully rotate in both directions (right shown here), and then observes the quality and quantity of the ROM.

Figure 17.17

Assessment	The clinician assesses for ROM, side-to-side asymmetry, and overall limited mobility. They should assess C1-C2 segmental mobility regardless of whether or not a limitation was determined.
Note	The clinician should make sure that the client maintains cervical flexion.

SEGMENTAL MOBILITY TESTING

C1-C2 ROTATION: FLEXION–ROTATION TEST (PPIVM)

 Video 17.18 in the web resource shows a demonstration of this test.

Client Position	Supine with head at top of table
Clinician Position	Standing at head of table facing client
Movement	The clinician fully flexes the client's head (to help eliminate movement coming from the lower cervical spine) and then rotates it fully both to the right (as shown) and to the left, assessing for available motion and end-feel.

Figure 17.18

Assessment	Assessment is done for joint motion, client response, and end-feel.

- Loss of ≥10° is considered a positive test for cervicogenic headache: **SN 86 (NR), SP 100 (NR), +LR Inf, –LR 0.14**, QUADAS 12, in a study of 28 clients with side-dominant cervicogenic headache (mean age 43.3 years, 20 women, mean duration of symptoms not reported) matched with 28 asymptomatic clients and using a criterion reference.[24]
- SN 91 (NR), SP 90 (NR), +LR 9.1, –LR 0.1, QUADAS 8, in a study of 23 cervicogenic HA, 23 asymptomatic controls, and 12 migraine HA clients (aged 18-66 years, mean duration of symptoms not reported) matched with 28 asymptomatic clients, using a headache questionnaire and Visual Analogue Scale (VAS) as a reference for pain.[132]

Note	The full flexion of the cervical spine must be maintained throughout the assessment.

PRONE C0-C1, C1-C2, C2-3 PAIVM

It should be noted that these three prone techniques are distinctly PAIVMs due to the motion's being distinctly imparted through accessory joint play.

Statistics[133]
- SN 59, SP 82, +LR 3.3, –LR 0.49, at C0-C1, QUADAS 10
- SN 62, **SP 87**, **+LR 4.9**, –LR 0.43, at C1-C2
- SN 65, SP 78, +LR 2.9, –LR 0.44, at C2-C3

PRONE C0-C1 PAIVM

 Video 17.19 **in the web resource shows a demonstration of this test.**

Client Position	Prone with arms relaxed at sides of table, head in neutral
Clinician Position	Standing at head of table facing client
Movement and Direction of Force	The clinician palpates the suboccipital region, using thumb-over-thumb purchase contact on the C0-1 joint *(a, b)*. The clinician pushes the paraspinal musculature medially to avoid compressing through this tissue when performing this assessment. Keeping their elbows straight and leaning over the client as shown *(c)*, the clinician applies force in the direction of the client's orbit (eye). Initially, they should apply light pressure only. If the client tolerates this well, the clinician should repeat movements and reassess.
Assessment	Assessment is done for joint play/passive accessory motion, client response, and end-feel. Reproduction of concordant pain suggests dysfunction. Impaired joint mobility or end-feel may also suggest dysfunction if concordant pain is also reproduced.

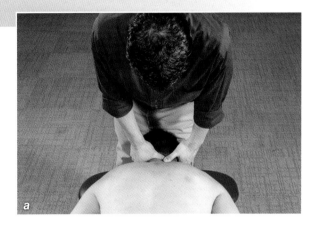

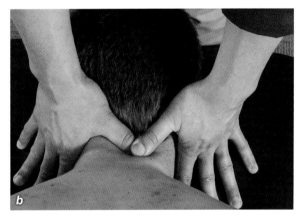

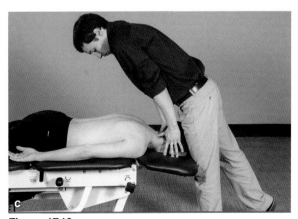

Figure 17.19

PRONE C1-C2 PAIVM

 Video 17.20 **in the web resource shows a demonstration of this test.**

Client Position	Prone with arms relaxed at side of table, head in neutral
Clinician Position	Standing at head of table facing client
Movement and Direction of Force	The clinician palpates the facet joint of the client's C2-3 (right side as shown) *(a)*, using thumb-over-thumb purchase contact on the joint *(b)*. The clinician rotates the client's head to the ipsilateral side (approximately 30°) (right rotation as shown). Keeping their elbows straight and standing on the opposite side *(c)*, the clinician applies force in the direction of the client's mouth. Initially, they apply light pressure. If the client tolerates this well, the clinician can repeat movements and reassess.
Assessment	Assessment is done for joint play/passive accessory motion, client response, and end-feel. Reproduction of concordant pain suggests dysfunction. Impaired joint mobility or end-feel may also suggest dysfunction if concordant pain is also reproduced.

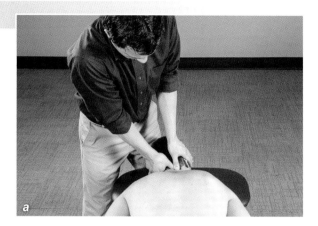

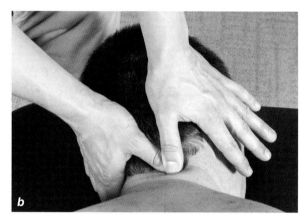

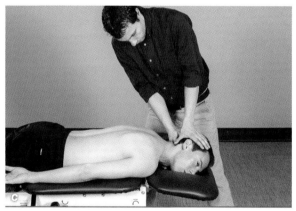

Figure 17.20

PRONE C2-C3 PAIVM

Video 17.21 in the web resource shows a demonstration of this test.

Client Position	Prone with arms relaxed at side of table, head in neutral
Clinician Position	Standing at head of table facing client
Movement and Direction of Force	The clinician palpates the facet joint of the client's C2-3 (right side as shown) *(a)*, using thumb-over-thumb purchase contact on the joint *(b)*. Keeping their elbows straight and leaning slightly over the client *(c)*, the clinician applies force in the direction of the table. Initially, they apply light pressure only. If the client tolerates this well, the clinician should repeat movements and reassess.
Assessment	Assessment is done for joint play/passive accessory motion, client response, and end-feel. Reproduction of concordant pain suggests dysfunction. Impaired joint mobility or end-feel may also suggest dysfunction if concordant pain is also reproduced.

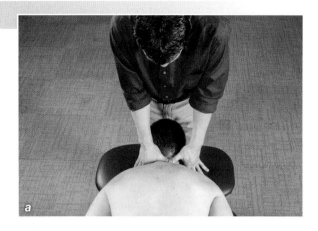

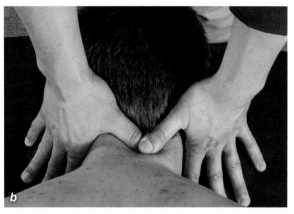

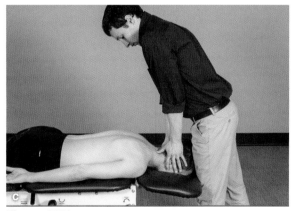

Figure 17.21

TYPICAL CERVICAL SPINE (C3-C7): SEGMENTAL MOBILITY TESTING

EXTENSION PAIVM

Client Position	Supine with head at top of table
Clinician Position	Standing at head of table facing client
Movement and Direction of Force	The clinician first ensures that the client's neck is in neutral since clients will often Figure 17.22 when lying supine. The clinician may need to place a towel or firm surface under the occiput to promote neutral spine posture. The clinician purchase involves placing the radial border of their index fingers along the lamina of the vertebra to be tested. The clinician lifts ventrally/anteriorly with both fingers until extension occurs

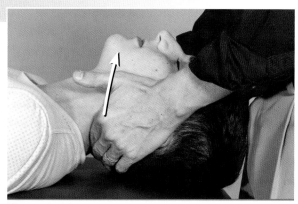

Figure 17.22

at the desired segment. The clinician starts their assessment cranially (at C3-C4) and moves caudally from segment to segment along the cervical spine. Initially, they apply light pressure and gradually increase the pressure if tolerated to properly assess the movement.

Assessment	Assessment is done for joint play/passive accessory motion, client response, and end-feel. Reproduction of concordant pain suggests dysfunction. Impaired joint mobility or end-feel may also suggest dysfunction if concordant pain is also reproduced.

- Restricted movement with this assessment can be either bilateral or unilateral with down and back (posterior and inferior, or extension) movement limitation of that level's facets.

- To determine if the restriction is bilateral or unilateral, the clinician will perform side-glide assessments.

SIDE-GLIDE PAIVM

Client Position	Supine with head at top of table
Clinician Position	Standing at head of table facing client
Movement and Direction of Force	With the anterior radial aspect of the MCP joint of the index finger (right hand as shown), the clinician purchases the articular pillar of the segment to be tested. The clinician will have to move to the side to be assessed and keep their forearms in line with the direction being assessed, extend the wrist, and gently cup their hands around the client's neck (no pressure on ventral/anterior surface of neck). The clinician side glides the segment to the opposite direction (left as shown), adding a little tilt at the end of the movement. (This makes it easier to feel what is going on.) In side gliding to the left, the clinician checks for movement down and back on the right, and up and forward on the left.
Assessment	Assessment is done for joint play/passive accessory motion, client response, and end-feel. Reproduction of concordant pain suggests dysfunction. Impaired joint mobility or end-feel may also suggest dysfunction if concordant pain is also reproduced.

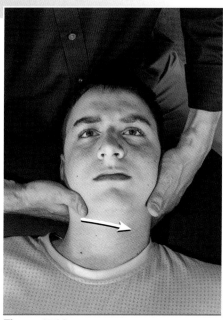

Figure 17.23

- The side glide is named for the direction the head moves.
- The left side glide is relatively the same as right side bending.
- Restricted side-glide movement either involves ipsilateral restricted down and back (posterior and inferior) movement or contralateral restricted up and forward (anterior and superior) movement.

ROTATION PAIVM

Client Position	Supine with head at top of table
Clinician Position	Standing at head of table facing client
Movement and Direction of Force	The clinician purchases the posterior portion of the transverse process with the radial portion of the index finger on the side contralateral to the direction of rotation (left side/hand as shown). With the other hand (clinician's right hand as shown), the clinician supports and stabilizes the client's head and spine. The clinician rotates the client's head (to the right as shown) by side bending their own body. The clinician should use a hand motion that is similar to sliding a hand around a cylinder.
Assessment	The clinician assesses for joint play/passive accessory motion, client response, and end-feel, looking for restricted contralateral up and forward (superior and anterior) movement and ipsilateral down and back movement (posterior and inferior). Restricted joint mobility or end-feel and/or reproduction of concordant pain suggest potential dysfunction at this level.

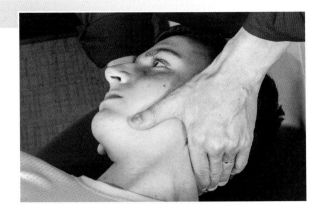

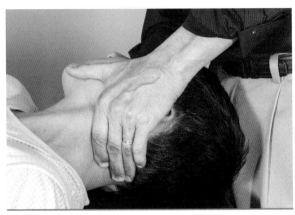

Figure 17.24

PRONE POSTERIOR-ANTERIOR (PA) MOBILIZATION (PAIVM)

Client Position	Prone with arms relaxed at sides of table, head in neutral
Clinician Position	Standing at head of table facing client
Movement and Direction of Force	The clinician palpates facet joint of respective levels of cervical spine using thumb-over-thumb purchase contact on the joint (spinous processes for central PAs and facet joints on each respective side for unilateral PAs). Initially, the clinician applies light pressure only in the posterior–anterior direction. If the client tolerates this well, the clinician should repeat the movements and reassess.
Assessment	Assessment is done for joint play motion/passive accessory motion, client response, and end-feel. Reproduction of concordant pain suggests dysfunction. Impaired joint mobility or end-feel may also suggest dysfunction if concordant pain is also reproduced.

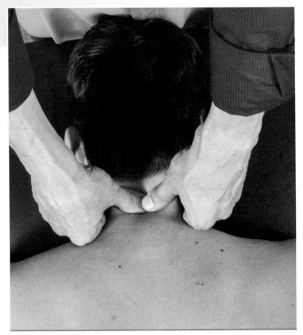

Figure 17.25

Statistics
- SN 88 (76-95), SP 39 (23-58), +LR 1.5, −LR 0.30, at C2-C3
- SN 89 (79-96), SP 50 (37-63), +LR 1.8, −LR 0.21, at C5-C6, QUADAS 5 in a study of 173 clients with neck pain in whom cervical zygapophyseal joint pain was suspected on clinical examination (median age 42 years; 95 women; duration of symptoms NR), using a controlled diagnostic block as a reference standard.[134]
- **SN 100 (NR), SP 100 (NR),** QUADAS 9, in a study of 20 clients with neck pain (mean age NR; 13 women; duration of symptoms at least 12 months), using a radiographically controlled diagnostic nerve block as a reference standard.[31]

Critical Clinical Pearls

When performing joint mobility assessment (PPIVM and PAIVM) for cervical and thoracic spine, keep the following in mind:

- Pain during segmental testing is associated with reports of neck pain: **SN 82**, SP 79, +LR 3.9, **−LR 0.23**, QUADAS 9.[135]
- Intertester reliability for this testing is poor[136] to good.[137]
- Assessment of pain intertester reliability is better than mobility assessment alone for both cervical and thoracic spine.[137]
- Isolating appropriate upper cervical spine level of pathology using the concordant sign was **100% SN** and **100% SP** in one high-quality study.[31]
- Segmental mobility testing for determination of C1-C2 contribution to cervicogenic headache is (**SN 86, −LR 0,14, SP 100, +LR Inf**).[24]
- Joint mobility assessment (PAIVM) of C0-1 (SP 82, +LR 3.3), C1-2 (**SP 87, +LR 4.9**), and C2-3 (SP 78, +LR 2.9) all had diagnostic capability in one high-quality study (QUADAS 10).[133]

PALPATION SIDE GLIDE TEST

Client Position	Sitting, head in neutral
Clinician Position	Standing to the side and facing the client
Movement and Direction of Force	The clinician places one hand on top of the client's head (left as shown). With the other hand (right as shown), the clinician purchases the respective levels to be assessed (e.g., C2-3, C3-4). The clinician imparts a side bending force as shown and assesses for availability of motion at the palpated segment.
Assessment	A (+) test is restricted joint play/passive accessory motion, suggesting potential dysfunction at this level.
Statistics	SN 98 (NR), SP 74 (NR), +LR 3.8, **−LR 0.03**, QUADAS 10, in a study of three clients with congenitally blocked vertebra (mean age and sex NR), using radiograph as a reference standard.[138]

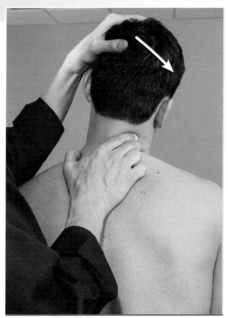

Figure 17.26

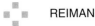

Critical Clinical Pearls

The clinician is reminded of the stronger diagnostic accuracy of the prone PA (PAIVM) examination. This examination is suggested, especially when concordant pain is reproduced. The sequence of testing in prone is as follows:

- Prone C0-C1 PAIVM (SN 59, SP 82, +LR 3.3, –LR 0.49)[133]
- Prone C1-C2 PAIVM (SN 62, **SP 87, +LR 4.9**, –LR 0.43)[133]
- Prone C2-C3 PAIVM (SN 65, SP 78, +LR 2.9, –LR 0.44)[133]
- Prone posterior–anterior (PA) mobilization (PAIVM) for typical cervical spine (C3-7)[31]

Flexibility

As detailed in chapter 8, flexibility concerns the motion that a particular joint is capable of. Assessment of flexibility can assist the clinician in determination of the potential presence of soft-tissue dysfunction.[139] The primary muscles of concern relative to the cervical spine are listed in tables 17.5 and 17.6.

TABLE 17.5 Cervical Musculature

Muscle	Origin	Insertion	Action	Innervation
Levator scapulae	Transverse processes of C1-C4	Superomedial border of scapula	Elevation of scapula, scapular adduction, and downward rotation	Dorsal scapular nerve C3-C5
Trapezius	Superior nuchal line, occipital protuberance, nuchal ligament	Lateral clavicle, acromion, spine of scapula	Elevation of scapula	Spinal root of accessory nerve C3-C4
Sternocleidomastoid	Mastoid process and lateral superior nuchal line	Sternal head: anterior manubrium Clavicular head: superior medial clavicle	Neck flexion, ipsilateral side bending, and contralateral rotation	Spinal root of accessory nerve C2-C3

TABLE 17.6 Suboccipital Muscles

Muscle	Origin	Insertion	Action	Innervation
Obliquus capitis inferior	C2 spinous process	C1 transverse process	Rotation of atlas (turning head to same side)	Dorsal ramus of C1
Obliquus capitis superior	C1 transverse process	Occipital bone	Extension and lateral flexion of head	Dorsal ramus of C1
Rectus capitis posterior major	C2 spinous process	Occipital bone	Extension of head, rotation of head to same side	Dorsal ramus of C1
Rectus capitis posterior minor	Posterior tubercle of C2	Occipital bone	Extension of head	Dorsal ramus of C1

LEVATOR SCAPULAE ASSESSMENT

Client Position
Supine with arms initially at side or resting on their stomach

Clinician Position
Sitting at the head of the table

Movement
Clinician stabilizes the shoulder girdle with one hand, while supporting the occiput with the other hand. The clinician then introduces flexion, side bending away, and rotation toward side to be tested to the resistance barrier *(a)*. In an alternative option, the clinician places the client's arm above the head and exerts caudad compression on the elbow with the same head position *(b)*.

Assessment
The clinician assesses the muscle length and compares it to the opposite side. Asymmetry implicates restricted muscle length and excursion.

Statistics
There are no known normative or statistical data for this flexibility measure.

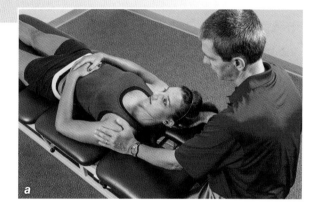

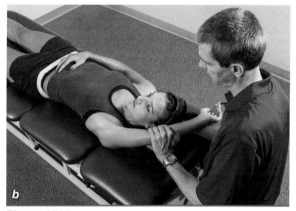

Figure 17.27

UPPER TRAPEZIUS ASSESSMENT— SITTING

Client Position	Upright posture
Clinician Position	Standing just behind the side to be tested
Movement	The clinician side bends the client's cervical spine (laterally flexed) away and rotates it toward the side to be tested *(a)*. The clinician then elevates the shoulder girdle on the side being tested by lifting up on the ipsilateral elbow as shown *(b)* without allowing trunk movement.
Assessment	• If additional ROM is achieved with shoulder girdle elevation, especially with cervical rotation, tightness in the upper trapezius is implicated.
	• Asymmetry from side to side also implicates upper trapezius tightness or restriction.
	• No additional ROM, or improvement in ROM, might suggest cervical spine joint restriction(s).
Statistics	There are no known normative or statistical data for this flexibility measure.

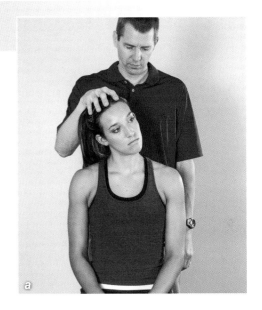

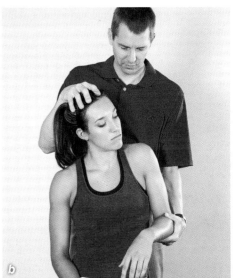

Figure 17.28

STERNOCLEIDOMASTOID ASSESSMENT

Client Position	Supine with arms at their side or resting comfortably on their stomach
Clinician Position	Sitting at the head of the table, directly facing the client
Movement	The clinician stabilizes the client's shoulder girdle with one hand (left as shown) while supporting the client's occiput with the other hand (right as shown). The clinician introduces cervical spine side bending away from and rotation toward the side to be assessed.

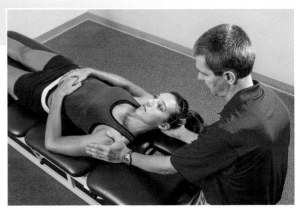

Figure 17.29

Assessment Muscle length is assessed and compared to the other side.

Statistics There are no known normative or statistical data for this flexibility measure.

SUBOCCIPITAL MUSCLES ASSESSMENT

Client Position Supine with arms resting at side or comfortably on their stomach

Clinician Position Standing or sitting at the head of the table, directly facing the client

Movement The clinician supports the client's head with one hand and places the other hand on the client's forehead *(a)*. The clinician flexes the client's upper cervical spine (right hand as shown) (chin tuck) while applying gentle traction (left hand as shown). The clinician rotates the client's head 30° to focus the assessment on that side *(b)*.

Assessment Muscle length is assessed and compared to the opposite side.

Statistics There are no known normative or statistical data for this flexibility measure.

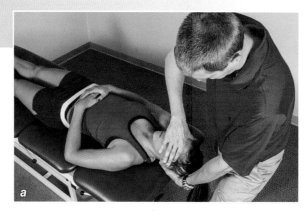

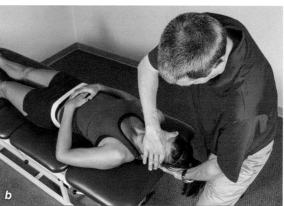

Figure 17.30

MUSCLE PERFORMANCE TESTING

In cervical radiculopathy, manual muscle testing is thought by some to be the most important component of the examination for localizing the involved nerve root.[68, 140, 141] Upper extremity weakness could be caused by cervical radiculopathy, brachial plexopathy, peripheral nerve entrapment neuropathy (e.g., median neuropathy, radial neuropathy, or ulnar neuropathy), poor client effort, or pain from a tendinopathy (e.g., shoulder impingement or lateral epicondylopathy). Manual muscle testing will assist the clinician in interpretation of whether or not the muscle weakness is myotomal, involving peripheral nerve root, a single muscle, and so on. Bono and colleagues suggested that the diagnosis of cervical radiculopathy be considered in clients with atypical findings such as deltoid weakness, scapular winging, weakness of the intrinsic muscles of the hand, chest or deep breast pain, and headaches.[68]

The clinician should also be cognizant of muscle performance impairments presenting in clients with various pathologies or treatment-based classifications. Coordination, strength, and endurance deficits of neck and upper quarter muscles (longus colli, middle trapezius, lower trapezius, and serratus anterior) are common in clients with movement coordination impairments.[11]

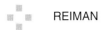

CAPITAL EXTENSION

Client Position	Prone, arms at their sides, with head off edge of table
Clinician Position	Standing directly to the side of the client
Movement and Assessment	The clinician provides resistance over the client's occiput (superior region) while placing their other hand beneath the client's head. The clinician should be prepared to provide support if the head gives way with resistance. The client is instructed to look at the wall directly in front of them as clinician provides resistance.

- Grade 5: completes motion against maximum resistance without substituting cervical extension
- Grade 4: completes motion against strong resistance
- Grade 3: completes motion without resistance (The clinician will have to support the client's head in their hand to start testing.)

The client position for grades lower than 3 is supine with the head on table. The clinician sits directly cranial to the client's head and supports it with both hands under the occiput. The clinician instructs the client to look back at them.

- Grade 2: completes limited ROM without resistance
- Grade 1: muscle activity without movement
- Grade 0: no muscle activity

Primary Muscles	Rectus capitis posterior major and minor
	Obliquus capitis superior and inferior
	Longissimus capitis
	Splenius capitis
	Spinalis capitis
	Upper trapezius
Primary Nerves	Suboccipital nerve (C1)
	Greater occipital nerve (C2-3)

CERVICAL EXTENSION

Client Position	Prone, arms at their sides, with head off edge of table
Clinician Position	Standing directly to the side of the client
Movement and Assessment	The clinician places one hand over the back of the client's head (superior region) for resistance and their other hand under the client's chin, prepared to provide support if the head gives way with resistance. The clinician instructs the client to push their head into the clinician's hand while looking at floor as clinician provides resistance.

- Grade 5: completes motion against maximum resistance
- Grade 4: completes motion against strong resistance
- Grade 3: completes motion without resistance (The clinician will have to support the client's head in their hand to start testing.)

The client position for grades lower than 3 is supine with the head on the table. The clinician supports the client's head with both hands under the occiput and instructs the client to push their head into the clinician's hands.

- Grade 2: completes small ROM pushing into clinician's hands
- Grade 1: muscle activity without movement
- Grade 0: no muscle activity

Primary Muscles	Longissimus cervicis
	Semispinalis cervicis
	Iliocostalis cervicis
	Upper trapezius
Secondary Muscles	Levator scapulae
	Multifidi
	Rotatores cervicis
Primary Nerves	C2-T5

CAPITAL FLEXION

Client Position	Supine with head supported on table, arms at side
Clinician Position	Standing directly in front of the client
Movement and Assessment	The clinician places both hands around the client's mandible to give resistance in a cranial and posterior direction. The clinician instructs the client to tuck their chin.

- Grade 5: completes motion against maximum resistance
- Grade 4: completes motion against strong resistance
- Grade 3: completes motion without resistance
- Grade 2: completes partial ROM without resistance
- Grade 1: muscle activity without movement
- Grade 0: no muscle activity

Primary Muscles	Rectus capitis anterior and lateralis
	Longus capitis
Secondary Muscles	Stylohyoid
	Mylohyoid
	Digastric muscle
Primary Nerve	C1-3

CERVICAL FLEXION

Client Position	Supine with head supported on table, arms at sides
Clinician Position	Standing directly to the side of the client
Movement and Assessment	The clinician places two fingers on the client's forehead for resistance and the other hand on the client's chest for stabilization. The clinician instructs the client to lift their head from the table, still looking at ceiling.

- Grade 5: completes motion against moderate two-finger resistance
- Grade 4: completes motion against mild resistance
- Grade 3: completes motion without resistance

For grades below 3, the clinician palpates each sternocleidomastoid muscle as the client rolls their head in each direction.

- Grade 2: completes partial motion without resistance
- Grade 1: muscle activity without movement
- Grade 0: no muscle activity

(continued)

Cervical Flexion *(continued)*

Primary Muscles	Sternocleidomastoid
	Scalenus anterior
	Longus colli
Secondary Muscles	Scalenus medius
	Scalenus posterior
	Infrahyoid muscles
Primary Nerves	C2-6
	Accessory nerve

CERVICAL ROTATION

Client Position	Supine with head supported on table, arms at sides
Clinician Position	Standing directly to the side of the client
Movement and Assessment	The client's face is rotated as far as possible to one side. The clinician places one hand over the side of the head above the client's ear for grades 5 and 4 and uses it for resistance. The clinician instructs the client to rotate their head to neutral rotation against the resistance. Repeat for rotators on the other side.

- Grade 5: completes motion against maximal resistance
- Grade 4: completes motion against moderate resistance
- Grade 3: completes motion without resistance

For grades below 3, the client is sitting. The clinician palpates each sternocleidomastoid and instructs the client to turn their head in each direction.

- Grade 2: completes partial motion without resistance
- Grade 1: muscle activity without movement
- Grade 0: no muscle activity

Primary Muscles	Sternocleidomastoid
	Scalenus anterior
Secondary Muscles	Scalenus medius
	Scalenus posterior
	Trapezius
	Rotatores cervicis
Primary Nerves	C2-6
	Accessory nerve

SPECIAL TESTS

As mentioned in chapter 10 (Special Tests), in many cases the clinician is overly dependent on the performance and interpretation of special test findings with respect to differential diagnosis of the client's presenting pain. Utilization of special tests for ruling in (or helping to diagnose) a particular pathology should occur at this point in the examination process. It is also hoped that the clinician has a much clearer picture of the client's presentation prior to this point in the examination and will therefore depend minimally on special test findings with respect to diagnosis of the client's pain.

The pathologies of the cervical spine have various methods of determination for their presence or absence. As with all regions of the body, special tests are one such component. Also, as with other regions of the body, these special tests are but one small component of the examination process. Additionally, respective to the cervical spine, mobility assessments are distinct components of pathology diagnosis (e.g., joint mobility assessment for cervicogenic headache and mechanical neck pain). The special tests relative to the cervical spine are listed and described here.

Index of Special Tests

Cervicogenic Headache

Flexion–Rotation Test (C1-C2)
C0-1, C1-2, C2-3 Joint Mobility Assessment

Cervical Radiculopathy

Shoulder Abduction Test (Bakody's Sign)
Spurling's Test
Neck Hyperextension Test (Jackson's Test)
Cervical Distraction Test
Brachial Plexus Compression Test
Upper Limb Neurodynamic Test, Median Nerve Bias
Cervical Radiculopathy Test Item Cluster
Lhermitte's Sign (also refer to the musculoskeletal screening section of chapter 7, Orthopedic Screening and Nervous System Examination)

Cervical Nerve Root Compression

Arm Squeeze Test
Abduction Extension Cervical Nerve Root Stress Test

Cervical Spine Mechanical Neck Pain

Joint Mobility Assessment (PAIVM; refer to Segmental Mobility Testing under Motion Tests earlier in the chapter)

First Rib Mobility (refer to chapter 18, Thoracic Spine)

Cervical Rotation Lateral Flexion Test (associated with brachialgia and TOS; refer to chapter 18, Thoracic Spine)

Case Studies

Go to www.HumanKinetics.com/OrthopedicClinicalExamination and complete these case studies for chapter 17:

- Case study 1 discusses a 48-year-old female who is experiencing head, neck, and upper shoulder pain after a car accident.
- Case study 2 discusses a 46-year-old female nurse who experiences headaches while changing IV lines.

Abstract Links

Go to www.HumanKinetics.com/OrthopedicClinicalExamination to access abstract links on these issues:

Alar ligament test

Brachial plexus compression test

C1-C2 rotation—flexion-rotation test

Cervical rotation statistics

Cervicogenic headache

Diagnostic accuracy of the Dix-Hallpike test

Modified sharp purser test

Neck hyperextension text (Jackson test)

Palpation slide glide test

Prone posterior-anterior mobilization

Shoulder abduction test (Brody's Sign)

Spurling's test

CERVICOGENIC HEADACHE

FLEXION–ROTATION TEST (C1-C2)

See the description of the flexion–rotation test (C1-C2) in the prior Motion Tests section. As mentioned in that section, loss of $\geq 10°$ is considered a positive test for cervicogenic headache: **SN 86, SP 100.**[24]

C0-1, C1-2, C2-3 JOINT MOBILITY ASSESSMENT

The clinician should assess the respective levels as described in the Motion Tests section. The test was considered (+) for both pain reproduction and restricted mobility.

Statistics[133]
- SN 59 (NR), SP 82 (NR), +LR 3.3, –LR 0.49, at C0-C1, QUADAS 10, in a study of 77 female clients (25 control clients, mean age 22.9 ± 3.5 years; 27 cervicogenic headache clients, mean age 25.3 ± 3.9 years; and 25 migraine with aura clients, mean age 22.9 ± 3.5 years; duration of symptoms ranged from 9 months to >10 years), using an assessment rating on a 0-7 mobility scale and client assessment of pain rating on a VAS with comparison among groups
- SN 62 (NR), **SP 87 (NR)**, **+LR 4.9**, –LR 0.43, at C1-C2
- SN 65 (NR), SP 78 (NR), +LR 2.9, –LR 0.44, at C2-C3

CERVICAL RADICULOPATHY

SHOULDER ABDUCTION TEST (BAKODY'S SIGN)

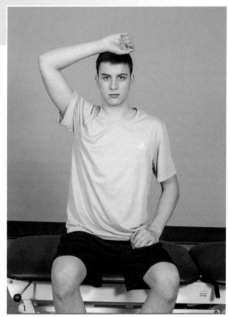

Figure 17.31

Client Position	Sitting with arms relaxed
Clinician Position	Standing directly to the side or behind the client
Movement	The client actively places their involved hand on top of their head.
Assessment	A (+) test is a reduction of the client's concordant pain.
Statistics	• SN 43-50, SP 80-100, +LR 2.2, –LR 0.50–0.71 in a literature review of provocative tests of the cervical spine[142]
	• SN 31-42 (NR), **SP 100 (NR)**, **+LR Inf**, –LR 0.58–0.69, QUADAS 10, in a study of 69 clients with cervical disc disease (median age was 52 years; 16 women; duration of symptoms NR), using a reference standard of cervical myelography[140]
	• SN 17 (0-34), SP 92 (85-99), +LR 2.1, –LR 0.91, QUADAS 10, in a study of 82 clients suspected to have cervical radiculopathy or carpal tunnel syndrome (mean age 45 ± 12 years, 41 women, duration of symptoms NR), using a reference standard of electromyography and nerve conduction study[18]

SPURLING'S TEST

 Video 17.32 **in the web resource shows a demonstration of this test.**

Figure 17.32

Client Position	Sitting with bilateral arms relaxed at sides
Clinician Position	Standing directly behind client
Movement	The clinician stabilizes the client's shoulder. The clinician then performs passive side bending of the client's cervical spine with 7 kg of overpressure. A common variation of this test involves side bending and rotation, combined with extension. Overpressure is applied at end-range.
Assessment	A (+) test is reproduction of concordant pain.
Reliability	The version involving side bending, rotation, and extension with overpressure has (κ) of 0.62.[18]

(continued)

Spurling's Test *(continued)*

Statistics
- SN 50 (27-73), SP 86 (77-94), +LR 3.5, –LR 0.6, QUADAS 10, in a study of 82 clients suspected to have cervical radiculopathy or carpal tunnel syndrome (mean age 45 ± 12 years; 41 women; duration of symptoms NR), using a reference standard of electromyography and nerve conduction study.[18]
- SN 50 (27-73), SP 74 (63-85), +LR 1.9, –LR 0.7 for the version involving side bending, rotation, and extension.[18]
- SN 36-39 (NR), **SP 92 (NR)**, **+LR 4.5–4.9**, –LR 0.7, QUADAS 10, in a study of 69 clients with cervical disc disease (median age was 52 years; 16 women; duration of symptoms NR), using a reference standard of cervical myelography.[140]
- **SN 93 (77-99), SP 95 (76-100), +LR 19.6, –LR 0.07**, QUADAS 9, in a study of 50 clients with neck and arm pain (mean age 42 years; 13 women; mean duration of symptoms 7.2 months), using a reference standard of surgical or MRI findings on 50 clients with neck and arm pain.[122]
- SN 11(NR), SP 100 (NR), +LR Inf, –LR 0.11, QUADAS 8, in a study of 65 clients (mean age 53.1 years; 27 women; duration of symptoms NR), using MRI as a reference standard.[143]

Whenever cervical radiculopathy is suspected, clinicians should include the following staged provocative maneuvers in the physical evaluation: extension and side bending first, followed by the addition of axial compression in cases with an inconclusive effect.[144]

NECK HYPEREXTENSION TEST (JACKSON'S TEST)

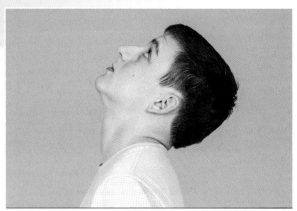

Figure 17.33

Client Position	Sitting with bilateral arms relaxed at sides
Clinician Position	Standing directly behind the client
Movement	The client actively hyperextends the neck. If no symptoms are produced, the clinician applies overpressure into cervical extension.
Assessment	A (+) test is reproduction of concordant pain into shoulder or arm.
Statistics	SN 25 (NR), SP 90 (NR), +LR 2.5, –LR 0.83, QUADAS 8, in a study of 65 clients (mean age 53.1 years; 27 women; duration of symptoms NR), using MRI as a reference standard.[143]

CERVICAL DISTRACTION TEST

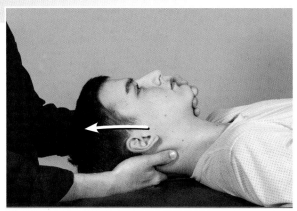

Figure 17.34

Client Position	Supine with arms relaxed
Clinician Position	Sitting, directly facing client
Movement	The clinician grasps the back of the client's head (particularly the occipital condyles bilaterally) with one hand (right as shown) and places the other hand (left as shown) just below the client's chin. The clinician applies a traction force with bilateral arms and reassesses the client's symptoms.

Assessment	A (+) test is reduction of concordant pain during distraction.
Reliability	(κ) 0.88
Statistics	

- SN 44 (21-67), **SP 90 (82-98)**, **+LR 4.4**, –LR 0.63, QUADAS 10, in a study of 82 clients suspected to have cervical radiculopathy or carpal tunnel syndrome (mean age 45 ± 12 years; 41 women; duration of symptoms NR), using a reference standard of electromyography and nerve conduction study.[18]
- SN 40 (NR), **SP 100 (NR)**, **+LR Inf**, –LR 0.40, QUADAS 10, in a study of 69 clients with cervical disc disease (median age was 52 years; 16 women; duration of symptoms NR), using a reference standard of cervical myelography.[140]

BRACHIAL PLEXUS COMPRESSION TEST

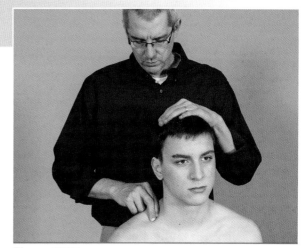

Figure 17.35

Client Position	Sitting with arms relaxed
Clinician Position	Standing directly behind client
Movement	The clinician applies firm compression to the client's brachial plexus by squeezing the plexus under the thumb or fingers.
Assessment	A (+) test is reduction of concordant pain into the shoulder or arm.
Statistics	SN 69 (NR), SP 83 (NR), +LR 4.1, –LR 0.4, QUADAS 8, in a study of 65 clients (mean age 53.1 years; 27 women; duration of symptoms NR) with symptoms suggestive of a cervical cord lesion, and using MRI as a reference standard.[143]

UPPER LIMB NEURODYNAMIC TEST: MEDIAN NERVE BIAS

Refer to chapter 7 (Orthopedic Screening and Nervous System Examination) for more detail on this test.

Critical Clinical Pearls

When performing a neural dynamic assessment (in this example, the upper limb tension test, or ULTT), it is important to keep the following in mind:

- The client who truly has neurodynamic dysfunction could be easily provoked with these tests. Therefore, it is important to try to ascertain their level of symptom irritability prior to testing and to take this into account during testing.
- This type of testing should be performed sequentially.
- Each preceding maneuver must be maintained when performing the next movement in the sequence (assuming no previous concordant symptoms have already been reproduced).
- More provoking movements are not required once symptoms are reproduced.
- Remember the criteria for a (+) test.

CERVICAL RADICULOPATHY TEST ITEM CLUSTER

Four criteria: cervical rotation < 60°, (+) Spurling's test, (+) distraction test, and (+) upper limb neurodynamic test (median nerve bias).[18]

- 2 of 4 (+) tests: SN 39, SP 56, +LR 0.9, −LR 1.1
- 3 of 4 (+) tests: SN 39, **SP 94, +LR 6.1**, −LR 0.64
- 4 of 4 (+) tests: SN 24, **SP 99, +LR 30.3**, −LR 0.76

LHERMITTE'S SIGN

This test is also thought to signify the possible presence of spinal cord conditions, including multiple sclerosis, tumors, or other space-occupying lesions,[145] and it should be considered part of the screening examination.

Client Position	Sitting with arms relaxed
Clinician Position	Standing directly to the side of the client
Movement	The clinician introduces lower cervical flexion.
Assessment	A (+) test is production of an electrical-type response or sensation of pins and needles near the end of motion.
Statistics	SN 3 (NR), SP 97 (NR), +LR 1.0, −LR 1.0, QUADAS 8, in a study of 65 clients (mean age 53.1 years; 27 women; duration of symptoms NR) with symptoms suggestive of a cervical cord lesion, and using MRI as a reference standard.[143]

CERVICAL NERVE ROOT COMPRESSION

ARM SQUEEZE TEST

Client Position	Sitting with arms relaxed
Clinician Position	Standing directly behind the client
Movement	The clinician applies a firm squeeze with the hand (right as shown) (simultaneous thumb and fingers compression, thumb from posterior [triceps muscle] and fingers from anterior [biceps muscle]) to the middle third of the client's upper arm with approximately 6 to 8 kg force.
Assessment	A test was considered (+) when the VAS pain rating was 3 points higher on pressure at this location compared with digital pressure on the acromioclavicular joint and anterolateral subacromial areas of the shoulder.
Statistics	SN 95 (85-99), SP 96 (87-99), +LR 24, −LR 0.05, QUADAS 8, in a study of 1,567 clients (mean age 57 ± 15 years; 930 women; duration of symptoms NR) with complaints of shoulder pain and clinical examination of the cervical spine, the shoulder, and the upper limb; using electromyography (for C5 to T1 roots), X-rays (AP and lateral view), and MRI of the cervical spine as a reference standard; 350 asymptomatic clients were also assessed (mean age 55 years, 200 women).[123]

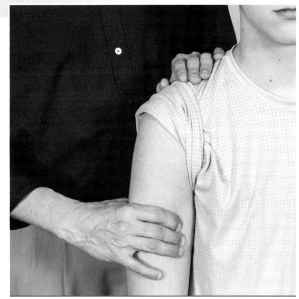

Figure 17.36

ABDUCTION EXTENSION CERVICAL NERVE ROOT STRESS TEST

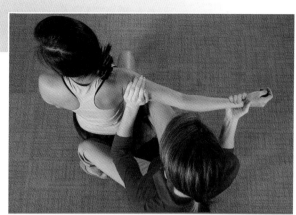

Figure 17.37

Client Position	Standing with arms relaxed
Clinician Position	Standing directly behind the client to the side of the arm to be tested
Movement	The clinician abducts the client's shoulder (not exceeding 90°), slightly flexes the elbow, and asks the client to turn their head away from the side being assessed. The clinician then applies a moderate posterior to anterior pressure on the posterior humeral head (with left hand as shown) while simultaneously horizontally abducting the arm 30°. The clinician holds this position for a few seconds and then asks the client about new or exacerbating pain or paresthesia along a dermatome.
Assessment	A test was considered (+) if the client reported new pain or paresthesia, or exacerbation of preexisting pain or paresthesia along a dermatome.
Statistics	SN 79 (NR), SP 98 (NR), +LR 40, –LR 0.21, QUADAS 8, in a study of 24 clients (mean age 51 ± 13 years; gender and duration of symptoms NR) with cervical radiculopathy; using MRI of the cervical spine as a reference standard; 65 control group clients seen for reasons other than cervical radiculopathy were also assessed (mean age 56 ± 16 years; gender and duration of symptoms NR).[146]
Note	This study assessed nerve root tension and compression on cadavers as a correlation in this study.

Critical Clinical Pearls

When examining the client for the potential presence or absence of cervical radiculopathy, keep the following in mind:

- Various cervical spine levels, when involved, will likely have different presentations (e.g., dermatomal pain and sensory distribution, myotomal level weakness reflecting the level).

- Utilization of tests with the highest diagnostic accuracy is suggested (cervical rotation < 60°, (+) ULTT (median nerve bias), (+) Spurling's test, and (+) distraction test).

- The arm squeeze test and the abduction extension cervical nerve root stress test are relatively newly described. Although they demonstrate potentially strong diagnostic accuracy, they were performed in studies of higher bias.

- As with all pathologies, the entire funnel examination should provide the clinician with findings to support or refute the presence of cervical radiculopathy.

PALPATION

Palpation of the cervical spine requires practice and special attention to detail of the structure being palpated. Due to the fact that several of the structures are deep, in close proximity to major vessels anteriorly, and small in size, caution and detail is necessary when palpating these structures. Reference to more easily palpable landmarks (table 17.7) may assist the clinician in determination of appropriate spinous level. Additionally, determination of the exact level of the spine being palpated may have limited clinical utility.

Posterior Aspect

The posterior aspect of the cervical spine is most likely what the clinician considers when performing palpation assessment of this region of the body. This section describes the bony and soft-tissue structures that the clinician may want to consider regarding palpation of the posterior cervical spine.

Bony Structures

- **Inion (external occipital protuberance):** The clinician places their fingers on the medial aspect of the base of the client's skull, then moves the hands slightly superiorly into the hairline and feels for a rounded prominence. This structure is sometimes referred to as the *bump of knowledge*.
- **Superior nuchal line:** From the inion, the clinician can move their fingers laterally and inferiorly diagonally toward the mastoid process. They will then feel the ridge of the superior nuchal line under their fingers.
- **Occiput:** The clinician places their hands under the base of the client's head and allows their fingertips to rest on the most inferior aspect.
- **Mastoid process:** The clinician places their fingers directly under the client's earlobes, feeling a rounded prominence on each side under their fingers (figure 17.38).
- **Transverse process of C1:** The clinician should place their fingers just inferior and posterior to the mastoid process (figure 17.39). Although this structure can be deep, the clinician should be careful not to press too firmly since it is often tender to palpation.

TABLE 17.7 Identification of Specific Vertebral Levels

Vertebral level	Identification
C1	2 finger widths below occipital protuberance
C2	3 finger widths below occipital protuberance
C3-4	C3: level of hyoid bone posteriorly; C4: top of thyroid cartilage
C5	Bottom of thyroid cartilage
C6	Cricoid cartilage
C7	Base of neck (prominent posterior spinous process)
	Use palpation of C6-C7-T1 technique (described below).
T2	Superior angle of scapula
T3	Scapular spine
T7	Inferior angle of scapula
T10	Xiphoid process
T12	12th rib

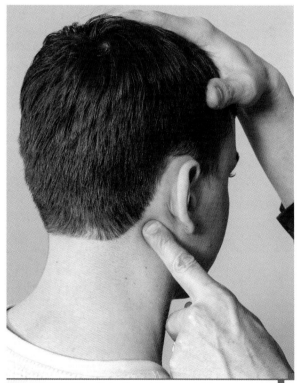

Figure 17.38 Palpation of the mastoid process.

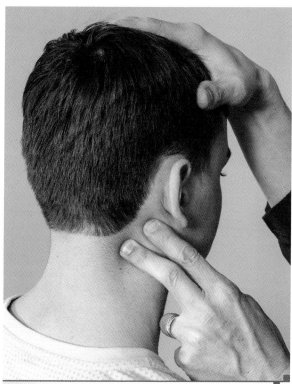

Figure 17.39 Palpation of the transverse process of C1.

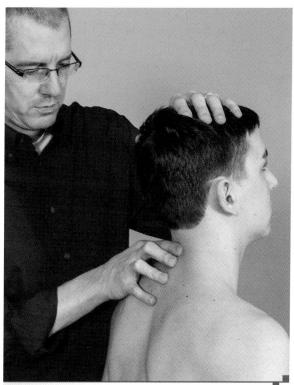

Figure 17.40 Palpation of the spinous process of C7.

- **Spinous process of C2:** The clinician places their fingers on the inion and moves inferiorly into an indentation. As the clinician continues to move inferiorly, the first rounded prominence that they will feel is the spinous process of C2.

- **Spinous processes:** The clinician places their middle fingers in the upper portion of the midline of the posterior aspect of the neck. They will feel blunt prominences under their fingers. They can start counting the spinous processes from C2 caudally. The normal spine has a natural lordosis. Note that the spinous processes of C3, C4, and C5 are deeper and closer together, making them difficult to differentiate individually.

- **Spinous process of C7:** This is normally the longest of all the cervical spinous processes. It is referred to as the *prominens*. Sometimes it can be of the same length as T1. To determine C7, the clinician places one finger on the presumed C7, one over C6, and a third finger over T1, and then has the client extend their head slightly (figure 17.40). The C6 vertebra will drop off slightly at the beginning of the

movement, followed by C7 with a slight increase in extension, and T1 will not drop off at all. T1 is immobilized by the first ribs bilaterally.

- **Articular pillar (facet joints):** The clinician moves their fingers laterally approximately 2 cm from the spinous processes, over the erector spinae until they find a depression—this is the articular pillar. As the clinician palpates in a caudal direction, they will be able to differentiate the joint lines of the facet joints because they feel like a stick of bamboo. If the joints have deteriorated due to osteoarthritis, they become enlarged and are not as clearly delineated. These facet joints can be normally tender to palpation.

- **Transverse processes of cervical spine:** The clinician moves their fingers to the most lateral aspect of the client's neck, where they will feel a series of blunt prominences. These are the transverse processes, which are often referred to the as the *anterior* and *posterior tubercles*. These also are often normally tender to palpation.

- **Spinous processes of thoracic spine:** These are longer and more slender than those of the cervical spine. They are usually prominent enough to palpate in respect to each other from cranial to caudal. Landmarks from the table can be used as described previously.

- **Transverse processes of the thoracic spine:** These are slightly lateral to the facet joints.

- **Spine of scapula:** The clinician can palpate the posterior aspect of the acromion and follow it medially along the ridge of the spine of the scapula as it tapers and ends at the level of the spinous process of the 3rd thoracic vertebra.

- **Medial border of the scapula:** The clinician can move superiorly from the medial aspect of the spine of the scapula until they palpate the superior angle, which is located at the level of the 2nd thoracic vertebra. The levator scapula is attached here, and this area is often tender to palpation. The inferior angle of the scapula is located at the level of T7.

Soft-Tissue Structures

- **Trapezius:** See chapter 18.

- **Suboccipital muscles:** To palpate this group of muscles, the clinician can place their fingertips at the base of the occiput while the client is supine. These muscles are very deep, and the clinician is most likely palpating the fascia and superficial muscles. These muscles can also often be in spasm and are often very tender to palpation.

- **Ligamentum nuchae:** Its superficial portion has its attachment to the external occipital protuberance and C7. The clinician can have the client flex their neck before attempting palpation. This structure is easily palpable directly over the spinous processes. This ligament continues caudally as the supraspinous and interspinous ligaments.

- **Levator scapulae:** This is attached to the transverse processes of C1-4 and the superior medial aspect of the scapula. Tenderness is often noted over its distal attachment on the superior medial border of the scapula. The clinician can palpate along the superior medial border of the scapula with the client in the supine or prone position. The clinician should have the client turn their head in the opposite direction to increase the tension on the muscle.

Anterior Aspect

The anterior aspect of the cervical spine is less likely what the clinician considers when performing palpation assessment of this region of the body. This section describes the bony and soft-tissue structures that the clinician may want to consider regarding palpation of the anterior cervical spine.

Bony Structures

- **Hyoid bone:** This is located at the anterior aspect of C3-4. It is often used as a landmark for locating the C3 spinous process. Using their thumb and index finger, the clinician can surround the most superior aspects of the structure and move it from side to side. The clinician may have to ask the client to slightly extend their neck in order to more easily palpate this structure (figure 17.41).

- **Thyroid cartilage:** This is commonly referred to as the *Adam's apple*. It is located at the anterior aspect of the C4 vertebral body and is partially covered by the thyroid gland.

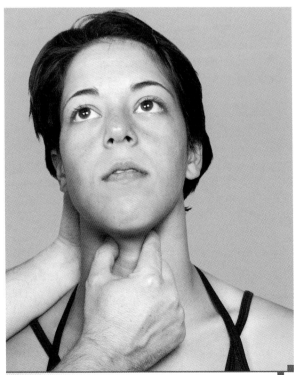

Figure 17.41 Palpation of the hyoid bone.

- **First cricoid ring:** The clinician can continue to palpate inferiorly until they reach a slightly softer tissue at the level of the C6 vertebrae. Palpation of this area can often be naturally unpleasant.

- **Suprasternal notch:** The clinician can stand directly facing client and use their index finger to locate the triangular notch between the two clavicles.

- **Sternal angle (angle of Louis):** The clinician may continue inferiorly approximately 5 cm until they locate a transverse ridge where the manubrium joins the sternum.

- **Second rib:** If the clinician continues directly laterally from this location, they will find the attachment of the second rib.

- **First rib:** This structure can be difficult to palpate because it is located behind and inferior to the clavicle. If the clavicle is elevated, the clinician can move their fingers posterior and inferior from the middle one-third of the clavicle, where they will locate the 1st rib just anterior to the trapezius (figure 17.42). It is normally tender to palpation.

- **First costal cartilage:** The clinician can place their index finger immediately below the clavicle and in contact with the lateral border of the manubrium. If necessary, the clinician can ask the client to perform rapid, repeated high costal inspirations to make it easier to palpate this structure.

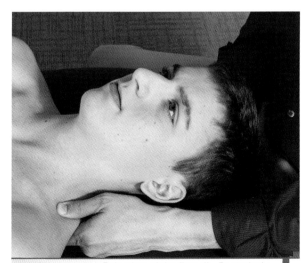

Figure 17.42 Palpation of the first rib. Posteriorly, the clinician pushes back the superior fibers of the trapezius muscle.

- **Ribs:** The second rib is the most superior rib palpable on the anterior part of the chest. The clinician should locate the second rib as previously described. They can then proceed inferiorly and count the ribs by placing their fingers in the intercostal spaces. The 5th rib is located at the xiphisternal junction. The clinician should note the symmetry of alignment and movement.

- There are seven true ribs, three false ribs (ribs 8, 9, and 10), and two floating ribs (ribs 11 and 12).

Soft-Tissue Structures

- **Sternocleidomastoid muscle:** The clinician can ask the client to side bend the head toward and rotate away (against slight resistance from the clinician) from the side of the muscle they are palpating. The clinician then palpates the distal attachments on the manubrium of the sternum and the medial aspect of the clavicle. They next follow the muscle superiorly and laterally up to the mastoid process, then move just medial from here to feel the occipital pulse just distal to the superior nuchal line.

- **Scalene muscles:** Both the anterior and medial scalene attach distally to the 1st rib. Compression of the subclavian artery and brachial plexus between these structures can be noted in TOS. The posterior scalene attaches distally to the 2nd rib. The clinician can place their fingers over the lateral aspect of the client's neck in the anterior triangle and ask the client to side bend away to put these muscles on a stretch. Inhalation can also make these muscles more prominent for palpation.

- **Lymph node chain:** These are present as several nodes throughout neck. They are not normally palpable except if enlarged due to disease. The clinician can use their thumb and finger to surround the SCM for palpation.

- **Subclavian artery:** The clinician may locate the clavicular portion of the SCM by asking the client to turn the head away. They next place a large digital grip on the medial one-third of the clavicle on the SCM muscle, and then they will feel the pulse of this artery.

- **Carotid pulse:** The clinician can locate the SCM and place their index and middle fingers medial to the midsection of the muscle belly, and then carefully press toward the transverse processes of the cervical spine. Having the client rotate the head toward the side being palpating to decrease the tension on the muscles in this area will help with palpation.

- **Brachial plexus:** This approach is identical to that of the subclavian artery. This structure can be felt as a full cylindrical cord. To tighten this structure and thus make it more perceptible, the clinician can ask the subject to perform a contralateral lateral flexion of the head and place the upper limb of the subject in ER and extension.
- **Parotid gland:** This gland is not normally palpable. If it is enlarged, it can be palpated in the area of the mandibular angle and anterior to the SCM.

PHYSICAL PERFORMANCE MEASURES

The craniocervical flexion test (CCFT) is a clinical test of the anatomical action of the deep cervical flexor muscles, the longus capitis, and longus colli. The CCFT could be described as a test of neuromotor control. The features assessed are the activation and isometric endurance of the deep cervical flexors as well as their interaction with the superficial cervical flexors during the performance of five progressive stages of increasing craniocervical flexion range of motion. It is a low-load test performed in the supine position with the client guided to each stage by feedback from a pressure sensor placed behind the neck. While the test in the clinical setting provides only an indirect measure of performance, the construct validity of the CCFT has been verified in a laboratory setting by direct measurement of deep and superficial flexor muscle activity. Specifically, the client performs a head nod (craniocervical flexion) in five progressive stages of increasing range. Feedback to the client is provided by the pressure sensor positioned behind the neck and, targeted 2 mmHg increases in pressure are made from a baseline of 20 to 30 mmHg.

Clients with neck pain disorders, compared to controls, have an altered neuromotor control strategy during craniocervical flexion characterized by reduced activity in the deep cervical flexors and increased activity in the superficial flexors, usually accompanied by altered movement strategies. These

clients also display reduced isometric endurance of the deep cervical flexor muscles. The muscle impairment identified with the CCFT appears to be generic to neck pain disorders of various etiologies.[147]

A similar test for the cervical spine is the deep neck flexor endurance test. The client lies supine and performs craniocervical flexion. Next, the clinician draws a line across the skin folds in the neck that are created due to this motion. Additionally, the clinician places their hand just below the posterior occiput. The client is instructed to hold this position for as long as possible. The test is terminated if the edges of the lines no longer approximate each other or if the client's head touches the clinician's hand for more than 1 second. Mean endurance time has been investigated in two separate studies. The mean endurance for women without neck pain was 14.5 ± 4.3 seconds; for men without neck pain, it was 18.2 ± 3.3 seconds.[148] Neck flexor muscle endurance test results for the group without neck pain (mean = 38.95 ± 26.4 s) and the group with neck pain (mean = 24.1 ± 12.8 s) were significantly different.[149]

The endurance test of the short neck flexors can be regarded as appropriate instruments for measuring different aspects of neck muscle function in clients with nonspecific neck pain.[150] Refer to chapter 21 (Shoulder) for additional regionally related physical performance tests.

COMMON ORTHOPEDIC CONDITIONS OF THE CERVICAL SPINE

While it is impossible to distinctly describe various pathological presentations of the cervical spine, there are evidence-based findings supportive of particular pathologies of this region of the body. Therefore, the intent of this section of the chapter is to present current evidence-supported findings suggestive of cervical spine pathologies. As previously described in chapter 4 (Evidence-Based Practice and Client Examination), though, not all examination findings are absolutely supported with clinical evidence, and the clinician should also rely on clinical experience and input from the client when performing differential diagnosis of a client's presentation of pain and dysfunction.

Various cervical spine pain causes have been described in the literature including, but not limited to, osteoarthritis, disc disorders, trauma, myofascial pain syndrome, torticollis, and whiplash. Clearly defined diagnostic criteria have not been established for these conditions. As in the case for LBP, a patho-anatomical cause is not discernible in the majority of clients presenting with complaints of neck pain and neck-related symptoms of the upper quarter.[151]

Clarification on specific terminology of similar types of pathologies in the spine is necessary prior to investigating the examination for each of these pathologies. General definitions are given here and additional detail is given for each pathology in the sections that follow. Stenosis is an abnormal narrowing in a blood vessel or other tubular organ or structure. With respect to the cervical spine, this would include the central canal (where the spinal cord runs) and the intervertebral foramen bilaterally (where the nerve roots exit the spine). Spondylosis is degenerative osteoarthritis of the joints between spinal vertebral levels. Spondylolysis is a defect of the pars interarticularis of a vertebra, and spondylolisthesis is the anterior displacement or posterior displacement (retrolisthesis) of a vertebra or the vertebral column in relation to the vertebra below.

Cervical spine degeneration (spondylosis) can involve various forms of stenosis and (dependent on the location of this stenosis) can have different clinical presentation. Figure 17.43 helps delineate these differences. Degeneration of the spine involving the spinal canal will result in central canal stenosis and the potential for myelopathy and upper motor neuron signs, since it involves encroachment on part of the central nervous system (spinal cord). Lateral foraminal stenosis (due to various reasons including radiculopathy, bone spurs, etc.) can result in nerve root involvement and the potential for lower motor neuron signs and symptoms (since it involves encroachment on the peripheral nervous

system). Spinal degeneration can also result in axial cervical pain without true or hard neurological findings (e.g., reflex changes, abnormal sensation, abnormal myotomes). In such cases, the client may have a combination of neck and arm pain (radiculitis).

Cervical Spine Spondylosis (Degenerative Disc Disease, Spinal Arthritis)

ICD-9: 721.0 (cervical spondylosis without myelopathy); 721.1 (cervical spondylosis with myelopathy)

ICD-10: M48 (spinal stenosis); M50 (cervical disc disorders); M50.3 (cervical disc degeneration)

Spondylosis is a degenerative osteoarthritis of the joints between the center of the spinal vertebrae and neural foramina. If this condition occurs in the facet joints, it can be considered facet syndrome. If severe, it may cause pressure on nerve roots with subsequent sensory or motor disturbances, such as pain, paresthesia, or muscle weakness in the limbs.

When the space between two adjacent vertebrae narrows, compression of a nerve root emerging from the spinal cord may result in radiculopathy (sensory and motor disturbances, such as severe pain in the neck, shoulder, arm, back, or leg, accompanied by muscle weakness). Less commonly, direct pressure on the spinal cord (typically in the cervical spine) may result in myelopathy, characterized by global weakness, gait dysfunction, loss of balance, and loss of bowel or bladder control. The client may experience a phenomenon of tingling or burning (paresthesia) in hands and legs because of nerve compression and lack of blood flow. If vertebrae of the neck are involved, it is referred to as *cervical spondylosis*. Lower back spondylosis is termed *lumbar spondylosis*.

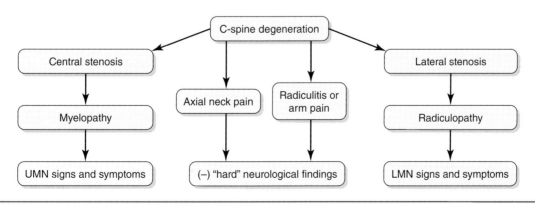

Figure 17.43 Cervical spine degeneration. UMN = upper motor neuron; LMN = lower motor neuron; (−) negative.

I. Client Interview

Subjective History

- The client frequently complains of general, diffuse neck pain, as well as stiffness and limited ROM.

- In more severe cases, the client will complain of radiating pain down one arm (nerve root impingement) or bilateral arms (in cases of spinal canal impingement), as well as sensory or motor disturbances (such as pain, paresthesia, or muscle weakness in the arms).

- Looking up overhead (into extension) and turning the head to the involved side are commonly painful.

- Clients are typically older adults with forward head and poor posture.[11, 152]

- Clients may report radiculopathy or myelopathy-related symptoms.

Outcome Measures

- Any relevant clinical outcome measure can be used.

- The MDC for the PSFS in cervical radiculopathy clients has been reported to be 2.1 points, with an MCID of 2.0.[42]

- Pain drawing is helpful for determining the distribution of symptoms.[153]

Diagnostic Imaging

- Radiographic findings include joint space narrowing, bone sclerosis, periarticular cysts, and osteophytes. Refer to chapter 6 for a definition of OA according to Kellgren and Lawrence.[154]

II. Observation

- Forward head posture is more likely in older clients.[152]

- Reduced cervical flexion and rotation were found with clients demonstrating forward head posture and thoracic kyphosis.[152]

III. Triage and Screening

- All nonmusculoskeletal causes, as well as causes from related joints, should be ruled out.

- An alert, asymptomatic client without distracting injury or neurological deficit who is able to complete a functional ROM examination may be safely cleared from cervical spine immobilization without radiographic evaluation (SN 98).[60]

- Canadian C-Spine Rule: demonstrated better diagnostic accuracy (SN range 90-100) than either the NEXUS criteria (SN range 83-100)[58] or physician clinical judgment alone (SN 92)[59] and, therefore, an improved ability to **rule out** an actual fracture.

- Alar ligament testing:

  - Significant variability in diagnostic accuracy (SN 69-100, −LR 0.29–0.31; SP 72-96, +LR 18-Inf) with improved ability to **rule in** versus **rule out** alar ligament insufficiency with less complex testing.[107]

  - Better ability to **rule in** (SP 96-100, +LR 18-Inf) versus rule out (SN 72, −LR 0.30) alar ligament insufficiency with more complex testing.[107]

- Sharp-Purser test: demonstrates stronger ability to **rule in** (SP 96, +LR 17.3) than rule out (SN 69, −LR 0.32) transverse ligament insufficiency.[108]

- More complex transverse ligament testing is also better able to **rule in** (SP 99, +LR 65) than rule out (SN 65, −LR 0.35) transverse ligament insufficiency.[107]

- Cervical rotation is helpful for **ruling in** (SP 100, +LR 83.3) potential vertebrobasilar ischemia.[115]

- Combined cervical extension and rotation is helpful for **ruling in** (SP 98, +LR 4.2) a potential upper cervical neurovascular compromise.[117]

- Clinical examinations for myelopathy are mostly SP, and lack SN; the majority of current studies are of poor to moderate quality.[81] The clinician should then be cautious with interpretation of (+) or (−) clinical examination findings when testing for myelopathy.

IV. Motion Tests

- Assessment of cervical spine ROM is reliable across various clients and measurement devices.[124-126]

- Decreased cervical rotation (<60°) toward involved side is common for those with radiculopathy.[18]

- Elderly clients have been shown to have decreased ROM in all planes compared to their younger counterparts, for both men and women.[130, 131] The elderly group also had a wider variation of cervical ROM values as compared to the younger group. Women were found to have greater ROM in all cohort age groups.[130]

V. Muscle Performance Testing

- Coordination, strength, and endurance deficits of neck and upper quarter muscles (longus colli, middle trapezius, lower trapezius, and serratus anterior) are common in clients with movement coordination impairments.[11]

- Chronic neck pain clients, on average, have lower neck muscle strength compared with controls.[35]

VI. Special Tests

- Spurling's test: A (+) test had less than good ability to help **rule in** (SP 86, +LR 3.5) cervical radiculopathy in one study[18] and a good ability to help **rule out** (SN 92, −LR 0.07) and **rule in** (SP 95, +LR 18.6) cervical radiculopathy in another study.[122]

- PA glides: Lack of a mobility restriction or concordant pain with PA glides of the cervical spine helps **rule out** (SN 100,[31] SN 89[134]) facet joint involvement.

  - A detected mobility restriction or concordant pain helps **rule in** (SP 100) facet joint involvement.[31]

  - Hypomobility and reproduction of concordant pain demonstrates greater diagnostic accuracy (**SN 100, SP 100**) than detection of hypomobility alone.[31, 134]

VII. Palpation

- Localized tenderness over the facet joints without other root tension signs or neurologic signs may indicate facet joint pain.[155]

- If the muscle (strain) or ligament (sprain) is palpable, it likely will be tender to palpation.

VIII. Physical Performance Measures

- The CCFT, deep neck flexor endurance test, and progressive isoinertial lifting evaluation (if appropriate) can be used.

- Clients with chronic neck pain may perform less well on certain functional tests (e.g., lifting, reaching).[35]

POTENTIAL TREATMENT-BASED CLASSIFICATIONS

- Pain control (if client is pain dominant), mobility, and exercise and conditioning may be used.

Cervical Spine Myelopathy

ICD-9: 336.9 (unspecified disease of spinal cord); 721.1 (cervical spondylosis with myelopathy)

ICD-10: G95; M48 (spinal stenosis); M50 (cervical disc disorder with myelopathy); M50.3 (cervical disc degeneration)

Myelopathy is a pathology of the spinal cord. When this pathology is due to trauma, it is referred to as a *spinal cord injury*. Myelopathy can be due to anything creating pressure or insult to the spinal cord. In the musculoskeletal client, this is most likely due to the intervertebral disc, nerve root adhesions or scar tissue, or the surrounding bone, muscle, cartilage, or tendon. It is characterized by a variable distribution pattern and may involve clinical findings in the legs initially, with subsequent gait changes, leg weakness, and spasticity.[156, 157] Clinical signs and symptoms are dependent on the level of spinal cord involvement (cervical, thoracic, or lumbar). These signs and symptoms are also dependent on the extent of the pathology (anterior, posterior, or lateral portion of the spinal cord).

I. Client Interview

Subjective History

- The lack of the presence of at least one clinical finding helped rule out myelopathy (SN 94, −LR 0.18), while the presence of three out of five (+) findings helped rule in myelopathy (SP 99, +LR 30.9), QUADAS 8:[33]

  - Gait deviation

  - (+) Hoffmann's sign

- (+) Inverted supinator sign
- (+) Babinski test
- Age > 45 years

- Signs and symptoms of clinical myelopathy of the cervical spine may include the following:

  - Sensory deficits are typically inconsistent and typically occur later on, and occur more typically in the arms than in the leg.[157]

  - Upper motor neuron signs (weakness, increased muscle tone, spasticity, clumsiness, altered gait due to balance dysfunction).[157]

  - Clients may describe bowel or bladder symptoms and sexual dysfunction.

  - Clumsiness in gait.[158, 159]

  - Neck and shoulder stiffness.[160, 161]

  - Paresthesia in one or both arms or hands.[162]

  - Leg stiffness or weakness preceding bowel and bladder symptoms.[157]

  - Spasticity or hyperreflexia.[157, 159]

  - The client with cervical myelopathy (CM) may actually present with hyperreflexia below the affected level and hyporeflexia at the level specifically involved.[156]

  - Uncommon symptoms can include restless legs. Other symptoms that may be attributed to compression of the vertebral artery may include nausea, dizziness, and dysphagia.[156]

Outcome Measures

- Subjective pain ratings and pain constancy scores were not helpful for ruling in or ruling out myelopathy.[33]

- The Japanese Orthopaedic Association Score is effective at measuring changes in a client's condition. It measures physical function constructs and sensory involvement.[163, 164]

- The European Myelopathy Score is a disease-specific, physician-oriented scale that measures a number of constructs of function.[163, 164]

II. Observation

- Due to decreased intervertebral and spinal canal space with extension and side bending, the client may be unwilling or hesitant to perform activities involving these motions.

- Since these clients are more likely to be older adults, poor posture may be a common presentation. Reduced cervical flexion and rotation were found with clients demonstrating forward head posture and thoracic kyphosis.[152]

- Gait changes may include trembling and cramping of thigh and calf muscles, difficulty negotiating steps or curbs, as well as difficulty getting into and out of a vehicle.[158, 159]

III. Triage and Screening

- All nonmusculoskeletal causes, as well as causes from related joints, should be ruled out.

- History is used for triage, during which red flags should be identified and yellow flags assessed.[53]

- All nonmusculoskeletal causes, as well as causes from related joints, should be ruled out.

- An alert, asymptomatic client without distracting injury or neurological deficit who is able to complete a functional ROM examination may be safely cleared from cervical spine immobilization without radiographic evaluation (SN 98).[60]

- Canadian C-Spine rule: demonstrated better diagnostic accuracy (SN range 90-100) than either the NEXUS criteria (SN range 83-100)[58] or physician clinical judgment alone (SN 92)[59] and, therefore, an improved ability to **rule out** an actual fracture.

- Alar ligament testing:

  - Significant variability in diagnostic accuracy (SN 69-100, −LR 0.29–0.31; SP 72-96, +LR 18-Inf) with improved ability to **rule in** versus **rule out** alar ligament insufficiency with less complex testing.[107]

- Better ability to **rule in** (SP 96-100, +LR 18-Inf) versus rule out (SN 72, −LR 0.30) alar ligament insufficiency with more complex testing.[107]

- Sharp-Purser test: demonstrates stronger ability to **rule in** (SP 96, +LR 17.3) than rule out (SN 69, −LR 0.32) transverse ligament insufficiency.[108]

- More complex transverse ligament testing is also better able to **rule in** (SP 99, +LR 65) than rule out (SN 65, −LR 0.35) transverse ligament insufficiency.[107]

- Cervical rotation is helpful for **ruling in** (SP 100, +LR 83.3) potential vertebrobasilar ischemia.[115]

- Combined cervical extension and rotation is helpful for **ruling in** (SP 98, +LR 4.2) potential upper cervical neurovascular compromise.[117]

- Clinical examinations for myelopathy are mostly SP and lack SN; the majority of current studies are of poor to moderate quality.[81] The clinician should then be cautious with interpretation of (+) or (−) clinical examination findings when testing for myelopathy.

- Clients are likely to present with increased reflexes, muscle tone, and potential for pathological reflexes (e.g., Babinski, clonus, Hoffman's).[165]

IV. Motion Tests

- Assessment of cervical spine ROM is reliable across various clients and measurement devices.[124-126]

- Elderly clients have been shown to have decreased ROM in all planes compared to their younger counterparts, for both men and women.[130, 131] The elderly group also had a wider variation of cervical ROM values as compared to the younger group. Women were found to have greater ROM in all cohort age groups.[130]

- Both active and passive ROM are often limited.

- ROM limitations in arms were inconsistently found.

- Cervical spine extension may produce symptoms down the spine.

V. Muscle Performance Testing

- Coordination, strength, and endurance deficits of neck and upper quarter muscles (longus colli, middle trapezius, lower trapezius, and serratus anterior) are common in clients with movement coordination impairments.[11]

- Chronic neck pain clients, on average, have lower neck muscle strength compared with controls.[35]

VI. Special Tests

- Overall, myelopathic signs are not highly SN in diagnosing the presence of cervical myelopathy, since 21% of clients with cervical myelopathy failed to demonstrate any myelopathic signs.[166]

- No correlation exists between the presence of myelopathic signs and diabetes. However, those with cord signal changes on MRI were significantly more likely to demonstrate myelopathic signs.[166]

- Tests such as single leg stance, tandem gait, and balance exercises are often very difficult for clients with cervical myelopathy.

- Hoffman's reflex: has demonstrated the ability to **rule out** (SN 94) cervical myelopathy, although this study was performed on 16 clients without cervical pain or radiculopathy and with a positive Hoffmann's reflex.[167] Hoffman's reflex demonstrated less impressive ability to **rule in** CM or UMN disorder (SP 84, +LR 3.7) in a poorly designed study of 39 clients with CM and 37 controls.[166]

- Babinski test: demonstrated the strongest diagnostic value of all tests for confirmation of CM in one well-designed study comparing multiple tests (**SP 92, +LR 4.0**).[168]

- Inverted supinator sign: has limited ability to rule in (SP 78) or rule out (SN 61) CM or UMN disorder.[168]

- Clonus: is a very poor screening test, but it has demonstrated better ability to **rule in** CM or UMN disorder in two fairly well-designed studies (SP 99, +LR 5.4, QUADAS 7;[33] SP 96, +LR 2.7, QUADAS 11[168]).

- Suprapatellar reflex (a quick striking reflex hammer to the suprapatellar tendon): A (+) test (hyperreflexive knee extension) helps **rule in** (SP 97, +LR 6.9) CM or UMN disorder.[33]

- Achilles tendon reflex (hyperreflexia): A (+) test helps **rule in** (SP 98, +LR 7.8) CM or UMN disorder.[33]

- No improvement in posttest probability was determined after clustering findings such as clumsiness in hands, gait problems, clonus, the Babinski test, Hoffman's reflex, and others.[168]

VII. Palpation

- Stiffness in legs, spasticity, and widespread numbness to palpation may be noted.

VIII. Physical Performance Measures

- The CCFT, deep neck flexor endurance test, and possibly the progressive isoinertial lifting evaluation may be used.

- Clients with chronic neck pain may perform less well on certain functional tests (e.g., lifting, reaching).[35]

- The Tally counter (pushing the button of a tally counter as many times as possible in 10 seconds),[169] foot tapping (tapping foot as many times as possible in 10 seconds with heel on ground and sitting in a chair), and grip and release (repeatedly flexing and releasing their fingers as fast as possible in sitting)[170] tests are suggested for these clients as an assessment that is objective, quantitative, simple, reliable, and capable of detecting small functional changes.

POTENTIAL TREATMENT-BASED CLASSIFICATIONS

- Pain (if client is pain dominant), exercise and conditioning, and possibly mobility or stability (dependent on clinical presentation) may be used.

Cervical Radiculopathy

ICD-9: 723.4 (brachial neuritis or radiculitis)

ICD-10: G54; M54.1 (radiculopathy)

Radiculopathy is an encompassing term referring to a set of conditions in which one or more nerves are affected, most significantly at the nerve root. The insult to the nerve occurs at or near the root of the nerve (nerve root) as the peripheral nerve exits the spinal cord via the lateral foramina. The affected nerve may be inflamed, compressed, or symptomatic due to improper blood flow. Common causes of nerve root compression are from part of the intervertebral disc, nerve root adhesions or scar tissue, or the surrounding bone, muscle, cartilage, or tendon. Although the insult is at the nerve root, the symptoms are often felt distal to that point because the entire length distal to the insult location is affected. This can result in pain (radicular pain), weakness, numbness, or difficulty controlling specific muscles. Therefore, in the cervical spine, symptoms will often be encountered distally in the arms. Since this is a nerve root insult, cervical radiculopathy is a lower motor neuron dysfunction.

As with examination of all pathologies, a comprehensive examination is suggested. The combination of history, physical examination, modern imaging techniques, and needle EMG has been suggested for diagnosing the cause and site of cervical radiculopathy.[35] Regarding the clinical examination for nerve root compression and radiculopathy, consistent evidence suggests that testing is generally stronger for ruling out versus ruling in the pathology.[35]

I. Client Interview

Subjective History

- Clients with cervical radiculopathy do have a loss of feeling (SP 92). Their most bothersome location of symptoms is in the neck (SP 90) and arm above the elbow (SP 93), greater than in the shoulder and scapula or below the elbow (SP 83 for both).[18]

- None of the subjective history showed the ability to rule out cervical radiculopathy.[18]

- Pain with the Valsalva maneuver helps rule in (SP 94, +LR 3.7) the possibility of cervical radiculopathy.[18]

Outcome Measures

- The MDC for the NDI has been reported to range from 14 percentage points[42] up to 20 percentage points for cervical radiculopathy.[37]

- The MDC for the PSFS in these clients has been reported to be 2.1 points, with an MCID of 2.0.[42]

- Pain drawing is helpful for determining the distribution of symptoms.[153]

Diagnostic Imaging

- Evidence exists against the use of electrodiagnostic testing in clients with neck pain without suspected radiculopathy.[35]

II. Observation

- Reduced cervical flexion and rotation were found with clients demonstrating forward head posture and thoracic kyphosis.[152]

- Clients will often hold their head away from the involved side, avoiding rotation to that side.[171]

- A client may have decreased arm swing or display guarded posturing of involved arm; they may cradle the arm or place it behind or on top of their head to reduce the tension on the nerve root.[172]

III. Triage and Screening

- All nonmusculoskeletal causes, as well as causes from related joints, should be ruled out.

- History is used for triage, during which red flags should be identified and yellow flags assessed.[53]

- Radiculopathy typically presents with diminished deep tendon reflexes.

- An alert, asymptomatic client without distracting injury or neurological deficit who is able to complete a functional ROM examination may be safely cleared from cervical spine immobilization without radiographic evaluation (SN 98).[60]

- Canadian C-Spine Rule: demonstrated better diagnostic accuracy (SN range 90-100) than either the NEXUS criteria (SN range 83-100)[58] or physician clinical judgment alone (SN 92)[59] and, therefore, an improved ability to **rule out** an actual fracture.

- Alar ligament testing:
  - Significant variability in diagnostic accuracy (SN 69-100, −LR 0.29–0.31; SP 72-96, +LR 18-Inf) with

improved ability to **rule in** versus **rule out** alar ligament insufficiency with less complex testing.[107]

  - Better ability to **rule in** (SP 96-100, +LR 18-Inf) versus rule out (SN 72, −LR 0.30) alar ligament insufficiency with more complex testing.[107]

- Sharp-Purser test: demonstrates stronger ability to **rule in** (SP 96, +LR 17.3) than rule out (SN 69, −LR 0.32) transverse ligament insufficiency.[108]

- More complex transverse ligament testing is also better able to **rule in** (SP 99, +LR 65) than rule out (SN 65, −LR 0.35) transverse ligament insufficiency.[107]

- Cervical rotation is helpful for **ruling in** (SP 100, +LR 83.3) potential vertebrobasilar ischemia.[115]

- Combined cervical extension and rotation is helpful for **ruling in** (SP 98, +LR 4.2) a potential upper cervical neurovascular compromise.[117]

- Sensitivity to light touch and pinprick are more reproducible than examinations demonstrating decreased sensation.[35]

- Clinical examinations for myelopathy are mostly SP and lack SN; the majority of current studies are of poor to moderate quality.[81] The clinician should then be cautious with interpretation of (+) or (−) clinical examination findings when testing for myelopathy.

IV. Motion Tests

- Assessment of cervical spine ROM is reliable across various clients and measurement devices.[124-126]

- Elderly clients have been shown to have decreased ROM in all planes compared to their younger counterparts, for both men and women.[130, 131] The elderly group also had a wider variation of cervical ROM values as compared to the younger group. Women were found to have greater ROM in all cohort age groups.[130]

- Decreased cervical rotation (<60°) toward involved side is common for those with radiculopathy.[18]

V. Muscle Performance Testing

- Coordination, strength, and endurance deficits of neck and upper quarter muscles (longus colli, middle trapezius, lower trapezius, and serratus anterior) are common in clients with movement coordination impairments.[11]

- Chronic neck pain clients, on average, have lower neck muscle strength compared with controls.[35]

- Neurological symptoms may lead to pain, motor weakness, or sensory deficits along the affected nerve root.[165]

- Advanced cervical radiculopathy cases may present with muscle wasting and fasciculations.[165]

- Manual muscle testing affords greater SP than either reflex or sensory testing, and single-root-level involvement can be detected clinically 75% to 80% of the time.[173]

VI. Special Tests

- Deep tendon reflexes: Loss of these reflexes is typically thought to be the most reliable clinical finding for cervical radiculopathy.[174]

- Upper limb tension test median nerve bias: A (−) test has ideal ability to help **rule out** (SN 97, −LR 0.12) cervical radiculopathy.[18]

- Spurling's test: A (+) test had good ability to help **rule in** (SP 86, +LR 3.5) cervical radiculopathy in one study,[18] and a good ability to help **rule out** (SN 92, −LR 0.07) and **rule in** (SP 95, +LR 18.6) cervical radiculopathy in another study.[122]

- Distraction test: A (+) test has good (**SP 90, +LR 4.4**)[18] and ideal ability to help rule in (**SP 100, +LR Inf**) cervical radiculopathy.[140]

- Valsalva test: A (+) test has good ability to help **rule in** (SP 94, +LR 3.5) cervical radiculopathy.[18]

- CPR variables include upper limb tension test (median nerve), Spurling's test, distraction test, and cervical rotation < 60° to ipsilateral side; posttest probabilities are as follows:[18]

  - 2 (+) tests = 21%
  - 3 (+) tests = 65%
  - 4 (+) tests = 95%

- A recent systematic review suggests that, when consistent with the history and other physical findings, a positive Spurling's test, traction or neck distraction, and Valsalva maneuver might be indicative of a cervical radiculopathy, while a negative ULTT might be used to rule it out. However, the lack of evidence precludes any firm conclusions regarding their diagnostic value, especially when used in primary care.[175]

- Bakody's sign or shoulder abduction test: A (+) test for reduction of pain has good ability to help **rule in** (SP 80, +LR 1.9–2.2;[140] SP 92, +LR 2.1[18]) cervical radiculopathy.

- Brachial plexus compression test: A (+) test has good ability to help **rule in** (SP 83, +LR 4.1) cervical radiculopathy.[143]

- Neck hyperextension test: A (+) test has less than good ability to help rule in (SP 90, +LR 2.5) cervical radiculopathy.[143]

- Cervical hyperflexion: A (−) test (not reproducing the client's concordant pain) has good ability to help **rule out** (SN 89) cervical radiculopathy.[18]

- Biceps brachii deep tendon reflex: An absent or reduced response with this test was the single best traditional neurologic test to help **rule in** (SP 95, +LR 4.8) cervical radiculopathy.[18]

- Decreased triceps reflex (SP 92, 93) and decreased brachioradialis reflex (SP 94, 95) have good ability to help rule in radiculopathy, although the +LRs are all <3 for these tests.[18, 176]

- Abduction extension cervical nerve root test: A (−) test has only fair ability to rule out (SN 79, −LR 0.21) cervical radiculopathy or cervical nerve root compression, and a (+) test also has only fair ability to help rule in (SP 98, +LR 40) the condition in a study of moderate bias (QUADAS 8).[146]

- Arm squeeze test: has only fair ability to help rule out (SN 95, −LR 0.05) cervical nerve root compression with a (−) test and rule in (SP 96, +LR 24) the condition with a (+) test (especially as compared to arm pain), although the study was of moderate bias (QUADAS 8).[123]

- PA glides: Lack of a mobility restriction or concordant pain with PA glides of the cervical spine helps **rule out** (SN 100,[31] SN 89[134]) facet joint involvement.

  - A detected mobility restriction or concordant pain helps **rule in** (SP 100) facet joint involvement.[31]

  - Hypomobility and reproduction of concordant pain demonstrate greater diagnostic accuracy (**SN 100, SP 100**) than detection of hypomobility alone.[31, 134]

VII. Palpation

- Tenderness or pain as noted with the brachial plexus compression test helps **rule in** (SP 83, +LR 4.1) more than **rule out** (SN 69, −LR 0.4) cervical radiculopathy.[143]

VIII. Physical Performance Measures

- The CCFT, deep neck flexor endurance test and progressive isoinertial lifting evaluation may be used.

- Clients with chronic neck pain may perform less well on certain functional tests (e.g., lifting, reaching).[35]

POTENTIAL TREATMENT-BASED CLASSIFICATIONS

- Pain control and mobility (most likely primary TBCs)
- Exercise and conditioning

Cervical Spine Instability/CAD

ICD-9: 728.4 (laxity of a ligament); 443.24 (desiccation of vertebral artery)

ICD-10: M24.2 (disorder of a ligament, unspecified site); 167.0 (dissection of cerebral arteries, nonruptured); 160.7 (subarachnoid hemorrhage from intracranial artery, unspecified)

Instability in the cervical spine is a condition of significant concern for the client and clinician. Signs and symptoms are suggestive of potential ligamentous tear or cervical artery dysfunction. These conditions most likely result from trauma or significant pathological sequelae. These clients should be treated with significant caution.

I. Client Interview

Subjective History

- Clients can report signs or symptoms suggestive of instability and CAD:

Differential Diagnosis of Cervical Spine Myelopathy and Cervical Spine Radiculopathy

- Myelopathy will present with upper motor neuron signs, while radiculopathy will present with lower motor neuron signs.
- Myelopathy is more likely to present with lower extremity involvement.
- Myelopathy is more likely to present with multiple dermatomal level symptoms or presentation versus radiculopathy, which is more likely to have a single dermatomal level.
- Myelopathy is more likely to present with bilateral extremity involvement versus the unilateral level involvement seen with radiculopathy.
- Myelopathy is more likely to present with signs and symptoms such as clumsiness in gait, spasticity, and bowel or bladder symptoms.
- Older age is more likely a variable to consider in those clients with myelopathy versus radiculopathy.
- Both pathologies are likely to present with neck stiffness or pain and pain radiating away from the cervical spine.

dizziness, diplopia, drop attacks, dysphagia, dysarthria, diaphoresis, ataxia, numbness (around the lips), nystagmus, and nausea.

- Clients can report significant or minor mechanism or trauma related to onset of symptoms.

Outcome Measures

- Any appropriate clinical outcome measure can be used; the NDI and PSFS are most likely.

Diagnostic Imaging

- Transcranial Doppler (TCD) may be a useful screening method in clients with VBI for the detection of large vessel occlusive disease of the intracranial vertebrobasilar system. Remember that proximal vertebral artery stenoses will be missed by TCD.[47]

II. Observation

- The clinician should be especially cognizant of the client who is unwilling to move their head independent of their body (i.e., the client that turns their whole body to look at something versus just turning their head).

- Reduced cervical flexion and rotation were found with clients demonstrating forward head posture and thoracic kyphosis.[152]

III. Triage and Screening

- All nonmusculoskeletal causes, as well as causes from related joints, should be ruled out.

- History is used for triage, during which red flags should be identified and yellow flags assessed.[53]

- The potential for cervical spine instability should be examined with the use of tools such as NEXUS and the Canadian C-Spine Rules, as well as stability testing discussed in this chapter.

- An alert, asymptomatic client without distracting injury or neurological deficit who is able to complete a functional ROM examination may be safely cleared from cervical spine immobilization without radiographic evaluation (SN 98).[60]

- Canadian C-Spine Rule: demonstrated better diagnostic accuracy (SN range 90-100) than either the NEXUS criteria (SN range 83-100)[58] or physician clinical judgment alone (SN 92)[59] and, therefore, an improved ability to **rule out** an actual fracture.

- Alar ligament testing:
  - Significant variability in diagnostic accuracy (SN 69-100, −LR 0.29–0.31; SP 72-96, +LR 18-Inf) with improved ability to **rule in** versus **rule out** alar ligament insufficiency with less complex testing.[107]
  - Better ability to **rule in** (SP 96-100, +LR 18-Inf) versus **rule out** (SN 72, −LR 0.30) alar ligament insufficiency with more complex testing.[107]

- Sharp-Purser test: demonstrates stronger ability to **rule in** (SP 96, +LR 17.3) than rule out (SN 69, −LR 0.32) transverse ligament insufficiency.[108]

- More complex transverse ligament testing is also better able to **rule in** (SP 99, +LR 65) than rule out (SN 65, −LR 0.35) transverse ligament insufficiency.[107]

- Cervical rotation is helpful for **ruling in** (SP 100, +LR 83.3) a potential vertebrobasilar ischemia.[115]

- Combined cervical extension and rotation is helpful for **ruling in** (SP 98, +LR 4.2) a potential upper cervical neurovascular compromise.[117]

- Clinical examinations for myelopathy are mostly SP and lack SN; the majority of current studies are of poor to moderate quality.[81] The clinician should then be cautious with interpretation of (+) or (−) clinical examination findings when testing for myelopathy.

IV. Motion Tests

- Assessment of cervical spine ROM is reliable across various clients and measurement devices.[124-126]

- The client will likely be very guarded and limited in ROM and will occasionally have complaints of nausea or vomiting, dizziness, and so on.[11]

- Elderly clients have been shown to have decreased ROM in all planes compared to their younger counterparts, for both men and women.[130, 131] The elderly group also had a wider variation of cervical ROM values as compared to the younger group. Women were found to have greater ROM in all cohort age groups.[130]

V. Muscle Performance Testing

- Coordination, strength, and endurance deficits of neck and upper quarter muscles (longus colli, middle trapezius, lower trapezius, and serratus anterior) are common in clients with movement coordination impairments.[11]

- Chronic neck pain clients, on average, have lower neck muscle strength compared with controls.[35]

VI. Special Tests

- Both side bending and rotation stress testing result in a measurable increase in length of the contralateral alar ligament.[177]

- Testing produces a consistent direct effect on the transverse ligament (anterior shear testing) and the tectorial membrane (distraction testing) that is consistent with their theorized mechanism for clinical use.[178]

- Sharp-Purser Test: A (+) test has good ability to help **rule in** (SP 96, +LR 17) cervical instability.[108]

- Despite the fact that there are various tests for cervical spine stability or CAD, this is an area of underwhelming investigation. It is likely that several other well-designed studies will be required prior to comprehension of the clinical utility of these various tests.

- Refer to the Triage and Screening section of this chapter to more fully elucidate these tests, their current clinical utility, and overall comprehension of this diagnosis.

VII. Palpation

- Careful palpation of the cervical spine with this diagnosis (if palpation is necessary at all) is suggested.

VIII. Physical Performance Measures

- These tests are not suggested if this diagnosis is a potential suspicion.

POTENTIAL TREATMENT-BASED CLASSIFICATIONS

- Stability

Whiplash-Associated Disorder (WAD)

ICD-9: 847.0 (sprain of neck)

ICD-10: S13.4 (sprain and strain of cervical spine); S13.4XXA (sprain of ligaments of spine)

Whiplash-associated disorder (WAD), more commonly termed *whiplash*, is a broad term encompassing variable signs and symptoms related to cervical spine dysfunction caused by or related to distortion of the cervical spine associated with cervical extension and possibly with other directions of movement. The mechanism of injury is most frequently associated with motor vehicle accidents (MVA) or high-speed collision contact injuries. A wide variety of signs and symptoms are associated with whiplash injuries.[24, 179-193] The variability in signs and symptoms led to the use of the term *whiplash-associated disorder*. The greatest levels of improvement in pain and disability post injury occur within 3 months, with little if any improvement after this period.[192]

I. Client Interview

Subjective History

- Poor prognostic factors for recovery:[192]
  - High neck pain intensity
  - Neurological symptoms
  - Women 2.7 times as likely to be unrecovered at 3 months
  - Older age
  - No seat belt used
  - Rear impact in MVA
  - Reduced cervical ROM
  - Prior neck pain or headache
  - Anxiety or depression

- Can have complaints of dizziness and unsteadiness.[194]

- Central hypersensitivity.[195]

- Complaints of sensory hypersensitivity.[195]

- Psychological factors can potentially include pain catastrophizing, fear avoidance, lower pain self-efficacy, and distress.[195]

Outcome Measures

- Numerical pain rating scale.[192]
- Neck Disability Index.[192]
- Any appropriate clinical outcome measure may be used; the NDI and PSFS are most likely.

Diagnostic Imaging

- Fatty infiltration of the cervical extensor musculature was found in female clients with WAD and not in clients with chronic neck pain or in healthy controls.[196]

II. Observation

- Chronic neck pain due to WAD is associated with abnormal cervical spine motion and gait patterns.[32]
- The clinician should be especially cognizant of the client who is unwilling to move their head independent of their body (i.e., the client who turns their whole body to look at something versus just turning their head). This should alert the clinician to the possibility of cervical spinal instability or CAD.
- Reduced cervical flexion and rotation were found with clients demonstrating forward head posture and thoracic kyphosis.[152]

III. Triage and Screening

- All nonmusculoskeletal causes, as well as causes from related joints, should be ruled out.
- History is used for triage, during which red flags should be identified and yellow flags assessed.[53]
- Due to the high frequency of whiplash in traumatic injury mechanisms, such as motor vehicle accidents, dives, falls, and sporting injuries, as well as correlation between head and cervical spine injuries, cervical spine fractures, instability, and CAD testing should be ruled out when appropriate.

- An alert, asymptomatic client without distracting injury or neurological deficit who is able to complete a functional ROM examination may be safely cleared from cervical spine immobilization without radiographic evaluation (SN 98).[60]
- Canadian C-Spine Rule: demonstrated better diagnostic accuracy (SN range 90-100) than either the NEXUS criteria (SN range 83-100)[58] or physician clinical judgment alone (SN 92)[59] and, therefore, an improved ability to **rule out** an actual fracture.
- Alar ligament testing:
  - Significant variability in diagnostic accuracy (SN 69-100, −LR 0.29–0.31; SP 72-96, +LR 18-Inf) with improved ability to **rule in** versus **rule out** alar ligament insufficiency with less complex testing.[107]
  - Better ability to **rule in** (SP 96-100, +LR 18-Inf) versus **rule out** (SN 72, −LR 0.30) alar ligament insufficiency with more complex testing.[107]
- Sharp-Purser test: demonstrates stronger ability to **rule in** (SP 96, +LR 17.3) than rule out (SN 69, −LR 0.32) transverse ligament insufficiency.[108]
- More complex transverse ligament testing is also better able to **rule in** (SP 99, +LR 65) than rule out (SN 65, −LR 0.35) transverse ligament insufficiency.[107]
- Cervical rotation is helpful for **ruling in** (SP 100, +LR 83.3) a potential vertebrobasilar ischemia.[115]
- Combined cervical extension and rotation is helpful for **ruling in** (SP 98, +LR 4.2) a potential upper cervical neurovascular compromise.[117]
- Clinical examinations for myelopathy are mostly SP and lack SN; the majority of current studies are of poor to moderate quality.[81] The clinician should then be cautious with interpretation of (+) or (−) clinical examination findings when testing for myelopathy.

- Cold hyperalgesia or cold intolerance and impaired sympathetic vasoconstriction have been described.[197]
- These clients have demonstrated lower reflex thresholds (spinal cord hyperexcitability) than healthy subjects.[195]
- These clients have demonstrated slower reaction times than healthy controls.[193]

IV. Motion Tests

- Assessment of cervical spine ROM is reliable across various clients and measurement devices.[124-126]
- Increased cervical spine translational and rotational motion in women with WAD was found at levels C3-4, C4-5, and C5-6.[198]
- Chronic neck pain due to WAD is associated with abnormal cervical spine motion.[32] These clients have less mobility compared to controls, as well as less volitional ROM.[35]
- Limited cervical spine ROM is likely and is prognostic for poor recovery.[192]
- Elderly clients have been shown to have decreased ROM in all planes compared to their younger counterparts, for both men and women.[130, 131] The elderly group also had a wider variation of cervical ROM values as compared to the younger group. Women were found to have greater ROM in all cohort age groups.[130]

V. Muscle Performance Testing

- Changes in muscle and motor function have been synthesized to potentially include loss of movement, altered muscle recruitment patterns, morphological changes in neck muscles, disturbed eye movement control, loss of balance and joint repositioning errors, and decreased muscle strength of neck and upper quarter muscles.[195]
- Coordination, strength, and endurance deficits of neck and upper quarter muscles (longus colli, middle trapezius, lower trapezius, and serratus anterior) are common in clients with movement coordination impairments.[11]
- Chronic neck pain clients, on average, have lower neck muscle strength compared with controls.[35]

VI. Special Tests

- PA glides: A lack of a mobility restriction or concordant pain with PA glides of the cervical spine helps **rule out** (SN 100,[31] SN 89[134]) facet joint involvement.
  - A detected mobility restriction or concordant pain helps **rule in** (SP 100) facet joint involvement.[31]
  - Hypomobility and reproduction of concordant pain demonstrate greater diagnostic accuracy than detection of hypomobility alone.[31, 134]
- Dizziness and unsteadiness can cause joint reposition errors in cervical spine.[194]

VII. Palpation

- Muscle guarding, spasm, and tenderness are likely in the upper cervical spine with chronic WAD and generally in the upper quarter with acute WAD.[195]

VIII. Physical Performance Measures

- Several studies have demonstrated deep neck flexor endurance dysfunction, dysfunction on the CCFT, and other performance measures.
- Clients with chronic neck pain may perform less well on certain functional tests (e.g., lifting, reaching).[35]

POTENTIAL TREATMENT-BASED CLASSIFICATIONS

- Pain and mobility (if appropriate) can be used for acute WAD; stability may also be appropriate.
- Mobility and pain control are also likely appropriate for chronic WAD.

Cervicogenic Headaches or Cervicocranial Syndrome

ICD-9: 339.0 (other headache syndromes); 784.0 (headache)

ICD-10: G44 (other headache syndromes); R51 (headache)

Variously described types of headaches exist, and cervicogenic headache is one such type. This type of headache is typically attributed to mechanical causes. Therefore, the clinician should be able to reproduce some of the signs and symptoms the client presents with during a thorough examination. The most frequently described region of the spine attributable to cervicogenic headaches is the upper cervical spine. Upper cervical spine arthropathy at the levels of C0 through C3 have been most frequently described in the literature, with restrictions of C1-C2 being the most common.[20-24]

I. Client Interview

Subjective History[11, 125]

- Unilateral headache (HA) associated with cervical or suboccipital area symptoms is aggravated by neck movements or positions.

- Headache is produced or aggravated with provocation of the ipsilateral posterior cervical myofascia and joints.

- 70% of clients with frequent intermittent HA report cervical symptoms associated with HA.[199]

- It had been estimated that only 14% to 18% of chronic HAs were cervicogenic in nature.

- Major criteria for cervicogenic HA include the following:[200]

  - Signs and symptoms of head pain are precipitated either by neck movement and sustained awkward head positioning or by external pressure over the upper cervical or occipital region on the symptomatic side.

  - Clients may have restriction of ROM in the neck.

  - Ipsilateral neck, shoulder, or arm pain are of a rather vague nonradicular nature or, occasionally, arm pain is of a radicular nature.

- Head pain features include the following: (1) typically moderate to severe, nonthrobbing, and non-lancinating pain, usually starting in the neck, (2) episodes of varying duration, and (3) fluctuating, continuous pain.

- Clients are more likely to be female.

- Less likely features include nausea, photophobia, phonophobia, dizziness, ipsilateral blurred vision, difficulty swallowing, and ipsilateral periocular edema.

Outcome Measures

- Any appropriate clinical outcome measure may be used; the NDI and PSFS are most likely.

- A headache questionnaire has been suggested.[201]

Diagnostic Imaging

- No evidence exists supporting the validity of facet joints or medial branch blocks as diagnosing cervical facet joint pain as the primary cause of serious neck pain.[35]

- No evidence exists that common degenerative changes on cervical MRI are associated with pain in clients with supposed cervicogenic headache.[35]

II. Observation

- Forward head posture has been suggested.[202]

- Reduced cervical flexion and rotation were found with clients demonstrating forward head posture and thoracic kyphosis.[152]

III. Triage and Screening

- All nonmusculoskeletal causes, as well as causes from related joints, should be ruled out.

- History is used for triage, during which red flags should be identified and yellow flags assessed.[53]

- An alert, asymptomatic client without distracting injury or neurological deficit who is able to complete a functional ROM examination may be safely cleared from cervical spine immobilization without radiographic evaluation (SN 98).[60]

- Canadian C-Spine Rule: demonstrated better diagnostic accuracy (SN range 90-100) than either the NEXUS criteria (SN range 83-100)[58] or physician clinical judgment alone (SN 92)[59] and, therefore, an improved ability to **rule out** an actual fracture.

- Alar ligament testing:
  - Significant variability in diagnostic accuracy (SN 69-100, −LR 0.29–0.31; SP 72-96, +LR 18-Inf) with improved ability to **rule in** versus **rule out** alar ligament insufficiency with less complex testing.[107]
  - Better ability to **rule in** (SP 96-100, +LR 18-Inf) versus rule out (SN 72, −LR 0.30) alar ligament insufficiency with more complex testing.[107]

- Sharp-Purser test: demonstrates stronger ability to **rule in** (SP 96, +LR 17.3) than rule out (SN 69, −LR 0.32) transverse ligament insufficiency.[108]

- More complex transverse ligament testing is also better able to **rule in** (SP 99, +LR 65) than rule out (SN 65, −LR 0.35) transverse ligament insufficiency.[107]

- Cervical rotation is helpful for **ruling in** (SP 100, +LR 83.3) a potential vertebrobasilar ischemia.[115]

- Combined cervical extension and rotation is helpful for **ruling in** (SP 98, +LR 4.2) a potential upper cervical neurovascular compromise.[117]

- Clinical examinations for myelopathy are mostly SP and lack SN; the majority of current studies are of poor to moderate quality.[81] The clinician should then be cautious with interpretation of (+) or (−) clinical examination findings when testing for myelopathy.

IV. Motion Tests

- Cervical AROM and segmental mobility have been suggested as useful measures for classifying clients in this category.[11]

- Painful or limited restrictions (joint arthropathy found at C0 through C3 levels, with restrictions of C1-C2 being the most common)[20-24] may exist for cervicogenic HAs, but there is no evidence of these restrictions in migraine HAs.[133]

- Limited and painful upper cervical spine mobility with manual examination were noted.[133]

- A 10° or greater ROM loss with the cervical flexion–rotation test suggests C1-C2 involvement in cervicogenic-related headaches. This test is better at **ruling in** (SP 100) versus **ruling out** (SN 86) cervicogenic headaches attributable to a C1-C2 dysfunction.[24]

- Cervical flexion, extension, and rotation ROM were significantly less in these clients than in clients with migraine HA or tension HA, or in controls.[133, 203]

- Mean cervical spine ROM was reduced in clients with cervicogenic headache.[129]

- Cervicobrachial muscle tightness is common for these clients.[133, 202, 204] In fact, this muscle tightness was significantly higher in cervicogenic HA clients than in clients with migraine HA or in the control group.[133]

- Elderly clients have been shown to have decreased ROM in all planes compared to their younger counterparts, for both men and women.[130, 131] The elderly group also had a wider variation of cervical ROM values as compared to the younger group. Women were found to have greater ROM in all cohort age groups.[130]

V. Muscle Performance Testing

- Coordination, strength, and endurance deficits of neck and upper quarter muscles (longus colli, middle trapezius, lower trapezius, and serratus anterior) are common in clients with movement coordination impairments.[11]

- Cervical flexor muscle dysfunction has been identified.[133, 147, 202]

- Chronic neck pain clients, on average, have lower neck muscle strength compared with controls.[35]

VI. Special Tests

- Accessory motion: Lack of mobility restriction or concordant pain with PA glides of the cervical spine helps **rule out** (SN 100,[31] SN 89[134]) facet joint involvement.

    - A detected mobility restriction or concordant pain helps **rule in** (SP 100) facet joint involvement.[31]

    - Hypomobility and reproduction of concordant pain demonstrate greater diagnostic accuracy (**SN 100, SP 100**) than detection of hypomobility alone.[31, 134]

- Cervical flexion–rotation test: Not having a loss of ≥10° has good ability to help **rule out** (SN 86, −LR 0.14), while having a loss of ≥10° had excellent ability to help **rule in** (SP 100, +LR Inf), cervicogenic HAs.[24] In an additional study, this test had good ability to help **rule out** (SN 91, −LR 0.1) and rule in (SP 90, +LR 9.1) cervicogenic HA and movement impairment of C1-C2 in these clients.[132]

- Rotation ROM was significantly reduced in the cervicogenic HA group compared to the migraine and multiple HA form clients.[205]

VII. Palpation

- Headache is often produced or aggravated with provocation of the ipsilateral posterior cervical myofascia and joints.[11]

- Tenderness is noted in the suboccipital region, although pain pressure threshold testing was lower in these clients than in clients with migraine and tension HAs.[23]

VIII. Physical Performance Measures

- Clients may have substandard performance on the CCFT.[11]

- Clients with chronic neck pain may perform less well on certain functional tests (e.g., lifting, reaching).[35]

POTENTIAL TREATMENT-BASED CLASSIFICATIONS

- Headache

- Pain control or mobility as potential secondary categories

Cervical Spine Mechanical Neck Pain

ICD-9: 723.1 (cervicalgia); 847.0 (sprain of neck)

ICD-10: M54.2 (cervicalgia); S13.4 (sprain and strain of cervical spine); S13.4XXA (sprain of ligaments of spine)

Mechanical neck pain has had various definitions, including "non-specific pain in the area of the cervico-thoracic junction that is exacerbated by neck movements"[206] and "pain primarily confined in the area on the posterior aspect of the neck that can be exacerbated by neck movements or sustained postures."[207] Mechanical neck pain typically has a characteristic pattern of limited motion and may worsen with active and passive motions into the directions of restricted movement.

I. Client Interview

Subjective History

- Reported prevalence of pain related to the facet joints has ranged from 36% to 67% of clients with chronic neck pain.[208]

- The main distribution of referred pain was as follows: Pain in the occipital region was referred from C2-C3 and C3, while pain in the upper posterolateral cervical region was referred

Differential Diagnosis of Most Common Headache Types

Refer to chapter 15 (Face and Head) for this information.

from C0-C1, C1-C2, and C2-C3. Pain in the upper posterior cervical region was referred from C2-C3, C3-C4, and C3; that in the middle posterior cervical region from C3-C4, C4-C5, and C4; and that in the lower posterior cervical region from C4-C5, C5-C6, C4, and C5. In addition, pain in the suprascapular region was referred from C4-C5, C5-C6, and C4; that in the superior angle of the scapula from C6-C7, C6, and C7; and that in the midscapular region from C7-T1 and C7.[19]

- Clients are more likely to be younger (age < 50 years).[11]

- Reported symptoms are isolated to the neck region.[11]

- Symptoms are more than likely acute in nature (duration < 12 weeks).[11]

- Women consistently reported neck pain 83% more often than men.[209]

- Risk factors for mechanical neck pain include the following:[210-213]
  - Previous musculoskeletal pain
  - Low physical capacity
  - Awkward work postures
  - Physical or repetitive work
  - Prior neck pain
  - Blue collar versus white collar work
  - Middle age
  - Additional health complaints
  - Psychological factors
  - Passive coping mechanisms

Outcome Measures

- The suggested MCID for the NDI is 9.5 (19 percentage points) for clients with mechanical neck disorders,[40] while others have suggested a MDC of 10.2 and MCID of 7.5.[41]

- The MCID for the numerical pain rating scale is a change in score of 1.3 points or higher.[40]

- Any appropriate clinical outcome measure may be used; the NDI and PSFS are most likely.

Diagnostic Imaging

- No evidence exists supporting the validity of facet joints or medial branch blocks as diagnosing cervical facet joint pain as the primary cause of serious neck pain.[35]

II. Observation

- The client may present with a specific pattern of restriction (e.g., the inability to perform motions requiring closing of a facet joint that will not close, such as extension, ipsilateral side bending, and rotation).

- Reduced cervical flexion and rotation were found with clients demonstrating forward head posture and thoracic kyphosis.[152]

III. Triage and Screening

- All nonmusculoskeletal causes, as well as causes from related joints, should be ruled out.

- History is used for triage, during which red flags should be identified and yellow flags assessed.[53]

- An alert, asymptomatic client without distracting injury or neurological deficit who is able to complete a functional ROM examination may be safely cleared from cervical spine immobilization without radiographic evaluation (SN 98).[60]

- Canadian C-Spine Rule: demonstrated better diagnostic accuracy (SN range 90-100) than either the NEXUS criteria (SN range 83-100)[58] or physician clinical judgment alone (SN 92)[59] and, therefore, an improved ability to **rule out** an actual fracture.

- Alar ligament testing:
  - Significant variability in diagnostic accuracy (SN 69-100, −LR 0.29–0.31; SP 72-96, +LR 18-Inf) with improved ability to **rule in** versus **rule out** alar ligament insufficiency with less complex testing.[107]
  - Better ability to **rule in** (SP 96-100, +LR 18-Inf) versus rule out (SN 72, −LR 0.30) alar ligament insufficiency with more complex testing.[107]

- Sharp-Purser test: demonstrates stronger ability to **rule in** (SP 96, +LR 17.3) than rule out (SN 69, −LR 0.32) transverse ligament insufficiency.[108]

- More complex transverse ligament testing is also better able to **rule in** (SP 99, +LR 65) than rule out (SN 65, −LR 0.35) transverse ligament insufficiency.[107]

- Cervical rotation is helpful for **ruling in** (SP 100, +LR 83.3) a potential vertebrobasilar ischemia.[115]

- Combined cervical extension and rotation is helpful for **ruling in** (SP 98, +LR 4.2) a potential upper cervical neurovascular compromise.[117]

- Clinical examinations for myelopathy are mostly SP and lack SN; the majority of current studies are of poor to moderate quality.[81] The clinician should then be cautious with interpretation of (+) or (−) clinical examination findings when testing for myelopathy.

IV. Motion Tests

- Assessment of cervical spine ROM is reliable across various clients and measurement devices.[124-126]

- PA glides: Lack of a mobility restriction or concordant pain with PA glides of the cervical spine helps **rule out** (SN 100,[31] SN 89[134]) facet joint involvement.

  - A detected mobility restriction or concordant pain helps **rule in** (SP 100) facet joint involvement.[31]

  - Hypomobility and reproduction of concordant pain demonstrates greater diagnostic accuracy (**SN 100**, **SP 100**) than detection of hypomobility alone.[31, 134]

  - Hypomobility and reproduction of concordant pain demonstrates greater diagnostic accuracy than detection of hypomobility alone in upper cervical spine.[133]

    SP 82, +LR 3.3, at C0-C1

    SP 87, **+LR 4.9**, at C1-C2

    SP 78, +LR 2.9, at C2-C3

- Palpation side glide test has ideal ability to help **rule out** (SN 98, −LR 0.03) radiographically verified congenitally blocked vertebrae.[138]

- Elderly clients have been shown to have decreased ROM in all planes compared to their younger counterparts, for both men and women.[130, 131] The elderly group also had a wider variation of cervical ROM values as compared to the younger group. Women were found to have greater ROM in all cohort age groups.[130]

V. Muscle Performance Testing

- Clients are likely to have both limited ROM and strength in cervical spine region, especially deep neck flexor weakness.[11]

- Due to the close relationship of this pathology with cervical sprain and strain pathology, these clients can also demonstrate coordination, strength, and endurance deficits of neck and upper quarter muscles (longus colli, middle trapezius, lower trapezius, serratus anterior).[11]

- Chronic neck pain clients, on average, have lower neck muscle strength compared with controls.[35]

VI. Special Tests

- See Motion Tests section.

- Pain during segmental testing has moderate ability to rule in (SP 79, +LR 3.9) and **rule out** (SN 82, −LR 0.23) facet joint involvement.[135]

- Intertester reliability for this testing is poor[136] to good.[137]

- Assessment of pain intertester reliability is better than mobility assessment alone for both cervical and thoracic spine.[137]

- Isolating appropriate upper cervical spine level of pathology using concordant sign has good ability to both **rule out** (SN 100) and **rule in** (SP 100) facet joint involvement in one high-quality study.[31]

- Joint mobility assessment (PAIVM) of C0-C1 (SP 82, +LR 3.3), C1-C2 (**SP 87**, **+LR 4.9**), and C2-C3 (SP 78, +LR 2.9) all have fair to good ability to rule in facet joint involvement in one high-quality study (QUADAS 10).[133]

VII. Palpation

- Local tenderness with 30 kPa of pressure helps **rule in** (SP 95) cervical facet joint pain, although caution is suggested by the authors.[214]

VIII. Physical Performance Measures

- The endurance test of the short neck flexors and the cervical PILE test can be regarded as appropriate instruments for measuring different aspects of neck muscle function in clients with nonspecific neck pain.[150]

- Clients with chronic neck pain may perform less well on certain functional tests (e.g., lifting, reaching).[35]

POTENTIAL TREATMENT-BASED CLASSIFICATIONS

- Mobility is most likely unless client is pain dominant. Exercise and conditioning may also be used.

Cervical Spine Sprain or Strain

ICD-9: 847.0 (sprain of neck)

ICD-10: S13.4 (sprain and strain of cervical spine); S13.4XXA (sprain of ligaments of spine)

Sprains and strains of the cervical spine (as with any sprain and strain) are pain attributed to ligamentous and muscular or soft-tissue causes, respectively. Unlike cervical instability and mechanical neck pain, sprains and strains of the cervical spine will not have corresponding instability or joint dysfunctions. Sprains and strains of the cervical spine, though, can be commonly associated with other dysfunctions. Therefore, a comprehensive examination is required to ascertain the exact extent of the client's dysfunction.

I. Client Interview

Subjective History

- Longstanding neck pain (duration > 12 weeks)[11]

- Likely to report specific mechanism of onset

- Pain likely to be motion related and worse with motions that stress the involved structures

Outcome Measures

- Any appropriate clinical outcome measure may be used; the NDI and PSFS are most likely.[11]

Diagnostic Imaging

- No evidence exists supporting the validity of facet joints or medial branch blocks as diagnosing cervical facet joint pain as the primary cause of serious neck pain.[35]

II. Observation

- Reduced cervical flexion and rotation were found with clients demonstrating forward head posture and thoracic kyphosis.[152]

- If acute, the client may hold the head in a position of least stress to the involved structures.

III. Triage and Screening

- All nonmusculoskeletal causes, as well as causes from related joints, should be ruled out.

- History is used for triage, during which red flags should be identified and yellow flags assessed.[53]

- An alert, asymptomatic client without distracting injury or neurological deficit who is able to complete a functional ROM examination may be safely cleared from cervical spine immobilization without radiographic evaluation (SN 98).[60]

- Canadian C-Spine Rule: demonstrated better diagnostic accuracy (SN range 90-100) than either the NEXUS criteria (SN range 83-100)[58] or physician clinical judgment alone (SN 92)[59] and, therefore, an improved ability to **rule out** an actual fracture.

- Alar ligament testing:
  - Significant variability in diagnostic accuracy (SN 69-100, −LR 0.29–0.31; SP 72-96, +LR 18-Inf) with improved ability to **rule in** versus **rule out** alar ligament insufficiency with less complex testing.[107]

- Better ability to **rule in** (SP 96-100, +LR 18-Inf) versus rule out (SN 72, −LR 0.30) alar ligament insufficiency with more complex testing.[107]

- Sharp-Purser test: demonstrates stronger ability to **rule in** (SP 96, +LR 17.3) than rule out (SN 69, −LR 0.32) transverse ligament insufficiency.[108]

- More complex transverse ligament testing is also better able to **rule in** (SP 99, +LR 65) than rule out (SN 65, −LR 0.35) transverse ligament insufficiency.[107]

- Cervical rotation is helpful for **ruling in** (SP 100, +LR 83.3) a potential vertebrobasilar ischemia.[115]

- Combined cervical extension and rotation is helpful for **ruling in** (SP 98, +LR 4.2) a potential upper cervical neurovascular compromise.[117]

- Clinical examinations for myelopathy are mostly SP and lack SN; the majority of current studies are of poor to moderate quality.[81] The clinician should then be cautious with interpretation of (+) or (−) clinical examination findings when testing for myelopathy.

IV. Motion Tests

- Assessment of cervical spine ROM is reliable across various clients and measurement devices.[124-126]

- Muscle–tendon involvement is typically concordant with passive lengthening and active muscle contraction of the involved muscle groups.[215]

- Flexibility deficits of upper quarter muscles (scalenes, upper trapezius, levator scapulae, pectoralis minor, and pectoralis major) are common.[11]

- Elderly clients have been shown to have decreased ROM in all planes compared to their younger counterparts, for both men and women.[130, 131] The elderly group also had a wider variation of cervical ROM values as compared to the younger group. Women were found to have greater ROM in all cohort age groups.[130]

V. Muscle Performance Testing

- Coordination, strength, and endurance deficits of neck and upper quarter muscles (longus colli, middle trapezius, lower trapezius, and serratus anterior) are common in clients with movement coordination impairment.[11]

- Chronic neck pain clients, on average, have lower neck muscle strength compared with controls.[35]

VI. Special Tests

- PA glides: Lack of a mobility restriction or concordant pain with PA glides of the cervical spine helps **rule out** (SN 100[31] SN 89[134]) facet joint involvement.

  - A detected mobility restriction or concordant pain helps **rule in** (SP 100) facet joint involvement.[31]

  - Hypomobility and reproduction of concordant pain demonstrates greater diagnostic accuracy (**SN 100, SP 100**) than detection of hypomobility alone.[31, 134]

- Pain during segmental testing has moderate ability to rule in (SP 79, +LR 3.9) and **rule out** (SN 82, −LR 0.23) facet joint involvement.[135]

VII. Palpation

- If the ligament (sprain) or muscle (strain) is palpable, it likely will be tender to palpation.

VIII. Physical Performance Measures

- Clients may have ergonomic inefficiencies with performing repetitive activities.[11]

- The endurance test of the short neck flexors and the cervical PILE test can be regarded as appropriate instruments for measuring different aspects of neck muscle function in clients with nonspecific neck pain.[150]

- Clients with chronic neck pain may perform less well on certain functional tests (e.g., lifting, reaching).[35]

POTENTIAL TREATMENT-BASED CLASSIFICATIONS

- Pain, mobility, and exercise and conditioning are the most likely, dependent on client impairments.

Differential Diagnosis of Cervical Spine Mechanical Neck Pain and Cervical Spine Sprain or Strain

- A lack of a mobility restriction or concordant pain with PA glides of the cervical spine helps **rule out** (SN 100,[31] SN 89[134]) facet joint involvement (mechanical neck pain).

- Concordant pain with prone PA glides in the upper cervical spine helps rule in facet joint involvement (mechanical neck pain).

- Assessment of pain during PA glides demonstrates stronger diagnostic accuracy than determination of joint mobility.

- Both conditions may have insidious or traumatic onset.

- Both conditions are likely to have restricted motion presentation. Muscle strains will be limited in motions when the involved muscle is elongated.

- Muscle soft-tissue (strain) dysfunction is most likely going to be painful when stretched or elongated and actively contracted or shortened (especially against resistance), while mechanical dysfunction will be painful with joint play motion testing of that particular joint.

- It is not likely that either condition will have hard neurological findings (e.g., reflex changes, altered sensation, or myotomal weakness).

Cervicogenic Dizziness

ICD-9: 780.4 (cervicogenic dizziness)

ICD-10: R42 (cervicogenic dizziness)

Cervicogenic dizziness (CGD) tends to be a controversial diagnosis because there are no diagnostic tests to confirm that it is the cause of the dizziness. CGD is a diagnosis that is provided to people who have neck injury or pain as well as dizziness and in whom other causes of dizziness have been ruled out.[216] CGD has been defined as "a non-specific sensation of altered orientation in space and disequilibrium originating from abnormal afferent activity from the neck."[216] Clients with CGD typically describe their dizziness as vertigo, lightheadedness, blurry vision, disequilibrium, or nausea. Several proposed mechanisms leading to cervicogenic dizziness exist, including mechanical compression of the vertebral artery system, irritation of the cervical sympathetic nervous system, and abnormal proprioceptive input from the upper cervical spine.[216, 217]

Reported suggestions for subjective examination include past medical history, differentiation of dizziness symptoms (e.g., disequilibrium, lightheadedness, and vague dizziness), dizziness circumstances (e.g., symptoms usually have a causal symptomatic relationship to neck position and pain), dizziness intensity (a modified VAS rating of 0-10 out of 10 for current and recent range of pain level), and length of dizziness (typically lasts from several minutes to hours).[217]

Suggestions for physical examination include medical screening (e.g., upper cervical spine stability, CAD, and CNS testing), vestibular system exam (e.g., benign paroxysmal positional vertigo, vestibulo-ocular reflex, dynamic visual acuity), cervical spine posture, AROM, accessory motion, and palpation. For cervicogenic dizziness, the authors suggested the neck torsion nystagmus test, neck torsion smooth pursuit test, cervical spine joint position error test, and cervical spine manual traction or distraction test.[217]

Klippel-Feil Syndrome

ICD-9: 756.16 (Klippel-Feil syndrome)

ICD-10: Q76.1 (Klippel-Feil syndrome)

This rare condition is characterized by the congenital fusion of any two of the seven cervical vertebrae. The syndrome occurs in a heterogeneous group of clients unified only by the presence of a congenital defect in the formation or segmentation of the cervical spine. Klippel-Feil syndrome can be identified by shortness of the neck. Those with the syndrome have a very low hairline and limited ability to move the neck. These clients appear to have no neck.

Torticollis

ICD-9: 723.5 (torticollis, unspecified)

ICD-10: M43.6 (torticollis)

Torticollis (commonly referred to as *wryneck*) is one of a broader category of disorders that exhibit flexion, extension, or twisting of muscles of the neck beyond their normal position. In torticollis, the neck tends to twist to one side, causing head tilt to the same side and tightness of the sternocleidomastoid, but rotation in the opposite direction.

CONCLUSION

The cervical spine has a strong, interdependent relationship with the shoulder and thoracic spine. Thus, these areas should be ruled out. Additionally, face and head as well as TMJ-related involvement should be considered in the differential diagnosis. As with the face and head, clients presenting with acute trauma onset of symptoms should be ruled out for the potential for serious pathological involvement. Using the CCSR, subjective history, observation of the client, and triage screening mechanisms, the clinician can help rule out the concerns for serious pathology. Once serious pathology has been ruled out, the clinician should utilize the systematic, evidence-based approach advocated by this text. As with all sections of the body, a systematic approach involves ruling out competing diagnoses with SN tests followed by using SP tests to help rule in potential pathology. However, remember the importance of the entire examination sequence's funnel approach and all of its components, not simply special tests.

18

THORACIC SPINE

Michael P. Reiman, PT, DPT, OCS, SCS, ATC, FAAOMPT, CSCS

Thoracic spine pain (TSP) is experienced across the lifespan by healthy people and is a common presentation in primary health care clinical practice. However, the epidemiological characteristics of thoracic spine pain are not well documented compared to neck and low back pain.[1] Thoracic spine pain interfering with school or leisure ranged from 3.5% to 9.7% for 1-year prevalence. Generally, studies reported a higher prevalence for TSP in child and adolescent populations, and particularly for females. The 1-month, 6-month, 1-year, and 25-year incidences were 0% to 0.9%, 10.3%, 3.8% to 35.3%, and 9.8%, respectively. Pain in the thoracic spine was found to be significantly associated with concurrent musculoskeletal pain, backpack use, posture, lifestyle, growth, and physical, social, psychological, and environmental factors. Risk factors identified for thoracic spine pain in adolescents include age (being older) and poorer mental health.[1] Prevalence of pain in the thoracic spine varied with occupational group and time period. One-year prevalence of pain in the thoracic spine ranged from 3.0% to 55.0%, with most occupational groups having medians around 30%.[2] Other findings suggest the prevalence of thoracic pain to be 15% of the general population and up to 22% of the population in interventional pain management settings.[3]

CLINICALLY APPLIED ANATOMY

The thoracic spine has several unique characteristics. The upper thoracic spine has characteristics of the typical cervical spine, while the lower thoracic spine has characteristics of the lumbar spine. The vertebral body in the thoracic spine is larger than those in the cervical spine, yet smaller than those in the lumbar spine. Transverse processes in the thoracic spine are true transverse processes like those in the lumbar spine (not anterior and posterior tubercles as in the cervical spine). Most of the transverse processes in the thoracic spine articulate with a rib (figure 18.1).

The spinous processes in the thoracic spine are like those in the lumbar spine, with single projections posteriorly (unlike the bifid spinous processes in the cervical spine). The spinous processes slope inferiorly and are the longest of any region of the spine. The extent of inferior slope of these spinous processes is not universally described. Typically, the upper thoracic spinous processes have a more horizontal orientation, similar to the cervical spine, and the lower thoracic spinous processes (particularly T11 and T12) are shorter than the other vertebrae with more posterior projections, similar to the lumbar spine. The first and last three spinous processes are almost horizontal, while those in the mid-thoracic spine are steeply inclined.

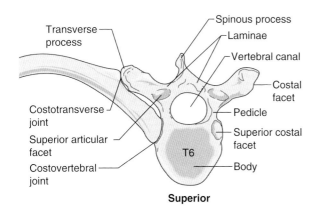

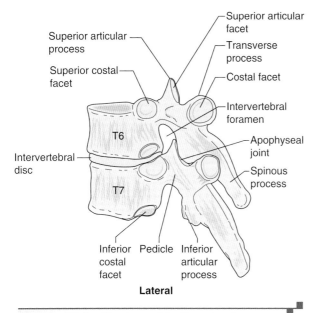

Figure 18.1 Structures of the thoracic spine.

The facet (zygapophyseal) joints in this region of the spine are plane synovial joints, like those of the cervical and lumbar spine. The orientation of these joints is approximately 10° to 20° from the frontal or vertical plane or approximately 70° to 80° from the transverse or horizontal plane. The frontal plane orientation of the thoracic and cervical spine facets allows for mobility with rotation and side bending. The more vertical orientation of the thoracic spine facets limits flexion mobility to an extent.

The typical thoracic vertebra has 12 separate articulations. These include 4 zygapophyseal articulations (a superior and inferior surface on each side of the vertebra), 2 costotransverse articulations, 4 costovertebral articulations, and 2 vertebral body–intervertebral disc–vertebral body articulations. Anteriorly the typical rib has a costochondral and a chondral sternal joint. Ribs 8 through 10 are considered false ribs because they articulate indirectly with the sternum anteriorly via the costal cartilage of rib 7 (figure 18.2). Ribs 11 and 12 are floating ribs and do not articulate anteriorly.

The spinous processes are no longer bifid as they are in the cervical spine. Additionally, the transverse processes also are true transverse processes; they do not have anterior and posterior tubercles for the nerve root. The spinous processes, for the most part, project posteriorly and distally (see figure 18.1). This is particularly the case in the mid-thoracic spine. The extent that the spinous process projects distally varies depending on the level of the spine and the individual client.

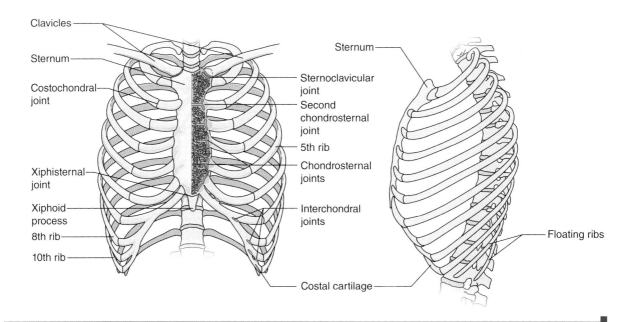

Figure 18.2 Anterior and lateral view of rib cage demonstrating true and false ribs.

The thoracic spine articulates with both the cervical and lumbar spine. An additional unique characteristic of the thoracic spine is that it articulates with the rib cage and therefore requires interdependent motion between all of these structures. Articulation with the rib cage limits thoracic spinal mobility. The thoracic spine has the least mobility of all three sections of the spine. Spinal stability and internal organ protection are primary functions of the thoracic spine.

Articulation of the thoracic spine with the rib cage encompasses multiple joints and ligaments. The first rib articulates with the first thoracic vertebra (T1). The 1st, 11th, and 12th ribs articulate fully with their own vertebrae. The typical ribs articulate with the vertebral body of the same level, as well as with the superior vertebra and the interposed disc (figure 18.3). Movement of the trunk region requires movement not only of the thoracic spine, but of the ribs as well. Thoracic spine flexion is correlated with rib superior glide and anterior roll, while thoracic extension corresponds with rib inferior glide and posterior roll (figure 18.4). These combined motions allow for rib cage elevation and depression.

CLIENT INTERVIEW

This interview is typically the first encounter the clinician will have with the client. As previously

discussed in chapter 5 (Client Interview and Observation), this component of the examination can

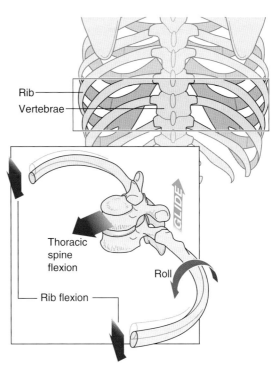

Figure 18.4 Flexion and extension of the thoracic spine and corresponding rib movement.

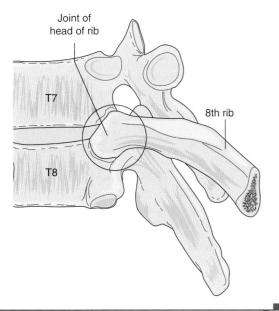

Figure 18.3 A typical rib articulating with vertebra of the same level, vertebra of the level above, and the interposed intervertebral disc.

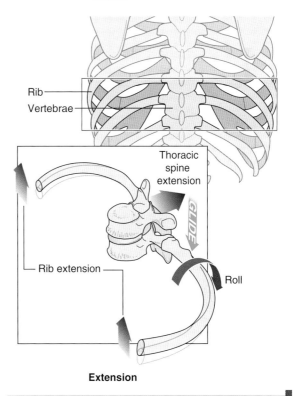

provide the clinician with a significant amount of information relevant to the probability of the client's presenting diagnosis. For purposes of this text, the interview is described relative to each body part or section but generally includes subjective reports by the client, as well as findings from their outcome measures. Additionally included in this section is radiographic imaging. While clinicians should avoid biasing their examination by interpreting findings of radiographic imaging prior to seeing the client (in most cases without concerns for red flags and major medical-related issues), this point in the examination is most likely where clinicians will encounter radiographic imaging. Additionally, in some instances, clinicians must interpret radiographic imaging early in the examination to rule out serious pathology prior to continuing with other components of the examination sequence.

The examination process of the thoracic spine begins with the client interview. It allows the clinician to gather information from the client about the chief complaint, the mechanism of injury, and the location and irritability of pain associated with the injury. The clinician uses data gathered from the client interview to generate an initial set of hypotheses concerning the underlying cause of impairments, functional deficits, and injured structures. From this, the clinician can generate client-identified problem lists that can be used to guide and formulate an examination strategy.

Subjective

The subjective interview on a client with thoracic-spine-related pain requires questioning of cervical and (possibly) lumbar spine, depending on the location of the pain. As noted in figure 18.5, thoracic-related pain can have a variable presentation that involves structures other than the thoracic spine. Additionally, the clinician must consider pain in the rib regions. For example, costochondritis is thought to be a self-limiting condition of unknown etiology that typically presents with pain around the second to fifth costochondral joints.[4] Rib dysfunction, shingles, and thoracic spine discogenic pathology have also been reported to present around the ribs.

Of initial importance in subjective inquiry (as with any other area of the body) is determining the potential for the existence of nonmusculoskeletal pain. Visceral pain has the tendency to be vague and dull in nature and may be accompanied by nausea and vomiting and similar symptoms (refer to chapter 6, Triage and Differential Diagnosis).

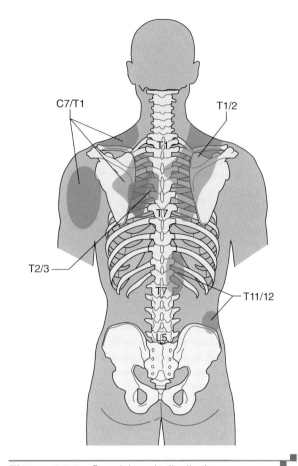

Figure 18.5 Facet joint pain distribution.

Pain in the thoracic spine and trunk area requires careful differential diagnosis of visceral structures as pain generators, due in part to their anatomical proximity. The mechanism of injury will also assist clinicians in determining the potential presence of red flags. A nonspecific, insidious onset that is progressively worsening and is not relieved should alert the clinician for the potential of nonmusculoskeletal pain.

The clinician should be cognizant of thoracic-spine-related pathology of typical nature that is of insidious onset, such as osteoarthritis, scoliosis, Scheuermann's disease, and occasionally costochondritis. Costochondritis is typically thought to result from a physical strain. Tietze syndrome, which is very similar in presentation, can often have an insidious onset. The pain with costochondritis is typically unilateral and intermittent.[5]

Serious pathology of a musculoskeletal nature most typically involves vertebral compression fractures of the thoracic spine. Reported mechanisms of onset for these fractures include falls, lifting even light objects, bending, jogging, and previous history of trauma.[6, 7] Pain for these clients is typically more intense, but of shorter duration; more often it occurred suddenly and persisted during the night.[8] These clients are typically elderly women, and they may not present with any specific mechanism of onset. Previous literature suggests a two- to threefold increase of risk in American women over 60 years of age.[6] Clients with at least one vertebral fracture have a four- to fivefold increase in the risk of having additional vertebral fractures, as well as a threefold increase in the risk of hip fracture.[9]

Age is also a variable to consider for other thoracic-spine-related pathologies. Posture abnormalities are quite common in older adults due to osteoporosis and compression fractures, as described previously. An additional age cohort to consider for poor posture is teenagers. Teenagers are typically going through large growth spurts. Additionally, other specific pathologies such as scoliosis and Scheuermann's disease are noted in this age group. Scoliosis is present in 2% to 4% of children between 10 and 16 years of age and is more likely to occur in girls.[10, 11]

Female clients are also more likely to present with costochondritis[5, 12, 13] and thoracic outlet syndrome.[14-20] Costochondritis was also found to be more common in Hispanics.[5]

Due to the close proximity to the cervical and lumbar spine, the client presenting with pain in the thoracic spine area should be questioned regarding relevant cervical- or lumbar-related potential pathologies. For additional detail in this regard, refer to chapters 17 (Cervical Spine) and 19 (Lumbar Spine).

Outcome Measures

Outcome measures in the thoracic spine are likely to include those described in the cervical and lumbar spines. Generic measures, including the Patient-Specific Functional Scale and such, would also be appropriate measures for the thoracic spine. This section describes additional outcome measures that are specific to the thoracic-spine-related pathology in greater detail.

Outcomes from psychosocial and health-related quality of life (HRQL) studies indicate that body image is a significant issue for clients with scoliosis and their clinicians. Scoliosis literature reveals that self-report measures of body image and HRQL share unreliable correlations with radiographic measures and clinician recommendations for surgery. However, current body image and HRQL measures do not indicate which aspects of scoliosis deformity are the most distressing for clients.[21]

Scoliosis Outcome Measures

• **Scoliosis Research Society: SRS-22 Questionnaire.** The SRS-22 is a modified version[22] of the original questionnaire.[23] It is a general questionnaire relative to scoliosis. The SRS-22 has been shown to be a valid and reliable instrument for assessing clients with adolescent idiopathic scoliosis that is sensitive to changes following surgery. Its metric properties were also found to be appropriate for evaluating adults with spinal deformities.[24]

• **Walter Reed Visual Assessment Scale (WRVAS).** More specific questionnaires relative to scoliosis that assess body image include the WRVAS and Spinal Appearance Questionnaire (SAQ). The WRVAS scale features seven items addressing visual aspects of scoliosis: body curve, head pelvis, rib prominence, shoulder level, flank prominence, scapula rotation, and head rib pelvis.[25-27] Each item consists of five illustrations scaled to indicate worsening deformity with higher scores. This scale assesses the client's perception of their deformity without cognitive or emotional connotations.[25] It has been suggested that the WRVAS is a more accurate reflection of the effect of scoliosis deformity on client body image and HRQL than radiographic imaging is.[21]

• **Trunk Appearance Perception Scale (TAPS).** The TAPS is based on simplicity and ease of completion and scoring. It includes three sets of drawings corresponding to three views of the torso: posterior view, anterior view, and posterior view with client bending forward (Adam's test). It is a reliable instrument with satisfactory discrimination according to the severity of the deformity.[28]

Thoracic Outlet Syndrome

• **Brief Pain Inventory (BPI).** The BPI characterizes acute or chronic pain based on pain severity and interference scores calculated by the arithmetic mean of four severity and seven interference items, respectively, both reported on a scale from 0 to 10, with higher scores being more unfavorable. Additional BPI assessment areas include pain location, measured by body diagram, and pain medication usage and associated relief.

• **Cervical Brachial Symptom Questionnaire (CBSQ).** The CBSQ is the most specific for neck, arm, and shoulder impairment. It quantifies the extent of symptoms related to thoracic outlet syndrome (TOS), such as pain, fatigue, swelling, paresthesia, and numbness, in the upper extremity with certain activities.

Diagnostic Imaging

Imaging of the thoracic spine, with respect to musculoskeletal dysfunction, primarily involves vertebral fractures and scoliosis (table 18.1). Vertebral fractures can have various contributing causes such as malignancy, osteoporosis, and trauma. Additional detail regarding this diagnosis is given at the end of this chapter. Scoliosis is also described at the end of this chapter, as well as in chapter 14 (Posture).

Radiographs

Similar to the cervical spine, established guidelines suggest when radiographic imaging should be implemented for the possibility of a thoracolumbar (TL) spine fracture. The presence of one or more of these criteria in a client with blunt multitrauma is an indication for thoracolumbar spine X-ray screening.[33]

High-Risk Mechanism of Injury

- Motor vehicle or motorbike accident at a speed of at least 70 kmph (45 mph)
- A fall from 3 m (10 ft)
- Ejection from motor vehicle or motorcycle
- Any mechanism of injury outside these criteria that could cause TL fracture

Painful Distracting Injury

- Painful torso or long-bone injury sufficient to distract client from the pain of TL injury

New Neurological Signs or Back Pain or Tenderness

- Clinical findings suspicious of new vertebral fracture: back pain, back tenderness, a palpable step in vertebral palpation, midline thoracolumbar bruising, and any neurological signs consistent with spinal cord injury

Cognitive Impairment

- Glasgow Coma Scale < 15
- Any abnormal mentation or clinical intoxication

Known Cervical Spine Fracture

- Evidence of new traumatic cervical spine fracture

Weight-bearing entire spine anteroposterior (coronal) and lateral (sagittal) views are typically utilized for clients with scoliosis to assess the scoliosis curves, as well as the kyphosis and lordosis curvature. These full-length spine radiographs are standard for assessment of scoliosis. In clients who are still growing, serial radiographs are suggested at 3- to 12-month intervals to follow curve progression. The standard method for quantitatively assessing the scoliosis curvature is measurement of the Cobb angle. Refer to chapter 14 (Posture) for description and detail regarding this measurement.

TABLE 18.1 Diagnostic Accuracy of Various Imaging Modalities for the Thoracic Spine

Pathology	Diagnostic test	Gold standard	SN/SP
Vertebral fracture	CT	SQ-Rx	Moderate fx: 81/87[29]
			Severe fx: **96/92**[29]
	DEXA	Conventional radiography	70/98[30]
		SQ-Rx	**98/99.8**[31]
Scoliosis	Chest radiographs	Standing thoracolumbar radiographs	**94**/62 (thoracic curves)
			38/**97** (thoracolumbar)
			20/**99** (lumbar)
			26/**98** (double major curve)[32]

SN = sensitivity; SP = specificity; CT = computed tomography; DEXA = dual-energy X-ray absorptiometry; SQ-Rx = semi-quantitative grading method of radiography; fx = fracture

The color coding for suggestion of **good** and **ideal** diagnostic accuracy values reported in this table are without quality scoring (QUADAS), a very important aspect of determination of the clinical utility of such values. Therefore, it is suggested that the reader keep this in mind when interpreting such values.

A consensus recommendation on radiographic parameters that should be used routinely to assess thoracolumbar fractures should include the Cobb angle, to assess sagittal alignment; vertebral body translation percentage, to express traumatic anterolisthesis; anterior vertebral body compression percentage, to assess vertebral body compression, the sagittal-to-transverse canal diameter ratio, and canal total cross-sectional area (measured or calculated); and the percent canal occlusion, to assess canal dimensions.[34]

Vertebral fractures, especially those due to osteoporosis, are suggested to be underreported. Although more advanced imaging, such as computed tomography (CT), has demonstrated improved diagnostic capability, radiographic imaging is still considered the standard by some due to its lower cost and radiation exposure.[9]

Magnetic Resonance Imaging

MRI is typically not utilized for clients with scoliosis, except when it is necessary to look at the spinal cord. This likely would be in cases where the potential for neurological pathology may exist (or potentially exist). Indications for MRI in a client with scoliosis include the following:[35]

- Age < 10 years
- Signs of neurologic deterioration
- Rapid progression
- Foot deformity
- Back pain, neck pain, or headache
- Radiographic features suggestive of nonosseous lesion: wide spinal canal, thin pedicles, and wide neural foramina

Computed Tomography

Clinical examination alone cannot detect significant fractures of the thoracolumbar spine. It should be combined with CT imaging to reduce the risk of missed injury.[36] A review suggested the superior SN of reformatted visceral CT for detecting thoracolumbar spine injury. Clients undergoing visceral CT could have their thoracolumbar spine promptly evaluated. However, further prospective evaluation of the CT protocols to optimize visualization of both the viscera and the bone was suggested.[37] Regarding fractures specifically, a study suggests that dual-energy X-ray absorptiometry (DEXA) of the spine done for assessing bone mineral density may detect vertebral fractures in asymptomatic clients.

They suggested that standard radiography remains the reference standard for diagnosing vertebral fractures in clients with suggestive symptoms.[9]

Review of Systems

Refer to chapter 6 (Triage and Differential Diagnosis) for detail on review of systems relevant to the thoracic spine.

OBSERVATION

As with all regions of the body, and most relevant to each region of the spine, a multiview assessment of the client is necessary for observation. Multiview observation includes viewing from different positions, as well as with different activities. The thoracic spine is an area that can present with common postural dysfunctions, including scoliosis and Scheuermann's disease (see Posture, chapter 14). Observation of the client with thoracic-spine-related pain includes general observation of their presentation in the waiting room, presentation in the clinic, their posture in natural sitting and standing positions, and their presentation with correction for normal posture. Clients with a forward head, for example, demonstrated increased thoracic kyphosis and limited cervical rotation and flexion.[38]

Clients with upper crossed syndrome (tight pectorals and suboccipital muscles with weak antagonists) will present with forward head and bilaterally rounded shoulders. Increased tensile load stresses on the antagonists of these muscle groups (scapula retractors and deep neck flexors, respectively) as well as on the joints involved can lead to dysfunctions in the upper cervical spine and cervicothoracic junction, although many people have this posture without pain or dysfunction.

The clinician can assess the client's trunk and thoracic posture with general observation from anterior, posterior, and side views. With the anterior and posterior views, the clinician is determining if there are any side-to-side, or frontal plane, asymmetries. The side view is to assess for sagittal plane dysfunction, such as excessive kyphosis.

A more detailed observation can include an open-hand palpation of the client's thoracic spine (figure 18.6) assessing for postural curvature, symmetry of the rib cage from side to side and cranial to caudal, as well as skin and soft-tissue mobility. The clinician can also have client sit in an upright,

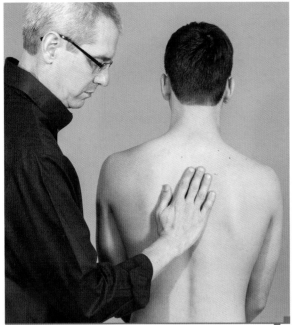

Figure 18.6 Palpation assessment of thoracic posture.

normal posture position to assess for differences in the previously mentioned characteristics in the normal position versus client's natural position.

The clinician should be especially cognizant of how the client presents with movement, looking for pain posturing or compensations with transfer activities, gait, and so on. The client with painful thoracic extension, for example, will likely sit in a slouched or stooped manner to avoid pain. These clients will also likely have pain with overhead reaching since thoracic extension and side bending are needed for this activity.[39] Pain with rotation of the thoracic spine (rib cage) will be noted with activities such as reaching for objects in the back seat of the car and turning over in bed.

Clients with rib dysfunction, or costochondritis, can have pain with normal, nonlabored breathing that worsens when breathing is labored. Additionally, since gait requires the trunk to rotate slightly in the transverse plane (see Gait, chapter 13), the more irritable or involved client may have pain with this activity.

As with examination of other areas of the body, the clinician should be cognizant of potential correlations to other impairments. For example, subjects with hyperkyphotic postures demonstrated higher depression scores and less hamstring flexibility than clients with normal thoracic posture.[40]

TRIAGE AND SCREENING

Triage and screening is a necessary component of the examination process that should be done prior to continuing with the examination. Ruling out serious pathology (refer to chapter 6, Triage and Differential Diagnosis) and pain generation from other related (or close-proximity) structures helps the clinician more accurately determine the necessity of continuing with the other examination components to identify the actual source of the client's pain. Additionally, implementing strong screening tests (tests of high SN and low –LR) at this point in the examination is suggested for narrowing down the competing diagnoses of the respective body region (cervical and lumbar spine in this case) when this is applicable.

Ruling Out Serious Pathology: Red Flags

Triage and screening for the thoracic spine should rule out the cervical and lumbar spines as potential pain generators, as well as the potential for fractures and for other nonmusculoskeletal contributors to the client's pain. Since pain in the thoracic spine and rib cage area has the potential for visceral (and other nonmusculoskeletal) contributors, the clinician is referred to chapter 6 as well.

Vertebral Compression Fracture

One of the more serious musculoskeletal related pathologies of the thoracic spine is vertebral compression fractures. While these should always be suspected in cases of trauma to the thoracic spine, other variables are worthy of consideration (e.g., age, loss of body height, thoracic localized pain) with the strongest predictors of fracture being sudden occurrence of pain (odds ratio = 3.3) and height loss >6 cm (odds ratio = 3.1).[8] Study consisted of 410 postmenopausal women with osteoporosis, mean age 74.3 ± 5.5 years, and used spine radiography as a reference standard.[8]

Two other separate studies have investigated predictor variables for vertebral compression fracture.[41, 42]

Study 1

- Female sex
- Age> 70 years
- Significant trauma

- Prolonged use of corticosteroids
  - SN 88, SP 50, +LR 1.8, −LR 0.24 when 1 of 4 variables present
  - SN 38, **SP 100, +LR 218**, −LR 0.62, QUADAS 9 when 3 of 4 variables present in a study of 1,172 clients with acute LBP (mean age 44 ± 15.1 years, 546 women), reference standard not reported (NR)[41]

Study 2

- Age > 52 years
- No presence of leg pain
- Body mass index ≤ 22

- Does not exercise regularly
- Female gender
  - SN 95 (83-99), SP 34 (33-34), +LR 1.4, −LR 0.16 when 1 of 5 variables present
  - SN 37 (24-51), **SP 96 (3.7-14.9), +LR 9.6**, −LR 0.65, QUADAS 9 when 4 of 5 variables present in a retrospective study of 38 clients with fracture (mean age 66.9 ± 10.9 years, 34 women) and 1,410 without compression fracture or wedge deformity, but spinal pain (mean age 54.9 ± 16 years, 827 women), using a reference standard of standard radiography or CT scan[42]

CLOSED-FIST PERCUSSION SIGN

Client Position	Standing or sitting (as shown) facing a mirror so that the clinician can gauge their reaction
Clinician Position	Standing behind the client
Movement	Clinician uses a firm, closed-fist percussion along the entire length of the client's spine.
Assessment	A (+) test is when the client complains of a sharp, sudden fracture pain.
Statistics	SN 88 (75-95), SP 90 (73-98), +LR 8.8, −LR 0.14, QUADAS 10, in a study of 83 consecutive clients with a suspected symptomatic osteoporotic vertebral compression fracture (mean age 78.4 years, 75 women, acute onset of back pain of varying duration), using MRI as a reference standard[43]

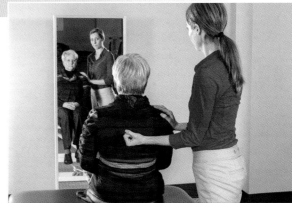

Figure 18.7

SUPINE SIGN

Client Position	Lying supine, bilateral arms and legs relaxed with only one pillow under head
Clinician Position	Standing to the side to observe client's response
Assessment	A (+) test is when the client is unable to lie supine due to severe pain in their spine.
Statistics	SN 81 (67-91), SP 93 (83-99), +LR 11.6, −LR 0.20, QUADAS 10, in a study of 83 consecutive clients with a suspected symptomatic osteoporotic vertebral compression fracture (mean age 78.4 years, 75 women, acute onset of back pain of varying duration), using MRI as a reference standard[43]

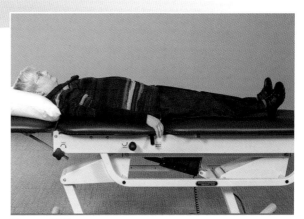

Figure 18.8

WALL TO OCCIPUT DISTANCE

The client stands against a vertical surface, heels and buttocks touching the surface. With the client's head facing forward in Frankfurt plane (head positioned so that the inferior orbital ridge is in the same horizontal plane with the notch above the tragus of the ear), the clinician uses a tape measure to quantify the distance between the occiput and the wall to the closest 0.5 cm, then repeats the drill and takes the average of three measurements. A study of 280 women referred for assessment of osteoporosis (mean age 54.5 years, 75 women, symptom duration NR), using radiography as a reference standard, found the following results.[44]

- 0 cm distance from wall: **SN 100 (95-100)**, SP 0 (0-3)
- 4.1–6.0 cm distance from wall: SN 41 (31-52), **SP 92 (87-95), +LR 5.1**, –LR 0.64
- >6.0 cm distance from wall: SN 28 (20-39), **SP 96 (92-98), +LR 7**, –LR 0.30, QUADAS 10

KYPHOSIS ANGLE

The client stands with head facing forward in Frankfurt plane (head positioned so that the inferior orbital ridge is in the same horizontal plane with the notch above the tragus of the ear). The clinician positions a handheld digital inclinometer over T12 and zeroes it, then moves it to T4 and records the angle between the two positions. The clinician repeats the drill and takes the average of three measures. A study of 280 women referred for assessment of osteoporosis (mean age 54.5 years, 75 women, symptom duration NR), using radiography as a reference standard, found the following results.[44]

- 0° to 20°: **SN 100 (95-100)**, SP 0 (0-3)
- 21° to 30°: **SN 89 (81-94)**, SP 23 (18-31), +LR 1.3, **–LR 0.5**
- 31° to 40°: SN 67 (57-76), SP 75 (69-81), +LR 2.7, –LR 0.31
- >40°: SN 31 (22-41), **SP 93 (88-96), +LR 4.4**, –LR 0.74, QUADAS 10

Critical Clinical Pearls

Clinicians must remember the following when performing the preceding described ruling-out measures for vertebral compression fracture:

- As always, tests and measures such as these are performed when there is suspicion of a fracture in the first place.
- These tests and measures are not necessarily performed as a standard measure for ruling out the thoracic spine as a potential pain generator when there is little suspicion of the presence of vertebral compression fracture (in such cases, ROM with or without overpressure are suggested).
- With the closed-fist percussion test, the clinician should start with lighter pressure.
- The clinician may be able to gather from the subjective history whether or not the supine sign would be positive (e.g., they cannot lie supine at home).

Ruling Out Pain Generation From Other Related Structures: Cervical and Lumbar Spines

The cervical and lumbar spines can be pain generators for the thoracic spine. The upper quarter screen will determine cervical spine ROM and the potential for the cervical spine as a pain generator to the client's complaints of thoracic pain. The lower quarter screen (described in chapter 7, Orthopedic Screening and Nervous System Examination) will determine lumbar spine ROM and the potential for the lumbar spine as a pain generator. Additional considerations for these sections of the spine are presented in the following sections.

Rule Out Cervical Spine

The upper quarter screen involving ROM with or without overpressure to the cervical spine will assist the clinician with ruling out the cervical spine. Specifically relevant to the cervical spine is discogenic-related pathology. To help rule out this pathology, clinicians can use a combination of Spurling's test and the upper limb neurodynamic test (median nerve bias).

- Spurling's test: **SN 93 (77-99), SP 95 (76-100), +LR 19.6, −LR 0.07**, QUADAS 9[45]
- Median nerve upper limb neurodynamic test: **SN 97 (90-100)**, SP 22 (12-33), +LR 1.3, **−LR 0.12**, QUADAS 10[46]

Rule Out Lumbar Spine

The lower quarter screen involving ROM with or without overpressure to the lumbar spine will assist the clinician with ruling out the lumbar spine. The following section lists suggested special tests the clinician can use to rule out the lumbar spine as a potential pain generator for the client with presentation of hip pain. The details of each of these tests can be found in chapter 7. Radiculopathy or discogenic-related pathology is ruled out with a combination of ROM and special tests assessments.

Repeated Motions (Range of Motion)

- Centralization or peripheralization: 5 to 20 reps
  - **SN 92 (NR)**, SP 64 (NR), +LR 2.6, **−LR 0.12**, QUADAS 12[47]
  - SN 40 (28-54), **SP 94 (73-99), +LR 6.7**, QUADAS 13[48]

Special Tests

- Straight leg raise test
  - **SN 97 (NR)**, SP 57 (NR), +LR 2.2, **−LR 0.05**, QUADAS 10[49]
  - Pooled analysis: **SN 92 (87-95)**, SP 28 (18-40), +LR 2.9, **−LR 0.29;**[50] **SN 91 (82-94)**, SP 26 (16-38), +LR 2.7, **−LR 0.35**[51]
- Slump test
  - **SN 83 (NR)**, SP 55 (NR), +LR 1.8, **−LR 0.32**, QUADAS 11[52]
  - SN 84 (NR), SP 83 (NR), +LR 4.9, −LR 0.19, QUADAS 7[53]

Facet joint dysfunction is ruled out with the seated extension–rotation test. As noted in chapter 19 (Lumbar Spine), facet joint dysfunction is ruled in with posterior–anterior spinal joint play assessments eliciting stiffness and concordant pain.

Seated Extension and Rotation

- **SN 100 (NR)**, SP 22 (NR), +LR 1.3, **−LR 0.0**, QUADAS 11[54]
- **SN 100 (NR)**, SP 12 (NR), +LR 1.1, **−LR 0.0**, QUADAS 10[55]

Additionally, as with any joint, clearing AROM with or without overpressure is necessary. AROM of all motions as per the lower quarter screen described in chapter 7 should be implemented. In order to fully clear the lumbar and cervical spines (in this case), full AROM (with overpressure if pain-free) must be present.

Sensitive Tests: Thoracic Spine

Sensitive tests of the thoracic spine consist of two tests already listed: closed-fist percussion test and supine sign. See the previous sections for details. Another SN test for scoliosis includes the following:

Adam's Forward Bending or Flexion Test

- Thoracic curves: **SN 92 (85-100)**, SP 60 (47-74), +LR 2.3, **−LR 0.13**
- Lumbar curves: SN 73 (60-86), SP 68 (57-80), +LR 2.3, −LR 0.40, QUADAS 9[56]

Additionally, as with any joint, clearing AROM with or without overpressure is necessary. In order to fully clear the thoracic spine, full AROM (with overpressure if pain-free) must be present. Detail in this regard is described in the following section.

MOTION TESTS

Gravina and colleagues demonstrated a strong correlation between radiological and goniometer evaluation of thoracic kyphosis and lumbar lordosis.[57] Therefore, this showed that measurements of ROM are reliable and also confirmed the clinical utility of goniometer assessment for the quantification of thoracic kyphosis and lumbar lordosis. The positions, ROM normal values, and end-feels for the thoracic spine are listed in table 18.2.

Passive and Active ROMs

Refer to chapter 19 (Lumbar Spine) for specific goniometric ROM measurements of the lumbar and thoracic spine. The following sections provide general tests of thoracic spine ROM and mobility that the clinician can additionally use to assess movement and potential for pain provocation of thoracic spine. Moreover, clinicians can use these movements to screen for potential thoracic spine contribution to clients' pain when assessing cervical and thoracic spines, as well as the shoulder joint.

TABLE 18.2 Thoracic Spine Arthrology

Joint	Close-packed position	Resting position	Capsular pattern	ROM norms	End-feel
Intervertebral joint	Not a synovial joint		Greater limitation of extension, side bending, and rotation than of forward bending	Flexion: 60° Extension: 25° Side bending: 25° Left side bending: 25° Rotation: 30° for the thoracic and lumbar spine	Firm for side bending and rotation and as tissue stretch for extension and flexion
Zygapophyseal (facet) joint	Full extension	Midway between flexion and extension			

GENERAL ACTIVE ROM TESTING OF THE TRUNK AND THORACIC SPINE

EXTENSION ACTIVE ROM TESTING

Client Position	In long-sitting to produce counter curve locking of the lumbar spine (eliminating movement from the lumbar spine); grasping opposite elbows in overhead position
Clinician Position	Standing directly behind or to the side of the client to assess movement
Movement	The clinician asks the client to bring their elbows posterior without extending at the shoulders or moving their arms off of the head. Verbal cueing may be required to ensure this extension movement is performed at the thoracic spine.
Assessment	The clinician assesses for areas of the spine that do not extend or that remain in kyphosis. They can apply overpressure at end ROM to discern presence (or lack) of concordant pain.
Note	This particular technique is not suggested for the client with shoulder pathology. The client with shoulder girdle pathology can cross arms across chest, but the clinician should monitor for excessive shoulder girdle motion/compensation (e.g., shoulder girdle elevation).

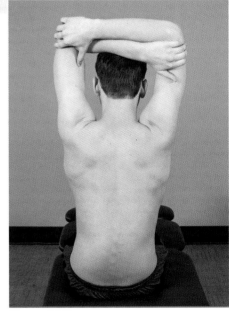

Figure 18.9

FLEXION ACTIVE ROM TESTING

Client Position	Standing
Clinician Position	Standing directly behind or to the side of the client to assess movement
Movement	The clinician asks the client to flex their spine one segment at a time from cranial to caudal as if they were curling around a horizontal round cylinder. Verbal cueing may be required to help the client perform this properly.
Assessment	The clinician monitors for areas of compensation or areas that are skipped during this movement. Movement should be symmetrical as the client flexes segmentally. The clinician can apply overpressure at end ROM to discern presence (or lack) of concordant pain.

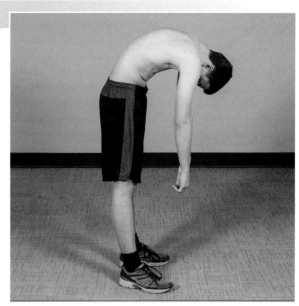

Figure 18.10

ROTATION ACTIVE ROM TESTING

Client Position	In long-sitting to produce counter curve locking of the lumbar spine (eliminating movement from the lumbar spine); interlacing hands behind their head
Clinician Position	Standing directly behind or to the side of the client to assess movement
Movement	The clinician asks the client to rotate in each direction (right rotation being shown), leading the movement with their chest versus rotating their shoulders only.
Assessment	The clinician assesses for areas of the spine demonstrating asymmetrical movement, specifically a lack of a symmetrical or gradually rounded curve of the thoracic spine. They can apply overpressure at end ROM to discern presence (or lack) of concordant pain.
Note	This particular technique is not suggested for the client with shoulder pathology. Clients with shoulder pathology can cross arms across chest, but the clinician should monitor for shoulder girdle motion compensation (e.g., scapular protraction/retraction) versus trunk rotation in these clients.

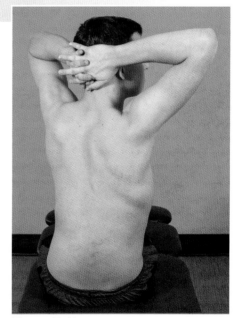

Figure 18.11

SIDE BENDING ACTIVE ROM TESTING

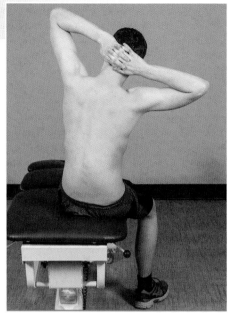

Client Position	In long-sitting with leg of the side to be assessed off the table and the foot on the floor; interlacing fingers behind their head
Clinician Position	Standing directly behind or to the side of the client to assess movement
Movement	The clinician asks the client to perform side bending to the side with the leg on the floor (right side being shown), leading with their shoulder blade to avoid side bending of the head.
Assessment	The clinician assesses for areas of asymmetrical movement, such as a lack of symmetrical curving of the spine. They can apply overpressure at end ROM to discern presence (or lack) of concordant pain.
Note	This particular technique is not suggested for the client with shoulder pathology. The client with shoulder pathology again can cross arms across chest, but monitor for shoulder girdle compensation (e.g., scapular depression and elevation).

Figure 18.12

GENERAL PASSIVE ROM TESTING OF THE TRUNK AND THORACIC SPINE

FLEXION PASSIVE ROM TESTING

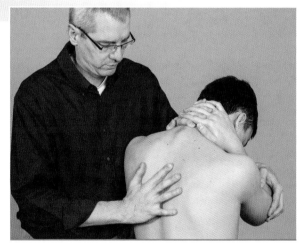

Client Position	Sitting with legs on floor and hands clasped behind head as shown. Long-sitting can be utilized if the clinician notices that the client moves excessively.
Clinician Position	Standing to the side of the client
Movement	The clinician stabilizes the distal thoracic or upper lumbar spine with one hand (right being shown) placed just distal to the segment of the thoracic spine to be assessed (upper thoracic being demonstrated) and grasps the client's arms (covering both the client's elbows) with the other hand (left hand in this example). The clinician then passively flexes the client's thoracic spine or upper trunk to end range flexion. To assess the middle and lower thoracic spine in this example, the clinician would move their right hand distal to the section of the thoracic spine to be assessed.
Assessment	The clinician assesses for asymmetrical or abnormal movement and pain provocation.

Figure 18.13

EXTENSION PASSIVE ROM TESTING

Client Position Sitting with legs on floor and hands clasped behind head as shown. Long-sitting can be utilized if the clinician notices that client moves excessively.

Clinician Position Standing to the side of the client

Movement The clinician stabilizes the distal thoracic or upper lumbar spine with one hand (right being shown) placed just distal to the segment of the thoracic spine to be assessed (upper thoracic being demonstrated) and grasps the client's arms under both elbows with other hand (left hand being shown). The clinician then passively extends client's thoracic spine or upper trunk to end range extension. As with flexion described previously, to assess the middle and lower thoracic spine in this example, the clinician would move their stabilizing right hand distal to the section of the thoracic spine to be assessed.

Assessment The clinician assesses for asymmetrical or abnormal movement and pain provocation.

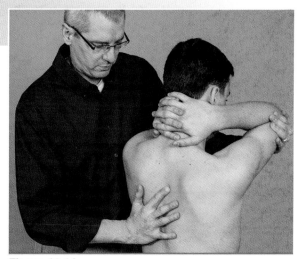

Figure 18.14

SIDE BENDING PASSIVE ROM TESTING

Client Position Sitting with legs on floor and hands clasped behind head as shown. Long-sitting can be utilized if the clinician notices that the client moves excessively.

Clinician Position Standing to the side of the client

Movement The clinician stabilizes the distal thoracic or upper lumbar spine with one hand and puts their other arm (left arm being shown) under the client's elbow closest to them and then grasps the client's opposite shoulder with other hand. The clinician then passively side bends the client's thoracic spine or upper trunk away from them (right side bending as shown) to end range side bending. The clinician would then need to go to the client's other side (standing on client's right side) and perform the same movement to be able to assess side bending in both directions. As described with both flexion and extension previously, to assess the middle and lower thoracic spine in this example, the clinician would move their right hand distal to the section of the thoracic spine to be assessed.

Assessment The clinician assesses for asymmetrical or abnormal movement and pain provocation.

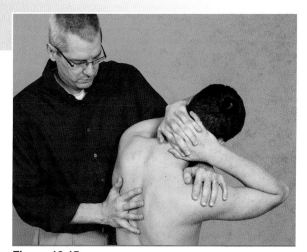

Figure 18.15

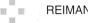
ROTATION PASSIVE ROM TESTING

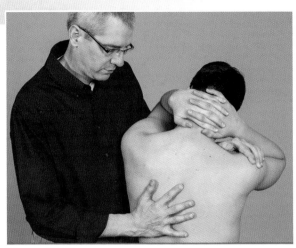

Figure 18.16

Client Position	Sitting with legs on floor and hands clasped behind head as shown. Long-sitting can be utilized if the clinician notices that the client moves excessively.
Clinician Position	Standing to the side of the client
Movement	The clinician stabilizes the distal thoracic or upper lumbar spine with one hand (clinician's right hand being shown) and places their other arm (left arm being shown) under the client's elbow closest to them and (crossing the client's chest) grasps the client's opposite shoulder (right shoulder in this example) with their hand. The clinician then passively rotates the client's thoracic spine or upper trunk away or toward them (shown in this example) to end range rotation. The clinician would then need to perform the movement in the opposite direction of rotation. As described with flexion, extension, and side bending previously, to assess the middle and lower thoracic spine in this example, the clinician would move their right hand distal to the section of the thoracic spine to be assessed.
Assessment	The clinician assesses for asymmetrical or abnormal movement and pain provocation.

Passive Accessories

Passive accessory motion assessment is essential for determining the potential for joint play dysfunction in the joints being examined. The following section details distinct component assessments of passive joint mobility for the thoracic joint.

PASSIVE ACCESSORY (OR ARTICULAR) INTERVERTEBRAL MOTION (PAIVM)

THORACIC SPINE CENTRAL PA MOBILIZATION

 Video 18.17 **in the web resource shows a demonstration of this test.**

Client Position	Lying prone with head supported in table opening, or using a towel or mobilization wedge to maintain cervical spine in neutral
Clinician Position	Standing to the side of the client
Movement and Direction of Force	The clinician places the mobilizing hand on the involved spinout process, making purchase via the pisiform on ulnar border of their hand. They place their supporting hand over the mobilizing hand or wrist (figure 18.17). Maintaining full extension of the elbows on both arms, the clinician moves the spinout process from posterior to anterior, imparting force from clinician's body.
Assessment	Assessment is done for joint play/passive accessory motion, client response, and end-feel. Reproduction of concordant pain suggests dysfunction. Impaired joint mobility or end-feel may also suggest dysfunction if concordant pain is also reproduced.
Notes	The clinician can also use pincer grip purchase with the thumb and index finger to perform the same mobilization technique (figure 18.18). The clinician purchases the upper segment involved and mobilizes it in an up and forward direction. They should make sure their forearm is in the line of the mobilizing force. The clinician can also assess the upper thoracic spine using bilateral pisiform purchase on the respective transverse processes (figure 18.19). Mobilization force is applied in posterior–anterior (and likely inferior/caudal) direction, again assessing for joint play/passive accessory motion, client response, and end-feel.

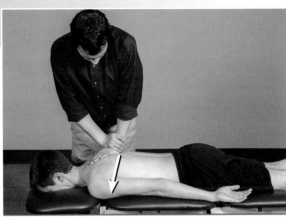

Figure 18.17

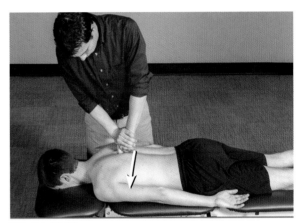

Figure 18.18

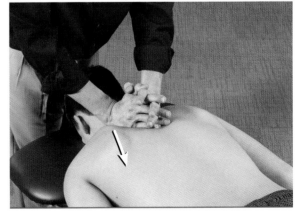

Figure 18.19

UNILATERAL PA MOBILIZATION

Client Position	Lying prone with head supported in table opening, or using towel or mobilization wedge to maintain cervical spine in neutral
Clinician Position	Standing to side of client
Movement and Direction of Force	The clinician can use a pincer grip or thumb side-to-side purchase (as shown in figure 18.20) over the involved transverse process to be mobilized. With extended elbows, the clinician imparts force and movement through their own body.
Assessment	Assessment is done for joint play/passive accessory motion, client response, and end-feel. Reproduction of concordant pain suggests dysfunction. Impaired joint mobility or end-feel may also suggest dysfunction if concordant pain is also reproduced.
Note	The clinician can also assess this region by placing purchase hand (right in example) as described: one finger (3rd digit) on the inferior or caudal transverse process and the other finger (2nd digit) on the superior or cephalad/cranial transverse process (figure 18.21). The mobilizing hand (not shown, and left hand in example) would lie flat over this hand with pisiform contact on 2nd finger and 5th metacarpal-phalangeal joint contact over 3rd finger (same as would be

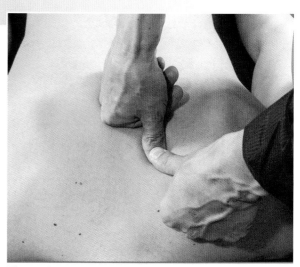

Figure 18.20

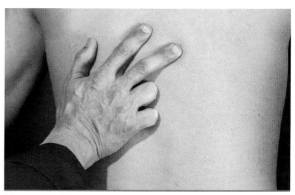

Figure 18.21

performed with a bilateral PA mobilization [the ulnar border of mobilizing hand provides anterior mobilization]). Superior vertebra will rotate to the right and inferior vertebra will rotate to the left; gapping occurs at the right facet joint of the assessed segment.

Critical Clinical Pearls

When performing PAIVM, it is important to keep the following in mind:

- The clinician should compare segments above and below the area being tested, as well as the joints on each side.
- The clinician is reminded of the low diagnostic accuracy and reliability for determination of the grading of joint mobility motion.
- Pain provocation with mobility testing is the suggested standard for determination of the potential presence of joint dysfunction.

FIRST RIB MOBILITY

CERVICAL ROTATION LATERAL FLEXION TEST (ASSOCIATED WITH BRACHIALGIA AND TOS)

 Video 18.22 **in the web resource shows a demonstration of this test.**

Client Position	Sitting with bilateral arms relaxed
Clinician Position	Standing directly behind client
Movement and Direction of Force	The clinician rotates the client's head contralaterally (right in this example) to the rib being assessed (left first rib in this example). From this rotated position, the clinician passively side bends the client's ipsilateral ear (clients left ear in this example) toward their chest.
Assessment	A (+) test is a bony restriction blocking lateral flexion.
Statistics	SN/SP NR; reliability was (κ) of 1.0 in a study of 23 clients with brachialgia and thoracic outlet syndrome, with cineradiographic examination as a reference standard.

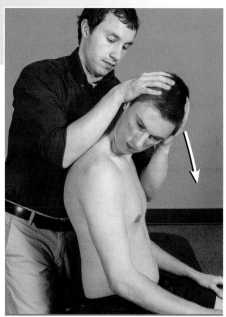

Figure 18.22

FIRST RIB SPRING TEST

Client Position	Supine with bilateral arms and head relaxed
Clinician Position	Sitting at the top of the table, directly facing the client's head
Movement and Direction of Force	The clinician passively rotates the client's head toward the side to be assessed (left in this example). They place their hand (clinician's left hand in this example) posterior to the first rib and then apply a downward force on the first rib in a caudal and ventral direction toward the client's opposite hip (right hip in this example).
Assessment	A (+) test is if the rib appears hypomobile compared to the contralateral side, or if concordant pain is reproduced.

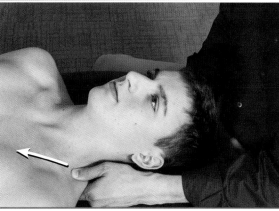

Figure 18.23

Statistics	SN/SP NR, reliability (κ) 0.35, in a study of 61 clients with nonspecific neck pain (age range 20-71 years, 46 women, mean duration of symptoms NR) and with comparison among two clinicians, each with more than 25 years of experience.[58]

Flexibility

Refer to chapter 17 (Cervical Spine), chapter 19 (Lumbar Spine), and chapter 21 (Shoulder) for details on flexibility assessments relevant to the thoracic spine.

MUSCLE PERFORMANCE TESTING

Refer to chapter 19 (Lumbar Spine) for details on muscle performance testing of the thoracic spine.

SPECIAL TESTS

As mentioned in chapter 10 (Special Tests), in many cases the clinician is overly dependent on the performance and interpretation of special test findings with respect to differential diagnosis of the client's presenting pain. Utilization of special tests for ruling in (or helping to diagnose) a particular pathology should occur at this point in the examination process. It is also hoped that the clinician has a much clearer picture of the client's presentation prior to this point in the examination and will therefore depend minimally on special test findings with respect to diagnosis of the client's pain.

Clinical special tests employed for the thoracic spine are poorly investigated. One of the more common pathologies in the thoracic spine, thoracic outlet syndrome (TOS), utilizes clinical special tests with limited diagnostic accuracy. Thoracic outlet syndrome testing is traditionally based on assessment of pain reproduction and distal arm pulse changes. Since only 5% to 10% of reported TOS cases are vascular related,[59-62] pulse changes as a positive response may not be appropriate.

Index of Special Tests

Thoracic Compression Fracture

Predictor Variables	Supine Sign	Kyphosis Angle
Closed-Fist Percussion Sign	Wall to Occiput Distance	

Scoliosis

Adam's Forward Bending or Flexion Test

Thoracic Outlet Syndrome

Adson's Test	Hyperabduction Test	Roos Test
Costoclavicular Test	Wright Test	Supraclavicular Pressure Test

First Rib Restriction

Cervical Rotation Lateral Flexion Test
First Rib Spring Test

Thoracic Spine General Mobility

Structural versus Flexible Kyphosis Test

Disc Pathology and Neural Tension

Slump Test (refer to chapter 7, Orthopedic Screening and Nervous System Examination)

Case Studies

Go to www.HumanKinetics.com/OrthopedicClinicalExamination and complete these case studies for chapter 18:

- Case study 1 discusses a 13-year-old female with mid- and upper-thoracic spine pain.
- Case study 2 discusses a 73-year-old female with mid-thoracic spine pain.

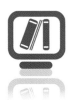

Abstract Links

Go to www.HumanKinetics.com/OrthopedicClinicalExamination to access abstract links on these issues:

Adams forward bending/flexion test	First rib spring test
Adson's test	Kyphosis angle
Cervical rotation lateral flexion test	Roos test
Closed-fist percussion sign	Vertical compression fracture

THORACIC COMPRESSION FRACTURE

Please refer to the Triage and Screening section for details on all of these tests.

SCOLIOSIS

ADAM'S FORWARD BENDING OR FLEXION TEST

Client Position	Standing with legs shoulder-width apart, equal weight on both legs, and arms relaxed at side
Clinician Position	Standing either directly in front of or behind the client (as shown)
Movement	The client bends slowly forward and reaches their hands toward the floor.
Assessment	A (+) test is asymmetry of the trunk, specifically a rib hump on one side.
Statistics	• Thoracic curves: **SN 92 (85-100)**, SP 60 (47-74), +LR 2.3, **–LR 0.13**, QUADAS 9, in a study of 105 consecutive clients referred for adolescent idiopathic or congenital scoliosis (87 girls, mean age 15.5 ± 4.8 years, mean duration symptoms NR), using the Cobb angle as a reference standard[56]

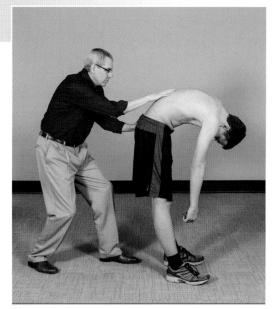

Figure 18.24

- Lumbar curves: SN 73 (60-86), SP 68 (57-80), +LR 2.3, –LR 0.40, QUADAS 9, in a study of 105 consecutive clients referred for adolescent idiopathic or congenital scoliosis (87 girls, mean age 15.5 ± 4.8 years, mean duration symptoms NR), using Cobb angle as a reference standard[56]
- SN 87 (NR), SP 93 (NR), +LR, –LR, QUADAS 5 in a study of 2,700 clients from the island of Samos, Greece (ages 8-16 years, other demographic data NR), using Cobb angle as a reference standard[63]

THORACIC OUTLET SYNDROME

ADSON'S TEST

 Video 18.25 in the web resource shows a demonstration of this test.

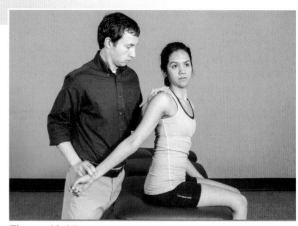

Figure 18.25

Client Position	Sitting, bilateral arms relaxed
Clinician Position	Standing directly behind the client's arm to be assessed
Movement	The clinician assesses the client's pulse for pulse rate and strength. The clinician then has the client rotate their head to the side to be assessed, tuck the chin, and extend the head slightly. The clinician externally rotates and extends the client's arm, while the client inhales and holds their breath for 10 seconds as the clinician monitors the radial pulse.
Assessment	A (+) test occurs with reproduction of symptoms and change in radial pulse. This test is thought to implicate the scalene muscles as the symptom generator.
Statistics	• SN not tested (NT), SP 89 (NR) for vascular changes and paresthesia; 100 for pain, QUADAS 9, in a study of 53 asymptomatic clients (mean age 29.7 ± 6.4 years, 27 women, mean duration symptoms NR), with symptom reproduction as a reference standard[64]
	• SN 50 (NR), SP NR, QUADAS 5, in a study of 16 clients with nonspecific TOS (mean age, gender, and duration of symptoms NR), with Doppler duplex imaging as a reference standard[65]
	• SN 79 (NR), SP 76 (NR), +LR 3.3, –LR 0.27, QUADAS 8 (pulse abolition), in a study of 48 clients (mean age 36 years for 26 women and 43 years for 5 men for those with TOS, 42 years for 13 women and 39 years for 4 men without TOS, symptom duration NR), with medical history, clinical examination, or angiography as a reference standard[66]

COSTOCLAVICULAR TEST

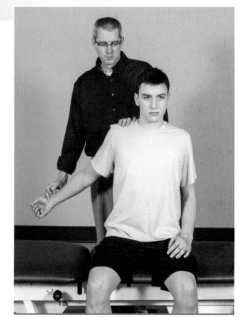

Figure 18.26

Client Position	Sitting, bilateral arms relaxed
Clinician Position	Standing directly behind the client, to the side of the arm to be assessed
Movement	The clinician palpates the client's radial pulse at rest. Once a pulse strength and rate have been determined in resting position, the clinician passively externally rotates and extends the client's arm, drawing it down and back. The clinician instructs the client to inhale and hold their breath for 10 seconds as the clinician assesses pulse strength and rate.
Assessment	Test is (+) with reproduction of symptoms and disappearance of radial pulse. Clients with symptoms suggestive of TOS while wearing backpacks or a heavy coat should be assessed with this test. This test is thought to implicate the costoclavicular space as the symptom generator.
Statistics	SN not tested (NT), SP 89 (NR) for vascular changes and paresthesia; 100 for pain, QUADAS 9, in a study of 53 asymptomatic clients (mean age 29.7 ± 6.4 years, 27 women, mean duration symptoms NR), with symptom reproduction as a reference standard[64]

HYPERABDUCTION TEST

Client Position	Sitting, bilateral arms relaxed
Clinician Position	Standing directly behind the client to the side to be assessed
Movement	The clinician assesses the client's radial pulse in resting position. The clinician places the client's arm to be assessed in full elevation and external rotation, and then holds it there for 1 minute, monitoring the client's radial pulse in the hyperabducted position.
Assessment	A test is (+) with reproduction of symptoms and disappearance of radial pulse.

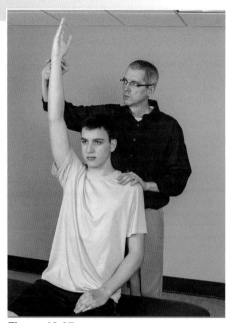

Figure 18.27

Statistics
- SN NT, SP 64 (NR) for paresthesia and 79 for pain, QUADAS 9, in a study of 53 asymptomatic clients (mean age 29.7 ± 6.4 years, 27 women, mean duration of symptoms NR), using symptom reproduction as a reference standard[64]
- SN 52 (NR), SP 90 (NR), +LR 5.2, –LR 0.53, QUADAS 8 (pulse abolition), in a study of 48 clients (mean age 36 years for 26 women and 43 years for 5 men for those with TOS, 42 years for 13 women and 39 years for 4 men without TOS, symptom duration NR), using medical history, clinical examination, or angiography as a reference standard[66]
- SN 84 (NR), SP 40 (NR), +LR 1.4, –LR 0.4 (symptom reproduction)[66]

WRIGHT TEST

Client Position	Sitting, bilateral arms relaxed
Clinician Position	Standing directly behind the client to the side to be assessed
Movement	The clinician assesses the client's radial pulse in resting position. The clinician turns the client's head to the unaffected side and places the arm to be assessed in full elevation and external rotation. The clinician holds the arm in the hyperabducted position for 1 minute, monitoring the radial pulse.
Assessment	A test is (+) with reproduction of symptoms and disappearance of radial pulse.
Statistics	• SN 70 (NR), SP 53 (NR), +LR 1.5, –LR 0.56, QUADAS 8 (pulse abolition), in a study of 48 clients (mean age 36 years for 26 women and 43 years for 5 men with TOS, 42 years for 13 women and 39 years for 4 men without TOS, symptom duration NR), using medical history, clinical examination, or angiography as a reference standard[66]
	• SN 90 (NR), SP 29 (NR), +LR 1.3, –LR 0.34, QUADAS 8 (pulse abolition)[66]

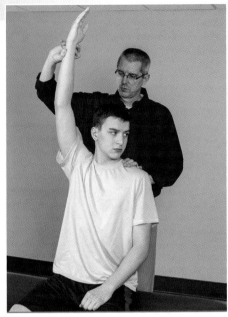

Figure 18.28

ROOS TEST

Client Position	Sitting, bilateral arms relaxed
Clinician Position	Standing, monitoring client
Movement	The clinician instructs the client to abduct both arms to 90°, with elbows bent to 90°, then to slowly open and close their hands for up to 3 minutes while maintaining this position.
Assessment	A (+) test is if the client's arms feel heavy, or if client complains of ischemia pain, paresthesia, or reproduction of other symptoms.
Statistics	• SN 84 (NR), SP 30 (NR), +LR 5.2, –LR 0.53, QUADAS 8, in a study of 48 clients (mean age 36 years for 26 women and 43 years for 5 men for those with TOS, 42 years for 13 women and 39 years for 4 men without TOS, symptom duration NR), using medical history, clinical examination, or angiography as a reference standard[66]

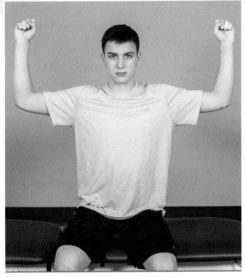

Figure 18.29

• SN 82 (NR), SP 100 (NR), +LR Inf, –LR 0.18, QUADAS 5, in a study of 41 clients symptomatic for brachial plexus compression (mean age 41 years) and 16 control clients, using surgery as a reference standard[67]

SUPRACLAVICULAR PRESSURE TEST

Client Position	Sitting, bilateral arms relaxed
Clinician Position	Standing directly facing client; placing their fingers on the client's upper trapezius and their thumbs on the lowest portion of anterior scalene near the first ribs
Movement	Clinician squeezes their thumbs and fingers together for 30 seconds.
Assessment	A test is (+) with reproduction of symptoms and disappearance of radial pulse.
Statistics	SN NT, SP 79 (NR) for vascular changes, 85 for paresthesia, 98 for pain, QUADAS 9, in a study of 53 asymptomatic clients (mean age 29.7 ± 6.4 years, 27 women, mean duration symptoms NR), using symptom reproduction as a reference standard[64]

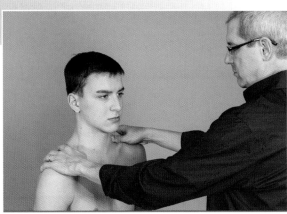

Figure 18.30

Critical Clinical Pearls

When performing TOS testing, keep the following in mind:

- The majority of TOS is neurogenic versus vascular.
- One of the suggested primary findings of this type of testing is the reduction in pulse, a vascular finding.
- TOS testing is likely to create diffuse symptoms when positive.
- The diagnosis of TOS has been suggested anecdotally by some as a diagnosis of exclusion.

FIRST RIB RESTRICTION

Please refer to the Motion Tests (Passive Accessories) section for details on all of these tests.

THORACIC SPINE GENERAL MOBILITY

STRUCTURAL VERSUS FLEXIBLE KYPHOSIS TEST

Client Position	Prone with bilateral hands on forehead
Clinician Position	Standing at the client's head, directly facing client
Movement	A belt is placed around the thoracic apex of kyphosis. The client actively lifts the trunk, or is passively lifted (as shown) into extension.
Assessment	Not being able to extend the thoracic spine (either actively or passively) suggests that the kyphosis is structural.
Statistics	NR

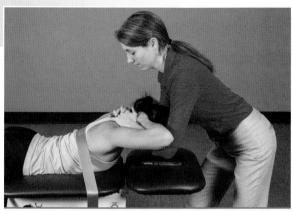

Figure 18.31

DISC PATHOLOGY AND NEURAL TENSION

Please refer to chapter 7 (Orthopedic Screening and Nervous System Examination) for the details of the slump test.

PALPATION

Refer to chapter 17 (Cervical Spine) for specific landmarks relevant to the thoracic spine. Palpate along the thoracic spine and rib cage for postural curvature, symmetry, and general mobility of the skin and soft tissue. Palpation of the thoracic spine spinous processes is similar to the process in the cervical and lumbar spine. Palpation of the transverse processes is similar to the process in the lumbar spine.

PALPATION OF RIB ANGLE

Client Position	Sitting, bilateral arms relaxed
Clinician Position	Standing next to the client, on the opposite side of the one to be assessed
Movement	The clinician reaches across the anterior portion of the client's body and grasps their posterior shoulder girdle on the side away from them (left as shown). Using this hand (left as shown), the clinician protracts the client's shoulder girdle to expose rib angles of rib cage. The clinician palpates along rib angles from cranial to caudal, feeling for symmetry, tenderness, and general mobility with breathing. Tenderness and asymmetry may be indicative of rib dysfunction.

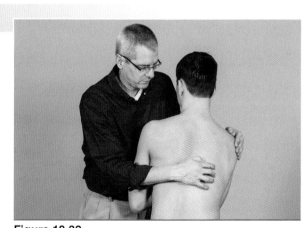

Figure 18.32

RIB CAGE POSTERIOR PALPATION

Client Position	Prone
Clinical Position	Standing to the side of client
Movement	The clinician assesses the symmetry of the paired ribs just lateral to the costochondral junction. The clinician should also have the client perform repeated normal inspiration and expiration and should assess for range and quality of movement below their fingertips. The clinician should make note of any increase or decrease in the intercostal space.

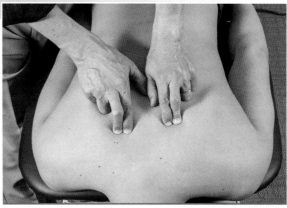

Figure 18.33

PHYSICAL PERFORMANCE MEASURES

Refer to chapters 17 (Cervical Spine) and 19 (Lumbar Spine) for appropriate physical performance measures.

COMMON ORTHOPEDIC CONDITIONS OF THE THORACIC SPINE

While it is impossible to distinctly describe various pathological presentations of the thoracic spine, there are evidence-based findings supportive of particular pathologies of this region of the body. Therefore, the intent of this section of the chapter is to present current evidence-supported findings suggestive of thoracic spine pathologies. As previously described in chapter 4 (Evidence-Based Practice and Client Examination), though, not all examination findings are absolutely supported with clinical evidence, and the clinician should also rely on clinical experience and input from the client when performing differential diagnosis of a client's presentation of pain and dysfunction.

The thoracic spine likely has the least common prevalence of pathology compared to the more commonly described pathologies of the cervical and lumbar spine. The clinician should however be cognizant of the potential for these pathologies in isolation or in combination with pathologies of the cervical and lumbar spine and shoulder predominantly.

Vertebral Compression Fracture

ICD-9: 733.13 (pathological fracture of vertebra)

ICD-10: M48.50 (collapsed vertebra)

A vertebral compression fracture is a collapse of a vertebra due to trauma or pathological decreased bone density of a vertebra. The decreased bone density can be due to osteoporosis, osteogenesis imperfecta, lytic lesions from tumors, or infection. Otherwise healthy people can also sustain this type of fracture due to excessive compressive loads on the spine. The anterior portion of the vertebral body is the most susceptible to this type of fracture due to the trabecular bone content in this area. These fractures have a characteristic wedge shape deformity, where there is a greater loss of vertebral body height anteriorly than posteriorly.

I. Client Interview

Subjective History

- Reported mechanisms of onset include falls, lifting even light objects, bending, jogging, and previous history of trauma.[6, 7]

- Pain was more intense, but of shorter duration; more often it occurred suddenly and persisted during the night.[8]

- Reported risk factors: history of fracture, history of osteoporosis, decreased height, physical activity.[6]

  - Reported risk factors for men: cigarette smoking, consumption of alcoholic beverages, previous history of trauma, tuberculosis, peptic ulcers.[6]

- Reported risk factors for women: late menarche, early menopause, increase in age, low consumption of cheese and yogurt, low physical activity.[6, 7]

- Most likely in elderly women and in clients with trauma.

- Two- to threefold increased risk in American women over 60 years of age.[6]

- Osteoporosis and vertebral compression fractures are prevalent in men aged 60-74 years; the majority of deformities were present in people without osteoporosis.[68]

- Male osteoporosis is reported to be markedly underdiagnosed.[68]

- Clients with at least one vertebral fracture have a four- to fivefold increase in the risk of having additional vertebral fractures, as well as a threefold increase in the risk of hip fracture.[9]

Outcome Measures

- Visual Analogue Scale, Oswestry Disability Index

- Any appropriate outcome measure that is clinically relevant

Diagnostic Imaging

- Little data support using plain film radiographs to diagnose thoracolumbar spine fractures, although this has remained the radiologic gold standard by default.[69]

- Most blunt trauma clients require CT to screen for other injuries. This has allowed the single admitting series of CT scans to also include screening for bony spine injuries.[69]

- A combination of both clinical examination and CT screening based on mechanism will likely be required to ensure adequate SN with an acceptable SP for the diagnosis of clinically significant injuries of the thoracolumbar spine.[70]

- Spinous process fractures one level above the osteoporotic compression fracture are infrequent (4% of cases), but they do occur.[71]

- CT has good ability to help **rule out** (SN 81) and **rule in** (SP 87) moderate vertebral fracture, but ideal ability to help **rule out** (SN 96) and **rule in** (SN 92) severe vertebral fractures.[29]

- DEXA has good to ideal ability to help **rule out** (SN 70-98) and an ideal ability to **rule in** (SP 98-99) vertebral fracture.[30, 31]

- Scoliosis: Chest radiographs have ideal ability to help **rule out** (SN 94) thoracic curves and ideal ability to **rule in** thoracolumbar (SP 97), lumbar (SP 99), and double major curves (SP 98).[32]

II. Observation

- Monitor for excessive kyphosis, particularly at 1-2 segments.

- See Triage and Screening section that follows.

III. Triage and Screening

- Rule out any potential visceral involvement (see chapter 6).

- All nonmusculoskeletal causes, as well as causes from related joints, should be ruled out.

- Assessment of thoracolumbar spine deformity, tenderness to palpation, and neurological deficits does little to rule out (SN 48) thoracolumbar spine fractures. Positive results on these assessments had good ability to help **rule in** (SP 85) thoracolumbar spine fractures.[70]

- Measurement of wall-to-occiput distance: If 0 cm, it has ideal ability to help **rule out** (SN 100) vertebral compression fracture, and if between 4.1 and 6.0 cm, it has good ability to help **rule in** (SP 93) vertebral compression fracture.[44]

- Kyphosis angle of 21° to 30° between wall and occiput has good ability to help **rule out** (SN 89) compression fracture.[44]

- Presence of only one variable has less than good ability to help rule out (SN 88, −LR 0.24) vertebral fracture, while presence of three or four variables has less than good ability to help rule in (SP 100, +LR 1.8) vertebral fracture.[41]

- Presence of only two variables present has good ability to help **rule out** (SN 95, −LR 0.16) vertebral fracture, while presence of four or five variables has good ability to help **rule in** (SP 96, +LR 9.6) vertebral fracture.[42]

- Closed-fist percussion sign has good ability to help **rule out** (SN 88, −LR 0.14) and ideal ability to help **rule in** (SP 90, +LR 8.8) vertebral fracture.[43]

- Supine sign has good ability to help **rule out** (SN 81, −LR 0.20) and ideal ability to help **rule in** (SP 93, +LR 11.6) vertebral fracture.[43]

- Assessment of thoracolumbar spine deformity, tenderness to palpation, and neurological deficits does little to rule out (SN 48) thoracolumbar spine fractures. Positive results on these assessments were helpful for **ruling in** (SP 85) thoracolumbar spine fractures.[70]

IV. Motion Tests

- Pain worsened by flexion of spine.[8]

- Moderate decrease in trunk ROM due to pain.

V. Muscle Performance Testing

- Muscle performance deficits probable due to pain and limitations.

VI. Special Tests

- See Triage and Screening section.

VII. Palpation

- In adults (mean age 63 years), the peak location for vertebral fractures were at T7-T8 and T12-L1. In pediatric clients (mean age 7.7 years), the peak location for vertebral fractures were T6-T7 and L1-L2.[72]

VIII. Physical Performance Measures

- Most likely, these are not appropriate at early stages of rehabilitation.

POTENTIAL TREATMENT-BASED CLASSIFICATIONS

- Pain control (most likely), exercise and conditioning, and possibly mobility may be appropriate.

Costochondritis

ICD-9: 733.6

ICD-10: M94 (chondrocostal junction syndrome [Tietze])

Costochondritis, also known as chest wall pain, costosternal syndrome, or costosternal chondrodynia is a benign and often temporary inflammation of the costal cartilage, which connects each rib to the sternum at the costosternal joint, and is a common cause of chest pain. Though costochondritis is often self-limited, it can be a recurring condition that can appear to have few or no signs of onset. Typically, refraining from physical activity will assist with preventing the onset of an attack. Costochondritis symptoms can be similar to the chest pain associated with a heart attack. Unexplained chest pain is considered a medical emergency until potentially life-threatening cardiac issues can be ruled out. Costochondritis is differentiated from Tietze syndrome by the finding of swelling of the costal cartilages (Tietze syndrome). The causes of Tietze syndrome are not well understood, but like costochondritis, the syndrome is thought to result from a physical strain.

I. Client Interview

Subjective History

- Prevalence rate of 30% in those clients complaining of chest pain[5]

- More common in women than men[5, 12, 13]

- More common in Hispanics[5]

- Thought to be self-limiting condition of unknown etiology that typically presents with pain around the second to fifth costochondral joints[4]

- Symptoms usually resolved by 1 year but can reoccur[5]

- Pain is typically unilateral and often intermittent[5]

- Role of inflammation has been suggested by a raised erythrocyte sedimentation rate and morning stiffness[5]

- Little evidence suggesting infection etiology[4]

Outcome Measures

- Patient-Specific Functional Scale[73]
- Any appropriate outcome measure that is relevant

Diagnostic Imaging

- Imaging is appropriate for ruling out fracture or stress fracture.

II. Observation

- Client may demonstrate pain posturing, avoidance of trunk rotation, and deep breathing when irritable.[5, 13, 73]

III. Triage and Screening

- Rule out any potential visceral involvement (see chapter 6).
- All nonmusculoskeletal causes, as well as causes from related joints, should be ruled out.
- Assessment of thoracolumbar spine deformity, tenderness to palpation, and neurological deficits does little to rule out (SN 48) thoracolumbar spine fractures. Positive results on these assessments had good ability to help **rule in** (SP 85) thoracolumbar spine fractures.[70]
- Measurement of wall-to-occiput distance: If 0 cm, it has ideal ability to help **rule out** (SN 100) vertebral compression fracture, and if between 4.1 and 6.0 cm, it has good ability to help **rule in** (SP 93) vertebral compression fracture.[44]
- Kyphosis angle of 21° to 30° between wall and occiput has good ability to help **rule out** (SN 89) compression fracture.[44]
- Presence of only one variable has less than good ability to help rule out (SN 88, −LR 0.24) vertebral fracture, while presence of three or four variables has less than good ability to help rule in (SP 100, +LR 1.8) vertebral fracture.[41]
- Presence of only two variables has good ability to help **rule out** (SN 95, −LR 0.16) vertebral fracture, while presence of four or five variables has good ability to help **rule in** (SP 96, +LR 9.6) vertebral fracture.[42]

- Closed-fist percussion sign has good ability to help **rule out** (SN 88, −LR 0.14) and ideal ability to help **rule in** (SP 90, +LR 8.8) vertebral fracture.[43]
- Supine sign has good ability to help **rule out** (SN 81, −LR 0.20) and ideal ability to help **rule in** (SP 93, +LR 11.6) vertebral fracture.[43]
- Assessment of thoracolumbar spine deformity, tenderness to palpation, and neurological deficits does little to rule out (SN 48) thoracolumbar spine fractures. Positive results on these assessments were helpful for **ruling in** (SP 85) thoracolumbar spine fractures.[70]

IV. Motion Tests

- Thoracic spine or rib cage mobility and ROM can be limited and painful.[13, 73]
- Clinicians should assess joint mobility of thoracic spine, first rib mobility, costovertebral, costosternal, and sternoclavicular joints.[13, 74, 75]

V. Muscle Performance Testing

- Muscle testing of associated thoracic spine and rib cage musculature can be limited and painful.[13, 73]

VI. Special Tests

- Cervical rotation lateral flexion test has been suggested to examine for influence of first rib elevation in brachialgia or TOS.[15]

VII. Palpation

- Clinicians should look for associated anterior chest wall tenderness that is localized to the costochondral junction of one or more ribs without notable swelling, heat, and erythema, which are indicative of Tietze syndrome.[76]

VIII. Physical Performance Measures

- Any appropriate physical performance measure (PPM)

POTENTIAL TREATMENT-BASED CLASSIFICATIONS

- Pain control (most likely), exercise and conditioning, and possibly mobility may be appropriate.

Posture Abnormality

ICD-9: 732.0 (juvenile osteochondrosis of spine)

ICD-10: M42.0 (juvenile osteochondrosis of spine)

Posture abnormality is a broad term for various forms of postural dysfunctions, including poor posture, scoliosis, and Scheuermann's disease primarily. Poor posture, often termed *upper crossed syndrome*, is a common postural dysfunction where the client demonstrates a forward head and bilaterally rounded shoulders. Scheuermann's disease is a self-limiting skeletal disorder of childhood. It is also known as Scheuermann's kyphosis, Calvé disease, and juvenile osteochondrosis of the spine. Scheuermann's disease describes a condition where the vertebrae grow unevenly with respect to the sagittal plane. This uneven growth results in the signature wedging shape of the vertebrae, causing the characteristic kyphosis. Scoliosis is specifically discussed in a subsequent section.

I. Client Interview

Subjective History

- Most commonly affects teenagers

Outcome Measures

- Any appropriate outcome measure

Diagnostic Imaging

- Imaging is typically utilized to rule out other pathologies

II. Observation

- Forward head posture and thoracic kyphosis are associated with reduced cervical ROM, specifically general cervical rotation and flexion.[38]

- Excessive lordotic curve in lumbar spine and excessive kyphotic curve in thoracic spine.

- Male clients with this condition often have broad, barrel chests.

- Clients have decreased height due to excessive thoracic kyphosis.

III. Triage and Screening

- Rule out any potential visceral involvement (see chapter 6).

- All nonmusculoskeletal causes, as well as causes from related joints, should be ruled out.

- Assessment of thoracolumbar spine deformity, tenderness to palpation, and neurological deficits does little to rule out (SN 48) thoracolumbar spine fractures. Positive results on these assessments had good ability to help **rule in** (SP 85) thoracolumbar spine fractures.[70]

- Measurement of wall-to-occiput distance: If 0 cm, it has ideal ability to help **rule out** (SN 100) vertebral compression fracture, and if between 4.1 and 6.0 cm, it has good ability to help **rule in** (SP 93) vertebral compression fracture.[44]

- Kyphosis angle of 21° to 30° between wall and occiput has good ability to help **rule out** (SN 89) compression fracture.[44]

- Presence of only one variable has less than good ability to help rule out (SN 88, −LR 0.24) vertebral fracture, while presence of three or four variables has less than good ability to help rule in (SP 100, +LR 1.8) vertebral fracture.[41]

- Presence of only two variables has good ability to help **rule out** (SN 95, −LR 0.16) vertebral fracture, while presence of four or five variables has good ability to help **rule in** (SP 96, +LR 9.6) vertebral fracture.[42]

- Closed-fist percussion sign has good ability to help **rule out** (SN 88, −LR 0.14) and ideal ability to help **rule in** (SP 90, +LR 8.8) vertebral fracture.[43]

- Supine sign has good ability to help **rule out** (SN 81, −LR 0.20) and ideal ability to help **rule in** (SP 93, +LR 11.6) vertebral fracture.[43]

- Assessment of thoracolumbar spine deformity, tenderness to palpation, and neurological deficits does little to rule out (SN 48) thoracolumbar spine fractures. Positive results on these assessments were helpful for **ruling in** (SP 85) thoracolumbar spine fractures.[70]

IV. Motion Tests

- Thoracic spine restricted mobility, most notably at the apex of the curve in thoracic spine.

V. Muscle Performance Testing

- Muscles that are in a shortened position are likely to demonstrate weakness.
- Muscles that are in a lengthened position are likely to demonstrate weakness.

VI. Special Tests

- No tests are specifically applicable for this pathology.
- Tests utilized are to rule out other pathologies described.

VII. Palpation

- Muscles that are tonically active (shortened) are likely to be tender to palpation (cervical suboccipital muscles, pectoral muscles, lower thoracic and lumbar paraspinals, and hip flexors).

VIII. Physical Performance Measures

- Any appropriate PPM may be used. Trunk endurance testing may be particularly worthy of assessment.

POTENTIAL TREATMENT-BASED CLASSIFICATIONS

- Mobility, exercise and conditioning, and pain control (less likely) may be appropriate.

Scoliosis

ICD-9: 737 (curvature of spine)

ICD-10: M41 (scoliosis)

Scoliosis is an abnormal curvature of the spine, most significantly involving the thoracic spine, and to a lesser degree, the lumbar spine. The Scoliosis Research Society has defined it as a lateral curvature of the spine greater than 10° as measured using the Cobb method on a standing radiograph.[77] Scoliosis is typically classified as either congenital, idiopathic (subclassified as infantile, juvenile, adolescent, or adult, according to when onset occurred), or neuromuscular (a secondary symptom of another condition, such as spina bifida, cerebral palsy, spinal muscular atrophy, or physical trauma). A lesser-known cause of scoliosis could be a condition called Chiari malformation.

The spine with scoliosis will have side bending in one direction and rotation in the opposite. The scoliotic spine will have a rib hump on the side opposite of the side bending or on the same side as the rotation of the vertebrae. The rib hump is due to the posterior displacement of the rib cage on that side. A single curve (thoracic scoliosis) will give the spine a *C* appearance, while a double curve (thoracic and lumbar scoliosis) will give an *S* appearance.

Curves in younger clients, as well as double curves, are more likely to progress than curves in older clients or single curves. Curves less than 30° at bone maturity are unlikely to progress, whereas curves measuring from 30° to 50° progress an average of 10° to 15° over a lifetime. Curves greater than 50° at maturity progress steadily at a rate of 1° per year.[10] The prevalence of curves greater than 30° is less than 1%.[10]

I. Client Interview

Subjective History

- Present in 2% to 4% of children between 10 and 16 years of age.[10, 11]
- Of adolescents diagnosed with scoliosis, only 10% have curve progression requiring medical intervention.[10]
- Often present with gradual, insidious onset of pain, if pain is even present. The scoliosis may be found with screening examination in school and so on.

Outcome Measures

- Scoliosis Research Society: SRS-22 questionnaire[22, 24, 28]
- Walter Reed Visual Assessment Scale (WRVAS)[21, 25, 28]
- Trunk Appearance Perception Scale (TAPS)[28]
- Any appropriate outcome measure

II. Observation

- Curves as described prior: *C* curve versus *S* curve

Diagnostic Imaging

- Weight-bearing full-spine anteroposterior, coronal and lateral, and sagittal radiographs are standard.
- Full-length standing spine radiographs are the standard method for evaluating the severity and progression of the scoliosis.

- In growing clients, serial radiographs are obtained at 3- to 12-month intervals to follow curve progression. In some instances, MRI investigation is warranted to look at the spinal cord.

- The standard method for assessing the curvature quantitatively is measurement of the Cobb angle, which is the angle between two lines drawn perpendicular to the upper end plate of the uppermost vertebra involved and the lower end plate of the lowest vertebra involved.

- Risser grading of 0 to 5 can also be assessed on the ilium. Grading is based on the degree of bony fusion of the iliac apophysis, from grade 0 (no ossification) to grade 5 (complete bony fusion).

- Risk of curve progression:[11, 78, 79]

  - Curves of 10° to 19° and Risser stage 2 to 4 (limited growth potential) are low risk.

  - Curves of 10° to 19° and Risser stage 0 to 1 (high growth potential) are moderate risk.

  - Curves of 20° to 29° and Risser stage 2 to 4 (limited growth potential) are low or moderate risk.

  - Curves of 20° to 29° and Risser stage 0 to 1 (high growth potential) are high risk.

  - Curves > 29° and Risser stage 2 to 4 (limited growth potential) are high risk.

  - Curves > 29° and Risser stage 0 to 1 (high growth potential) are very high risk.

III. Triage and Screening

- Rule out any potential visceral involvement (see chapter 6).

- All nonmusculoskeletal causes, as well as causes from related joints, should be ruled out.

- Assessment of thoracolumbar spine deformity, tenderness to palpation, and neurological deficits does little to rule out (SN 48) thoracolumbar spine fractures. Positive results on these assessments had good ability to help **rule in** (SP 85) thoracolumbar spine fractures.[70]

- Measurement of wall-to-occiput distance: If 0 cm, it has ideal ability to help **rule out** (SN 100) vertebral compression fracture, and if between 4.1 and 6.0 cm, it has good ability to help **rule in** (SP 93) vertebral compression fracture.[44]

- Kyphosis angle of 21° to 30° between wall and occiput has good ability to help **rule out** (SN 89) compression fracture.[44]

- Presence of only one variable has less than good ability to help rule out (SN 88, −LR 0.24) vertebral fracture, while presence of three or four variables has less than good ability to help rule in (SP 100, +LR 1.8) vertebral fracture.[41]

- Presence of only two variables has good ability to help **rule out** (SN 95, −LR 0.16) vertebral fracture, while presence of four or five variables has good ability to help **rule in** (SP 96, +LR 9.6) vertebral fracture.[42]

- Closed-fist percussion sign has good ability to help **rule out** (SN 88, −LR 0.14) and ideal ability to help **rule in** (SP 90, +LR 8.8) vertebral fracture.[43]

- Supine sign has good ability to help **rule out** (SN 81, −LR 0.20) and ideal ability to help **rule in** (SP 93, +LR 11.6) vertebral fracture.[43]

- Assessment of thoracolumbar spine deformity, tenderness to palpation, and neurological deficits does little to rule out (SN 48) thoracolumbar spine fractures. Positive results on these assessments were helpful for **ruling in** (SP 85) thoracolumbar spine fractures.[70]

IV. Motion Tests

- Client will likely have restricted side bending toward convexity and rotation toward concavity.

V. Muscle Performance Testing

- Client will likely have limited trunk muscle performance.

VI. Special Tests

- The use of the forward bending test alone in school screening for scoliosis is insufficient.[80]
- The forward bending test provides some assistance to help **rule out** scoliosis with an SN of 88 for a Cobb angle $\geq 20°$ and an SN of 80 for needing treatment, although caution is advised when using this tool alone as a screening procedure for scoliosis.[81]

VII. Palpation

- Paraspinal muscles on the concave side will feel taut due to the fact that they are shortened.
- Paraspinal muscles on the convex side will feel taut due to the fact that they are lengthened.

VIII. Physical Performance Measures

- Any appropriate PPM may be used.

POTENTIAL TREATMENT-BASED CLASSIFICATIONS

- Pain control (if pain dominant), exercise and conditioning, and mobility may be appropriate.

Thoracic Spine Osteoarthritis

ICD-9: 719.49 (pain in unspecified joint); 719.58 (stiffness of unspecified joint)

ICD-10: M25.5 (pain in unspecified joint); M25.6 (stiffness in unspecified joint)

Osteoarthritis of the thoracic region of the spine has characteristics similar to that of the cervical and lumbar spines. Refer to the cervical and lumbar spine chapters for additional detail.

I. Client Interview

Subjective History

- As with other spine osteoarthritis clients, sustained positions, especially weight bearing, can be particularly painful.

Outcome Measures

- Any relevant clinical measure is appropriate.

Diagnostic Imaging

- Radiographic findings include joint space narrowing, bone sclerosis, periarticular cysts, and osteophytes. Refer to chapter 6 for definition of osteoarthritis according to Kellgren and Lawrence.[82]
- Disc space narrowing and osteophytes are associated with a decreased vertebral fracture prevalence in postmenopausal women with osteoporosis.[83]

II. Observation

- Due to increased trabecular bone anteriorly and susceptibility to anterior vertebral collapse and wedging, as well as the fact that intervertebral foramen space is increased with flexion, these clients likely will have increased thoracic kyphosis.

Differential Diagnosis of Postural Abnormality Versus Scoliosis

- Scoliosis is a postural abnormality.
- Postural abnormality therefore includes various types of abnormalities.
- Structural scoliosis is an abnormality in the transverse (spine rotation toward the convex side prominence) and frontal planes (side bending toward the concave side) predominantly.
- Radiographic imaging will consistently demonstrate a structural spinal abnormality with structural scoliosis.
- Postural abnormality can be a static or dynamic (functional, position dependent, or temporary) dysfunction.

III. Triage and Screening

- Rule out any potential visceral involvement (see chapter 6).

- All nonmusculoskeletal causes, as well as causes from related joints, should be ruled out.

- Assessment of thoracolumbar spine deformity, tenderness to palpation, and neurological deficits does little to rule out (SN 48) thoracolumbar spine fractures. Positive results on these assessments had good ability to help **rule in** (SP 85) thoracolumbar spine fractures.[70]

- Measurement of wall-to-occiput distance: If 0 cm, it has ideal ability to help **rule out** (SN 100) vertebral compression fracture, and if between 4.1 to 6.0 cm, it has good ability to help **rule in** (SP 93) vertebral compression fracture.[44]

- Kyphosis angle of 21° to 30° between wall and occiput has good ability to help **rule out** (SN 89) compression fracture.[44]

- Presence of only one variable has less than good ability to help rule out (SN 88, −LR 0.24) vertebral fracture, while presence of three or four variables has less than good ability to help rule in (SP 100, +LR 1.8) vertebral fracture.[41]

- Presence of only two variables has good ability to help **rule out** (SN 95, −LR 0.16) vertebral fracture, while presence of four or five variables has good ability to help **rule in** (SP 96, +LR 9.6) vertebral fracture.[42]

- Closed-fist percussion sign has good ability to help **rule out** (SN 88, −LR 0.14) and ideal ability to help **rule in** (SP 90, +LR 8.8) vertebral fracture.[43]

- Supine sign has good ability to help **rule out** (SN 81, −LR 0.20) and ideal ability to help **rule in** (SP 93, +LR 11.6) vertebral fracture.[43]

- Assessment of thoracolumbar spine deformity, tenderness to palpation, and neurological deficits does little to rule out (SN 48) thoracolumbar spine fractures. Positive results on these assessments were helpful for **ruling in** (SP 85) thoracolumbar spine fractures.[70]

IV. Motion Tests

- Thoracic and trunk extension are limited and painful.[83]

- Limited joint mobility with PA assessment is likely.

V. Muscle Performance Testing

- Trunk muscle performance deficits are likely.

VI. Special Tests

- No tests are specifically designed for assessment of this pathology; other tests used in this (and other chapters) will help rule out potential contributing pathology.

VII. Palpation

- Clinicians should look for tenderness over the involved segments, specifically the involved joints.

VIII. Physical Performance Measures

- Any relevant PPM can be used.

POTENTIAL TREATMENT-BASED CLASSIFICATIONS

- Pain control (if pain dominant), mobility, and exercise and conditioning may be appropriate.

Thoracic Outlet Syndrome

ICD-9: 353.0 (brachial plexus lesions)

ICD-10: G54 (brachial plexus disorders)

This syndrome is characterized by a collection of signs and symptoms due to compression or irritation of the brachial plexus and subclavian vessels. There are three main types of thoracic outlet syndrome (TOS): neurogenic TOS (produced by compression of the brachial plexus, accounting for 95% of all TOS cases), arterial TOS (due to compression of the subclavian artery), and venous TOS (due to compression of the subclavian vein). Thoracic outlet syndrome is controversial with respect to characteristics, clinical presentation, and treatment.

I. Client Interview

Subjective History[14-20]

- The majority of cases are clients between the ages of 20 and 50 years; women are three or four times more likely than men to have the syndrome.

- The majority of TOS clients have vague complaints.

- The majority of TOS cases are neurogenic; only approximately 5% to 10% of all TOS cases are due to vascular causes. These vascular complaints, if present, would include pallor, weakness, and early fatigue in the arms.

- Pain and paresthesia in dermatomal distribution of nerve trunks may be present for neurogenic TOS.

- Clients may complain of loss of dexterity, muscle weakness, spasms in neck and scapular muscles, and feeling of heaviness and fatigue in the arms.

- Less than 5% of reported cases have true ischemia or atrophy.

- Clients may be intolerant to cold.

Outcome Measures

- Brief Pain Inventory and Cervical Brachial Symptom Questionnaire[84]

- Any questionnaire relevant to client

Diagnostic Imaging

- Low SN and SP of diagnostic examinations

II. Observation

- Presence of a cervical rib (rib articulating with C7) is rare (0.74%).[85]

- The presence of elongated C7 transverse processes (transverse apophysomegaly) is also rare (an overall prevalence of 2.21%).[85]

- Client may have posture with forward head and bilaterally rounded shoulders.[86]

III. Triage and Screening

- Rule out any potential visceral involvement (see chapter 6).

- All nonmusculoskeletal causes, as well as causes from related joints, should be ruled out.

- Assessment of thoracolumbar spine deformity, tenderness to palpation, and neurological deficits does little to rule out (SN 48) thoracolumbar spine fractures. Positive results on these assessments had good ability to help **rule in** (SP 85) thoracolumbar spine fractures.[70]

- Measurement of wall-to-occiput distance: If 0 cm, it has ideal ability to help **rule out** (SN 100) vertebral compression fracture, and if between 4.1 and 6.0 cm, it has good ability to help **rule in** (SP 93) vertebral compression fracture.[44]

- Kyphosis angle of 21° to 30° between wall and occiput has good ability to rule out (SN 89) compression fracture.[44]

- Presence of only one variable has less than good ability to help rule out (SN 88, −LR 0.24) vertebral fracture, while presence of three or four variables has less than good ability to help rule in (SP 100, +LR 1.8) vertebral fracture.[41]

- Presence of only two variables has good ability to help **rule out** (SN 95, −LR 0.16) vertebral fracture, while presence of four or five variables has good ability to help **rule in** (SP 96, +LR 9.6) vertebral fracture.[42]

- Closed-fist percussion sign has good ability to help **rule out** (SN 88, −LR 0.14) and ideal ability to help **rule in** (SP 90, +LR 8.8) vertebral fracture.[43]

- Supine sign has good ability to help **rule out** (SN 81, −LR 0.20) and ideal ability to help **rule in** (SP 93, +LR 11.6) vertebral fracture.[43]

- Assessment of thoracolumbar spine deformity, tenderness to palpation, and neurological deficits does little to rule out (SN 48) thoracolumbar spine fractures. Positive results on these assessments were helpful for **ruling in** (SP 85) thoracolumbar spine fractures.[70]

IV. Motion Tests

- The potential for restricted cervical spine joint and soft-tissue mobility should be assessed.
- Clients may have restricted mobility of first rib.[16, 19]
- Clients may have restricted flexibility of pectoralis major and minor, scalene muscles, and trapezius.[87]

V. Muscle Performance Testing

- Clinicians should look for weakness of rhomboids and serratus anterior muscles.[87]

VI. Special Tests

- TOS is most effectively diagnosed through diagnosis of exclusion of other more clinically supported diagnoses.
- TOS testing is marginally helpful for diagnosing or screening TOS, especially since only 5% to 10% of reported TOS cases are vascular related.[59-62]
- The supraclavicular pressure test has less than good ability to rule out (SN 98 when + test was pain) TOS.[64]
- Adson's test has a less than good ability to help rule in (SP 89 for vascular changes; SP 100 for pain) TOS.[64]
- The costoclavicular test is somewhat helpful for ruling in (SP 89 for vascular changes; SP 100 for pain) TOS.[64]
- The hyperabduction test has limited ability to help rule out or rule in TOS.
- Roos test: Diagnostic accuracy is undetermined.

VII. Palpation

- Supraclavicular tenderness[20]
- Tender to palpation pectoralis minor[86]
- Tender to palpation scalenes, first rib, potentially cervical facets[16-18]

VIII. Physical Performance Measures

- Any relevant physical performance measure can be used.
- Clinicians may want to consider closed chain kinetic test, upper extremity Y-balance test, and any overhead reaching test.

POTENTIAL TREATMENT-BASED CLASSIFICATIONS

- Pain control (if pain dominant), mobility, exercise and conditioning may be appropriate.

CONCLUSION

The thoracic spine is more stable (and hence, less mobile) than the cervical and lumbar spines. Despite this natural lack of mobility, joint dysfunction and pathology occur, and clinicians should be mindful of their presence. Clinical examination of the dysfunctional thoracic spine requires the clinician to take an effective history, to attempt to screen for serious medical pathology, and to examine the quality of motion and strength of the trunk and shoulder complex. This chapter indicates which of those exam tests have optimal SN and SP to offer clinicians the most evidence-based tests to incorporate into their examinations.

19

LUMBAR SPINE

Michael P. Reiman, PT, DPT, OCS, SCS, ATC, FAAOMPT, CSCS

Low back pain (LBP) is the most prevalent of all musculoskeletal conditions and is one of the primary reasons people visit their primary care physician. Low back pain affects nearly everyone at some time in their lives and about 4% to 33% of the population at any given point.[1] Low back pain is the most prevalent musculoskeletal dysfunction for both athletes (68% of athletes reporting LBP over past 1 year) and nonathletes (50% prevalence reporting).[2] It is the most prevalent form of musculoskeletal pain reported by adults 25 years of age and older.[3] In the vast majority of instances, LBP is either mechanical low back or leg pain (97%) or of the lumbar sprain and strain (70%) variety.[4]

Although many people experience at least one episode of LBP in their lives, in up to 85% of the clients, no specific pathology is identified.[5] Clearly delineating the pain generator in those clients with LBP can be difficult due to convergence.[6] The pain generator for clients presenting with pain in the low back and pelvis area has been variable. In fact, in 10% to 33% of these clients, the location of their pain generator was undefined. Additionally, when the pain generator could be determined in these studies, the prevalence of pain attributed to discogenic, facet, sacroiliac, and hip joint structures was quite variable.[7-11]

Recurrence of LBP is also an issue. Most people who experience activity-limiting LBP go on to have recurrent episodes. Estimates of recurrence at 1 year range from 24% to 84%.[12-14] A meta-analysis confirmed that most improvement in LBP occurs within the first 6 weeks post onset and that recovery after that time frame is much slower.[15] Therefore, while most LBP will resolve on its own, it frequently reoccurs.

CLINICALLY APPLIED ANATOMY

The lumbar spine is the largest portion of the spine. This portion of the spine consists of five lumbar vertebrae that gradually increase in size from lumbar vertebra one (L1) to lumbar vertebra five (L5). The fifth lumbar vertebra articulates with the sacroiliac joint (SIJ). The specific anatomical structures of the lumbar spine (figure 19.1)—vertebral bodies, spinous and transverse processes, and so on—are analogous to those of the cervical and thoracic spine.

Spinous processes project directly posterior and are larger than in any other portion of the spine. The transverse processes are also larger than those in the thoracic spine. Unlike the anterior and posterior tubercles in the cervical spine, the transverse processes in the lumbar spine (like those in the thoracic spine) are true transverse processes. Facet joint orientation in the lumbar spine favors sagittal plane motion predominantly in this region of the

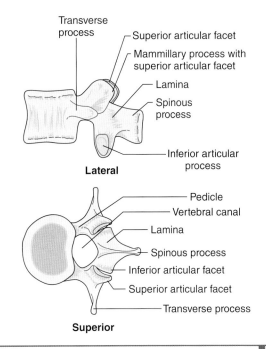

Figure 19.1 Structures of the lumbar vertebra.

spine. The facet joint orientation is 90° in the sagittal plane. Due to this facet joint orientation, rotation in this part of the spine is quite limited (figure 19.2).

The lumbar spine articulates cranially with the thoracic spine, caudally with the sacrum, and distally with the pelvic girdle. Due to the increased size of the vertebral bodies and intervertebral discs, as well as articulation with the pelvic girdle, this area of the spine is responsible for accommodating increased loads both from cranial to caudal and caudal to cranial.

The capsule around the facet joints is thickest posteriorly. It is also reinforced by the multifidus here. Anteriorly the capsule is absent, replaced by the ligamentum flavum. Flexion causes the capsule to get taut, while extension causes it to slacken.

The intervertebral disc in the lumbar spine (like that in the thoracic spine) has more distinct annulus fibrosis and nucleus pulposus. These discs have types 1 and 2 collagen, predominantly. The outer annulus has both types, but type 1 predominates. Type 1 collagen is in tissues that resist tensile forces. The nucleus also has both types, but type 2 is the primary type of collagen here. Type 2 collagen is in tissues that resist compressive forces.

The blood supply to these discs is mostly limited to the outer one-third of the annulus via small branches of the metaphyseal arteries. The remainder of nutrition to the disc is delivered through diffusion of material through the end plate (figure 19.3).

The clinician should be particularly concerned about the client who is weight-bearing sensitive. While this could include potentially several different pathologies (e.g., fracture, stress fracture, and disc pathology), one less commonly described pathology is Schmorl's node. While nutritional material can move from the vertebral body to the disc, material can also potentially move from the disc into the vertebral body. A Schmorl's node involves intrusion of the disc material into the end plate and body of the vertebrae.

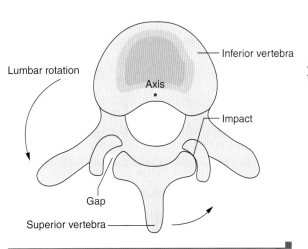

Figure 19.2 Facet joint orientation limiting rotation in the lumbar spine.

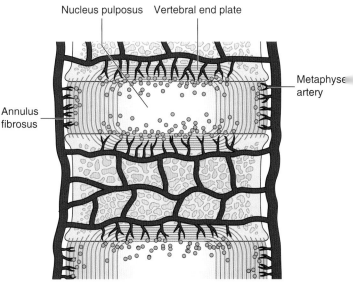

Figure 19.3 Disc nutrition.

CLIENT INTERVIEW

The interview is typically the first encounter the clinician will have with the client. As previously discussed in chapter 5 (Client Interview and Observation), this component of the examination can provide the clinician with a significant amount of information relevant to the probability of the client's presenting diagnosis. For purposes of this text, the interview is described relative to each body part or section but generally includes subjective reports by the client, as well as findings from their outcome measures. Additionally included in this section is radiographic imaging. While clinicians should avoid biasing their examination by interpreting findings of radiographic imaging prior to seeing the client (in most cases without concerns for red flags and major medical-related concerns), this point in the examination is most likely where clinicians will encounter radiographic imaging. Additionally, in some instances, radiographic imaging is necessary early in the examination for ruling out serious pathology prior to continuing with other components of the examination sequence.

Subjective

Subjective questioning for the client with LBP should be deliberate and focused. The ability to use different types of questions may also assist the client in describing the location of their pain.[16] As previously mentioned, the clinician should be cognizant of LBP coming from another source.[6-11] In light of the fact that only 10% to 15% of causes of LBP can reliably be attributed to a specific pathoanatomical finding, for the management of nonspecific LBP, the American College of Physicians (ACP) and the American Pain Society recommend that clinicians conduct a focused history and physical examination to help place clients with LBP into one of three broad categories:[17]

1. Nonspecific low back pain
2. Back pain potentially associated with radiculopathy or spinal stenosis
3. Back pain potentially associated with another specific spinal cause

Pain location for many clients with pain in the low back, pelvic girdle, or SIJ pain can vary from midline LBP to pain in the buttock, groin, and into the leg. Pain that is midline in the low back is more suggestive of disc disease.[8] Pain located along the paraspinals and relatively local to this area is more suggestive of facet joint or SIJ dysfunction, but clinicians cannot rule out discogenic sources of pain.[8] Pain referral related to facet joints (like discogenic and SIJ; see figure 19.4) can radiate into the proximal thigh, groin, or upper lumbar regions.[18-20] Pain

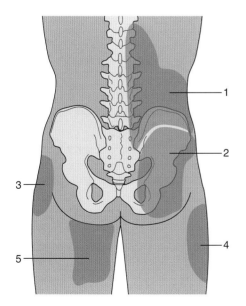 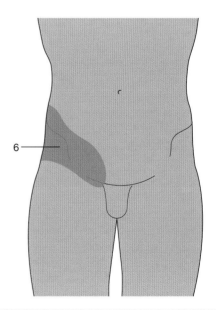

Figure 19.4 Potential referred pain pattern distributions for lumbar facet joints (in order of most to least frequent distribution): (1) lumbar spinal region, (2) gluteal region, (3) trochanter region, (4) lateral thigh region, (5) posterior thigh region, and (6) groin region.

Adapted from Fukui et al. 1997.

that radiates below the client's knee is suggestive of radiculopathy or sciatica due to a disc herniation[21, 22] and is less suggestive of facet joint dysfunction, SIJ dysfunction, or stenosis, although these conditions can present this way.[9, 20, 23]

The nature and degree of pain are important factors to investigate. Questions defining the depth and nature of the pain can assist the clinician in locating the pain-generating structure. Information to carefully consider is whether the pain is improving or not. Careful differential diagnosis should assist the clinician with determining the presence of red flags or deleterious consequences related to the client's LBP. Other questions related to red flag concerns could be as follows: Have they lost weight unexpectedly? Do they have bowel and bladder concerns that are new or that coincided with onset of back pain? Is the pain not relieved by position change or medication? Is their first onset of pain before the age of 20 or after age 55? Do they have significant other comorbidities? Red flag concerns are also discussed later in this chapter (see the section Triage and Screening), as well as in chapter 6 (Triage and Differential Diagnosis).

Description of muscle and sensory deficits would be more suggestive of neurological involvement, thereby most likely including pathologies such as stenosis, radiculopathy, and potentially instability and spondylolisthesis.[24-27] Mechanism of onset is an important variable to inquire about. If the clinician can identify a specific movement pattern or mechanism, they are more likely to be able to discern the structure from which the pain is emanating. For example, muscle strain or ligament strain injuries to the lumbar spine are frequently associated with a history of specific trauma to the involved area.[28]

Age is a variable for the clinician to consider. Intervertebral disc disease is more prevalent in younger clients,[29] while facet joint arthropathy, sacroiliac joint dysfunction, and stenosis are more prevalent as people age.[24, 29-32] Additionally, spinal malignancy is more common in adults over the age of 50.[5] Insidious onset of pain in a client under the age of 20 or over the age of 50 is a long-held concern as a red flag for nonmusculoskeletal pain.[5] Clients under the age of 20 have been thought to infrequently incur LBP, although with increasing sports participation, use of school backpacks, and so on, the clinician should be cognizant of the increased likelihood of LBP in those under the age of 20. An increase in age is associated with a higher prevalence of LBP.[33] The more severe forms of LBP increase with age, much as the prevalence of LBP does.[34] The prevalence of LBP has been shown to increase past 41 years of age, peak in the sixth decade of life, and then level off.[3]

The client's occupation is an important variable to consider in the interview. Occupational differences in the prevalence of LBP have been reported.[12] Occupations with a higher physical demand have a higher prevalence of LBP than those with lower physical demand. Sedentary occupations have a prevalence of 18.3% for those reporting LBP, while material workers have been reported to have a 39% prevalence of LBP.[35]

Prevalence of LBP does appear to be related to gender and educational status. Women tend to have a higher prevalence of LBP than men.[36-38] While both sexes should be asked about the possibility of reproductive organ involvement, inquiring women about the regularity of their menstrual cycle is important. Lower educational status is associated with increased prevalence of LBP.[33, 39]

Clients with specific lumbar dysfunctions have characteristic subjective reports. For example, clients with spinal instability will have some common characteristics. Some of these characteristics include[40-45] history of trauma, repeated, unprovoked episodes of the low back feeling unstable, inconsistent symptoms, reports of frequently self-manipulating their spine, and symptoms aggravated with sustained positions and then relieved with movement after these sustained positions. In one study, reporting of a feeling of lumbar collapse with ordinary tasks was specific (SP; SP 88) for lumbar spinal instability.[46] Pain immediately on sitting down and relieved by standing up is specific (SP 100) for lumbar spinal instability.[47]

Other pathologies will also have subjective reports specific to that particular pathology. Not having pain below the buttocks helps rule out stenosis with high sensitivity (SN) (SN 88)[24, 31] and sciatica (SN 90).[22] No pain with seated position (SP 93)[24] and symptoms being improved when seated are characteristic of stenosis (SP 83;[24] SP 86[48]). Pain with coughing or sneezing is often attributed to neurological involvement due to increases in intrathecal pressure.

The client's pain relationship to activity can also be informative. Pain first thing in the morning is often attributed to osteoarthritis, especially with movement at this time. Pain worse in the morning that is aggravated with rest and relieved with repeated motion has been attributed to mechanical-related lumbar spine pain.[49]

Risk factors for LBP are worthy of consideration. Current literature does not support a definitive cause for initial episodes of LBP. Risk factors are multifactorial and population specific and are only weakly associated with the development of LBP. However, development of recurrent pain risk factors does include the following:[50]

- History of previous episodes
- Excessive mobility in the spine
- Excessive mobility in other joints

Risk factors for the development of chronic LBP include the following:[50]

- Presence of symptoms below the knee
- Psychological distress or depression
- Fear of pain, movement, and reinjury or low expectations of recovery
- Pain of high intensity
- A passive coping style

Outcome Measures

Several outcome measures are utilized for the assessment of LBP. Validated self-report questionnaires, such as the Oswestry Disability Index (ODI) or the Roland-Morris Disability Questionnaire are useful tools for identifying a client's baseline status relative to pain, function, and disability and for monitoring a change in a client's status throughout the course of treatment. The ODI has long-standing recognition as an acceptable standard measure for capturing perceived disability in clients with LBP. Numerous studies have established its reliability, validity, and responsiveness. Originally described by Fairbank and colleagues,[51] there are also modified versions widely reported in the literature.[52, 53] This index contains 10 items: 8 related to activities of daily living and 2 related to pain. Each item is scored from 0 to 5, and the total score is expressed as a percentage, with higher scores corresponding to greater disability. Multiple studies have been undertaken to determine the error associated with the measure and the minimally important change, with the most recent international consensus conference determining that the minimally important change was 10 points (out of 100), or 30% from the baseline score.[54]

The Roland-Morris Disability Questionnaire was originally described by Roland and Morris.[55] It asks clients to gauge whether each of the 24 items

is possible to accomplish. The activities are led by the stem, "Because of my back pain," thus allowing it to be region specific. Like the ODI, the Roland-Morris Disability Questionnaire has excellent psychometrics. It is easy to administer and has been shown to be responsive in clinical trials. A minimally important change of 5 points (out of 24), or 30% from the baseline score, has been reported.[54] Baseline functional impairment (as demonstrated with the Roland Morris Index and ODI primarily) showed increasing likelihood of poor outcomes from the highest functional impairment at 3 to 6 months and at 1 year to the lowest functional impairment at 3 to 6 months and at 1 year.[56]

The assessment of biopsychosocial factors related to LBP is of particularly increasing relevance due to strong suggestions that these factors have stronger correlation with LBP, return to work after LBP, and other LBP-related variables than do biomedical variables.[57] In fact, it has been recommended that LBP examination include assessment of psychosocial risk factors.[17] Validated self-report questionnaires, such as the Modified ODI and the Roland-Morris are suggested as part of appropriate care and assessment. These measures are useful for identifying a client's baseline status relative to pain, function, and disability. Additionally, they are useful for monitoring a change in the client's status throughout the course of treatment.[50]

Diagnostic Imaging

Spinal imaging has been employed on a routine basis for clients with LBP[58-61] despite evidence-based recommendations for conducting imaging only for those clients who have severe or progressive neurologic deficits or signs or symptoms that suggest a serious or specific underlying condition (table 19.1).[17] It has even been suggested that in the absence of such features, radiographic imaging is of limited value and exposes clients to unnecessary harms.[62] Abnormal findings on lumbar spine imaging[63-69] in asymptomatic clients and on lack of correlation with function[70-72] also call into question the extent of standard practice diagnostic imaging. Therefore, routine imaging not only increases the client's exposure to radiation but also accelerates lumbar spine degeneration.[73] Table 19.2 outlines the diagnostic accuracy of various imaging modalities for the lumbar spine.

TABLE 19.1　Suggestions for Use of Imaging in Clients With Acute Low Back Pain

Clinical situation and imaging	Suggestions for initial imaging
IMMEDIATE IMAGING	
Radiography plus ESR; consider MRI if initial imaging result is negative, but high clinical suspicion for cancer remains	• Major risk factors for cancer (new onset of low back pain with history of cancer, multiple risk factors for cancer, or strong clinical suspicion for cancer)
MRI	• Risk factors for spinal infection (new onset of low back pain with fever and history of intravenous drug use or recent infection) • Risk factors for or signs of the cauda equina syndrome (new urine retention, fecal incontinence, or saddle anesthesia) • Severe neurologic deficits (progressive motor weakness or motor deficits at multiple neurologic levels)
DEFER IMAGING UNTIL AFTER THERAPY TRIAL	
Radiography with or without ESR	• Weaker risk factors for cancer (unexplained weight loss or age > 50 years) • Risk factors for or signs of ankylosing spondylitis (morning stiffness that improves with exercise, alternating buttock pain, awakening because of back pain during the second part of the night, or younger age [20 to 40 years]) • Risk factors for vertebral compression fracture (history of osteoporosis, use of corticosteroids, significant trauma, or older age [>65 years for women or >75 years for men])
MRI	• Signs and symptoms of radiculopathy (back pain with leg pain in an L4, L5, or S1 nerve root distribution or positive result on straight leg raise or crossed straight leg raise test) in clients who are candidates for surgery or epidural steroid injection • Risk factors for or symptoms of spinal stenosis (radiating leg pain, older age, or pseudoclaudication) in clients who are candidates for surgery
No imaging	• No criteria for immediate imaging and back pain improved or resolved after a 1-month trial of therapy • Previous spinal imaging with no change in clinical status

ESR = erythrocyte sedimentation rate; MRI = magnetic resonance imaging

Based on R. Chou et al., 2007, "Diagnosis and treatment of low back pain: A joint clinical practice guideline from the American College of Physicians and the American Pain Society," *Annals of Internal Medicine* 147(7): 478-491.

The use of imaging also has not improved determination of the client's need for surgery, or their long-term outcome status. Despite an increase in the number of magnetic resonance imaging (MRI) and computed tomography (CT) scans, the number of clients deemed as surgical candidates has not changed.[87] With respect to outcome status, psychosocial factors were more strongly predictive of functional disability than imaging findings were.[68] In typical clients with LBP or radiculopathy, MRI does not appear to have measurable value in terms of planning conservative care. In addition to these previously described concerns regarding diagnostic imaging is the potential psychological influence of

clients learning of their imaging findings. Modic and colleagues have suggested that MRI does not appear to have a measurable value in terms of planning conservative care. In fact, they suggested that sharing imaging findings with clients does not alter outcome; it may be counterproductive and is associated with a lesser sense of well-being in clients.[69, 88] Only when an imaging finding is concordant with the client's pain pattern or neurologic deficit can causation be considered.[68]

Although there may be an association between degenerative MRI changes and chronic LBP, strong recommendation against the routine use of MRI for clients with chronic LBP is made. Also, since there

TABLE 19.2 Diagnostic Accuracy of Various Imaging Modalities for the Lumbar Spine

Pathology	Diagnostic test	Gold standard	SN/SP
Lumbar disc herniation	MRI	Surgery	Pooled analysis: 75/77[74]
	CT		Pooled analysis: 77/74[75]
Lumbar spinal stenosis			Pooled analysis not possible[74]
	MRI	Surgery	96/67[76]
	US	Myelography or CT scan	90/96[77]
Malignant VCF	PET-CT	Biopsy or clinical follow-up	74-90/55-74 (dependent on location)[78]
	Bone scintigraphy	Vertebral biopsy or follow-up	29/93[79]
Benign VCF	PET-CT	Biopsy or clinical follow-up	100/29[78]
	MRI		64/83[78]
	DXA	Expert conventional radiography evaluation	70/98[80]
Vertebral metastasis	Bone SPECT	Clinical history and findings with other imaging techniques	91/93[81]
		Plain radiograph imaging	87/91[82]
			74/81[82]
Spondylolysis/ spondylolisthesis	MRI	MRI grading system	99.6/87[83]
Spondylolysis	Radiographs	Cadaver model	98/97[84]
Spondylarthritis	Ultrasonography	Clinical examination, pelvic radiograph, MRI of lumbar spine and sacroiliac joints, HLA-B typing	77/81[85]
Lumbar spine stress fracture	MRI	CT	99.6/87[83]
Inflammatory back pain	MRI	MRI standardized definitions from online data entry system	51/97[86]
	MRI (bone marrow edema)		67/88[86]

VCF = vertebral compression fracture; DXA = dual-energy X-ray absorptiometry; MRI = magnetic resonance imaging; CT = computed tomography; US = ultrasound; PET-CT = positron emission tomography-computed tomography; SPECT = single-photon emission computed tomography; HLA-B = human antigen leukocytes-B

The color coding for suggestion of **good** and **ideal** diagnostic accuracy values reported in this table are without quality scoring (QUADAS), a very important aspect of determination of the clinical utility of such values. Therefore, it is suggested that the reader keep this in mind when interpreting such values.

are no data evaluating the efficacy of the surgical treatment of degenerative MRI changes, a strong recommendation is made against the surgical treatment of chronic LBP based solely on degenerative MRI changes.[89]

Structural variables on both MRI and discography testing at baseline had only weak association with LBP episodes and no association with disability or future medical care.[90, 91] The strongest associations were noted for degenerative disc abnormalities, and associated LBP was found with Modic changes demonstrating a moderate association with anterolisthesis in one study.[92]

Interestingly, the development of serious LBP disability in a cohort of clients with both structural and psychosocial risk factors was strongly predicted by baseline psychosocial variables.[90] Additionally, depression was found to be a more important predictor of LBP than MRI.[93] It has been suggested that the use of advanced imaging should be reserved for those considering surgery or with suspicion of systemic disease.[30]

A final consideration for the acute LBP client is the representation of imaging findings. Findings on MRI within 12 weeks of serious LBP inception are highly unlikely to represent any new structural change. Most new changes (loss of disc signal, facet arthrosis, and end plate signal changes) represent progressive age changes not associated with acute events. Primary radicular syndromes may have new root compression findings associated with root irritation.[65]

The ACP recommendations suggest that clinicians perform diagnostic imaging and testing for clients with LBP when severe or progressive neurologic deficits are present or when serious underlying conditions are suspected on the basis of history and physical examination. Additional recommendations are listed in table 19.1.[17]

Radiographs

Plain spinal radiography in combination with standard laboratory tests is useful for identifying pathology but is not advisable for nonspecific neck or low back pain.[27] Suspicion of fracture, compression fracture (figure 19.5), and serious pathology warrant radiographic imaging in most cases.

Although 45° oblique views have long been regarded as the best projections for the detection of spondylolysis (figure 19.6), they can be insensitive. Radiography of the pars interarticularis is difficult because of the oblique orientation of the pars to all

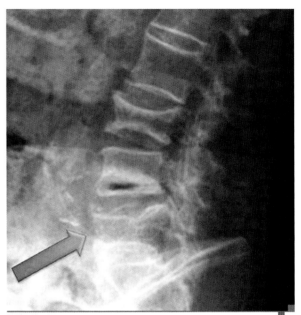

Figure 19.5 Plain lateral radiograph of an osteoporotic vertebral compression fracture.

© Michael Reiman

three orthogonal planes. Moreover, fractures are well shown only when the X-ray beam is tangential to the plane of the fracture. Therefore, a 45° oblique view demonstrates a pars defect well only if it is perpendicular to the pars.[94] In spondylolisthesis, forward displacement of the vertebra is determined on the lateral view (figure 19.7).

Magnetic Resonance Imaging

Magnetic resonance imaging is increasingly used as the primary imaging method in clients with LBP

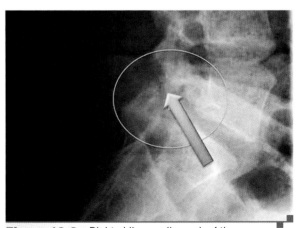

Figure 19.6 Right oblique radiograph of the lumbosacral spine shows spondylolysis of L5.

© Michael Reiman

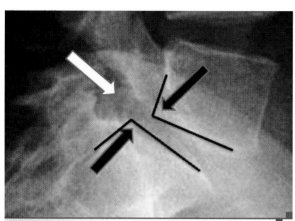

Figure 19.7 Right oblique radiograph demonstrating L5–S1spondylolisthesis (black arrows) and the wide osseous gap of the L5 pars interarticularis (white arrow).

© Michael Reiman

and radiculopathy due to its ability to delineate bone and soft tissue. Magnetic resonance imaging should be used as the primary investigation for adolescents with LBP and suspected stress reactions of the lumbar pars interarticularis. Moreover, MRI is the imaging modality of choice for identifying associated nerve root and spinal canal (figure 19.8) compression.[94]

In a systematic review, clear recommendations were given regarding the use of MRI for LBP. These recommendations stated that there was insufficient evidence to support the routine use of MRI in clients with chronic LBP. The other recommendation was that surgical treatment of chronic LBP based exclusively on MRI findings of degenerative changes was not recommended.[89] More recent findings question the accuracy of MRI findings for some pathologies. Wassenaar and colleagues suggested that a considerable proportion of clients may be classified incorrectly by MRI for herniated nucleus pulposus and spinal stenosis.[74]

Computed Tomography

Computed tomography has long been suggested to delineate fracture and show the presence of spinal stenosis or tumor. Computed tomography is the best procedure for clearly visualizing spondylolysis when a pars fracture is present, although it cannot reliably distinguish between a recent active fracture and a chronic, nonunion of a fracture.[94]

Multislice CT with multiplanar reformats is the most accurate modality for detecting the bony defect, and it may also be used for assessment of osseous healing. However, as with radiographs, it is not sensitive for detection of the early edematous stress response without a fracture line, and it exposes the client to ionizing radiation. Single-photon emission computed tomography (SPECT) use has been suggested to be limited by a high rate of false-positive and false-negative results and by considerable ionizing radiation exposure.[94] Early stress reactions can be detected with SPECT. Single-photon emission computed tomography nuclear medicine scan also differentiates active spondylolysis from inactive. It has been suggested that multiple imaging studies may have a role in the diagnosis of a pars lesion.[95]

Radionuclide Imaging: Bone Scan

Bone scan is often advocated for the detection of active bone disease and areas of high bone turnover. Such bone diseases might include pathologies of cancer and bone stress fracture.

Review of Systems

Refer to chapter 6 (Triage and Differential Diagnosis) for details on review of systems relevant to the lumbar spine.

OBSERVATION

Observation for the client with LBP starts with the client in the waiting room. Observing the client's

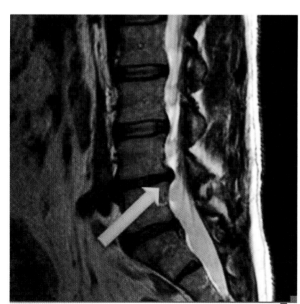

Figure 19.8 Magnetic resonance imaging demonstrating encroachment of spinal canal by intervertebral disc.

© Michael Reiman

sitting and movement posture when they are filling out paperwork and questionnaires can give the clinician a starting working hypothesis regarding diagnosis. Pain posturing may be noted with the client sitting (unequal weight distribution) and with sit-to-stand transfers. A systematic review found that multiple studies suggest that clients in acute distress, or fear-related behavior, from LBP often have a decreased willingness to move.[96] General client appearance can alert the clinician as to the extent of the pathology. Pain irritability will likely cause the client to demonstrate pain posturing. Additionally, the client may appear uncomfortable.

Although a weak correlation between sitting occupations and LBP exists,[97] the clinician should be cognizant of how the client sits, the extent of time they spend sitting during a day, and their activity while sitting. Clients sensitive to subtle changes in lumbar spine and pelvis position during sitting will likely try to compensate with pain-relieving positions that may or may not be helpful to their condition.

Sit-to-stand transfers and squatting and lifting movements should also be assessed. Despite the fact that the relationship between lifting and LBP has been found to be equivocal, the clinician should observe lifting movements to monitor for pain reproduction and compensated movement patterns.[98] Having the client demonstrate their normal movement patterns gives the clinician valuable information regarding what the client will do throughout the day. They should correct the compensated movement pattern and assess for changes in pain. Improvement in the client's pain level with the corrected movement patterns is not only helpful for the rehabilitation process, but it also educates the client on the necessity of proper, consistent movement.

Gait pattern should alert the clinician to lumbar pathology. A wide-based gait pattern presentation has a high positive likelihood ratio (+LR 13) and is therefore suggestive of spinal stenosis.[32] Clients in acute distress due to LBP are also likely to demonstrate an antalgic, slow, guarded gait pattern.

Observation of the client's posture should be performed (as with any other body area) from anterior, posterior, and both side views. Generally, the clinician is observing for asymmetrical differences from side to side or from anterior to posterior. Specific things to look for would be the amount of lumbar lordosis in the spine, iliac crest height levels, side-to-side symmetry of distance between each arm and side of trunk, the frontal, sagittal, and transverse plane orientation of the entire spine, and so on. As discussed in chapter 14 (Posture), lower crossed syndrome is a common posture presentation for clients with pain in the mid to low back, pelvis, and hip regions.

Some specific spinal positions the clinician should assess for are the amount of lordosis in the lumbar spine and the symmetry of the spine alignment in the frontal plane. Decreased lumbar lordosis, or flattened back posture appearance, can indicate an inflamed intervertebral disc, spinal stenosis, and possible facet or sacroiliac joint dysfunction. Flexion positioning decreases the compression on the posterior elements of the intervertebral disc and increases the cross-sectional area of the intervertebral foramen by 12%, while extension increases the posterior disc compression and decreases the intervertebral foramen by 15%.[99] Ipsilateral side bending and rotation also significantly decrease the intervertebral foramen.[100] Therefore, acutely inflamed discogenic clients and clients with stenosis involving the intervertebral foramen may avoid (or have pain with) ipsilateral side bending and rotation. These clients will occasionally present with a lateral shift (figure 19.9). The assessment for the

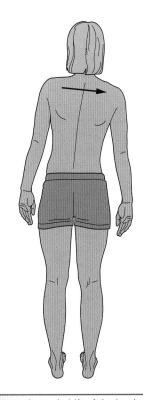

Figure 19.9 Lateral shift of the lumbar spine.

presence of a lateral shift is of particular importance in identifying and appropriately classifying clients with low back pain. The original treatment-based classification scheme proposed that clients with such a shift should be their own classification.[101] Correction of a lateral shift is generally accepted as a first step in the treatment process for a client presenting with it. Of concern though is the fact that detecting a lateral shift with observation has only moderate reliability, even when trained raters judge stable stimuli.[102]

Nerve root compression in the foramen was found to be 21.0% in neutral, 15.4% in flexion, and 33.3% in extension.[99] Thus, while the compression on the nerve root is less in flexion, the tension on the nerve root is increased. Clients with nerve root adhesions and adverse neural tension (or adverse neurodynamic movement) tend to avoid forward flexion and demonstrate poor posture. This compensated posture is to avoid increased tension on the nerve root.

Clients with radiographic instability in the lumbar spine likely will demonstrate an excessive lordotic posture, which with prolonged positioning can produce pain. These clients have been suggested to have a lack of neutral spine stability;[103, 104] therefore, they have to posture in increased lordosis (increasing compression on the facet joints) to provide stability. If these clients demonstrate such a compensated posture statically, this posture will likely worsen with dynamic movement due to the increasing demands for stabilization with movement.[103-105] The clinician should make sure to observe for any scars or skin markings on the client. Previous surgical scars should be examined

for potential pain contribution. Unusual skin markings or skin lesions may indicate the potential of underlying mesodermal and neural abnormalities.

TRIAGE AND SCREENING

Triage and screening is a necessary component of the examination process that should be done prior to continuing with the examination. Ruling out serious pathology (refer to chapter 6, Triage and Differential Diagnosis) and pain generation from other related (or close-proximity) structures helps the clinician more accurately determine the necessity of continuing with the other examination components to identify the actual source of the client's pain. Additionally, implementing strong screening tests (tests of high SN and low –LR) at this point in the examination is suggested for narrowing down the competing diagnoses of the respective body region (thoracic spine, sacroiliac joint, and hip in this case) when this is applicable.

Ruling Out Serious Pathology: Red Flags

As with examining all regions of the body, in the examination, the clinician attempts to determine if the client is presenting with serious pathology. In the large majority of clients with LBP, symptoms will be attributed to nonspecific mechanical factors. In fact, in clients presenting to a primary care provider with LBP, previously undiagnosed serious pathology prevalence was 0.9%.[106] Eighty percent of clients in primary care settings with acute LBP

Critical Clinical Pearls

When performing differential diagnosis of various lumbar spine pathologies, it is important to utilize observational findings:

- Clients presenting with lateral shift of the lumbar spine are likely shifting away from where they have symptoms. This could be due to various reasons, including
  - Nerve root compression in the foramen
  - Muscle spasm, guarding, or protection from pain
- Increased lordosis posture may suggest lumbar spine instability (or more appropriately termed lack of neuromuscular control) and/or tight hip flexors.
- A flexed lumbar spine posture may suggest spinal stenosis, especially if present in an older adult.

were found to have at least one red flag.[106] Additionally, it is suggested that individual red flags do not necessarily mean the presence of serious pathology; however, the presence of multiple red flags should raise the clinical suspicion and indication for further investigation.[106-110] Specific pathological concerns relevant to LBP include cancer,[5, 107] spinal infection,[111] cauda equina syndrome,[5, 112] spinal compression and stress fractures,[106, 108] ankylosing spondylitis,[113] and abdominal aortic aneurysm.[114] Refer to chapter 6 for details and diagnostic accuracy on specific red flag concerns relevant to LBP.

Failure to improve with conservative care can also be a sign of a serious medical condition or misdiagnosis. As a general guideline, failure of a client to demonstrate improvement in less than 30 days can be interpreted as a red flag.[115]

Cancer

The subjective history was found to be of stronger diagnostic accuracy than the physical examination when ruling in or out the presence of cancer. Additionally, the same study found that cancer could be ruled out (SN 100) if they had the following four factors present:[116]

- <50 years of age
- No previous history of cancer
- No unexplained weight loss
- Had not failed 1 month of conservative therapy

The most recent findings also suggest the presence of multiple red flag presence for ruling in cancer. The single red flag with the highest posttest probability (33%) for detection of spinal malignancy was history of malignancy.[117]

Cauda Equina Syndrome

Cauda equina syndrome (CES) is discussed in greater detail in chapter 6. CES is a medical referral. One or more of the following must be present for the diagnosis of CES:[118]

- Bladder or bowel dysfunction
- Reduced sensation in saddle area
- Sexual dysfunction
- Possible neurological deficit in the lower limb (motor or sensory loss, reflex change)

Bladder and sensory disturbances are believed to be the strongest predictors by some, especially saddle sensory deficits. Any client suspected of CES

must undergo immediate MRI to exclude this diagnosis.[118, 119] Signs and symptoms helpful for ruling out CES include the following:[120-122]

- History of back pain (**SN 94**)
- Urinary retention (**SN 90**)
- Rapid symptom onset within 24 hours (**SN 89**)
- Sacral sensation loss (**SN 85**)
- Lower extremity weakness or gait loss (**SN 84**)
- Loss of sphincter tone (**SN 80**)

Spinal Fracture

While serious pathology prevalence is quite low, spinal fracture is pathology of particular concern for the client presenting with LBP, since it was the most common serious pathology found.[106] In a systematic review of 12 studies, five clinical features were useful for raising or lowering the probability of vertebral fracture: age > 50 years (SN 79, SP 64, +LR 2.2, −LR 0.34), female gender (SN 47, SP 80, +LR 2.3, −LR 0.67), major trauma (SN 65, **SP 95**, **+LR 12.8**, −LR 0.37), pain or tenderness (SN 60, **SP 91**, **+LR 6.7**, −LR 0.44), and a distracting painful injury (SN 41, SP 75, +LR 1.7, −LR 0.78).[108]

Most recent findings suggest that older age, prolonged corticosteroid use, severe trauma, and the presence of a contusion or abrasion increased the likelihood of spinal fracture. The probability (90%) of spinal fracture was higher with multiple red flags.[117]

The status of a diagnostic prediction rule containing four features (female sex, age > 70 years, significant trauma, and prolonged use of corticosteroids) was moderately associated with the presence of fracture.[106] A study of 1,172 clients presenting to primary care physician for care of acute LBP (mean age 43.9 ± 15.1 years; 546 women; mean duration off work or school prior to consultation 1.5 days) that used radiography as a reference standard had the following statistics: The presence of 1 positive features: **SN 88** (not reported, or NR), SP 50 (NR); ≥2 positive features: SN 63 (NR), **SP 96 (NR)**; ≥3 positive features: SN 38 (NR), **SP 100 (NR)**.[106]

Another clinical prediction rule for compression fracture has also been reported. The variables included age > 52 years, no presence of leg pain, body mass index < 22, client not regularly exercising, and female gender.[123]

- ≤1 of 5 variables present: **SN 97 (89-99)**, SP 6 (6-7), +LR 1.4, **−LR 0.16**, QUADAS 8, in 1,448 consecutive clients seen at a spine surgery center (mean age range 55-67 years; 861 women; mean duration of symptoms NR), and using radiography as a reference standard.

- ≥4 of 5 variables present: SN 37 (24-51), **SP 96 (95-97)**, +LR 9.6, −LR 0.65 in the same study.

Additionally, there are clinical examination testing methods to discern the potential presence of a fracture. These tests are described next.

VERTEBRAL COMPRESSION FRACTURE

CLOSED-FIST PERCUSSION TEST

Client Position	Stands or sits (as shown) facing a mirror so that the clinician can gauge their reaction
Clinician Position	Standing directly behind the client
Movement	The clinician provides firm pressure over each level of the vertebral spine using a firm, closed-fist percussion.
Assessment	A test is considered (+) when the client complains of a sharp, sudden, fracture pain in the spine.
Statistics	**SN 88 (75-95)**, **SP 90 (73-98)**, **+LR 8.8**, **LR −0.14**, QUADAS 11, in a study of 83 clients with suspected acute osteoporotic vertebral compression fractures (mean age 78.4 years; 75 women; all had acute onset of pain of varying duration), and using MRI as a reference standard.[124]

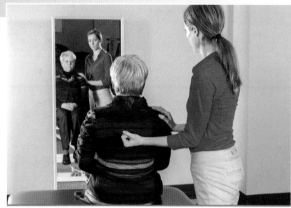

Figure 19.10

SUPINE SIGN

Client Position	Supine, legs extended, and arms relaxed; only one pillow under the head
Clinician Position	Standing directly to the side of the client
Movement	The clinician monitors and inquires of the client's response to the position.
Assessment	A test is considered (+) when the client complains of a sharp, sudden, fracture pain in the spine and is unable to lie supine.
Statistics	**SN 81 (67-91)**, **SP 93 (78-99)**, **+LR 11.6**, **−LR 0.20**, QUADAS 11, in a study of 83 clients with suspected acute osteoporotic vertebral compression fractures (mean age 78.4 years; 75 women; all had acute onset of pain of varying duration), and using MRI as a reference standard.[124]

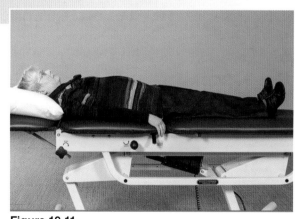

Figure 19.11

In short, clinicians should consider diagnostic classifications associated with serious medical conditions or psychosocial factors and should initiate referral to the appropriate medical practitioner in the following cases: (1) the client's clinical findings are suggestive of serious medical or psychological pathology, (2) the reported activity limitations or impairments of body function and structure are not consistent with those presented in the diagnosis or classification section of these guidelines, or (3) the client's symptoms are not resolving with interventions aimed at normalization of their impairments of body function.[50] A neurological screen should also be performed at this time, especially if the clinician suspects serious pathology or neurological involvement. Reflexes and myotome- and dermatome-level testing are recommended. Additionally, if warranted, upper motor neuron testing would be employed at this point in the examination. Refer again to chapter 7 (Orthopedic Screening and Nervous System Examination) for specific details on these tests, as well as the performance of the lower quarter screen.

Ruling Out Pain Generation From Nonorganic or Psychological Sources

These cognitive factors may manifest themselves clinically as abnormal illness behavior, defined by Waddell and colleagues[125] as "maladaptive overt illness related behavior which is out of proportion to the underlying physical disease and more readily attributable to associated cognitive and affective disturbances." Waddell and colleagues[125] have developed clinical tools that indicate the presence of abnormal illness behavior by identifying physical signs or symptom descriptions that are nonorganic in nature. Nonorganic signs and symptom descriptors (table 19.3) have been identified and recommended for use in the evaluation of clients with LBP. These signs and symptoms are believed to be more highly associated with aspects of distress and illness behavior than physical pathology in clients with chronic LBP. They offer only a psychological yellow flag and not a complete psychological assessment. These signs and symptoms have demonstrated correlation with other illness behaviors related to pain.[126] While Waddell's signs and symptoms have demonstrated clinical utility for determining pain related to nonorganic sources, they demonstrated poor predictive validity for determining clients who would not return to full-duty work within 4 weeks of initiating physical therapy in a group of acutely injured workers.[127]

An additional examination procedure that may be of benefit to the clinician trying to ascertain the presence of nonorganic LBP is the Hoover test. The client is supine with bilateral legs extended and the

TABLE 19.3   Waddell's Signs of Nonorganic Signs and Symptoms for Low Back Pain

Sign	Definition
Superficial or nonanatomic tenderness	Pain with light or superficial palpation of the skin, or widespread deep tenderness that is not localized to 1 structure, does not follow an anatomic distribution, and often extends to the thoracic spine, sacrum, or pelvis.
Overreaction	Exaggerated painful response to a stimulus that is not reproduced when the same stimulus is given later, or exaggerated response to a stimulus that should not cause back pain (e.g., gently pinching the skin on the back in the area of pain).
Nonreproducibility of pain when client is distracted	A positive physical finding is found on routine formal assessment but is not present when the client is distracted and it is checked again (e.g., pain with a standard straight leg raise test [passive flexion at the hip while the client is lying on the back with knee extended] but not when the clinician passively extends the leg while the client is sitting and plantar reflex is being checked).
Regional weakness or sensory change	Regional sensory change (stocking sensory loss or sensory loss in an entire extremity or side of the body) or regional weakness (weakness that is jerky, with intermittent resistance such as cogwheeling or catching). Organic weakness can be overpowered smoothly.
Pain on axial loading or simulated rotation	Pain with vertical pressure applied to the standing client's head, or back pain when the shoulders and pelvis are passively rotated in the same plane as the client stands relaxed with the feet together.

Adapted from Waddell et al. 1980.

clinician is at the client's feet with their hands under the client's heels. The client is asked to lift one leg off the table while keeping the knees straight. Even if the client is unable to lift the leg, the clinician should feel increased pressure under the heel of the leg not being lifted due to increased stabilizing effort from this leg in an attempt to lift the assessed leg.[128]

Ruling Out Pain Generation From Other Related Structures

The lower quarter screen (chapter 7) is a global assessment of the lower quarter that determines the potential for other areas of the body to contribute to the client's pain. If warranted, additional examination may be part of the screen on an individual basis. Suggestions of additional testing that may be warranted for ruling out other areas of the body as potential pain generators are described in the following sections.

Rule Out SIJ Dysfunction

Assistance in ruling out SIJ dysfunction can be accomplished with the use of pain provocation cluster testing:[10] **SN 91 (62-98)**, **SP 83 (68-96)**, **+LR 6.97**, **−LR 0.11**, QUADAS 13

- Thigh thrust test: **SN 88 (64-97)**, SP 69 (47-82), +LR 2.80, **−LR 0.18**, QUADAS 12[129]

- Gaenslen's test: SN 50-53, SP 71-77, +LR 1.8–2.2, −LR 0.66, QUADAS 12[129]

- Distraction test: SN 60 (36-80), SP 81 (65-91), +LR 3.20, −LR 0.49, QUADAS 12[129]

- Compression test: SN 69 (44-86), SP 69 (51-79), +LR 2.20, −LR 0.46, QUADAS 12[129]

- Sacral thrust test: SN 63 (39-82), SP 75 (58-87), +LR 2.50, −LR 0.50, QUADAS 12[129]

Laslett and colleagues assessed the diagnostic utility of the McKenzie method of mechanical assessment combined with the following sacroiliac tests: distraction, thigh thrust, Gaenslen, sacral thrust, and compression. The McKenzie assessment consisted of flexion in standing, extension in standing, right and left side gliding, flexion in lying, and extension in lying. The movements were repeated in sets of 10, and centralization and peripheralization were recorded. If it was determined that repeated movements resulted in centralization, the client was considered to present with pain of discogenic origin. If discogenic origin of pain was ruled out, the cluster of tests exhibited the following (3 out of 5 required to be positive):

- **SN 94 (72-99)**, SP 78 (61-89), +LR 4.29, **−LR 0.80**, QUADAS 12[129]

The test with the strongest diagnostic capability of ruling out SIJ-related dysfunction is the thigh thrust test:

- Thigh thrust test: **SN 88 (64-97)**, SP 69 (47-82), +LR 2.80, **−LR 0.18**, QUADAS 12[129]

- Utilization of thigh thrust test alone is likely most efficient for screening SI dysfunction

Rule Out Hip Joint

- **Hip fracture:** Ruling out hip fracture with clinical examination is best achieved with the patellar-pubic percussion test. Pooled analysis: **SN 95 (92-97)**, **SP 86 (78-92)**, **+LR 6.11**, **−LR 0.07**, across 3 studies with 782 clients.[130]

- **Hip osteoarthritis:** The gold standard clinical diagnosis for hip osteoarthritis (OA) is that clients with hip pain and hip internal rotation (IR) range of motion (ROM) $\leq 15°$ who experienced pain with IR, had morning stiffness ≤ 60 min., and were ≥ 50 years old could be identified as having hip OA (SN 86).[131]

- **Hip impingement or labral tear and potential intra-articular involvement:** Other hip-related pathologies should also be considered, dependent on client presentation. Refer to chapter 24 for more detail. It is worth mentioning here, though, the necessity to rule out the potential for hip impingement (femoroacetabular impingement) and labral tear. The flexion-adduction-internal rotation (FADDIR) test has been described for both pathologies. The diagnostic accuracy of this test in a recent meta-analysis is as follows:

Flexion-Adduction-Internal Rotation (FADDIR) Test

- Pooled **SN 94 (88-97)**, SP 8 (2-20), +LR 1.02, **−LR 0.48**, across four studies with 128 clients (MRA reference standard).[130]

- Pooled **SN 99 (95-100)**, SP 7 (0-34), +LR 1.06, **−LR 0.15**, across two studies with 157 clients (arthroscopy reference standard).[130]

Flexion-Internal Rotation Test

- Pooled analysis: **SN 96 (82-100)**, SP 17 (12-54), +LR 1.12, **−LR 0.27**, across three studies with 42 clients.[130]

Critical Clinical Pearls

Differential diagnosis of presenting pain from the lumbar spine, pelvis, and hip complex is complicated by several variables:

- Presence of at least one red flag in multiple clients without serious pathology
- The convergence of pain generated in one of these areas presenting symptoms in another area
- The interdependent biomechanical relationship between each of these areas

Additionally, as with all joints, assessment of joint motion assists in ruling out the hip as a potential pain generator. Pain-free active and passive ROM with overpressure will help the clinician rule out the hip joint as a potential contributor to the client's hip pain.

The use of fluoroscopically guided intra-articular hip injection has been suggested to differentiate pain source in clients with concomitant hip and lumbar spine arthritis. This technique demonstrated as follows: SN 100, SP 81, +LR 11.1, −LR 0.[132]

Sensitive Tests: Lumbar Spine

Ruling out particular pathologies in the lumbar spine can be complicated. Once competing pain-generating joints have been ruled out as outlined previously, clinicians should implement SN tests of the lumbar spine to narrow down the potential diagnoses. The use of special tests can be of assistance (as well as all other components of the funnel examination approach). These tests, along with their correlation with pathology, are presented here. Additionally, the diagnostic accuracy of these tests relative to the pathology investigated is also presented. Ruling out radiculopathy or discogenic pathology can be assisted with low-bias studies examining repeated motions, a search for centralization or peripheralization responses, and straight leg raise and slump testing. To assist in ruling out facet joint dysfunction, the clinician should integrate the seated extension–rotation testing. The diagnostic accuracy of each of these tests is listed in the following section.

Radiculopathy or Discogenic-Related Pathology

Centralization and Peripheralization: 5-20 reps

- **SN 92 (NR)**, SP 64 (NR), +LR 2.6, **−LR 0.12**, QUADAS 12[133]
- SN 40 (28-54), **SP 94 (73-99), +LR 6.7**, −LR 0.64 QUADAS 13[134]

Special Tests

Straight Leg Raise Test

- **SN 97 (NR)**, SP 57 (NR), +LR 2.2, **−LR 0.05**, QUADAS 10[21]
- Pooled analysis: **SN 92 (87-95)**, SP 28 (18-40), +LR 2.9, **−LR 0.29**;[135] **SN 91 (82-94)**, SP 26 (16-38), +LR 2.7, **−LR 0.35**[136]

Slump Test

- **SN 83 (NR)**, SP 55 (NR), +LR 1.8, **−LR 0.32**, QUADAS 11[137]
- SN 84 (NR), SP 83 (NR), +LR 4.9, −LR 0.19, QUADAS 7[138]

Facet Joint Dysfunction

Ruled out with the seated extension–rotation test

Seated Extension–Rotation

- **SN 100 (NR)**, SP 22 (NR), +LR 1.3, **−LR 0.0**, QUADAS 11[139]
- **SN 100 (NR)**, SP 12 (NR), +LR 1.1, **−LR 0.0**, QUADAS 10[20]

Additionally, as with any joint, clearing AROM with or without overpressure is necessary. In order to fully clear the lumbar spine, full AROM (with overpressure if pain-free) must be present. Details in this regard are described in the following section.

MOTION TESTS

Motion assessment is a very important aspect of the examination for the orthopedic client. Motion dysfunction can be used to differentiate contractile versus noncontractile tissue (see chapters 8 and 9). Assessment of end-feel, potential capsular patterns, and ROM norm values (table 19.4) can give the clinician an appreciation of the potential impairments for the orthopedic client they are assessing. Active ROM, PROM, and joint play assessments are necessary to determine not only the presence or absence of joint dysfunction but also the precise aspects of the motion that are dysfunctional.

Passive and Active ROMs

Active ROM should be assessed in all planes. If AROM is full and pain-free, overpressure can be applied at end ROM to assess response. Repeated ROM can be employed if pain is reproduced with a particular motion in order to assess client response to repeated motions, directional preference,[142] and the potential for centralization or peripheralization[133, 134] of symptoms. Additionally, the clinician should assess for changes in the lumbar and thoracic curves of the spine, presence of any deviations in motion, provocation of pain in general, location of such pain, and any compensatory movements.

Clients with excessive trunk AROM, especially with complaints of catching and giving way, should have suspicion of lumbar spinal instability. This is particularly the case if they have a high score on Beighton's generalized ligamentous laxity scale.[41-43, 45, 46]

There was a high degree of correlation ($r = 0.93$ overall) in a study comparing inclinometer measurement with radiographic measures for lumbar flexion and extension.[143] Therefore, the following techniques (whether using goniometers or inclinometers) are reliable measures. Other techniques, such as using tape measures, have also been described. Range-of-motion testing in the spine can be utilized to determine not only the amount of motion available, but also the potential that that portion of the spine is a pain generator. After checking the client's AROM, the clinician can assess AROM with overpressure and potentially PROM to determine if there is a reproduction of concordant pain with these movements.

TABLE 19.4 Lumbar Spine Arthrology

Joint	Close-packed position	Resting position	Capsular pattern[140]	ROM norms[141]	End-feel
Intervertebral joint	Not a synovial joint		Capsular pattern for the lumbar spine is a marked and equal restriction of side bending followed by restriction of flexion and extension	Flexion: 60° Extension: 25° Right side bending: 25° Left side bending: 25° Rotation: 30° for the thoracic and lumbar spine	Firm for side bending and rotation and as tissue stretch for extension and flexion
Zygapophyseal (facet) joint	Full extension	Midway between flexion and extension			

LUMBAR FLEXION AND EXTENSION

Client Position	Standing on bilateral feet, arms relaxed at side
Clinician Position	Standing directly to either side of the client
Goniometer Alignment	The fulcrum is over the lateral aspect of the greater trochanter, the proximal arm is aligned with the lateral midline of the trunk, and the distal arm is aligned with the lateral midline of the femur, using the lateral epicondyle of knee as a reference.

(continued)

Lumbar Flexion and Extension *(continued)*

Movement	The client flexes at the trunk (keeping the knees straight) to bend as far forward as they can go. If no pain is elicited, the clinician can apply overpressure at end range of motion. Lumbar extension: The client extends backward at the waist (keeping the knees straight) to extend as far backward as they can go. If no pain is elicited, the clinician can apply overpressure at end range of motion. The clinician can also assess for change in symptoms (particularly centralization and peripheralization or a directional preference on part of the client). These motions can also be assessed passively on the part of the clinician by passively moving the client in the desired direction.
Assessment	Clinician assesses for amount of ROM, end-feel, quality of the movement, client response, potential difference between AROM and PROM, and so on. Reproduction of the client's concordant pain is a (+) response, implicating the lumbar spine as a potential pain generator. If no pain is elicited with full AROM and overpressure, it helps eliminate the lumbar spine as a potential pain generator.
Note	Active range of motion should be performed prior to PROM and/or overpressure to determine the client's willingness to move.

LUMBAR ROTATION

Client Position	Sitting on table, feet off the end of the table and arms crossed over chest
Clinician Position	Standing directly to the side of the client, on the side to be assessed
Goniometer Alignment	The fulcrum is over the center of the cranial aspect of the client's head, the proximal arm is parallel to an imaginary line between the ASIS on each side, and the distal arm is aligned with an imaginary line between the two acromion processes.
Movement	The client rotates the trunk (from the waist) to their side as far as they can go. If no pain is elicited, the clinician can apply overpressure at end range of motion. The clinician can also assess for change in symptoms (particularly centralization and peripheralization or a directional preference on part of the client). These motions can also be assessed passively on the part of the clinician by passively moving the client in the desired direction.
Assessment	Clinician assesses for amount of ROM, end-feel, quality of the movement, client response, potential difference between AROM and PROM, and so on. Reproduction of the client's concordant pain is a (+) response, implicating the lumbar spine as a potential pain generator. If no pain is elicited with full AROM and overpressure, it helps eliminate the lumbar spine as a potential pain generator.
Note	Active range of motion should be performed prior to PROM and/or overpressure to determine the client's willingness to move.

LUMBAR SIDE BENDING

Client Position	Standing on bilateral feet, arms relaxed at side
Clinician Position	Standing directly to the side of the client, on the side to be assessed
Goniometer Alignment	The fulcrum is over the spinous process of S1, the proximal arm is perpendicular to the ground, and the distal arm is aligned with the posterior aspect of the spinous process of C7.
Movement	The client side bends the trunk (from the waist) to their side as far as they can go. If no pain is elicited, the clinician can apply overpressure at end range of motion. The clinician can also assess for any change in symptoms (particularly centralization and peripheralization or a directional preference on part of the client). These motions can also be assessed passively on the part of the clinician by passively moving the client in the desired direction.
Assessment	Clinician assesses for amount of ROM, end-feel, quality of the movement, client response, potential difference between AROM and PROM, and so on. Reproduction of the client's concordant

pain is a (+) response, implicating the lumbar spine as a potential pain generator. If no pain is elicited with full AROM and overpressure, it helps eliminate the lumbar spine as a potential pain generator.

Note Active range of motion should be performed prior to PROM and/or overpressure to determine the client's willingness to move.

In the cervical and lumbar spine, it may be particularly beneficial to also perform combined motions (figure 19.12). These are often referred to as quadrant positions. Therefore, if the single-plane movements were unremarkable for reproduction of the client's pain, the clinician may want to also implement these combined motions to further test these regions of the spine. Posterior quadrants

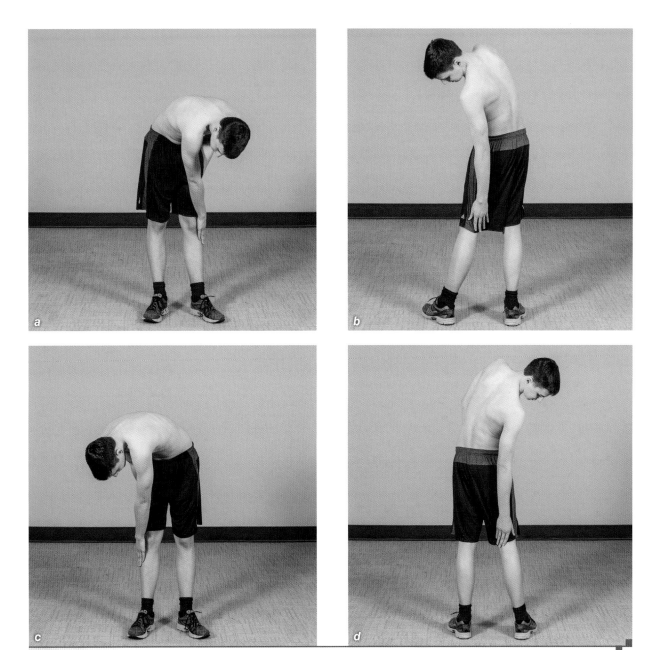

Figure 19.12 Combined motion assessment of the trunk: *(a)* flexion, left side bend, and rotation, *(b)* extension, left side bend, and rotation, *(c)* flexion, right side bend, and rotation, and *(d)* extension, right side bend, and rotation.

would involve the motions of extension, side bending, and rotation to the same side, while anterior quadrants would involve the combined active motions of flexion, side bending, and rotation to the same side. Additionally, combined with assessment of the client's ability to perform a squat, these measures provide the clinician with a nice big-picture assessment of the client's functional status, degree of irritability, willingness to move, and so on.

Passive Accessories

Passive accessory motion assessment is essential for determining the potential for joint play dysfunction in the joints being examined. The following section details distinct component assessments of both PPIVM and PAIVM motion assessments relative to the lumbar spine.

PASSIVE PHYSIOLOGICAL INTERVERTEBRAL MOTION (PPIVM)

FLEXION AND EXTENSION

Client Position	Lying on either side
Clinician Position	Standing directly in front of the client, at the level of the lumbar spine
Movement	The clinician palpates the interspace between the adjacent spinous processes of the target motion segment with one finger, while moving the lumbar spine from neutral into flexion or extension via the client's uppermost limb (right as shown). The clinician will start at the L5-S1 level and move cranially to the next segment as movement is detected at each respective level. For flexion, the clinician will move the client's hip further into hip flexion when assessing each respective

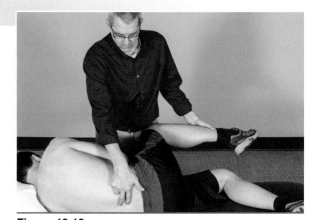

Figure 19.13

segment (from caudal to cranial). When assessing extension, the clinician will move the client's hip further into hip extension when assessing each respective level.

Assessment PPIVMs were rated on a 5-point ordinal scale, with 0 and 1 indicating hypomobility, normal anchored at 2, and 3 and 4 indicating hypermobility. Pain response can also be utilized, although its diagnostic utility is unknown.[45]

Statistics

Flexion PPIVMs
- SN 5 (1-22), **SP 99 (97-100)**, **+LR 8.7**, –LR 0.96, QUADAS 11, in a study of 138 consecutive clients with recurrent or chronic LBP (mean age 40 ± 11.2 years; gender NR; mean duration of symptoms 8.3 ± 8 years), using flexion–extension radiographs as a reference standard (to diagnose translation radiographic instability).[45]

- SN 5 (1-36), **SP 99 (97-100)**, **+LR 4.1**, –LR 0.96, QUADAS 11, in a study of 138 consecutive clients with recurrent or chronic LBP (mean age 40 ± 11.2 years; gender NR; mean duration of symptoms 8.3 ± 8 years), using flexion–extension radiographs as a reference standard (to diagnose rotation radiographic instability).[45]

Extension PPIVMs
- SN 16 (6-38), **SP 98 (94 -99)**, **+LR 7.1**, –LR 0.86, QUADAS 11, in a study of 138 consecutive clients with recurrent or chronic LBP (mean age 40 ± 11.2 years; gender NR; mean duration 8.3 ± 8 years), using flexion–extension radiographs as a reference standard (to diagnose translation radiographic instability).[45]

- SN 22 (6-55), **SP 97 (94-99)**, **+LR 8.4**, –LR 0.80, QUADAS 11, in a study of 138 consecutive clients with recurrent or chronic LBP (mean age 40 ± 11.2 years; gender not reported; mean duration 8.3 ± 8 years), using flexion–extension radiographs as a reference standard (to diagnose rotation radiographic instability).[45]

SIDE BENDING

Client Position	Side lying
Clinician Position	Standing directly in front of client at the level of the lumbar spine

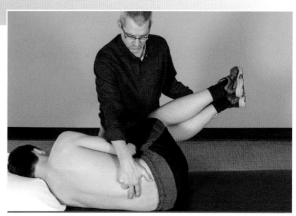

Figure 19.14

Movement	The clinician places the client's bilateral knees resting on the front of their hip and palpates the interspace between the adjacent spinous processes of the target motion segment with one finger, while moving the lumbar spine from neutral into side bending by moving both the client's legs up toward the ceiling (for top-side side bending) (right side bending as shown) or down toward the floor (for downside side bending). The clinician will start at the L5-S1 level and move cranially to the next segment as movement is detected at each respective level.
Assessment	Side bending PPIVMs can be rated on a hypomobile, normal, or hypermobility scale. Assessment is done for joint motion, client response, and end-feel. Reproduction of concordant pain suggests dysfunction. Impaired joint mobility or end-feel may also suggest dysfunction if concordant pain is also reproduced.

PASSIVE ACCESSORY (ARTICULAR) INTERVERTEBRAL MOTION (PAIVM)

POSTERIOR TO ANTERIOR GLIDES

This is useful for identifying an impaired segment.

Client Position	Prone, with bilateral arms and legs relaxed
Clinician Position	Standing directly over the client
Movement and Direction of Force	The clinician directly purchases the vertebra to be assessed. The clinician is directly over the contact area, elbow extended. Soft-tissue slack is taken up as the clinician performs a bilateral or central posterior to anterior (PA) glide to end range in order to assess joint mobility. The clinician assesses each level of the lumbar spine and lower thoracic spine. Additionally, unilateral assessments are implemented with contact over the ipsilateral facet joints of both sides respectively and the entire lumbar spine and lower thoracic spine as detailed previously.
Assessment	Assessment is done for joint play/passive accessory motion (hypomobility, normal mobility, or hypermobility in most studies below), client response, and end-feel. Reproduction of concordant pain suggests dysfunction. Impaired joint mobility or end-feel may also suggest dysfunction if concordant pain is also reproduced.

- SN 43 (27-61), **SP 95 (77-91)**, +LR 8.6, –LR 0.6, QUADAS 12, in a study of 49 clients with LBP (33.9 ± 10.9 years; 42% were female; median duration of symptoms 27 days), using flexion–extension radiographs as a reference standard (for the detection of lack of hypomobility for the diagnosis of radiographic instability).[43]

- SN 46 (30-64), SP 81 (60-92), +LR 2.4, –LR 0.7, QUADAS 12, in a study of 49 clients with LBP (33.9 ± 10.9 years; 42% were female; median duration of symptoms 27 days), using flexion–extension radiographs as a reference standard (for the detection of hypermobility for the diagnosis of radiographic instability).[43]

- SN 82 (64-92), **SP 81 (60-92, +LR 4.3**, –LR 0.22 (at least one variable [lack of hypomobility and lumbar flexion ROM > 53°] present); SN 29 (13-46), SP 98 (91-100), +LR 12.8, –LR 0.72 (both variables present).[43]

- SN 33 (12-65), SP 88 (83-92), +LR 2.8, –LR 0.8, QUADAS 11, in a study of 138 consecutive clients with recurrent or chronic LBP (mean age 40 ± 11.2 years; gender NR; mean duration 8.3 ± 8 years), using flexion–extension radiographs as a reference standard (rotational PA to diagnose radiographic instability).[45]

(continued)

Posterior to Anterior Glides *(continued)*

- SN 29 (14-50), SP 89 (83-93), +LR 2.5, –LR 0.8, QUADAS 11, in a study of 138 consecutive clients with recurrent or chronic LBP (mean age 40 ± 11.2 years; gender NR; mean duration 8.3 ± 8 years), using flexion–extension radiographs as a reference standard (transitional PA to diagnose radiographic instability).[45]

Note   There are multiple ways to perform central PA glides (CPAs) and unilateral PA glides (UPAs).

Video 19.15 **in the web resource shows a demonstration of pisiform purchase, manipulator dip purchase, and bilateral facet joint purchase.**

CPAs

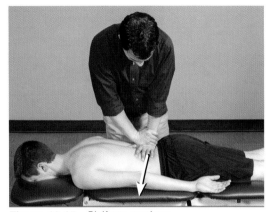

Figure 19.15   Pisiform purchase.

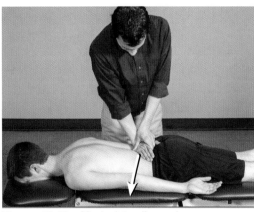

Figure 19.16   Manipulator dip purchase.

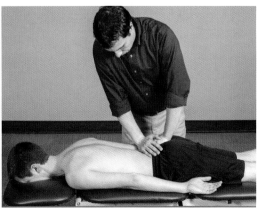

Figure 19.17   Bilateral facet joint purchase.

UPAs

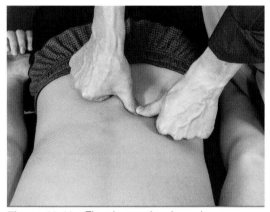

Figure 19.18   Thumb-over-thumb purchase.

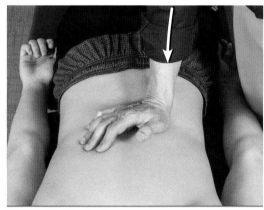

Figure 19.19   Pisiform purchase.

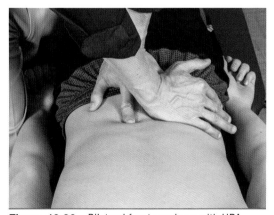

Figure 19.20   Bilateral facet purchase with UPA ipsilateral.

Critical Clinical Pearls

The clinician is reminded of the importance of the movement examination in each respective body part. In the lumbar spine, for example, motion testing has high diagnostic ability or ruling in assistance with the following tests:

- Repeated motion testing for centralization or peripheralization of symptoms (**SP 94 (73-99), +LR 6.7**)
- Posterior-to-anterior (PA) glides for the diagnosis of radiographic instability when there is a lack of hypomobility (**SP 95 (77-91), +LR 8.6**)
- Posterior-to-anterior (PA) glides for the diagnosis of radiographic instability when at least one variable (lack of hypomobility and lumbar flexion ROM > 53°) is present (**SP 81 (60-92), +LR 4.3**)

Flexibility

As detailed in chapter 8, flexibility is the motion that a particular joint is capable of. Assessment of flexibility can assist the clinician in determining the potential presence of soft-tissue dysfunction of any of the listed muscles in table 19.5.

TABLE 19.5 Muscles of the Lumbar Spine

Muscle	Origin	Insertion	Action	Innervation
LUMBAR ERECTOR SPINAE MUSCLES				
Erector spinae Iliocostalis lumborum	Iliac crest, sacrum	Lower borders of lowest seven ribs	Bilateral action: extension of trunk Unilateral action: lateral trunk flexion ipsilaterally	Dorsal rami of spinal nerves in corresponding area
Longissimus thoracis	Intermediate part of extensor aponeurosis	Lower 10 ribs and adjacent vertebral transverse processes		
Quadratus lumborum	Medial part of iliac crest	12th rib, lower lumbar vertebrae	Lateral flexion of vertebral column; fixes last rib to form stable base for contraction of diaphragm	Branches from T12 and L1-L3
Latissimus dorsi	Spinous processes of lower 6 thoracic and all lumbar and sacral vertebrae; posterior part of iliac crest	Medial lip (crest of lesser tubercle) and floor of intertubercular groove of humerus	Extension, adduction, and medial rotation of arm	Thoracodorsal nerve

LUMBAR ERECTOR SPINAE ASSESSMENT

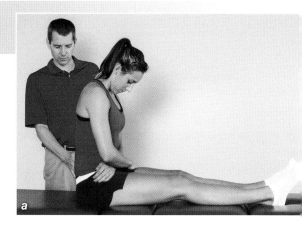

Client Position	Long-sitting on a testing surface, keeping the pelvis as vertical as possible
Clinician Position	Standing to the side of the client
Movement	The client is instructed to bend forward at the lumbopelvic region and move the forehead toward the knees *(a)*. For the second part of the assessment, the clinician should have the client sit at the end of the table with bilateral knees flexed. The client forward bends as far as possible, moving the forehead toward the knees without moving the pelvis *(b)*.
Assessment	Posterior tilting of the pelvis *(a)* is a sign of adaptive shortening of the hamstrings. In this position, an adult should achieve a distance of 10 cm or less between the forehead and knees, as well as demonstrate a smooth, even curve of the spine. If the forward bending of the trunk is greater in the second position than in the first position, this is usually the result of an increased tilt of the pelvis and adaptive shortening of the hamstrings versus adaptive shortening of the erector spinae.
Statistics	There are no known reliability data for this flexibility measure.[144]

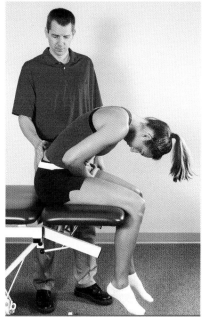

Figure 19.21

QUADRATUS LUMBORUM ASSESSMENT I

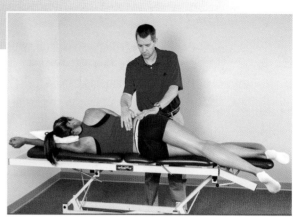

Figure 19.22

Client Position	Lying on the nontest side with the bottom leg bent slightly at the hip and knee for stability
Clinician Position	Standing in front of the client
Movement	The clinician should have the client extend the top leg beyond the edge of the table and allow the top (test) leg to drop toward the floor.
Assessment	The clinician should measure the distance from the epicondyle of the medial femoral condyle of the knee to the floor and compare it to the other side. Shortness and tightness are present if the ROM is asymmetric. The clinician should also assess for the development of tension in the quadratus lumborum, as well as for reduced caudad motion of the iliac crest being assessed.
Statistics	There are no known normative or reliability data for this flexibility measure.[145]

QUADRATUS LUMBORUM ASSESSMENT II

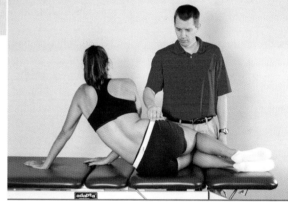

Figure 19.23

Client Position	Side-lying with the hips and knees flexed at about 45°
Clinician Position	Monitoring from behind the client. (Photo shows clinician in front of client so that view of client position is unobstructed.)
Movement	The clinician should ask the client to push up sideways from the table to a point where the pelvis begins to move. They should monitor the client to avoid trunk flexion or rotation during the assessment.
Assessment	Tightness can be less accurately assessed during lumbar side-bending to the contralateral side in standing. Normal movement would be smooth, symmetrical curving of the spine in both directions. Shortness and tightness are present if the ROM is asymmetric.
Statistics	There are no known reliability data for this flexibility measure.[144, 145]

LATISSIMUS DORSI ASSESSMENT

Client Position	Sitting in a neutral spine position, arms resting at the side
Clinician Position	Standing behind the client
Movement	The clinician should instruct the client to rotate the trunk to the left *(a)* and then to the right. They should note the quantity and quality of the motion through the thoracic and lumbar spine. The clinician will next instruct the client to flex the upper extremities to 90°, then fully externally rotate and adduct the client's shoulders and approximate the hypothenar eminences of bilateral upper extremities. The clinician should instruct the client to rotate the trunk to the left *(b)* and to the right. Again, they will observe the quantity and quality of the motion through the thoracic and lumbar spine.
Assessment	The clinician will compare the quantity and quality of the client's motion with the arms at the side in bilateral directions, as well as with the arms elevated, externally rotated, and adducted. Comparisons are of side-to-side differences, as well as between arms at the side and arms when elevated. The motion is markedly reduced in the second position when the latissimus dorsi muscle is tight because this position increases the tension through this muscle.
Statistics	There are no known reliability data for this flexibility measure.[146]

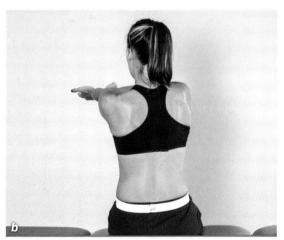

Figure 19.24

MUSCLE PERFORMANCE TESTING

Specific movements and strength grading of the trunk muscles are detailed in the following tests.

The clinician should also consider myotomal weakness. This assessment is typically performed in the lower quarter screen section of the examination. Therefore, at this point in the examination, the clinician has already performed myotomal assessment, and is more focused on specific trunk movements and muscle weakness.

TRUNK FLEXION

Client Position	Supine, arms clasped behind head
Clinician Position	Standing directly to the side of the client, stabilizing the client just above the ankle
Movement and Assessment	The client flexes the trunk through curl-up ROM until their scapulae clear the table.
Grading for Trunk Flexion	• Grade 5: completes ROM with hands clasped behind head
	• Grade 4: completes ROM with arms crossed over chest

- Grade 3: completes ROM with arms outstretched, reaching toward toes
- Grade 2: depression of rib cage toward pubic symphysis
- Grade 1: muscle activity without movement
- Grade 0: no muscle activity

Primary Muscles	Rectus abdominis
	Internal oblique
	External oblique
Secondary Muscles	Psoas major and minor
Primary Nerve	Nerve to rectus abdominis (T7-12)

TRUNK EXTENSION

Client Position	Prone with hands clasped behind head
Clinician Position	Standing directly to the side of the client
Movement and Assessment	The client raises their trunk into end-range extension.

- Grade 5: holds position without wavering
- Grade 4: may waver or display signs of effort during testing

   Thoracic spine strength for grades 5 and 4 is the same, but the position is different. For assessing thoracic spine extension strength, the starting position is the same as that for lumbar, except the client is aligned so that the nipple line of the client is at the edge of the table.

- Grade 3: for the lumbar and thoracic spine is with the client starting for the thoracic spine, arms at side of body, and extending to end ROM
- Grade 2: completes partial ROM from full body on table position
- Grade 1: muscle activity without movement
- Grade 0: no muscle activity

Primary Muscles	Iliocostalis thoracis and lumborum
	Longissimus thoracis
	Spinalis thoracis
	Multifidi
	Rotatores and interspinales
	Quadratus lumborum
Secondary Muscles	Gluteus maximus
Primary Nerve	T1-L5

TRUNK ROTATION

Client Position	Supine with hands clasped behind head
Clinician Position	Standing directly to the side of the client
Movement and Assessment	The client rotates to one side with the upper trunk.

- Grade 5: scapula contralateral to direction of rotation; clears the table
- Grade 4: scapula contralateral to direction of rotation; clears the table with arms crossed across chest

(continued)

Trunk Rotation *(continued)*

- Grade 3: scapula contralateral to direction of rotation; clears the table with arms outstretched, reaching toward toes
- Grade 2: client unable to complete motion, but clinician observes depression of rib cage
- Grade 1: muscle activity without movement
- Grade 0: no muscle activity

Primary Muscles	External oblique (ipsilateral)
	Internal oblique (contralateral)
Primary Nerve	T7-12

ELEVATION OF PELVIS

Client Position	Supine or prone with hip in extension, grasping the table for stabilization
Clinician Position	Standing at the client's feet, directly facing them
Assessment	The client hikes up the pelvis, bringing the iliac crest toward the ribs as the clinician attempts to pull their leg down by grasping just above their ankle.

- Grade 5: completes motion against maximum resistance
- Grade 4: completes motion against very strong resistance
- Grade 3: completes motion without resistance
- Grade 2: completes partial motion without resistance
- Grade 1: muscle activity without movement
- Grade 0: no muscle activity

Primary Muscles	Quadratus lumborum
	External oblique
	Internal oblique
Secondary Muscles	Iliocostalis lumborum
Primary Nerve	Nerve to quadratus lumborum (T12-L)

SPECIAL TESTS

As mentioned in chapter 10 (Special Tests), in many cases the clinician is overly dependent on the performance and interpretation of special test findings with respect to differential diagnosis of the client's presenting pain. Utilization of special tests for ruling in (or helping to diagnose) a particular pathology should occur at this point in the examination process. It is also hoped that the clinician has a much clearer picture of the client's presentation prior to this point in the examination and will therefore depend minimally on special test findings with respect to diagnosis of the client's pain.

As with other regions of the body, special testing for the lumbar spine has limitations. For example, straight leg raise (SLR) testing has undergone significant investigation. Most of these studies were performed on surgical populations, and therefore their diagnostic accuracy values are interpretable to only these types of clients. In these studies, the SLR showed high SN (and variable SP), whereas the cross-legged SLR showed high SP (coupled with low SN). However, these results were found in populations with a very high prevalence of disc herniation (mostly above 75%) and likely a severe spectrum of disease bias, and they cannot be generalized to other populations. The diagnostic performance of physical examination tests in primary care populations and other general, unselected client groups is still unclear because evidence from these settings is scarce. Better performance may be obtained when combinations of tests are evaluated, including information from both client history and physical examination, but this requires further study.[135]

Special tests are not the only part of the examination procedure. For example, when used in isolation, diagnostic performance of most physical tests (scoliosis, paresis or muscle weakness, muscle wasting, impaired reflexes, and sensory deficits) was poor. Some tests (forward flexion, hyperextension test, and slump test) performed slightly better, but the number of studies was small. In the one primary care study, most tests showed higher SP and lower SN compared to other settings. As mentioned previously when used in isolation, current evidence indicates poor diagnostic performance of most physical tests used to identify lumbar disc herniation.[135]

Index of Special Tests

Lumbar Radiculopathy or Discogenic Related Symptoms

Centralization and Peripheralization

Extension Loss

Vulnerability in the Neutral Zone

Lumbar Radiculopathy, Discogenic Symptoms, and Neurodynamic Tests

Slump Test

Straight Leg Raise Test

Well-Leg Raise Test (Cross Straight Leg Raise)

Flip Sign (Sitting SLR)

Femoral Nerve Tension Test

Femoral Nerve Tension in Side Lying Test

Zygapophyseal Joint–Related Pain

Extension–Rotation Test

Posterior-to-Anterior Glides

Passive Physiological Intervertebral Motion

Lumbar Spinal Stenosis

Two-Stage Treadmill Test

Quadrant Test (Extension Biased)

Flexion Dysfunction

Quadrant Test (Flexion Biased)

Spondylolisthesis

One-Legged Hyperextension (Stork) Test

Kemp Test

Palpation for Spinous Process Step-Off

Radiographic Lumbar Spinal Instability

Passive Lumbar Extension Test

Instability Catch Sign

Painful Catch Sign

Apprehension Sign

Shear Test

Prone Instability Test

Passive Physiological Intervertebral Movements (PPIVMs): Extension

Passive Physiological Intervertebral Movements (PPIVMs): Flexion

Neuromuscular Control

Active Hip Abduction Test

Ankylosing Spondylitis

Chest Expansion Test

Case Studies

Go to www.HumanKinetics.com/OrthopedicClinicalExamination and complete these case studies for chapter 19:

- Case study 1 discusses a 36-year-old female with lower back and buttock pain.
- Case study 2 discusses a 62-year-old female with localized lower back pain.

Abstract Links

Go to www.HumanKinetics.com/OrthopedicClinicalExamination to access abstract links on these issues:

Active hip abduction test

Chest expansion test

Closed fist percussion test

Extension loss

Extension-rotation test

Femoral nerve tension test

Flexion/Extension

Flip test (sitting SLR)

Kemp test

One-legged hyperextension test (stork test)

Passive lumbar extension test

Posterior to anterior glides

Prone instability test

Quadrant test (extension biased)

Repeated range of motions

Seated extension-rotation

Shear test

Slump test

Straight leg raise test

Two stage treadmill test

LUMBAR RADICULOPATHY OR DISCOGENIC-RELATED SYMPTOMS

CENTRALIZATION AND PERIPHERALIZATION

Video 19.25 **in the web resource shows a demonstration of this test.**

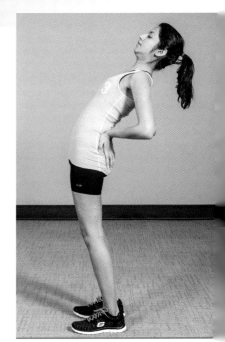

Client Position	Standing with bilateral hands on hips (for loaded assessment). The test can also be performed in supine for flexion and prone for extension (see figure 19.26) if an unloaded assessment is preferred.
Clinician Position	Monitoring client from the side
Movement	The clinician asks the client to perform repeated lumbar spine movements to end range. The range of repetitions described was 5 to 20 repetitions until a definitive centralization or peripheralization of symptoms occurred. The motions assessed included extension, flexion, and side bending.
Assessment	A (+) test is when symptoms centralize or peripheralize with repeated motions. Ideally, one motion would centralize symptoms and the opposite motion would peripheralize symptoms.

Figure 19.25

Statistics	• **SN 92 (NR)**, SP 64 (NR), **+LR 2.6**, **–LR 0.12**, QUADAS 12, in a study of 63 clients with chronically disabling LBP (mean age 39.6 ± 11.1 years; 22 women; mean duration of symptoms 15.3 months), using discography as a reference standard[133]

- SN 40 (28-54), **SP 94 (73-99)**, **+LR 6.7**, –LR 0.63, QUADAS 13, in a study of 107 clients with persistent LBP (mean age 42.5 ± 11.8 years; 44.9% were female; mean duration of symptoms 165.2 weeks), using discography as a reference standard[134]

EXTENSION LOSS

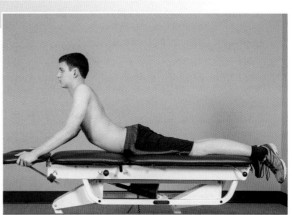

Client Position	Prone with bilateral hands grasping each side of the table at their head level
Clinician Position	Monitoring client from the side
Movement	The clinician asks the client to perform a press-up, extending bilateral elbows (and therefore their lumbar spine) as far as they can go (keeping their pelvis in contact with the table).
Assessment	A (+) test is defined as a moderate or major loss of extension.
Statistics	Any two of the variables (centralization of symptoms with repeated motions, persistent pain between LBP episodes, vulnerable in the neutral zone, and extension loss) resulted in diagnostic accuracy of the following:

Figure 19.26

- SN 30 (21-42), **SP 95 (78-99)**, **+LR 6.5**, –LR 0.77, QUADAS 11, in a study of 107 clients with disabling LBP and high levels of psychological distress (mean age 42.9 ± 11.8 years; 47.7% were female; mean duration of symptoms 170.1 weeks), using discography as a reference standard[139]

VULNERABILITY IN THE NEUTRAL ZONE

Client Position	Standing with bilateral arms at side
Clinician Position	Monitoring client from the side
Movement	Client is asked to move into a slightly flexed, slightly extended, or slightly side-bent position.
Assessment	A (+) test is worsening of symptoms at neutral ranges.
Statistics	• SN 31 (NR), SP 82 (NR), +LR 1.7, –LR 0.84, QUADAS 12, in a study of 63 clients with chronically disabling LBP (mean age 39.6 ± 11.1 years; 22 women; mean duration of symptoms of 15.3 months), using discography as a reference standard[133]
	• See diagnostic accuracy values listed previously for extension loss as a variable.[139]

LUMBAR RADICULOPATHY, DISCOGENIC SYMPTOMS, AND NEURODYNAMIC TESTS

Refer to chapter 7 for descriptions and diagnostic accuracy of these tests:

- Slump Test
- Straight Leg Raise (SLR) Test
- Well-Leg Raise Test (Cross Straight Leg Raise)
- Flip Sign (Sitting SLR)
- Femoral Nerve Tension Test
- Femoral Nerve Tension in Side Lying Test

ZYGAPOPHYSEAL JOINT–RELATED PAIN

EXTENSION–ROTATION TEST

 Video 19.27 in the web resource shows a demonstration of this test.

Client Position	Sitting, bilateral distal legs off the edge of the table and feet on the floor if possible
Clinician Position	Sitting to the side of the client, blocking their knees
Movement	The clinician passively moves the client into full extension and (while maintaining end-range extension) rotates the client's trunk to end-range motion in both directions (one at a time).
Assessment	A (+) test is reproduction of concordant pain.

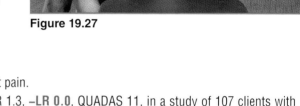

Figure 19.27

Statistics

- SN 100 (NR), SP 22 (NR), +LR 1.3, –LR 0.0, QUADAS 11, in a study of 107 clients with disabling LBP and high levels of psychological distress (mean age 42.9 years; 48% female; mean duration of symptoms NR, but mean duration off work was 119 weeks), using discography as a reference standard[139]

- SN 100 (NR), SP 12 (NR), +LR 1.1, –LR 0.0, QUADAS 10, in a study of 167 consecutive clients with chronic LBP and no previous history of lumbar spine surgery, and using zygapophyseal joint blocks as a reference standard[20]

POSTERIOR-TO-ANTERIOR GLIDES

Refer to the Passive Accessories section under Motion Tests for details on these tests.

PASSIVE PHYSIOLOGICAL INTERVERTEBRAL MOTION

Refer to the Passive Physiological Intervertebral Motion (PPIVM) section under Motion Tests for details on these tests.

LUMBAR SPINAL STENOSIS

TWO-STAGE TREADMILL TEST

Client Position	Standing on the treadmill in straddle stance until the belt moves
Clinician Position	Monitoring the client from the side of the treadmill, raising and lowering the treadmill height
Movement	Once the treadmill is started very slowly, the clinician asks the client to walk on the treadmill at a comfortable walking pace with the treadmill at a height level to the floor and a 15° elevation for a maximum of 10 minutes. The client rests for 10 minutes after each bout.
Assessment	The client is queried regarding when symptoms increased above baseline and when (if they needed) to stop testing. If symptoms worsen with walking on a level treadmill compared to the elevated treadmill, this is considered a (+) test for stenosis. An earlier onset of symptoms with level walking, increased total walking time on an inclined treadmill, and prolonged recovery time after level walking are significantly associated with stenosis.[31] Although the distance reached in the treadmill test predicted the grade of stenosis in MRI, it had a limited diagnostic importance for the level of clinical symptoms in lumbar spinal stenosis.[147]

Statistics

- Longer total walking time during inclined walking: SN 50 (38-63), **SP 92 (78-100)**, **+LR 6.5**, –LR 0.54, QUADAS 9, in a study of 45 clients (26 stenotic [mean age 64.6 ± 8.7] and 19 nonstenotic [mean age 49.3 ± 14.4]; gender and duration of symptoms NR), using MRI or CT scan as a reference standard[31]

- Earlier onset of symptoms with level walking: SN 68 (50-86), **SP 83 (66-100)**, **+LR 4.1**, –LR 0.39, QUADAS 9, in a study of 45 clients (26 stenotic [mean age 64.6 ± 8.7] and 19 nonstenotic [mean age 49.3 ± 14.4]; gender and duration of symptoms NR), using MRI or CT scan as a reference standard[31]

- Required prolonged recovery after level walking: **SN 82 (66-98)**, SP 68 (48-89), +LR 2.6, **–LR 0.26**, QUADAS 9, in a study of 45 clients (26 stenotic [mean age 64.6 ± 8.7] and 19 nonstenotic [mean age 49.3 ± 14.4]; gender and duration of symptoms NR), and using MRI or CT scan as a reference standard[31]

QUADRANT TEST (EXTENSION BIASED)

Client Position	Standing, arms relaxed at side
Clinician Position	Standing behind and to the side of the client on the side for the movement being performed
Movement	The client actively extends, side bends, and rotates the spine to the ipsilateral side, sliding their hand down the ipsilateral leg. The clinician can guide the client in this motion and provide overpressure if no pain is reported with their active movement. The client holds the position for up to 3 seconds if no pain.
Assessment	A (+) test is client reports pain or numbness or tingling in the area of the back or lower extremities.
Statistics	SN 70 (NR), QUADAS 9, in a study of 24 men and 50 women with chronic LBP (mean age 66.8 ± 12.4 years; duration of symptoms > 6 months), using physician diagnosis as a reference standard[25]

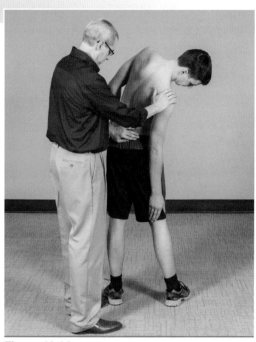

Figure 19.28

FLEXION DYSFUNCTION

QUADRANT TEST (FLEXION BIASED)

Client Position	Standing with weight equally distributed on bilateral legs
Clinician Position	Standing to the side of client, monitoring client response
Movement	Client actively flexes, side bends, and rotates the spine to the ipsilateral side, sliding their hands down the leg on each side, respectively.
Assessment	A (+) test is reproduction of concordant pain.
Statistics	NR

SPONDYLOLISTHESIS

ONE-LEGGED HYPEREXTENSION (STORK) TEST

Client Position	Standing on bilateral legs, arms across abdomen
Clinician Position	Monitoring the client from the side
Movement	The clinician asks the client to lift one leg slightly (right as shown) and hold it against their weight-bearing leg. While maintaining this position, the client hyperextends the lumbar spine to their end ROM. Some have advocated the use of end ROM rotation as well.
Assessment	A reproduction of concordant pain is a (+) response.
Statistics	SN 50-55 (32-71), SP 46-58 (18-64), +LR 1.0-1.6, –LR 0.8-1.0, QUADAS 8, in a study of 71 clients with LBP (age range 10-30 years; gender NR; symptom duration < 6 months), using radiological investigation (including SPECT, MRI, and CT) as a reference standard[148]

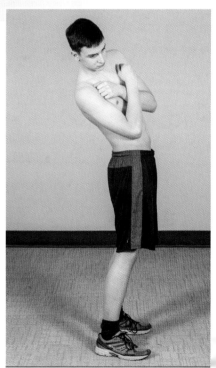

Figure 19.29

KEMP TEST

Client Position	Standing on bilateral legs, arms across abdomen or chest
Clinician Position	Monitoring client from the side
Movement	The client is asked to hyperextend and rotate the lumbar spine to their end ROM in both directions (one direction at a time) as tolerated.
Assessment	A reproduction of concordant pain is a (+) response.
Statistics	A positive prevalence of 74% to 77% in those clients with MRI (reference standard) and 76% prevalence in those clients without MRI confirmed spondylolisthesis in a study of 200 consecutive clients (56 females; mean age 14.1 ± 1.5 years; mean duration of symptoms not reported) with LBP[149]

Figure 19.30

PALPATION FOR SPINOUS PROCESS STEP-OFF

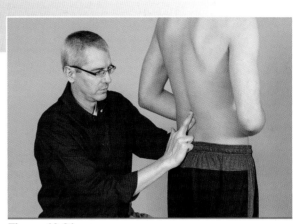

Figure 19.31

Client Position	Standing in a relaxed position with feet comfortably side by side
Clinician Position	Seated and facing the client to the side
Movement	The clinician maintains a side view of the client's lumbar spine. The clinician applies and maintains firm contact on the lumbosacral spinous processes while sliding the examining fingertips from the upper lumbar region to the sacrum.
Assessment	A (+) test is palpating one spinous process anterior to the levels above and below.
Statistics	SN 60 (NR), SP 87 (NR), +LR 4.6, –LR 0.45, QUADAS 8, in a study of 30 clients with LBP, using radiography as a reference standard[150]

RADIOGRAPHIC LUMBAR SPINAL INSTABILITY

PASSIVE LUMBAR EXTENSION TEST

Video 19.32 in the web resource shows a demonstration of this test.

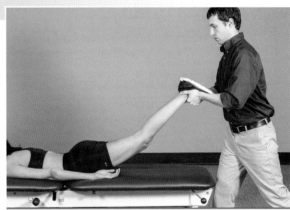

Figure 19.32

Client Position	Prone with bilateral legs at the end of the table, bilateral arms relaxed at side
Clinician Position	Standing at the end of the table, directly facing the client's legs
Movement	The clinician lifts the client's bilateral lower extremities (LEs) concurrently to a height of about 30 cm from the table while maintaining the bilateral knees extended and gently pulling the legs.
Assessment	A (+) test is the client complaining of pain in lumbar region, including LBP, a heavy feeling in the low back, and feeling as if the low back were coming off, and symptoms disappearing when the client's legs were returned to the table.
Statistics	**SN 84 (69-94), SP 90 (82-96), +LR 8.8, –LR 0.17**, QUADAS 12, in a study of 38 clients positive for lumbar instability (mean age 68.3 ± 12.3 years, 9 women) and 84 clients negative for lumbar instability (mean age 69.1 ± 10.5 years, 50 women), using radiological evaluation as a reference standard[46]

INSTABILITY CATCH SIGN

Client Position	Standing with bilateral hands on hips
Clinician Position	Standing, monitoring client response
Movement	The client is instructed to perform trunk flexion as far as possible and then return to an erect upright position.
Assessment	A (+) test is an inability to return to full upright or erect position.
Statistics	SN 26 (13-43), SP 86 (79-94), +LR 1.8, –LR 0.86, QUADAS 12, in a study of 38 clients positive for lumbar instability (mean age 68.3 ± 12.3 years, 9 women) and 84 clients negative for lumbar instability (mean age 69.1 ± 10.5 years, 50 women), using radiological evaluation as a reference standard[46]

PAINFUL CATCH SIGN

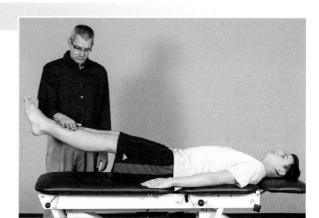

Figure 19.33

Client Position	Supine with bilateral legs extended, bilateral arms relaxed at side
Clinician Position	Standing at the side of the table, directly facing the client's legs
Movement	The client is instructed to lift their legs (keeping knees straight) about 30 cm high. The client is then asked to lower their legs back to the table.
Assessment	A (+) test is when the legs fall down instantly during the lowering of the legs back to the table.
Statistics	SN 37 (22-54), SP 73 (62-82), +LR 1.4, –LR 0.87, QUADAS 12, in a study of 38 clients positive for lumbar instability (mean age 68.3 ± 12.3 years, 9 women) and 84 clients negative for lumbar instability (mean age 69.1 ± 10.5 years, 50 women), using radiological evaluation as a reference standard[46]

APPREHENSION SIGN

Clients were asked whether they had felt a sensation of lumbar collapse because of sudden LBP when they performed ordinary tasks, including bending back and forth or from side to side and sitting down or standing up.

Assessment	A (+) test was when the client affirmed that they had experienced such episodes.
Statistic	SN 18 (8-34), SP 88 (79-94), +LR 1.6, –LR 0.93, QUADAS 12, in a study of 38 lumbar instability positive clients (mean age 68.3 ± 12.3 years, 9 women) and 84 lumbar instability negative clients (mean age 69.1 ± 10.5 years, 50 women), using radiological evaluation as a reference standard[46]

SHEAR TEST

Client Position	Standing with weight equally on bilateral legs, bilateral crossed hands over the lower abdomen
Clinician Position	Standing to the side of the client. The clinician places one hand over the client's bilateral hands and the other hand vertically over the lumbar spine and then palpates the level to be tested with the index finger.
Stabilization	The clinician uses the hand that is placed vertically over the lumbar spine (clinician's left hand as shown). While the index finger palpates the interspinous level to be tested, the rest of the hand provides posterior stability to the levels distal to the interspinous segment being tested. The test is to be repeated at each lumbar level.
Mobilization	The clinician provides an anterior-to-posterior force (with right hand as shown) against the stabilization force provided posteriorly.
Assessment	A (+) test occurs when symptoms are provoked; it is not based on the amount of intersegmental motion detected.[41]
Statistics	• Diagnostic accuracy NR • Reliability coefficient (κ) = 0.35 (0.20–0.51)[41]

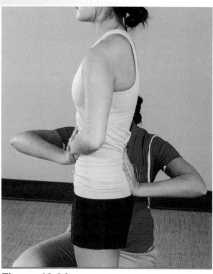

Figure 19.34

PRONE INSTABILITY TEST

Client Position	Prone with legs off the edge of the table and bilateral feet on the floor, grasping onto the sides of the table as shown
Clinician Position	Standing to the side of the client. The clinician places the hypothenar region of the wrist over a specific level spinous process of the lumbar vertebrae.
Mobilization	The clinician provides posterior-to-anterior intervertebral (IV) motion testing (PA glide) at each respective level of the lumbar spine and assesses for reproduction of the client's symptoms *(a)*. The client then lifts both legs off the floor *(b)*. Posterior-to-anterior IV motion testing is reapplied to any segments that were identified as painful.
Assessment	A (+) test occurs when pain is provoked during the first part of the test (legs on floor) but disappears when the test is repeated with the legs off the floor.
Statistics	• SN 61 (NR), SP 57 (NR), +LR 1.4, –LR 0.69, QUADAS 12, in a study of 49 clients with suspicion of instability (mean age 39.2 ± 11.3 years; 57% were women; median duration of symptoms 78 days), using flexion–extension radiographs as a reference standard[43] • Reliability coefficient (κ) = 0.87 (0.80–0.94);[41] (κ) = 0.69[43]

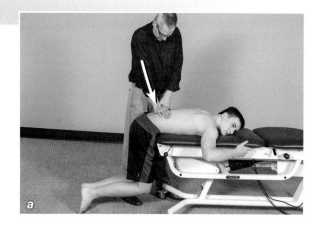

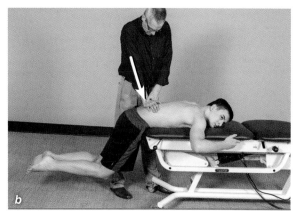

Figure 19.35

PASSIVE PHYSIOLOGICAL INTERVERTEBRAL MOVEMENTS (PPIVMS): EXTENSION

Refer to the Passive Physiological Intervertebral Motion (PPIVMs) section under Motion Tests for details on these tests.

PASSIVE PHYSIOLOGICAL INTERVERTEBRAL MOVEMENTS (PPIVMS): FLEXION

Refer to the Passive Physiological Intervertebral Motion (PPIVMs) section under Motion Tests for details on these tests.

NEUROMUSCULAR CONTROL

ACTIVE HIP ABDUCTION TEST

Client Position	Side lying, maintaining frontal plane alignment and keeping legs in alignment with trunk
Clinician Position	Standing, observing client in the frontal plane
Movement	The client is instructed to perform a single active abduction of the hip, keeping the knee extended and in line with the trunk.
Assessment	The client is asked to rate the difficulty of the task.

- 0 = no difficulty
- 5 = unable to perform
- Scores summed for both legs

The clinician rates the performance also.

- 0 = no loss of frontal plane position
- 1 = minimal loss of frontal plane
- 2 = moderate loss of frontal plane
- 3 = severe loss of frontal plane

The worst score from two sides is used.

Statistics

- Examiner scoring (cutoff score ≥ 2): SN 41 (23-67), SP 85 (68-94), +LR 2.7, –LR 0.70, QUADAS 9, in a study of 43 previously asymptomatic clients prior to a 2-hour standing protocol designed to induce LBP (mean age 42 years; mean disease duration 18.1 years), using rating of pain (pain developers or nonpain developers) as a reference standard[151]
- Client self-rated scoring (cutoff score ≥ 4): SN 35 (17-59), **SP 92 (76-98)**, **+LR 4.6**, –LR 0.70, QUADAS 9, in a study of 43 previously asymptomatic clients prior to a 2-hour standing protocol designed to induce LBP (mean age 42 years; mean disease duration 18.1 years), using rating of pain (pain developers or nonpain developers) as a reference standard[151]

Critical Clinical Pearls

Other related lumbar spine pathologies (e.g., stenosis, facet joint arthropathy) that have poor tolerance for extension or extension–rotation movement could also have pain with the following tests advocated for lumbar spine spondylolisthesis:

- Stork Test
- Kemp Test
- Passive Lumbar Extension Test
- Prone Instability Test

ANKYLOSING SPONDYLITIS

CHEST EXPANSION TEST

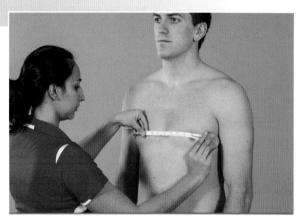

Figure 19.36

Client Position	Standing, arms relaxed at side
Clinician Position	Standing directly in front of client, facing them
Movement	The clinician uses a cloth tape measure to measure the circumferential distance around the client's chest (at nipple line), both at rest and at the end of a deep breath.
Assessment	A (+) test is a change in the two measurements of <2.5 cm.
Statistics	SN 9 (NR), SP 99 (NR), +LR 9, –LR 0.92, QUADAS 7, in a study of 449 clients with pain or stiffness in their back (mean age 42 years; mean disease duration 18.1 years), using the New York criteria (definitive radiographic changes in SIJ) as a reference standard[113]

PALPATION

Assessment of landmarks can be used to guide the clinician with palpation of the lumbar spine and pelvic girdle. As with observation (and as for all body areas to be assessed), the clinician should observe the client from the front, back, and each side for general symmetry, obvious deformities, and so on. Table 19.6 lists some important landmarks to assist the clinician with palpation.

Posterior Aspect

Palpation of the posterior aspect of the lumbar spine includes palpation of the bony and soft-tissue structures. The primary bony and soft-tissue structures available to be palpated posteriorly are listed here.

Bony Structures

• **Iliac crest:** This is very prominent and easy to palpate. The clinician can extend their fingers and place their index fingers of each hand at the level of the client's waist on each side laterally. The clinician should press medially and inferiorly until they feel a firm ridge under their index fingers. Following this level around posteriorly corresponds with the L4-L5 interspace level posteriorly.

• **Posterior superior iliac spine (PSIS):** The clinician can follow the iliac crest around posteriorly and inferiorly until they reach this structure. It is usually slightly prominent and slightly inferior to the normal dimple in this region (figure 19.37).

• **Spinous processes:** From the PSIS, the clinician can move their fingers in a medial

TABLE 19.6 Landmarks for Lumbar Spine

Landmark	Location
Anterior superior iliac spine (ASIS)	At the level of the sacral promontory
Posterior superior iliac spine (PSIS)	At the level of the second sacral spinous process (S2)
Iliac crest	At the level of the L4-L5 interspace
L3 transverse processes	Will be the widest lateral transverse process in the lumbar spine
Umbilicus	L3 spinous level
Ischial tuberosities	Tip of coccyx

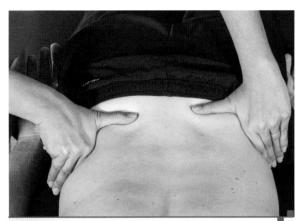

Figure 19.37 Palpation of the PSIS.

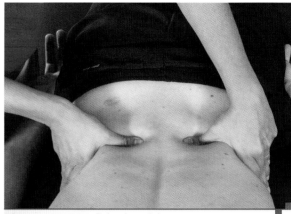

Figure 19.38 Palpation of the transverse processes.

and superior direction at a 30° angle. They will then be on the L5 spinous process. They can also use the L4-5 interspace as previously described and count accordingly. The clinician can locate the L1 by first finding the 12th rib and moving their fingers medially and down one level. Side-to-side asymmetry of the spinous processes from one level to the next may indicate the presence of a rotational dysfunction.[145] Palpation of the interspace between corresponding spinous processes can give the clinician an appreciation for the vertical height between corresponding vertebral levels. If two spinous processes have very little to no space between them, the clinician should suspect decreased size of the intervertebral disc or increased lumbar lordosis (which would approximate the spinous processes). Observation and palpation from the side would give an appreciation for the extent of lumbar lordosis.

- **Transverse processes:** This is typically positioned in a horizontal position (figure 19.38). Typically L3 is the longest and L1 is the shortest. These are typically more difficult to palpate in the lumbar spine due to the amount of muscle mass in this area. They are most easily identified in the trough located between the spinalis and longissimus muscles. The clinician can locate L5 by starting at the PSIS and moving again in a 30° to 45° angle superiorly and medially.

- **Zygapophyseal (facet) joints:** Between the spinous and transverse processes, the clinician should palpate the facet joints. They are approximately 2 to 3 cm lateral from the

spinous process. Localized tenderness over the facet joints without other root tension signs or neurologic signs may indicate facet joint pain.[18]

- **Sacroiliac (SI) joint:** The joint line is not palpable due to the posterior aspect of the innominate bone covering it. The PSIS is typically located at the level of S2.

- **Sacral base:** The clinician should start at the PSIS and move their thumbs medially and anteriorly until they contact the sacral base.

- **Sacral sulcus:** Starting at the PSIS, the clinician can palpate slightly above and medial to it on the sacrum adjacent to the ilium. The depth of the right side should be compared to that of the left side. If one side is deeper than the other, sacral torsion or rotation on the ilium around the horizontal plane may be indicated (as proposed by osteopathic literature).

- **Inferior lateral angle (ILA):** This is located approximately 1 in. (2.5 cm) lateral and slightly superior to the sacrococcygeal junction. The clinician should palpate on the inferior ILAs on both sides to determine relative superior or inferior position. A difference of 1/4 in. (6 mm) or more may suggest that the sacrum is side bent.

- **Ischial tuberosity:** The clinician should have the client lie on the contralateral side with their knee slightly flexed. They will palpate with their thumbs at the level of the client's gluteal folds until they feel a prominence. The clinician can also perform this at the level of the gluteal folds with the client in prone position, palpating for height (superior–inferior) and for depth (anterior–posterior). An anterior iliac rotation (as proposed by osteopathic literature) moves the ischial tuberosity posterior and vice versa. An upslip (as proposed by osteopathic literature but demonstrating little supporting evidence) moves the ischial tuberosity superior and vice versa.

- **Coccyx:** The tip of the coccyx can be found in the gluteal cleft.

Soft-Tissue Structures

- **Skin and soft tissue:** In general, these should be palpated for texture and pliability. Normally the skin in the lumbar spine and gluteal area can be pin rolled between the fingers without difficulty. Tightness or pain produced with this maneuver may indicate underlying pathology.[145]

- **Erector spinae muscles:** These are easily palpable just lateral to the spinous processes. Their lateral border appears to be a groove. They are often tender and in spasm in clients with acute low back pain. This group consists of spinalis (most medial), longissimus, and iliocostalis (most lateral) muscles. The clinician should ask the client to extend their trunk to make these muscles more prominent.

- **Sacrotuberous ligament:** From the ischial tuberosity, the clinician can move their thumbs in a medial and superior direction until they feel resistance against their thumbs. This is the sacrotuberous ligament running from the ischial tuberosity to the sacrum. Hypertrophy, increased firmness, and decreased spring indicate a problem. A posterior iliac rotation can cause sacrotuberous ligament irritation (as proposed by osteopathic literature).

- **Sacrospinous ligament:** This is located deep to the sacrotuberous ligament, slightly more than halfway between the PSIS and the ischial tuberosity and slightly medial.

Side Lying Position

Various-soft tissue structures relative to the lumbar spine and pelvis can be palpated in the side-lying position. The primary structures are the piriformis and sciatic nerve. Descriptions of how to palpate these structures in side-lying position are listed here.

Soft-Tissue Structures

- **Piriformis:** This is located between the anterior inferior aspect of the sacrum and the greater trochanter. This muscle is very deep and difficult to palpate. If the muscle is in spasm, the clinician can detect a cordlike structure under their fingers as they palpate the length of the muscle from the lateral border of the middle of the sacrum to the greater trochanter. It will be deep to the gluteus maximus, at the intersection of two lines. One line extends from the ASIS to the ischial tuberosity, while the other runs from the PSIS to the greater trochanter.

- **Sciatic nerve:** The clinician can locate the mid-position between the ischial tuberosity and the greater trochanter (figure 19.39). They may be able to roll the nerve under their fingers if they take up the soft tissue slack. This nerve typically exits under the piriformis muscle, except for in 12% of the population, with whom it pierces the piriformis muscle and in 0.5% of the population with whom the nerve runs superficial to the piriformis.

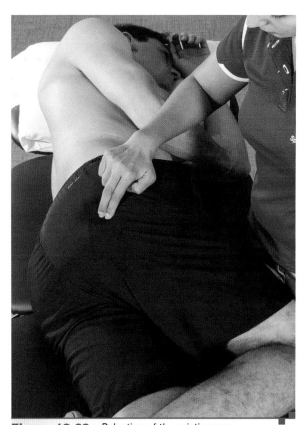

Figure 19.39 Palpation of the sciatic nerve.

Supine Position

Palpation of the anterior aspect of the lumbar spine includes palpation of the bony and soft-tissue structures. The primary bony and soft-tissue structures available to be palpated anteriorly are listed here.

Bony Structures

- **Anterior-aspect anterior superior iliac spine (ASIS):** The clinician can start along the iliac crest and move anteriorly and inferiorly diagonally toward the pubic ramus until they feel the most prominent protuberance anteriorly. They should use their thumbs to check for symmetry of location bilaterally (figure 19.40).

- **ASIS and PSIS:** A superior or inferior difference indicates possible leg length discrepancy or innominate rotation.

  - Medial or lateral difference indicates a possible iliac internal or external rotation.

  - Inclination angle of PSIS to ASIS: The clinician should palpate the ASIS and PSIS together from the side view. It has been suggested that there should be an 8° to 10° angle to the horizontal plane.

- **Pubic tubercles:** The clinician can start with the heel of their hand at the umbilicus. Applying slightly firm pressure, they gradually slide the heel of their hand inferiorly until they feel a hard resistance. The clinician should move their finger pads (one from each hand) on either side of the midline of the client's body to determine the relative position of the right

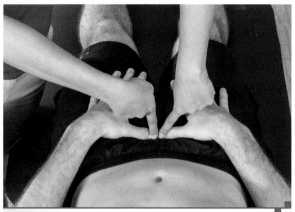

Figure 19.41 Palpation of the pubic tubercles.

and left sides. Another method is to have the client palpate this structure themselves (with their own thumbs) and the clinician then palpates the client's thumbs (or fingers) as shown (figure 19.41).

Soft-Tissue Structures

- **Abdominal muscles:** The clinician can make the rectus abdominis more prominent by asking the client to perform a curl-up. They should palpate along the length of the muscle from the pubic tubercle to the medial portion of the distal rib cage.

- **Abdominal aorta:** (See chapter 6 for palpation assessment.) This structure continues the thoracic aorta below the diaphragm. It descends in front and to the left of the spine before it divides into two terminal branches at the level of the L4-5 disc.

PHYSICAL PERFORMANCE MEASURES

Physical performance measures relevant to the lumbar spine can range from lower-level balance exercises to sit-to-stand tasks and sport-related tasks (jumping, speed, agility tests) dependent on the needs of the client. The Roland-Morris Disability Questionnaire correlated moderately (Pearson's product-moment correlation ranging from 0.29–0.41) with a physical performance test battery (lumbar flexion ROM, a 50-foot [15 m] walk at fastest speed, a 5-min. walk, 5 repetitions of sit-to-

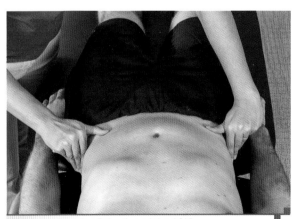

Figure 19.40 Palpation of the ASIS.

stand, 10 repetitions of trunk flexion, and loaded reach tasks). For the clients in the study, mean duration of symptoms was 108.12 ± 127.9 months with an average age of 45.6 years (48 women and 35 men). The loaded reach involved the clients reaching forward while holding a weight of 5% of their body weight.[152]

Another common measure in clients with LBP is trunk endurance. College-aged clients with both pain (P = 0.019) and disability (P = 0.006) differed in trunk endurance from age-matched colleagues without LBP. These pain and disability clients also scored lower (P = 0.01) than their age-matched colleagues.[153]

Fear-avoidance beliefs and physical activity levels were closely associated with trunk endurance testing as well. In a study of 68 clients post single-level microdiscectomy of 4 to 6 weeks, it was demonstrated that high fear-avoidance belief scores, as well as low levels of physical activity, correlated directly with lower endurance scores for trunk endurance.[154]

The utilization of physical performance measures for the lumbar spine is becoming more popularly described in the literature. Some of the more commonly utilized physical performance measures (as well as the discrete physical parameter they measure) relative to the lumbar spine are listed in table 19.7.

TABLE 19.7 Physical Performance Measure Suggestions for the Lumbar Spine

Discrete physical parameter	Potential physical performance measurements for the lower-level client (if appropriate)	Potential physical performance measurements for the higher-level client (if appropriate)
Balance	Single-leg stance test Romberg test Four square step test Functional reach test Side-step test Tandem walking Tinetti test	Any of the tests appropriate for the lower-level client Star excursion balance test Multiple single-leg hop stabilization test
Fundamental movement	Deep squat test Sock test Sit-to-stand test Self-paced walking test Timed up and go test	Any of the tests appropriate for the lower-level client Rotational stability Trunk stability push-up
Strength and power	1RM leg press Lunge test Knee bending in 30 s	Any of the tests appropriate for the lower-level client Jump and hop tests
Lower extremity anaerobic power	Only if appropriate and necessary	Any of the tests appropriate for the lower-level client Wingate anaerobic power test Lower extremity functional test
SAQ	Only if appropriate and necessary	Any of the tests appropriate for the lower-level client Edgren side-step test Illinois agility test Pro agility test Zigzag run test
Trunk endurance	Supine bridge test	Trunk flexion, extension, and lateral flexion bilaterally Repetitive box lifting task Loaded forward reach test

SAQ = speed, agility, and quickness

COMMON ORTHOPEDIC CONDITIONS OF THE LUMBAR SPINE

While it is impossible to distinctly describe various pathological presentations of the lumbar spine, there are evidence-based findings supportive of particular pathologies of this region of the body. Therefore, the intent of this section of the chapter is to present current evidence-supported findings suggestive of lumbar spine pathologies. As previously described in chapter 4 (Evidence-Based Practice and Client Examination), though, not all examination findings are absolutely supported with clinical evidence, and the clinician should also rely on clinical experience and input from the client when performing differential diagnosis of a client's presentation of pain and dysfunction.

Clarification on specific terminology of similar types of pathologies in the lumbar spine is necessary prior to investigating the examination for each of these pathologies. General definitions are given here and (when necessary) additional detail is given in subsequent sections for each pathology. *Spinal stenosis* is an abnormal narrowing in a blood vessel or other tubular organ or structure. With respect to the lumbar spine, this would include the central canal (where the spinal cord runs) and the intervertebral foramen bilaterally. *Spondylosis* is degenerative osteoarthritis of the joints between spinal vertebral levels. Spondylolysis is a defect of the pars interarticularis of a vertebra, and *spondylolisthesis* is the anterior displacement or posterior displacement (retrolisthesis) of a vertebra or the vertebral column in relation to the vertebra below.

Lumbar spine degeneration (spondylosis) can involve various forms of stenosis and (dependent on the location of this stenosis) can have different clinical presentation. Figure 19.42 helps delineate these differences. Degeneration of the spine involving the spinal canal will result in central canal stenosis and the potential for myelopathy and upper motor neuron signs. Lateral foraminal stenosis (due to various reasons including radiculopathy and bone spurs) can result in nerve root involvement and the potential for lower motor neuron signs and symptoms. Spinal degeneration can also result in axial lumbar pain without true or hard neurological findings. In such cases the client may have a combination of low back and leg pain (radiculitis).

Lumbar Spinal Stenosis

ICD-9: 723.0, 724.0

ICD-10: M48 (spinal stenosis); M54.5 (low back pain)

Lumbar spinal stenosis (LSS) is a medical condition in which the spinal canal narrows and compresses the spinal cord and nerves at the level of the lumbar vertebra. This is usually due to the common occurrence of spinal degeneration that occurs with aging. It can also sometimes be caused by spinal disc herniation, osteoporosis, or a tumor. In the cervical (neck) and lumbar (low back) region, it can be a congenital condition to varying degrees. Lumbar spinal stenosis is a result of degenerative, developmental, or congenital disorders. Neurogenic claudication (ischemia of the lumbosacral nerve roots secondary to compression from surrounding structures, hypertrophied facets, scar tissue, and discs) is a common symptom of LSS.

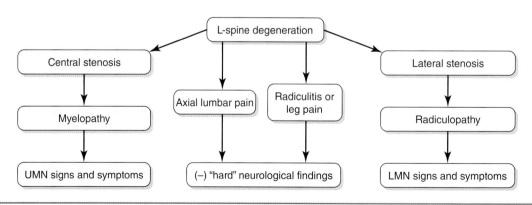

Figure 19.42   Lumbar spine degeneration. UMN = upper motor neuron; LMN = lower motor neuron; (−) = negative

Spinal stenosis may affect the cervical or thoracic region, in which case it is known as *cervical spinal stenosis* or *thoracic spinal stenosis*. In some cases, it may be present in all three places in the same client. Lumbar spinal stenosis may occur at different localizations in the spinal canal, sometimes at more than one location at the same time. In central canal stenosis, nerve roots in the cauda equina may be compressed. Lateral recess stenosis and foraminal stenosis may cause compression of the nerve roots leaving the spine.

Lumbar spinal stenosis results in LBP as well as pain or abnormal sensations in the legs, thighs, feet, or buttocks, or loss of bladder and bowel control. Central canal stenosis can result in upper motor neuron symptoms, while lateral stenosis is more likely to result in lower motor neuron symptoms.

Lumbar Spine Spondylosis (Degenerative Disc Disease, Spinal Arthritis)

Spondylosis is a degenerative osteoarthritis of the joints between the center of the spinal vertebrae or neural foramina. If this condition occurs in the facet joints, it can be considered facet syndrome. If severe, it may cause pressure on nerve roots with subsequent sensory or motor disturbances, such as pain, paresthesia, or muscle weakness in the limbs. Spondylosis can contribute to spinal stenosis.

When the space between two adjacent vertebrae narrows, compression of a nerve root emerging from the spinal cord may result in radiculopathy (sensory and motor disturbances, such as severe pain in the neck, shoulder, arm, back, or leg, accompanied by muscle weakness). Less commonly, direct pressure on the spinal cord (typically in the cervical spine) may result in myelopathy, characterized by global weakness, gait dysfunction, loss of balance, and loss of bowel or bladder control. The client may experience a phenomenon of shocks (paresthesia) in the hands and legs because of nerve compression and lack of blood flow. If vertebrae of the neck are involved, it is referred to as *cervical spondylosis*. Lower back spondylosis is termed *lumbar spondylosis*.

Clinical differentiation between neurogenic-related and vascular-related claudication can be difficult to ascertain. The following sidebar on differential diagnosis provides some clinical information relative to each of these conditions for the purpose of differentially diagnosing these two similar pathologies.

I. Client Interview

- Requires both the presence of a characteristic clinical presentation, including neurogenic claudication, radicular pain, or both, and radiographic or anatomic lumbar spinal stenosis (LSS).[32]

Differential Diagnosis of Neurogenic and Vascular Claudication

Description	Neurogenic	Vascular
Quality of pain	Cramping	Burning, cramping
LBP	Frequently present	Absent
Sensory symptoms	Frequently present	Absent
Muscle weakness	Frequently present	Absent
Reflex changes	Frequently present	Absent
Bicycle test	Symptoms only when sitting upright	Symptoms not position dependent (e.g., symptoms in upright, flexed, and extended postures)
Arterial pulses	Normal	Decreased or absent
Skin/dystrophic changes	Absent	Frequently present
Aggravating factors	Upright posture, extension of trunk	Any leg activity
Relieving factors	Sitting, bending forward	Rest; no leg activity
Walking uphill	Symptoms produced later	Symptoms typically not position dependent
Walking downhill	Symptoms produced earlier	

Subjective History[25, 26, 155, 156]

- It is one of the most common degenerative spinal diseases.
- It can be complicated by the range of possible clinical presentations.[32]
- Complaints can include low back and leg pain.
- The most common symptom associated with LSS is neurogenic claudication, a variable pain or discomfort with walking or prolonged standing that radiates beyond the spinal area into one or both buttocks, thighs, lower legs, or feet.[32]
- Neurogenic claudication should be differentiated from vascular claudication (see Special Tests section).
- Muscle weakness
- Sensory disturbances
- Not being over the age of 65 years helps rule out stenosis (SN 77).[24, 30, 31]
- Not having pain below buttocks helps **rule out** stenosis (SN 88).[24, 31]
- Not having leg symptoms get worse with walking or get better with sitting helps **rule out** stenosis (SN 81).[24, 31]
- Having bilateral buttock or leg pain helps **rule in** stenosis (SP 92).[157]
- If the client has bilateral leg pain, but it is not relieved by sitting, it helps **rule out** stenosis (SN 81).[31]
- No pain with seated position helps **rule in** stenosis (SP 93).[24]
- Symptoms being improved when seated helps **rule in** stenosis (SP 83;[24] SP 86[48]).
- Symptoms being improved with bending forward helps **rule in** stenosis (SP 92).[158]
- If the client's best posture is not sitting, it helps **rule out** stenosis (SN 89).[31]
- If the client's worst posture is not standing or walking, it helps **rule out** stenosis (SN 89).[31]
- Walking improved with holding onto shopping cart provides limited help with ruling out (SN 63) or ruling in (SP 67) stenosis.[31]

- Clinical prediction rule (variables) for lumbar spinal stenosis:[48]
  - Bilateral symptoms, leg pain > back pain, pain during walking or standing, pain relief when sitting, and age > 48 years
  - <1 (+) finding helps to rule out stenosis: SN 96, SP 20, +LR 1.2, −LR 0.19, QUADAS 8, in a study of 1,448 clients who presented with a primary complaint of back pain with or without leg pain, and using clinical findings and imaging as a reference standard
  - 4 out of 5 (+) findings helps to rule in stenosis: SN 6, SP 98, +LR 4.6, −LR 0.95, QUADAS 8 in the same study

Outcome Measures[26]

- The Physical Function Scale has demonstrated construct validity for the measurement of walking in a lumbar spinal stenosis population.
- The Swiss Spinal Stenosis Questionnaire can be used to measure walking capacity.
- Oxford Claudication Score
- ODI
- Other common measures may be clinically applicable, including the FABQ, SF-36, Roland-Morris, and the Quebec Back Pain Disability Scale.[50]

Diagnostic Imaging

- There is a need for consensus on well-defined, unambiguous radiological criteria to define lumbar spinal stenosis in order to improve diagnostic accuracy and to formulate reliable inclusion criteria for clinical studies.[71]
- Radiographic findings include joint space narrowing, bone sclerosis, periarticular cysts, and osteophytes. Refer to chapter 6 for a definition of osteoarthritis according to Kellgren and Lawrence.[159]
- Imaging characteristics of spinal stenosis showed moderate to substantial reliability.[160]

- No superior accuracy for myelography was seen compared with CT or MRI.[72]

- No indication exists that any of the imaging tests has superior accuracy.[72]

- MRI findings failed to show a major clinical relevance when evaluating the walking distance, pain level, function, and subjective report of function with lumbar spinal stenosis; therefore, they should be treated with some caution.[70, 147, 161, 162]

- MRI helps **rule out** (SN 96) stenosis.[76]

II. Observation

- Clients with more pronounced stenosis tend to have a more severe reduction of walking ability,[163] potentially with a wide-based gait.[72]

- A wide-based gait helps **rule in** (SP 97, +LR 13) the likelihood of spinal stenosis.[24]

- Clinicians should look for lumbar flexion and decreased lumbar lordosis.[31]

III. Triage and Screening

- All nonmusculoskeletal causes, as well as causes from related joints, should be ruled out.

- Clients may have decreased leg sensation in dermatomal pattern.[31]

- Clients may have diminished pedal pulse.[156]

- 62% of clients had abnormal reflexes.[25]

- 58% had abnormal vibration sense, while 50% had abnormal pinprick sense.[25]

- Clinicians should rule out other potential symptom contributors, such as diabetes mellitus and vascular claudication.

- The following signs and symptoms helpful for **ruling out** CES:[120-122]
  - History of back pain (SN 94)
  - Urinary retention (SN 90)
  - Rapid symptom onset within 24 hours (SN 89)
  - Sacral sensation loss (SN 85)
  - Lower extremity weakness or gait loss (SN 84)
  - Loss of sphincter tone (SN 80)

- A diagnostic prediction rule helps **rule out** (SN 95) a vertebral fracture when ≤1 of 5 variables were present and helps **rule in** (SP 96) a vertebral fracture when ≥4 of 5 variables were present.[123]

- Another diagnostic prediction rule helps **rule out** (SN 88) a vertebral fracture when only 1 of 4 variables were present and helps **rule in** (SP 96 when ≥ 2 of 4 variables present and SP 100 when ≥ 3 of 4 variables were present) a vertebral fracture.[106]

- The closed-fist percussion test has good ability to help **rule out** (SN 88, −LR 0.13) and ideal ability to help **rule in** (SP 90, +LR 8.8) vertebral compression fracture.[124]

- The supine sign has good ability to help **rule out** (SN 81, −LR 0.2) and ideal ability to help **rule in** (SP 93, +LR 11.6) vertebral compression fracture.[124]

IV. Motion Tests

- 61% of clients had pain with lumbar extension, while 54% had pain with side bending.[25]

V. Muscle Performance Testing

- Clients may have decreased leg strength, especially of extensor hallucis longus.[156]

- 64% of clients demonstrated leg weakness.[25]

VI. Special Tests

- Romberg test: A (+) test or abnormal result has good ability to help **rule in** (SP 91, +LR 4.2) spinal stenosis.[32]

- Quadrant test: A (−) test has less than good ability to help rule out (SN 70) spinal stenosis.[25]

- The quadrant test was the strongest predictor of symptom severity.[25]

- Neurogenic claudication should be differentiated from vascular claudication. The signs and symptoms described previously, the two-staged treadmill test, and walking uphill or downhill can assist with differential diagnosis. Clients with LSS are more likely to have more pain or difficulty with walking downhill than uphill (which may be pain relieving).

- Two-stage treadmill test:[31]
    - Earlier onset of symptoms with level walking helps **rule in** stenosis (SP 83, +LR 4.1).
    - Longer walking time during inclined walking helps **rule in** stenosis (SP 92, +LR 6.5).
    - Not requiring a prolonged recovery after level walking helps **rule out** (SN 82, −LR 0.26) stenosis.

VII. Palpation

- Localized tenderness over the facet joints without other root tension signs or neurologic signs may indicate facet joint pain.[18]

VIII. Physical Performance Measures

- Shuttle walking test (SWT) demonstrated very good test–retest reliability (ICC 0.92)[164]
- The mean SWT was 150 m among 32 clinic clients with lumbar spinal stenosis.[164]

POTENTIAL TREATMENT-BASED CLASSIFICATIONS

- Specific exercise direction, pain control (if pain dominant), mobility (if limited mobility), and exercise and conditioning may be appropriate.
- Traction may be applicable if distraction relieves symptoms.

Sciatica

ICD-9: 724.3

ICD-10: G57; M51.1; M54.3; M54.4 (sciatica)

Sciatica is a set of symptoms including pain that may be caused by general compression or irritation of one of the spinal nerve roots that gives rise to each sciatic nerve, or by compression or irritation of one or both sciatic nerves. In addition to pain, the client may have numbness, muscular weakness, or an abnormal sensation including a tingling or prickly feeling (paresthesia) and difficulty in moving or controlling the leg. Typically, the symptoms are unilateral.

Although sciatica is a relatively common form of low back pain and leg pain, the true mean-ing of the term is often misunderstood. Sciatica is a set of symptoms rather than a true diagnosis. Sciatica can be caused by nerve irritation (radiculitis), disc pathology (radiculopathy), bony impingement of the nerve, spondylolisthesis, spinal stenosis, and compression from the piriformis muscle primarily.

I. Client Interview

Subjective History

- Presence and distribution of pain.[21]
    - Pain drawing in a surgical cohort: SN 46 and **SP 84**
    - Sciatic pain in a nonsurgical cohort: **SN 99** and SP 6
    - Pain below the knee in a surgical cohort: **SN 90** and SP 15
- Sensory symptoms in a nonsurgical cohort: SN 30 and SP 58.[21]
- Not having pain below the knee helps **rule out** sciatica (SN 90).[22]
- Both centralization of pain and pain when rising from sitting were significantly associated with discogenic source of pain.[49]
- Possible risk factors for sciatica:[165]
    - Male sex
    - Age 30-50 years
    - Obesity
    - Multiple pregnancies
    - History of back pain
    - Mental stress
    - Long-term smoking
    - Work-related twisting

Outcome Measures

- Common outcome measures may be clinically applicable, including the FABQ, SF-36, Roland-Morris, and the Quebec Back Pain Disability Scale.[50]

Diagnostic Imaging

- MRI has a less than good ability to rule out (pooled SN 75) and rule in (pooled SP 77)[74] lumbar disc pathology and sciatica, while CT also has fair ability to rule out (SN 77) and rule in (SP 74)[75] lumbar disc pathology and sciatica.

II. Observation

- Atrophy of calf muscle:[21]
  - Nonsurgical clients: SN 29 and **SP 97**
  - Surgical clients: SN 38 and SP 50

III. Triage and Screening

- All nonmusculoskeletal causes, as well as causes from related joints, should be ruled out.

- The following signs and symptoms are helpful for **ruling out** CES:[120-122]
  - History of back pain (SN 94)
  - Urinary retention (SN 90)
  - Rapid symptom onset within 24 hours (SN 89)
  - Sacral sensation loss (SN 85)
  - Lower extremity weakness or gait loss (SN 84)
  - Loss of sphincter tone (SN 80)

- A diagnostic prediction rule helps **rule out** (SN 95) a vertebral fracture when ≤1 of 5 variables were present and helps **rule in** (SP 96) a vertebral fracture when ≥4 of 5 variables were present.[123]

- Another diagnostic prediction rule helps **rule out** (SN 88) a vertebral fracture when only 1 of 4 variables were present and helps **rule in** (SP 96 when ≥ 2 of 4 variables present and SP 100 when ≥ 3 of 4 variables were present) a vertebral fracture.[106]

- The closed-fist percussion test has good ability to help **rule out** (SN 88, −LR 0.14) and ideal ability to help **rule in** (SP 90, +LR 8.8) vertebral compression fracture.[124]

- The supine sign has good ability to help **rule out** (SN 81, −LR 0.20) and ideal ability to help **rule in** (SP 93, +LR 11.6) vertebral compression fracture.[124]

- Depressed reflexes:[21]
  - Ankle or knee jerk in a surgical cohort: SN 54 and SP 68
  - Ankle jerk in nonsurgical clients: SN 48 and **SP 89**
  - Ankle jerk in surgical clients: SN 54 and SP 60
  - Knee jerk in surgical clients: SN 4-14 and SP 65-92

- Sensory deficits in surgical clients: SN 28-60 and SP 57-65.[21]

IV. Motion Tests

- Repeated motions to centralize pain helps **rule in** (SP 100) discogenic source of LBP.[49]

- Centralization or peripheralization of radiating pain (using between 5 and 20 repetitions) helps **rule in** (SP 94, +LR 6.7)[134] and **rule out** (SN 92, −LR 0.12)[133] a discogenic source of LBP.

V. Muscle Performance Testing

- Paresis:[21]
  - Iliopsoas in nonsurgical clients: SN 10 and **SP 97**
  - Tibialis anterior in nonsurgical clients: SN 54 and **SP 89**
  - Gastrocnemius in nonsurgical clients: SN 13 and **SP 100**
  - Gastrocnemius in surgical clients: SN 47 and SP 52
  - Extensor hallucis longus in surgical clients: SN 62 and SP 50

VI. Special Tests

- When used in isolation, current evidence indicates poor diagnostic performance of most physical tests used to identify lumbar disc herniation. However, most findings arise from surgical populations and may not apply to primary care or nonselected populations.[135]

- Straight leg raise test:
  - In surgical populations, characterized by a high prevalence of disc herniation (58–98%), the SLR had good ability to help **rule out** (pooled SN 92, +LR 0.29) radiculopathy or discogenic symptoms with widely varying SP (10-100).[135]
  - It had good (**pooled SN 91, −LR 0.35**)[136] and ideal ability (**SN 97, −LR 0.05**) to help rule out radiculopathy and discogenic symptoms.[21]

- The SLR is the only sign consistently reported to be SN for sciatica due to disc herniation, but it is limited by its low SP.[27]

• Crossed leg, or well leg, raise test: In pooled analysis it had good ability to help **rule in** (SP 90) lumbar radiculopathy and discogenic symptoms.[135]

• Slump test: A (−) test helps **rule out** (SN 83, −LR 0.32) lumbar radiculopathy and discogenic symptoms.[137]

• A client self-rating of ≥4 on the side-lying active hip abduction test is helpful for **ruling in** (SP 92) a neuromuscular control deficit of the trunk musculature or inability to maintain postural control in the frontal plane and potential for developing pain.[151]

• A clinician rating of ≥2 on the side-lying active hip abduction test is helpful for **ruling in** (SP 85) a neuromuscular control deficit of the trunk musculature or inability to maintain postural control in the frontal plane and potential for developing pain.[151]

VII. Palpation

• The piriformis may be tender to palpation.

• Clinicians should palpate for muscle spasm and guarding of lumbar spine and pelvic girdle musculature (particularly paraspinals).

• Localized tenderness over the facet joints without other root tension signs or neurologic signs may indicate facet joint pain involvement.[18]

VIII. Physical Performance Measures

• Any appropriate physical performance measure may be used.

• Trunk endurance testing has been utilized in clients post lumbar laminectomy and has been found to correlate strongly with FABQ scores.[154]

• Lumbar radiculopathy physical performance measures may be clinically applicable.

POTENTIAL TREATMENT-BASED CLASSIFICATIONS

• Specific exercise direction, pain control (if pain is dominant), mobility (if limited mobility), and exercise and conditioning may be appropriate.

• Traction may be applicable if not centralizing or if client does not have a directional preference.

Lumbar Radiculopathy

ICD-9: 724.4 (thoracic or lumbosacral neuritis or radiculitis, unspecified); 729.2 (neuralgia, neuritis, and radiculitis, unspecified)

ICD-10: G54, M54.1 (radiculopathy); M54.5 (low back pain)

Radiculopathy is an encompassing term referring to a set of conditions in which one or more nerves are affected, most significantly at the nerve root. The insult to the nerve occurs at or near the root of the nerve (nerve root) as the peripheral nerve exits the spinal cord via the lateral foramina. The affected nerve may be inflamed, compressed, or symptomatic due to improper blood flow. Common causes of nerve root compression are from part of the intervertebral disc, nerve root adhesions or scar tissue, and surrounding bone, muscle, cartilage, or tendons.

Although the insult is at the nerve root, the symptoms are often felt distal to that point because the entire length of the nerve distal to the insult location is being affected. This can result in pain (radicular pain), weakness, numbness, or difficulty controlling specific muscles. Therefore, in the lumbar spine, symptoms will often be encountered distally in the legs. Since this is a nerve root insult, lumbar radiculopathy is a lower motor neuron dysfunction.

Clinical differentiation of lumbar spinal stenosis and radiculopathy due to disc herniation can also be difficult. The following differential diagnosis provides some clinical information relative to each of these conditions for the purpose of differentially diagnosing these two similar pathologies.

Differential Diagnosis of Lumbar Spinal Stenosis and Radiculopathy Due to Disc Herniation

Description	Lumbar spinal stenosis	Radiculopathy due to disc herniation
Age	Usually >50 years old	Usually <50 years old
Onset	Usually more insidious	Usually more sudden
Position change: sitting (flexion)	Better	Worse
Position change: extension	Worse	Better
Focal muscle weakness	Less common	Can be common
Dural tension	Less common	Common
Upper motor neuron (UMN) or lower motor neuron (LMN) involvement	Central stenosis: UMN Lateral foraminal stenosis: LMN	LMN

I. Client Interview

Subjective History

- Complaints could potentially include radicular pain, weakness, numbness in legs, and difficulty controlling specific muscles affected by the involved nerve root.

- Clients are typically in the 30- to 45-year age range.

- Mechanism of injury is most often a component of flexion and rotation.

- With increasing age, lumbar disc herniation is more cranially localized. Mean ages of the clients with disc herniation at L5-S1, L4-5, L3-4, and L2-3 were 44.1 ± 0.5 years, 49.5 ± 0.6 years, 59.5 ± 0.9 years, and 59.6 ± 2.7 years, respectively.[166]

Outcome Measures

- Common outcome measures may be clinically applicable, including the FABQ, SF-36, Roland-Morris, and the Quebec Back Pain Disability Scale.[50]

Diagnostic Imaging

- MRI has a less than good ability to rule out (pooled SN 75) and rule in (pooled SP 77)[74] lumbar disc pathology or sciatica, while CT scan also has fair ability to rule out (SN 77) and rule in (SP 74)[75] lumbar disc pathology or sciatica.

- Based on a recent systematic review, lumbar provocation discography may be a useful tool for evaluating chronic lumbar discogenic pain.[167]

II. Observation

- Atrophy of calf muscle:[21]

  - Nonsurgical clients: SN 29 and **SP 97**

  - Surgical clients: SN 38 and SP 50

III. Triage and Screening

- All nonmusculoskeletal causes, as well as causes from related joints, should be ruled out.

- The following signs and symptoms are helpful for **ruling out** CES:[120-122]

  - History of back pain (SN 94)

  - Urinary retention (SN 90)

  - Rapid symptom onset within 24 hours (SN 89)

  - Sacral sensation loss (SN 85)

  - Lower extremity weakness or gait loss (SN 84)

  - Loss of sphincter tone (SN 80)

- A diagnostic prediction rule helps **rule out** (SN 95) a vertebral fracture when ≤1 of 5 variables were present and helps **rule in** (SP 96) a vertebral fracture when ≥4 of 5 variables were present.[123]

- Another diagnostic prediction rule helps **rule out** (SN 88) a vertebral fracture when only 1 of 4 variables were present and helps **rule in** (SP 96 when ≥ 2 of 4 variables present and SP 100 when ≥ 3 of 4 variables were present) a vertebral fracture.[106]

- The closed-fist percussion test has good ability to help **rule out** (SN 88, −LR 0.14) and ideal ability to help **rule in** (SP 90, +LR 8.8) vertebral compression fracture.[124]

- The supine sign has good ability to help **rule out** (SN 81, −LR 0.20) and ideal ability to help **rule in** (SP 93, +LR 11.6) vertebral compression fracture.[124]

- Refer to the preceding section Sciatica for additional information.

IV. Motion Tests

- Repeated motions to centralize pain helps **rule in** (SP 100) discogenic source of LBP.[49]

- Centralization or peripheralization of radiating pain (using between 5 and 20 repetitions) helps **rule in** (SP 94, +LR 6.7)[134] and **rule out** (SN 92, −LR 0.12)[133] a discogenic source of LBP.

V. Muscle Performance Testing

- Decreased muscle strength and sensory loss are relatively well correlated in lumbar radiculopathy clients.[27]

- Refer to the preceding section Sciatica for additional information.

VI. Special Tests

- When used in isolation, current evidence indicates poor diagnostic performance of most physical tests used to identify lumbar disc herniation. However, most findings arise from surgical populations and may not apply to primary care or nonselected populations.[135]

- Straight leg raise test:
  - In surgical populations characterized by a high prevalence of disc herniation (58–98%), the SLR had good ability to help **rule out** (pooled SN 92, +LR 0.29) radiculopathy or discogenic symptoms with widely varying SP (10-100).[135]
  - The test had good (**pooled SN 91, −LR 0.35**)[136] and ideal ability (**SN 97, −LR 0.05**) to help rule out radiculopathy or discogenic symptoms.[21]
  - The SLR is the only sign consistently reported to be SN for sciatica due to disc herniation, but it is limited by its low SP.[27]

- Crossed straight leg, or well-leg, raise test: In pooled analysis, it had good ability to help **rule in** (SP 90) lumbar radiculopathy or discogenic symptoms.[135]

- Slump test: A (−) test helps **rule out** (SN 83, −LR 0.32) lumbar radiculopathy or discogenic symptoms.[137]

- A client self-rating of ≥4 on the side-lying active hip abduction test is helpful for **ruling in** (SP 92) a neuromuscular control deficit of the trunk musculature or inability to maintain postural control in the frontal plane and potential for developing pain.[151]

- A clinician rating of ≥2 on the side-lying active hip abduction test is helpful for **ruling in** (SP 85) a neuromuscular control deficit of the trunk musculature or inability to maintain postural control in the frontal plane and potential for developing pain.[151]

- Refer to the preceding section Sciatica for additional information.

VII. Palpation

- Palpate facet joints for tenderness. Localized tenderness over the facet joints without other root tension signs or neurologic signs may indicate facet joint pain.[18]

- Palpate paraspinal musculature for muscle guarding or spasm.

- The piriformis muscle may be tender.

- Refer to the preceding section Sciatica for additional information.

VIII. Physical Performance Measures

- A 10 m course shuttle walk test has been suggested.

- In L3 and L4 radiculopathies, unilateral quadriceps weakness was best detected by a single-leg sit-to-stand test. Clients of similar age with radicular pain caused by L5 or S1 radiculopathies could perform this test.[168]

- Trunk endurance testing has been utilized in clients post lumbar laminectomy and has been found to correlate strongly with FABQ scores.[154]

POTENTIAL TREATMENT-BASED CLASSIFICATIONS

- Specific exercise direction, pain control (if pain is dominant), mobility (if limited mobility), and exercise and conditioning may be appropriate.

- Traction may be applicable if distraction relieves symptoms.

Lumbar Spondylolysis and Spondylolisthesis

ICD-9: 738.4, 756.12 (spondylolysis, spondylolisthesis)

ICD-10: G; M43, M43.1 (spondylolysis, spondylolisthesis); M53.2 (spinal instabilities); M54.5 (low back pain); Q76.2 (congenital spondylolisthesis)

Spondylolysis and spondylolisthesis are among the various causes of LBP attributed to instability.

Spondylolysis is described as a bony defect, possibly a stress fracture, of one or both pars interarticularis, and it most commonly occurs in the lower lumbar spine.[169] Spondylolisthesis is displacement of a corresponding higher vertebra, often occurring as the result of a defect in the pars.[170] More recently, a consensus definition of spondylolisthesis is an acquired anterior displacement of one vertebra over the subjacent vertebra, associated with degenerative changes, without an associated disruption or defect in the vertebral ring.[171] Spondylolysis has been reported as a precipitating factor for this condition, which can be classified as isthmic, dysplastic, degenerative, traumatic, and pathologic.[172-174] Spondylolisthesis can further be graded I to IV to indicate severity. Grade I describes displacement of 0% to 25%, grade II describes displacement of 26% to 50%, whereas in grade III the displacement may be up to 75%. Displacement of 75% to 100% is classed as grade IV.[175]

I. Client Interview

Subjective History

- Reported prevalence of spondylolysis ranges from approximately 6% to 11.5% in the general population,[176] and approximately 7% to 8% in elite athletes only, although this percentage is likely grossly underreported.[95, 177-178]

- Nearly 50% of LBP cases in adolescent athletes have been attributed to spondylolysis.[179]

Differential Diagnosis of L3 Lumbar Radiculopathy Versus Degenerative Medial Meniscus Tear

- Clients with L3 radiculopathy are more likely to have a potential decrease in patella tendon reflexes or sensation to medial knee.

- Radiculopathy is more likely to respond to centralization or peripheralization with repeated trunk motions.

- Both pathologies could have muscle weakness.

- Both pathologies could present from an insidious onset.

- Repeated knee motions are more likely to provoke a medial meniscus tear.

- Radiculopathy may cause decreased lumbar ROM and a positive SLR and slump tests.

- Radiculopathy may present with alterations in sensation and reflexes.

- Degenerative medial meniscus tear more likely to be provoked with weight bearing knee flexion movements (e.g., stairs, squatting) with trunk in relatively neutral position.

- Higher incidence of these injuries has been documented in dancers, gymnasts, figure skaters, weightlifters, and football players,[95, 178] although active spondylolysis has been reported in almost every sport.[148]

- The incidence of spondylolysis in the pediatric population was found to be 8.2% at an average age of 7.5 years. The incidence of spondylolisthesis was 10.9% at an average age of 6.5 years, with 75% being isthmic type.[180]

- Repetitive microtrauma leading to spondylolysis has been attributed to specific movements or activities, particularly hyperextension combined with rotation and loading.[95, 148, 178]

- If the client has lumbar spine instability, symptoms can include the following:[40-46, 181]

  - History of trauma

  - Repeated, unprovoked episodes of the low back feeling unstable

  - Inconsistent symptoms

  - Frequent self-manipulation

  - Symptoms aggravated with sustained positions and relieved with movement after these sustained positions

  - Aberrant motion with trunk flexion–extension

  - Gower's sign (full-trunk AROM without difficulty and having to use hands on their thighs to attain an upright trunk position when returning from full-trunk flexion)

  - Excessive trunk AROM

  - Possible high Beighton ligamentous laxity score (see chapter 8, Range of Motion Assessment)

- Reporting of a feeling of lumbar collapse with ordinary tasks helps **rule in** (SP 88) lumbar spinal instability.[46]

- Pain immediately on sitting down that is relieved by standing up helps **rule in** (SP 100) lumbar spinal instability.[47]

- Age < 37 years old helps **rule in** (SP 81) radiographic instability.[43]

Outcome Measures

- The Oswestry Disability Index, General Function Score, and Disability Rating Index have been reported in a recent systematic review.[182]

- Common outcome measures may be clinically applicable, including the FABQ, SF-36, Roland-Morris, and the Quebec Back Pain Disability Scale.[50]

Diagnostic Imaging

- Controversy surrounds limitations in computed tomography, single-photon computed tomography, and magnetic resonance imaging techniques in the accurate diagnosis of spondylolysis and spondylolisthesis.

- MRI is the imaging modality of choice for identifying associated nerve root compression. Single-photon emission computed tomography (SPECT) use is limited by a high rate of false-positive and false-negative results and by considerable ionizing radiation exposure.[94]

- MRI results suggest a high rate of active spondylolysis in young athletes with low back pain who test negative for spondylolysis on plain radiography. Magnetic resonance imaging appears to be useful in the early diagnosis of active spondylolysis.[183]

- The oblique view radiograph is designed to show a fracture in the region of the pars interarticularis (Scotty dog collar fracture).

- Radiographs and CT have ideal ability to help **rule out** (SN 98) and **rule in** (SP 97) spondylolysis.[84]

- MRI has ideal ability to **rule out** (SN 100) and good ability to **rule in** (SP 87) spondylolysis or spondylolisthesis.[83]

II. Observation

- Excessive lumbar lordosis posture can be commonly present (especially with instability) as the client compensates for lack of stability.

- Clinicians should monitor for observable signs of instability:[41, 42]

- Full-trunk flexion with difficulty recovering to upright posture (Gower's sign)
- Aberrant trunk AROM
- Spinal angulation on full-trunk AROM
- Creases on abdomen or low back

• A high score on the Beighton ligamentous laxity test should increase suspicion of lumbar spinal instability.[41] A Beighton score > 2 was suggested to help **rule in** (SP 86) radiographically confirmed instability of the lumbar spine.[43]

III. Triage and Screening

• All nonmusculoskeletal causes, as well as causes from related joints, should be ruled out.

• The following signs and symptoms are helpful for **ruling out** CES:[120-122]

- History of back pain (SN 94)
- Urinary retention (SN 90)
- Rapid symptom onset within 24 hours (SN 89)
- Sacral sensation loss (SN 85)
- Lower extremity weakness or gait loss (SN 84)
- Loss of sphincter tone (SN 80)

• A diagnostic prediction rule helps **rule out** (SN 95) a vertebral fracture when ≤1 of 5 variables were present and helps **rule in** (SP 96) a vertebral fracture when ≥4 of 5 variables were present.[123]

• Another diagnostic prediction rule helps **rule out** (SN 88) a vertebral fracture when only 1 of 4 variables were present and helps **rule in** (SP 96 when ≥ 2 of 4 variables present and SP 100 when ≥ 3 of 4 variables were present) a vertebral fracture.[106]

• The closed-fist percussion test has good ability to help **rule out** (SN 88, −LR 0.14) and ideal ability to help **rule in** (SP 90, +LR 8.8) vertebral compression fracture.[124]

• The supine sign has good ability to help **rule out** (SN 81, −LR 0.20) and ideal ability to help **rule in** (SP 93, +LR 11.6) vertebral compression fracture.[124]

IV. Motion Tests

• Clients with instability can demonstrate a catching sensation when returning to upright posture from trunk-flexed posture.[40]

• Pain with the sit-to-stand test (pain immediately on sitting down and relieved by standing up) helps **rule in** (SP 100, +LR Inf) lumbar instability.[47]

• Clients demonstrate Gower's sign with AROM of trunk.[41]

• Clients have pain during lateral trunk flexion and trunk extension motions.[184]

• Lumbar spine flexion of >53° (SP 86) was more helpful than total lumbar spine extension of >26° (SP 76) for **ruling in** radiographically confirmed lumbar spine instability.[43]

V. Muscle Performance Testing

• Muscle performance deficits should be noted, especially of trunk musculature.[185]

VI. Special Tests

• Passive lumbar extension test: has good ability to **rule out** (SN 84, −LR 0.17) and ideal ability to **rule in** (SP 90, +LR 8.8) radiographic instability. The interesting finding of this study is the average age of the clients investigated (68- to 69-year-old men and women; women were more prevalent in client number). Therefore this test may have more clinical utility for either degenerative spondylolisthesis or stenosis.

• Instability catch sign, painful catch sign, and apprehension sign: have limited ability to help rule in or out instability.[46]

• Single-leg stork (one-legged hyperextension) test: provides little help to rule out (SN 50-55) or rule in (SP 46-68) spondylolisthesis.[148]

- Kemp test: also provides little help to rule out or rule in spondylolisthesis (74–77% prevalence of positive findings in those with, but 76% prevalence positive finding in those without spondylolisthesis).[149]

- Percussion of spinous process: reproduced concordant pain in 58% of those with and 66% of those without MRI confirmed spondylolisthesis. Therefore, this assessment is of little clinical utility for this diagnosis.[149]

- Prone instability test: Although highly reliable, it has less than good ability to rule out (SN 61) or rule in (SP 57) radiographic instability.[43]

- Shear test: has been utilized for this diagnosis (unknown diagnostic accuracy).

- Lack of hypomobility during PA glides: as long as one variable (lack of hypomobility or lumbar flexion > 53°) was present, it had good ability to help **rule in** (SP 81, +LR 4.3) radiographic instability.[43]

- Lack of hypomobility during PA glides is helpful for **ruling in** (SP 95, +LR 8.6) radiographic instability.[43]

- Extension PPIVMs have good ability to help **rule in** (SP 81, +LR 4.3)[43] radiographic instability and ideal ability to help rule in (**SP 98**, **+LR 7.1**) translation and (**SP 97**, **+LR 8.4**) rotation radiographic instability.[45]

- Client self-rating of ≥4 on the side-lying active hip abduction test has good ability to help **rule in** (SP 92, +LR 4.6) a neuromuscular control deficit of the trunk musculature or inability to maintain postural control in the frontal plane and potential for developing pain.[151]

- Clinician rating of ≥2 on the side-lying active hip abduction test has less than good ability to help rule in (SP 85, +LR 2.7) a neuromuscular control deficit of the trunk musculature or inability to maintain postural control in the frontal plane and potential for developing pain.[151]

VII. Palpation

- Clinicians should use palpation of malalignment.[41]

- Clinicians should use palpation of step-off or one vertebra anterior.[150, 184]

- Palpation of spinous process anterior to the other (step-off) helps **rule in** (SP 87, +LR 4.7) spondylolisthesis.[150]

- Clients may have paravertebral muscle hypertrophy or spasm.[184]

- Clients may have hamstring spasm.[184]

- Localized tenderness over the facet joints without other root tension signs or neurologic signs may indicate facet joint pain.[18]

VIII. Physical Performance Measures

- Physical performance measures are appropriate for client status and required functional requirements.

POTENTIAL TREATMENT-BASED CLASSIFICATIONS

- Stability, exercise and conditioning, pain control (if client is pain dominant), and specific exercise direction may be used.

Lumbar Spine Mechanical-Related Pain

ICD-9: 724.2

ICD-10: G; M54.5 (low back pain); M99 (lumbosacral segmental or somatic dysfunction); S33.5, S33.7 (sprain of lumbar spine joint and ligament)

Low back pain of a mechanical nature is typically described as back pain related to facet joint dysfunction, segmental dysfunction, or somatic dysfunction. Mechanical LBP can often involve strain and sprain pathology.

I. Client Interview

Subjective History

- Clients have absence of pain when rising from sitting for facet joint–related pain.[49]

- Back pain is worse with extension from a flexed position.[186]

- Pain not being relieved by recumbent position helps **rule out** facet joint–related pain.[187, 188]

- Pain is worse in morning, aggravated with rest, and relieved with repeated motions.[49]

- Prevalence of low back pain is related to facet-joint dysfunction ranges from 15% to 40% of clients with diagnosis of double facet joint anesthesia.[186, 188, 189]

- Pain can be nonspecific with deep, achy quality, and usually occurs either unilaterally or bilaterally in the low back.[190, 191]

- Pain radiates across the low back and often into the proximal thigh, groin, and upper lumbar region.[18, 19]

- No symptoms occur with the Valsalva maneuver.[191]

- This condition is associated with post-traumatic facet synovitis.[19]

- Facet joint arthrosis most commonly affects the L4-L5 level, then L3-L4.[192]

- Facet joint arthrosis most commonly affects men, and the prevalence of this finding ranges from 57% of those in the 20- to 29-year-old age range to 100% of those over the age of 60 years.[192]

Outcome Measures

- Any appropriate lumbar spine–related outcome measure (Oswestry Disability Index, Fear Avoidance Beliefs Questionnaire, Global Rating of Change, Patient-Specific Functional Scale, Roland-Morris, and so on) may be used.

Diagnostic Imaging

- Diagnostic imaging is most likely necessary only in cases of concern for red flags or pathology warranting physician referral.

- Clinicians should use the imaging methods (as appropriate) listed in table 19.2 to assist with ruling out other pathology.

II. Observation

- Clients may have a normal gait pattern.[191]

- Clinicians should observe for compensated movements that clients use to avoid either a closing pattern (extension and ipsilateral side bending or rotation) or an opening pattern (flexion and contralateral side bending or rotation).

III. Triage and Screening

- All nonmusculoskeletal causes, as well as causes from related joints, should be ruled out.

- The following signs and symptoms are helpful for **ruling out** CES:[120-122]
  - History of back pain (SN 94)
  - Urinary retention (SN 90)
  - Rapid symptom onset within 24 hours (SN 89)
  - Sacral sensation loss (SN 85)
  - Lower extremity weakness or gait loss (SN 84)
  - Loss of sphincter tone (SN 80)

- A diagnostic prediction rule helps **rule out** (SN 95) a vertebral fracture when ≤1 of 5 variables were present and helps **rule in** (SP 96) a vertebral fracture when ≥4 of 5 variables were present.[123]

- Another diagnostic prediction rule helps **rule out** (SN 88) a vertebral fracture when only 1 of 4 variables were present and helps **rule in** (SP 96 when ≥ 2 of 4 variables present and SP 100 when ≥ 3 of 4 variables were present) a vertebral fracture.[106]

- The closed-fist percussion test has good ability to help **rule out** (SN 88, −LR 0.14) and ideal ability to help **rule in** (SP 90, +LR 8.8) vertebral compression fracture.[124]

- The supine sign has good ability to help **rule out** (SN 81, −LR 0.20) and ideal ability to help **rule in** (SP 93, +LR 11.6) vertebral compression fracture.[124]

IV. Motion Tests

- Combined motions of trunk hyper-extension and extension–rotation increase pain.[188]

V. Muscle Performance Testing

- Pain or limited muscle performance may be present in the surrounding muscles.
- Clinicians should assess myotomes to assist with ruling out more serious pathology.

VI. Special Tests

- Extension–rotation test: A (–) test had ideal ability to help **rule out** (SN 100, –LR 0) zygapophyseal joint–related pain.[20, 139]
- The following variables in the clinical prediction rule help to rule out or rule in zygapophyseal joint syndrome using zygapophyseal joint block as a reference standard:[193]
  - Age ≥ 50 years
  - Symptoms best when walking
  - Symptoms best when sitting
  - Onset of pain is paraspinal
  - (+) lumbar extension–rotation test

  ≥3 variables present: SN 85, **SP 91**, **+LR 9.7**, –LR 0.17

≥2 variables present: **SN 100**, SP 50, +LR 2.0, **–LR 0.0**

- Client self-rating of ≥4 on the side-lying active hip abduction test is helpful for **ruling in** (SP 92) a neuromuscular control deficit of the trunk musculature or inability to maintain postural control in the frontal plane and potential for developing pain.[151]
- Clinician rating of ≥2 on the side-lying active hip abduction test is helpful for **ruling in** (SP 85) a neuromuscular control deficit of the trunk musculature or inability to maintain postural control in the frontal plane and potential for developing pain.[151]

VII. Palpation

- Localized tenderness over the facet joints without other root tension signs or neurologic signs may indicate facet joint pain.[18]

VIII. Physical Performance Measures

- Any physical performance measure relevant to the physical demands of the client's hobbies or occupation may be used.

POTENTIAL TREATMENT-BASED CLASSIFICATIONS

- Mobility (if joint hypomobility is detected)

Differential Diagnosis of Spondylolisthesis and Lumbar Mechanical (Facet Joint) Pain

- A spondylolisthesis may have a palpable step deformity or depression over the spinous process, although diagnostic accuracy of this measure is somewhat limited.
- The stork test with extension will be positive for a spondylolisthesis and has been investigated in this pathology. This test likely could also be positive for facet joint pathology. The diagnostic accuracy for this measure is also limited.
- A spondylolisthesis is more common in younger athletes, whereas facet joint pain is more common in middle-aged to aging adults.
- An oblique view X-ray will show fracture of the pars interarticularis and possible translation of the lamina.

- Stabilization (if joint hypermobility is detected)
- Other potential TBCs: pain control (only if client is pain dominant), exercise and conditioning, specific exercise direction

Lumbar Spine Strain or Sprain

ICD-9: 724.2

ICD-10: M54.5 (low back pain); S33.5 (sprain and strain of lumbar spine)

Pathology or dysfunction of the lumbar spine involves muscle (strain) or ligament (sprain) injury of one or more muscles relative to the lumbar spine or associated regions. As mentioned previously, this dysfunction is often associated with mechanical LBP.

I. Client Interview

Subjective History

- Sprain or strain injury rates were significantly higher in football and gymnastics, and 80% of the injuries occurred in practice, 6% in competition, and 14% during preseason conditioning.[194]
- Muscle strains occurred with much greater frequency than other types of injuries, and acute back injuries were much more prevalent (59%) than overuse injuries (12%) or injuries associated with pre-existing conditions (29%).[194]
- Pain is often described as occurring in a broad area.[28, 195, 196]
- Clients will typically describe a history of trauma to the area.[28]

Outcome Measures

- Any appropriate lumbar spine–related outcome measure (Oswestry Disability Index, Fear Avoidance Beliefs Questionnaire, Global Rating of Change, Patient-Specific Functional Scale, Roland-Morris, and so on) may be used.

Diagnostic Imaging

- Diagnostic imaging is most likely necessary only in cases of concern for red flags or pathology warranting physician referral.
- Clinicians should use the imaging methods (as appropriate) listed in table 19.2 to assist with ruling out other pathology.

II. Observation

- If pain is acute, the client may display pain posturing and avoidance of positions that tensile load or stretch the involved soft-tissue structures.
- If pain is acute, the client may demonstrate compensation or guarding with activities of daily living.

III. Triage and Screening

- All nonmusculoskeletal causes, as well as causes from related joints, should be ruled out.
- The following signs and symptoms are helpful for **ruling out** CES:[120-122]
  - History of back pain (SN 94)
  - Urinary retention (SN 90)
  - Rapid symptom onset within 24 hours (SN 89)
  - Sacral sensation loss (SN 85)
  - Lower extremity weakness or gait loss (SN 84)
  - Loss of sphincter tone (SN 80)
- A diagnostic prediction rule helps **rule out** (SN 95) a vertebral fracture when ≤1 of 5 variables were present and helps **rule in** (SP 96) a vertebral fracture when ≥4 of 5 variables were present.[123]
- Another diagnostic prediction rule helps **rule out** (SN 88) a vertebral fracture when only 1 of 4 variables were present and helps **rule in** (SP 96 when ≥ 2 of 4 variables present and SP 100 when ≥ 3 of 4 variables were present) a vertebral fracture.[106]

- The closed-fist percussion test has good ability to help **rule out** (SN 88, −LR 0.14) and ideal ability to help **rule in** (SP 90, +LR 8.8) vertebral compression fracture.[124]

- The supine sign has good ability to help **rule out** (SN 81, −LR 0.20) and ideal ability to help **rule in** (SP 93, +LR 11.6) vertebral compression fracture.[124]

IV. Motion Tests

- Motion is restricted when muscle (strain) or ligament (sprain) involved is stressed.[28] A muscle strain is more likely to be stressed with muscle contraction and/or muscle stretch versus a ligament sprain, which is more likely to be stressed with any activity that stresses its integrity (usually any activity that causes it to lengthen).

- Clients may have muscle length deficits. These muscle length deficits may or may not be relevant to their pain and/or dysfunction.

V. Muscle Performance Testing

- Resistance to muscle involved (strain) or across ligament involved (sprain) will elicit pain.

VI. Special Tests

- Special testing likely will be (−) unless other pathology coexists.

- Extension–rotation test: A (−) test had ideal ability to help **rule out** (SN 100, −LR 0) zygapophyseal joint–related pain.[20, 139]

- Refer to the section Lumbar Spine Mechanical-Related Pain

- Client self-rating of ≥4 on the side-lying active hip abduction test is helpful for **ruling in** (SP 92) a neuromuscular control deficit of the trunk musculature or inability to maintain postural control in the frontal plane and potential for developing pain.[151]

- Clinician rating of ≥2 on the side-lying active hip abduction test is helpful for **ruling in** (SP 85) a neuromuscular control deficit of the trunk musculature or inability to maintain postural control in the frontal plane and potential for developing pain.[151]

VII. Palpation

- If the muscle (strain) or ligament (strain) is palpable, it likely will be tender to palpation.

- Localized tenderness over the facet joints without other root tension signs or neurologic signs may indicate facet joint pain.[18]

VIII. Physical Performance Measures

- Any physical performance measure relevant to the physical demands of the client's hobbies or occupation may be used.

POTENTIAL TREATMENT-BASED CLASSIFICATIONS

- Mobility (if joint hypomobility is detected)

- Stabilization (if joint hypermobility is detected)

- Other potential TBCs: pain control (only if client is pain dominant), exercise and conditioning, specific exercise direction

Ankylosing Spondylitis

Refer to chapter 20 (Sacroiliac Joint and Pelvic Girdle).

Differential Diagnosis of Lumbar Spine Instability
Versus Noninstability Pathologies

- Instability clients will more likely complain of an unprovoked feeling of the low back being unstable, history of trauma, and inconsistent symptoms than noninstability clients do.
- Instability clients will more likely be frequent manipulators of their spine.
- Instability clients will more likely be involved in higher-level activities or daily activities that could provoke their symptoms (e.g., they are more likely involved in sport activities).

CONCLUSION

The lumbar spine can present with multiple complex presentations and various clinical pathologies that are difficult to differentially diagnose. A systematic, detailed funnel approach utilizing best clinical evidence, as outlined in this chapter, affords the clinician the utmost opportunity to most accurately ascertain the client's impairments and potential diagnoses and thereby most appropriately treat the client.

20

SACROILIAC JOINT AND PELVIC GIRDLE

Michael P. Reiman, PT, DPT, OCS, SCS, ATC, FAAOMPT, CSCS

Sacroiliac joint (SIJ) dysfunction, more commonly referred to as pelvic girdle pain (PGP), is one of the most controversial dysfunctions in orthopedic medicine. Part of the controversy is encompassed in such variables as the actual prevalence of the dysfunction, the type of joint, the extent of movement at the joint, the diagnostic accuracy of imaging, and clinical examination of this region of the body. Due to its structure and function, the SIJ is highly dependent on ligamentous stabilization. Palpation of these ligaments may reveal potential pathology in cases where the ligament is stressed. The posterior sacroiliac and sacrotuberous ligaments are of particular vulnerability to such dysfunction. The sacrotuberous ligament is more vulnerable to sacral flexion (nutation) and innominate posterior ilial rotation.

The European guidelines for pelvic musculoskeletal pain, excluding gynecological or urological disorders, define it as follows:

Pelvic girdle pain generally arises in relation to pregnancy, trauma, arthritis, and osteoarthritis. Pain is experienced between the posterior iliac crest and the gluteal fold, particularly in the vicinity of the SIJ. The pain may radiate in the posterior thigh and can also occur in conjunction with, or separately in, the symphysis. The endurance capacity for standing, walking, and sitting is diminished. The diagnosis of PGP can be reached after exclusion of lumbar causes. The pain or functional disturbances in relation to PGP must be reproducible by specific clinical tests.[1]

Due to the controversial nature of this area, as well as limited evidence and agreement among experts examining this region, this chapter takes the approach that the diagnosis of the client with PGP is a diagnosis of exclusion.[1, 2]

CLINICALLY APPLIED ANATOMY

The sacrum is a wedge-shaped bone from superior to inferior, as well as posterior to anterior, held in suspension by ligamentous support with limited joint articulation (figure 20.1). The sacroiliac joint (SIJ) is described as a true diarthrodial-type synovial joint consisting of matching articular surfaces separated by a joint space (figure 20.2). This joint space contains synovial fluid, as do all synovial joints, enveloped by a fibrous capsule. The SIJ, although a synovial joint, is quite different from any other synovial joint due to some unique characteristics. The articulation between the wedge-shaped sacrum and the bilateral innominate bones is between

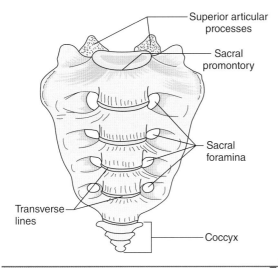

Figure 20.1 Anterior aspect of the sacrum.

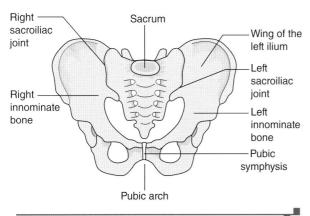

Figure 20.2 Anterior aspect of the pelvis showing the sacroiliac joint.

macroscopic ridges on each surface. These macroscopic ridges develop as adaptations to forces exerted on the joint. The SIJ has fibrocartilage in addition to hyaline cartilage. The articular surfaces of the SIJ are covered with hyaline cartilage. The iliac cartilage has the appearance of fibrocartilage. Significant variability in the size and shape of the SIJ has been described.

The SIJ must support the weight of the upper body as well as tolerate ground reaction forces with gait. Therefore, the SIJ is supported by multiple ligaments that limit its mobility and provide stability to the joint (figure 20.3). These ligaments are stressed with sacral and innominate motions. Additionally, these ligaments provide stability to the entire pelvic girdle.

CLIENT INTERVIEW

The interview is typically the first encounter the clinician will have with the client. As previously discussed in chapter 5 (Client Interview and Observation), this component of the examination can provide the clinician with a significant amount of information relevant to the probability of the client's presenting diagnosis. For purposes of this text, the interview is described relative to each body part or section, but the client interview generally includes subjective reports by the client, as well as findings from their outcome measures. Additionally included in this section is radiographic imaging. While clinicians should avoid biasing their examination by interpreting findings of radiographic imaging prior to seeing the client (in most cases without concerns for red flags and major medically related concerns), this point in the examination is most likely where clinicians will encounter radiographic imaging. Additionally, in some instances, radiographic imaging is necessary early in the examination for ruling out serious pathology prior to continuing with other components of the examination sequence.

Subjective

In a diagnostic study, Slipman and colleagues found a wide variability of pain referral patterns for the SIJ. While 94% of the pain was located in the buttock, pain also radiated to the thigh (48%) and to the lower leg, ankle, and foot (54% of the pain referral).[3] SIJ pain has been described as occur-

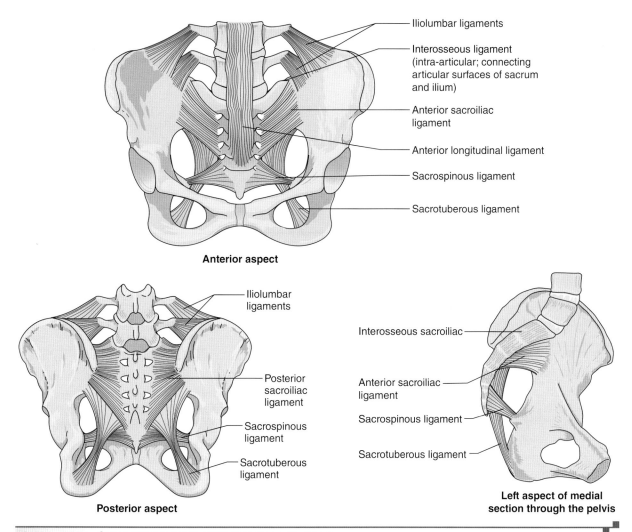

Iliolumbar ligaments

Interosseous ligament
(intra-articular; connecting
articular surfaces of sacrum
and ilium)

Anterior sacroiliac
ligament

Anterior longitudinal ligament

Sacrospinous ligament

Sacrotuberous ligament

Anterior aspect

Iliolumbar
ligaments

Posterior
sacroiliac
ligament

Sacrospinous
ligament

Sacrotuberous
ligament

Posterior aspect

Interosseous sacroiliac

Anterior sacroiliac
ligament

Sacrospinous ligament

Sacrotuberous ligament

**Left aspect of medial
section through the pelvis**

Figure 20.3   Supporting ligaments of the sacroiliac articulations.

ring anywhere from the lumbar paraspinals (from around L1 distally) to the entire leg.[3-5] As mentioned in chapter 19 (Lumbar Spine), convergence of pain in the low back, pelvis, and hip region makes it difficult to discern the true pain generator based solely on pain location.[6] The reported prevalence of SIJ dysfunction ranges from 7% to 45% of those with pain in the lumbar spine, pelvis, and hip region.[3, 7, 8] More recently, SIJ pain has been described as "an underappreciated source of mechanical low back pain, affecting between 15% and 30% of individuals with chronic, nonradicular pain."[9] It has been suggested that clients with SIJ dysfunction, especially acutely, will describe their pain location as directly over the posterior superior iliac spine (PSIS) in what has been described as the Fortin finger test (figure 20.4).[4] The point of maximum discomfort was described within 10 cm caudal and 3 cm lateral

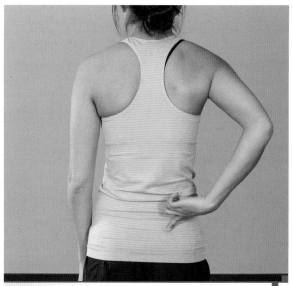

Figure 20.4   Fortin finger test.

to the PSIS in two studies[4, 10] and within 3 cm from PSIS in another study.[11] The pain referral patterns of the SIJ are extremely variable, though.

Mechanism of pain onset can be variable for the client with SIJ dysfunction. This is particularly the case since there are multiple types of SIJ dysfunction (sacroiliac joint dysfunction, symphysiolysis, and pregnancy-related posterior pelvic pain). The most frequently described mechanism is a combination of axial loading and rotation of the trunk.[9] If the mechanism was due to trauma, the client should be asked if it was a one-time macrotraumatic episode, or if it is a repetitive microtraumatic mechanism. The latter is likely suggestive of instability. As with the lumbar spine, other indicators of instability would include subjective reports of unprovoked episodes of feeling unstable or giving way, inconsistent symptoms, symptoms aggravated by prolonged positioning, and frequent self-manipulating.

Clinicians should also ask about aggravating factors. As referenced previously, there are specific indicators of lumbosacral instability. Clients with SIJ dysfunction due to hypomobility are generally accepted to have more pain with the larger excursion of movement of the pelvic girdle. Running would then be more painful than walking, which would be more painful than standing. Clients with SIJ dysfunction, whether it be from hypo- or hypermobility, will likely have pain with transitional movements. Such activities would include turning over in bed and rising from a seated position.[12] Clients with piriformis syndrome are likely to have increased pain when sitting with increased weight on that buttock (especially with a wallet) and decreased pain with a gait pattern where the hip is externally rotated.

Specific questions for potential SIJ instability would include questions related to pregnancy. Such questions might include the following: Is this their first pregnancy? If not, how many pregnancies have they had, and have they had previous similar episodes of pain and dysfunction with these pregnancies? Did the pain or dysfunction resolve after child birth? Have they had previous interventions for the pain or dysfunction? If so, were these interventions helpful? Pregnancy can result in SIJ pain due to altered posture (increased lordosis), weight gain, and third-trimester hormone-induced ligamentous relaxation.[9] Prevalence of low back pain (LBP) of 49% to 62% has been reported in pregnant women.[13, 14] Symptoms for the client with pregnancy-related posterior pelvic pain (PRPPP) are the following:[15] stabbing, aching pain between the posterior iliac crests and gluteal folds, with or without radiation down the leg; pain in symphysis pubis, as well as from other areas of pelvic girdle, typically increasing in intensity from weight-bearing activity; and pain in the pubic bone that can sometimes radiate to the pelvic floor and down the thigh. The peak time frame of symptom exacerbation for the pregnant client is typically between the 24th and 36th weeks of pregnancy.[16] Although questions regarding these issues should be asked, contraceptive pills, body mass index (BMI), height, and weight increase during pregnancy do not appear to be risk factors for the development of PRPPP. Risk factors shown to be correlative of PRPPP are young age, a previous history of LBP, heavy workload, and a history of previous trauma to the pelvic girdle region.[1]

The client's age may be indicative of specific low back and pelvic girdle dysfunctions. Clients with younger age were more likely to have intervertebral disc disease than pain of sacroiliac origin.[17] Young age was a risk factor for clients with PRPPP.[1] Younger age onset is also predictive of ankylosing spondylitis (AS). An age of onset ≤ 40 years was 100% SN for AS.[18]

As with other areas of the body relative to subjective examination, other questions of importance should include the following: What aggravates or relieves the symptoms? What is the nature of the pain? What is the intensity of the pain (pain level on a 0-10 scale)? Is pain noted with sleep? Is the pain significant with job or recreational activities? What medications is the client taking? Do these medications help with the pain or dysfunction? What, if any, diagnostic imaging has been done? What were the results of such imaging? Additionally, questions relative to red flags, or nonmusculoskeletal causes, should be addressed.

Other potential questions more specific to SIJ pain may include the presence of a leg length discrepancy and previous surgical fusion. In one study clients with chronic LBP were significantly more likely to have a leg length discrepancy of ≥5 mm than were the asymptomatic controls.[19] Increased SIJ stress, including degeneration, has been reported post lumbar spine fusion.[20-24]

Outcome Measures

Outcome measures are often body-part specific and are suggested to be used in that manner. Due to the significant overlapping in pain presentation, pain location, and objective measures between the low back and SIJ, the outcome measures discussed in chapter 19 (Lumbar Spine) are suggested for SIJ dysfunction when appropriate. The Oswestry Disability Index (ODI), Fear-Avoidance Beliefs Questionnaire (FABQ), Global Rating of Change (GROC), and the Patient-Specific Functional Scale (PSFS) are some of the more appropriate measures for clients with SIJ dysfunction. These measures are likely appropriate for PRPPP as well. The principal measures suggested for PRPPP are the Quebec Back Pain Disability Scale and the ODI.[1] The principal measures suggested for AS include the Visual Analogue Scale (VAS) for measuring spinal and night pain and the Bath AS Global score (BASG).[25]

Diagnostic Imaging

Diagnostic imaging for the SIJ, like other components of the examination process for this region, has some controversy (table 20.1). As with other areas of the body, namely closely associated areas of the lumbar spine and hip, abnormal findings on imaging of the sacroiliac joint have been found in asymptomatic clients. As with these related areas, these findings call into question the extent of standard practice diagnostic imaging.[26]

Radiographs

In stable and alert trauma clients, a thorough clinical examination will detect pelvic fractures with nearly 100% sensitivity (SN), thus rendering initial

TABLE 20.1 Diagnostic Accuracy of Various Imaging Modalities for the Sacroiliac Joint and Pelvic Girdle

Pathology	Diagnostic test	Gold standard	SN/SP
Spondylarthritis and SIJ dysfunction	Scintigraphy	Rheumatologist diagnosis	Any (unilateral or bilateral) 65/51 Bilateral, isolated, unilateral, and sacroiliitis SN were 65, 40, and 25, respectively/Respective SP 51, 58, and 93[27]
	Bone scan	Diagnostic block	13/100[28] 46/89[29]
	CT	Diagnostic block	58/69[30]
	MRI	Standardized definitions	26/100[31]
AS	MRI	NI	NI; reliability among 4 independent radiologists (κ) was 0.63 to 0.72, 0.73 for detection of erosion on the joint. ICC for erosion was 0.79. For comparison, the (κ) and ICC values for bone marrow edema were 0.61 and 0.93, respectively.[32]
	MRI	MRI standardized definitions from online data entry system	90/97[33]
Sacroiliitis in clients with confirmed AS	Scintigraphy	MRI	52/78[34]

SIJ = sacroiliac joint; NI = not investigated; CT = computed tomography; MRI = magnetic resonance imaging; AS = ankylosing spondylitis; ICC = interclass correlation coefficient

The color coding for suggestion of **good** and **ideal** diagnostic accuracy values reported in this table are without quality scoring (QUADAS), a very important aspect of determination of the clinical utility of such values. Therefore, it is suggested that the reader keep this in mind when interpreting such values.

radiography unnecessary.[35] Among all of the studies, the variables that were most predictive of a pelvic fracture included history of trauma, swelling, pain with compression of pelvis, complaints of instability, neuropathy, pain with hip range of motion (ROM), and pain during a rectal examination.[35]

Magnetic Resonance Imaging

Currently, MRI is the most sensitive imaging modality available for detection of sacroiliitis, often enabling detection of axial inflammation long before structural lesions are observed radiographically, thus facilitating early diagnosis of axial spondylarthritis (SpA). However, MRI will never capture all facets of SpA, and the expert opinion of a rheumatologist will remain the crucial step in recognition of this disease.[36] The imaging modality of choice is typically MRI. Bony erosions are more likely conclusively indicative of SpA over bony edema, since asymptomatic and nonspecific LBP clients can have bony edema, and these clients are less likely to have bony erosions shown on MRI.[37]

Computed Tomography

Computed tomography is generally accepted as the gold standard for already established bone changes. A limitation of CT scan is the inability to detect inflammation, which can be a common presentation in those with SIJ dysfunction.

Ultrasound

Ultrasound, as with its use in other areas of the body, is best for detection of soft-tissue pathology. It is particularly useful for detection of posterior ligamentous pathology. Ultrasound imaging can also be particularly helpful for pregnant women due to the lack of radiation.

Review of Systems

Refer to chapter 6 (Triage and Differential Diagnosis) for details on review of systems relevant to the sacroiliac joint and pelvic girdle.

OBSERVATION

Careful observation of the client's transfers and gait can be informative to the clinician. These tasks require optimal function of the lumbar spine, pelvis, and hip complex. Compensation or pain posturing during these tasks can alert the clinician to dysfunc-

tion in this region. Simple observation of whether or not the client sits with weight equally distributed on both buttocks could alert the clinician to the possibility of s dysfunctional side. For example, clients with piriformis syndrome are less likely to fully weight bear on the involved side.

Clients with a hypomobile SIJ will have observable dysfunction, more so with running gait than walking gait due to the increased demands on the pelvic girdle.[38] Alterations in stride length and timing can be indicative of mobility or stability dysfunction within the lumbo-pelvic-hip complex.[38] Pain during transitional movements is often a characteristic of pelvic girdle pain but is not usually characteristic of one particular dysfunction.[1]

Observation of posture is a necessary component of the examination for the client with pelvic girdle dysfunction. Deviations in the sagittal, frontal, and transverse planes should be noted both with static and dynamic postures.

Potentially observable signs of lumbar spine or SIJ instability can include creases posteriorly or on the abdomen, a step-off sign as with spondylolisthesis, full-trunk active range of motion (ROM), spinal angulation (lack of a rounded spine) on full-spine ROM, inability to recover from full-trunk flexion ROM without compensation (such as in Gower's sign, where the client puts their hands on their thighs to position the spine in an upright position), and deviation away from normal plane of movement with spine ROM. Decreased lumbar lordosis, increased thoracic kyphosis, and cervical hyperextension postures have been described in clients with AS.[39-41] Additionally, these clients have demonstrated muscle spasm and pain posturing with transitional movements.[40, 42]

Refer to chapter 19 (Lumbar Spine) for additional detail regarding observation.

TRIAGE AND SCREENING

Triage and screening is a necessary component of the examination process that should be done prior to continuing with the examination. Ruling out serious pathology (refer to chapter 6, Triage and Differential Diagnosis) and pain generation from other related (or close-proximity) structures helps the clinician more accurately determine the necessity of continuing with the other examination components to identify the actual source of the client's pain. Additionally, implementing strong screening tests (high SN and low –LR) at this point in the examination is suggested for narrowing down the competing diagnoses of the respective body region (lumbar spine and hip in this case) when this is applicable.

Ruling Out Serious Pathology: Red Flags

The clinician should be cognizant of red flags relevant to the lumbar spine and hip for the client with pathology related to the SIJ and pelvic girdle since these areas can refer pain here. Refer to chapters 19 and 24 for review of the relevant red flags for each of these areas.

Specific recommendations for the pelvic girdle include MRI, anteroposterior pelvis inlet and outlet, and flamingo radiographic views for ruling out sequestration of bone, bone and joint infections, and bone tumors. Blood tests and urinalysis are suggested laboratory tests. A (+) response from a guided local anesthetic injection is suggestive of ruling out nonmusculoskeletal causes of pelvic pain.[16]

A noncapsular pattern and gluteal swelling of unknown origin have also been suggested as red flags for the client with pelvic girdle–related pain.[43] The capsular pattern for the hip joint is flexion, abduction, and internal rotation as the most restricted motions. Gluteal swelling should be of insidious onset and not induced by trauma, for example.

Some specific red flag concerns for the SIJ and pelvic girdle include sign of the buttock and pelvic fracture. *Sign of the buttock* is a clinical assessment indicating a high suspicion of nonmusculoskeletal pain origin for the client's pain. The clinical examination is performed as follows:

- With the client lying supine, the clinician passively performs a straight leg raise to the point of restriction.
- The clinician then passively bends the client's knee, while keeping the thigh in the same position (same degree of hip flexion).
- The clinician then passively performs further hip flexion.
- A (+) test is indicated if hip flexion is still restricted or results in the same extent of pain as found with the knee extended.[44]

Pelvic fractures are most likely associated with trauma. Signs and symptoms of pelvic fracture include trauma, pain with pelvic palpation, pubic compression test, swelling, pain with compression of pelvis, complaints of instability, neuropathy, pain with hip ROM, and pain during a rectal examination.[35, 45, 46]

Vertebral fractures must be ruled out when examining for pelvic girdle pain, especially in the acutely injured or highly irritable client.

- A diagnostic prediction rule helps rule out (**SN 95, –LR 0.16**) a vertebral fracture when ≤1 of 5 variables were present and helps rule in (**SP 96, +LR 9.6**) a vertebral fracture when ≥4 of 5 variables were present.[47]
- The closed-fist percussion test helps rule out (**SN 88, –LR 0.14**) and rule in (**SP 90, +LR 8.8**) vertebral compression fracture.[48]
- The supine sign helps rule out (**SN 81, –LR 0.20**) and rule in (**SP 93, +LR 11.6**) vertebral compression fracture.[48]

Refer to chapter 18 for additional details on the preceding tests.

POSTERIOR PELVIC PALPATION

Client Position	Prone or sitting with bilateral upper and lower extremities relaxed
Clinician Position	Standing to client's side
Movement	The clinician carefully palpates the client's bilateral SIJ and sacrum (refer to Palpation section of this chapter).
Assessment	A (+) test is noted when local tenderness occurs with moderately deep palpation.
Statistics	SN 98 (not reported, or NR), SP 94 (NR), +LR 16.3, –LR 0.02, QUADAS 7, in a study of 66 clients with pelvic fractures (median age was 34 years, 32 women) presenting to emergency room within 24 hours of injury onset, using reference standard of CT scan[45]

ANTEROPOSTERIOR AND LATERAL COMPRESSION TEST

Client Position	Supine with bilateral upper and lower extremities relaxed
Clinician Position	Standing at client's side, directly facing them
Movemen	The clinician applies an anterior-to-posterior compression force and a lateral compression force to the iliac wings.
Assessment	A (+) test is reproduction of pain during compression.
Statistics	SN 98 (NR), SP 24 (NR), +LR 1.3, –LR 0.08, QUADAS 7, in a study of 66 clients with pelvic fractures presenting to emergency room within 24 hours of injury onset (median age was 34 years, 32 women), using reference standard of CT scan[45]

Video 20.1 **in the web resource shows a demonstration of this test.**

HIP FLEXION TEST

Client Position	Supine with bilateral lower extremities extended
Clinician Position	Standing to the client's side, directly facing them
Movement	The client performs an active hip flexion.
Assessment	A (+) test is reproduction of pain during the active movement, or the inability to perform such movement.
Statistics	**SN 90 (NR), SP 95 (NR), +LR 18, –LR 0.10**, QUADAS 9, in a study of 20 clients with pelvic fracture (mean age 57 years, 9 women, acute duration of symptoms), using a reference standard of radiologic examination[46]

PUBIC COMPRESSION TEST

Client Position	Supine with bilateral lower extremities extended
Clinician Position	Standing at client's side, directly facing them
Movement	The clinician applies a downward pressure on the client's pubic bones.
Assessment	A (+) test is reproduction of pain during compression.
Statistics	SN 55 (NR), SP 84 (NR), +LR 3.4, –LR 0.53, QUADAS 9, in a study of 20 clients with pelvic fracture (mean age 57 years, 9 women, acute duration of symptoms), using a reference standard of radiologic examination[46]

PASSIVE HIP MOTION

Client Position	Supine with bilateral lower extremities extended
Clinician Position	Standing at client's side, directly facing them
Movement	The clinician performs passive hip flexion, abduction, adduction, internal, and external rotation of the client's hip (refer to chapter 24, Hip).
Assessment	A (+) test is reproduction of pain during passive movement.
Statistics	SN 53 (NR), SP 76 (NR), +LR 2.2, –LR 0.62, QUADAS 7, in a study of 66 clients with pelvic fractures presenting to emergency room within 24 hours of injury onset (median age was 34 years, 32 women), using reference standard of CT scan[45]

Ruling Out Pain Generation From Other Related Structures

Sacroiliac joint dysfunction, with its complexity and controversial nature, has often been suggested as a diagnosis of exclusion. The examination component would thus begin with a focus primarily, but not exclusively, on ruling out more common diagnoses that refer pain to this region, eventually focusing on SIJ dysfunction as the only diagnosis left standing. This process, called *diagnosis by exclusion*, has been advocated in other difficult-to-diagnose syndromes.[49]

Rule Out Lumbar Spine

The following section lists suggested special tests for ruling out the lumbar spine as a potential pain generator for the client with presentation of hip pain. The details of each of these tests can be found in chapter 19. Additionally, as with any joint, clearing active range of motion (AROM) with or without overpressure is necessary. AROM of all motions as per the lower quarter screen described in chapter 7 should be implemented. In order to fully clear the lumbar spine and peripheral joints, full AROM (with overpressure if pain-free) must be present.

Radiculopathy or Discogenic-Related Pathology
This pathology can be ruled out with a combination of ROM and special tests assessments.

- Repeated Motions (Range of Motion)
  - Centralization or peripheralization: 5-20 reps
    - **SN 92 (NR)**, SP 64 (NR), +LR 2.6, **−LR 0.12**, QUADAS 12[50]
    - SN 40 (28-54), **SP 94 (73-99)**, **+LR 6.7**, −LR 0.64, QUADAS 13[51]
- Special Tests
  - Straight leg raise test
    - **SN 97 (NR)**, SP 57 (NR), +LR 2.2, **−LR 0.05**, QUADAS 10[52]
    - Pooled analysis: **SN 92 (87-95)**, SP 28 (18-40), +LR 2.9, **−LR 0.29**[53]

      SN 91 (82-94), SP 26 (16-38), +LR 2.7, **−LR 0.35**[54]
  - Slump test

- **SN 83 (NR)**, SP 55 (NR), +LR 1.8, **−LR 0.32**, QUADAS 11[55]
- **SN 84 (NR)**, SP 83 (NR), +LR 4.9, −LR 0.19, QUADAS 7[56]

Facet Joint Dysfunction
This is ruled out with the seated extension–rotation test. As noted in the lumbar spine chapter, facet joint dysfunction is ruled in with posterior–anterior spinal joint play assessments eliciting stiffness and concordant pain.

- Seated Extension–Rotation
  - **SN 100 (NR)**, SP 22 (NR), +LR 1.3, **−LR 0.0**, QUADAS 11[57]
  - **SN 100 (NR)**, SP 12 (NR), +LR 1.1, **−LR 0.0**, QUADAS 10[58]

Rule Out Hip Joint

The hip joint should be ruled out as a potential pain generator for the client presenting with pain in the SIJ and pelvic girdle region. The patellar–pubic percussion test can help clinicians rule out the potential for hip fracture. When ruling out hip osteoarthritis and intra-articular pathology, they can also use a combination of age, limitations in ROM, subjective complaints, and the flexion–adduction internal rotation test.

Hip Fracture
During clinical examination, this is best ruled out with the patellar–pubic percussion test.

- Patellar–Pubic Percussion Test
  - Pooled analysis: **SN 95 (92-97)**, **SP 86 (78-92)**, **+LR 6.11**, **−LR 0.07**, across three studies with 782 clients[59]

Hip Osteoarthritis
The gold standard clinical diagnosis for hip osteoarthritis is as follows: People with hip pain and hip internal rotation (IR) ROM of ≥15° who experienced pain with IR, had morning stiffness for ≤60 minutes, and were 50 years old or older could be identified as having hip osteoarthritis (OA; SN 86).[60]

Femoroacetabular Impingement, Labral Tear, or Intra-Articular Pathology
Other hip-related pathologies should also be considered, dependent on client presentation. Refer to chapter 24 for more detail. The potential for hip impingement (femoroacetabular impingement)

or labral tear must also be ruled out. The flexion-adduction-internal rotation (FADDIR) test has been described for both pathologies. The diagnostic accuracy of this test in a recent meta-analysis is as follows:

- Pooled **SN 94 (88-97)**, SP 8 (2-20), +LR 1.02, **−LR 0.48**, across four studies with 128 clients (MRA reference standard)[59]

- Pooled **SN 99 (95-100)**, SP 7 (0-34), +LR 1.06, **−LR 0.15**, across two studies with 157 clients (arthroscopy reference standard)[59]

Additionally, as with any joint, clearing AROM with or without overpressure is necessary. AROM of all motions, as per the lower quarter screen described in chapter 7, should be implemented. In order to fully clear the hip joint and lumbar spine (in this case), full AROM (with overpressure if pain-free) must be present.

Sensitive Tests: Sacroiliac Joint

Laslett and colleagues assessed the diagnostic utility of the McKenzie method of mechanical assessment combined with the following sacroiliac tests: distraction, thigh thrust, Gaenslen's test, sacral thrust, and compression.[2] The McKenzie assessment consisted of flexion in standing, extension in standing, right and left side gliding, flexion in lying, and extension in lying. The movements were repeated in sets of 10, and centralization and peripheralization were recorded. If it was determined that repeated movements resulted in centralization, the client was considered to present with pain of discogenic origin.

- Cluster of tests: If discogenic origin of pain was ruled out, the cluster of tests exhibited the following (3 out of 5 required to be positive):
  - SN 94 (72-99), SP 78 (61-89), +LR 4.29, −LR 0.80, QUADAS 12, in a study of 48 clients (mean age 42.1 ± 12.3 years, 32 women, mean duration of symptoms 31.8 ± 38.8 months) with symptomatic SIJ pain, and using fluoroscopically guided contrast-enhanced SIJ arthrography as a reference standard[2]

The test with the strongest diagnostic capability of ruling out SIJ-related dysfunction is the thigh thrust test:

- Thigh Thrust Test
  - **SN 88 (64-97)**, SP 69 (47-82), +LR 2.80, **−LR 0.18**, QUADAS 12[2]

MOTION TESTS

The motion at the SIJ, while limited, is interdependent on motion at the hip and lumbar spine joints. Movement at one of these regions affects motions at the others. Additionally, at the SIJ, sacral flexion (nutation) and sacral extension (contranutation) stress the sacrotuberous and long dorsal ligaments, respectively (figure 20.5). Nutation of the sacrum

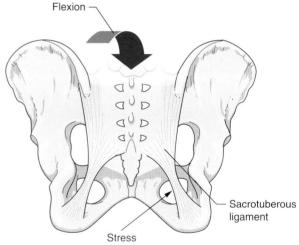

Sacral nutation

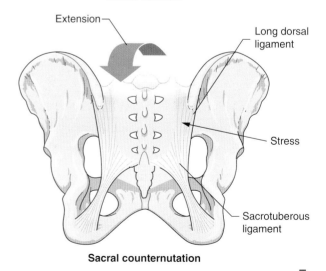

Sacral counternutation

Figure 20.5 Stress on the sacrotuberous ligament due to sacral nutation of the long dorsal ligament due to sacral counternutation.

(flexion of the sacrum relative to the ilia) results in the superior aspect of the sacrum moving anterior (figure 20.6). This motion is generally the result of load bearing and a functional adaptation to stabilize the pelvic girdle. Counternutation or contranutation (extension of the sacrum relative to the ilia), on the other hand, results in the superior aspect of the sacrum moving posterior (figure 20.6).

It has been suggested that pregnant and postpartum women are likely to have excessive joint play or arthrokinematics at the SIJ.[9, 38, 61-63] On the other hand, limited joint play should be expected for those clients presenting with spondylarthritis or AS. In those clients with piriformis syndrome, the combined motions of flexion, adduction, and internal rotation of the involved hip are suggested to be provocative.[64, 65]

Motion assessment is a very important aspect of the examination for the orthopedic client. Motion dysfunction can be used to differentiate contractile versus noncontractile tissue (chapter 9 and some content in chapter 1). Assessment of end-feel, potential capsular patterns, and ROM norm values (table 20.2) can give the clinician an appreciation of the potential impairments for the orthopedic client they are assessing. AROM, PROM, and joint play assessments are necessary for determining not only the presence or absence of joint dysfunction but also the precise aspects of the motion that are dysfunctional.

Passive and Active ROMs

Refer to chapters 19 (Lumbar Spine) and 24 (Hip) for goniometry testing relevant to the SIJ and pelvic girdle. The SIJ and pelvic girdle do not have independent goniometric measurement.

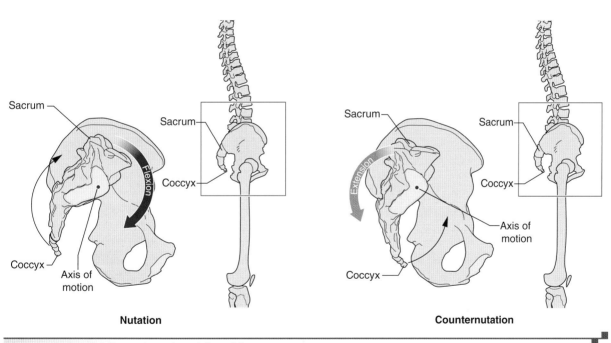

Nutation   **Counternutation**

Figure 20.6 Nutation and counternutation of the sacrum.

TABLE 20.2   Sacroiliac Joint and Pelvic Girdle Arthrology

Joint	Close-packed position	Resting position	Capsular pattern	ROM norms	End-feel
Sacroiliac	Not described	Not described	Pain when the joint is stressed	Motion of the SIJ is in three planes of movement, albeit limited in all three planes:[66] • Rotation around the X-axis corresponds with sagittal plane movement (sacral flexion–extension) and ranges from –1.1° to 2.2° with translation in this plane ranging from –0.3 to 8 mm. • Rotation around the Y-axis corresponds with horizontal or transverse plane of movement (rotation) and ranges from –0.8° to 4° with translation in this plane from –0.2 to 7 mm. • Rotation around the Z-axis corresponds with coronal or frontal plane movement (side bending) and ranges from –0.5° to 8° with translation in this plane from –0.3 to 6 mm.	Firm
Pubic symphysis	Not described	Not described	Pain when the joint is stressed	3° of rotation and 2° of translation have been described.[67] During single-leg stance, 2.6 mm of vertical and 1.3 mm of sagittal movement have been demonstrated on the weight-bearing side. During walking, the pubic symphysis can piston up and down, up to 2.2 mm vertically and 1.3 mm sagittally.[68]	Firm

PASSIVE ACCESSORIES

POSTERIOR-ANTERIOR GLIDE: SACRUM

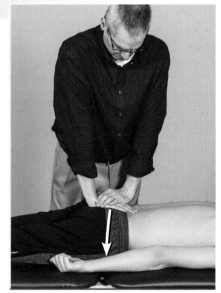

Client Position	Prone, legs extended
Clinician Position	Standing at the client's side
Stabilization	The rest of the client's body on the table serves as the stabilizing force.
Movement and Direction of Force	Clinician places hand over hand purchase with purchasing fingers pointing cranially. Keeping bilateral elbows straight, clinician imparts force directly anterior to assess overall SIJ mobility. Force directed at the superior part of the sacrum assesses only sacral flexion or nutation movement; force directed at the inferior part of the sacrum assesses only sacral extension or counter-nutation movement.
Assessment	Assessment is done for joint play/passive accessory motion, client response, and end-feel. Reproduction of concordant pain suggests dysfunction. Impaired joint mobility or end-feel may also suggest dysfunction if concordant pain is also reproduced.

Figure 20.7

ANTERIOR ROTATION GLIDE OF INNOMINATE

 Video 20.8 in the web resource shows a demonstration of this test.

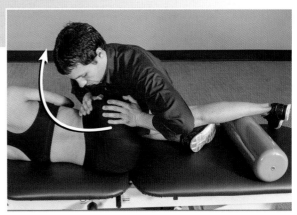

Figure 20.8

Client Position	Lying on their side with the top leg (leg to be assessed) (right as shown) resting on a pillow or bolster, in neutral extension, and parallel to the table
Clinician Position	Standing directly in front of the client
Stabilization	The client's body resting on the table serves as the stabilizing force. The clinician purchases their cranial hand (right as shown) over the client's anterior superior iliac spine (ASIS) and anterior iliac crest and their caudal hand (left as shown) over the client's ischial tuberosity.
Movement and Direction of Force	The clinician anteriorly rotates the innominate so that the ASIS moves toward the anterior femur/thigh in an anterior rotation direction (in a clockwise direction [for right innominate as shown]).
Assessment	Assessment is done for joint play/passive accessory motion, client response, and end-feel. Reproduction of concordant pain suggests dysfunction. Impaired joint mobility or end-feel may also suggest dysfunction if concordant pain is also reproduced.

POSTERIOR ROTATION GLIDE OF INNOMINATE

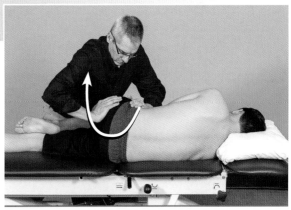

Figure 20.9

Client Position	Lying on their side with the side to be assessed on top or facing toward ceiling (left as shown) and in end available range hip flexion. Client's knee rests on clinician's anterior hip.
Clinician Position	Standing directly in front of the client
Stabilization	The client's body resting on the table serves as the stabilizing force. The clinician purchases their cranial hand (left as shown) over the client's ASIS and anterior iliac crest and their caudal hand (right as shown) over the ischial tuberosity.
Movement and Direction of Force	The clinician posteriorly rotates the innominate so that the ASIS moves away from the anterior femur/thigh, or in the posterior rotation direction (in a counterclockwise direction [for left innominate as shown]).
Assessment	Assessment is done for joint play/passive accessory motion, client response, and end-feel. Reproduction of concordant pain suggests dysfunction. Impaired joint mobility or end-feel may also suggest dysfunction if concordant pain is also reproduced.

The anterior and posterior rotation glides of the innominate are a general assessment of overall joint mobility of the SIJ and pelvic girdle. As with other mobility assessment techniques, clinicians should employ repeated movements of these techniques to determine client response. If the client's symptoms improve with repeated movement, the clinician should implement that particular movement as a potential intervention as part of the client's multimodal treatment approach.

Flexibility

Refer to chapters 19 (Lumbar Spine) and 24 (Hip) for flexibility assessments relevant to the SIJ.

MUSCLE PERFORMANCE TESTING

Refer to chapters 19 (Lumbar Spine) and 24 (Hip) for details on muscle performance testing for pelvic girdle–related musculature. The client with pelvic girdle dysfunction is likely to have muscle performance deficits. Resisted hip abduction and rotation are suggested to be provocative and likely weak for clients with piriformis syndrome.[64, 65, 69] Limited strength in the involved regions of the spine, hip, and shoulder is expected in clients with AS.[25] A positive direct correlation between hip muscle adductor weakness and the severity of pelvic girdle–related pain or dysfunction has been demonstrated.[70]

SPECIAL TESTS

As mentioned in chapter 10 (Special Tests), in many cases the clinician is overly dependent on the performance and interpretation of special test findings with respect to differential diagnosis of the client's presenting pain. Utilization of special tests for ruling in (or helping to diagnose) a particular pathology should occur at this point in the examination process. It is also hoped that the clinician has a much clearer picture of the client's presentation prior to this point in the examination and will therefore depend minimally on special test findings with respect to diagnosis of the client's pain.

Pelvic girdle diagnosis has traditionally relied on various forms of assessment, including signs and symptoms, as well as special testing. Special testing for the pelvic girdle primarily includes static ana-

tomical position testing, motion palpation testing, and pain provocation testing. Static anatomical position testing can include palpation of the sacral sulcus, pubic symphysis, anterior superior iliac spine, and iliac crests to detect asymmetries from side to side. A systematic review determined that motion of the SIJ is limited to minute amounts of rotation and translation, suggesting that clinical methods utilizing position and motion palpation testing for the diagnosis of SIJ pathology may have limited clinical utility.[66] This same review revealed that multiple studies concluded that clinicians should use caution when performing these tests during assessment.[66]

Levangie investigated several anatomic landmark and motion testing assessments of the pelvic girdle.[71] Gillet's test (+LR 1.2), long-sitting test (+LR 1.1), standing flexion test (+LR 0.81), standing ASIS asymmetry > 3 mm (+LR 0.94), standing PSIS asymmetry > 3 mm (+LR 1.1), and seated PSIS asymmetry > 3 mm (+LR 0.88) all demonstrated less than impressive diagnostic capabilities. None of these tests demonstrated the ability to alter posttest probability of a diagnosis even to a minimal degree.[72]

Laslett and colleagues[2] assessed the diagnostic utility of the McKenzie method of mechanical assessment combined with the following pain provocation sacroiliac tests: distraction, thigh thrust, Gaenslen's test, sacral thrust, and compression. The McKenzie assessment employed in this study consisted of flexion in standing, extension in standing, right and left side gliding, flexion in lying, and extension in lying. The movements were repeated in sets of 10, and centralization and peripheralization were recorded. If it was determined that repeated movements resulted in centralization, the client was considered to present with pain of discogenic origin. A hip joint assessment was also employed.[73] If discogenic and hip joint origin of pain were ruled out, the cluster of tests exhibited the following (3 out of 5 required to be positive):[2]

- Three (+) tests: **SN 94 (72-99)**, SP 78 (61-89), +LR 4.29, **−LR 0.80**, QUADAS 12, in a study of 48 clients (mean age 42.1 ± 12.3 years, 32 women, mean duration of symptoms 31.8 ± 38.8 months) with symptomatic SIJ pain, and using fluoroscopically guided contrast-enhanced SIJ arthrography as a reference standard

- Two (+) tests: **SN 93 (72-99)**, SP 66 (48-80), +LR 2.7, **−LR 0.10**

- Two (+) tests of distraction, thigh thrust, compression and sacral thrust: **SN 88 (64-97), SP 78 (61-89), +LR 4.0, −LR 0.16**

Therefore, diagnostic accuracy for pain provocation testing is clearly stronger than that of other types of SIJ and pelvic girdle testing. The difficulty with reliance on pain provocation testing for this region is that it does not necessarily guide treatment or determine the specific dysfunction. This type of testing merely implicates the SIJ and pelvic girdle as the potential pain generator. Along these lines, though, SIJ provocation tests appear morphologically confounded; that is, they may challenge other potential pain-generating tissues in addition to the purported structure of interest.

The following is recommended for diagnosis of a particular SIJ dysfunction. First, anterior and posterior innominate rotations are the primary dysfunctions described in the literature. Biomechanically, an anterior innominate rotation correlates with a sacral extension motion, while a posterior innominate rotation correlates with a sacral flexion motion, and vice versa. Sacral dysfunctions are very difficult to diagnose due to limited motion and limitations in landmark testing. The suggested sequence for SIJ or pelvic girdle examination of a hypomobile joint is as follows:

- Rule out competing diagnoses and pain generators.
- Use the cluster of tests from Laslett and colleagues to determine presence of dysfunction.[2]
- Use the anterior and posterior rotation glide assessment as described previously to determine the direction of innominate restriction. Treat in the direction of improving symptoms (e.g., repeated mobilization anteriorly improves symptoms, treat with repeated anterior innominate mobilizations).

Index of Special Tests

Pain Provocation Testing

Posterior Shear Test (Thigh Thrust)
Gaenslen's Test
Distraction Test

Compression Test
Sacral Thrust Test

Pelvic Girdle Pain and Pregnancy-Related Posterior Pelvic Pain

Active Straight Leg Raise Test
Stork Test (March Test or Gillet's Test)

Self-Test P4

Movement Testing

Standing Stork or March Test
Standing Flexion Test (Standing Forward Bending Test)

Supine Long-Sitting Test
Prone Knee-Bending Test (Deerfield's Test)

Muscle Dysfunction: Piriformis Syndrome

FAIR Test

Case Studies

Go to www.HumanKinetics.com/OrthopedicClinicalExamination and complete these case studies for chapter 20:

- Case study 1 discusses a 28-year-old male with posterior pelvic girdle and low back pain.
- Case study 2 discusses a 28-year-old female who is pregnant and has low back pain.

Abstract Links

Go to www.HumanKinetics.com/OrthopedicClinicalExamination to access abstract links on these issues:

Active straight leg raise test

Hip flexion test

Hip osteoarthritis

Patellar-pubic-percussion test

Posterior pelvic palpation

Posterior shear test (thigh thrust)

Repeated motions, centralization or peripheralization

Seated extension-rotation

Slump test

Stork test

Straight leg raise test

PAIN PROVOCATION TESTING

POSTERIOR SHEAR TEST (THIGH THRUST)

 Video 20.10 in the web resource shows a demonstration of this test.

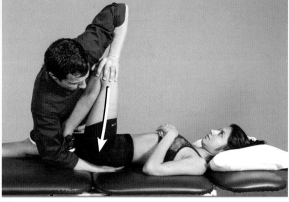

Figure 20.10

Client Position	Supine with both legs extended, arms relaxed
Clinician Position	Standing on the opposite side of leg to be tested, facing the client
Movement	The client flexes their hip to 90°, with neutral hip adduction. The clinician places their hand (right as shown) on the client's sacrum just medial to the PSIS on the test side (right as shown). The clinician applies an axial force through the femur at different angles of hip adduction or abduction and then applies a longitudinal force for up to 30 seconds, adding a bounce force at the end of the time frame if no pain has been reproduced prior. The clinician can perform up to five thrusts if no concordant pain is initially reproduced. If the first side is not painful, the other side should be tested in the same manner prior to determining the test is (−).
Assessment	A (+) test is indicated when the client's concordant SIJ-related pain is produced.
Statistics	This test was identified as a clinical test valuable for identifying clients who would likely benefit from placement into the stabilization treatment classification.[74]

- **SN 88 (64-97)**, SP 69 (82), +LR 2.80, **−LR 0.18**, QUADAS 12, in a study of 48 clients (mean age 42.1 ± 12.3 years, 32 women, mean duration of symptoms 31.8 ± 38.8 months) with symptomatic SIJ pain, and using fluoroscopically guided contrast-enhanced SIJ arthrography as a reference standard[2]

- Right side: SN 55 (22-84), SP 70 (51-85), +LR 1.9, −LR 0.62, QUADAS 10; Left side: SN 45 (18-75), SP 86 (67-95), +LR 3.3, −LR 0.63, in a study of 40 clients with chronic LBP for >3 months or active sacroiliitis (median age 26 years, 16 women), and using MRI with and without IV gadolinium as a reference standard[75]

- SN 17 (symphysiolysis), 84 (one-sided sacroiliac syndrome), 90 (pelvic girdle syndrome), and 93 (double-sided sacroiliac syndrome); SP 98, +LR 46.5, −LR 0.07, QUADAS 7, in a study of 2,269 pregnant female clients, 535 with pelvic joint pain (age NR, all in 33 weeks gestation), and using pathology definition as a reference standard[76]

- SN 62 (NR), SP 72 (NR), +LR 2.2, –LR 0.53, QUADAS 8, in a study of 123 pregnant clients (mean age range 29.6–32.5 years, 36 weeks gestation) with pregnancy-related pelvic pain, and using Doppler imaging vibration as a reference standard[77]
- SN 80 (NR), **SP 100, +LR Inf**, –LR 0.2, QUADAS 9, in a study of 40 clients with SIJ dysfunction (mean age 36 years, 30 women, mean duration symptoms NR), and using SIJ injection as a reference standard[78]
- SN 88 (NR), SP 89 (NR), +LR 8.0, –LR 0.13, QUADAS 7, in a study of 23 clients waiting for disc surgery (mean age 43 years, 14 women), 30 clients seen ≥6 weeks after disc surgery (mean age 45 years, 18 women), 25 clients with pelvic girdle pain in pregnancy (mean age 29 years), and 32 clients with pelvic girdle pain postpartum, and using CT scan as a reference standard for disc clients and pelvic girdle pain classification as a reference standard for pregnancy-related clients[79]

Critical Clinical Pearls

When performing the thigh thrust test, clinicians should keep the following in mind:

- The original description of the test is with the hand on the sacrum.
- The hand should be placed medial to the PSIS of the side being assessed.
- A gradual, progressive load is applied longitudinally through the femur for up to 30 seconds (assuming no pain reproduction) prior to thrust application.
- Assessment of bilateral sides should be pain-free in order for the test to be considered negative.
- The painful side and the side of test application should not be correlated.

GAENSLEN'S TEST

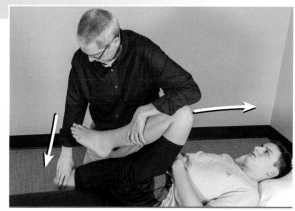

Figure 20.11

Client Position	Supine with both legs extended, arms relaxed
Clinician Position	Standing at client's side of the lower extremity to be tested, directly facing client
Movement	The clinician brings one of the client's legs into full hip and knee flexion, while the client maintains the hip closest to them (right as shown) in an extended position off the side of the table. The clinician initially applies overpressure to the flexed extremity, then to both extremities simultaneously if no reproduction of pain occurs. The clinician applies 3 to 5 torsions of overpressure (or stops if pain is reproduced) in order to rule out the potential for pelvic girdle pathology. If this sequence is not painful, the clinician has the client move to the other side of the table and performs an alternate leg movement sequence prior to determining the test is (–).
Assessment	A (+) test is noted when pain is reproduced in either SIJ region with performance of the test.
Statistics	• Right: SN 53 (30-75), SP 71 (53-84), +LR 1.84, –LR 0.66, QUADAS 12[2] • Left: SN 50 (27-73), SP 77 (60-89), +LR 2.21, –LR 0.65, QUADAS 12, in a study of 48 clients (mean age 42.1 ± 12.3 years, 32 women, mean duration of symptoms 31.8 ± 38.8 months) with symptomatic SIJ pain, and using fluoroscopically guided contrast-enhanced SIJ arthrography as a reference standard[2]

DISTRACTION TEST

Client Position	Supine with bilateral legs straight, arms relaxed
Clinician Position	Standing at side of leg to be tested, directly facing client
Movement	The clinician applies pressure to the client's ASIS on both sides (crossing arms over) in a posterolateral direction. The clinician applies the distraction force for up to 30 seconds, adding a bounce force at the end of the time frame if no pain has been reproduced prior.
Assessment	A (+) is indicated by reproduction of client's symptoms.
Statistics	SN 60 (36-80), SP 81 (65-91), +LR 3.20, –LR 0.49, QUADAS 12, in a study of 48 clients (mean age 42.1 ± 12.3 years, 32 women, mean duration of symptoms 31.8 ± 38.8 months) with symptomatic SIJ pain, and using fluoroscopically guided contrast-enhanced SIJ arthrography as a reference standard[2]
Note	Both distraction and compression test are named according to the description of what is happening to the anterior SIJ and respective ligamentous structures.

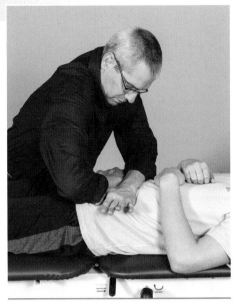

Figure 20.12

COMPRESSION TEST

Client Position	Side lying with hip and knees slightly bent
Clinician Position	Standing directly behind client at the level of their hips
Movement	The clinician compresses the client's pelvis, applying pressure over the anterior portion of the iliac crest and directed at the opposite iliac crest. The clinician applies force for up to 30 seconds, adding a bounce force at the end of the time frame if no pain has been reproduced prior. If the first side is not painful, the other side should be tested in the same manner by having the client lie on their other side prior to determining the test is (–).
Assessment	A test is (+) if symptoms are reproduced.
Statistics	SN 69 (44-86), SP 69 (51), +LR 2.20, –LR 0.46, QUADAS 12, in a study of 48 clients (mean age 42.1 ± 12.3 years, 32 women, mean duration of symptoms 31.8 ± 38.8 months) with symptomatic SIJ pain, and using fluoroscopically guided contrast-enhanced SIJ arthrography as a reference standard[2]
Note	Both distraction and compression tests are named according to the description of what is happening to the anterior SIJ and respective ligamentous structures.

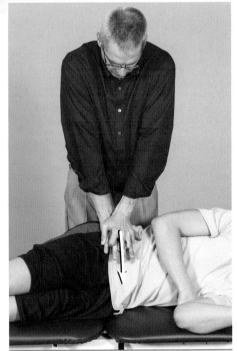

Figure 20.13

SACRAL THRUST TEST

Client Position	Prone with bilateral legs extended, arms relaxed
Clinician Position	Standing, facing the client's legs
Movement	The clinician delivers an anteriorly directed thrust directly over the client's sacrum. The clinician applies three to five hard thrusts at the level of the client's third sacral spinous level.
Assessment	A test is (+) if pain is reproduced in the SI region.
Statistics	SN 63 (39-82), SP 75 (58-87), +LR 2.50, –LR 0.50, QUADAS 12, in a study of 48 clients (mean age 42.1 ± 12.3 years, 32 women, mean duration of symptoms 31.8 ± 38.8 months) with symptomatic SIJ pain, and using fluoroscopically guided contrast-enhanced SIJ arthrography as a reference standard[2]

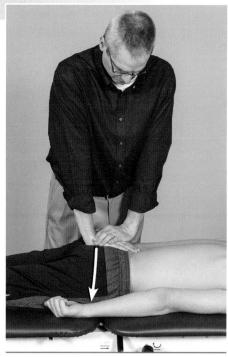

Figure 20.14

PELVIC GIRDLE PAIN AND PREGNANCY-RELATED POSTERIOR PELVIC PAIN

See the end of the chapter for the definition of posterior pelvic pain in pregnancy.[80] The active straight leg raise test and the stork test together have been suggested to measure the presence of a pelvic ring instability and poor neuromuscular control during loading.

ACTIVE STRAIGHT LEG RAISE TEST

Client Position	Supine with bilateral legs extended and placed 20 cm apart, arms relaxed
Clinician Position	Standing at client's side, facing the client
Movement	The clinician asks the client, "Try to raise your legs, one after the other, above the couch for 20 cm without bending the knee." The client scores the impairment on a 6-point scale:

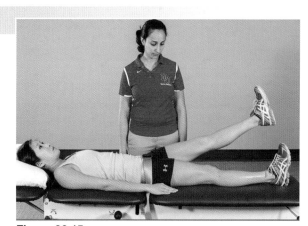

Figure 20.15

- 0 = not difficult at all
- 1 = minimally difficult
- 2 = somewhat difficult
- 3 = fairly difficult
- 4 = very difficult
- 5 = unable to do

The scores of both legs are added, so the summed score ranges from 0 to 10.

An additional comparison for this test can be done if the test was difficult or painful the first time. The leg-lift process is repeated with a belt, placed securely around the pelvis (as shown). The client is asked to compare the lift with the belt to the previous one without: more difficult, as difficult, or easier?

Assessment   A test is (+) if the lift was easier with the belt secured on the pelvis. This test has also been described with the clinician providing lateral to medial compression on each side of the pelvic girdle in lieu of a belt.

Statistics
- SN 87 (NR), SP 94 (NR), +LR 14.5, –LR 0.13, QUADAS 8, in a study of 200 pregnant clients with pelvic girdle pain (mean age 32.7 ± 3.5 years, median postpartum period of 1.7 years) and 50 female controls (mean age 47.7 ± 8.1 years), and using disability as measured on the Quebec Back Pain Disability Scale as a reference standard[63]
- SN 76 (NR) for clients with any difficulty for this test and sacral thrust test; SN 98 (NR) for clients with at least fair difficulty for this test and sacral thrust test in a study of 178 women with peripartum pelvic pain (mean age 32.7 ± 3.4 years, postpartum period median was 1.7 years)[81]
- SN 77 (NR), SP 55 (NR), +LR 2.2, –LR 0.42, QUADAS 8, in a study of 123 pregnant clients (mean age range 29.6–32.5 years, 36 weeks gestation) with pregnancy-related pelvic pain, and using Doppler imaging vibration as a reference standard[77]

Critical Clinical Pearls

When performing the active straight leg raise test, clinicians should keep the following in mind:

- Using a belt is more likely to provide consistent compression of the pelvis versus using their hands.
- Clinician utilization of hands provided uneven force, and success of this method is dependent on the size of the clinician and client.
- Investigation of diagnostic accuracy of this test is limited to women with peripartum-related pelvic pain.
- Testing interpretation (numerical rating versus ease rating) should be consistently utilized with repeated testing.

STORK TEST (MARCH TEST OR GILLET'S TEST)

Client Position   Standing with arms relaxed at side, weight evenly distributed on both feet

Clinician Position   Kneeling behind client; placing one thumb (right as shown) under the client's PSIS on the same side being tested and the other thumb (left as shown) over the S2 spinous process

Movement   The client stands on the contralateral leg only and flexes the ipsilateral (right as shown) hip and knee to 90°, bringing the knee toward the chest.

Assessment   If the ipsilateral PSIS fails to move posterior and inferior with respect to S2, it is considered a (+) test, suggesting hypomobility on that side.

Statistics
- SN 8 (4-13), SP 93 (85-97), +LR 1.1, –LR 0.99, QUADAS 10, in a study of 144 clients with LBP and 137 clients without LBP (mean age range of 35.2 ± 7.8 years to 35.5 ± 8.5 years, 60% were female, 60% of clients had acute LBP of <3 months), and measured innominate torsion with a crest level tester as a reference standard[71]

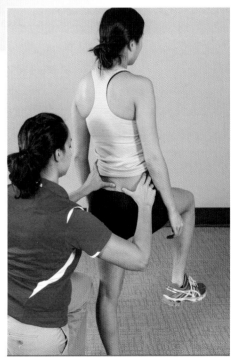

Figure 20.16

- SN 43 (NR), SP 68 (NR), +LR 1.3, –LR 0.84, QUADAS 10, in a study of 85 clients with complaints of sacroiliac joint pain (median age 44.5 years, 61 women, duration of symptoms was variable), and using sacroiliac joint blocks as a reference standard[5]

SELF-TEST P4

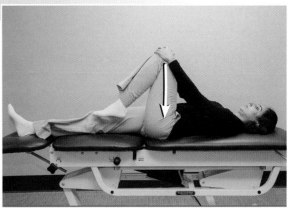

Client Position	Supine, flexing thigh to be assessed to 90°
Clinician Position	Monitoring client from the side
Movement	The client applies a self-directed downward force through their own hip, applying force at the knee and vertically through the femur.
Assessment	A (+) test is reproduction of concordant pain with test.
Statistics	SN 90 (NR), SP 92 (NR), +LR 11.3, –LR 0.11, QUADAS 4, in a study of 175 clients (100 pregnant women with pelvic girdle pain, 25 pregnant women without pain, and 50 nonpregnant women; mean age ranged from 28.2 to 30.5 years of age, mean gestational time was 24.6 weeks), using diagnosis of pelvic girdle pain as a reference standard[82]

Figure 20.17

MOVEMENT TESTING

Remember that this type of testing has poor diagnostic accuracy and reliability. The findings from these tests are likely inaccurate; therefore, their use should be questioned.

STANDING STORK OR MARCH TEST

See the description of this test earlier in the chapter.

STANDING FLEXION TEST (STANDING FORWARD BENDING TEST)

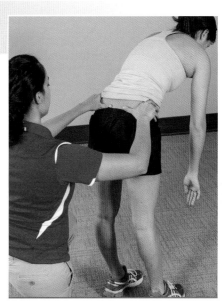

Client Position	Standing with arms relaxed at side, weight evenly distributed on both feet
Clinician Position	Kneeling behind client
Movement	The clinician assesses the relative heights of the client's bilateral PSIS by palpation. The client flexes forward as far as possible as the clinician continues to palpate the bilateral PSIS.
Assessment	A change in the relative relationship of the PSIS in the fully flexed position is considered a (+) test. The PSIS that elevates to a greater degree is suggested as the hypomobile side of the pelvis.
Statistics	SN 17 (12-24), SP 79 (70-87), +LR 0.8, –LR 1.04, QUADAS 10, in a study of 144 clients with LBP and 137 clients without LBP (mean age range of 35.2 ± 7.8 years

Figure 20.18

(continued)

Standing Flexion Test *(continued)*

to 35.5 ± 8.5 years, 60% were female, 60% of clients had acute LBP of <3 months), and using measured innominate torsion with a crest level tester as a reference standard[71]

Note The sitting flexion test (performed in the same manner, except the client is sitting throughout the test versus standing) has been suggested to discriminate between ilial dysfunction (standing flexion test) and sacral (sitting) and has the following statistics: SN 9 (6-14), SP 93 (85-98), +LR 1.3, –LR 0.97, QUADAS 10, in the Levangie study.[71]

SUPINE LONG-SITTING TEST

Client Position Supine with hips and knees extended

Clinician Position Standing at client's feet, directly facing client

Movement Clinician grasps each of the client's ankles, placing their thumbs below the medial malleoli *(a)*. The clinician makes a visual estimation of leg length, and then assists the client into a long-sitting position. The clinician then re-examines the relative leg lengths *(b)*.

Assessment A change in relative position of the medial malleoli is considered a (+) test with the suggestion that a leg that was longer in supine and is now even with the other leg is anteriorly rotated (or the leg that was short to start with and now even with the other leg is posteriorly rotated). This test alone does not determine the involved side.

Statistics SN 44 (36-52), SP 64 (53-74), +LR 1.7, –LR 0.9, QUADAS 10, in a study of 144 clients with LBP and 137 clients without LBP (mean age range of 35.2 ± 7.8 years to 35.5 ± 8.5 years, 60% were female, 60% of clients had acute LBP of <3 months), and using measured innominate torsion with a crest level tester as a reference standard[71]

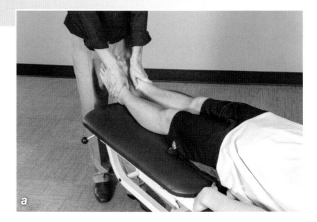
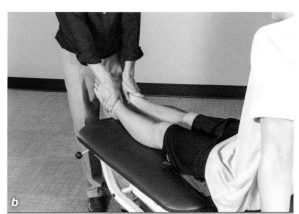

Figure 20.19

Note The clinician must maintain the client's entire body in midline alignment throughout the test to avoid false positive and negative results of testing.

PRONE KNEE-BENDING TEST (DEERFIELD'S TEST)

Client Position	Prone with bilateral legs straight and feet hanging off the end of the table
Clinician Position	Standing at client's feet, directly facing client
Movement	The clinician palpates the bottom of the client's bilateral heels to assess for relative leg lengths *(a)*. The clinician passively flexes the client's knees to approximately 90° *(b)*, and then again assesses the relative leg lengths in this position.
Assessment	A change in relative lengths occurring between the two positions is considered a (+) test. The interpretation with respect to the supine long-sitting test has also been suggested for this test. Again, this test alone would not determine the involved side.
Statistics	NR

Figure 20.20

Note
- The clinician must maintain the client's entire body in midline alignment throughout the test to avoid false positive and negative results of testing.

- Specific interpretation of test has been suggested as follows:

  - Negative: No relative change in lengths occur between the two test positions.

  - Posterior innominate on the right: Symptoms are on right side, the right leg appears shorter than the left in prone knee-extended position, and the right leg appears to be about equal to or longer than the left leg in prone knee-flexed position.

  - Posterior innominate on the left: symptoms are on left side, the left leg appears shorter than the right in prone knee-extended position, and the left leg appears to be about equal to or longer than the right leg in the prone knee-flexed position.

  - Anterior innominate on the right side: Symptoms are on the right side; the right leg appears to be longer than the left leg in the prone knee-extended position, and the right leg appears to be about equal to or shorter than the left leg in the prone knee-flexed position.

  - Anterior innominate on the left: Symptoms are on the left side, the left leg appears longer than the right leg in the prone knee-extended position, and the left leg appears to be about equal to or shorter than the right leg in the prone knee-flexed position.

  - The reader is cautioned (with all movement tests as described earlier) regarding making diagnostic decisions based on movement or palpation tests and based on the side of symptoms.

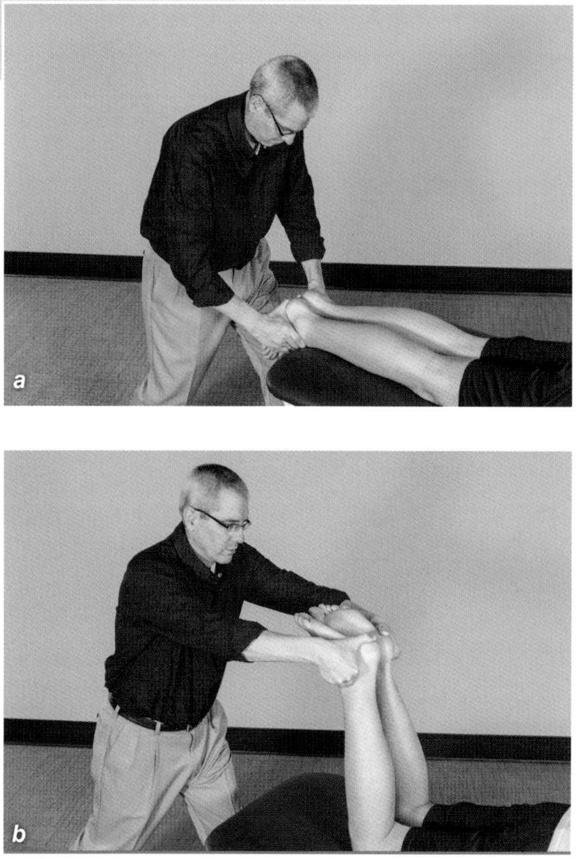

MUSCLE DYSFUNCTION: PIRIFORMIS SYNDROME

FAIR (FLEXION, ADDUCTION, AND INTERNAL ROTATION) TEST

Client Position	Side lying
Clinician Position	Standing behind the client, stabilizing iliac crest
Movement	The clinician passively brings the lower extremity into the combined motions of approximately 90° of hip flexion, maximal adduction, and knee flexion to 9° degrees. The clinician then applies upward and lateral pressure to the shin of the lower extremity to be tested (right as shown), passively internally rotating the thigh to 45°, or as near to 45° as client can tolerate.
Assessment	Pain elicited at the intersection of the sciatic nerve and the piriformis is considered a (+) test.
Statistics	**SN 88 (NR)**, **SP 83 (NR)**, **+LR 5.2**, **−LR of 0.14** in a sample of 918 consecutive clients (1,014 legs; (age 54-57 years, gender and mean duration symptoms NR) with follow-up on 733 legs and a reference standard of H reflex testing[64, 65]

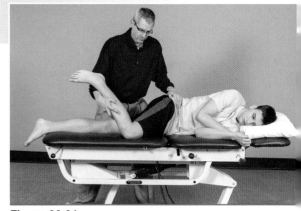

Figure 20.21

PALPATION

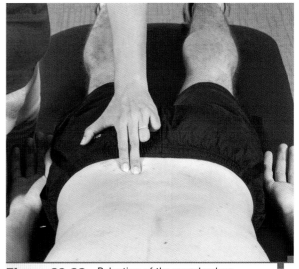

Figure 20.22 Palpation of the sacral sulcus.

Palpation for the diagnosis of pelvic girdle pain has limited clinical utility. Despite these limitations, palpation has been demonstrated to be useful for extraarticular disorders,[83] as well as for implicating the long dorsal ligament as a contributor to pelvic girdle pathology.[81] Refer to chapter 19 (Lumbar Spine) for palpation of landmarks in the pelvic girdle, as well as those that follow here.

Prone

Many landmarks for palpation of the SIJ and pelvic girdle are accessible in the prone position. The following are such landmarks.

- **Sacral base:** The clinician should start at the client's PSIS and move their thumbs medially and anteriorly until they contact the sacral base.

- **Sacral sulcus:** Starting at the PSIS, the clinician palpates slightly above (left index finger as shown) and medial (left 3rd finger as shown) to it on the sacrum adjacent to the ilium (figure 20.22). They should compare the depth of the right side to that of the left side. If one side is deeper than the other, sacral torsion or rotation on the ilium around the horizontal plane may be indicated.

- The long dorsal ligament can be palpated in the region of the sacral sulcus and just distal to the PSIS. This ligament was shown to frequently be tender in clients with peripartum pelvic pain, with a SN of 76.[81]

- **Inferior lateral angle (ILA):** This is located approximately 1 in. (2.5 cm) lateral and slightly superior to the sacrococcygeal junction (figure 20.23). The clinician palpates on

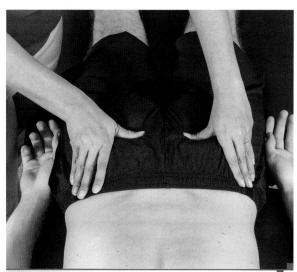

Figure 20.23   Palpation of the inferior lateral angle.

the ILAs on both sides to determine relative superior or inferior position. A difference of 1/4 in. (6 mm) or more has been suggested that the sacrum is side bent.

- **Ischial tuberosity:** The clinician should have the client lie on the contralateral side with their knee slightly flexed. They will palpate with their thumbs at the level of the client's gluteal folds until they feel a prominence. The clinician can also perform this at the level of the gluteal folds with the client in prone position, palpating for height (superior–inferior) and for depth (anterior–posterior). An anterior iliac rotation moves the ischial tuberosity posterior and vice versa. An upslip moves the ischial tuberosity superior and vice versa.

- **Coccyx:** The tip of the coccyx can be found in the superior gluteal cleft.

PHYSICAL PERFORMANCE MEASURES

Please refer to those listed in chapter 19 (Lumbar Spine).

COMMON ORTHOPEDIC CONDITIONS OF THE SACROILIAC JOINT AND PELVIC GIRDLE

While it is impossible to distinctly describe various pathological presentations of the sacroiliac joint, there are evidence-based findings supportive of particular pathologies of this region of the body. Therefore, the intent of this section of the chapter is to present current evidence-supported findings suggestive of sacroiliac joint pathologies. As previously described in chapter 4 (Evidence-Based Practice and Client Examination), though, not all examination findings are absolutely supported with clinical evidence, and the clinician should also rely on clinical experience and input from the client when performing differential diagnosis of a client's presentation of pain and dysfunction.

As previously mentioned in this chapter, due to the controversial nature of this area, as well as limited evidence and agreement among experts examining this region, it is suggested that diagnosis of the client with PGP is a diagnosis of exclusion.[1,2] Clinicians should use the previously proposed definition of PGP.[1] Therefore, more salient points proposed by this definition are suggested:

- A diagnosis of exclusion of lumbar causes (This text also suggests excluding hip joint potential pain generators.)
- Pain arising in relation to pregnancy, trauma, arthritis, or osteoarthritis
- Pain located in the vicinity of the SIJ that may radiated into posterior thigh
- Decreased endurance capacity for standing, walking, and sitting
- Pain or dysfunction should be reproduced with specific clinical tests.

Pain of Sacroiliac Origin

ICD-9: 724.6 (disorders of sacrum)

ICD-10: M33.6 (sprain and strain of sacroiliac joint)

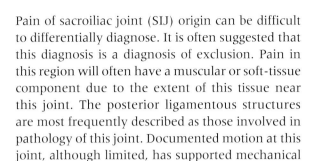

Pain of sacroiliac joint (SIJ) origin can be difficult to differentially diagnose. It is often suggested that this diagnosis is a diagnosis of exclusion. Pain in this region will often have a muscular or soft-tissue component due to the extent of this tissue near this joint. The posterior ligamentous structures are most frequently described as those involved in pathology of this joint. Documented motion at this joint, although limited, has supported mechanical dysfunction in this joint.

I. Client Interview

Subjective History

- 10% to 25% of clients with persistent mechanical low back pain below L5 have pain secondary to sacroiliac joint pathology.[84]

- Commonly described groin pain has little diagnostic value (SP 63). No other historical feature examined provided worthwhile diagnostic value.[5]

- SIJ has a variable pain description, including multiple locations. The most prevalent location is the buttocks (94%). Twenty-six percent of the pain-referral patterns included foot and ankle pain. Eighteen patterns of pain referral were observed in 50 consecutive clients who satisfied clinical criteria and demonstrated a positive diagnostic response to a fluoroscopically guided sacroiliac joint injection.[3]

- Prevalence rates for internal disc disruption (IDD), facet joint pain (FJP), and sacroiliac joint pain (SIJP) have been estimated to be 42%, 31%, and 18%, respectively.[85]

- Mechanism of injury can be repeated torsional stresses.[3, 8]

- Clients reported aggravated pain with sitting or lying on affected side, riding in the car, weight bearing on affected side when standing or walking, Valsalva maneuver, and trunk flexion.[8]

- Clients with SIJ pain exhibit no characteristic feature (such as pain with standing, walking, sitting, lying down) of diagnostic value,[5, 86] although more recently it has been suggested these clients have reduced endurance capacity for standing, walking, and sitting.[1]

- The presence or absence of thigh pain possesses a significant correlation with the source of chronic LBP for varying ages, whereas the presence of hip or girdle pain or leg pain did not significantly discriminate among IDD, FJP, or SIJP as the etiology of chronic LBP. Younger age was predictive of intervertebral disc disease regardless of the presence or absence of thigh pain.[17]

- Pain is typically unilateral, produced or increased on rising from sitting, and rarely at or above the level of L5.[12]

- It is suggested that clients with SIJ hypomobility have more pain with increased excursion of the pelvic girdle. Therefore, running is more painful than walking, walking is more painful than standing, and standing is more painful than sitting.

Outcome Measures

- The ODI, FABQ, GROC, and PSFS are recommended when appropriate.

Diagnostic Imaging

- In most cases of nonankylosing spondylitis PGP, there is limited value for imaging.[1]

- Local SIJ injections have not been recommended by some.[1]

- Indications are limited for use of radiography due to poor SN in detecting early stages of degeneration and arthritis of SIJ.[1]

- CT scan is established for bony changes, not inflammation. There is limited clinical utility for ruling out (SN 58) and ruling in (SP 69) SIJ pathology.[30]

- MRI is helpful for **ruling in** (SP 100) SIJ pathology.[31]

- Bone scan is helpful for **ruling in** (SP 100,[28] SP 89[29]) SIJ pathology.

II. Observation

- Clients with sacral flexion lesions are thought to have increased lumbar lordotic posture, while those with sacral extension lesions are thought to have relatively flat lumbar spine posture due to the fact that when the sacrum flexes, the lumbar spine extends, and vice versa.

- Since the SIJ is a stress-relieving joint, these clients will likely have pain in weight-bearing positions (e.g., running worse than walking, walking worse than standing).[8]

III. Triage and Screening

- All nonmusculoskeletal causes, as well as causes from related joints, should be ruled out.

- Sign of the buttock, when suspected, should be ruled out with hip flexion both with knee extended and flexed as previously described.

- Palpation of the posterior pelvis has less than good ability to help rule out (SN 98, −LR 0.02) and rule in (SP 94, +LR 16.3) pelvic fractures due to study bias.[45]

- Compression test: A (−) compression of the pelvis has less than good ability to help rule out (SN 98, −LR 0.08) pelvic fractures due to study bias.[45]

- Hip flexion test: A (−) test has good ability to help **rule out** (SN 90, −LR 0.10) pelvic fractures and a (+) test has good ability to help **rule in** (SP 95, +LR 18) pelvic fractures.[46]

- Spine fractures, when suspected, should be ruled out as described in the section Ankylosing Spondylitis.

IV. Motion Tests

- Limited adduction and flexion may be noted due to the stress on the joint.

V. Muscle Performance Testing

- Clinicians should assess for muscle performance deficits for pelvic girdle musculature, especially gluteal and small stabilizer musculature.

VI. Special Tests

- The following tests were recommended by the European guidelines for diagnosis of pelvic girdle pain:[1]
  - Posterior pelvic pain provocation test (P4/thigh thrust)
  - Patrick's (FABER) test
  - Palpation of the long dorsal SIJ ligament and pubic symphysis
  - Gaenslen's test
  - Modified Trendelenburg test

- 3 out of 5 tests (after discogenic origin of symptoms ruled out) when (−) are more helpful for **ruling out** (SN 94, −LR 0.80) than when (+) are helpful in **ruling in** (SP 78, +LR 4.3) SIJ-related dysfunction.

- Thigh thrust test: This is the most SN of the provocation tests. A (−) thigh thrust test helps **rule out** (SN 88, −LR 0.18;[2] SN 80, −LR 0.2[78]) SIJ-related dysfunction and a (+) test helps **rule in** (SP 100, +LR Inf;[78] SP 70-86, +LR 1.9–3.3[75]) SIJ-related dysfunction.

- The active straight leg raise (ASLR) test is recommended as a functional test of pelvic girdle stability and motor control, especially in pregnant or postpartum women.[1] The diagnostic accuracy of this test was good to ideal (SN 87 [NR], SP 94 [NR], +LR 14.5, −LR 0.13), but the QUADAS was 8.[63]

- All pelvic girdle movement and palpation asymmetry tests have poor diagnostic accuracy.

VII. Palpation

- No tenderness to palpation of the long dorsal (posterior sacroiliac) ligament helps **rule out** pelvic girdle–related pain: overall SN 76, SN 86 when both the ASLR and thigh thrust tests were (−), SN 98 when only severe pelvic clients were included.[81]

- Tenderness to palpation of the ipsilateral long dorsal SIJ ligament (compared to the contralateral ligament) is suggestive of a sacral extension or anterior innominate rotation dysfunction on that side.

- Tenderness to palpation of the ipsilateral sacrotuberous ligament (compared to the contralateral ligament) is suggestive of a sacral flexion or posterior innominate rotation dysfunction on that side.

- Palpation of torsions is strongly suggested to be of limited clinical utility,[66] but the following have been described:
  - Anterior torsions of the sacrum (left on left, right on right dysfunctions) are flexion dysfunctions with the sacral sulcus deeper on the contralateral side to the direction of rotation and the inferior lateral angle of the sacrum prominently posterior on

the side of the direction of rotation. These lesions are suggested to also correspond with increased lumbar extension posture and sacral mobility to a PA glide (as compared to posterior torsions).

- Posterior torsions of the sacrum (right on left; left on right dysfunctions) are extension dysfunctions with the sacral sulcus more posterior (or shallow) on the ipsilateral side to the direction of rotation and the inferior lateral angle of the sacrum prominently posterior on the side of the direction of rotation. These lesions are suggested to also correspond with decreased lumbar lordosis, or flat back type, of lumbar spine posture and lack of sacral mobility to a PA glide (as compared to anterior torsions).

VIII. Physical Performance Measures

- Any physical performance measure relevant to the physical demands of the client's hobbies or occupation may be used.
- Refer to chapter 19 (Lumbar Spine) for additional suggestions.

POTENTIAL TREATMENT-BASED CLASSIFICATIONS

- Mobility (if joint hypomobility is detected)
- Stabilization (if joint hypermobility is detected)
- Other potential TBCs: pain control (only if pain is dominant), exercise and conditioning, specific exercise direction

Pregnancy-Related Posterior Pelvic Pain (PRPPP)

ICD-9: 724.6 (disorders of sacrum)

ICD-10: M33.6 (sprain and strain of sacroiliac joint)

Posterior pelvic pain in pregnancy has the following definition:[80]

- A history of time- and weight bearing–related pain in the posterior pelvis, deep in the gluteal area
- A pain drawing with well-defined markings of pain in the buttocks distal and lateral to the L5-S1 area, with or without radiation to the posterior thigh or knee, but not into the foot
- A (+) posterior pelvic pain provocation (thigh thrust) test
- Free movements in the hips and spine and no nerve-root syndrome
- Pain when turning in bed

Additionally, Albert and colleagues further classify these clients into subgroups:[76]

Differential Diagnosis of Pain of Sacroiliac Origin and Lumbar Spine Origin

- Both conditions are likely to present with pain in lower back or buttock region.
- Lumbar spine–related pain due to discogenic origin is more likely to cause radiating pain that is responsive to repeated movements (centralization or peripheralization).
- Reported prevalence of pain of lumbar spine origin is greater than that of sacroiliac origin.
- The thigh thrust test is the most SN test to assist in ruling out potential sacroiliac origin pain.
- Assessment of sacroiliac pain origin should not rely on palpation of landmarks or movement discrimination tests due to their suggested limited clinical utility.[66]
- Clinicians should use highly SN tests for each respective body section to help rule it out as a potential pain generator due to the close relationship between these two areas.
- Although both areas can have variable pathologies, the lumbar spine is more likely to have variable pathological presentation. Refer to chapter 19 (Lumbar Spine) for greater detail in this regard.

- Pelvic girdle syndrome: daily pain in all three pelvic joints, confirmed with positive pain provoked by the tests from the equivalent joints.
- Symphysiolysis: daily pain in the pubic symphysis only, confirmed with positive pain provoked by the tests from the symphysis. Symphysiolysis does not imply an actual lysis, but the nomenclature is used by the Danish Health Authorities as a classification of pregnant women with pelvic pain.
- One-sided sacroiliac syndrome: daily pain from one sacroiliac joint, confirmed with positive pain provoked by the tests from the same joint.
- Double-sided sacroiliac syndrome: daily pain from both sacroiliac joints, confirmed with positive pain provoked by the tests from both joints.
- Miscellaneous: daily pain in one or more pelvic joints but with inconsistent objective findings (e.g., pain history from the pubic symphysis and objective findings from one sacroiliac joint). This category also included findings indicating inflammatory rheumatic diseases.

I. Client Interview

Subjective History

- Significant symptoms of pregnancy-related pubic symphysis dysfunction were pubic bone pain on walking, turning over in bed, climbing stairs, and standing on one leg, as well as previous damage to back or pelvis. Using a score of 1 for each of the preceding symptoms, a score of 2 and above was considered diagnostic of symphysis pubis dysfunction.[87]
- In 75% to 83% of cases, lumbopelvic pain in pregnant women is PRPPP.[15]
- Overall, about 45% of pregnant women and 25% of postpartum women suffer from PRPPP.[15]
- Symptoms:[15] stabbing, aching pain between the posterior iliac crests and gluteal folds, with or without radiation down the leg; pain in symphysis pubis, as well as from other areas of pelvic girdle, typically increases in intensity from weight-bearing activity; pain in the pubic bone that can sometimes radiate to the pelvic floor and down the thigh.

- Peak of symptoms reported to be closer to third trimester between 24th and 36th weeks of pregnancy.[16]
- Risk factors for development of pain during pregnancy are a history of previous LBP, young age, heavy workload, and previous trauma to the pelvis.[1]
- Contraceptive pills, BMI, height, and weight increase during pregnancy are not suggested as risk factors for pregnancy-related SIJ pain.[1]
- Sick leave due to back pain during pregnancy is a risk factor for postpartum pelvic girdle pain.[88]

Outcome Measures

- The Quebec Back Pain Disability Scale and ODI are recommended.[1]
- The FABQ, GROC, and PSFS are recommended when appropriate.

Diagnostic Imaging

- Scintigraphy, CT, and local SIJ injections are not recommended.[1]
- In most cases of nonankylosing spondylitis PGP, there is limited value for imaging.[1]
- Indications are limited for use of radiography due to poor SN in detecting early stages of degeneration and arthritis of SIJ.[1]
- MRI is recommended for excluding ankylosing spondylitis and severe traumatic (postpartum) injuries.[1]

II. Observation

- Pregnant women will demonstrate hyperlordotic posture and bilaterally externally rotated gait.[9, 61]

III. Triage and Screening

- All nonmusculoskeletal causes, as well as causes from related joints, should be ruled out.
- Sign of the buttock, when suspected, should be ruled out as described in the section Pain of Sacroiliac Origin.

- Pelvic fractures, when suspected, should be ruled out as described in the section Pain of Sacroiliac Origin.
- Spine fractures, when suspected, should be ruled out as described in the section Ankylosing Spondylitis.

IV. Motion Tests

- Pregnant and postpartum pregnant women are likely to have excessive joint play or arthrokinematics at the SIJ.[9, 38, 61-63]

V. Muscle Performance Testing

- A positive direct correlation between hip muscle adductor weakness and the severity of pelvic girdle–related pain or dysfunction has been demonstrated.[70]

VI. Special Tests

- Thigh thrust: A (−) thigh thrust test helps rule out (SN 84-93;[76] SN 88, −LR 0.13[79]) and a (+) test helps rule in (SP 98, +LR 46.5; SP 89, +LR 8.0) pregnancy-related pelvic girdle pain, although both studies suffer from bias.
- Active straight leg raise: The active straight leg raise (ASLR) test is recommended as a functional test of pelvic girdle stability and motor control, especially in pregnant or postpartum women.[1]
  - A (−) ASLR test helps rule out (SN 87, −LR 0.13;[63] SN 76-98;[81] SN 77, −LR 0.42[77]) and a (+) test helps rule in (SP 94, +LR 14.5)[63] pregnancy-related pelvic girdle pain, although the studies again suffer from bias.
  - All pelvic girdle movement and palpation asymmetry tests have poor diagnostic accuracy.

VII. Palpation

- Pain to palpation of pubic symphysis >5 seconds after palpation.[76]
- Pubic symphysis is often very painful.[82]
- No tenderness to palpation of the long dorsal (posterior sacroiliac) ligament helps **rule out** pelvic girdle–related pain: overall SN 76, SN 86 when both the ASLR and thigh thrust test were (−); SN 98 when only severe pelvic clients were included.[81]

VIII. Physical Performance Measures

- Any physical performance measure relevant to the physical demands of the client's hobbies or occupation may be used.
- Refer to chapter 19 (Lumbar Spine) for additional suggestions.

POTENTIAL TREATMENT-BASED CLASSIFICATIONS

- Mobility (if joint hypomobility is detected)
- Stabilization (if joint hypermobility is detected)
- Other potential TBCs: pain control (only if pain is dominant), exercise and conditioning, specific exercise direction

---

Differential Diagnosis of Pain of Sacroiliac Origin and Pregnancy-Related Posterior Pelvic Pain (PRPPP)

- Both conditions are pathologies of the SIJ or pelvic girdle.
- 75% to 83% of cases of lumbopelvic pain in pregnant women are PRPPP.[15]
- Pain of sacroiliac origin can present in both men and women, although it is more prevalent in women.
- An ASLR test is suggestive of motor control dysfunction, and it has been exclusively investigated in women (either those who are pregnant or who have a history of PRPPP). This test is recommended as a functional test of pelvic girdle stability and motor control, especially in pregnant or postpartum women.[1]

Spondylarthritis and Spondyloarthropathy

ICD-9: 720 (ankylosing spondylitis); 721 (spondylosis); 724.6 (disorders of the sacrum)

ICD-10: M53.3 (sacrococcygeal disorders, not elsewhere classified)

This broad terminology has been described on the one end as any joint disease of the vertebral column. Spondyloarthropathy with inflammation is termed *spondylarthritis*. Spondylarthritic conditions have been specifically termed *seronegative spondyloarthropathies*. They have increased incidence of HLA-B27 and a negative rheumatoid factor. Conditions such as ankylosing spondylitis, reactive arthritis (Reiter's syndrome), and psoriatic arthritis are typical seronegative spondyloarthropathies. Other less commonly included conditions are Behçet's disease and Whipple's disease. These clients may also suffer from extra-articular manifestations. Such previously described manifestations include, but are not limited to, low bone mineral density, inflammatory bowel, and atherosclerotic diseases.[89, 90]

I. Client Interview

Subjective History

- Nonvertebral symptoms can include asymmetric peripheral arthritis, plantar fasciitis, costochondritis, and toe interphalangeal joint arthritis.
- LBP is the most commonly described symptom. Typically the client's LBP decreases with activity.

Outcome Measures

- The ODI, FABQ, GROC, and PSFS are recommended when appropriate.
- Any relevant measure, when appropriate, is recommended.

Diagnostic Imaging

- Radiographic findings include joint space narrowing, bone sclerosis, periarticular cysts, and osteophytes. Refer to chapter 6 for definition of osteoarthritis according to Kellgren and Lawrence.[91]
- MRI is helpful for **ruling out** (SN 90) and **ruling in** (SP 97) AS.[33]
- Bone marrow edema is commonly found not only for these clients, but also for those with nonspecific LBP

and for healthy subjects, while erosions are rarely observed in the latter two groups.[37]

II. Observation

- As with other arthropathies, transitional movements are often painful (e.g., sitting to standing, turning over).
- Stiffness and guarding of movement may be noted when the client first moves from a static position.

III. Triage and Screening

- All nonmusculoskeletal causes, as well as causes from related joints, should be ruled out.
- Sign of the buttock, when suspected, should be ruled out as described in the section Pain of Sacroiliac Origin.
- Spine fractures, when suspected, should be ruled out as described in the section Ankylosing Spondylitis.
- Pelvic fractures, when suspected, should be ruled out as described in the section Pain of Sacroiliac origin.

IV. Motion Tests

- As with other arthropathies, limited joint play (arthrokinematic motion) and ROM of the pelvic girdle may be found.

V. Muscle Performance Testing

- Due to significant correlations of gluteal muscle weakness in arthropathies of the lumbar spine and hip, it is suggested that these may also be present in these clients (and therefore should be examined for).
- In those with suggestion of AS, limited strength in involved regions of the spine, hip, and shoulder is expected.[25]

VI. Special Tests

- Special testing as described in the section Ankylosing Spondylitis should be employed to rule out the possibility of that pathology.
- Thigh thrust test is suggested as described in the section Pain of Sacroiliac Joint Origin.
- All pelvic girdle movement and palpation asymmetry tests have poor diagnostic accuracy.

VII. Palpation

- Tenderness directly over SI joint.[39]

- Localized tenderness over the facet joints without other root tension signs or neurologic signs may indicate facet joint pain.[92]

- No tenderness to palpation of the long dorsal (posterior sacroiliac) ligament helps **rule out** pelvic girdle–related pain: overall SN 76, SN 86 when both the active SLR and thigh thrust test were (−), SN 98 when only severe pelvic clients were included.[81]

VIII. Physical Performance Measures

- Any physical performance measure relevant to the physical demands of the client's hobbies or occupation may be used.

- Refer to chapter 19 (Lumbar Spine) for additional suggestions.

POTENTIAL TREATMENT-BASED CLASSIFICATIONS

- Mobility (if joint hypomobility is detected)

- Stabilization (if joint hypermobility is detected)

- Other potential TBCs: pain control (only if pain is dominant), exercise and conditioning, specific exercise direction

Ankylosing Spondylitis

ICD-9: 720 (ankylosing spondylitis)

ICD-10: M08.1 (juvenile ankylosing spondylitis); M45 (ankylosing spondylitis)

Ankylosing spondylitis (AS) is a common inflammatory rheumatic disease that predominantly affects the sacroiliac joints and spine, leading to structural damage and functional impairments and a decrease in quality of life. Incidence of ankylosing spondylitis is between 0.5 and 14 per 100,000 people per year.[93] Ankylosing spondylitis almost always affects SIJ and usually progresses to the thoracic spine. Average onset of symptoms for AS is 25 years old. There is a higher incidence of AS in men. There is a hereditary factor involved with AS.

I. Client Interview

Subjective History[39-42, 75, 93]

- Prevalence of symptoms are two to three times greater for men than women.

- Onset of the syndrome typically occurs in the second or third decade of life.

- Symptom onset typically occurs in late adolescence or early adulthood.

- If age of onset is not ≤40 years of age, it helps **rule out** (SN 100) ankylosing spondylitis.[18]

- If pain is not relieved by lying down, it helps **rule out** (SN 80) ankylosing spondylitis.[18]

- Women may have a slightly earlier onset than men.

- Pain typically starts in the sacrum, buttock, or low back; accompanied with morning stiffness in the same area for a few hours.

- Clients have arthritic complaints in hips and low back early in disease; with disease progression they will describe neck stiffness and difficulty with activities requiring rib cage expansion (e.g., deep breath).

- Clients may complain of fatigue.

- Screening questions for ankylosing spondylitis:

  - Has the discomfort ever gone on for 3 months or more?

  - Has the back been stiff, especially in the morning?

  - Did you discover your back discomfort before the age of 40 years old?

  - Did the problem begin slowly?

  - Has the problem been improved by exercise?

At least four (+) responses yielded a SN of 95 and a SP of 85 in a study of 138 clients (63 of whom were attending rheumatology clinics for low back pain and 75 healthy controls) with a reference standard of HLA-B27 testing.[94]

Outcome Measures

- VAS to measure spinal and night pain and the BASG are recommended.[25]

Diagnostic Imaging

- MRI helpful for **ruling out** (SN 90) and **ruling in** (SP 97) AS.[33]

- The Stoke Ankylosing Spondylitis Spine Score (SASSS) is a useful, valid score that correlates with clinical outcomes measures, and has identified specific patterns of radiographic progression in ankylosing spondylitis.[95]

- Men have more severe radiographic changes.[96]

- Radiographic findings include joint space narrowing, bone sclerosis, periarticular cysts, and osteophytes. Refer to chapter 6 for definition of osteoarthritis (OA) according to Kellgren and Lawrence.[91]

II. Observation

- Decreased lumbar lordosis and increased kyphotic thoracic spine appearance[39-41]

- Cervical spine hyperextension[39]

- Gluteal muscle atrophy[39-41]

- Muscle spasms and pain posturing or limited mobility with transitioning movements are likely.[40, 42]

III. Triage and Screening

- All nonmusculoskeletal causes, as well as causes from related joints, should be ruled out.

- A diagnostic prediction rule helps **rule out** (SN 95) a vertebral fracture when ≤1 of 5 variables were present and helps **rule in** (SP 96) a vertebral fracture when ≥4 of 5 variables were present.[47]

- The closed-fist percussion test helps **rule out** (SN 88) and **rule in** (SP 90) vertebral compression fracture.[48]

- The supine sign helps **rule out** (SN 81) and **rule in** (SP 93) vertebral compression fracture.[48]

- Sign of the buttock, when suspected, should be ruled out as described in the section Pain of Sacroiliac Origin.

- Pelvic fractures, when suspected, should be ruled out as described in the section Pain of Sacroiliac Origin.

IV. Motion Tests

- The modified Schober flexion test can be used to measure the increase in the distance between two skin marks on the first sacral spinous process (S1) and 10 cm above S1 after maximal forward bending.[41]

- Lumbar hypomobility: Clients may have restricted spinal mobility in flexion and extension of the lumbar spine.[41, 42, 95, 96]

- Presentation can vary from mild stiffness to fused spine.[41]

- Decreased chest expansion occurs with disease progression.[41, 42, 95, 96]

V. Muscle Performance Testing

- Limited strength in involved regions of the spine, hip, and shoulder is expected.[25]

VI. Special Tests

- Chest expansion test helps **rule out** (SN 91, −LR 0.09) and **rule in** (SP 99, +LR 91) ankylosing spondylitis.[18]

- 4 out of 5 (+) tests on the SI joint provocation tests (Gaenslen, FABER, Mennell, thigh thrust, and sacral thrust tests) helps **rule in** (SP 84-93) AS.[75]

VII. Palpation

- Clients may have tenderness directly over the SI joint.[39]

- Localized tenderness over the facet joints without other root tension signs or neurologic signs may indicate facet joint pain.[92]

VIII. Physical Performance Measures

- Any physical performance measure relevant to the physical demands of the client's hobbies or occupation may be used.

- Refer to chapter 19 (Lumbar Spine) for additional suggestions.

POTENTIAL TREATMENT-BASED CLASSIFICATIONS

- Pain control (if pain is dominant), exercise and conditioning, and mobility for soft-tissue restrictions are the most likely to be used.

Piriformis Syndrome

ICD-9: 355.0 (lesion of sciatic nerve); 724.3 (sciatica)

ICD-10: M54.3 (sciatica); M62.9 (disorder of muscle, unspecified)

Piriformis syndrome is a neuromuscular order that occurs when the sciatic nerve is compressed or otherwise irritated by the piriformis muscle, causing pain, tingling, and numbness in the buttocks and along the path of the sciatic nerve descending down the lower thigh and into the leg. Diagnosis is often difficult due to few validated and standardized diagnostic tests. Piriformis syndrome has been suggested as a diagnosis of exclusion, as with other SIJ dysfunctions. In fact, it has also been suggested that piriformis muscle–related pain is a result of other dysfunction as the pain generator. The syndrome may be due to anatomical variations in the muscle–nerve relationship, or from overuse or strain. The client can complain of, and present with, pain radiating into the lower extremity.

I. Client Interview

Subjective History

- Reported prevalence of piriformis syndrome among chronic low back pain clients varies widely, between 5% and 36%.[69, 97, 98]

- Pain in the gluteal region may radiate into the buttocks and legs.

- Pain can be more significant with the hip internally rotated during ADLs (e.g., client may state less pain with hip externally rotated during gait).

- Pain with sitting can be noted, especially if increased weight is on that buttock (e.g., wallet in that back pocket).

Outcome Measures

- Any appropriate clinical measure can be used; the ODI and FABQ are suggested when appropriate.

Diagnostic Imaging

- Usually none is applicable because this is often a diagnosis of exclusion.

- Diagnostic modalities such as CT, MRI, ultrasound, and EMG are mostly useful in excluding other conditions.

- Magnetic resonance neurography is a medical imaging technique that can show the presence of irritation of the sciatic nerve.

II. Observation

- Sitting on the involved side may be irritable to the client, especially if a wallet is in the back pocket on that side.

III. Triage and Screening

- All nonmusculoskeletal causes, as well as causes from related joints, should be ruled out.

- Sign of the buttock, when suspected, should be ruled out as described in the section Pain of Sacroiliac Origin.

- Pelvic fractures, when suspected, should be ruled out as described in the section Pain of Sacroiliac Origin.

- Spine fractures, when suspected, should be ruled out as described in the section Ankylosing Spondylitis.

IV. Motion Tests

- Combined motions of flexion, adduction, and internal rotation of the involved hip are suggested to be provocative.[64, 65]

V. Muscle Performance Testing

- Resisted hip abduction and rotation are suggested to be provocative and likely weak.[64, 65, 69]

VI. Special Tests

- The FAIR test helps **rule out** (SN 88, −LR 0.14) and **rule in** (SP 83, +LR 5.2) piriformis syndrome.[65]

VII. Palpation

- Clients may have tenderness over piriformis or sciatic notch, with or without neurologic signs.[69, 98]

- Surrounding soft tissue may also be tender, but not as concordant as piriformis muscle.

VIII. Physical Performance Measures

- Any physical performance measure relevant to the physical demands of the client's hobbies or occupation may be used.
- Refer to chapter 19 (Lumbar Spine) for additional suggestions.

POTENTIAL TREATMENT-BASED CLASSIFICATIONS

- Mobility (if joint hypomobility is detected)
- Stabilization (if joint hypermobility is detected)
- Other potential TBCs: pain control (only if pain is dominant), exercise and conditioning, specific exercise direction

CONCLUSION

The SIJ and pelvic girdle is a limited mobility structure that has an interdependent relationship with the lumbar spine and hip joint. Thus, those joints should be ruled out when examining this area. The clinician should be cognizant of the controversial nature of this area in general. Significant debate relates to the amount of available motion and the importance of special testing for differential diagnosis. As always, the clinician should utilize a sequential, evidence-based examination as described in this chapter (and all chapters of this text). All components of the examination sequence are important to the differential diagnosis, particularly in areas of the body such as the SIJ and pelvic girdle due to the controversy. As such, the clinician need not perform an examination that is overly reliant on clinical special tests.

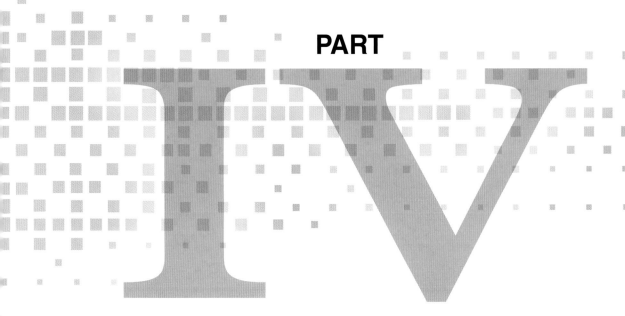

Examination of the Extremities

In part IV, the clinician is introduced to the funnel examination process as it applies to the extremities. As in part III, each of the eight components are described in detail respective to the body part. Additionally, as in part III, the end of each chapter has a section titled Common Orthopedic Conditions that provides great detail on each of the eight primary components of the funnel examination and the supporting evidence (or lack thereof) for each component, as well as ICD-9 and ICD-10 coding (with links) for each of these pathologies. At the end of each pathology, the text lists suggested treatment-based classifications for guiding appropriate interventions. Great, detailed evidence, with color-code scheme, is provided here as well so that the clinician can quickly discern if the evidence supporting the testing measures is **ideal**, **good**, or less than good.

SHOULDER

Michael P. Reiman, PT, DPT, OCS, SCS, ATC, FAAOMPT, CSCS
Christopher Fiander, PT, DPT, OCS, CSCS

In the United States, 33.2% of physician office visits for musculoskeletal pain are for shoulder pain. Men and younger adults (≤52 years old) more often associated their shoulder pain with previous injury, but there were no racial differences in injury status. Injury-related shoulder pain was related to work in more than one-fifth (21.3%) of visits.[1] The prevalence of shoulder pain is 7% to 27% for adults, and it is increasing for women and older people.[1, 2] Shoulder pain prevalence in those over the age of 25 years is 20.9%, second only to low back pain.[3] The most frequent cause of shoulder pain is subacromial impingement syndrome (SAIS); however, no consensus exists for the syndrome's diagnostic criteria.[4] The physical examination tests used to diagnose SAIS vary widely in clinical trials. This lack of consensus for diagnosing SAIS is an obstacle to investigating treatment interventions and arriving at a prognosis for this disorder. Several reasons exist for the lack of diagnostic consensus, including the multifactorial nature of this disorder along with the limited and conflicting evidence as to the diagnostic capability of physical tests for SAIS.

CLINICALLY APPLIED ANATOMY

The shoulder joint, composed of five bones and four different articulations, allows for a large range of motion (ROM). Part of the reason for increased ROM at the shoulder is that it is a ball-and-socket joint. Unlike the hip, though, it is not typically a weight-bearing joint. The depth of the glenoid fossa is not nearly as deep as that of the acetabular fossa in the hip. Additionally, the synovial capsule in the shoulder is not as taut as that in the hip joint. The anatomical relationship between the humeral head and glenoid fossa has been described as similar to the relationship between a golf ball and the golf tee it sits on.

The shoulder is the most proximal link of the upper extremity to the axial skeleton. It must work in cooperation with the elbow and hand for efficient human function. A complex joint, the shoulder has three true joints in the glenohumeral (GH; figure 21.1), acromioclavicular (figure 21.2), and

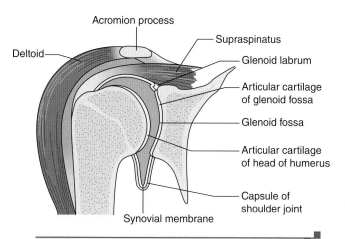

Figure 21.1 Glenohumeral joint.

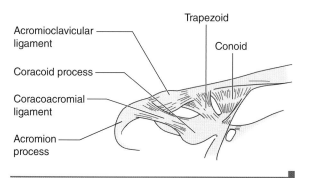

Figure 21.2 Acromioclavicular joint.

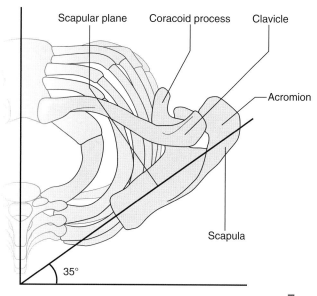

Figure 21.4 Scapulothoracic joint.

sternoclavicular joints (figure 21.3), and a pseudojoint in the scapulothoracic joint (figure 21.4). Articulations of this complex include the humerus, clavicle, scapula, and dorsal surface of the ribs. The

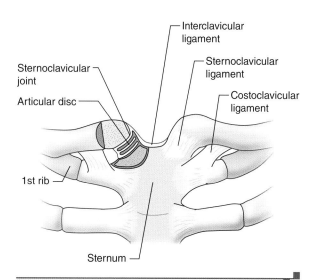

Figure 21.3 Sternoclavicular joint.

shoulder complex is the most mobile of any joint in the human body. This multiplanar joint has increased ROM and relative laxity that can lead to multiple injuries.

This mobility of the shoulder complex allows for the use of the arm in large ranges and in all planes of movement. The stability of the shoulder complex is provided by multiple ligaments. The different portions of the capsule itself restrain the humeral head in various ranges. Due to the complex nature of the multiple articulations in the shoulder complex, these ligaments are also necessary for providing stabilization (figure 21.5). The glenohumeral ligaments provide stability at different points in humeral abduction, with the superior elements restraining external rotation and extension with the humerus in 0° of abduction, the middle ligaments restraining external rotation and abduction at approximately 45° of abduction, and the anteroinferior band resisting external rotation at 90° of abduction.[5]

The glenohumeral ligaments blend into the labrum, the fibrous cartilage on the periphery of the glenoid surface. The labrum functionally acts as a passive stability component to the glenohumeral joint by increasing the glenoid depth by 75% vertically and 50% horizontally. The long head of the biceps is a significant muscle attachment to the labrum that may offer a dynamic level of stability to the labrum and anterior aspect of the glenohumeral joint. This also means that the labrum needs to be a stable anchor for the long head of the biceps.[6]

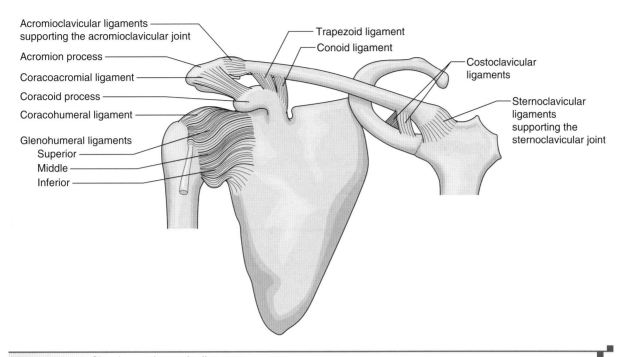

Figure 21.5   Glenohumeral capsular ligaments.

Acromioclavicular ligaments supporting the acromioclavicular joint
Acromion process
Coracoacromial ligament
Coracoid process
Coracohumeral ligament
Glenohumeral ligaments
Superior
Middle
Inferior
Trapezoid ligament
Conoid ligament
Costoclavicular ligaments
Sternoclavicular ligaments supporting the sternoclavicular joint

Dynamic stability is produced by the force coupling of the rotator cuff and deltoid, as well as by force couples with the periscapular muscles. The rotator cuff works to maintain centricity of the humeral head in the glenoid, while the deltoid contracts to produce an abduction movement (figure 21.6). To achieve full shoulder elevation, the scapula needs to upwardly rotate. This is done with the force couple produced by the serratus anterior, upper trapezius, and lower trapezius. Additionally, contraction of the rotator cuff muscles (figure 21.7) provides a compressive force to the glenohumeral joint and applies tension to the capsule and ligaments to enhance passive stability as well. The scapular muscles (figure 21.8) also stabilize the scapula against the rib cage.

The acromioclavicular (AC) joint forms the roof of the shoulder joint. While the glenohumeral joint exhibits the most motion in the shoulder girdle, the AC joint and clavicular motion move normally to contribute to shoulder girdle stability and prevent impingement during overhead motion. The clavicle must rotate posteriorly and the AC joint must tip posteriorly, along with the scapular posterior tilt and upward rotation that occur.[7] Another consideration in the AC joint is the shape of the acromion. The acromion is often described as being type I (flat), II (smooth curve), or III acromion (anterior hook).[8] The type of acromion a client has may dictate how much subacromial space is available, and thus may be associated with subacromial impingement. The sternoclavicular (SC) joint connects the shoulder girdle to the rib cage through the manubrium. The SC joint is a saddle joint, and it has a stable ligamentous system and inherent bony stability, seemingly for the important vascular structures in

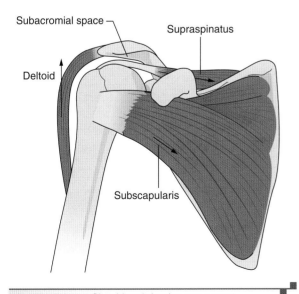

Subacromial space
Supraspinatus
Deltoid
Subscapularis

Figure 21.6   Shoulder abduction movement.

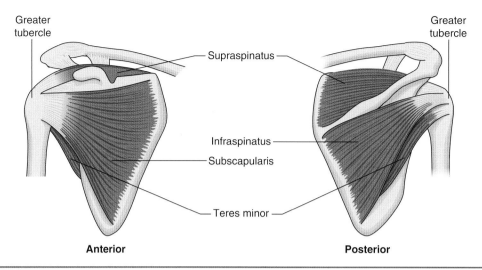

Figure 21.7   Rotator cuff muscles.

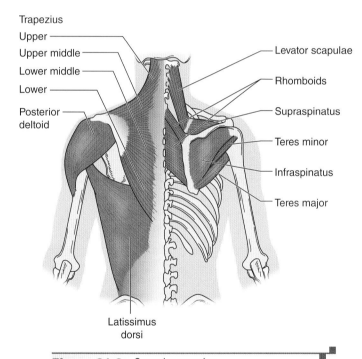

Figure 21.8   Scapular muscles.

its proximity. The SC joint moves into elevation and depression, as well as protraction and retraction, all of which are necessary for full shoulder girdle movement.

The scapulothoracic (ST) joint is a pseudojoint, not a true synovial joint. The ST joint is considered the articulation of the scapula on the thorax and is controlled proximally by the various scapular muscles that attach to it and distally by the AC joint. Proper and efficient motion is thought to be necessary for preventing impingement. This idea is discussed further later in this chapter.

CLIENT INTERVIEW

This interview is typically the first encounter the clinician has with the client. As previously discussed in chapter 5, this component of the examination can provide the clinician with a significant amount of information relevant to the probability of the client's presenting diagnosis. For purposes of this text, the interview is described relative to each body part or section, but it generally includes subjective reports by the client, as well as findings from their outcome measures. Additionally included in this section is radiographic imaging. While clinicians should avoid biasing their examination by interpreting findings of radiographic imaging prior to seeing clients (in most cases without concerns for red flags and major medical-related issues), this point in the examination is most likely where clinicians will encounter radiographic imaging. Moreover, in some instances, clinicians must interpret radiographic imaging early in the examination to rule out serious pathology prior to continuing on with other components of the examination sequence.

Subjective

Clinicians interview clients for a detailed background regarding the onset and nature of their concordant pain and chief complaint. They should encourage clients to specify any areas of pain in the shoulder girdle, along with any associated neck or arm pain. Clinicians must be able to differentially diagnose shoulder pain from cervical spine dysfunction. Clinicians should query for hand dominance, location and severity of symptoms, and the mechanism of injury. Specifically, a history of trauma versus insidious onset of symptoms may assist the clinician in identifying a traumatic tear versus a degenerative process, respectively. In a cohort by Wofford and colleagues, approximately one-third of clients presenting to a primary care office for shoulder pain had injury related to a traumatic event.[1] Additionally, an insidious onset may require the clinician to screen adjacent anatomical areas for possible sources of referred pain to the shoulder.

Clinicians must recognize prognostic factors that are obtained in the client history. For example, gradual onset of pain, longer duration of symptoms (>3 months), and higher pain rating scores are associated with poorer outcomes. The presence of psychosocial stressors has also been negatively correlated with outcomes.[9] Age and the presence of night pain are associated with the presence of rotator cuff tears.[10]

A history of trauma in combination with complaints of popping, clicking, or catching may be associated with a SLAP (superior labrum, anterior to posterior) tear, but this hypothesis is strengthened further by clinical examination.[11] Reports of trauma and apprehension may be associated with glenohumeral instability. Instability may also be indicated in a client who reports a history of multiple spontaneous or volitional subluxations and relocations. Trauma may also cause a rotator cuff tear, most commonly in men in their mid-50s.[12]

The type and nature of pain should always be assessed. Many shoulder pathologies may have similar pain presentations. For example, biceps tendinopathy clients often complain of anterior shoulder pain or pain with reaching or lifting, similar to the complaint of clients with subacromial impingement syndrome.[13] Clients with several different pathologies may complain of a pain with nonspecific location in the shoulder. While clients with both rotator cuff tear (RCT) and labral injury have been described to have vague shoulder pain, those with RCT often state that pain is the most common complaint and that it leads to a reduction in their shoulder strength (pain inhibition) and functional impairment,[14] whereas clients with labral tear are more likely to have complaints of clicking, catching, locking, or popping in the shoulder despite

the nonspecific daily activities.[15, 16] These clients are likely unable to perform activities related to high-level sports.[16] Clients with adhesive capsulitis likely have activity limitations along with their nonspecific pain. Activity limitations include pain during sleep, pain and difficulty with grooming and dressing, and pain with reaching activities.[17]

Not all shoulder pain is nonspecific in nature. Clients with AC joint pathologies typically complain of pain on the top of the shoulder near the AC joint. The distribution of pain can be into the trapezius or anterior shoulder, but it is typically local to the AC joint.[18] These clients may also report a history of direct trauma to the AC joint or repetitive activity that overloads the AC joint (e.g., push-ups).[18]

Subjective history related to scapular dyskinesis is not well defined because the dyskinesis itself has been found in both symptomatic and asymptomatic people.[19] Symptom report for the client with instability may also be variable. These may range from generalized shoulder pain to reports of multiple dislocations or episodes of joint instability.[20]

As in all areas of the body, the clinician should query the client for a description of their typical function and any repetitive activities that may be contributing to the client's symptoms. Clients who utilize their upper extremity for repetitive lifting and reaching should describe the nature of their employment and any recreational activity that requires lifting and reaching. If there is no specific mechanism of injury, the clinician needs to consider systemic areas that can refer pain to the shoulder such as the cardiovascular system, the lungs, intra-abdominal organs, and diaphragm. Clinicians should also explore any possible neurological symptoms that may be referred from the cervical spine or indicative of other central or peripheral nerve lesions. This is discussed further in the Triage and Screening section of this chapter.

Outcome Measures

As with other areas of the body, several outcome measures have been utilized for shoulder dysfunction. While some outcome measures are specifically for a particular pathology or condition, others have a broader focus.

A systematic review investigated the quality and content of the psychometric evidence relating to four shoulder disability scales: the Disabilities of the Arm, Shoulder, and Hand (DASH) questionnaire, the Shoulder Pain and Disability Index (SPADI), the

American Shoulder and Elbow Surgeons (ASES) score, and the Simple Shoulder Test (SST). Most studies suggested that all four questionnaires have excellent reliability (intraclass correlation coefficient [ICC] ≥ 0.90). The four questionnaires are strongly correlated ($r > 0.70$) with each other and with a number of similar indices, and the questionnaires were able to differentiate between different populations and disability levels. The psychometric properties of the ASES, DASH, and SPADI were shown to be acceptable for clinical use. Conversely, some properties of the SST still need be evaluated, particularly the absolute errors of measurement.[21]

A more recent critical appraisal of the literature investigated several questionnaires for their development process, validity, reliability, responsiveness, and clinical application.[22] Five common shoulder client-based scores were identified: DASH, Oxford Shoulder Score (OSS), Shoulder Disability Questionnaire (SDQ-UK), SPADI, and the Shoulder Rating Questionnaire (SRQ). Based on this critical appraisal, the authors stated that the DASH received the best ratings for its clinimetric properties, followed by the OSS.[22]

The ASES, DASH, SPADI, and SST have been studied the most regarding psychometric properties. The DASH, ASES, or SPADI are currently recommended to be used prior to and after interventions, particularly for clients with adhesive capsulitis.[17]

While several outcomes measures have been proposed for shoulder instability, the Western Ontario Shoulder Instability (WOSI) index has been validated the most in the literature, and has been correlated with DASH scores.[23] The Western Ontario Osteoarthritis of the Shoulder (WOOS) index has been validated as an outcomes measure for clients with primary osteoarthritis in the shoulder; it relates to clients' symptoms, recreation and work, lifestyle, and emotions.[24]

As with other areas in orthopedic examination, patient-specific functional scale (PSFS) is a measure of clients' specific functional tasks that are measurable and repeatable. The global rating of change (GROC) is also a measure that can be used for multiple areas in orthopedic examination to measure clients' perception of the change in status of their pain or disability.

Diagnostic Imaging

Diagnostic imaging may be necessary for clients presenting with shoulder pain or dysfunction. Table 21.1 indicates the sensitivity and specificity of the various imaging modalities. Sensitivity and specificity values are provided and categorized based on a given shoulder pathology. The imaging modalities included are radiographs, magnetic resonance imaging (MRI), magnetic resonance arthrography (MRA), computed tomography arthrography (CTA), and ultrasonography (US).

Radiographs

A conventional anteroposterior radiograph cannot provide any predictive information on the clinical status of the client.[36] The most common views that are examined for shoulder radiographs are anteroposterior (AP; figure 21.9*a*) and axial views (figure 21.9*b*). AP views may be done with the client's humerus prepositioned into either internal or external rotation to view different aspects of the humeral head, or with the client's arm holding a weight in their hand to assess for gapping of the AC joint (figure 21.9*c*). The axillary view allows for visualization of the bony position of the humerus, superior scapula, and the acromion and distal clavicle as they form the AC joint. Other views are available, such as the Stryker AP (humerus positioned in 90° of both aB and ER) view, which may indicate a Hill-Sachs lesion associated with glenohumeral instability.[37]

Magnetic Resonance Imaging

In a systematic review, the accuracy for detection of full-thickness tears was found to be equally diagnostic for MRI compared to MRA (figure 21.10) in some studies, and MRA was found to be better at identifying partial-thickness tears overall. Other studies found MRA to perform better than MRI for all outcomes.[26] For detection of partial tears, although the accuracy was low, MRI was more accurate than ultrasound in both studies.[26]

For shoulder impingement syndrome and rotator cuff tears, MRI and US have a comparable accuracy for detection of full-thickness rotator cuff tears. MRA and US might be more accurate for the detection of partial-thickness tears than MRI. Given the large difference in the cost of MR and US, ultrasound may be the most cost-effective diagnostic method for identification of full-thickness tears in a specialist hospital setting (Evidence level 3).

Both MRA and CTA are effective methods for the detection of labrum tears. More recently, multidetector CTA has offered the advantages of thinner slices than with MRA in a shorter examination time.

TABLE 21.1 Diagnostic Accuracy of Imaging Modalities for the Shoulder

Pathology	Diagnostic test	Reference standard	SN/SP
RCT full thickness	US	Surgery, MRI, radiography	Pooled analysis: **95/96**[25]
			Pooled analysis: **84/98**[26]
		Arthroscopy/open surgical findings	Pooled analysis: **96/93**[27]
			Pooled analysis: **92/94**[28]
RCT partial thickness	US	Surgery, MRI, radiography	Pooled analysis: 72/93[25]
		Arthroscopy/open surgical findings	Pooled analysis: **84/89**[27]
			Pooled analysis: 67/94[28]
RCT full thickness	MRI	Surgery	Pooled analysis: 67/95[26]
			Pooled analysis: **91/97**[29]
			Pooled analysis: **92/93**[28]
RCT partial thickness	MRI	Surgery	Pooled analysis: 44/90[26]
			Pooled analysis: **80/95**[29]
			Pooled analysis: 64/92[28]
RCT full thickness	MRA	Surgery	Pooled analysis: **95/93**[26]
	CTA		Pooled analysis: **95/99**[28]
			100/94[30]
			89/98[30]
RCT partial thickness	MRA	Surgery	Pooled analysis: 62/92[26]
			Pooled analysis: **86/96**[28]
	CTA		74/**100**[30]
			22/87[30]
RCT all tears (subscapularis)	MRI		73/94[31]
AC joint arthropathy	Radiographs	AC joint injection	41/90[32]
	Bone scan		82/70[32]
	MRI		85/50[32]
Tendinopathy	US	Surgery, MRI, radiography	Pooled analysis: 67-93/**88-100**[25]
Calcifying tendinitis	US	Surgery, MRI, radiography	Pooled analysis: **100**/85-98[25]
Subacromial bursitis	US	Surgery, MRI, radiography	Pooled analysis: 79-81/**94-98**[25]
Glenoid labrum injury	MRI	Surgery	Pooled analysis: 76/87[33]
	MRA		Pooled analysis: **88/93**[33]
SLAP tear	MRI	Surgery	86/13[34]
	MRA		72/**95**[30]
	CTA		**86/90**[30]
Bankart lesion	MRA	Surgery	**90/100**[30]
	CTA		**86/95**[30]
Hill-Sachs lesion	MRA	Surgery	75/**98**[30]
	CTA		**93/90**[30]
Instability/ labroligamentous tears	MRA	Surgery	**88/91**[35]

US = ultrasonography; MRI = magnetic resonance imaging; MRA = magnetic resonance arthrography; CTA = computed tomography arthrography; RCT = rotator cuff tear

The color coding for suggestion of **good** and **ideal** diagnostic accuracy values reported in this table are without quality scoring (QUADAS), a very important aspect of determination of the clinical utility of such values. Therefore, it is suggested that the reader keep this in mind when interpreting such values.

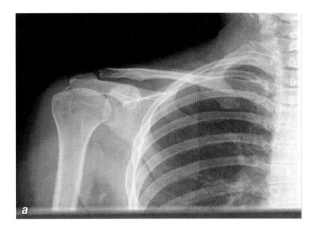
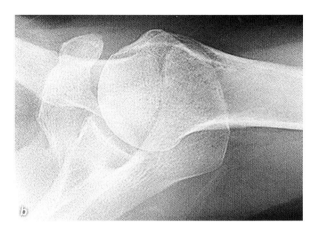
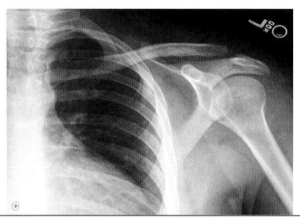

Figure 21.9 Shoulder radiographs: *(a)* anterior to posterior, *(b)* axial view, and *(c)* AP weight-bearing view of AC joint separation.

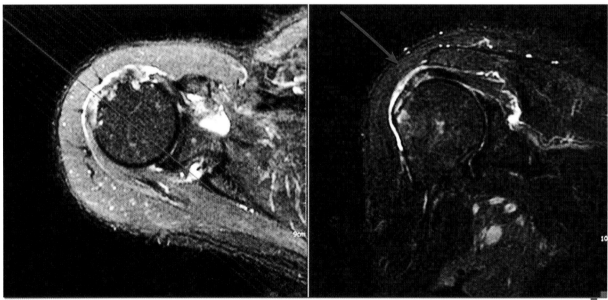

Figure 21.10 Supraspinatus tear shown in an MRI (left) and MRA (right).

Still, MRA has the advantage over CTA to directly visualize the affected structures with a better evaluation of extent and location and to detect associated capsuloligamentous injuries.[38]

It has been suggested that SLAP tears (figure 21.11) are often incorrectly diagnosed based on MRI evaluation, with MRI providing a high level of sensitivity and low level of specificity. On the basis of the results of this study, conventional MRI is not a suitable test for accurately evaluating the biceps labral complex for the presence of a SLAP tear.[34]

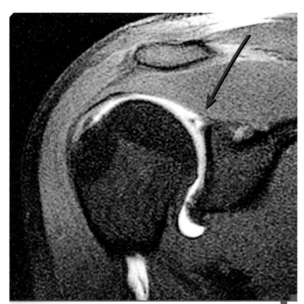

Figure 21.11   MRA: glenoid labrum SLAP tear.
© MedPix

Pain relief with intra-articular injection to the AC joint was significantly related to capsular hypertrophy identified on MRI. The SN in diagnosing a successful injection (range, 9–82%) was highest for caudal osteophytes (82%) and capsular hypertrophy (73%). The specificity (range, 51–97%) was highest for subchondral cysts (97%), subchondral bone marrow edema (95%), and joint effusion (92%). MRI findings have a reasonable SN and a high SP in predicting relevant short-term pain relief after intra-articular injection.[39]

Computed Tomography

As has been mentioned in the MRI section, CT is a useful diagnostic modality in diagnosing labral pathology.[38] It is also useful in appreciating details of the bony anatomy, particularly in examples where trauma may cause a fracture that is not readily seen on standard radiographs. CT also has the benefit of generating three-dimensional reconstruction of the shoulder for diagnosis and operative planning.[37] CTA also offers diagnostic capabilities for RCTs, since it has SN of 89 and SP of 98. While MRA had better SN and SP (100 and 94, respectively), the reported values of CTA suggest that it is an alternative to MRA.[30]

Diagnostic Ultrasound

Diagnostic ultrasound (US) has demonstrated strong SN and SP values in screening and diagnosing RCTs. Diagnostic US may provide less utility in diagnosing other subacromial disorders such as bursitis and tendinopathy.[25, 26] Regarding RCTs, US may be as effective as MRI in diagnosing any RCTs in cohorts of clients with suspected RCT pathology who are being evaluated for surgical intervention. Both MRI and US exhibit lower sensitivity in ruling out partial-thickness tears.[40] The effectiveness of US as a diagnostic or screening modality may be dependent on the experience of the clinician.[37]

Review of Systems

Refer to chapter 6 (Triage and Differential Diagnosis) for details on review of systems relevant to the shoulder.

OBSERVATION

The client with shoulder pain with active ROM will likely have guarded posturing of the involved shoulder, including limited upper extremity swing during gait. The client may hold the involved upper extremity in an internally rotated, adducted position, with the forearm held against the abdomen. The clinician can determine the client's willingness to move and use the shoulder early in the examination process when they introduce themselves to the client. A client with a highly irritated right shoulder is less likely to shake the clinician's hand during the introduction than a client with a low or moderately irritated shoulder.

Forward head, rounded shoulder posture (FHRSP) has been associated with decreased subacromial space. FHRSP is also associated with increased thoracic kyphosis, altered scapular muscle activity, and altered mechanics and scapular position in clients with shoulder pain from impingement and rotator cuff disease. However, asymptomatic clients with FHRSP also exhibit alterations in muscle activity with increased anterior tilt and limitations in upward rotation with shoulder elevation, suggesting that the posture is as much of a cause of altered mechanics as the pain may be.[41]

Static postural assessment is often implored because components of posture such as increased kyphosis or FHRSP are thought to be associated with a lack of shoulder elevation. However, static postural assessment is not consistently indicative of ability to move in clients with SAIS because clients may be able to move themselves out of the less-than-ideal postures.[42] Similarly, clinicians will commonly query the client for hand dominance. From an observational standpoint, hand dominance may be associated with a depressed scapula. This apparent asymmetry may not be indicative of dysfunction.[43]

TRIAGE AND SCREENING

Triage and screening is a necessary component of the examination process that should be done prior to continuing with the examination. As with all specific body part examinations, at this point the clinician must decide whether or not to continue with the examination. Specifically, they should determine whether to continue examining the client or refer them to a physician. Ruling out serious pathology (refer to chapter 6, Triage and Differential Diagnosis) and pain generation from other related (or close-proximity) structures helps the clinician more accurately determine the necessity of continuing with the other examination components to identify the actual source of the client's pain. Additionally, implementing strong screening

tests (tests of high SN and low –LR) at this point in the examination is suggested for narrowing down the competing diagnoses of the respective body region (cervical spine and elbow joint in this case) when this is applicable.

Ruling Out Serious Pathology: Red Flags

Signs, symptoms, and conditions that must be screened relevant to the shoulder include constant, progressive nonmechanical pain; history of drug abuse, cancer, or HIV; weight loss of 10% body mass or more in a time period of 10 to 21 days; violent trauma; widespread neurological signs and symptoms; a soft-tissue mass on clinical examination; acute coronary syndrome; and the suspected presence of a shoulder fracture.

Several prediction rules are applicable to acute coronary syndrome (see chapter 6 for greater detail). Twenty of these studies have been derived, while 10 have been validated at least one time.[44] The study with the strongest SN (98) and lowest false negative rate (<2%) was performed by Selker and colleagues.[45] This was a time-insensitive predictive instrument utilizing electrocardiography as a gold standard. The predictor variables included the presence of the following:

- Chest pain
- Shortness of breath
- Upper abdominal pain or dizziness
- Men > 30 years and women > 40 years of age

All other remaining prediction rules had SN of <95% in follow-up validation studies.[44] Tests for fractures and serious pathology from trauma include the olecranon-manubrium percussion test and bony apprehension test.

OLECRANON-MANUBRIUM PERCUSSION TEST

 Video 21.12 **in the web resource shows a demonstration of this test.**

The olecranon-manubrium percussion test is a useful clinical examination assessment for shoulder trauma.[46]

Client Position	Sitting with upper extremities crossed and the upper extremity to be assessed supported
Clinician Position	Standing directly in front of and facing the client

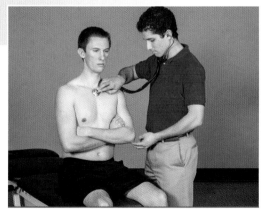

Figure 21.12

Movement	The clinician places a stethoscope over the manubrium. The clinician then taps the olecranon of the upper extremity to be assessed (left as shown).
Assessment	A normal response or negative test is a crisp sound equal to the sound elicited on the non-involved upper extremity. A (+) test is a lack of crisp sound equal to the noninvolved upper extremity.
Statistics	• **SN 84 (76-95)**, **SP 99 (87-100)**, **+LR 84**, **−LR 0.3**, QUADAS 12, in a prospective study of 96 clients (age, gender and mean duration of symptoms not reported [NR]), using shoulder trauma with radiography as a reference standard.[46]
	• This test provided useful clinical utility for anterior shoulder dislocations, clavicle fractures, and humerus fractures, but it was not clinically useful for AC joint abnormalities.
	• A similar type of testing (using a stethoscope and tuning fork on opposite sides of a suspected fracture or stress fracture) has been implemented for multiple locations; the one most appropriately related to the shoulder was the clavicle and humerus.[47]

BONY APPREHENSION TEST

  Video 21.13 **in the web resource shows a demonstration of this test.**

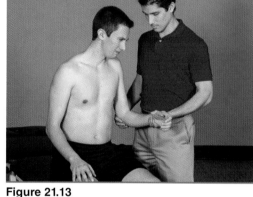

Client Position	Seated or standing
Clinician Position	Standing directly behind the client
Movement	The clinician grasps the client's forearm (with the elbow flexed to 90°) to be assessed with one hand (left as shown) and stabilizes the humerus/elbow and shoulder girdle with the other hand (right as shown). The clinician abducts and externally rotates the arm to ≤45°.

Figure 21.13

Assessment	A (+) test for anterior instability due to a bony lesion is the client demonstrating or stating apprehension during the test.
Statistics	• **SN 94 (NR)**, **SP 84 (NR)**, **+LR 5.9**, **−LR 0.07**, QUADAS 9, in 29 consecutive clients (average age 24 years, 7 female, mean duration symptoms NR) with symptomatic shoulder instability, and using arthroscopy as a reference standard.[48]
	• Bony lesion: **SN 100 (NR)**, **SP 86 (NR)**, **+LR 7.1**, **−LR 0.0**, QUADAS 9, for 8 cases of bony lesions that were positive and 3 of the soft-tissue lesions. Compared to preoperative radiographs: SN 50, **SP 100**, **+LR Inf**, −LR 0.5.[48]
	• This test had a higher SN than plain radiographs for osseous lesions.[48]

Ruling Out Pain Generation From Other Related Structures

As with all joints, screening the joints above and below for potential contribution to pain generation should be employed. Ruling out the cervical spine is of particular importance due not only to its close proximity to the shoulder but also to its potential for referral into the shoulder and entire upper extremity.

Rule Out Cervical Spine

Suspicion of cervical instability or cervical artery dysfunction should be addressed as discussed in chapter 17 (Cervical Spine) prior to proceeding with the examination. The upper quarter screen will determine cervical spine ROM and the potential for the cervical spine as a pain generator to the client's complaints of shoulder pain. Additionally, assessment of pain generation due to radiculopathy or discogenic-related pathology can be ruled out with a combination of Spurling's test and the upper limb neurodynamic test (median nerve bias):

- Spurling's test: **SN 93 (77-99), SP 95 (76-100), +LR 19.6, −LR 0.07, QUADAS 9**[49]

- Median nerve upper limb neurodynamic test: **SN 97 (90-100)**, SP 22 (12-33), +LR 1.3, **−LR 0.12**, QUADAS 10[50]

- Arm squeeze test (described for cervical nerve root compression): SN 95 (85-99), SP 96 (87-99), +LR 24, −LR 0.05, QUADAS 8[51]

As noted in chapter 17 (Cervical Spine), facet joint dysfunction can be ruled in with reproduction of concordant pain with posterior-anterior spinal joint-play assessment or facet joint block.

Rule Out Elbow Joint

The elbow joint should be incorporated into the triage as discussed in chapter 22 (Elbow) prior to proceeding with the examination. This is particularly true for clients who have sustained trauma, such as a fall on an outstretched hand. ROM of the elbow may indicate its contribution to pain generation in the upper arm. ROM may also help to rule out the presence of a fracture as is indicated in the following sensitive tests for the elbow.

Fracture

- Elbow extension test
  - **SN 97 (85-100)**, SP 69 (57-80), +LR 3.1, **−LR 0.04**, QUADAS 10[52]
  - **SN 100, SP 100, +LR Inf, −LR 0**, QUADAS 11[53]

- Overall active range of motion (AROM)
  - **SN 100 (93-100), SP 97 (88-100), +LR 33, −LR 0**, QUADAS 11[53]

- Overall AROM and tenderness to palpation
  - **SN 100 (93-100)**, SP 67 (53-78), +LR 3, **−LR 0**, QUADAS 11[53]

Additionally, as with any joint, clearing AROM with or without overpressure is necessary. AROM of all motions as per the upper quarter screen described in chapter 7 should be implemented. In order to fully clear the cervical spine, full AROM (with overpressure if pain-free) must be present.

Sensitive Tests: Shoulder

The shoulder joint is incorporated into any upper quarter triage. Many clinical examination tests are described for various pathologies of the shoulder girdle. However, there is a paucity of clinical tests that have strong SN and (−) LR values to help rule out shoulder pathologies this early in the examination. Appropriate screening clinical exam findings are described in the following section.

Fracture

- The clinician should perform the olecranon-manubrium and bony apprehension tests as described earlier.

Impingement

- Hawkins-Kennedy test
  - Pooled analysis: SN 74 (57-85), SP 57 (46-67), +LR 1.7, −LR 0.5, in six studies with 1,029 clients[54]
  - Pooled analysis: **SN 80 (72-86)**, SP 56 (45-67), +LR 1.84, **−LR 0.35**, in seven studies with 944 clients[55]

Additionally, as with any joint, clearing AROM with and without overpressure is necessary. In order to fully clear the shoulder joint, full AROM (with overpressure if pain-free) must be present. Detail in this regard is described in the following section.

MOTION TESTS

Motion at the shoulder is complex due to the multiple joints involved. Glenohumeral motion in the open kinetic chain involves a convex surface (humeral head) moving on a relatively stationary concave glenoid. Therefore, the proposed roll and glide will be in opposite directions except for flexion and extension, which are described as the axis of rotation spinning the humeral head around a point in the glenoid (figure 21.14). Abduction, for example, would involve a superior roll and inferior glide of the humeral head on the glenoid. Based on these mechanics and the shape of the joints that make up the shoulder girdle, theoretical capsular patterns, closed pack and resting positions have been described (indicated in table 21.2). Table 21.2 also describes typical ROM values for each motion and suspected normal end-feels of each motion.

While the convex–concave rule and construct provide a theoretical basis with which to visualize the glenohumeral arthrokinematics, the clinician must recognize that evidence indicates more variability in arthrokinematics than this construct would suggest. This variability is seen in both asymptomatic clients and in those with dysfunction.[56, 57]

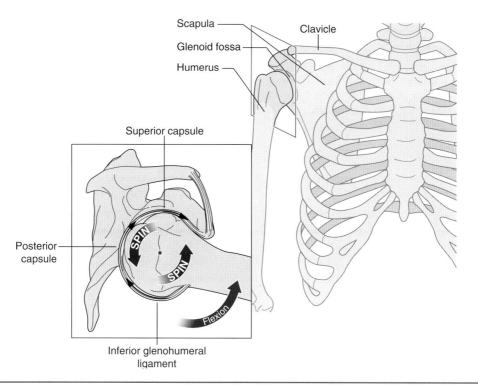

Scapula

Glenoid fossa

Humerus

Clavicle

Superior capsule

Posterior capsule

SPIN

SPIN

Flexion

Inferior glenohumeral ligament

Figure 21.14 Glenohumeral joint flexion in the sagittal plane.

TABLE 21.2 Shoulder Arthrology

Joint	Close-packed position	Resting position	Capsular pattern	ROM norms	End-feel
Glenohumeral	Abduction, ER	50° abduction, 30° horizontal adduction	ER, abduction, IR	Flexion: 0–180° Extension: 0–60° Abduction: 0–180° Internal rotation: 0–70° External rotation: 0–90°	All motions are firm end-feel
Sternoclavicular	Full elevation and protraction	Arm at side	Pain at extreme ROM, especially full elevation and protraction	10–15° of elevation; approximately 15–30° of both protraction and retraction; 15–31° of posterior rotation[60]	Firm for all motions
Acromioclavicular	90° abduction	Arm at side	Pain at extreme ROM	30° of upward rotation and approximately 17° of downward rotation[60]	Firm for all motions

(continued)

Table 21.2 *(continued)*

Joint	Close-packed position	Resting position	Capsular pattern	ROM norms	End-feel
Scapulothoracic	Pseudojoint without close- or loose-packed position, capsular pattern, and end-feel				
	Motions are referenced to the glenoid fossa. The motions at this joint include elevation and depression, upward and downward rotation, abduction and adduction, internal and external rotation, and anterior and posterior tipping.				

ER = external rotation; IR = internal rotation; ROM = range of motion

Similarly, the theoretical capsular pattern described for the glenohumeral joint does not have concrete evidence, with no specific pattern evident in clients with capsular dysfunction. Clinicians may instead observe limitation in all planes of glenohumeral motion with a capsular dysfunction (such as adhesive capsulitis), with a restriction into one plane possibly suggesting a dysfunction in only one portion of the capsule (the posterior capsule restricting internal rotation, for example).[58, 59]

The clinician is reminded of the relationship of movement between the glenohumeral and scapulothoracic joints. Scapulohumeral rhythm states that for every 2° of glenohumeral abduction or flexion, there is a corresponding 1° of upward rotation occurring at the scapulothoracic joint. Therefore, for every 3° of shoulder elevation, two-thirds of the motion comes from the humerus and one-third comes from the scapula.

The sternoclavicular joint is a saddle joint where elevation and depression motions involve a convex medial clavicle moving on a concave sternum (figure 21.15). Therefore, when assessing medial clavicular inferior glide, the clinician is assessing for sternoclavicular joint elevation. Protraction and retraction, on the other hand, occur in the transverse plane, in which the concave medial end of the clavicle glides on the convex sternum.

Passive and Active ROMs

Shoulder ROM measurements with a standard goniometer demonstrate good to excellent reliability (ICC: 0.80–0.99).[61] Measures of PROM for external rotation in clients with adhesive capsulitis has shown excellent reliability (ICC: 0.98–0.99).[62]

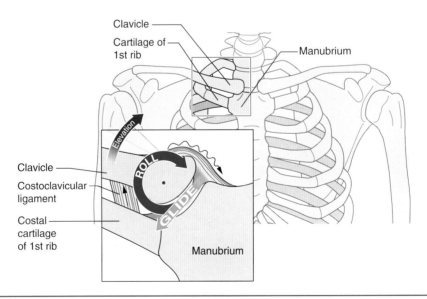

Figure 21.15 Arthrokinematics of sternoclavicular elevation.

SHOULDER FLEXION

Client Position	Supine with knees flexed to flatten lumbar spine, arms at side
Clinician Position	Standing directly to the side of the client
Goniometer Alignment	The clinician positions the fulcrum over the lateral aspect of the greater tubercle, with the proximal arm aligned parallel to the midaxillary line of the thorax and the distal arm aligned with the lateral midline of humerus, using the lateral epicondyle for reference.
Movement	The clinician stabilizes the client's scapula primarily via their weight on the table. The clinician passively lifts the client's arm overhead, maintaining the extremity in neutral abduction or adduction. End ROM of glenohumeral flexion occurs when resistance to further motion is felt or compensation of trunk movement is noted. The clinician can also monitor for excessive scapular motion. End-feel is firm due to soft-tissue restraints. This motion can be performed similarly actively by the client (without assistance from the clinician). Active range of motion should be performed prior to PROM to determine the client's willingness to move and so on.
Assessment	Clinician assesses for amount of ROM, end-feel, quality of the movement, client response, potential difference between AROM and PROM, and so on.

SHOULDER EXTENSION

Client Position	Prone with head rotated to the other side, arm relaxed
Clinician Position	Standing directly to the side of the client
Goniometer Alignment	The clinician positions the fulcrum over the lateral aspect of the greater tubercle and aligns the proximal arm parallel to the midaxillary line of the thorax and the distal arm with the lateral midline of the humerus, using the lateral epicondyle for reference.
Movement	The clinician's proximal hand stabilizes the ipsilateral scapula if necessary. The clinician passively moves the arm to be assessed to end range extension, with firm end-feel due to soft-tissue restraints. The elbow can be bent if necessary. This motion can be performed similarly actively by the client (without assistance from the clinician). Active range of motion should be performed prior to PROM to determine the client's willingness to move and so on.
Assessment	Clinician assesses for amount of ROM, end-feel, quality of the movement, client response, potential difference between AROM and PROM, and so on.

SHOULDER INTERNAL ROTATION

Client Position	Supine with arm to be assessed in 90° abduction. The forearm is perpendicular to the table (elbow 90° flexion) and is in neutral supination or pronation. The full length of the upper arm is placed on the table, with a pad under it to keep the humerus level with the acromion.
Clinician Position	Standing directly to the side of the client
Goniometer Alignment	The clinician positions the fulcrum over the olecranon process and aligns the proximal arm perpendicular to or parallel with the floor and the distal arm with the midline of the ulna (ulnar styloid for reference).
Movement	The clinician's proximal hand stabilizes the proximal humerus or distal clavicle. The clinician, purchasing the client's wrist, passively moves the arm to be assessed to end range internal rotation, with firm end-feel due to soft-tissue restraints. The clinician must monitor for shoulder girdle elevation. This motion can be performed similarly actively by the client (without assistance from the clinician). Active range of motion should be performed prior to PROM to determine the client's willingness to move and so on.
Assessment	Clinician assesses for amount of ROM, end-feel, quality of the movement, client response, potential difference between AROM and PROM, and so on.

SHOULDER EXTERNAL ROTATION

Client Position	The client is supine, with the arm to be assessed in 90° abduction. The forearm is perpendicular to the table (elbow 90° flexion) and in neutral supination or pronation. The full length of the upper arm is placed on the table with a pad under it to keep the humerus level with the acromion.
Clinician Position	Standing directly to the side of the client
Goniometer Alignment	The clinician positions the fulcrum over the olecranon process and aligns the proximal arm perpendicular to or parallel with the floor and the distal arm with the midline of the ulna (ulnar styloid for reference).
Movement	The clinician's proximal hand stabilizes the proximal humerus or distal clavicle. The clinician, purchasing the client's wrist, passively moves the arm to be assessed to end range external rotation, with firm end-feel due to soft-tissue restraints. The clinician must monitor for shoulder girdle elevation. This motion can be performed similarly actively by the client (without assistance from the clinician). Active range of motion should be performed prior to PROM to determine the client's willingness to move and so on.
Assessment	Clinician assesses for amount of ROM, end-feel, quality of the movement, client response, potential difference between AROM and PROM, and so on.

SHOULDER ABDUCTION

Client Position	Supine with arm relaxed at side
Clinician Position	Standing directly to the side of the client
Goniometer Alignment	The clinician positions the fulcrum over the ipsilateral anterior aspect of the acromion process and aligns the proximal arm so that it is parallel to the midline of the anterior aspect of sternum and the distal arm with the anterior midline of humerus (mid elbow as a reference).
Movement	The clinician's proximal hand stabilizes the trunk when passively assessing the ROM. The clinician's other hand grasps the client's wrist and moves the arm to end range abduction (normal end-feel is firm owing to soft tissue stretch). This motion can be performed similarly actively by the client (without assistance from the clinician). Active range of motion should be performed prior to PROM to determine the client's willingness to move and so on.
Assessment	Clinician assesses for amount of ROM, end-feel, quality of the movement, client response, potential difference between AROM and PROM, and so on.

Passive Accessories

Passive accessories are meant to evaluate the inert structures of the joint being assessed. The clinician will impart a force to replicate the proposed normal glides of the joints in the shoulder. Assessment of the client's response to the glide (i.e., report of concordant pain, relief of pain) during the glide is considered a significant finding. The clinician should also attempt to assess the mobility by detecting any obvious hypomobility or hypermobility by comparing it to that of the asymptomatic side. The following section describes passive accessory assessment for all components of the shoulder complex.

GLENOHUMERAL JOINT INFERIOR GLIDE

Client Position	Supine
Clinician Position	Standing at the client's arm to be tested
Stabilization	The clinician uses the hand farthest from the shoulder (right as shown) to hold the arm against their trunk. The scapula is stabilized by the client's lying on the plinth.
Movement and Direction of Force	The clinician purchases the client's proximal humerus as close to the joint as possible, with the assessing arm (left as shown) locked at the clinician's side. They apply assessing force via their entire body. The clinician uses their assessing hand to glide the proximal humerus inferior and slightly lateral along the plane of the joint.
Assessment	Assessment is done for joint play/passive accessory motion, client response, and end-feel. Reproduction of concordant pain suggests dysfunction. Impaired joint mobility or end-feel may also suggest dysfunction if concordant pain is also reproduced.

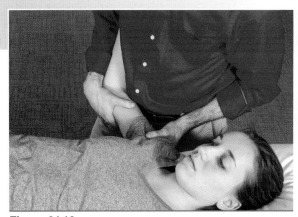

Figure 21.16

GLENOHUMERAL JOINT ANTERIOR GLIDE

Client Position	Prone
Clinician Position	Standing directly to the side of the supine client's arm to be tested
Stabilization	The clinician uses the hand farthest from the shoulder (right as shown) to hold their arm. The scapula is stabilized by the client's lying on the plinth.
Movement and Direction of Force	The clinician uses the assessing hand (left as shown) to purchase the proximal humerus as close to the joint as possible, applying primary force from the web space between the thumb and index finger. The clinician uses the assessing hand to glide the humerus in a posterior to anterior–medial direction along the plane of the joint.
Assessment	Assessment is done for joint play/passive accessory motion, client response, and end-feel. Reproduction of concordant pain suggests dysfunction. Impaired joint mobility or end-feel may also suggest dysfunction if concordant pain is also reproduced.

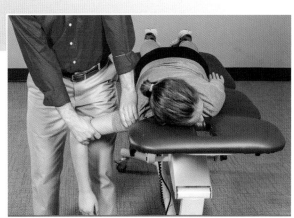

Figure 21.17

GLENOHUMERAL JOINT POSTERIOR GLIDE

 Video 21.18 in the web resource shows a demonstration of this test.

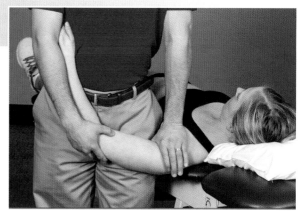

Client Position	Supine
Clinician Position	Standing directly to the side of the supine client's arm to be tested
Stabilization	The clinician uses the hand farthest from the shoulder (right as shown) to stabilize the client's arm between their arm and the side of their body.
Movement and Direction of Force	The clinician uses the assessing hand (left as shown) to purchase the proximal humerus such that the primary force is coming from the web space between the thumb and index finger. The clinician uses the assessing hand to glide the humerus in a posterior to posterior–lateral direction along the plane of the joint.
Assessment	Assessment is done for joint play/passive accessory motion, client response, and end-feel. Reproduction of concordant pain suggests dysfunction. Impaired joint mobility or end-feel may also suggest dysfunction if concordant pain is also reproduced.

Figure 21.18

Critical Clinical Pearls

When performing assessment of accessory glides, keep the following in mind:

- The clinician may need to accommodate their direction of force based on their client's posture. For example, a clinician may have to produce a more posterior–lateral glide (versus mostly posterior glide) on a client with significantly rounded shoulders who is lying supine.

- In a client with low irritability, the clinician should consider producing glides at the point of restriction or concordant symptoms.

- The clinician is reminded that the concave–convex rule is inconsistent in clinical scenarios and that consistent assessment and reassessment of the effect of manual therapy should guide them in the optimal direction of gliding for treatment purposes.

STERNOCLAVICULAR JOINT POSTERIOR GLIDE

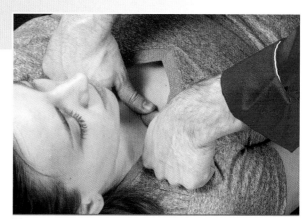

Client Position	Supine
Clinician Position	Standing directly to the side of the client's arm to be tested
Stabilization	The client's body resting on the table serves as a stabilizing force.
Movement and Direction of Force	The clinician should use both thumbs to purchase the anterior sternal end of the clavicle, approximately 3 cm from the medial end. Using thumb-over-thumb

Figure 21.19

purchase, the clinician glides the clavicle at the purchase site directly posterior and along the plane of the joint.

Assessment   Assessment is done for joint play/passive accessory motion, client response, and end-feel. Reproduction of concordant pain suggests dysfunction. Impaired joint mobility or end-feel may also suggest dysfunction if concordant pain is also reproduced.

STERNOCLAVICULAR JOINT ANTERIOR GLIDE

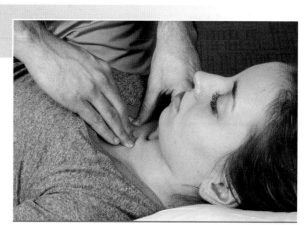

Figure 21.20

Client Position	Supine
Clinician Position	Standing directly to the side of the client's arm to be tested
Stabilization	The client's body resting on the table serves as a stabilizing force. The clinician's stabilizing hand (right as shown) holds the sternum.
Movement and Direction of Force	The clinician uses the mobilizing hand (left as shown) to purchase around the posterior surface of the clavicle with their fingers. The clinician uses their fingers to glide the clavicle anteriorly along plane of the joint.
Assessment	Assessment is done for joint play/passive accessory motion, client response, and end-feel. Reproduction of concordant pain suggests dysfunction. Impaired joint mobility or end-feel may also suggest dysfunction if concordant pain is also reproduced.

STERNOCLAVICULAR JOINT SUPERIOR GLIDE

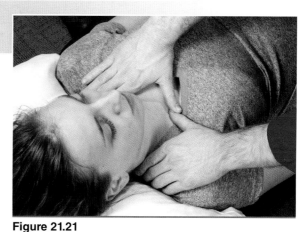

Figure 21.21

Client Position	Supine
Clinician Position	Standing directly to the side of the client's arm to be tested
Stabilization	The client's body resting on the table serves as a stabilizing force.
Movement and Direction of Force	Both thumbs purchase the inferior sternal end of clavicle approximately 3 cm from the medial (sternal) end. The clinician uses both thumbs (thumb-over-thumb purchase) to glide the clavicle superior and medial along the plane of the joint.
Assessment	Assessment is done for joint play/passive accessory motion, client response, and end-feel. Reproduction of concordant pain suggests dysfunction. Impaired joint mobility or end-feel may also suggest dysfunction if concordant pain is also reproduced.

STERNOCLAVICULAR JOINT INFERIOR GLIDE

Client Position	Supine
Clinician Position	Standing directly to the side of the client's arm to be tested
Stabilization	The client's body resting on the table serves as a stabilizing force.
Movement and Direction of Force	Both thumbs purchase the superior sternal end of the clavicle approximately 3 cm from the medial end. The clinician uses both thumbs (thumb-over-thumb purchase) to glide the clavicle inferior and lateral along the plane of the joint.
Assessment	Assessment is done for joint play/ passive accessory motion, client response, and end-feel. Reproduction of concordant pain suggests dysfunction. Impaired joint mobility or end-feel may also suggest dysfunction if concordant pain is also reproduced.

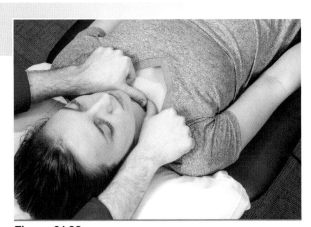

Figure 21.22

ACROMIOCLAVICULAR JOINT POSTERIOR GLIDE

Client Position	Supine
Clinician Position	Standing directly to the side of the client's arm to be tested
Stabilization	The client's body resting on the table serves as a stabilizing force.
Movement and Direction of Force	Both thumbs purchase the anterior surface of the lateral (acromial) end of the clavicle at the joint. The clinician uses both thumbs (thumb-over-thumb purchase) to glide the distal clavicle posteriorly along the plane of the joint.
Assessment	Assessment is done for joint play/passive accessory motion, client response, and end-feel. Reproduction of concordant pain suggests dysfunction. Impaired joint mobility or end-feel may also suggest dysfunction if concordant pain is also reproduced.

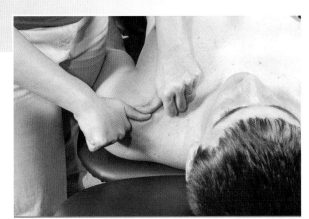

Figure 21.23

ACROMIOCLAVICULAR JOINT ANTERIOR GLIDE

Client Position	Supine
Clinician Position	Standing directly to the side of the client's arm to be tested
Stabilization	The client's body resting on the table serves as a stabilizing force.
Movement and Direction of Force	Both thumbs purchase the posterior surface of the lateral end of the clavicle at the joint. The clinician uses both thumbs

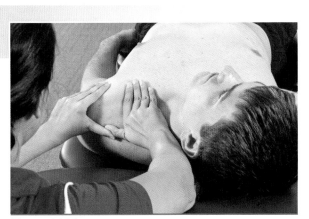

Figure 21.24

(thumb-over-thumb purchase) to glide the distal clavicle anteriorly along the plane of the joint.

Assessment   Assessment is done for joint play/passive accessory motion, client response, and end-feel. Restricted joint mobility or end-feel and/or reproduction of concordant pain suggest potential dysfunction.

SCAPULOTHORACIC JOINT GLIDES

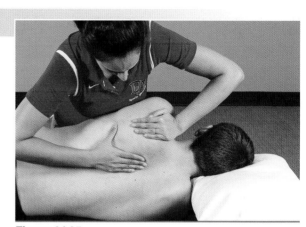

Figure 21.25

Client Position   Side lying

Clinician Position   Standing directly in front of the client

Stabilization, Movement, and Direction of Force   The clinician places one hand (left as shown) over the acromion and uses the other hand (right as shown) to purchase the inferior border of the scapula. Both hands perform the glides. The clinician uses both hands to glide the scapula in the direction to be assessed (described in the following list).

- Distraction: Fingertips from both hands purchase the medial border of the scapula and distract it posteriorly (away) from rib cage.
- Medial glide: Both hands glide the scapula toward the spine.
- Lateral glide: Both hands glide the scapula away from the spine.
- Inferior glide: Both hands glide the scapula inferiorly toward the iliac crest.
- Superior glide: Both hands glide the scapula superiorly toward the head.

Assessment   Assessment is done for joint play/passive accessory motion, client response, and end-feel. Reproduction of concordant pain suggests dysfunction. Impaired joint mobility or end-feel may also suggest dysfunction if concordant pain is also reproduced.

Flexibility

Muscle length may be a component of an initial examination in the shoulder or may be completed at subsequent follow-up visits in managing a client with shoulder pain, depending on the priority of other impairment findings during the clinical exam.[64] Table 21.3 describes common muscles that can contribute to altered mechanics of the shoulder girdle if flexibility impairments exist. Illustrations and descriptions of the flexibility assessment are provided as follows.

TABLE 21.3 Shoulder Musculature

Muscle	Origin	Insertion	Action	Innervation
Pectoralis major	Medial 1/4 of clavicle, sternum, costal cartilage of ribs 2-6	Crest of greater tubercle	Humerus adduction and internal rotation	Medial and lateral pectoral nerve
Pectoralis minor	Ribs 3-5	Medial portion of coracoid process	Scapular protraction	Medial and lateral pectoral nerve
Biceps brachii	Short head: tip of coracoid process of scapula; long head: supraglenoid tubercle of scapula	Radial tuberosity and bicipital aponeurosis into fascia of forearm	Flexion and supination of forearm; flexion of the arm	Musculocutaneous nerve
Triceps brachii	Long head: infraglenoid tubercle of scapula; lateral head: posterior surface of humerus above and lateral to groove of radial nerve and lateral intermuscular septum; medial head: posterior surface of humerus below and medial to groove of radial nerve and both intermuscular septa	Proximal end of olecranon of ulna	Extension of forearm; extension of arm (long head)	Radial nerve

POSTERIOR SHOULDER TIGHTNESS

Client Position	Side lying with the side to be tested on top and the head and trunk in a neutral position
Clinician Position	Standing in front of the client and supporting the testing arm with one hand while concurrently blocking the lateral border of the scapula
Movement	The clinician maintains the client's testing arm in neutral rotation and brings the arm to 90° of abduction. While maintaining neutral rotation by supporting the distal humerus, the clinician passively lowers the testing arm into horizontal adduction.

The clinician's stabilizing hand (right as shown) maintains pressure along the scapular border for the duration of the test. Of note, some studies describe this assessment performing the same movement while maintaining the client's elbow in full extension. Otherwise, the assessment is performed as described here.

Assessment	The clinician measures the angle of horizontal adduction relative to the horizontal plane. The client's end range is determined as either the point in the ROM where terminal horizontal adduction is reached or where the client's arm starts to internally rotate. The posterior shoulder is considered restricted if the client's arm is unable to drop below a 0° point relative to the horizontal plane.
Statistics	There are no known normative data for this flexibility measure. One study indicates good intra-rater reliability (0.79) in a sample of clients with postoperative ROM impairments. A clinically significant change in this population was found to be 8°.

Figure 21.26

PECTORALIS MAJOR ASSESSMENT

Client Position	Supine with hands clasped behind their head
Clinician Position	Standing (or sitting) directly to the side to be assessed
Movement	Keeping the cervical spine in neutral, the client is instructed to let the elbows move toward the table while keeping the lumbar spine flat.
Assessment	Using a tape measure, the clinician measures the distance between the olecranon process of the humerus and the table surface.
Statistics	There are no known normative data for this flexibility measure.

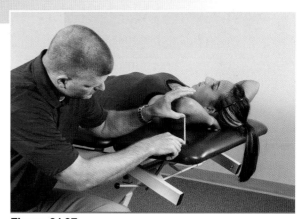

Figure 21.27

PECTORALIS MINOR ASSESSMENT

Client Position	Supine with arms resting in anatomical position, with the legs and lumbar spine flat against the evaluating surface
Clinician Position	At the head of the examination table and either sitting or kneeling to visualize the superior shoulder girdle
Movement	The client relaxes their shoulders to a resting position.
Assessment	The clinician measures the distance from the posterior aspect of the acromion to the examination table.
Statistics	There are no known normative data for this flexibility measure.

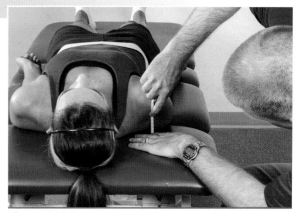

Figure 21.28

TRICEPS ASSESSMENT

Client Position	Sitting with the shoulder and elbow at end range flexion, and the forearm in full supination
Clinician Position	Standing alongside or behind the client, depending on the best view of the client's arm
Movement	The clinician flexes the client's elbow to the end range while maintaining the arm in shoulder flexion.
Assessment	The clinician measures the angle of elbow flexion with a goniometer using the axis at the lateral epicondyle, with the arms of the goniometer along the humerus proximally and along the forearm distally.
Statistics	There are no known normative data for this flexibility measure.

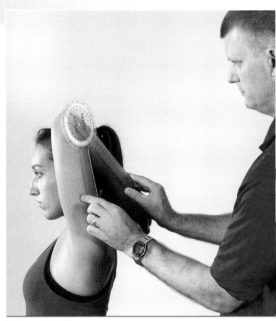

Figure 21.29

BICEPS ASSESSMENT

Client Position	Supine and lying close to the edge of the examination table
Clinician Position	Siting or kneeling alongside the client
Movement	The clinician brings the client's arm off the table to allow shoulder and elbow extension, along with forearm pronation.
Assessment	The clinician centers a goniometer with the axis of rotation in the glenohumeral joint. The measurement arm of the goniometer is along the midline of the humeral shaft while the stable arm of the goniometer is either perpendicular or parallel to the thorax.
Statistics	There are no known normative data for this flexibility measure.

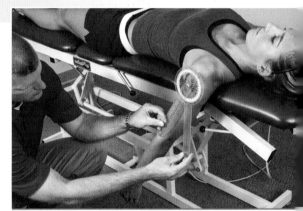

Figure 21.30

Critical Clinical Pearls

Glenohumeral internal rotation deficit (GIRD) is not described as a flexibility assessment previously. When assessing for GIRD, keep the following in mind:

- This assessment should be a normal part of the motion assessment.

- The acromion should be blocked to isolate glenohumeral motion.

- GIRD may be a result of soft-tissue restriction, capsular restriction, or both.

- The clinician should be sure to assess for the total arc of rotational motion from one limb to the other, since a client may have an apparent lack of IR but have compensatory excessive ER and relatively equal total rotation bilaterally.

- The clinical finding of GIRD and its relation to pathology or dysfunction is debatable, with recent studies suggesting that differences in total range of motion in the shoulder are more correlated with upper extremity dysfunction in overhead athletes.[65]

- Posterior shoulder tightness may be easier to change than GIRD.[63]

MUSCLE PERFORMANCE TESTING

Appreciating strength throughout the rotator cuff and scapular muscles has been proposed in clients with shoulder dysfunction. Muscle dysfunction in the rotator cuff may be implicated through several clinical special tests (the infraspinatus test, for example). Several special tests have also been suggested for identifying scapular dyskinesis due to inefficient strength or motor control of the scapular muscles (the scapular assistance test, for example). All of these tests will be referenced later in this chapter, including descriptions of their respective diagnostic value.

A review of the EMG studies to delineate muscle strength difference in clients with and without SAIS suggested that the most significant differences between groups involve an overactivity of the upper trapezius and decreased activity of the lower trape-zius in clients with SAIS when performing elevation in the scapular plane.[66] Handheld dynamometry (HHD) has been shown to be reliable when using manual muscle testing (MMT) for the upper, lower, and middle trapezius and serratus anterior. However, concurrent surface EMG suggested that only the upper and lower trapezius muscle test position truly engaged the respective muscles for a valid assessment. As such, the supine serratus test and prone middle trapezius test may lack validity in their assessment.[67]

Handheld dynamometry and surface EMG have been used in healthy subjects to exhibit construct validity of traditional MMT positions for assessing RC strength, though true isolation without synergistic muscle activity was not possible.[68] Another study used EMG to identify optimal testing positions for the RC and recommended the following: resisting elevation at 90° of elevation, with 45° of external rotation in the scapular plane for the supraspinatus; resisting external rotation at 0° of humeral elevation, with 45° of internal rotation.[69, 70]

SCAPULAR ABDUCTION AND UPWARD ROTATION

Client Position	Seated with bilateral knees flexed over the edge of the table
Clinician Position	Standing directly to the side of the client
Movement and Assessment	The clinician palpates the client's inferior angle of the scapula between the web spaces of one hand. The client raises the arm to 130° of flexion. The clinician's other hand provides resistance proximal to the elbow.

- Grade 5: scapula maintains abducted and rotated position against maximal resistance just above the elbow
- Grade 4: scapular muscles yield against maximal resistance and scapula moves in direction of adduction and downward resistance
- Grade 3: scapula moves through full ROM without winging, but cannot tolerate resistance
- Grade 2: scapula abducts and upwardly rotates, trying to maintain arm above 90°
- Grade 1: muscle activity without movement
- Grade 0: no muscle activity

Primary Muscles	Serratus anterior
Secondary Muscles	Pectoralis minor
Primary Nerve	Long thoracic nerve (C5-7; serratus anterior)

SCAPULAR ELEVATION

Client Position	Seated with bilateral knees flexed over the edge of the table
Clinician Position	Standing directly behind the client
Assessment	The client shrugs bilateral shoulders and attempts to maintain their position as the clinician pushes down on their shoulders.

- Grade 5: completes motion against maximal resistance
- Grade 4: completes motion against strong resistance
- Grade 3: completes motion without resistance
- Grade 2: completes full ROM in prone gravity-minimized position
- Grade 1: muscle activity without movement
- Grade 0: no muscle activity

Primary Muscles	Trapezius
	Levator scapulae
Secondary Muscles	Rhomboid major and minor
Primary Nerves	Spinal accessory and C3-4 (trapezius)
	Dorsal scapular nerve and C3-4 (levator scapulae)
	C5 (levator scapulae)

SCAPULAR DEPRESSION AND ADDUCTION

Client Position	Prone with arm overhead and externally rotated approximately 145°, with the thumb pointing to the ceiling
Clinician Position	Standing directly beside the client

Movement and Assessment	The clinician asks the client to lift their arm to the ceiling and then provides resistance over the distal humerus with one hand and palpates the middle and lower trapezius with the other hand.

- Grade 5: completes motion against maximal resistance
- Grade 4: completes motion against strong resistance
- Grade 3: completes motion without resistance
- Grade 2: completes full scapular ROM without weight of arm (clinician supporting client's arm at elbow)
- Grade 1: muscle activity without movement
- Grade 0: no muscle activity

Primary Muscles	Middle and lower trapezius
Secondary Muscles	Pectoralis major and minor
	Latissimus dorsi
Primary Nerve	Accessory nerve

SHOULDER FLEXION

Client Position	Sitting with arm at side, elbow flexed and forearm pronated
Clinician Position	Standing directly beside the client
Movement and Assessment	The clinician asks the client to hold their arm in a position of 90° flexion, then provides resistance just above the client's elbow with one hand. The clinician can use the other hand to stabilize the client's shoulder.

- Grade 5: completes motion against maximal resistance
- Grade 4: completes motion against strong resistance
- Grade 3: completes motion to 90° without resistance
- Grade 2: completes partial ROM to 90° against gravity without resistance
- Grade 1: muscle activity without movement
- Grade 0: no muscle activity

Primary Muscles	Anterior deltoid
	Coracobrachialis
Secondary Muscles	Middle deltoid
	Pectoralis major
Primary Nerves	Axillary nerve (C5-6; deltoid)
	Musculocutaneous nerve (C5-7; coracobrachialis)

SHOULDER EXTENSION

Client Position	Prone, arm at side and internally rotated
Clinician Position	Standing directly to the side of the client
Assessment	The clinician asks the client to keep their elbow straight and raise their arm to the ceiling. The clinician provides resistance just above the elbow.

- Grade 5: completes motion against maximal resistance
- Grade 4: completes motion against strong resistance
- Grade 3: completes motion without resistance

(continued)

Shoulder Extension *(continued)*

- Grade 2: completes partial ROM against gravity without resistance
- Grade 1: muscle activity without movement
- Grade 0: no muscle activity

Primary Muscles	Latissimus dorsi
	Posterior deltoid
	Teres major
Secondary Muscles	Triceps brachii
Primary Nerves	Subscapular nerve (C5-6; teres major)
	Axillary (C5-6; deltoid)
	Thoracodorsal nerve (C6-8; latissimus dorsi)

SHOULDER ABDUCTION

Client Position	Sitting, arm at side with elbow slightly flexed
Clinician Position	Standing directly behind the client
Movement and Assessment	The clinician asks the client to hold their arm at 90° shoulder abduction as they resist just above the elbow with one hand. The clinician can use the other hand to stabilize the client's shoulder.

- Grade 5: completes motion against maximal resistance
- Grade 4: completes motion against strong resistance
- Grade 3: completes motion to 90° without resistance
- Grade 2: completes partial ROM to 90° against gravity without resistance
- Grade 1: muscle activity without movement
- Grade 0: no muscle activity

Primary Muscles	Middle deltoid
	Supraspinatus
Primary Nerves	Axillary (C5-6; deltoid)
	Suprascapular (C5-6; supraspinatus)

SHOULDER HORIZONTAL ABDUCTION

Client Position	Prone, shoulder abducted 90° with elbow flexed and forearm off the edge of the table
Clinician Position	Standing directly to the side of the client
Movement and Assessment	The clinician asks the client to lift their elbow up to ceiling as they provide resistance just above the elbow.

- Grade 5: completes motion against maximal resistance
- Grade 4: completes motion against strong resistance
- Grade 3: completes motion without resistance

A sitting position is used for grades below 3. The clinician supports the arm to be tested under the forearm and places the arm in similar position as described previously. The clinician palpates the posterior deltoid superior to the axilla.

- Grade 2: completes full ROM without resistance and with the arm supported
- Grade 1: muscle activity without movement
- Grade 0: no muscle activity

Primary Muscles	Posterior deltoid

Secondary Muscles	Infraspinatus
	Teres minor
Primary Nerve	Axillary (C5-6)

SHOULDER HORIZONTAL ADDUCTION

Client Position	Supine, arm abducted 90° with elbow flexed 90°
Clinician Position	Standing directly to the side of the client
Movement and Assessment	The clinician asks the client to pull their arm across their chest while they provide resistance just proximal to the wrist.

- Grade 5: completes motion against maximal resistance
- Grade 4: completes motion against strong resistance
- Grade 3: completes motion without resistance

A sitting position is used for grades below 3. The clinician supports the arm to be tested under the forearm and places it in a similar position to the one described previously. The clinician palpates the pectoralis major just medial to the shoulder joint.

- Grade 2: completes full ROM against gravity without resistance and with the arm supported
- Grade 1: muscle activity without movement
- Grade 0: no muscle activity

Primary Muscles	Pectoralis major
Secondary Muscles	Anterior deltoid
Primary Nerves	Medial pectoral nerve (C6-T1; sternocostal portion)
	Lateral pectoral nerve (C5-6; clavicular portion)

SHOULDER EXTERNAL ROTATION

Client Position	Prone, head turned to the side to be assessed. Shoulder abducted 90°, with towel under the humerus and forearm hanging off the edge of the table.
Clinician Position	Standing directly to the side of the client
Movement and Assessment	The clinician asks the client to raise their forearm up and forward toward the ceiling as they provide resistance with two fingers just proximal to wrist. The clinician uses the other hand to support the client's elbow, providing counterpressure at end of ROM.

- Grade 5: completes motion against maximal resistance
- Grade 4: completes motion against strong resistance
- Grade 3: completes motion without resistance

For grades below 3, the client should be prone, with their entire arm off the edge of the table, maintaining a neutral rotation position. The client is instructed to turn their palm up and outward.

- Grade 2: completes full ROM (e.g., palm faces up) without resistance
- Grade 1: muscle activity without movement
- Grade 0: no muscle activity

Primary Muscles	Infraspinatus
	Teres minor
Secondary Muscles	Posterior deltoid
Primary Nerves	Axillary nerve (C5-6; teres minor)
	Suprascapular nerve (C5-6; infraspinatus)

SHOULDER INTERNAL ROTATION

Client Position	Prone, head turned to the side to be assessed. Shoulder abducted 90°, with a towel under the humerus and forearm hanging off the edge of the table.
Clinician Position	Standing directly to the side of the client
Movement and Assessment	The clinician asks the client to raise their forearm up and back toward the ceiling as they provide resistance with two fingers just proximal to the wrist. The clinician uses their other hand to support the client's elbow, providing counterpressure at end of ROM.

- Grade 5: completes motion against maximal resistance
- Grade 4: completes motion against strong resistance
- Grade 3: completes motion without resistance

For grades below 3, the client should be prone, with the entire arm off the edge of the table and in a neutral rotation position. The client is instructed to turn their palm down and inward.

- Grade 2: completes full ROM (e.g., palm faces down) without resistance
- Grade 1: muscle activity without movement
- Grade 0: no muscle activity

Primary Muscles	Subscapularis
	Pectoralis major
	Latissimus dorsi
	Teres major
Secondary Muscles	Anterior deltoid
Primary Nerves	Subscapularis (C5-6; subscapularis)
	Medial and lateral pectoral nerve (C5-T1; pectoralis major)
	Thoracodorsal nerve (C6-8; latissimus dorsi)

SPECIAL TESTS

As mentioned in chapter 10 (Special Tests), in many cases the clinician is overly dependent on the performance and interpretation of special test findings with respect to differential diagnosis of the client's presenting pain. Utilization of special tests for ruling in (or helping to diagnose) a particular pathology should occur at this point in the examination process. It is also hoped that the clinician has a much clearer picture of the client's presentation prior to this point in the examination and will therefore depend minimally on special test findings with espect to diagnosis of the client's pain.

Clinicians can choose from an extensive selection of special tests that are purported to assist in diagnosing pathology and dysfunction in the shoulder complex. Despite the abundance of available special clinical tests, review of the literature reveals significant limitations in shoulder testing. For example, a variety of tests are described to potentially diagnose RCT. However, multiple systematic reviews have indicated that rotator cuff clinical tests have poor accuracy in diagnosing the location and extent of an RCT.[55, 71, 72] Several other reviews indicate similar limitations in the diagnostic and screening abilities of shoulder special tests.[4, 55, 70, 71, 73-80]

This section discusses the evidence related to special tests of the shoulder complex. Statistical values indicate those tests with stronger quality in contributing to either helping to rule in or rule out a diagnosis. In multiple cases, recent evidence has indicated that combining these tests may be more effective.[55] However, even combining tests for a common dysfunction such as SAIS does not offer definitive information with regard to pathology. As such, special tests should not be the crux of the examination. Refer to the Triage and Screening section of this chapter to review concepts in screening for ruling out areas, such as the cervical spine, that may mimic shoulder dysfunction and pain.

Index of Special Tests

Subacromial Impingement Syndrome (SAIS)

Neer's Sign
Hawkins-Kennedy Test
Painful Arc

Internal Rotation Resisted
   Strength Test
Cross-Body Adduction Test

Infraspinatus or External Rotation
   Resistance Test
Clusters of Tests

Rotator Cuff Tear

Rent Test
Lateral Jobe Test

Supine Impingement Test
Empty Can Test

Supraspinatus Tear or SAIS

Drop Arm Test

Full Can Test

Supraspinatus and Infraspinatus Tear

External Rotation Lag Sign

Infraspinatus and Teres Minor Tear

Drop Sign

Hornblower's Sign

Subscapularis Tear

Lift-Off Test
Internal Rotation Lag Sign

Belly Press Test
Bear Hug Test

Rotator Cuff Tear or Posterior Labral Tear

Posterior Impingement Sign

Labral Pathology and Shoulder Instability

Biceps Load I
Crank Test
Biceps Load II
Active Compression Test

Speed's Test
Anterior Slide Test
Yergason's Test
Compression Rotation Test

Passive Compression Test
Passive Distraction Test
Cluster Testing for Labral Tears

Posteroinferior Labral Lesion

Kim Test

Jerk Test

Instability

Surprise Test or Anterior
   Release Test

Anterior Apprehension Test
Relocation Test

Hyperabduction Test
Sulcus Sign

Biceps Tendinopathy

Biceps Tendon Palpation
Upper Cut Test

Speed's Test
Clusters

(continued)

AC Joint Pathology

Paxinos Sign	Cross-Body Adduction Test	Active Compression Test
AC Joint Palpation	AC Resisted Extension Test	Cluster Testing

Adhesive Capsulitis

Shoulder Shrug Sign   Coracoid Pain Test

Tests for Scapular Dyskinesis

Scapular Assistance Test	Lateral Scapular Slide Test	SICK Scapula
Scapular Dyskinesis Test	Scapular Retraction Test	

Nerve Palsies

Deltoid Extension Lag Sign   Triangle Sign
Active Elevation Lag Sign

Case Studies

Go to www.HumanKinetics.com/OrthopedicClinicalExamination and complete these case studies for chaper 21:

- Case study 1 discusses a 23-year-old male baseball pitcher with pain in is his right anterior shoulder.
- Case study 2 discusses a 52-year-old female artist with pain in her right shoulder with overhead painting.

Abstract Links

Go to www.HumanKinetics.com/OrthopedicClinicalExamination to access abstract links on these issues:

AC joint palpation	External rotation lag sign	Passive distraction test
Active compression test	Full can test	Paxinos sign
Anterior apprehension test	Hawkins-Kennedy	Rent test
Anterior slide test	Hornblower's sign	Scapular assistance test
Arm squeeze test	Internal rotation resisted strength test	Scapular dyskinesis test
Biceps load I		Scapular retraction test
Biceps load II	Kim test	Shoulder shrug sign
Biceps tendon palpation	Lateral Jobe test	Speeds test
Bony apprehension test	Lateral scapular slide test	Spurling's test
Coracoid pain test	Lift-off test	Supine impingement test
Crank test	Neer's sign	Surprise test (anterior release test)
Cross body adduction test	Olecranon manubrium percussion test	
Drop arm test		Upper cut test
	Passive compression test	Yergason's test

SUBACROMIAL IMPINGEMENT SYNDROME (SAIS)

The single tests of painful arc, external rotation resistance, and Neer's sign are useful screening tests for ruling out SAIS. The single tests of painful arc, external rotation resistance, and empty can are helpful for confirming SAIS. The reliability of all tests was acceptable for clinical use. Based on reliability and diagnostic accuracy, the single tests of the painful arc, external rotation resistance, and empty can have the best overall clinical utility. The cutoff point of ≥3/5 (+) tests can help confirm the diagnosis of SAIS, while ≤2/5 (+) tests help to rule out SAIS.[4]

Neer impingement sign, Hawkins-Kennedy impingement test, Patte maneuver, and Jobe supraspinatus test are highly reproducible and therefore reliable to use in clinical practice to identify clients with subacromial pain with an impingement phenomenon, but the maneuvers are limited as structural discriminators. All four maneuvers have an almost perfect agreement (κ coefficients 0.91–1.00), if performed with suggested standardizations.[74]

NEER'S SIGN

Client Position	Sitting or standing
Clinician Position	Standing alongside the client, stabilizing the scapula in an attempt to block scapulothoracic movement
Movement	The clinician brings the client's involved arm into passive forward flexion with glenohumeral internal rotation.[70, 74] This is also described as having the client actively forward flex the involved arm until the point of pain or until end range of motion is achieved.[54]
Assessment	A test is (+) if pain is reproduced,[54] particularly along the anterior or lateral aspect of the shoulder.[70]

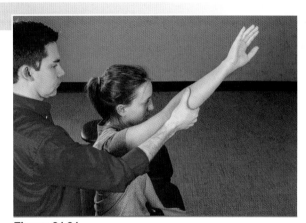

Figure 21.31

Statistics

- Pooled analysis: SN 78 (68-71), SP 58 (46-67), +LR 1.9, –LR 0.4, in five studies with 1,127 clients.[54]

- Pooled analysis: SN 72 (60-81), SP 60 (40-77), +LR 1.79, –LR 0.47, in seven studies with 946 clients.[55]

- SN 89 (NR), SP 30 (NR), +LR 1.02 NR, –LR 0.94 NR, QUADAS 8, in a study of 120 clients presenting to an orthopedic surgeon with shoulder pain (mean age of 52 years; 72 women; mean duration of symptoms NR), using subacromial injection as a reference standard.[81]

- SN 75 (NR) and SP 30 (NR), QUADAS 7, in 85 clients with shoulder pain (mean age of 40 years; 27% females; mean duration of symptoms NR), using a reference standard of bursitis diagnosed on arthroscopy.[82]

- **SN 81 (62-100)**, SP 54 (38-69), +LR 1.76, **–LR 0.35**, QUADAS 10, in a study of 55 clients (ranging in age from 18-83; 8 women; mean duration of symptoms 49 months), using shoulder pain and surgery as a reference standard. Surgical findings for SAIS included evidence of supraspinatus degeneration or involvement of the bursa.[4]

- SN 62 (NR), SP 0 (NR), QUADAS 10, in a study of 34 clients (mean age of 57; 14 women; median duration of symptoms 2 years), using chronic shoulder pain and diagnostic US as a reference standard.[70]

- SN 60 (47-73), SP 35 (22-48), +LR 0.92, –LR 1.14, QUADAS 13, in a study of 52 clients with acute shoulder pain and inability to abduct shoulder >90° (age range 18-75 years old; 14 women; < 2 week onset of shoulder pain), using diagnostic US and response to lidocaine injection as reference standards.[78]

- Reliability has been calculated as (κ) = 1.0 in 33 subjects with shoulder pain in a primary care clinic, mean age of 32, and duration of symptoms ranging from 2 to 14 weeks.[74]

HAWKINS-KENNEDY TEST

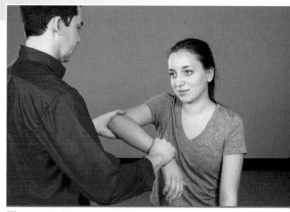

Figure 21.32

Client Position	Sitting upright
Clinician Position	Standing in front of or to the side of the client
Movement	The clinician grasps the client's elbow with one hand (left as shown) and wrist with the other hand (right as shown). If the client demonstrates significant shoulder girdle elevation during test, the clinician stabilizes the client's shoulder girdle with one hand and grasps the client's elbow or proximal forearm with the other hand. The client's arm is flexed to 90° with the elbow in flexion. The arm is then internally rotated while maintaining the 90° of flexion. The internal rotation continues until the client reports provocation of their concordant pain or until the clinician observes elevation of the scapula.[54, 70]
Assessment	A (+) test is if the client's pain is reproduced.
Statistics	• Pooled analysis: SN 74 (57-85), SP 57 (46-67), +LR 1.7, –LR 0.5, in six studies with 1,029 clients.[54]
	• Pooled analysis: **SN 80** (72-86), SP 56 (45-67), +LR 1.84, **–LR 0.35**, in seven studies with 944 clients.[55]
	• SN 74 (NR), SP 50 (NR), +LR 1.48, –LR NR, QUADAS 10, in a study of 34 clients with chronic shoulder pain (mean age of 57; 14 women; median duration of symptoms 2 years), using diagnostic US as a reference standard.[70]
	• SN 63 (39-86), SP 62 (46-77), +LR 1.63, –LR 0.61, QUADAS 10, in a study of 55 clients with presenting shoulder pain (ranging in age from 18-83; 8 women; mean duration of symptoms for at least 1 week), using surgery as a reference standard.[4]
	• SN 77 (66-88), SP 26 (14-38), +LR 1.0, –LR 0.88, QUADAS 13, in a study of 52 clients with acute shoulder pain and inability to abduct shoulder >90° (age range 18-75 years old; 14 women; <2-week onset of shoulder pain), using diagnostic US and response to lidocaine injection as reference standards.[78]
	• Reliability has been calculated as (κ) = 0.91 in 33 subjects with shoulder pain in a primary care clinic, average age of 32, and duration of symptoms ranging from 2 to 14 weeks.[74]

PAINFUL ARC

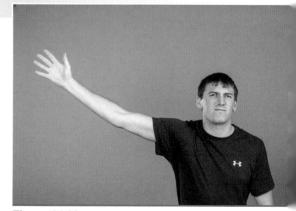

Figure 21.33

Client Position	Sitting or standing upright
Clinician Position	Facing the client to monitor for quality of movement or for client reactions that indicate pain
Movement	The client actively abducts the arm while maintaining anatomical position (palm facing forward).
Assessment	A test is (+) if the client reports pain from approximately 60° to 120° but does not report pain outside of this range of abduction.[70]

Statistics
- Pooled analysis: SN 53 (31-74), SP 76 (68-84), +LR 2.3, –LR 0.62, in four studies with 756 clients[55]
- SN 29.6 (NR), SP 50 (NR), +LR 0.59, –LR 1.40, QUADAS 10, in a study of 34 clients (mean age of 57; 14 women; median duration of symptoms 2 years), using chronic shoulder pain and diagnostic US as reference standards[70]
- SN 75 (54-96), SP 67 (52-81), +LR 2.25, –LR 0.38, QUADAS 10, in a study of 55 clients with presenting shoulder pain (age ranging in age from 18-83 years of age; 8 women; pain for at least 1 week), using surgery as a reference standard[4]
- SN 96 (90-100), SP 4 (1-9), +LR 1.0, –LR 1.0, QUADAS 13, in a study of 52 clients with acute shoulder pain and inability to abduct shoulder >90° (age range 18-75 years old; 14 women; <2-week onset of shoulder pain), using diagnostic US and response to lidocaine injection as reference standards[78]

INTERNAL ROTATION RESISTED STRENGTH TEST

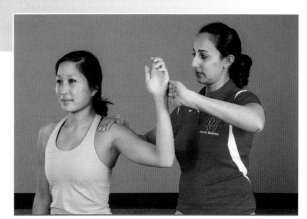

Client Position	Sitting or standing upright with arm positioned into 90° of abduction and 80° of ER. The elbow is maintained in 90° of flexion throughout the test.
Clinician Position	Standing behind the client, with one hand stabilizing the humerus or scapula (right as shown) and the opposite hand placed at the distal end of the forearm (left as shown)
Movement	The clinician has the client resist both internal rotation (IR) and external rotation (ER) in this position.

Figure 21.34

Assessment A test is (+) if there is weakness in IR relative to ER.

Statistics SN 88 (NR), SP 96 (NR), +LR 22, –LR 0.12, QUADAS 8 in a study of 110 clients with chronic shoulder pain with average of 16 weeks failed conservative measures including cortisone injection and physical therapy (mean age NR; 35 females; average duration of symptoms 10.9 months), using arthroscopic findings as a reference standard[83]

CROSS-BODY ADDUCTION TEST

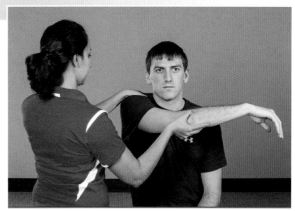

Client Position	Sitting or standing upright with the arm in 90° of shoulder flexion with the elbow slightly bent
Clinician Position	Standing in front of the client
Movement	The clinician stabilizes the client's trunk and shoulder girdle with one hand (left as shown) and grasps the client's elbow with the other hand (right as shown). The clinician moves the client's arm across their body toward the opposite shoulder while maintaining the initial amount of flexion.

Figure 21.35

Assessment A test is (+) if it reproduces pain in the anterior or superior shoulder.

(continued)

Cross-Body Adduction Test *(continued)*

Statistics
- SN 82 (NR), SP 27.7 (NR), +LR 1.13, –LR 0.64, QUADAS 7, in a study of 120 clients with complaints of shoulder pain (mean age NR; 72 female; mean duration of symptoms NR), using cortisone injection into the AC joint as a reference standard[81]
- SN 22.5 (NR), SP 82 (NR), +LR 1.25, –LR 0.93, QUADAS 10, in a study of 552 clients with shoulder pain (mean age, gender, and mean duration of symptoms NR), using arthroscopic findings as a reference standard[77]

INFRASPINATUS OR EXTERNAL ROTATION RESISTANCE TEST

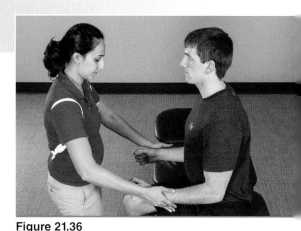

Figure 21.36

Client Position   Sitting with the elbows flexed to 90° and the elbows maintained against the body

Clinician Position   Standing in front of the client

Movement   The client provides resistance into ER while the clinician offers resistance at the distal forearm.

Assessment   A test is (+) if the client is unable to maintain the resistance due to either weakness or pain.

Statistics
- SN 56 (32-81), **SP 87 (77-98)**, **+LR 4.4**, –LR 0.50, QUADAS 10, in a study of 55 clients presenting with shoulder pain (mean age 40.6 ± 15.1 years; 8 women; mean symptom duration of 33.8 ± 48.9 months), using surgical findings as a reference standard[4]
- When *pain* is the finding: SN 34 (NR), **SP 100 (NR)**, **+LR Inf**, –LR 0.66, QUADAS 10, in a study of 34 clients with chronic shoulder pain (mean age of 57 years; 14 women; median duration of symptoms 2 years), using diagnostic US as a reference standard
- When *weakness* is the finding: SN 55 (NR), SP 25 (NR), +LR 0.74, –LR 1.8[70]

CLUSTERS OF TESTS

Hawkins-Kennedy, Painful Arc, and Infraspinatus Test

Statistics
- All three tests (+): SN (NR), SP (NR), **+LR 10.56**, **–LR 0.17**, QUADAS 10, in a study of 552 clients (mean age, gender, and mean duration of symptoms NR), using bursitis, partial- or full-thickness RCT, and arthroscopic findings as reference standards[77]
- Two of three tests (+): SN (NR), SP (NR), **+LR 5.06**, **–LR 0.17**, QUADAS 10[77]

Hawkins-Kennedy, Painful Arc, Neer's Sign, External Rotation Resistance Test, and Empty Can Test

Statistics   Three of any five tests (+): SN 75 (54-96), SP 74 (61-88), +LR 2.93, –LR 0.34, QUADAS 10, in a study of 55 clients presenting with shoulder pain (mean age 40.6 ± 15.1 years; 8 women; mean symptom duration of 33.8 ± 48.9 months), using surgical findings as a reference standard[4]

ROTATOR CUFF TEAR

RENT TEST

Client Position	Sitting with bilateral arms relaxed at side. The arm being tested is brought into passive shoulder extension.
Clinician Position	Standing directly behind the client; palpating the humeral head immediately anterior to the acromion while supporting the arm at the olecranon to maintain humeral extension
Movement	The clinician moves the humerus into internal and then external rotation. The clinician palpates for a depression, described as approximately one finger width, after passing over the greater tuberosity.
Assessment	A test is (+) if a *rent* (the depression) is palpable during the passive rotation of the humerus.
Statistics	**SN 96 (NR), SP 97 (NR), +LR 32, –LR 0.04**, QUADAS 10, in a study with 109 clients with rotator cuff tear (mean age NR; 42 females; mean duration symptoms NR), using surgery as a reference standard[84]

LATERAL JOBE TEST

Video 21.37 in the web resource shows a demonstration of this test.

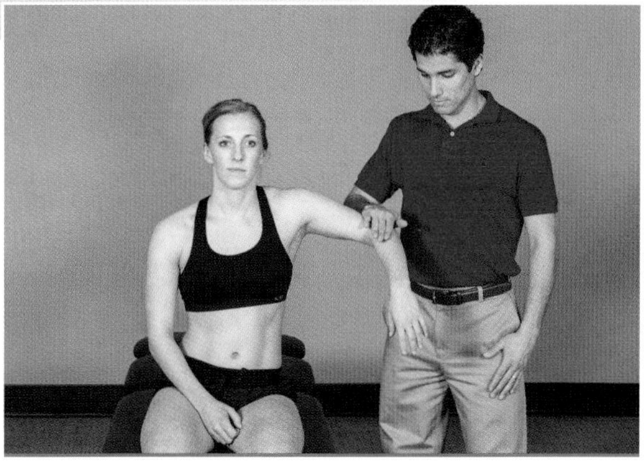

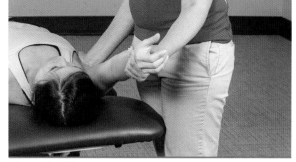

Client Position	Sitting or standing in an upright position with the arms abducted to 90° and placed in full glenohumeral internal rotation
Clinician Position	Standing to the side of or directly behind the client
Movement	The clinician applies an inferior force to the distal humerus while the client resists this motion.

Figure 21.37

Assessment	A test is (+) if the client reports pain or exhibits weakness.
Statistics	**SN 81 (72-88), SP 89 (79-95), +LR 7.36, –LR 0.10**, QUADAS 10 in 175 clients with shoulder pain (mean age NR; 78 females; mean duration symptoms NR) undergoing arthroscopy as a reference standard for suspected rotator cuff tear[85]

SUPINE IMPINGEMENT TEST

Client Position	Supine with arms resting by their side
Clinician Position	Standing right beside the client
Movement	Stabilizing the lateral shoulder girdle, the clinician passively moves the client's arm into end-range humeral elevation, then externally rotates the humerus and adducts the arm toward the client's ear. Once this position is achieved, the clinician internally rotates the client's arm.
Assessment	A test is (+) if the client reports pain with this position.

Figure 21.38

Statistics	**SN 97 (NR)**, SP 9 (NR), +LR 1.07, **–LR 0.33**, QUADAS 10, in a study with 448 clients (mean age NR; 166 females; mean duration of symptoms NR), using shoulder pain and arthrogram for suspected rotator cuff tear as a reference standard[10]

EMPTY CAN TEST

Client Position	Standing or sitting in an upright position with the arms positioned in 90° of elevation
Clinician Position	Standing in front of the client, offering resistance at the distal arm
Movement	The clinician offers resistance at the distal arm in an attempt to push the arm out of the elevated position (pushing arm down toward floor as shown), initially with the arms in the thumb-up position. The client then moves their arm into the scapular plane and full internal rotation, as if pouring out a can (as shown). The clinician again offers resistance to the distal forearm.

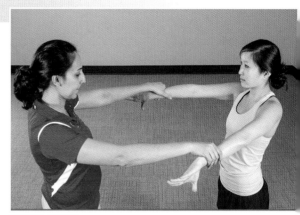

Figure 21.39

Assessment	A test is (+) if pain is reproduced or if there is obvious weakness compared to the initial thumb-up position.
Statistics	• Pooled analysis: SN 69 (54-81), SP 62 (38-81), +LR 1.8, –LR 0.5, in six studies with 695 clients.[54]
	• Pain as the (+) finding: SN 52 (NR), SP 33 (NR), +LR 0.78, –LR NR, QUADAS 10, in a study of 34 clients (mean age 57 years; 14 women; mean duration of symptoms 2 years), using chronic shoulder pain and diagnostic US as reference standards. Findings on US could include full-thickness or partial-thickness tears.[70]
	• *Weakness* as the (+) finding: SN 52 (NR), SP 67 (NR), +LR 1.56, –LR (NR).[70]
	• SN 50 (26-75), SP 87 (77-98), +LR 3.90, –LR 0.57, QUADAS 10, in a study of 55 clients presenting with shoulder pain (age ranging from 18-83 years; 8 women; mean duration of symptoms NR), using surgery as a reference standard.[4]
	• SN 44 (NR), **SP 90 (NR)**, **+LR 4.37**, –LR 0.62, QUADAS 10, in a study of 552 clients presenting with shoulder pain (mean age, gender, and mean duration of symptoms NR), using arthroscopy as a reference standard.[77]
	• Reliability has been calculated as (κ) = 0.94 in 33 subjects with shoulder pain (mean age 32 years, gender NR, and mean duration of symptoms ranging from 2 to 14 weeks) in a primary care clinic.[74]

SUPRASPINATUS TEAR OR SAIS

DROP ARM TEST

Client Position	Sitting or standing upright
Clinician Position	Standing behind the client using one hand to support the scapula and the opposite hand to hold the distal arm
Movement	The clinician brings the client's involved arm into passive abduction *(a)*. The clinician asks the client to maintain the abducted position and then releases the distal end of the arm *(b)*. They then ask the client to slowly lower the arm back to the side.

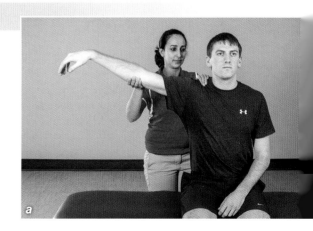

Assessment	A test is (+) if the client is unable to control the lowering of the arm.
Statistics	• Pooled analysis: SN 21 (14-30), SP 92 (86-96), +LR 2.6, –LR 0.86, in five studies with 1,213 clients[54]

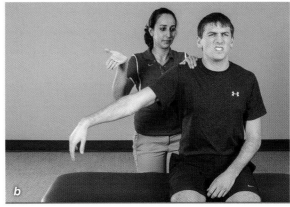

Figure 21.40

• SN 41 (28-54), SP 83 (73-93), +LR 2.41, –LR 0.71, QUADAS 13, in a study of 52 clients with acute shoulder pain and inability to abduct the shoulder >90° (age range 18-75 years old; 14 women; mean duration of symptoms <2 weeks), using diagnostic US and response to lidocaine injection as reference standards[78]

• SN 10 (NR), SP 98 (NR), +LR 5.0, –LR 0.92, QUADAS 5, in a study of 400 clients (age, gender, and mean duration of symptoms NR), using suspected RCT and surgery as reference standards[86]

• SN 27 (NR), SP 88 (NR), +LR 2.3, –LR 0.83, QUADAS 10, in a study of 552 clients (age, gender, and mean duration of symptoms NR), using suspected RCT and surgery as reference standards[77]

FULL CAN TEST

Client Position	Standing with the arms abducted to 90° and their thumbs pointing to the ceiling
Clinician Position	Standing directly in front of the client
Movement	The clinician applies an inferior force to the distal forearms bilaterally.
Assessment	A test is (+) if the clinician notes more significant weakness in the symptomatic arm, or if pain is provoked.
Statistics	• SN 86 (NR), SP 57 (NR), +LR 2.01, –LR 0.25, QUADAS 8, in a study of 136 clients presenting with shoulder pain (mean age 43 years; 31 women; mean duration symptoms NR), using MRI and surgery as reference standards[87]

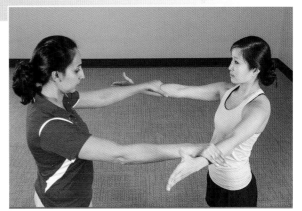

Figure 21.41

• SN 80-83, SP 50-53, +LR 1.6–1.78, –LR 0.4–0.32, QUADAS 8, in a study of 149 clients presenting with shoulder pain (mean age 53 years; gender and mean duration symptoms NR), using MRI and surgery as reference standards[88]

SUPRASPINATUS AND INFRASPINATUS TEAR

EXTERNAL ROTATION LAG SIGN

 Video 21.42 **in the web resource shows a demonstration of this test.**

Client Position	Sitting in an upright position with the arm positioned passively into 20° of abduction and full ER. The elbow is flexed to 90°.
Clinician Position	Standing directly behind the client
Movement	The clinician initially moves the client's arm into abduction and external rotation (as described previously) *(a)*. The clinician continues to support the elbow at the olecranon, and then releases the support at the wrist *(b)*. The clinician asks the client to maintain this position of ER.
Assessment	The test is considered (+) if the client is unable to maintain the ER in the 20° of abduction, as evidenced by the arm falling into IR.
Statistics	• SN 42 (NR), **SP 90 (NR)**, **+LR 4.20**, –LR 0.65, QUADAS 10, in 552 clients (age, gender, and mean duration of symptoms NR), using an RCT of any severity and arthroscopy as reference standards[77]

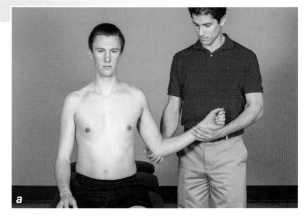

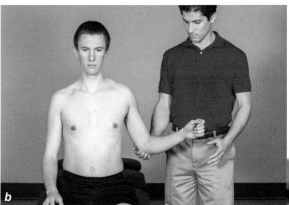

Figure 21.42

• SN 45 (31-59), **SP 91 (83-79)**, **+LR 5.0**, –LR 0.6, QUADAS 13, in a study of 52 clients presenting with acute shoulder pain and inability to abduct shoulder >90° (age range 18-75 years old; 14 women; mean duration of symptoms <2 weeks), using diagnostic US and response to lidocaine injection as reference standards[78]

• SN 46 (NR), **SP 94 (NR)**, **+LR 7.2**, –LR 0.60, QUADAS 11, in 37 clients presenting with chronic shoulder pain (mean age 55.5 years; 21 women; mean duration of shoulder pain 37.5 months), using diagnostic US as a reference standard[79]

INFRASPINATUS AND TERES MINOR TEAR

DROP SIGN

Client Position	Sitting in an upright position with the arm positioned passively into 90° of both abduction and external rotation
Clinician Position	Standing to the side of the client, supporting the client's arm at the olecranon and wrist
Movement	The clinician initially moves the client's arm into abduction and external rotation (as described previously) *(a)*. The clinician continues to support the elbow at the olecranon, and then releases the support at the wrist *(b)*. The clinician asks the client to maintain the position of ER in the abducted position.
Assessment	The test is considered (+) if the client is unable to maintain the external rotation as evidenced by the arm falling back into IR.
Statistics	• SN 73 (NR), SP 77, +LR 3.2, –LR 0.3, QUADAS 11, in 37 clients presenting with chronic shoulder pain (mean age of 55.5 years; 21 women; mean duration of shoulder pain 37.5 months), using diagnostic US as a reference standard[79]

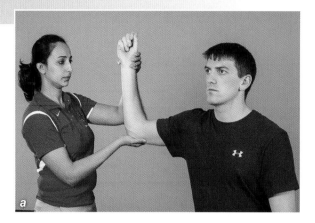

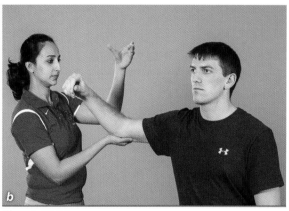

Figure 21.43

• SN 45 (31-59), SP 70 (58-82), +LR 1.5, –LR 0.79, QUADAS 13, in a study of 52 clients presenting with acute shoulder pain and inability to abduct shoulder >90° (age range 18-75 years old; 14 women; mean duration of symptoms <2 weeks), using diagnostic US and response to lidocaine injection as reference standards[78]

HORNBLOWER'S SIGN

Client Position	Sitting in an upright position with the arm positioned passively into 90° of both ER and abduction. The elbow is flexed to 90°.
Clinician Position	Standing to the side of the client, supporting the arm at the olecranon and wrist initially
Movement	The clinician applies resistance at the wrist into IR and asks the client to maintain the externally rotated position against the resistance *(a)*.
Assessment	The test is considered (+) if the client fails to maintain the externally rotated and abducted position against the clinician's resistance *(b)*.
Statistics	SN 100 (NR), SP 93 (NR), +LR 12, –LR 0.05, QUADAS 7, in 54 clients presenting with suspected RCT (mean age 66 years; 21 women; mean duration of symptoms 5.6 years), using surgery as a reference standard[89]

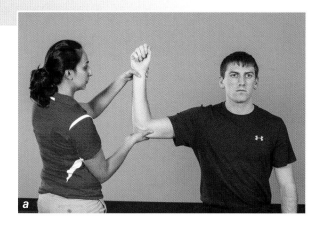

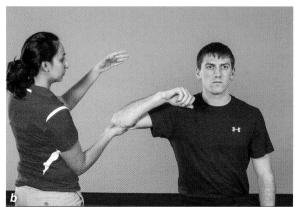

Figure 21.44

SUBSCAPULARIS TEAR

LIFT-OFF TEST

 Video 21.45 **in the web resource shows a demonstration of this test.**

Client Position	Sitting or standing upright with the arm positioned into a posterior reach position of GH extension, adduction, and IR, with the hand resting on their back
Clinician Position	Standing behind or to the side of the client to observe the arm
Movement	The client is cued to attempt to lift their hand off their back.
Assessment	The test is (+) if the client is unable to bring their hand off their back.
Statistics	• Pooled SN 42 (19-69), pooled **SP 97 (79-100)**, **+LR 16.47**, –LR 0.6, in four studies with 267 clients[54]
	• SN 17.6 (NR), **SP 100 (NR)**, +LR (NR), –LR 0.82, QUADAS 11, in a study of 68 clients (mean age 45 years; 19 women; mean duration symptoms NR), using a diagnosis of RCT and surgery as reference standards[90]

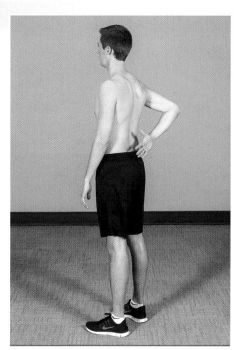

Figure 21.45

INTERNAL ROTATION LAG TEST

Client Position	Sitting in an upright position with the arm positioned passively behind the back into an internally rotated and extended position
Clinician Position	Standing directly behind the client, supporting the arm at the elbow and wrist
Movement	The clinician releases the wrist and asks the client to maintain the arm in the internally rotated position.
Assessment	The test is considered (+) if the client fails to maintain the internally rotated position, as evidenced by the hand falling toward the spine.
Statistics	• **SN 100 (NR), SP 84 (NR)**, +LR 6.2, –LR 0.0, QUADAS 11, in 37 clients presenting with shoulder pain (mean age 55.5 years; 21 women; mean duration of symptoms 37.5 months), using diagnostic US as a reference standard[79]
	• SN 31 (18-41), SP 87 (78-96), +LR 2.38, –LR 0.79, QUADAS 13, in a study of 52 clients presenting with acute shoulder pain and inability to abduct shoulder >90° (age range 18-75 years old; 14 women; mean duration of symptoms <2 weeks), using diagnostic US and response to lidocaine injection as reference standards[78]

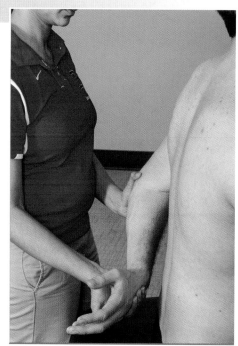

Figure 21.46

BELLY PRESS TEST

Client Position	Sitting in an upright position with the involved arm placed into 90° of elbow flexion and with full internal rotation such that their hand is resting on their stomach and their elbow is pointing straight out to the side
Clinician Position	Standing to the side of the client
Movement	The client is asked to press their hand into their stomach, inducing an internal rotation force *(a)*.
Assessment	The test is considered (+) if the client's shoulder moves into external rotation and/or extension as evidenced by the elbow drifting posteriorly *(b)*.
Statistics	SN 40 (NR), **SP 98 (NR)**, +LR 20, –LR 0.61, QUADAS 11, in a study of 68 clients presenting with a diagnosis of RCT (mean age 45 years; 19 women; mean duration of symptoms NR), using surgery as a reference standard[90]

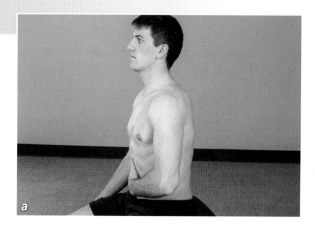

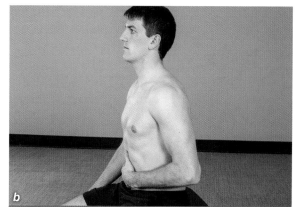

Figure 21.47

BEAR HUG TEST

Client Position	Sitting in an upright position with the involved arm reaching across the body so that the hand is resting on the opposite shoulder. The shoulder is also flexed so that the elbow is pointing straight out in front of the body.
Clinician Position	Standing in front of the client
Movement	The clinician attempts to pull the client's hand off their shoulder.
Assessment	The test is (+) if the client is unable to keep their hand on the opposite shoulder.
Statistics	SN 60 (NR), **SP 92 (NR), +LR 7.2**, –LR 0.44, QUADAS 11, in a study of 68 clients presenting with a suspected RCT (mean age 45 years; 19 women; mean duration of symptoms NR), using surgery as a reference standard[90]

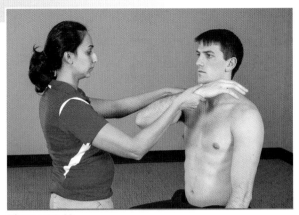

Figure 21.48

ROTATOR CUFF TEAR OR POSTERIOR LABRAL TEAR

POSTERIOR IMPINGEMENT SIGN

Client Position	Supine with the shoulder positioned in 90° to 110° of abduction, full external rotation, and 10° to 15° of horizontal abduction
Clinician Position	Immediately to the side of the client, supporting the arm at the elbow and the wrist into the previously mentioned position
Movement	The clinician passively moves the client into the abducted, externally rotated, and horizontally abducted position.
Assessment	A test is (+) if the client reports pain in the posterior aspect of the shoulder.
Statistics	SN 76 (NR), SP 85 (NR), +LR 5.06, –LR 0.29, QUADAS 7, in a study of 69 clients with suspected RCT and with RCT or a posterior labral tear (mean age 22.7; gender and mean duration of symptoms NR), using surgery as a reference standard[91]

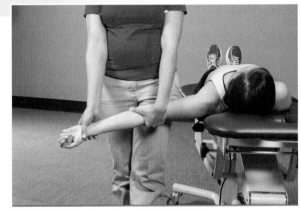

Figure 21.49

LABRAL PATHOLOGY AND SHOULDER INSTABILITY

BICEPS LOAD I

Client Position	Supine with the arm maintained in 90° of abduction, 90° of elbow flexion, and full supination
Clinician Position	Standing to the side of the involved arm, with one hand supporting the client's elbow (left as shown) and the opposite hand at the distal forearm (right as shown)
Movement	The clinician maintains the abducted and externally rotated position of the client's arm. The clinician then asks the client to resist elbow flexion while maintaining the glenohumeral position.
Assessment	A test is (+) if pain or apprehension is noted during the resistance.
Statistics	**SN 91 (NR), SP 97 (NR), +LR 30.3, –LR 0.09**, QUADAS 9, in a study of 75 clients presenting with suspected labral tear (mean age 25 years; 11 females; mean duration symptoms NR), using surgery as a reference standard[92]

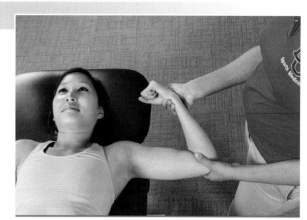

Figure 21.50

CRANK TEST

Client Position	Supine, placing the arm into 160° of abduction and full external rotation. The elbow is flexed to 90°.
Clinician Position	Standing immediately to the side of the client, supporting the arm at the olecranon (as shown)
Movement	The clinician applies compression at the olecranon directly through the humerus (with right arm as shown) while repeatedly moving the client's arm through internal and external rotation at the shoulder. Compression through the humerus is maintained throughout the rotational movement.
Assessment	A test is (+) if the client reports pain or if the clinician hears sounds of clicking, clunking, or popping.
Statistics	• Pooled analysis: SN 34 (19-53), SP 75 (65-83), +LR 1.36 (0.84–2.21), –LR 0.88 (0.69–1.12) in 282 clients across four studies with a SLAP tear[55] • SN 40 (NR), SP 73 (NR), +LR 1.48, –LR 0.82, QUADAS 11, in a study of 61 clients presenting with a suspected labral tear (mean age 38 years; 11 women; mean duration symptoms NR), using arthroscopy as a reference standard[93] • SN 58 (NR), SP 72 (NR), +LR 2.1, –LR 0.58, QUADAS 9, in a study of 54 clients presenting with a suspected labral tear (mean age 23 years; 2 females; mean duration of symptoms NR), using arthroscopy as a reference standard[94]

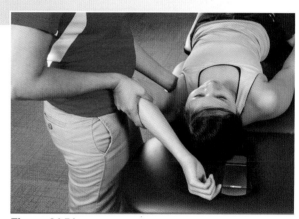

Figure 21.51

(continued)

Crank Test *(continued)*

- SN 46 (NR), SP 56 (NR), +LR 1.1, –LR 0.96, QUADAS 11, in a study with 65 clients presenting with suspected labral tear (mean age 46 years; 20 women; mean duration of symptoms 12 months), using surgery as a reference standard[95]
- **SN 91 (NR), SP 93 (NR), +LR 13.6** and **6.5, –LR 0.1** and 0.22, QUADAS 10, in a study with 62 clients presenting with failed conservative treatment consisting of medication and physical therapy for 3 months (mean age 28 years; 22 women; mean duration of symptoms NR), using arthroscopy as a reference standard[96]

BICEPS LOAD II

 Video 21.52 **in the web resource shows a demonstration of this test.**

Client Position	Supine with the arm maintained in 120° of abduction and 90° of elbow flexion. The forearm is in full supination. The shoulder is brought into maximal external rotation.
Clinician Position	Standing to the side of the involved arm, with one hand supporting the client's elbow and the opposite hand at the distal forearm

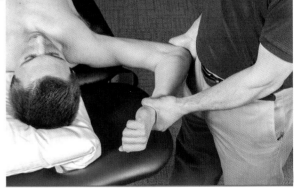

Figure 21.52

Movement	The clinician maintains the abducted and externally rotated position of the client's arm. The clinician then asks the client to resist elbow flexion while maintaining the glenohumeral position.
Assessment	A test is (+) if pain is noted during the resistance.
Statistics	• SN 30 (NR), SP 78 (NR), +LR 1.36, –LR 0.90, QUADAS 10, in a study of 297 clients, 146 presenting with suspected labral tear (mean age 45 years; 52 women; mean duration of symptoms NR), using surgery as a reference standard.[97]
	• **SN 90 (NR), SP 97 (NR), +LR 30.3, –LR 0.11**, QUADAS 11, in a study of 127 clients presenting with suspected labral tear (mean age 31 years; 38 females; mean duration of symptoms NR), using surgery as a reference standard.[98] Another systematic review calculated a slightly lower +LR at 26.3 with regard to this same study,[73] though both +LRs would suggest that this test has some diagnostic benefit based on this one study.

ACTIVE COMPRESSION TEST

Client Position	Sitting or standing in the upright position. The arm is brought into 90° of shoulder flexion with elbow extension, full internal rotation and 10° of horizontal adduction.
Clinician Position	Standing immediately to the side of the client
Movement	The client maintains the starting position of the arm. The clinician has the client resist at the distal aspect of the arm, maintaining the initial position *(a)*. The clinician then brings the client's arm into full external rotation, while maintaining

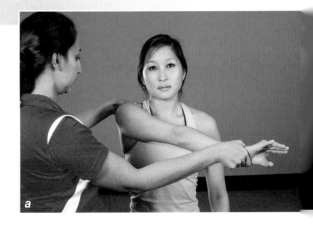

the other components of the initial position *(b)*. The clinician again offers resistance to the distal arm while the client maintains the flexed, externally rotated, horizontally adducted position.

Assessment   A test is (+) for labral pathology if the client reports deep joint pain with resistance during the internally rotated position of the test. The test is also described as being (+) for AC joint pathology if the client reports pain on the top of the shoulder.

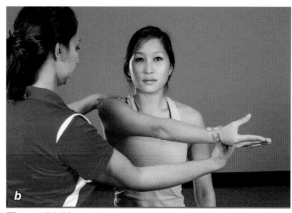

Figure 21.53

Statistics   • Pooled analysis: SN 67 (51-80), SP 37 (22-54), +LR 1.1, –LR 0.89, in six studies with 782 clients[55]

• SN 63 (NR), SP 50 (NR), +LR 1.25, –LR 0.75, QUADAS 10, in a study of 132 clients with a suspected labral tear (mean age 45 years; 34 women; mean duration of symptoms NR), using surgery as a reference standard[99]

• SN 47 (NR), SP 55 (NR), +LR 1.04, –LR 0.96, QUADAS 11, in a study of 426 clients (mean age 45 years; 174 women; mean duration of symptoms NR), using surgery as a reference standard[100]

• **SN 85 (NR)**, SP 41 (NR), +LR 1.44, **–LR 0.36**, QUADAS 10, in a study with 102 clients with a suspected labral tear (mean age of 33 years; 53 overhead athletes and 49 nonathletes who sustained a single-event trauma; gender and mean duration of symptoms NR), using surgery as a reference standard[101]

• SN 63 (NR), SP 53 (NR), +LR 1.34, –LR 0.70, QUADAS 10, in a study 297 clients, 146 with suspected labral tear (mean age 45 years; 52 women; mean duration of symptoms NR), using surgery as a reference standard[97]

SPEED'S TEST

Client Position   Sitting or standing upright with the arm positioned into shoulder external rotation, elbow extension, and forearm supination

Clinician Position   Standing in front of the client, with one hand (left as shown) supporting the proximal end of the arm and the opposite hand (right as shown) positioned at the distal forearm

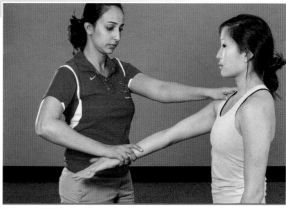

Figure 21.54

Movement   The clinician offers resistance at the distal forearm to simultaneously challenge the elbow and shoulder flexion position as the client flexes the shoulder through 60° of motion.

Assessment   A test is (+) if the client's shoulder pain is reproduced.

Statistics   • Pooled analysis: SN 20 (5-53), SP 78 (58-90), +LR 0.9 (0.43–1.9), –LR 1.03 (0.86–1.23), in four studies with 327 clients[55]

• SN 18 (NR), SP 87 (NR), +LR 1.4, –LR 0.94, QUADAS 11, in a study of 60 clients with a suspected labral tear (mean age 38 years; 11 women; mean duration of symptoms NR), using surgery as a reference standard[93]

• SN 90 (NR), SP 14 (NR), +LR 1.04, –LR 0.72, QUADAS 10, in a study of 46 clients with suspected labral tear (mean age 64 years; 14 women; mean duration of symptoms NR), using surgery as a reference standard[102]

• SN 32 (NR), SP 66 (NR), +LR 0.94, –LR 1.03, QUADAS 10, in a study of 297 clients, 146 with suspected labral tear (mean age 45 years; 52 women; mean duration of symptoms NR), using surgery as a reference standard[97]

ANTERIOR SLIDE TEST

Client Position	Sitting upright with their hand resting on their iliac crest and the forearm in a pronated position
Clinician Position	Standing behind the client with one hand (right as shown) stabilizing proximally over the scapula and clavicle. The opposite hand (left as shown) is supporting the elbow over the olecranon.
Movement	The clinician produces an anterior force directed through the humerus while the client resists this movement.
Assessment	A test is (+) if pain or clicking symptoms are reproduced.

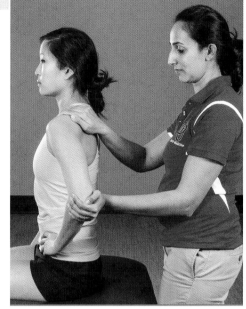

Figure 21.55

Statistics
- Pooled analysis: SN 17 (3-55), SP 86 (81-89), +LR 1.2, −LR 0.97, in four studies with 831 clients[55]
- SN 78 (NR), **SP 92 (NR)**, **+LR 4.3**, −LR 0.24, QUADAS 5, in a study of 226 clients presenting with suspected labral tear (age ranging from 18-38 years; 73 women; mean duration of symptoms NR), using arthroscopy as a reference standard[103]
- SN 8 (NR), SP 84 (NR), +LR 0.49, −LR 1.1, QUADAS 11, in a study of 426 clients presenting with suspected labral tear (mean age 45 years; 174 women; mean duration of symptoms NR), using arthroscopy as a reference standard[100]
- SN 5 (NR), SP 93 (NR), +LR 0.71, −LR 1.0, QUADAS 9, in a study of 54 clients presenting with suspected labral tear (mean age 23 years; 2 women; mean duration of symptoms NR), using arthroscopy as a reference standard[94]

YERGASON'S TEST

Client Position	Sitting or standing in an upright position, with their arm in 90° of flexion
Clinician Position	Standing beside the client
Movement	The client starts with the arm in a fully pronated position. The clinician offers resistance at the distal forearm while the client attempts to supinate the arm.
Assessment	A test is (+) if the client reports pain over the origin of the biceps.

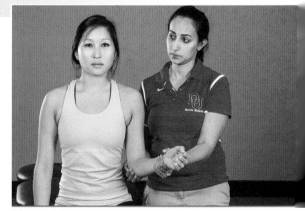

Figure 21.56

Statistics
- Pooled analysis: SN 12 (7-21), SP 95 (91-98), +LR 2.49, −LR 0.91, in 246 clients across three studies with a SLAP tear[55]
- SN 13 (NR), SP 94 (NR), +LR 1.9, −LR 0.94, QUADAS 10, in 132 clients presenting with suspected labral tear (mean age 45 years; 34 women; mean duration of symptoms NR), using surgery as a reference standard[99]
- SN 12 (NR), **SP 98 (NR)**, **+LR 6**, −LR 0.9, QUADAS 9, in a study of 54 clients presenting with suspected labral tear (mean age 23 years; 2 women; mean duration of symptoms NR), using surgery as a reference standard[94]

- SN 43 (NR), SP 79 (NR), +LR 2.1, –LR 0.72, QUADAS 11, in a study of 50 clients presenting with suspected labral tear (mean age 50 years; 16 women; mean duration of symptoms NR), using surgery as a reference standard[104]
- SN 12 (NR), SP 96 (NR), +LR 3.0, –LR 0.92, QUADAS 11, in a study of 60 clients presenting with suspected labral tear (mean age 38 years; 11 females; mean duration of symptoms NR), using surgery as a reference standard[93]

COMPRESSION ROTATION TEST

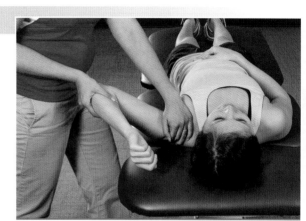

Client Position	Supine
Clinician Position	Standing beside the client with one hand (right as shown) stabilizing the shoulder girdle and the opposite hand (right as shown) supporting the elbow. The clinician retains the client's elbow in flexion and initially places the shoulder in 90° of abduction.
Movement	The clinician produces compression of the humerus into the glenoid by loading through the olecranon/elbow. While maintaining the compression, the clinician moves the client's arm passively from external rotation to internal rotation.

Figure 21.57

Assessment	A test is (+) if the client's shoulder pain or clicking is reproduced.
Statistics	• Pooled analysis: SN 25 (14-38), SP 78 (73-82), +LR 2.8, –LR 0.87, in 355 clients across two studies with a SLAP tear[55]
	• SN 25 (NR), SP 100, +LR (NR), –LR (NR), QUADAS 9, in a study of 54 clients presenting with suspected labral tear (mean age 23 years; 2 women; mean duration of symptoms NR), using arthroscopy as a reference standard[94]
	• SN 24 (NR), SP 75 (NR), +LR 0.98, –LR 1.0, QUADAS 11, in a study of 426 clients presenting with suspected labral tear (mean age 45 years; 174 women; mean duration of symptoms NR), using arthroscopy as a reference standard[100]
	• SN 61 (NR), SP 54 (NR), +LR 1.33, –LR 0.72, QUADAS 10, in a study of 297 clients, 146 presenting with suspected labral tear (mean age 45 years; 52 women; mean duration of symptoms NR), using surgery as a reference standard[97]

PASSIVE COMPRESSION TEST

 ***Video 21.58** in the web resource shows a demonstration of this test.*

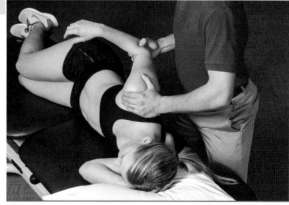

Client Position	Side lying with the side to be tested on top. The arm is resting along the client's side with the elbow flexed to 90°.
Clinician Position	Standing directly behind the client with one hand (right as shown) supporting at the elbow and the second hand (left as shown) stabilizing over the top of the scapula

Figure 21.58

(continued)

Passive Compression Test *(continued)*

Movement The clinician compresses through the humerus, passively externally rotates the client's arm with 30° of abduction, and extends the shoulder, while maintaining the ER and compression. This results in passive compression of the superior labrum on to the glenoid.

Assessment A test is (+) if the client reports pain or if catching in the shoulder is noted.

Statistics **SN 82 (NR), SP 86 (NR), +LR 5.7, –LR 0.21**, QUADAS 9, in a study with 61 clients presenting with suspected labral tear (mean age 33 years; 4 women; mean duration of symptoms NR) and 2 months failed conservative care, using surgery as a reference standard[105]

PASSIVE DISTRACTION TEST

Client Position Supine

Clinician Position Beside the client on the side to be tested

Movement The clinician passively moves the client's arm into 150° of abduction, with full elbow extension and forearm supination *(a)*. The clinician places one hand (right as shown) on the distal forearm and passively pronates the forearm while the clinician's opposite hand (left as shown) holds the distal humerus to prevent any humeral rotation during the forearm movement *(b)*.

Assessment A test is (+) if the client reports pain during the passive pronation component of the test.

Statistics SN 53 (NR), SP 94 (NR), +LR (8.8), –LR (0.5), QUADAS 8, in a study of 246 clients presenting with a SLAP tear (mean age 44 years; 86 women; mean duration of symptoms NR), using surgery as a reference standard[106]

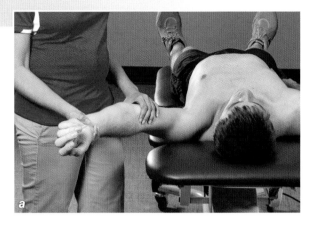

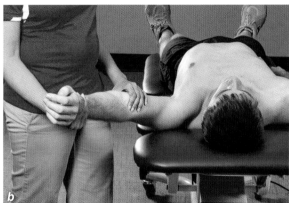

Figure 21.59

CLUSTER TESTING FOR LABRAL TEARS

The cluster of tests with the best SN, SP, or both in studies with the least amount of bias are as follows:

- For a type II SLAP tear, a (+) finding on the apprehension test (described in the Instability Tests section later in this chapter), the compression rotation test, and the Speed's test provided SN 25 (NR), SP 92 (NR), +LR 3.13, –LR 0.82.

- For any labral tear, a (+) finding on the crank test and the anterior slide test offered SN 34 (NR), SP 91 (NR), +LR 3.75, –LR 0.73.

- For any labral tear, a (+) finding on the apprehension and relocation tests (both described in the Instability Tests section later in this chapter) offered SN 38 (NR), **SP 93 (NR)**, **+LR 5.43**, –LR 0.67.[55]

POSTEROINFERIOR LABRAL LESION

KIM TEST

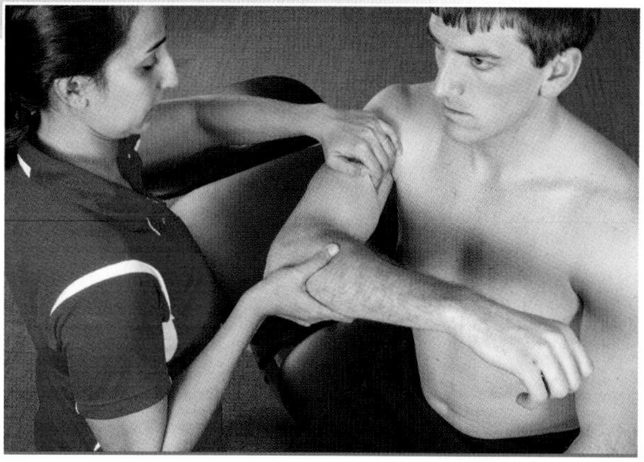

Client Position	Sitting or standing in an upright position
Clinician Position	Standing in front of and to the outside of the client's arm. The clinician uses one hand (right as shown) to support at the elbow and the second hand (left as shown) to support at the humerus.
Movement	The clinician passively moves the client's arm into 90° of abduction. The clinician then brings the client's shoulder diagonally across the body. The hand supporting the elbow (right as shown) provides a compression force throughout the motion, while the opposite hand (left as shown) simultaneously provides a posterior and inferior glide to the glenohumeral joint.

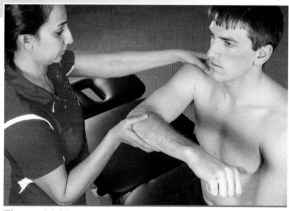

Figure 21.60

Assessment	A test is (+) for a posterior labral tear if posterior shoulder pain is reproduced.
Statistics	**SN 80 (NR)**, **SP 94 (NR)**, **+LR 12.6**, **–LR 0.21**, QUADAS 11, in 172 clients with suspected labral tear (mean age 43 years; 67 women; mean duration of symptoms NR), using surgery as a reference standard[107]

JERK TEST

Client Position	Sitting in an upright position
Clinician Position	Standing in front of the client and to the outside of the arm being tested. One hand (left as shown) stabilizes the scapula and the opposite hand (right as shown) supports the elbow and maintains the client's arm in 90° of abduction and internal rotation.
Movement	The clinician provides compression through the humerus and maintains the compression while moving the client's arm through horizontal adduction.

Figure 21.61

Assessment	A test is (+) if shoulder pain or clicking is reproduced.
Statistics	• SN 25 (NR), SP 80 (NR), +LR 1.3, –LR 0.94, QUADAS 9, in a study of 54 clients with suspected labral tear (mean age 23 years; 2 women; mean duration of symptoms NR), using surgery as a reference standard[94] • SN 73 (NR), **SP 98 (NR)**, **+LR 34.7**, –LR 0.27, QUADAS 11, in 172 clients with suspected labral tear (mean age 43 years; 67 women; mean duration of symptoms NR), using surgery as a reference standard[107]

INSTABILITY

SURPRISE TEST OR ANTERIOR RELEASE TEST

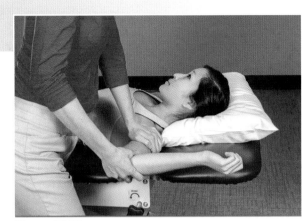

Figure 21.62

Client Position	Supine
Clinician Position	Immediately to the side of the client, supporting the arm being tested at the elbow with one hand (right as shown), while placing the opposite hand (left as shown) over the anterior aspect of the humeral head to maintain a posterior force on the anterior aspect of the shoulder.
Movement	The clinician passively moves the client's arm into 90° of abduction and full external rotation, while maintaining the posterior force over the anterior joint line of the shoulder. After achieving this position, the clinician will remove their hand (left as shown) from the anterior aspect of shoulder without prompting the client.
Assessment	A test is (+) if the client reports shoulder pain after the posterior force is removed.

Statistics
- Pooled analysis: **SN 82 (69-91)**, **SP 86 (72-95)**, **+LR 5.42**, **–LR 0.25**, in 128 clients across two studies with anterior instability[55]
- **SN 92 (NR)**, **SP 84 (NR)**, **+LR 5.6**, **–LR 0.1**, QUADAS 10, in 169 clients with history of traumatic dislocation (mean age 38 years; 53 women; mean duration of symptoms NR), using MRA as a reference standard[20]
- SN 64 (NR), **SP 99 (NR)**, **+LR 58.6**, –LR 0.37, QUADAS 10, in 46 clients with anterior instability (mean age, gender, and mean duration of symptoms NR), using a combination of clinical examination and radiographs as a reference standard[108]

ANTERIOR APPREHENSION TEST

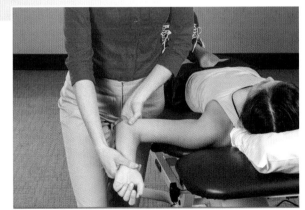

Figure 21.63

Client Position	Supine, with the elbow flexed to 90°
Clinician Position	Standing directly to the side of the client while supporting the arm at the elbow and the distal forearm
Movement	The clinician passively moves the client's arm into 90° of abduction and full external rotation. If the client is not apprehensive or having concordant pain, the clinician then applies an anterior force to the posterior proximal humerus, attempting to glide the humerus anterior.
Assessment	A test is (+) if the client reports pain or exhibits apprehension about having their arm in that position.

Statistics
- Pooled analysis: SN 66 (53-77), **SP 95 (93-98)**, **+LR 17.2**, –LR 0.39, in 409 clients across two studies with anterior instability[55]
- **SN 98 (NR)**, SP 72 (NR), +LR 3.5, **–LR 0.02**, QUADAS 10, in 169 clients presenting with history of traumatic dislocation (mean age 38 years; 53 women; mean duration of symptoms NR), using MRA as a reference standard[20]

- SN 72 (NR), **SP 96 (NR)**, **+LR 20.2**, –LR 0.29, QUADAS 11, in 363 clients presenting with a history of traumatic dislocation (mean age 29 years; 166 women; mean duration of symptoms NR), using surgery as a reference standard[109]
- SN 53 (NR), **SP 99 (NR)**, **+LR 53**, –LR 0.47, QUADAS 10, in 46 clients presenting with anterior instability (mean age, gender, and mean duration of symptoms NR), using a combination of clinical examination and radiographs as a reference standard[108]

RELOCATION TEST

 Video 21.64 in the web resource shows a demonstration of this test.

Client Position	Supine with the arm prepositioned passively into 90° of abduction and full ER. The elbow remains flexed at 90°.
Clinician Position	Standing immediately to the side of the client
Movement	The clinician passively moves the client's arm into the abducted, externally rotated position described. The clinician then applies an anterior force to the posterior aspect of the humeral head. After assessing the client's response, a posterior force is applied to the anterior aspect of the humeral head to effectively relocate the glenohumeral joint.

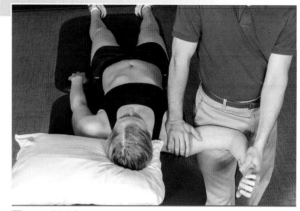

Figure 21.64

Assessment	A test is (+) if the client reports pain or apprehension when an anterior force is applied and then reports relief of symptoms when the posterior relocation force is applied.
Statistics	• Pooled analysis: SN 65 (55-73), **SP 90 (87-93)**, **+LR 5.5**, –LR 0.55, in 509 clients across three studies with anterior instability[55]
	• **SN 92 (NR)**, SP 84 (NR), **+LR 4.4**, **–LR 0.02**, QUADAS 10, in 169 clients presenting with history of traumatic dislocation (mean age 38 years; 53 women; mean duration of symptoms NR), using MRA as a reference standard[20]
	• **SN 81 (NR)**, **SP 92 (NR)**, **+LR 10.4**, **–LR 0.2**, QUADAS 11, in 363 clients presenting with history of traumatic dislocation (mean age 29 years old; 166 women; mean duration of symptoms NR), using surgery as a reference standard[109]
	• SN 46 (NR), SP 54 (NR), +LR 1.0, –LR 0.99, QUADAS 10, in 46 clients presenting with anterior instability (mean age, gender, and mean duration of symptoms NR), using a combination of clinical examination and radiographs as a reference standard[108]

HYPERABDUCTION TEST

Client Position	Sitting or standing
Clinician Position	Sitting next to the client on the side to be tested
Movement	The clinician passively moves the client's arm into abduction while maintaining a stable scapula with the opposite hand, effectively creating isolated glenohumeral abduction. The client's elbow remains in 90° of flexion. Neutral rotation is maintained.
Assessment	A test is (+) if the client reports or displays apprehension or if the client's arm is abducted past 105°.
Statistics	SN 67, SP 89, +LR 6.06, –LR 0.37 in 169 clients, 60 of whom presented with instability post trauma (mean age 30 years old; 53 women; mean duration of symptoms NR), using MRA as a reference standard[20]

SULCUS SIGN

Client Position	Sitting or standing upright
Clinician Position	Standing either behind or immediately to the side of the arm being tested
Movement	The clinician holds the distal humerus and stabilizes the trunk with the opposite hand. The clinician delivers a distraction force to the humerus.
Assessment	A test is (+) if the clinician denotes the presence of a sulcus at the glenohumeral joint.
Statistics	SN 17, SP 93, +LR 2.4, −LR 0.89, QUADAS 10, in 54 throwing athletes with a history of shoulder pain during throwing (mean age 23 years old; 2 women; average duration of symptoms NR), using arthroscopic surgery as a reference standard[94]

Critical Clinical Pearls

When assessing a client for anterior instability, keep the following in mind:

- Clients may have neural tension either concurrently with instability or as a differential diagnosis.
- Clinicians should ensure that the client can achieve close to the end range of normal or excessive ER.
- A neurological assessment may be appropriate if the client has instability from dislocation or subluxation unless the clinician already performed a neurological exam as part of an upper quarter triage.
- A Beighton scale may help suggest generalized laxity that may be contributing to the client's shoulder instability.

BICEPS TENDINOPATHY

BICEPS TENDON PALPATION

Client Position	Sitting or lying supine with the arm resting by their side
Clinician Position	In front of or to the side of the client
Movement	The clinician palpates the origin of the long head of the biceps.
Assessment	A test is (+) if the palpation reproduces the client's pain.

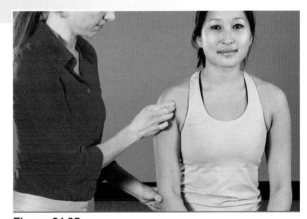

Figure 21.65

Statistics
- Palpating the biceps tendon has also been suggested for examining clients with SLAP tears. Pooled analysis related on palpating the biceps for SLAP tear reveals SN 39 (26-52), SP 67 (53-79), +LR 1.06, −LR 0.95, in 114 clients across two studies with a SLAP tear.[55]
- SN 53 (NR), SP 54 (NR), +LR 1.13, −LR (NR), QUADAS 12, in 40 of 847 clients presenting with suspected biceps tendon tear (mean age 59 years; 16 women; mean duration of symptoms NR), using arthroscopy as a reference standard.[110]

UPPER CUT TEST

Client Position	Sitting in an upright position with the arm being tested flexed to 90° at the elbow with the hand closed in a fist and the forearm supinated
Clinician Position	Standing to the side of the client with one hand on top of the client's fist (right as shown).
Movement	The clinician provides resistance downward and asks the client to flex their arm upward as if producing a boxing uppercut.
Assessment	A test is (+) if shoulder pain or painful clicking are reproduced.
Statistics	SN 73 (NR), SP 78 (NR), +LR 2.10, –LR 0.81, QUADAS 8, in 325 clients presenting with shoulder pain (mean age 43.2 years old; 93 women; mean duration of symptoms NR), using arthroscopy as a reference standard[111]

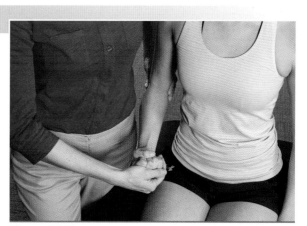

Figure 21.66

SPEED'S TEST

This has been previously described within the section on labral tear tests. Please refer to that section for details on how to perform this test.

- SN 69 (NR), SP 60 (NR), +LR 1.7, –LR 0.5, QUADAS 12, in 58 clients presenting with long head of the biceps tendinitis (prevalence rate of 61%; mean age of 56 years old; 45 women; mean duration of symptoms 11.8 months), using a reference standard of diagnostic US[112]

- SN 50 (NR), SP 67 (NR), +LR 1.51, –LR (NR), QUADAS 12, in 40 of 847 clients presenting with suspected biceps tendon tear (mean age 59 years; 16 women; mean duration of symptoms NR), using arthroscopy as a reference standard[110]

CLUSTERS

Gill and clients report that combining a positive Speed's test and painful palpation of the long head of the biceps offers SN 68 (NR), SP 49 (NR), +LR 1.31, –LR (NR) in 40 of 847 clients (mean age 59 years; 16 women; mean duration of symptoms NR), using suspected biceps tendon tear and arthroscopy as reference standards.[110]

AC JOINT PATHOLOGY

PAXINOS SIGN

Client Position	Sitting with arms relaxed at their side
Clinician Position	The clinician stands directly behind client, to the side of the shoulder to be assessed. The clinician places their hand over the affected shoulder such that the thumb rests under the posterolateral aspect of the acromion and the index and long fingers of the same or contralateral hand are placed superior to the mid-part of the ipsilateral clavicle.
Movement	The clinician applies pressure to the acromion with the thumb, in an anterosuperior direction, and inferiorly to the mid-part of the clavicular shaft with the index and long fingers.
Assessment	A (+) test is if pain was reported or increased in the region of the AC joint.
Statistics	SN 79 (NR), SP 50 (NR), +LR 1.6, –LR 0.42, QUADAS 13, in a study of 38 consecutive clients (mean age NR; 22 women; mean duration of symptoms NR) with shoulder pain bounded by the mid-part of the clavicle and the deltoid insertion, and using ≥50% pain relief from AC joint injection as a reference standard[32]

AC JOINT PALPATION

Client Position	Sitting with bilateral arms relaxed at sides
Clinician Position	Standing directly behind the client, facing the shoulder to be assessed
Movement	The clinician palpates the AC joint.
Assessment	A (+) test is reproduction of concordant pain localized to the AC joint.
Statistics	• **SN 96 (NR)**, SP 10 (NR), +LR 1.1, **–LR 0.40**, QUADAS 13, in a study of 38 consecutive clients presenting with shoulder pain bounded by the mid-part of the clavicle and the deltoid insertion (mean age NR; 22 females; mean duration of symptoms NR), using ≥50% pain relief from AC joint injection as a reference standard[32]

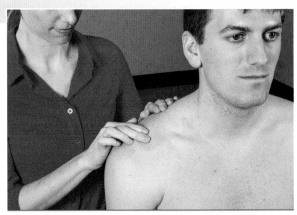

Figure 21.67

• SN 36 (20-57), SP 73 (65-80), +LR 1.37, –LR 0.87, QUADAS 13, in a study of 188 clients presenting to a primary care physician with an initial onset of shoulder pain (mean age of 42 years old; 90 women; mean duration of symptoms 7 weeks), using an injection under fluoroscopy to the AC joint as a reference standard[113]

CROSS-BODY ADDUCTION TEST

Client Position	Seated with bilateral arms relaxed at their sides
Clinician Position	Standing directly to the side or in front of the shoulder to be assessed, facing the client
Movement	The clinician places one hand (left as shown) on the client's trunk to provide stability and prevent the trunk from rotating. With the other hand (right as shown), the clinician grasps the client's elbow. The clinician passively horizontally adducts the client's arm across their chest to end range or pain production.

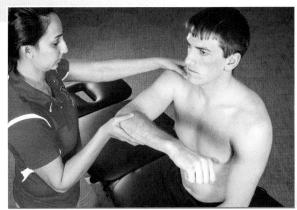

Figure 21.68

Assessment	A (+) test is reproduction of concordant pain localized to the AC joint.
Statistics	• SN 77 (NR), SP 79 (NR), +LR 3.6, –LR 0.29, QUADAS 11, in a study of 35 clients (mean age 45 years; 14 women; average duration of symptoms NR, but 21 clients had a traumatic onset reported), using surgery as a reference standard[18]
	• SN 64 (43-80), SP 26 (19-35), +LR 0.86, –LR 1.39, QUADAS 13, in a study of 188 clients presenting to a primary care physician with an initial onset of shoulder pain (average mean age 42 years; 90 women; mean duration of symptoms 7 weeks), using an injection under fluoroscopy to the AC joint as a reference standard[113]

AC RESISTED EXTENSION

Client Position	Sitting with the arm to be assessed in 90° of flexion and internal rotation
Clinician Position	Standing directly to the side of the shoulder to be assessed and facing the client. They place one hand (left as shown) on the client's shoulder for stabilization and the other (right as shown) on the distal elbow of the arm to be assessed.
Movement	The clinician stabilizes the client's trunk and resists the client's isometric attempt to horizontally extend (or horizontally abduct) their arm.
Assessment	A (+) test is reproduction of concordant pain localized to the AC joint.
Statistics	SN 72 (NR), **SP 85 (NR)**, **+LR 4.8**, –LR 0.32, QUADAS 11, in a study of 35 clients (mean age 45 years; 14 women; mean duration of symptoms NR, but 21 clients had a traumatic onset reported) diagnosed with AC joint pathology (local tenderness and significant pain relief with diagnostic injection), using surgery as a reference standard[18]

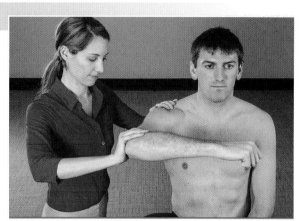

Figure 21.69

ACTIVE COMPRESSION TEST

This test has previously been described regarding labral pathology. Please refer to test description in that section.

Assessment	A (+) test with respect to AC joint pathology is reproduction of localized AC joint concordant pain.
Statistics	SN 14 (5-33), SP 92 (86-96), +LR 1.73, –LR 0.94, QUADAS 13, in a study of 188 clients presenting to a primary care physician with an initial onset of shoulder pain (mean age 42 years; 90 women; mean duration of symptoms 7 weeks), using an injection under fluoroscopy to the AC joint as a reference standard[113]

CLUSTER TESTING

Cluster testing consists of the cross-body adduction test, the AC resisted extension test, and the active compression test.

Statistics
- All 3 tests (+): SN 25 (NR), **SP 97 (NR)**, **+LR 8.3**, –LR 0.77, QUADAS 11, in a study of 35 clients diagnosed with AC joint pathology (mean age of 45 years old; 14 women; mean duration of symptoms NR, but 21 clients had a traumatic onset reported), using surgery as a reference standard[18]
- Any 2 of the 3 tests (+): **SN 81 (NR)**, **SP 89 (NR)**, **+LR 7.4**, **–LR 0.21**, QUADAS 11, in a study of 35 clients diagnosed with AC joint pathology (mean age of 45 years old; 14 women; mean duration of symptoms NR, but 21 clients had a traumatic onset reported), using surgery as a reference standard[18]

Additional cluster testing is comprised of the cross-body adduction test, active compression test, Hawkins-Kennedy test, and AC joint tenderness to palpation.

Statistics
- All 4 tests (+): SN 5 (1-24), **SP 99 (95-100)**, **+LR 5.70**, –LR 0.96, QUADAS 13, in a study of 188 clients presenting to a primary care physician with an initial onset of shoulder pain (mean age of 42 years old; 90 women; mean duration of symptoms 7 weeks), using an injection under fluoroscopy to the AC joint as a reference standard[113]

(continued)

Cluster Testing *(continued)*

- At least 3 tests (+): SN 30 (15-52), SP 81 (73-87), +LR 1.57, –LR 0.87, QUADAS 13, in a study of 188 clients presenting to a primary care physician with an initial onset of shoulder pain (mean age of 42 years old; 90 women; mean duration of symptoms 7 weeks), using an injection under fluoroscopy to the AC joint as a reference standard[113]

ADHESIVE CAPSULITIS

SHOULDER SHRUG SIGN

Client Position	Upright position
Clinician Position	Either in front of or behind the client for a view of the client's scapula
Movement	The client is asked to raise their arm into maximal shoulder flexion.
Assessment	The test is (+) if the client allows the shoulder girdle to shrug prior to achieving 90° of active flexion.
Statistics	• When related to adhesive capsulitis: **SN 90 (NR)**, SP 50 (NR), +LR 1.9, **–LR 0.1**, QUADAS 11
	• When related to glenohumeral arthritis: **SN 91 (NR)**, SP 57 (NR), +LR 2.1, **–LR 0.17**, in 982 clients (mean age 57 years; 267 women; mean duration of symptoms NR), using radiography and intra-operative findings as reference standards[114]

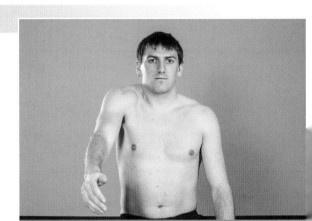

Figure 21.70

CORACOID PAIN TEST

Client Position	Sitting, arms relaxed at their sides
Clinician Position	Standing directly behind the client and to the side to be assessed
Movement	The clinician palpates the coracoid, AC joint, and the anterolateral subacromial region. The clinician asks the client to rate their pain on a scale of 0 (no pain) to 10 (most severe pain).
Assessment	A (+) test is when the pain with palpation of the coracoid is 3 points or greater above the score of the other two palpated areas.
Statistics	SN 96 (90-99), SP 89 (86-91), +LR 8.7, –LR 0.04, QUADAS 7, in a study of 85 clients presenting with primary adhesive capsulitis, 465 with rotator cuff tear, 48 with calcifying tendonitis, 16 with glenohumeral arthritis, 66 with AC arthropathy, and 150 asymptomatic clients (age range 43-64 years, gender and mean duration of symptoms NR), using comparison to those with the other conditions and to the controls as a reference standard[115]

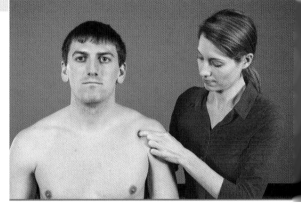

Figure 21.71

TESTS FOR SCAPULAR DYSKINESIS

SCAPULAR ASSISTANCE TEST

Client Position	Sitting, arms relaxed at their sides
Clinician Position	Standing directly behind the client
Movement	The client is asked to elevate their arm in the scapular plane and to rate their pain on a 0-10 scale (0 = no pain, 10 = worst pain). The clinician also observes to see if a painful arc is present. The client then repeats the elevation while the clinician manually assists the scapula into upward rotation and posterior tilting.
Assessment	The test is (+) if the client reports decreased pain with elevation when the clinician is providing the assistance.
Statistics	The scapular assistance test has not been assessed for diagnostic value. It has been studied for reliability in 46 clients presenting for physical therapy for various shoulder dysfunctions. (κ) coefficient was 0.53 in the scapular plane and 0.62 in the sagittal plane.[116]

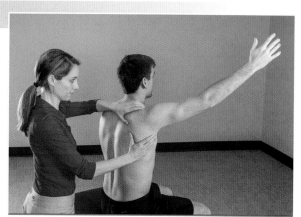

Figure 21.72

SCAPULAR DYSKINESIS TEST

Client Position	Upright position
Clinician Position	Standing directly behind the client to observe the scapula
Movement	The client is asked to perform up to five repetitions of shoulder flexion and abduction.
Assessment	The test is considered (+) if the clinician notes winging or abnormal movement. This may be quantified as normal movement, subtle dyskinesis, or obvious dyskinesis.
Statistics	Shoulder pain is >3/10, SN 24, SP 71, +LR 0.83, −LR 1.07. When shoulder pain is >6/10, SN 21, SP 72, +LR 0.75, −LR 1.1, QUADAS 10, with 66 collegiate athlete clients presenting with shoulder pain (mean age 21 years old; 16 women; mean duration of symptoms NR), using a reference standard of self-reported shoulder pain via the Penn Shoulder Scale.[117]

LATERAL SCAPULAR SLIDE TEST

Client Position	Sitting, arms relaxed at their sides
Clinician Position	Standing directly behind the client
Movement	The clinician measures from the inferior angle of the scapula to the thoracic spinous process at the same level. This measurement occurs with the client keeping their shoulder at 0°, 45°, and 90° of abduction. It is performed on both the symptomatic and asymptomatic sides.
Assessment	The test is considered (+) if there is >1 to 1.5 cm of distance difference in scapular position from one side to the other.

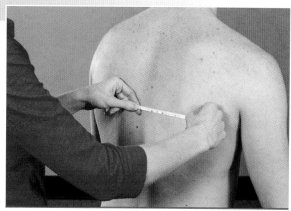

Figure 21.73

(continued)

Lateral Scapular Slide Test *(continued)*

Statistics When attempting to identify any shoulder dysfunction, Odom and colleagues calculated the following statistics with a QUADAS 8 in 20 of 46 clients with various shoulder pathologies (mean age of 30 years, gender and mean duration of symptoms were NR). Confidence intervals were not reported for the statistical analysis.[118]

At the 1 cm threshold:

- SN 35 (0°), 41 (45°), 43 (90°)
- SP 48 (0°), 54 (45°), 56 (90°)
- + LR 0.67 (0°), 0.89 (45°), 0.98 (90°)
- –LR 1.35 (0°), 1.09 (45°), 1.02 (90°)

At the 1.5 cm threshold:

- SN 28 (0°), 50 (45°), 34 (90°)
- SP 53 (0°), 58 (45°), 52 (90°)
- +LR 0.60 (0°), 1.19 (45°), 0.71 (90°)
- –LR 1.36 (0 °), 0.86 (45 °), 1.27 (90 °)

When attempting to identify shoulder diagnosis, Shadmehr and colleagues calculated the following statistics with a QUADAS of 7 in 27 of 57 clients with various shoulder pathologies (mean age of 48 years old, gender and mean duration of symptoms were not reported). Confidence intervals were not calculated for the statistical analysis.[119]

At the 1 cm threshold:

- SN 93-100 (0°), 90-93 (45°), 86-96 (90°)
- SP 8-23 (0°), 4-23 (45°), 4-15 (90°)
- + LR 1.01–1.3 (0°), 0.94–1.21 (45°), 0.90–1.13 (90°)
- –LR 0.88–0 (0°), 2.5–0.3 (45°), 3.5–0.27 (90°)

At the 1.5 cm threshold:

- SN 90-96 (0°), 83-93 (45°), 80-90 (90°)
- SP 12-26 (0°), 15-26 (45°), 4-19 (90°)
- +LR 1.02–1.3 (0°), 0.98–1.26 (45°), 0.83–1.11 (90°)
- –LR 0.15–0.83 (0°), 0.27–1.13 (45°), 0.52–5.0 (90°)

SCAPULAR RETRACTION TEST

Client Position Upright position in a natural posture

Clinician Position Standing in front of the client

Movement The clinician asks the client to bring their arm into elevation within the scapular plane. The clinician then attempts to push the arm inferiorly, asking the client to resist the movement. Next, the clinician cues the client to correct their scapular position by actively retracting the scapula. The first step is repeated with the client maintaining the retracted position.

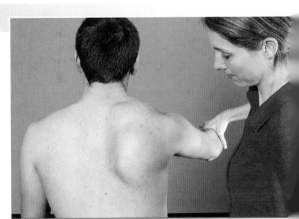

Figure 21.74

Assessment The test is (+) if the client's strength is better in the scapular retracted position versus the natural resting position.

Statistics SN 100, SP 33 (NR), +LR 1.49, –LR 0, QUADAS 3, in a study of 20 clients presenting with shoulder pain (mean age of 43 years, gender and mean duration of symptoms NR), using a reference standard of clinical or MRI diagnosis of labral injury, instability, impingement, decreased supraspinatus strength, and scapular dyskinesis on clinical exam[120]

SICK SCAPULA

Client Position	Sitting, arms relaxed at their sides
Clinician Position	Standing directly behind the client
Movement	The clinician palpates the coracoid and the contours of the scapula.
Assessment	*SICK* scapula is an acronym for *S*capular malposition, *I*nferior medial border prominence, *C*oracoid pain, and dys*K*inesis of scapula movement. A client exhibiting these attributes would be considered to have SICK scapula findings.
Statistics	SN 41 (NR); SP, +LR, and −LR (NR); QUADAS 11, in 34 clients (mean age 47 years; 2 women; mean duration of symptoms 28 months since time of AC joint grade III dislocation) when attempting to identify clients with SICK scapula in the presence of a chronic grade III AC dislocation, using clinical or radiographic examination as a reference standard[121]

NERVE PALSIES

The following tests have been purported to assess nerve palsies of axillary and spinal accessory nerves. These tests have been analyzed only in small samples,[122, 123] with only one of the studies reporting SN and SP numbers[122] (the triangle sign: SN 100, SP 95). Generalizability of these tests based on the current literature is limited at this time.

DELTOID EXTENSION LAG SIGN

Client Position	Sitting in an upright position
Clinician Position	Standing behind the client, grasping the client's arm at the wrist
Movement	The clinician passively moves the client's arm into full shoulder extension. The clinician then asks the client to maintain the arm in an extended position and releases the client's wrist.
Assessment	The test is (+) for axillary nerve palsy if a lag is noted (client is unable to maintain the extended position).

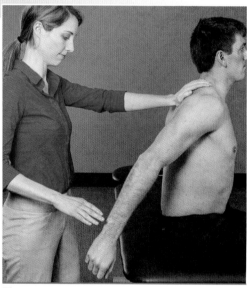

Figure 21.75

ACTIVE ELEVATION LAG SIGN

Client Position	Upright position
Clinician Position	The clinician stands behind the client and initially moves the client's arm passively through shoulder flexion to ensure that full elevation is available. After ensuring that full elevation is available, the clinician returns the client's arm to their side. Finally, the clinician places their hand on the client's lumbar spine.
Movement	The clinician continues to palpate the lumbar spine and asks the client to actively elevate the arm through as much range of motion as they are able. The clinician defines the amount of motion by the amount of flexion produced prior to lumbar hyperextension occurring. The movement is produced on the asymptomatic side three times and then on the symptomatic side three times.
Assessment	The test is (+) for spinal accessory nerve palsy if less shoulder elevation is noted on the symptomatic side compared to the asymptomatic side.

TRIANGLE SIGN

Client Position	The client sits in an upright position initially. After shoulder flexion range of motion has been assessed, the client is positioned in prone with the arms in a flexed position.
Clinician Position	The clinician stands behind the client when they are in the upright position. When the client is prone, the clinician stands alongside the client and monitors the lumbar spine.
Movement	The clinician initially moves the client's arm into shoulder flexion to assess if full shoulder flexion is available. If full flexion is available, the client is asked to lay prone with the shoulder flexed to end range. The client then attempts to actively flex the arm off the table.
Assessment	The test is (+) for spinal accessory nerve palsy if the client uses lumbar hyperextension to achieve active arm flexion on the symptomatic side.

PALPATION

The clinician should potentially palpate the entire shoulder complex, cervical spine, upper thoracic spine, and upper ribs when assessing the shoulder joint, dependent on the particular client presentation. Refer to chapters 17 (Cervical Spine) and 18 (Thoracic Spine) to review palpation of these structures.

Anterior Aspect

Bony Structures

- **Bicipital groove:** The clinician holds the client's arm in mid-position. They will move their fingers laterally from the coracoid process, past the lesser tuberosity and into the bicipital groove. It contains the tendon of the long head of the biceps. This groove is covered by the transverse humeral ligament, which can sometimes be lax and allow the biceps tendon to sublux. If this occurs, it will generally sublux medially as the humerus is rotated laterally. The clinician should have the client internally rotate, and their finger will roll onto the greater tuberosity. This structure is generally tender if the client has had an anterior dislocation of the shoulder.

- **Sternoclavicular joint:** The clinician palpates laterally to the head of the clavicle into the depression.

- **Clavicle:** The clinician can move medial to the acromion until a bulge is felt. Generally the clavicle will sit slightly higher than the acromion. The clinician may have the client abduct the shoulder in order to feel the clavicle rotate posteriorly. The clavicle is convex anterior medially and concave anterior laterally.

- **Coracoid process:** A very important structure, the coracoid process is the attachment of several structures. If the clinician can find the acromiocla-

vicular joint and drop about 2 cm medial and inferior, they will palpate the coracoid. This structure is almost always tender to palpation, even without pathology.

- **Acromioclavicular joint:** The clinician can palpate laterally along the clavicle to the most lateral aspect of the clavicle. They will feel where the clavicle is slightly superior to the acromion. The area will be tender with sprains of the AC ligament or with degeneration of the AC joint, which is common in weightlifters. Clients may also get crepitus from this location if there are any degenerative changes.

- **Lateral border of the scapula:** The clinician can find the inferior medial angle of the scapula and move superolaterally along scapula. As they move superior and laterally, they will first palpate the teres major and then the teres minor.

Soft-Tissue Structures

- **Short head of biceps:** This is the proximal attachment to the coracoid process (figure 21.76),

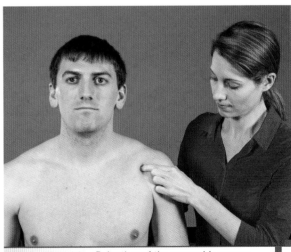

Figure 21.76 Palpation of the coracoid process.

while the distal attachment is the conjoined tendon of the biceps brachii.

- **Long head of biceps:** This structure is palpable proximally in the bicipital groove, as described before.

- **Supraspinatus:** To palpate its insertion, the clinician slightly extends the client's shoulder and palpates just the anterior lateral end of the acromion. There they should have the area of the top of the greater tubercle.

- **Infraspinatus:** The infraspinatus insertion is on the middle of the greater tubercle of the humerus.

- **Teres major:** This muscle has an origin along the dorsal surface of the lateral border of the scapula, while its insertion is on the lower portion of the greater tubercle.

- **Subscapularis:** The origin is along the entire costal surface of the scapula except for a small space near the glenohumeral joint. The insertion is along the lesser tubercle of the humerus. This can be a difficult structure to palpate. Clinicians may be able to palpate a portion of the subscapularis muscle belly by bringing the arm into approximately 45° of abduction and slight external rotation to expose the costal surface, though this may not be easily palpable on all clients.

- **Pectoralis major:** To palpate, the clinician may begin at the sternal attachment, then follow along the clavicle to palpate the upper fibers. They can follow these along to the crest of the greater tubercle of humerus. This muscle creates the anterior wall of axilla.

- **Deltoid:** The insertion is on the deltoid tuberosity of the humerus. To palpate the deltoid, the clinician starts on distal third of the clavicle and moves laterally and inferiorly around its posterior portion.

- **Sternocleidomastoid muscle:** A long thin muscle, the SCM has an insertion at the mastoid process of the occiput, while its proximal origin has two portions, one attaching to the clavicle and one attaching to the sternum. The clinician can palpate along the clavicle until they reach the SC joint. The clinician should have the client laterally flex the neck toward them while the client rotates it away; this will make the SCM more easily stand out for palpation.

- **Axillary lymph nodes:** Normal lymph nodes should not be palpated in a normal adult. If they are palpable, this could indicate malignancy or infection.

Posterior Aspect

Bony Structures

- **Lateral border of the scapula:** The clinician can find the inferior medial angle of the scapula and move superolaterally along the scapula. As they move superior and laterally, they will first palpate the teres major and then the teres minor

- **Superior angle of scapula:** The attachment of the levator scapula is at this location. The clinician can follow the spine of the scapula as far as it will go medially, then move their fingers superior to find the superior angle of the scapula. This area is commonly tender.

- **Spine of scapula:** The clinician may locate the bony prominence three-fourths along the spine cranially. Superior to the spine of the scapula lies the supraspinous fossa, where the supraspinatus muscle resides. Inferior to the spine of the scapula is the infraspinatus fossa, where the infraspinatus muscle lies.

- **Medial border of scapula:** At the superior portion are the attachments of the rhomboids. The medial border of the scapula should be no more than 3 in. (8 cm) from midline. If the medial border is greater than approximately 3 in. from midline, it would be considered abducted. Along the medial border of the scapula, the clinician may palpate the rhomboid major and minor.

- **Inferior angle of scapula:** This is located at the tip of the inferior portion of the scapula. If the inferior medial angle of the scapula is elevated away from the thoracic cage, it is considered to be tipped.

Soft-Tissue Structures

- **Supraspinatus:** For palpation, the clinician can passively flex the shoulder 90°, with the elbow flexed 90° and some internal rotation of the shoulder. To palpate its insertion, the clinician can slightly extend the shoulder and palpate just the anterior lateral end of the acromion; there they should find the area of the top of the greater tubercle.

- **Infraspinatus:** For palpation, the clinician should have the client either seated or prone on the table. In prone, the client should grab the edge of the table to maintain lateral rotation. The clinician can palpate along the spine of the scapula laterally then move their fingers inferiorly to the infraspinatus fossa.

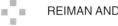

- **Teres minor:** For palpation, the clinician can follow the lateral angle of the scapula. The first muscle they will find is the teres major. As they palpate superiorly, the next muscle they come to will be the teres minor.

- **Latissimus dorsi:** This muscle is very palpable on the posterior lateral aspect of the trunk.

- **Rhomboids (major and minor):** To palpate the rhomboids, the clinician should locate the vertebral border of the scapula. The clinician should place the client's arm behind their waist to encourage scapular adduction, and the muscles will contract.

- **Trapezius muscle:** The upper part is a thin sheet running downward from the base of the skull and then curving downward and forward around the neck to insert on the clavicle. The second part extends from the ligaments of the neck to the acromion. It is much thicker and stronger. The middle portion includes fibers that arise from the 7th cervical vertebra to insert on the spine of the scapula. The lower portion of the trapezius fibers converge from their origin on the lower thoracic vertebrae and run superior and lateral to join a short tendon attached to a small tendon, which attaches to the inferior medial angle of the scapula. The clinician can follow the trapezius laterally and inferiorly from the external occipital protuberance to the clavicle. Also, they should follow the lower fibers from the medial aspect of the spine of the scapula, then move medially and inferiorly to the spinous processes of the lower thoracic vertebrae. The clinician can follow the middle fibers from the acromion to the spinous processes of the 7th cervical and upper thoracic vertebrae.

PHYSICAL PERFORMANCE MEASURES

Physical performance measures (PPMs) available for the shoulder are often appropriate for several areas of the upper quadrant, at times encompassing physical performance with issues that could include the cervical and upper thoracic spine, as well as any of the upper extremity joints. PPMs for the shoulder and upper quadrant have not been investigated as extensively as in the lower extremity; as such, there are fewer PPMs to select from. Table 21.4 includes lower-level balance

TABLE 21.4 Physical Performance Measure Suggestions for the Shoulder and Upper Quadrant

Discrete physical parameter	Potential physical performance measurements for the lower-level client (if appropriate)	Potential physical performance measurements for the higher-level client (if appropriate)
Balance and stability	Single-leg stance Tandem stance Romberg positions Traditional LE balance assessments may be necessary if the shoulder dysfunction is related to a fall.	Upper extremity Y balance test CKCUEST Any of the tests appropriate for the lower-level client
Fundamental movement	Any overhead reach or functional reach test	Overhead squat Any of the tests appropriate for the lower-level client
Strength	Only if appropriate and necessary	Flexed arm hang Pull-up test Push-up
Power	Only if appropriate and necessary	Overhead medicine ball throw Sidearm medicine ball throw Seated shot-put throw
Throwing accuracy	Only if appropriate and necessary	Functional Throwing Performance Index
Endurance	Scapular muscle endurance test	Scapular muscle endurance test

CKCUEST = closed kinetic chain upper extremity stability test

PPMs as well since balance may be a concern for clients who sustained a shoulder injury due to a fall or for clients who may have a shoulder dysfunction and a concurrent falls risk.

The Upper extremity Y balance test (UEYBT) has been correlated with a 2-minute timed push-up, lateral trunk endurance, and the closed kinetic chain upper extremity stability test (CKCUEST) in healthy, college-aged subjects. Additionally, there was no significant difference in measurements during the UEYBT from the dominant to non-dominant arm, which one may expect in a client with shoulder dysfunction.[124] The CKCUEST has similarly been investigated in healthy, college-aged baseball players and has been found to be a reliable measure of closed chain upper extremity function.[125] Both the UEYBT and the CKCUEST appear to be indicative of upper extremity closed chain stability as well as of general core and trunk strength and mobility.

The functional impairment test—hand, neck, shoulder, and arm (FIT-HaNSA) has been compared between clients with and without shoulder dysfunction. It has shown reliability and has correlated well with the DASH and SPADI, and moderately with strength and ROM measures at the shoulder.[126]

The overhead squat is a component of the Functional Movement Screen (previously discussed in chapter 12). This movement has not been researched in clients with shoulder pain, but it may have some utility as a PPM in this population due to the shoulder elevation that is incorporated in the overhead squat.

The flexed arm hang and pull-up test are used to quantify forearm and upper extremity flexor strength and endurance, though they have not been correlated with specific shoulder dysfunction. Similarly, the push-up test is used to assess general upper extremity strength and endurance, but it has not been correlated specifically with various shoulder dysfunctions.[127]

The backward overhead medicine ball throw, sidearm medicine ball throw, and seated shot-put throw have all been suggested as strength and power PPMs of the upper extremity. The backward overhead medicine ball throw has demonstrated reliability and validity with total-body power and vertical jump in both jumping and nonjumping athletes. The sidearm medicine ball throw has been correlated with isometric trunk rotational torque and 1RM on the bench press. The seated shot-put throw has been moderately correlated with power on the bench press in college football players.[127]

The Functional Throwing Performance Index (FTPI) has shown good reliability in small sample sets of overhead athletes and is a way to quantify proprioception.[128]

The scapular muscular endurance test has been investigated in clients with postural neck pain and has shown moderate reliability in this population. An average of 30.1 seconds is considered a clinically significant amount of change.[129] This has not been correlated in clients with isolated shoulder dysfunction, but it may be useful if considering the regional interdependence of scapulothoracic muscular endurance and shoulder pain.

COMMON ORTHOPEDIC CONDITIONS OF THE SHOULDER JOINT

While it is impossible to distinctly describe various pathological presentations of the shoulder, there are evidence-based findings supportive of particular pathologies of this region of the body. Therefore, the intent of this section of the chapter is to present current evidence-supported findings suggestive of shoulder pathologies. As previously described in chapter 4 (Evidence-Based Practice and Client Examination), though, not all examination findings are absolutely supported with clinical evidence, and the clinician should also rely on clinical experience and input from the client when performing differential diagnosis of a client's presentation of pain and dysfunction.

As with other regions of the body, and discussed in chapter 5, diagnostic labels for specific pathologies, although widely used, are not uniform. Therefore, since selection criteria for diagnostic conclusion could not uniformly be derived, it has been strongly suggested that the use of diagnostic labels be abolished.[130]

Rotator Cuff Tear or Tendinopathy

ICD-9: 726.1 (rotator cuff syndrome of shoulder and allied disorders); 726.9 (enthesopathy of unspecified site); 727.61 (complete rupture of rotator cuff)

ICD-10: M75.1 (rotator cuff syndrome); M75.2 (complete rotator cuff tear or rupture); M77.9 (enthesopathy, unspecified)

A rotator cuff injury can include any type of irritation or damage to the rotator cuff muscles or tendons of the shoulder.

I. Client Interview

Subjective History

- Rotator cuff tendinopathy affects 1 in 50 adults and is particularly common in athletes who throw repetitively and in laborers who have to work with their arms overhead.[131]

- Pain is the most common complaint, and it leads to a reduction in shoulder strength (pain inhibition) and functional impairment.[14]

- Onset is often insidious and can be due to falling on an outstretched hand or repetitive activities.[14, 26]

- Intrinsic degeneration within the rotator cuff is the principal factor in the pathogenesis of rotator cuff tears.[14, 26]

- Even without a report of pain, a client may have a chronic, degenerative full-thickness tear.[132]

- Description of a painful arc of motion has less than good ability to help rule in (SP 81, +LR 3.7) an RCT.[132]

Outcome Measures

- The DASH, ASES, SSI, and SPADI are all considered acceptable for use in clients with shoulder dysfunction related to rotator cuff tears.[21]

Diagnostic Imaging

- Hooked acromion is often present on radiographs.[133, 134]

- MRA demonstrates better diagnostic accuracy than either US or MRI (see table 21.1) for both ruling out and ruling in rotator cuff tears.

- US demonstrates better assistance for **ruling in** capability (SP 88-100) than **ruling out** (SN 67-95) capability.[25-28]

II. Observation

- The client may present with the arm held across the abdomen if it is highly irritable.[14, 26]

- Atrophy may be noted in the supraspinatus and infraspinatus fossa of the scapula on the involved side.[132]

III. Triage and Screening

- All nonmusculoskeletal causes, as well as causes from related joints, should be ruled out.

- The bony apprehension test demonstrates good diagnostic accuracy to help both **rule out** (SN 94, −LR 0.07) and **rule in** (SP 84, +LR 5.9) shoulder instability due to a bony lesion.[48]

- The olecranon-manubrium test demonstrates strong diagnostic accuracy to help both **rule out** (SN 84, −LR 0.3) and **rule in** (SP 99, +LR 84) anterior shoulder dislocations, clavicle fractures, and humerus fractures.[46]

IV. Motion Tests[132]

- Clients may be limited in overhead and reaching activities.

- They may report stiffness, weakness, or crepitus with attempted ROM.

- Clients may have painless lack of AROM when presenting with a full-thickness tear.

V. Muscle Performance Testing

- Increased pain and weakness with muscle testing of the involved tendon are predictive of increased tendon thickness and tendinopathy changes on US.[135]

- Pain or weakness may be present in internal rotation, external rotation, and glenohumeral elevation.[132]

- Optimal positions for strength testing include resisting elevation at 90° of elevation with 45° of external rotation in the scapular plane for the supraspinatus and resisting external rotation at 0° of humeral elevation with 45° of internal rotation.[69]

VI. Special Tests

- Painful arc: has less than good ability to help rule out (SN 71, −LR 0.36) and rule in (SP 81, +LR 3.7) an RCT.[132]

- Hawkins-Kennedy test: has less than good ability to help rule out (SN 66,

−LR 0.5) and rule in (SP 63, +LR 1.9) tendinopathy.

- Hawkins-Kennedy test: has less than good ability to help rule out (SN 76, −LR 0.51) and rule in (SP 48, +LR 1.5) an RCT in pooled analysis.[132]

- Neer's test: has less than good ability to help rule out (SN 64-68, −LR 0.60–1.1) and rule in (SP 30-61, +LR 0.98–1.6) an RCT in pooled analysis.[132]

- Rent test: A (+) test has ideal ability to help **rule in** (SP 97, +LR 32) and a (−) test also has ideal ability to help **rule out** (SN 96, −LR 0.04) an RCT.[71]

- Lateral Jobe test: A (+) test has good ability to help **rule in** (SP 89, +LR 7.36) and a (−) test has good ability to help **rule out** (SN 81, −LR 0.10) an RCT.[85]

- Supine impingement test: A (+) test has ideal ability to help **rule out** (SN 97, −LR 0.33) an RCT.[10]

- Empty can test: has less than good ability in pooled analysis to help either rule out or rule in an RCT. In two separate single studies, it had good ability to help **rule in** (SP 87-90, +LR 3.9–4.4) an RCT.[4, 77]

- Drop arm test: has poor ability to help rule out (SN 21, −LR 0.86) and less than good ability to help rule in (SP 92, +LR 2.6) an RCT in pooled analysis[54] and fair at best diagnostic ability in single studies.

- Full can test: has less than good ability to help rule out or rule in an RCT.

- External rotation lag sign: A (+) test has ideal ability to help **rule in** (SP 91-94, +LR 5–7.2)[78, 79] full-thickness supraspinatus or infraspinatus tears, while a (+) test has good ability to help **rule in** (SP 90, +LR 4.2)[77] an RCT of any severity.

- Drop sign and hornblower's signs: have less than good ability to help rule in or rule out an infraspinatus tear.

- Lift-off test: A (+) test has ideal ability to help **rule in** (SP 97, +LR 16.5) a

subscapularis tear according to pooled analysis,[54] as well as one single study (SP 100).[90]

- Internal rotation lag test: A (+) test has good ability to help **rule in** (SP 84, +LR 6.2) and a (−) test has ideal ability to help **rule in** (SN 100, −LR 0.0) a subscapularis tear.[79]

- Belly press test: A (+) test has ideal ability to help **rule in** (SP 98, +LR 20) a subscapularis tear.[90]

- Bear hug test: A (+) test has ideal ability to help **rule in** (SP 92, +LR 7.2) a subscapularis tear.[90]

VII. Palpation

- Palpation tends to elicit well-localized tenderness that is similar in quality and location to the pain experienced during activity.[136]

- (−) tenderness to palpation of the AC joint helps **rule out** (SN 96, −LR 0.40) AC joint pathology.[32]

- (−) tenderness of the supraspinatus helps **rule out** (SN 92) subacromial impingement.[137]

- (−) tenderness of the biceps tendon helps **rule out** (SN 85) subacromial impingement.[137]

- Increased tenderness to palpation of the involved tendon is predictive of increased tendon thickness and tendinopathy changes on US.[135]

VIII. Physical Performance Measures

- Scapular muscular endurance test
- Push-up test if the client can assume the position
- Considering the prevalence of RCTs in older people, clinicians may need to assess clients for a falls risk.

POTENTIAL TREATMENT-BASED CLASSIFICATIONS

- Exercise and conditioning, mobility if client has concurrent stiffness, and pain if client is highly irritable may be appropriate.

Differential Diagnosis of a Rotator Cuff Tear and C5 Radiculopathy

- RC pathology has a higher prevalence in older populations and frequently is associated with complaints of night pain and weakness in abduction.

- Both issues could present from an insidious onset.

- RC pathology may present after a fall on the outstretched arm or from overuse with repeated shoulder motions.

- A partial RCT will likely cause pain with resisted external rotation, abduction, or internal rotation.

- Both radiculopathy and a full-thickness tear could present with frank weakness in abduction and external rotation.

- Radiculopathy may cause decreased cervical ROM, a positive ULTT, and pain with Spurling's test.

- Radiculopathy may present with alterations in sensation and reflexes.

- Symptoms related to radiculopathy may be altered with repeated cervical ROM or traction.

Primary Shoulder Impingement

ICD-9: 726.2 (other affections of shoulder region, not elsewhere classified)

ICD-10: M75.4 (impingement syndrome)

Shoulder impingement syndrome is a clinical syndrome that occurs when the tendons of the rotator cuff muscles become impinged as they pass through the subacromial space. Primary impingement is due to lack of mobility in the shoulder joint. Subacromial bursitis and tendinopathy of the rotator cuff or biceps tendon can also cause symptoms of impingement.

I. Client Interview

Subjective History

- This syndrome is often associated with pain during repeated overhead activities.[132]

Outcome Measures

- The ASES, DASH, and SPADI were shown to be acceptable for clinical use.[21]

- The DASH was shown to require a 40% change from the initial score to be indicative of a substantial clinical benefit (SCB).[138]

Diagnostic Imaging

- Hooked acromion is often present on radiographs.[133, 134]

- MRI is better to help **rule out** (SN 85) AC joint arthropathy, while radiographs are better to help **rule in** (SP 90) AC joint arthropathy.[32]

- US demonstrates overall good diagnostic accuracy for calcifying tendinitis and subacromial bursitis.[25]

II. Observation

- FHRSP is associated with decreased subacromial space.[42]

- Scapular dyskinesis has been proposed as a dysfunction in clients with impingement and other shoulder disorders. However, dyskinesis is not associated with any singular diagnosis including impingement.[19]

III. Triage and Screening

- All nonmusculoskeletal causes, as well as causes from related joints, should be ruled out.

- The bony apprehension test demonstrates good diagnostic accuracy to help both **rule out** (SN 94, −LR 0.07) and **rule in** (SP 84, +LR 5.9) shoulder instability due to a bony lesion.[48]

- The olecranon-manubrium test demonstrates strong diagnostic accuracy to help both **rule out** (SN 84, −LR 0.3) and **rule in** (SP 99, +LR 84) anterior shoulder dislocations, clavicle fractures, and humerus fractures.[46]

IV. Motion Tests

- Clients may have posterior capsule mobility restriction.[139]

- Not having a painful arc of motion helps rule out (SN 75, −LR 0.38) shoulder impingement slightly better than having a painful arc of motion helps to rule it in (SP 67, +LR 2.3).[4]

V. Muscle Performance Testing

- Weakness may be present in shoulder abduction, rotation, and flexion.[140]

- Increased pain and weakness with muscle testing of the involved tendon are predictive of increased tendon thickness and tendinopathy changes on US.[135]

VI. Special Tests

- Hawkins-Kennedy test: A (−) test has good ability to help **rule out** (SN 80, −LR 0.35) but does not help rule in shoulder impingement in pooled analysis,[55] as well as in multiple single studies.

- Neer's sign: Across two meta-analyses and multiple single studies, the only strong diagnostic ability was a (−) test in one study that had good ability to help **rule out** (SN 81, −LR 0.35) SAIS.[4]

- Painful arc: Across one meta-analysis and multiple single studies, the only strong diagnostic ability was a (−) test in one study that had ideal ability to help **rule out** (SN 96, −LR 0.10) SAIS.[78]

- Internal rotation resisted strength and cross-body adduction tests: Have only less than good ability to help rule in or rule out SAIS.

- Infraspinatus or external rotation resistance test: A (+) test has good ability to help **rule in** (SP 87, +LR 4.4) SAIS.[4] When pain was the finding, this test had ideal ability to help **rule in** (SP 100, +LR Inf) SAIS.[70]

- Cluster tests:
  - Any combination of ≥3 (+) out of 5 tests (painful arc, external rotation resistance, empty can, Neer's test, and Hawkins-Kennedy test) has only fair ability to help rule in (SP 74, +LR 2.9) the diagnosis of SAIS, and <3 (+) out of 5 tests also has only fair ability to help rule out (SN 75, −LR 0.34) SAIS.[4]
  - (+) findings on the Hawkins-Kennedy, painful arc, and infraspinatus tests have ideal ability to help **rule in** (+LR 10.56) SAIS.[77]

- The majority of special tests for SAIS (used individually or combined) are limited in their abilities to diagnose or screen for the syndrome.

VII. Palpation

- Increased tenderness to palpation of the involved tendon is predictive of increased tendon thickness and tendinopathy changes on US.[135]

- (−) tenderness to palpation of the AC joint helps **rule out** (SN 96, −LR 0.40) AC joint pathology.[32]

- (−) tenderness of the supraspinatus helps **rule out** (SN 92) subacromial impingement.[137]

- (−) tenderness of the biceps tendon helps **rule out** (SN 85) subacromial impingement.[137]

VIII. Physical Performance Measures

- Scapular muscular endurance test.

- Push-up test if the client can assume the position.

- Work-, sport-, and activity-specific functions.

- The FIT-HaNSA may assist in quantifying activity-specific functions.

POTENTIAL TREATMENT-BASED CLASSIFICATIONS

- Mobility and exercise and conditioning are most likely to be used; pain control may also be used if client has high irritability.

Shoulder Secondary Impingement

ICD-9: 726.2 (other affections of shoulder region, not elsewhere classified)

ICD-10: M75.4 (impingement syndrome)

Shoulder impingement syndrome is a clinical syndrome that occurs when the tendons of the rotator cuff muscles become impinged as they pass through the subacromial space. Secondary impingement in the shoulder is attributed to weakness, laxity of the shoulder, scapular dysfunction, or the general lack of stability in the glenohumeral joint. The concept of internal impingement is also thought to be related to issues with laxity and a microinstability of the glenohumeral joint. Impingement may occur in the intra-articular space or posteriorly along the glenoid rim.[141]

I. Client Interview

Subjective History

- Symptoms may occur in the cocking position of throwing (approaching the 90° of external rotation or 90° of abduction position).[142]
- The client's chief complaint is often posterior shoulder pain with overhead sports (baseball, volleyball serving, and tennis).[142]

Outcome Measures

- The ASES, DASH, and SPADI can be used.[21]

Diagnostic Imaging

- Hooked acromion is possibly present on radiographs.[133, 134]
- MRI is better to help **rule out** (SN 85) AC joint arthropathy, while radiographs are better to help **rule in** (SP 90) AC joint arthropathy.[32]
- US demonstrates overall good diagnostic accuracy for calcifying tendinitis and subacromial bursitis.[25]

II. Observation

- Shoulder impingement is thought to be associated with scapular dyskinesis. However, dyskinesis is not associated with any specific pathology.[19]
- Lack of muscle efficiency associated with scapular dyskinesis may be more associated with resting posture than with any pathology.[41]

III. Triage and Screening

- All nonmusculoskeletal causes, as well as causes from related joints, should be ruled out.

- The bony apprehension test demonstrates good diagnostic accuracy to help both **rule out** (SN 94, −LR 0.07) and **rule in** (SP 84, +LR 5.9) shoulder instability due to a bony lesion.[48]
- The olecranon-manubrium test demonstrates strong diagnostic accuracy to help both **rule out** (SN 84, −LR 0.3) and **rule in** (SP 99, +LR 84) anterior shoulder dislocations, clavicle fractures, and humerus fractures.[46]

IV. Motion Tests

- Clients may have excessive ROM with external rotation.[139, 143]
- Not having a painful arc of motion helps rule out (SN 75, −LR 0.38) shoulder impingement slightly better than having a painful arc of motion helps to rule it in (SP 67, +LR 2.3).[4]
- Clients may have GIRD.[144]

V. Muscle Performance Testing

- Internal rotators may be weak.[139, 143]
- Decreased muscle endurance may occur in shoulder abductors and external rotators, especially in swimmers.[143]
- Increased pain and weakness with muscle testing of the involved tendon are predictive of increased tendon thickness and tendinopathy changes on US.[135]

VI. Special Tests

- See tests described previously for primary impingement.
- Internal-rotation resisted strength test showed good ability to help rule in (SP 96, +LR 22) and rule out (SN 88, −LR 0.12) internal impingement (although a QUADAS of only 8), which is thought to be associated with glenohumeral laxity.[83] This test has only been investigated by a single study.

VII. Palpation

- Increased tenderness to palpation of the involved tendon is predictive of increased tendon thickness and tendinopathy changes on US.[135]

- (−) tenderness to palpation of the AC joint helps **rule out** (SN 96, −LR 0.40) AC joint pathology.[32]

- (−) tenderness of the supraspinatus helps **rule out** (SN 92) subacromial impingement.[137]

- (−) tenderness of the biceps tendon helps **rule out** (SN 85) subacromial impingement.[137]

- Tenderness to palpation over the infraspinatus is associated with internal impingement.[142]

VIII. Physical Performance Measures

- Scapular muscular endurance test
- Push-up test
- CKCUEST for collegiate, overhead athletes
- Functional throwing performance index for overhead athletes

POTENTIAL TREATMENT-BASED CLASSIFICATIONS

- Exercise and conditioning are most likely to be used. Pain control may be used if the client has acute onset with high pain intensity. Mobility may be a secondary treatment if GIRD is present.

Labral Tear or Pathology (SLAP or Bankart)

ICD-9: 840.7 (superior glenoid labrum lesion)

ICD-10: S43.439A (superior glenoid labrum lesion)

The labrum in the shoulder partly functions to deepen the glenoid. The labrum can tear when the shoulder is subluxed or dislocated, as well as with repetitive microtrauma, which is common in repeated overhead activity. A superior labrum, anterior to posterior (SLAP) tear is a tear of the labrum on the superior portion of the labrum from anterior to posterior. A Bankart tear is a tear of the labrum in the anterior to inferior location of the labrum.

I. Client Interview

Subjective History

- Four types of SLAP tears (types I-IV) exist: Type I (labral fraying) is associated with rotator cuff tear. Types II (instability of labral–biceps complex) and IV (bucket handle tear of labrum extending into biceps tendon) are more symptomatic with reproduction of mechanism. Types III (bucket handle tear with stable labral–biceps complex) and IV are associated with traumatic instability. Type II is the most common.[16]

- Tears are more common in the dominant arm.[15, 34]

- Clinical history may involve a traction injury, direct trauma to the shoulder, or a fall on an outstretched arm. Frequently, no antecedent injury or activity is reported.[15]

- Clients may have complaints of clicking, catching, locking, or popping in the shoulder.[15, 16]

- Clients may have nonspecific complaints, but they are unlikely to be able to perform activities related to high-level sports.[16]

- If an associated anterior dislocation is present, a Hill-Sachs deformity and a Bankart lesion may occur with a SLAP tear.[145]

Outcome Measures

- The clinician can use the ASES, SPADI, and DASH.

- The clinician can use the WOSI if the client's labral tear is contributing to shoulder instability.

Diagnostic Imaging

- Concurrent shoulder injuries are often present with SLAP tears, including rotator cuff tears, cystic changes or marrow edema in the humeral head, capsular laxity, and Hill-Sachs or Bankart lesions.[15]

- MRI (SP 86)[34] and CTA (SP 86)[30] are both helpful for **ruling out** SLAP; MRA (SP 95) and CTA (SP 90) are helpful for **ruling in** SLAP.

- MRA (SN 90, SP 100) and CTA (SN 86, SP 95) both demonstrate strong diagnostic accuracy for both **ruling out** and **ruling in** Bankart lesions.[30]

II. Observation

- The clinician should monitor for apprehension if the labral tear is associated with shoulder instability.

III. Triage and Screening

- All nonmusculoskeletal causes, as well as causes from related joints, should be ruled out.

- The bony apprehension test demonstrates good diagnostic accuracy to help both **rule out** (SN 94, −LR 0.07) and **rule in** (SP 84, +LR 5.9) shoulder instability due to a bony lesion.[48]

- The olecranon-manubrium test demonstrates strong diagnostic accuracy to help both **rule out** (SN 84, −LR 0.3) and **rule in** (SP 99, +LR 84) anterior shoulder dislocations, clavicle fractures, and humerus fractures.[46]

IV. Motion Tests

- Labral tears are often associated with glenohumeral joint instability or impingement-like syndromes.[15, 16]

V. Muscle Performance Testing

- Increased pain and weakness with muscle testing of the involved tendon are predictive of increased tendon thickness and tendinopathy changes on US.[135]

VI. Special Tests

- Biceps load I: A (+) test (SP 97, +LR 30.3) and a (−) test (SN 91, −LR 0.09) have good ability to help **rule in** and **rule out** labral pathology and shoulder instability, respectively.

- Crank test: Across one meta-analysis and multiple single studies, the only strong diagnostic ability was one study that had a (+) test showing ideal ability to help **rule in** (SP 93, +LR 13.6) labral pathology or shoulder instability and a (−) test that also has ideal ability to help **rule out** (SN 91, −LR 0.1) labral pathology.[73]

- Biceps load II test: This was initially described as a strong test for helping **rule in** (SP 97, +LR 30.3) and **rule out** (SN 90, −LR 0.11) a SLAP tear,[98] but a second study with a larger sample size did not offer similarly strong statistics for this test.[97]

- Active compression test (O'Brien's test): has shown less than good ability to help rule in or rule out labral pathology.[55, 71, 97]

- Speed's test: less than good ability to help rule in or out labral pathology.

- Anterior slide test: Only one study had a (+) test demonstrating good ability to help **rule in** (SP 92, +LR 4.3) labral pathology.[103]

- Yergason's test: Only one study had a (+) test demonstrating ideal ability to help **rule in** (SP 95, +LR 2.5) SLAP tear.[55]

- Compression rotation test: less than good ability to help rule in or out labral pathology.[55, 94, 97, 100]

- In a single study with a small sample size, the passive compression test had good ability to help **rule out** (SN 82, −LR 0.21) labral pathology with a (−) test and **rule in** (SP 86, +LR 5.7) labral pathology with a (+) test.[105]

- Passive distraction test: less than good ability to help rule in (SP 94, +LR 8.8) or rule out (QUADAS 8) labral tear.[105] This study will need to be replicated to be more generalizable.[106]

- The jerk and Kim tests, with a (+) test, have good ability to help **rule in** (SP 98 and 94, +LR 34.7 and 12.6, respectively) posteroinferior instability and posterior labral tears.[107] Nakagawa and colleagues did not find similarly strong numbers for the jerk test (SN 25, SP 80, +LR 1.3, −LR 0.94).[94]

- While several clusters of findings for labral tears have been advocated, the cluster consisting of positive findings on both the apprehension and relocation tests offers the best numbers for helping to rule in a labral tear.[55] These tests are traditionally thought of as tests for glenohumeral instability, and a connection with these tests and labral pathology likely is related to the labrum's function in contributing to passive stability of the glenohumeral joint.

VII. Palpation

- Clients may have anterior joint tenderness.
- (–) tenderness to palpation of the AC joint helps **rule out** (SN 96, –LR 0.40) AC joint pathology.[32]
- (–) tenderness of the supraspinatus helps **rule out** (SN 92) subacromial impingement.[137]
- (–) tenderness of the biceps tendon helps **rule out** (SN 85) subacromial impingement.[137]
- Increased tenderness to palpation of the involved tendon is predictive of increased tendon thickness and tendinopathy changes on US.[135]
- Tenderness of the biceps does not offer any diagnostic benefit for labral tears.[55]

VIII. Physical Performance Measures

- Scapular muscular endurance test if the client is able to assume the position.
- Higher-level athletes may use PPMs such as the YBT or CKCUEST to assess for closed chain stability. The client would need to be further along in their recovery or rehabilitation and should not do these when pain or apprehension are limiting factors.
- Sport- or activity-specific assessments.
- Functional throwing performance index for overhead athletes.
- The clinician should consider performing a falls risk assessment if the client's instability is related to trauma from a fall.

POTENTIAL TREATMENT-BASED CLASSIFICATIONS

- Pain control and immobility may be used if the case is related to acute trauma; exercise and conditioning and possibly mobility may be used as a secondary category if the client presents with post-immobilization stiffness.

Shoulder Instability (With or Without Hill-Sachs or Reverse Hill-Sachs Lesion)

ICD-9: 831 (dislocation, sprain, and strain of shoulder)

ICD-10: S43 (dislocation, sprain, and strain of joints and ligaments of shoulder girdle)

Shoulder instability is related to laxity or disruption of the passive elements of the glenohumeral joint. The capsular ligaments may be lax from congenital laxity, systemic laxity, or a history of trauma. The ligamentous structures may also be torn from acute trauma, resulting in subluxation or dislocation.[146] Instability may be associated with other pathology such as labral tears, Bankart lesions (where the capsule avulses from the glenoid), or Hill-Sachs lesions of the humeral head from traumatic contact with the glenoid rim. Instability is often classified as TUBS (traumatic, unidirectional, Bankart, surgery) and AMBRI (atraumatic, multidirectional, bilateral, rehabilitation, inferior capsule shift).[147] Other classifications can include the presence or lack of trauma, direction of instability, or dislocation versus subluxation.[148]

I. Client Interview

Subjective History

- The most predictive client attributes related to shoulder instability are a reported history of dislocation, a younger age, a sudden onset of symptoms, and a positive finding on the release test of the shoulder.[20]
- Symptoms may range from generalized shoulder pain to reports of multiple dislocations or episodes of joint instability.[20]
- After a dislocation is reduced, pain is less likely to be the primary complaint, whereas clients will often report apprehension and decreased confidence in the use of their shoulder for normal lifestyle activities.[23]

Outcome Measures

- Western Ontario Shoulder Instability Index
- Simple shoulder test

- DASH
- SPADI

Diagnostic Imaging

- MRA (SN 75, **SP 98**) and CTA (**SN 93, SP 90**) both demonstrate strong diagnostic accuracy for detecting Hill-Sachs lesions.[30]
- MRA (**SN 88, SP 91**) demonstrates strong diagnostic accuracy for detecting labroligamentous tears or instability.[30]

II. Observation

- Sulcus signs may be present at the joint line.[148]
- Clients with instability often exhibit decreased scapular upward rotation and increased scapular internal rotation.[149]
- Assessment of scapular positioning does not correlate with the client's ability to move or with a specific pathology.[42]

III. Triage and Screening

- All nonmusculoskeletal causes, as well as related joints, should be ruled out.
- The bony apprehension test demonstrates good diagnostic accuracy to help both **rule out** (SN 94, −LR 0.07) and **rule in** (SP 84, +LR 5.9) shoulder instability due to a bony lesion.[48]
- The olecranon-manubrium test demonstrates strong diagnostic accuracy to help both **rule out** (SN 84, −LR 0.3) and **rule in** (SP 99, +LR 84) anterior shoulder dislocations, clavicle fractures, and humerus fractures.[46]

IV. Motion Tests

- Clients may have apprehension with active or passive motion during ADLs and in positions of instability.[23, 20, 55]
- They may have generalized laxity with glenohumeral motion.[147]

V. Muscle Performance Testing

- IR strength deficit is often present in clients with anterior shoulder instability.[146]
- General weakness of glenohumeral IR and ER is present in clients who have experienced recurrent dislocations.[146]

- Increased pain and weakness with muscle testing of the involved tendon are predictive of increased tendon thickness and tendinopathy changes on US.[135]

VI. Special Tests

- Anterior apprehension test: A (+) test had ideal ability to help **rule in** (SP 95-99, +LR 17.2–53) anterior shoulder instability.[55, 108, 109] This test also had good ability to **rule out** (SN 98, −LR 0.02) anterior instability in one study.[20]
- Relocation test: A (+) test has good (**SP 84, +LR 4.4**)[20] to ideal (**SP 90-92, +LR 5.5–10.4**)[55] ability to help **rule in** anterior shoulder instability and a (−) test has good (**SN 81, −LR 0.2**)[109] to ideal (**SN 92, −LR 0.02**)[20] ability to help **rule out** anterior shoulder instability.
- Surprise test: A (−) test has good ability to help **rule out** (SN 82, −LR 0.25) anterior shoulder instability and a (+) test also has good ability to help **rule in** (SP 86, +LR 5.4) anterior shoulder instability in pooled analysis.[55] In two single studies, a (−) test had ideal ability to help **rule out** (SN 92, −LR 0.1)[20] anterior instability and a (+) test had good (**SP 84, +LR 5.6**)[20] to ideal (**SP 99, +LR 58.6**)[108] ability to help **rule in** anterior instability.

VII. Palpation

- Increased tenderness to palpation of the involved tendon is predictive of increased tendon thickness and tendinopathy changes on US.[135]
- (−) tenderness to palpation of the AC joint helps **rule out** (SN 96, −LR 0.40) AC joint pathology.[32]
- (−) tenderness of the supraspinatus helps **rule out** (SN 92) subacromial impingement.[137]
- (−) tenderness of the biceps tendon helps **rule out** (SN 85) subacromial impingement.[137]

VIII. Physical Performance Measures

- Scapular muscular endurance test if the client is able to assume the position.

- Higher-level athletes may use PPMs such as the YBT or CKCUEST to assess for closed chain stability. The client would need to be further along in their recovery or rehabilitation and should not do these when pain or apprehension are limiting factors.

- Sport- and activity-specific assessments.

- Functional throwing performance index for overhead athletes.

- The clinician should consider performing a falls risk assessment if the client's instability is related to trauma from a fall.

POTENTIAL TREATMENT-BASED CLASSIFICATIONS

- Immobility and pain control may be used with acute onset.

- Clients presenting with acute, traumatic onset may require referral out because they could present with a positive olecranon-manubrium compression test or bony apprehension.

- If the client does not require immobilization or pain management, they will likely be in the exercise and conditioning category.

Shoulder Osteoarthritis

ICD-9: 715.11 (osteoarthrosis, localized, primary, shoulder region)

ICD-10: M19.019 (primary osteoarthritis, unspecified shoulder)

Shoulder osteoarthritis, like osteoarthritis of any synovial joint, involves a degenerative process of the joint. Articular cartilage breakdown, joint space narrowing, joint swelling, and pain are common characteristics of this condition.

I. Client Interview

Subjective History

- Clients may have complaints of general shoulder pain, limitations in shoulder function, and disability.

- This condition may be associated with concomitant RC pathology or impingement.

- It has a prevalence of 5% to 21% in Western countries.[150]

- Shoulder OA is more common in women and older people.[151]

Outcome Measures[150]

- ASES

- WOOS

Diagnostic Imaging

- Radiographic findings include joint space narrowing, bone sclerosis, periarticular cysts, and osteophytes. Refer to chapter 6 for a definition of osteoarthritis (OA) according to Kellgren and Lawrence.[152]

- MRI is better to help **rule out** (SN 85) AC joint arthropathy, while radiographs are better to help **rule in** (SP 90) AC joint arthropathy.[32]

- US demonstrates overall good diagnostic accuracy for calcifying tendinitis and subacromial bursitis.[25]

II. Observation

- Clients may present with a shrug sign during attempted shoulder elevation.[114]

III. Triage and Screening

- All nonmusculoskeletal causes, as well as related joints, should be ruled out.

- The bony apprehension test demonstrates good diagnostic accuracy to help both **rule out** (SN 94, −LR 0.07) and **rule in** (SP 84, +LR 5.9) shoulder instability due to a bony lesion.[48]

- The olecranon-manubrium test demonstrates strong diagnostic accuracy to help both **rule out** (SN 84, −LR 0.3) and **rule in** (SP 99, +LR 84) anterior shoulder dislocations, clavicle fractures, and humerus fractures.[46]

IV. Motion Tests

- Commonly motion tests are limited in all GH planes of motion in clients who are surgical candidates for total shoulder arthroplasty (TSA).[153]

V. Muscle Performance Testing

- Increased pain and weakness with muscle testing of the involved tendon are predictive of increased tendon thickness and tendinopathy changes on US.[135]

- Proprioception on joint repositioning tasks can be altered in clients with GH OA.[153]

VI. Special Tests

- Hawkins-Kennedy test: has good ability to help **rule out** (SN 80, −LR 0.35) but not rule in shoulder impingement.[55]
- The absence of the shrug sign during active elevation has ideal ability to help **rule out** (SN 91, −LR 0.17) glenohumeral arthritis.[114]

VII. Palpation

- (−) tenderness to palpation of the AC joint helps **rule out** (SN 96, −LR 0.40) AC joint pathology.[32]
- (−) tenderness of the supraspinatus helps **rule out** (SN 92) subacromial impingement.[137]
- (−) tenderness of the biceps tendon helps **rule out** (SN 85) subacromial impingement.[137]

VIII. Physical Performance Measures

- Scapular muscular endurance test.
- An older client may require PPMs to assess for falls risk.

POTENTIAL TREATMENT-BASED CLASSIFICATIONS

- Mobility or exercise and conditioning may be used. Pain control is possible if client has highly irritable symptoms.

Adhesive Capsulitis

ICD-9: 726.0 (adhesive capsulitis of shoulder)

ICD-10: M75.0 (adhesive capsulitis of shoulder)

Adhesive capsulitis, generically referred to as *frozen shoulder*, is a disorder of the shoulder joint capsule characterized by multiplanar restriction of ROM in the glenohumeral joint. It is marked by the presence of multiregional synovitis, creating limited motion or stiffness and pain in the joint. Primary adhesive capsulitis is generally believed to be of unknown cause. Secondary adhesive capsulitis is a result of another shoulder condition leading to limited use, and therefore limited motion and increased pain, of the shoulder. There are three or four stages of adhesive capsulitis. The three commonly accepted stages include freezing, frozen, and thawing.

I. Client Interview

Subjective History

- Suggested risk factors for adhesive capsulitis include clients with diabetes mellitus, thyroid disease, those between 40 and 65 years of age, women, and those with previous episode of adhesive capsulitis in the contralateral arm.[17]
- Activity limitations:[17]
  - Pain during sleep is common.
  - Pain and difficulty occur with grooming and dressing activities.
  - Pain with reaching activities occurs, such as behind the back, to shoulder level, and overhead.

Outcome Measures

- The clinician can use the DASH, ASES, or SPADI.[17]

Diagnostic Imaging

- Adhesive capsulitis is primarily diagnosed by history and physical examination; imaging is most likely useful for ruling out other or underlying pathology.[17]

II. Observation

- Commonly the client will demonstrate decreased arm swing with gait, pain posturing and compensated motion with reaching tasks, and unwillingness to move arm, dependent on their level of irritability.[17, 135, 137]

III. Triage and Screening

- All nonmusculoskeletal causes, as well as related joints, should be ruled out.
- The bony apprehension test demonstrates good diagnostic accuracy to help both **rule out** (SN 94, −LR 0.07) and **rule in** (SP 84, +LR 5.9) shoulder instability due to a bony lesion.[48]
- The olecranon-manubrium test demonstrates strong diagnostic accu-

racy to help both **rule out** (SN 84, −LR 0.3) and **rule in** (SP 99, +LR 84) anterior shoulder dislocations, clavicle fractures, and humerus fractures.[46]

IV. Motion Tests

- Loss of ROM in multiple planes, especially external rotation with the arm at client's side and in varying degrees of abduction, is common.[17]

- The capsular pattern proposed by Cyriax is inconsistent in clients with adhesive capsulitis and is limited in identifying capsular dysfunction.[17]

- Glenohumeral joint accessory motion is restricted.[17]

V. Muscle Performance Testing

- Increased pain and weakness with muscle testing of the involved tendon are predictive of increased tendon thickness and tendinopathy changes on US.[135]

VI. Special Tests

- Coracoid pain test: SN (96) and SP (89) are strong for helping to rule out and rule in (respectively) adhesive capsulitis, but QUADAS is only 7.[115]

- The absence of the shoulder shrug sign has ideal ability to help **rule out** (SN 90, −LR 0.1) adhesive capsulitis.[114]

VII. Palpation

- Increased tenderness to palpation of the involved tendon is predictive of increased tendon thickness and tendinopathy changes on US.[135]

- (−) tenderness to palpation of the AC joint helps **rule out** (SN 96, −LR 0.40) AC joint pathology.[32]

- (−) tenderness of the supraspinatus helps **rule out** (SN 92) subacromial impingement.[137]

- (−) tenderness of the biceps tendon helps **rule out** (SN 85) subacromial impingement.[137]

- Tenderness of the coracoid helps **rule out** (SN 96) and **rule in** (SP 89) adhesive capsulitis,[115] although the clinician should consider that 57% of clients with adhesive capsulitis also had acromioclavicular joint pain on examination due to believed compensatory movement at this joint.[154]

VIII. Physical Performance Measures

- No specific PPMs have been correlated to clients with AC. Clinicians are recommended to use client-reported activities as measures of function. For example, clinicians could have clients quantify reaching tasks (behind the back, across the body), self-care, or pain during sleep.[17]

Differential Diagnosis of AC Joint Pathology and Labral Pathology

- Both issues may result from traumatic injuries including blunt trauma to the shoulder or a fall on the outstretched hand.

- Both may cause anterior and superior shoulder pain.

- A labral tear may cause mechanical popping or clicking with glenohumeral movement.

- An AC joint disruption may cause elevation of the distal clavicle.

- A labral tear may have concurrent subjective and objective signs of glenohumeral instability, which may include a positive apprehension test.

- AC joint pathology will likely be tender to palpation immediately over the AC joint.

- A labral tear may have a positive biceps load I or biceps load II test.

- AC joint pathology may have at least two positive findings on the following cluster of tests: cross-body adduction, AC resisted extension, and active compression.

POTENTIAL TREATMENT-BASED CLASSIFICATIONS

- Mobility and pain control if client is highly irritable (freezing stage) may be used. Clinician can progress toward exercise and conditioning as ROM is restored.

AC Joint Pathology

ICD-9: 840.0 (acromioclavicular [joint or ligament] sprain)

ICD-10: S43.5 (sprain of acromioclavicular joint)

AC joint dysfunction encompasses painful disorders of the AC joint associated with traumatic sprains and dislocations. Clients could theoretically have osteoarthritic changes leading to pain at the AC joint. Additionally, AC joint dysfunction and motion abnormalities may be associated with SAIS.[7]

I. Client Interview

Subjective History

- Clients typically complain of pain on the top of the shoulder near the AC joint. The distribution of pain with AC pathologic lesions can be into the trapezius or anterior shoulder.[18]
- Clients may report history of direct trauma to the AC joint or repetitive activity that overloads the AC joint (e.g., push-ups).[18]

Outcome Measures

- The clinician can use the ASES, DASH, or SPADI.[21]

Diagnostic Imaging

- MRI is better to help **rule out** (SN 85) AC joint arthropathy, while radiographs are better to help **rule in** (SP 90) AC joint arthropathy.[32]
- US demonstrates overall good diagnostic accuracy for calcifying tendinitis and subacromial bursitis.[25]
- Radiographs may have findings of AC joint osteoarthritis that do not correlate with AC joint or subacromial pain.[155]

II. Observation

- Varying degrees of superior or posterior displacement of the distal clavicle may be observed.[156]

- Swelling or deformity of the AC joint may be noted.[18]

III. Triage and Screening

- All nonmusculoskeletal causes, as well as causes from related joints, should be ruled out.
- The bony apprehension test demonstrates good diagnostic accuracy to help both **rule out** (SN 94, −LR 0.07) and **rule in** (SP 84, +LR 5.9) shoulder instability due to a bony lesion.[48]
- The olecranon-manubrium test demonstrates strong diagnostic accuracy to help both **rule out** (SN 84, −LR 0.3) and **rule in** (SP 99, +LR 84) anterior shoulder dislocations, clavicle fractures, and humerus fractures.[46]

IV. Motion Tests

- Clients with painful shoulder elevation may lack posterior clavicular rotation and upward rotation of the scapula.[7]
- Scapular dyskinesis has been purported to be a common phenomenon in AC joint disruption,[157] though no one test for scapular dyskinesis is effective in ruling in or out AC joint dysfunction.[19]

V. Muscle Performance Testing

- Increased pain and weakness with muscle testing of the involved tendon are predictive of increased tendon thickness and tendinopathy changes on US.[135]

VI. Special Tests

- AC joint palpation: A (−) test helps **rule out** (SN 96, −LR 0.40) AC joint pathology in one well-designed study.[32]
- Paxinos sign,[32] cross-body adduction test,[18] and active compression test[113] had less than good ability to help rule out or rule in AC joint pathology.
- Clustering of multiple tests has good ability to help **rule out** (SN 81, −LR 0.21) AC joint pathology when two or more tests (cross-body adduction, AC resisted extension, and active compression) were (−).[18]
- Clustering of the same group of tests also has good ability to help **rule in** AC

joint pathology when two or more of these tests (SP 89, +LR 7.4) were (+). Having all three of these tests (+) has ideal ability to help **rule in** (SP 97, +LR 8.3) AC joint pathology.[18]

VII. Palpation

- See description of AC joint palpation in Special Tests.
- Increased tenderness to palpation of the involved tendon is predictive of increased tendon thickness and tendinopathy changes on US.[135]
- (−) tenderness to palpation of the AC joint helps **rule out** (SN 96, −LR 0.40) AC joint pathology.[32]
- (−) tenderness of the supraspinatus helps **rule out** (SN 92) subacromial impingement.[137]
- (−) tenderness of the biceps tendon helps **rule out** (SN 85) subacromial impingement.[137]

VIII. Physical Performance Measures

- Push-up test.
- Sport-, work-, or activity-specific tests: For example, power tests such as the backward overhead medicine ball throw may be appropriate for clients who play sports requiring upper extremity power, whereas the FIT-HaNSA may be appropriate for a client whose occupation could require repetitive reaching and lifting movements.

POTENTIAL TREATMENT-BASED CLASSIFICATIONS

- Immobility and pain control may be used if injury is related to acute trauma.
- Mobility and exercise and conditioning may be used if no acute pain is present or if the client is not pain dominant.

Scapular Dyskinesis

ICD-9: 719.41 (pain in joint, shoulder region)

ICD-10: M25.519 (pain in unspecified shoulder)

Altered scapular motion and position have been termed *scapular dyskinesis*, indicating an alteration of normal scapular kinematics. Dyskinesis has been hypothesized to relate to changes in glenohumeral and acromioclavicular dysfunction. Multiple factors have been suggested to cause dyskinesis, including (but likely not limited to) thoracic kyphosis, clavicle fracture, acromioclavicular joint dysfunction, glenohumeral joint internal derangement, cervical radiculopathy, long thoracic or spinal accessory nerve palsy, soft-tissue tightness, and scapular muscle dysfunction.

I. Client Interview

Subjective History

- Subjective history related to scapular dyskinesis is not well defined because the dyskinesis itself has been found in both symptomatic and asymptomatic people.[19] Scapular dyskinesis is a clinical manifestation that may be present in other shoulder dysfunction, such as AC joint dislocation and subacromial impingement syndrome. For more on subjective history, refer to previously mentioned sections related to these pathologies.

Outcome Measures

- No outcome measures are specific to scapular dyskinesis, but those related to SAIS and AC joint dislocation may be appropriate.

Diagnostic Imaging

- No imaging modalities are used for diagnosing scapular dyskinesis.

II. Observation

- The client's scapula may be observed in upright sitting or standing for static position or may be palpated during active shoulder girdle movements in these positions. However, asymmetry in scapular position, statically and dynamically, may be found in both symptomatic and asymptomatic clients. This asymmetry may suggest the need to further evaluate scapular muscle strength, but it neither independently diagnoses nor rules out shoulder dysfunction or pain.[19]

III. Triage and Screening

- All nonmusculoskeletal causes, as well as causes from related joints, should be ruled out.

- The bony apprehension test demonstrates good diagnostic accuracy to help both **rule out** (SN 94, −LR 0.07) and **rule in** (SP 84, +LR 5.9) shoulder instability due to a bony lesion.[48]
- The olecranon-manubrium test demonstrates strong diagnostic accuracy to help both **rule out** (SN 84, −LR 0.3) and **rule in** (SP 99, +LR 84) anterior shoulder dislocations, clavicle fractures, and humerus fractures.[46]

IV. Motion Tests

- Scapular kinematic abnormalities have been suggested in clients with shoulder pain.[7, 149]

V. Muscle Performance Testing

- Increased pain and weakness with muscle testing of the involved tendon are predictive of increased tendon thickness and tendinopathy changes on US.[135]

VI. Special Tests

- No examination test of the scapula was found to be useful in differentially diagnosing pathologies of the shoulder. Similarly, no special test for scapular dyskinesis has been shown to be effective in identifying symptomatic versus asymptomatic shoulders.[19]
- When the client presents with shoulder impingement symptoms, the scapular repositioning test and scapular assistance test are recommended for relating the client's symptoms to the position or movement of the scapula.[158]

VII. Palpation

- Increased tenderness to palpation of the involved tendon is predictive of increased tendon thickness and tendinopathy changes on US.[135]
- (−) tenderness of the supraspinatus helps **rule out** (SN 92) subacromial impingement.[137]
- (−) tenderness of the biceps tendon helps **rule out** (SN 85) subacromial impingement.[137]

VIII. Physical Performance Measures

- Scapular muscular endurance test
- Push-up test
- CKCUEST

POTENTIAL TREATMENT-BASED CLASSIFICATIONS

- Pain control can be used if the client is reporting high, constant levels of pain. Exercise and conditioning are highly likely because scapular dyskinesis is thought to be related to inefficient scapular stabilizer strength or coordination.

Biceps Tendinopathy

ICD-9: 840.8 (sprains and strains of other specified sites of shoulder and upper arm)

ICD-10: S46.119A (strain of muscle, fascia, and tendon of long head of biceps, unspecified arm, initial encounter)

Biceps tendinopathy can encompass tendinosis, subacromial impingement, or instability of the long head of the biceps in the bicipital groove.[13, 159] Given its attachment to the labrum, the biceps has also been associated with labral pathology, though clinical exams that stress the long head of the biceps are not diagnostic of labral tears.[112]

I. Client Interview

Subjective History

- Clients may have complaints of anterior shoulder pain or pain with reaching or lifting, similar to SAIS.[13]
- Clients may have chronic, degenerative tendon pathology versus post-traumatic pathology leading to instability of the long head in the bicipital groove.[13]
- The clinician should query the client for potential overuse by analyzing recreational and work activities.[159]

Outcome Measures

- The clinician can use the ASES, SPADI, or DASH.[21]

Diagnostic Imaging

- MR arthrogram provides the ability to help **rule in** (97-98) or **rule out** (SN 82-89) lesions of the long head of the biceps pulley.[13]
- Diagnostic US may have a role in diagnosing biceps tendon pathology.[159]

II. Observation

- FHRSP is associated with decreased subacromial space.[42]
- Scapular dyskinesis has been proposed as a dysfunction in clients with impingement and other shoulder disorders. However, dyskinesis is not associated with any singular diagnosis, including impingement.[19]

III. Triage and Screening

- All nonmusculoskeletal causes, as well as causes from related joints, should be ruled out.
- The bony apprehension test demonstrates good diagnostic accuracy to help both **rule out** (SN 94, −LR 0.07) and **rule in** (SP 84, +LR 5.9) shoulder instability due to a bony lesion.[48]
- The olecranon-manubrium test demonstrates strong diagnostic accuracy to help both **rule out** (SN 84, −LR 0.3) and **rule in** (SP 99, +LR 84) anterior shoulder dislocations, clavicle fractures, and humerus fractures.[46]

IV. Motion Tests

- Shoulder flexion and the palm-up position of the arm are components of the Speed's test and are thought to be associated with activity in the long head of the biceps.[55, 76]

V. Muscle Performance Testing

- Increased pain and weakness with muscle testing of the involved tendon are predictive of increased tendon thickness and tendinopathy changes on US.[135]

- Both Yergason's and Speed's tests are resisted tests that engage the biceps, and they have been theorized to be useful in diagnosing this pathology. However, the statistics at this point in time have not proven either to be of strong diagnostic utility.[55, 111]

VI. Special Tests

- The biceps tendon palpation,[55, 110] upper cut test,[111] and Speed's test[110, 112] have less than good ability to rule in or out biceps tendinopathy.
- Combining Speed's test with palpation of the biceps offers limited ability to rule out or in biceps tendon pathology.[55]

VII. Palpation

- Increased tenderness to palpation of the involved tendon is predictive of increased tendon thickness and tendinopathy changes on US.[135]
- (−) tenderness of the supraspinatus helps **rule out** (SN 92) subacromial impingement.[137]
- (−) tenderness of the biceps tendon helps **rule out** (SN 85) subacromial impingement.[137]
- Palpation of the biceps tendon can neither rule in nor rule out bicep tendon tears.[55, 110]

VIII. Physical Performance Measures

- No PPMs have been correlated specifically with biceps tendinopathy, but the pull-up test and flexed arm hang most directly challenge the elbow and shoulder flexors.[127]

POTENTIAL TREATMENT-BASED CLASSIFICATIONS

- Exercise and conditioning, mobility (if used as part of a concurrent primary SAIS), and pain control (if client is highly irritable) may be appropriate.

CONCLUSION

The shoulder girdle complex is a mobile structure that requires interaction of multiple joints and coordination of various muscle groups to achieve dynamic stability and allow the arm to move into functional positions. Clinical examination of the dysfunctional shoulder requires the clinician to take an effective history, to attempt to screen for serious medical pathology, and to examine the quality of motion and strength of the shoulder complex.

The clinician has an extensive amount of clinical exam tests that have been described for the shoulder girdle. This chapter indicates which of those exam tests have optimal sensitivity and specificity to offer clinicians the most evidence-based tests to incorporate into their examinations. The clinician should note that performing a fundamental sequential exam as described in all chapters in this text ends up replicating many of the better special tests for the shoulder girdle. For example, assessing strength frequently involves manual resistance in external rotation that is similar to the infraspinatus test. Similarly, basic PROM examination may replicate Neer's Anterior Apprehension test and the supine impingement test. These examples highlight the importance and utility of the fundamental parts of the clinical examination. As such, the clinician need not perform an examination that is overly reliant on clinical special tests. Additionally, the clinician does not need to use all of the clinical special tests described, even if multiple tests are strong from an evidence-based standpoint, because the client's history and the early components of the exam should indicate which tests are a priority in a given case.

22

ELBOW AND FOREARM

Dawn Driesner Kennedy, PT, DPT, OCS, COMT, FAAOMPT
Michael P. Reiman, PT, DPT, OCS, SCS, ATC, FAAOMPT, CSCS

Focused client history, clinical examination findings, and diagnostic imaging are important components in differential diagnosis of the elbow joint. Occupational and repetitive injuries are responsible for the majority of symptoms at the elbow joint, and they account for a variety of presentations.[1, 2] Typically the client is limited with activities of daily living (ADLs), lifestyle, sports, or work activities due to the chronic nature of dysfunction and symptoms in the elbow. The cervical spine as a potential pain generator for symptoms in this area should be ruled out to ensure symptoms are not the result of a more proximal origin. As with other body regions, limited and sometimes conflicting information is available for diagnostic values for client history, clinical examination results, and diagnostic imaging to confirm elbow and forearm pathologies. Lack of a golden (reference) diagnostic standard creates further difficulty in diagnosing elbow symptoms.[3]

CLINICALLY APPLIED ANATOMY

The elbow consists of three joints: The humerus (figure 22.1), radius, and ulna (figure 22.2) articulate with one another. Due to the more distal extension of the trochlea as compared to the capitulum, in full extension, the elbow has a valgus posture position. The angle between the humerus and radius and ulna is called the carrying angle (figure 22.3). A normal carrying angle is approximately 10° to 17°. This angle tends to keep objects away from the body. This is necessary to keep an object being carried in that arm from hitting the person's side; thus a woman's carrying angle is typically larger than a man's angle.[4, 5]

Three primary joint articulations exist at the elbow: the humeroulnar, humeroradial, and

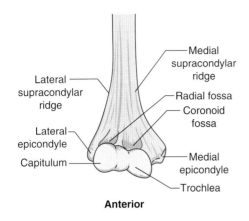

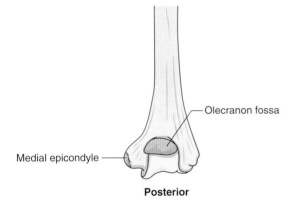

Figure 22.1 Anterior and posterior bony landmarks of the humerus.

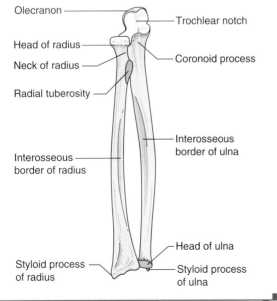

Figure 22.2 Bony anatomy of the forearm.

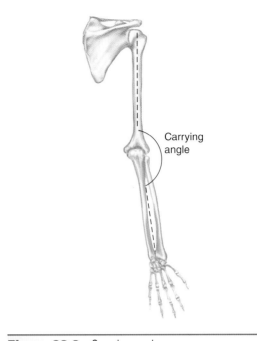

Figure 22.3 Carrying angle.

proximal radioulnar joints. (The distal radioulnar joint is an additional joint in the forearm connecting the radius and ulna, but it has more of an influence on wrist motions.) A synovial capsule surrounds the three joints and provides restraint to distraction forces in extension. Valgus and varus stresses at the elbow are primarily stabilized by the bony congruency, with little contribution from the capsule to resist these forces. At 90° of flexion, there is maximum instability of the bony alignment, so passive and active stabilizers are strongest near this range to assist in protection of the elbow.[6]

The primary motions of the elbow and forearm are flexion and extension, occurring at the humeroulnar and humeroradial joints, and pronation and supination, occurring at the humeroradial and proximal and distal radioulnar joints. The interosseous membrane (figure 22.4), along with the two radioulnar joints, connects the radius and ulna, allowing them to move on each other. The interosseous membrane is a thickened membranous tissue connecting the radius and ulna between the elbow and wrist. The membrane also transmits forces between the radius and ulna, as well as provides longitudinal stability of the forearm.[6]

The humeroulnar joint is classified as a diarthrodial modified hinge joint. It is formed by the

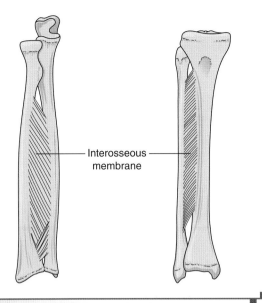

Figure 22.4 Interosseous membrane.

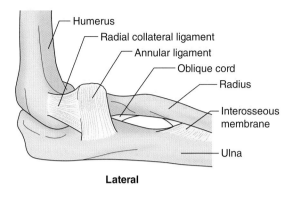

Lateral

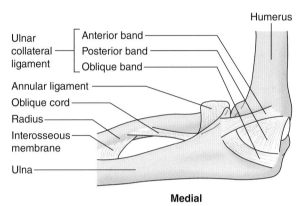

Medial

Figure 22.5 Lateral and medial ligaments of the elbow.

concave trochlear notch on the ulna moving on the convex trochlea of the humerus. The unique orientation of this joint, as well as the significant ligamentous support (figure 22.5), provides stabilization to the elbow. The ulnar collateral ligament (UCL), also referred to as the medial collateral ligament (MCL), has multiple bands and is the ligament of concern in baseball pitchers. In severe cases, instability of this ligament requires surgical intervention (Tommy John surgery). The elbow is more susceptible to valgus stress and torque, and it relies on the stronger UCL, especially the anterior band, to stabilize the elbow joint (compared to the weaker radial collateral ligament, RCL, or lateral collateral ligament, LCL). Contracture or tightness of the anterior musculature as a result of immobilization or neurological conditions can significantly reduce extension of the elbow, which can be challenging to restore.[6-8]

Another hinge joint in the elbow is the humeroradial joint, which allows the concave radial head to spin and glide on the convex capitulum. Pronation and supination are the primary motions that occur at the humeroradial joint, with contributions from the proximal and distal radioulnar joints (figure 22.6). During pronation, the radial head moves lateral and anteriorly as it spins at the humeroradial joint, with slight ulnar internal rotation. Conversely, the radial head moves

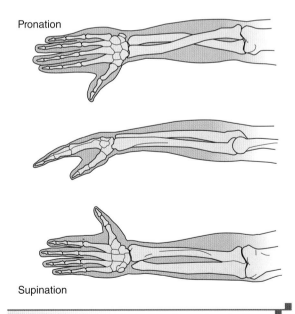

Figure 22.6 Open-chain pronation and supination.

medially and posteriorly during supination, with slight ulnar external rotation. A fulcrum is created at the biceps tuberosity on the radius that allows the radius to rotate over the ulna at the proximal radioulnar joint. The majority of supination and pronation motion occurs at the elbow joint, with more movement in the anterior–posterior direction compared to medial–lateral; however, the distal radioulnar joint accounts for about 17° of motion. The annular ligament, which surrounds the head of the radius, provides a little lateral stability but allows the rotation of the radial head. With disruption of the annular ligament, greater motion occurs in the medial and lateral direction with pronation and supination.[9] In closed kinetic chain movements, more supination and pronation occurs as a result of the ulna moving on a fixed radius. The humeroradial joint also allows the radial head to glide on the capitulum during flexion and extension.[6]

The medial and lateral epicondyles are the common origins for the forearm flexor and extensor muscles, respectively. It is these muscle groups and origin locations that are involved in medial and lateral epicondylalgia, and many have dual actions as two joint muscles (figure 22.7).

CLIENT INTERVIEW

This interview is typically the first encounter the clinician will have with the client. As previously discussed in chapter 5, this component of the examination can provide the clinician with a significant amount of information relevant to the probability of the client's presenting diagnosis. For purposes of this text, the interview is described relative to each body part or section but generally includes subjective reports by the client, as well as findings from their outcome measures. Additionally included in this section is radiographic imaging. While clinicians should avoid biasing their examination by interpreting findings of radiographic imaging prior to seeing clients (in most cases without concerns for red flags and major medical-related issues), this point in the examination is most likely where clinicians will encounter radiographic imaging. Additionally, in some instances, clinicians must interpret radiographic imaging early in the examination to rule out serious pathology prior to continuing with other components of the examination sequence.

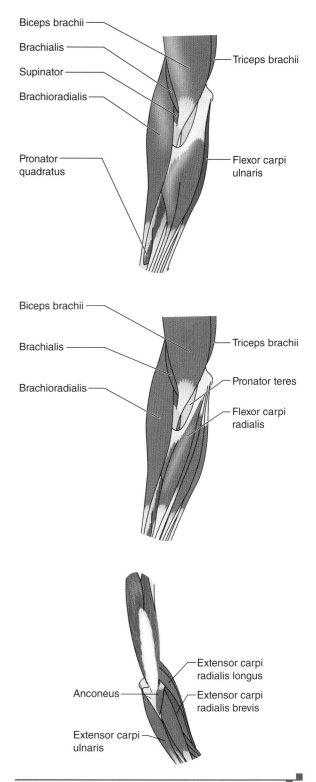

Figure 22.7 Muscles of the elbow and forearm.

Subjective

Detailed history including location and onset of symptoms should be investigated with clients who have elbow pain or dysfunction. First, clinicians should address traumatic versus overuse or repetitive onset of symptoms and determine if the onset was associated with work-related or sport-related activities. Acuity of symptoms is related to different pathologies than those pathologies with longer symptom duration. Typically with acute symptom onset, fractures, muscle strains, and ligamentous sprains are more likely to have occurred. Conversely, chronic issues typically result in soft-tissue dysfunction like tendinopathies and result in more time out of work or sport.[10]

The clinician should ask the client to provide details about typical movement patterns that might have contributed to repetitive stress. Certain injuries are more prevalent to the upper extremity due to the repetitive nature or forced grip required with some jobs. Hairdressers, secretaries or keyboardists, assembly line workers, machine operators, and electricians have a higher propensity for developing upper extremity dysfunction.[11, 12] Regarding work-related chronic conditions at the elbow, the client should be asked to comment on the amount of social support and stress related to work. Elevated perception of stress at work and poor support along with other psychosocial factors can influence pain intensity, prolong time out of work, and negatively affect outcomes.[13-17] The clinician should also ask the client if they have experienced similar symptoms before, which can also negatively affect prognosis.

Specific questions about previous history or current complaints of neck or shoulder pain will assist clinicians in eliminating other possible differential diagnoses of cervical radiculopathy or brachial plexopathy. Nerve compression and soft-tissue injuries of a more distal origin often have symptomology similar to conditions that are more proximally generated. Further questioning regarding neural symptoms including burning, tingling, and numbness in dermatomal distributions can help identify irritation. When these symptoms are present, and the cervical and shoulder regions have been cleared (active motion with overpressure is not reproductive of symptoms), then a peripheral nerve entrapment should be suspected, such as cubital tunnel syndrome.[18]

Further details about quality of pain, location of symptoms, duration of symptoms, and irritability (discussed in chapter 5, Client Interview and Observation) will help localize the source of potential pain generators. Sharp versus dull pain and the presence or absence of burning pain can help differentiate potential structures (muscle, tendon, bone, and nerve) as pain generators. Reports of popping, catching, or grinding should also be investigated to determine if degenerative changes or possible loose body or osteochondritis dissecans might be present.[19] Hand dominance will also provide greater insight to the degree of limitations on lifestyle and work-related activities, in addition to possible contribution to symptoms.

Questions regarding the age of the client and mechanism of injury will assist in diagnosis of more acute pathologies. Open growth plates and increased laxity of ligamentous structures result in different pediatric and adolescent pathologies, such as radial head subluxation (typical age less than 3 years) and supracondylar humerus fractures (most common between 5 and 7 years of age).[20] Adults, especially women, are more likely to sustain work-related repetitive stress resulting in tendinopathies; only in rare occasions do adults have isolated subluxation or dislocation of the radius.[21, 22] Mechanism of injury can also help isolate anatomical structures that are compromised. Repetitive pitching or playing overhead racquet sports puts greater strain on the structures at the medial elbow (higher reports of injury to the ulnar collateral ligament) compared to tennis, which increases lateral elbow demands.[23-25] Regarding elbow fractures, the mechanism can further indicate which structures are compromised; for example, falling forward on an outstretched arm will increase radial head fractures compared to falling backward on a flexed elbow, which puts the olecranon at greater risk. Typically fractures of the elbow occur in a specific pattern relating to the direction of fall.[26]

Addressing symptom progression (that is, whether pain and limitations are getting better or worse, or staying the same) will provide further information regarding expected outcome for the client. If a client's symptoms are improving, there might be a lessening effect on their daily activities, and the client should be further questioned to determine if any changes or interventions were required to reduce the level of irritation or if the

Potential Causes of Various Elbow Pathologies

Trauma or Repeated Microtrauma

Elbow dislocation

Radial subluxation or dislocation with or without fracture

Fracture: proximal humerus, radial, ulnar, or a combination

Avulsion injury of olecranon

Bony contusion (i.e., olecranon)

Soft-tissue contusion

Muscle strain or tear (most likely distal biceps)

Infectious

Osteomyelitis

Septic arthritis

Inflamed lymph nodes

Neurologic

Cervical radiculopathy

Increased neural tension

Shoulder instability

Thoracic outlet syndrome

Ulnar nerve entrapment

Neurovascular injury

Degenerative

Osteoarthritis

Osteolysis

Inflammatory

Rheumatoid arthritis

Juvenile rheumatoid arthritis

Bursitis

Systemic lupus erythematosus

Metabolic

Gout

Metabolic bone disease

Vascular

Osteonecrosis or avascular necrosis (osteochondritis dissecans)

Chondrolysis

Sickle cell disease

Neurovascular injury

Thrombosis

Neoplastic

Ulnar

Radial

Proximal humerus

symptoms spontaneously improved. Compiling information regarding the client's symptoms in a thorough subjective history should provide a working hypothesis for diagnosis that can be confirmed during the physical examination.

Outcome Measures

A variety of outcome measures exist in both research and clinical practice that can be used for the elbow and forearm. Both client and physical reports have been used with a variety of components to assess pain, strength, range of motion (ROM), function, and psychosocial aspects. A few elbow-specific outcomes are available in addition to regional questionnaires. Although some evidence supports several of the scales, it might be advantageous to use a combination, since there are benefits and limitations of using each of them and the combination creates a more comprehensive assessment approach. The Disability of the Arm, Shoulder and Hand (DASH); the Quick Disability of the Arm, Shoulder, and Hand (Quick-DASH); and the Oxford Elbow Score (OES) have demonstrated the greatest efficacy.[27]

The DASH is a client-reported outcome questionnaire that covers a large body region and encompasses a variety of symptoms and limitations that affect the entire upper extremity.[27-30] This outcome measure incorporates multiple dimensions and identifies the more challenging psychosocial factors that contribute to disability; it has been also validated in several countries.[31] Commonly the biggest limitation of the measure is the number of items and the time needed to complete the scale. Particular items of the full DASH were looked at in isolation, which led to the decreasing of items to create the Quick-DASH. The QuickDASH is the shortened version of the DASH; it consists of 11 of the original 30 DASH questions and addresses general function.[32] Similar to the DASH, the QuickDASH demonstrates good validity, reliability, and responsiveness to change in functional level, but it is about one-third the length and is suggested for assessment in clinical practice including initial assessment and routine follow-ups to indicate functional change.[33, 34]

Specific to the elbow, the Research Committee of the American Shoulder and Elbow Surgeons (ASES) developed an elbow assessment form to standardize functional evaluation.[35] By incorporating a self-evaluation of pain and function to be completed by the client and a physician section, components other than physical findings are assessed to address disability. The client uses a pain diagram to mark the location of their pain and a visual analogue scale to quantify its level. Ten activities of daily living are included on the function subscale, measured on a 4-point scale. If the client had previously undergone surgery, a 0- to 10-point satisfaction rating is also reported. Motion, stability, strength, and physical findings are reported by the clinician. Examples of physical findings are tenderness, special tests, scars, and crepitus, but currently this comprehensive assessment lacks adequate measurement qualities.

Studies have demonstrated good reliability, validity, and responsiveness for the original ASES upper extremity scale, and the ASES Elbow Evaluation has recently been validated for the elbow assessment.[36]

The Oxford Elbow Score (OES) is the only client-administered rating score specific to the elbow that has been validated in a high-quality study.[37, 38] Originally designed to be implemented after surgery, the score consists of 12 items that identify symptoms experienced in the last 4 weeks. Elbow function, pain, and psychosocial factors are also evaluated, with a separate domain for each factor. In contrast to the DASH and QuickDASH, the OES is not a disability score, so the best score is 100 and the worst is 0; it can account for specific limitations to the elbow that regional measures do not capture.[39]

An additional measure for the elbow joint and for a specific pathology is the Patient-Rated Tennis Elbow Evaluation (PRTEE). The PRTEE was developed for evaluation of lateral elbow pain (diagnosis-specific scale tendinopathy). This scale is based on the Patient-Rated Elbow Evaluation (PREE), and it combines pain and disability equally, each contributing to half of the total score.[40] The functional component includes specific activities (turning door knobs, lifting a glass, opening a jar) and usual activities (personal, work, housework, and sporting activities) for a total of 10 items. The pain subscale includes 5 items (pain at rest, best, worst, repeated activities, and carrying bag of groceries). Additional research of high quality is needed to determine the validity of the scale.[41]

Other important instruments exist for the elbow including the Visual Analogue Scale of pain and the handheld dynamometer. Since physical findings are not directly related to disability in clients with elbow pain, several of the scales incorporate psychosocial items in an attempt to explain the disparity, reinforcing that function is multifactorial.

Diagnostic Imaging

Depending on the type of pathology, different imaging techniques are recommended for elbow pathology. They have been affected by technological advancements and changes in clinical practice similar to physical examination techniques (table 22.1). Imaging techniques including ultrasound (US), magnetic resonance imaging (MRI), magnetic resonance arthrography (MRA), and radiography (X-rays), have been evaluated for effectiveness in

TABLE 22.1 Diagnostic Accuracy of Imaging Modalities for the Elbow and Forearm

Pathology	Diagnostic test	Reference standard	SN/SP
Fracture	MRI	Arthroscopy	90-100/67-89[43]
			Pooled analysis:
Distal humerus fracture	X-ray + 2DCT		43-80/75-87[44]
	X-ray + 3DCT		65-86/77-92[44]
	3D model		73-93/77-94[44]
Coronoid fracture	X-ray + 2DCT		40-95/67-100[45]
	X-ray + 3DCT	Radiography	80-100/67-100[45]
	3D model		**80-100/83-100**[45]
Pediatric fracture	US		86-98/70-85[46, 47]
Interobserver reliability	X-ray		$\kappa = 0.41$[46]
Ulnar collateral tear	MRI	Arthroscopy	57/100[48]
			79/NR[49]
	CTA		**86/91**[48]
			71/NR[49]
Osteochondritis dissecans	MRI	Arthroscopy	89/44[50]
			83/44[50]
Lateral epicondylalgia			Pooled analysis:
	MRI	Symptoms + clinical exam sign	**92-100/90**[51]
	US		76.5/76.2[52]
Medial epicondylalgia	US	Client symptoms and clinical exam signs	**95/92**[53]
Distal biceps rupture: Overall	MRI	Arthroscopy	**92/100**[54, 55]
Partial			59/100[54]
			92/85[56]
Complete			100/83[54]
Complete vs. normal	US		97/100[55]
Complete vs. partial			95/71[55]
Partial vs. normal			43/NR[55]
Ulnar neuropathy at elbow	US	Clinical exam, electrophysiological studies, and follow-up	
Largest CSA			95/71[57]
Distal largest CSA			**83/85**[57]
CSA at epicondyle			**83/81**[57]
Proximal LAPD			93/42[57]
Enlarged diameter > 1 level		Electrophysiological studies	58/78[58]
Enlarged CSA > 1 level			61/80[58]
Max diameter > 3.2 mm			44/85[58]
Max CSA > 10 mm			50/85[58]
Upper arm SR > 2.3			52/82[58]
Forearm SR > 2.9			42/87[58]
Nerve T2 signal	MRI	Clinical findings and nerve conduction	**83/85**[59]

MRI = magnetic resonance imaging; NR = not reported; CT = computed tomography; CTA = computed tomography arthrogram; 2DCT = two-dimensional CT; 3DCT = three-dimensional CT; US = ultrasound; SN = sensitivity; SP = specificity; CSA = cross-sectional area; LAPD = largest anteroposterior diameter; SR = swelling ratio

The color coding for suggestion of **good** and ideal diagnostic accuracy values reported in this table are without quality scoring (QUADAS), a very important aspect of determination of the clinical utility of such values. Therefore, it is suggested that the reader keep this in mind when interpreting such values.

diagnosis and how cost-effective each technique is for the examination of bony and soft-tissue disorders.[42]

Imaging is another component of the examination that can provide additional information regarding diagnosis and interventions, but it should be utilized in conjunction with client history and clinical examination. Difficulty visualizing landmarks due to complexity of the joints and discrepancy between physical findings and disability further emphasizes the importance of avoiding diagnosis based only on imaging.

Radiographs

Anteroposterior (AP) and lateral views are the standard views in plain film radiographs, with comparison made between sides to determine client-specific anatomy variations. AP views are performed in full extension compared to lateral views that place the elbow in 90° of flexion, each view allowing for different visualization of the joint. The client is positioned in sitting with the elbow and forearm supported on the cassette or table, the elbow fully extended and supinated for the AP view, and the beam perpendicular to the center of the joint. As with all extremity joints, comparison between sides is necessary, especially in pediatric clients and when evaluation can be limited secondary to range-of-motion limitations of the client.[60] Assessment of particular aspects on the AP view includes the following:

- Elbow dislocations and fractures are seen on AP and lateral views.
- Determine joint space and presence of osteoarthritis or osteophytes.
- If negative: Use conservative care and repeat X-rays in 7 to 10 days.

Lateral radiograph of the elbow is performed with the client in a sitting position with arm and forearm resting on table or cassette, elbow flexed at 90°, forearm in neutral, and thumb up.[60] The X-ray beam is at a 7° angulation distal to the center of the joint and allows for assessment of the following:

- Anterior humeral line; also listed as anterior humeral line: The line is parallel to anterior cortex of humerus at the intersection of distal, middle third of capitellum, and disruption can indicate supracondylar fractures.
- Radiocapitellar line; also listed as radiocapitellar line: The axis of the radial head and

neck is extended as the radiocapitellar line at the intersection of the midcapitellum (figure 22.8).[60]

- Demonstrated displacement of anterior or posterior fat pad, indicating fracture.
- Preferred for capitellum, olecranon, and radial fractures.
- Elbow dislocations and fractures are seen on AP and lateral views.
- Determine joint space and presence of osteoarthritis or osteophytes.
- If negative: Use conservative care and repeat X-rays in 7 to 10 days.
- Sail sign: The sail sign is a triangular displacement of the anterior fat pad. It is indicative of intracapsular fracture but is not always present. Not as common as the sail sign on radiographs is a posterior fat pad sign; similar to the sail sign, its presence should lead to further fracture work-up (figure 22.9).[60] Oblique views can provide additional information when a fat pad sign is present but AP and lateral images are negative for fracture.

Suspicion of fracture to deep intra-articular structures, especially the radial head, coronoid process, and capitellum, are better visualized on a variation of the lateral view, a radial head-capitellar

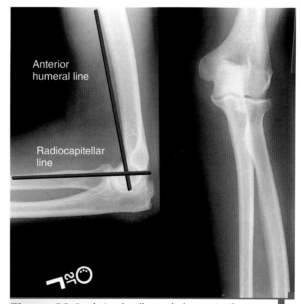

Figure 22.8 Lateral radiograph demonstrating anterior humeral and radiocapitellar lines.

© MedPix

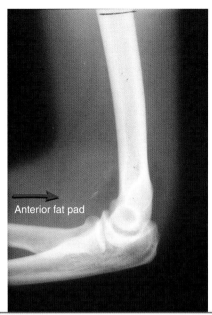

Figure 22.9 Anterior and posterior fat pad sign and secondary subtle radial head fracture.

© MedPix

view (figure 22.10). The client's forearm is positioned on the ulnar side (thumb up) with 90° of elbow flexion identical to the lateral view with a beam at 45° angle cephalad at radial head.

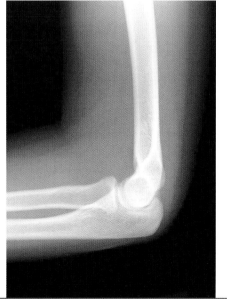

Figure 22.10 Radial head (radiocapitellar) view of normal elbow.

© MedPix

Plain radiographs have a number of limitations, including abilities of the radiology technician, client's willingness to move, and range-of-motion limitations due to injuries. Although no significant difference is present in radiographic evidence for clients with normal elbows or those with osteoarthritis, a classification system developed by Rettig and colleagues was successful at predicting postoperative outcomes.[61]

Magnetic Resonance Imaging and Magnetic Resonance Arthrography

Both MRI and MRA can be used in assessment of elbow pathology. Used clinically in the subacute setting, MRI has demonstrated benefit with osseous tissue, ligamentous tears, tendinopathies, and neurovascular conditions. Greater reliability in detecting bone injuries is found in plain MRI compared to CT, but MRA is superior for intra-articular fragments. Additionally, plain MRI can contribute to evaluation of epicondylopathy to rule out other tendon and ligamentous conditions, although typically imaging is not indicated.[42]

MRA can be used to determine complete versus partial tears of the ulnar collateral ligament, but evidence is lacking regarding sensitivity (SN) and specificity (SP) because most participants in studies are not clients with a known condition. MRI (along with US) can be used to evaluate biceps tendon tears or bursitis and nerve entrapment, but current research is limited without the ability to determine diagnostic accuracy values due to lack of a gold standard in evaluation.[42] However, MRA is being used more frequently to assess acute vascular injuries.

For ulnar neuropathy of the elbow, MRA can also be used to rule in and out the presence of the condition. A nerve T2 signal demonstrated good SN and SP (83% and 85%, respectively) for the diagnosis of neuropathy. Although the test statistics are positive, there is limited research to support the use of the costly MRA compared to US, which has also demonstrated good utility in the diagnosis of ulnar neuropathy with lower cost to the client. With higher SP, MRA could be used as a follow-up tool after ultrasound.[57, 59]

Computed Tomography

In both acute and subacute settings, computed tomography (CT) is used to identify osseous abnormalities, including fractures and location of loose bodies, although CT is typically not the first type of imaging performed.[44] Disruptions of the intra-articular cartilage of the elbow and osteochondral lesions can be identified with greater accuracy on CT compared to MRI.[42] Caution should be used in interpretation of CT findings in the elbow joint due to limitation of diagnostic accuracy values and studies comparing MRI, CT, and US. Most research is limited by the lack of a gold standard; therefore, CT shows greatest utility when applied after other initial screening techniques (active range of motion [AROM] or US).[44, 45, 47]

Ultrasound

High-frequency diagnostic ultrasound (US) of the hand, wrist, and elbow has significant potential to improve the quality of diagnosis and care provided by neuromuscular and musculoskeletal specialists. In clients with subjective reports of weakness, pain, and numbness of the hand, wrist, or elbow, diagnostic ultrasound can be an adjunct to electrodiagnosis and can help to identify ruptured ligaments and nerve compression. Clinicians should use a small high-frequency (>10 MHz) transducer, an instrument with a blunt-pointed tip to enhance sonopalpation of the elbow, for greater visualization of small anatomical structures and complex bony contours. With the client sitting and their arm resting on an examination table, clinicians should perform a standardized examination, which is suggested to include transverse and longitudinal images posteriorly, medially, laterally, and anteriorly in both flexed and extended positions.[62]

A range of conditions, including tendon and ligament ruptures, lateral epicondylopathy,

---

Critical Clinical Pearls

Ultrasound imaging can be utilized to evaluate common elbow pathologies.

Overuse syndromes are most likely to primarily include the following:

- Lateral epicondylopathy (tendon pathology of the common lateral forearm musculature; muscles performing wrist extension; common terminology is tennis elbow)
- Medial epicondylopathy (tendon pathology of the common medial forearm musculature; muscles performing wrist flexion; common terminology is golfer's elbow)
- Triceps tendon enthesopathy (tendon pathology of the triceps tendon musculature; muscle performing elbow extension)

Traumatic pathologies are most likely to include the following:

- Partial or total tendon rupture (partial or complete disruption in the continuity of the tendon)
- Ligament rupture (complete disruption in the continuity of the ligament)
- Fracture (break in the continuity of the bone)
- Dislocation (abnormal separation in the joint of two or more bones articulating joint surfaces)

Inflammatory disorders are most likely to include the following:

- Bursitis (inflammation of a bursa, a small sac of fluid that cushions and lubricates an area where tissues—including bone, tendon, ligament, muscle, or skin—rub against one another)
- Intra-articular effusion (swelling located within a joint, often causing it to be painful and have limited motion)

Entrapment neuropathies are most likely to include the following:

- Cubital tunnel syndrome (symptoms are a result of compression on the ulnar nerve as it travels on the medial aspect of the elbow in the cubital tunnel, characterized by pain and/or paresthesia and ulnar nerve involvement)
- Radial tunnel syndrome (symptoms are a result of compression on the radial nerve as it travels on the lateral aspect of the elbow, characterized by pain and/or paresthesia and radial nerve involvement)

neuropathies, and osteoarthritis, can be assessed with US evaluation.[63] Advantages of US include greater cost-effectiveness and convenience, less time spent, improved spatial resolution, and increased ability to perform dynamic movements to further stress elbow structures to improve accuracy of diagnosis. Difficulty with maintaining contact with curvy elbow landmarks and decreased ability to examine the deep structures due to bone shadowing are some obstacles with US to determine elbow pathologies.[64]

Only studies with small sample sizes have compared MRI and US for evaluation of epicondylopathy. Regarding SN, US was lower than MRI, but SP was comparable and could be used initially as a more cost-effective test with MRI follow-up for clients with normal US findings.[65] US (along with MRI) can be used to evaluate biceps tendon tears or bursitis and nerve entrapment, but current research is limited for determining diagnostic accuracy values to establish a gold standard in evaluation.[42]

Ultrasound has also been used for evaluation of ulnar neuropathy at the elbow with promising results, although the age, weight, body mass index, and sex of the client and elbow position can influence the clinician's ability to visualize the ulnar nerve.[66] Using cross-sectional area (CSA) measurements and the swelling ratio, studies have shown MRI and US are equally effective in the diagnosis of ulnar neuropathy at the elbow.[57, 58, 67, 68]

Review of Systems

Refer to chapter 6 (Triage and Differential Diagnosis) for details on review of systems relevant to the elbow and forearm.

OBSERVATION

Observation of the client with elbow pain is similar to that of other body regions. It includes general postural assessment (statically and dynamically), gait, transfers, and potential limitations in strength and mobility during activities of daily living. Clinicians should observe the client in sitting from both the anteroposterior and lateral vantage points, noting any asymmetries. Cervical, thoracic, and shoulder positions (i.e., forward head, rounded shoulders, slumped sitting position; see chapter 14) might indicate a more proximal origin of symptoms. Additionally, the attitude of the arm in a resting

position, carrying angle, or guarded position against the body can alert the clinician to the potential for greater structural pathology, to potential fracture or dislocation, and to the severity of symptoms. Presence of scars, swelling, ecchymosis, contractures, cysts, and atrophy are associated with different pathologies and are helpful in determining the locations of possible pain generators.

Dynamic activity for the elbow should also be assessed for the client. During gait, lack of normalized arm swing might indicate upper extremity pathologies, including the elbow, since the client might protect their arm to reduce irritation. Willingness to move during the examination, including transferring to or from a chair, shaking the hand, and writing tasks or completion of client-reported outcome measures, provides more information regarding movement and dysfunction during typical daily tasks, prior to a formal motion assessment. Functional ROM for the elbow during ADLs is 100° of total arc of motion for flexion and extension and 100° total arc of motion for rotation (supination and pronation).[69]

TRIAGE AND SCREENING

Triage and screening is a necessary component of the examination process that should be done prior to continuing with the examination. Ruling out serious pathology (refer to chapter 6, Triage and Differential Diagnosis) and pain generation from other related (or close-proximity) structures helps the clinician more accurately determine the necessity of continuing with the other examination components to identify the actual source of the client's pain. Additionally, implementing strong screening tests (tests of high SN and low –LR) at this point in the examination is suggested for narrowing down the competing diagnoses of the respective body regions (cervical spine, shoulder, and wrist in this case) when this is applicable.

Ruling Out Serious Pathology: Red Flags

The clinician should be cognizant of red flags relevant to other sinister pathology that would warrant immediate referral and stop the remainder of the examination sequence. Subjective history and observation of the client will help screen the client. Cervical spine and shoulder concerns and pathologies should be ruled out for the client with elbow pathology since these areas can refer pain here. Refer to chapters 17 and 21 for review of the relevant red flags for each of these areas.

Some specific red flag concerns for the elbow pathology client could include compartment syndrome and radial head fracture. With compartment syndrome, the clinician should assess for palpable tenderness and increased tension in the involved compartment, increased pain with stretching of that compartment, paresthesia, paresis, and sensory deficits related to that compartment, and the possibility of a diminished pulse relevant to that compartment. Additional symptoms expressed by the client that should prompt the clinician to determine the need for additional intervention or referral include tingling, burning, or numbness, forearm pain and tightness, a history of trauma or surgery, symptoms unchanged by position or movement, neurological diseases, unexplained weight loss,

history of corticosteroid exposure, or alcohol use (risk factors for avascular necrosis).[70, 71]

Of key importance with subjective history of trauma or falls is the need to rule out a fracture. The mechanism for fracture, including a radial head fracture, is likely a fall on an outstretched hand (FOOSH) injury. The client will likely present with elbow joint effusion, upper extremity held in a guarded posture, tenderness over the radial head, and restricted or painful pronation and supination AROM.[72]

Assessment for the potential of fractures in the upper and lower extremities has been utilized in previous studies.[73-75] Locations particular to the elbow that have been examined include the humerus, radius, and ulna, and they are commonly are associated with limitations of active ROM.[73] Several tests and examination findings are described here to rule in or out the presence of a fracture of the elbow region and to establish guidelines indicating which clients require referral for radiography.[76]

TUNING FORK AND STETHOSCOPE TO IDENTIFY FRACTURES

Client Position	Sitting with limb supported on their lap
Clinician Position	Sitting or standing facing the client
Movement	The clinician places a stethoscope on a more proximal aspect of the same bone that is injured or suspected for fracture. After striking the tuning fork against a rubber pad, the clinician places the vibrating tuning fork distal to the site of injury. The uninjured limb should be evaluated first. The clinician should listen for 6 to 8 seconds on each side.
Assessment	A (+) test indicated if sounds was diminished or absent from injured limb as compared to uninjured limb.

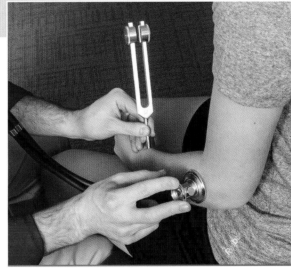

Figure 22.11

Statistics
- SN 83, SP 80, +LR 4.2, −LR 0.21, QUADAS 6, accuracy was 81% in a study of 37 clients (age 7-60 years; 18 females) with various locations and types of upper and lower extremity fractures less than 7 days old, using a criterion reference of radiography.[73]
- Placement over swelling area: SN 83, SP 92, +LR 10.4, −LR 0.2, in the same study

OLECRANON-MANUBRIUM PERCUSSION TEST

See figure 21.12 for a photo of this test.

Client Position	Sitting with upper extremities crossed and the upper extremity to be assessed supported
Clinician Position	Standing directly in front of and facing the client
Movement	The clinician places the stethoscope over the manubrium, and then taps the olecranon of the upper extremity to be assessed. As always, the uninjured or noninvolved limb should be evaluated first.
Assessment	A (+) test is a lack of crisp sound equal to that elicited on the noninvolved upper extremity. A normal response or (−) test is a crisp sound equal to the sound elicited on the noninvolved upper extremity.
Statistics	• **SN 84 (76-95)**, **SP 99 (87-100)**, **+LR 84**, **−LR 0.3**, QUADAS 12, in a prospective study of 96 clients with shoulder trauma, using radiography as a reference standard.[75]
	• This test provided useful clinical utility for anterior shoulder dislocations, clavicle fractures, and humerus fractures, but it was not clinically useful for AC joint abnormalities.
	• A similar type of testing (using stethoscope and tuning fork on opposite sides of suspected fracture or stress fracture) has been implemented for multiple locations; most appropriately related to the shoulder were the clavicle and humerus.[73]

BONY APPREHENSION TEST

See figure 21.13 for a photo of this test.

Client Position	Sitting or standing
Clinician Position	Standing directly behind the client
Movement	The clinician grasps the client's elbow or proximal forearm (with the elbow flexed at 90°) with one hand and uses their other hand to stabilize the shoulder girdle. The clinician abducts and externally rotates the client's arm (maximum of 45°).
Assessment	A (+) test for anterior instability due to a bony lesion is the client demonstrating or stating apprehension during the test.
Statistics	• **SN 94** (not reported, or NR), SP 84 (NR), +LR 5.9, **−LR 0.07**, QUADAS 9, in 29 consecutive clients, using symptomatic shoulder instability and arthroscopy as a reference standard.[77]
	• Bony lesion: **SN 100 (NR)**, **SP 86 (NR)**, **+LR 7.**, **−LR 0.0**, QUADAS 9. Eight cases of bony lesions were positive and three of the soft-tissue lesions. Compared to preoperative radiographs: SN 50, **SP 10**, +LR Inf, −LR 0.5.[77]
	• Higher SN than plain radiographs for osseous lesions.[77]

ELBOW EXTENSION TEST

Client Position	Supine or sitting and elbow fully extended and supported on a pillow
Clinician Position	Monitoring client from the side
Movement	The client attempts to fully extend their elbow.
Assessment	A (+) test is inability to fully extend the elbow, with comparison to unaffected side.

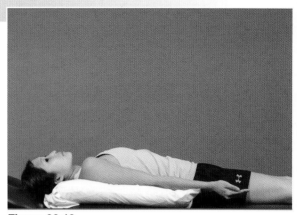

Figure 22.12

Statistics
- **SN 97 (85-100)**, SP 69 (57-80), +LR 3.1, **–LR 0.04**, QUADAS 10, in 114 consecutive clients, age > 14 years old, presenting to an urban emergency department with acute elbow injury within 24 hours (mean age 37 years; 61 women; mean duration of symptoms 3.75 hours after injury), using radiography as a reference standard[78]

- SN 96 (95-98), SP 48 (45-51), +LR 1.9, –LR 0.06, QUADAS 8, in 2,127 consecutive adults (>15 years old) and children (3-15 years) presenting to five emergency departments in England with acute elbow injury within 72 hours (960 adults: mean age 38, 49% female; 780 children: mean age 10 years old, 48% female; mean duration of symptoms NR), using radiography as reference standard[76]

- SN 98 (96-99), SP 48 (44-52), +LR 1.9, –LR 0.06, QUADAS 8, in 958 consecutive adults (>15 years old) presenting to five emergency departments in England with acute elbow injury within 72 hours (mean age 38; 49% female; mean duration of symptoms NR), using radiography as reference standard[76]

- SN 94 (91-97), SP 50 (45-54), +LR 1.9, –LR 0.06, QUADAS 8, in 778 children (3-15 years) presenting to five emergency departments in England with acute elbow injury within 72 hours (mean age 10 years old; 48% female; mean duration of symptoms NR), using radiography as reference standard[76]

- **SN 100 (93-100)**, **SN 100 (94-100)**, **+LR Inf**, **–LR 0**, QUADAS 11, in 115 consecutive clients (≥5 years of age) and subgrouped as adult (≥18 years) and children (<18 years) presenting to four emergency departments with acute elbow injury within 24 hours (mean age 29 years, 43% female; 71 adults: mean age 41 years, 45.5% female; 42 children: mean age 10.5 years, 41.5% female; mean duration of symptoms NR), using radiography as a reference standard[79]

OVERALL AROM

Client Position	Supine or sitting
Clinician Position	NA
Movement	The client attempts to actively flex to at least 90°, extend to full locked position of 0°, and actively pronate and supinate to full 180°.
Assessment	A (+) test is inability to flex to at least 90° or fully extend the elbow, with comparison to the unaffected side.
Statistics	**SN 100 (93-100)**, **SP 97 (88-100)**, **+LR 33**, **–LR 0**, QUADAS 11, in 115 consecutive clients (≥5 years of age) and subgrouped as adult (≥18 years) and children (<18 years) presenting to four emergency departments with acute elbow injury within 24 hours (mean age 29 years, 43% female; 71 adults: mean age 40.5 years, 45.5% female; 42 children: mean age 10.5 years, 40.5% female; mean duration of symptoms NR), using radiography as a reference standard[79]

OVERALL AROM AND TENDERNESS TO PALPATION

Client Position	Supine or sitting
Clinician Position	Standing or sitting to the side of the client's arm to be tested
Movement	The clinician palpates the olecranon, medial and lateral epicondyle, and radial head. The client attempts to actively flex to at least 90°, extend to a full locked position (0°), and actively pronate and supinate to full (180°).
Assessment	A (+) test is positive tenderness in addition to AROM limitations of inability to flex to at least 90° or fully extend the elbow, with comparison to unaffected side.
Statistics	**SN 100 (93-100)**, SP 67 (53-78), +LR 3.03, **–LR 0**, QUADAS 11, in 115 consecutive clients (≥5 years of age) and subgrouped as adults ≥18 years) and children (<18 years) presenting to four emergency departments with acute elbow injury within 24 hours (mean age 29 years, 43% female; 71 adults: mean age 40.5 years, 45.5% female; 42 children: mean age 10.5 years, 40.5% female; mean duration of symptoms NR), using radiography as a reference standard[79]

Ruling Out Pain Generation From Other Related Structures

As with all joints, screening the joints above and below for potential contribution to pain generation should be employed. Ruling out the cervical spine is of particular importance due not only to its close proximity to the shoulder but also to the potential for referral into the shoulder and entire upper extremity.[80] The upper quarter screen is a structured and traditional way to differentiate potential pain generators and consists of dermatomes, myotomes, deep tendon reflexes, and possible upper motor neuron involvement; refer to the upper quarter screen in chapter 7 (Orthopedic Screening and Nervous System Examination). A systematic approach is recommended for ruling out other regions. Refer to chapters 17 (Cervical Spine) and 21 (Shoulder) for greater detail regarding these examination procedures.

Rule Out Cervical Spine

The upper quarter screen will determine cervical spine ROM and the potential for the cervical spine as a pain generator. Additionally, see chapter 17 (Cervical Spine) for complete details on assessment of pain generation due to radiculopathy.

Radiculopathy or Discogenic-Related Pathology

This is ruled out with a combination of ROM and special tests, including Spurling's test and the upper limb neurodynamic test (median nerve bias).

- Spurling's test: **SN 93 (77-99), SP 95 (76-100), +LR 19.6, –LR 0.07**, QUADAS 9[81]
- Median nerve upper limb neurodynamic test: **SN 97 (90-100)**, SP 22 (12-33), +LR 1.3, **–LR 0.12**, QUADAS 10[82]
- Arm squeeze test (described for cervical nerve root compression): SN 95 (85-99), SP 96 (87-99), +LR 24, –LR 0.05, QUADAS 8[83]

Facet Joint Dysfunction

As noted in chapter 17 (Cervical Spine), facet joint dysfunction can be ruled in with reproduction of concordant pain with a posterior-to-anterior spinal joint-play assessment or facet joint block.

Rule Out Shoulder and Wrist Joints

The upper quarter screen will determine shoulder and wrist ROM and the potential for these joints as pain generators to the client's complaints of elbow pain. Full AROM and the application of overpressure for each motion at those joints (if pain-free) will help eliminate those motions and joints as contributors to the client's symptoms. Additionally, as with any joint, clearing AROM with or without overpressure is necessary. AROM of all motions as per the upper quarter screen described in chapter 7 should be implemented. In order to fully clear the cervical spine, full AROM (with overpressure if pain-free) must be present.

Fracture

The clinician can use the olecranon-manubrium and bony apprehension tests as described previously.

Impingement

Hawkins-Kennedy test

- Pooled analysis: SN 74 (57-85), SP 57 (46-67), +LR 1.7, −LR 0.5, in six studies with 1,029 clients[84]
- Pooled analysis: **SN 80 (72-86)**, SP 56 (45-67), +LR 1.84, **−LR 0.35**, in seven studies with 944 clients[85]

Additionally, as with any joint, clearing AROM with or without overpressure is necessary. In order to fully clear the elbow, full AROM (with overpressure if pain-free) must be present. Details in this regard are described in the following section.

MOTION TESTS

Motion assessment is a very important aspect of the examination for the orthopedic client. Motion dysfunction can be used to differentiate contractile versus noncontractile tissue (see chapter 9). Assessment of end-feel, potential capsular patterns, and ROM normative values can give the clinician an appreciation of the potential impairments for the orthopedic client they are assessing (table 22.2). Active ROM, PROM, and joint-play assessments are necessary to determine not only the presence or absence of joint dysfunction but also the precise aspects of the motion that are dysfunctional.

Passive and Active ROMs

Based on the potential pathology, the clinician can expect to find differences when assessing passive and active ROM. For example, clients with primary osteoarthritis will have initial reduction of flexion and extension at ends of motion that will progress as the disease process progresses.[69] Conversely, clients with trauma who are suspected of fracture might display limitations early in the ROM, with significant motion restrictions in one or all directions.[76, 78, 79]

Research has shown that intratester reliability is higher than intertester reliability both for AROM and PROM, indicating that the test–retest of motion should be performed by the same clinician. Higher intertester reliability has been seen with goniometric measurement when compared to the lower extremity.[86, 87] Experienced clinicians have demonstrated accuracy in estimating elbow range of motion with the human eye and were as good as those with a goniometer, intrarater reliability ranging from ICC of 0.9 to 0.97. Interestingly, intertester reliability increased with visual estimate by a highly trained clinician, interrater reliability of 0.96 for extension and 0.93 for flexion. All ROM should be rounded off to the nearest 5°, since more than 5° of motion are needed in order to be considered significant.[88]

TABLE 22.2 Elbow and Forearm Arthrology

Joint	Close-packed position	Resting position	Capsular pattern	ROM norms	End-feel
Humeroulnar	Full extension, forearm supination	70° (to 90°) of flexion, 10° supination	Flexion > extension	0–150°	Flexion: soft (soft-tissue approximation), hard (bony approximation in a thin person), or firm; extension is hard due to bony contact
Humeroradial	Flexed to 90°, 5° supination	Full extension, full supination	Flexion > extension		
Proximal radioulnar	5° supination	70° flexion, 35° supination	Supination = pronation	80–90° in both directions	Firm for both motions
Distal radioulnar	10° supination	5° supination	Supination = pronation		

ELBOW FLEXION

Client Position	Supine with the arm to be assessed lying straight on the table
Clinician Position	Standing directly to the side of the client
Goniometer Alignment	The clinician positions the fulcrum over the lateral epicondyle of the humerus and aligns the proximal arm with the lateral midline of the humerus and the distal arm with the lateral midline of the radius (radial styloid process for reference).
Movement	The clinician stabilizes the humerus to prevent shoulder flexion. The clinician passively moves the client's elbow to end range flexion. A normal end-feel is soft (or hard in the case of a thin person) or firm. This motion can be performed similarly actively by the client (without assistance from the clinician). Active range of motion should be performed prior to PROM to determine the client's willingness to move and so on.
Assessment	Clinician assesses for amount of ROM, end-feel, quality of the movement, client response, potential difference between AROM and PROM, and so on.

ELBOW EXTENSION

Client Position	Supine with arm to be assessed lying straight on table
Clinician Position	Standing directly to the side of the client
Goniometer Alignment	The clinician positions the fulcrum over the lateral epicondyle of humerus and aligns the proximal arm with the lateral midline of the humerus and the distal arm with the lateral midline of the radius (radial styloid process for reference).
Movement	The clinician stabilizes the humerus to prevent shoulder flexion. The clinician passively moves the elbow to end range extension. A normal end-feel is hard. This motion can be performed similarly actively by the client (without assistance from the clinician). Active range of motion should be performed prior to PROM to determine the client's willingness to move and so on.
Assessment	Clinician assesses for amount of ROM, end-feel, quality of the movement, client response, potential difference between AROM and PROM, and so on.

PRONATION

Client Position	Sitting with arm at side
Clinician Position	Standing directly to the side of the client
Goniometer Alignment	The clinician positions the fulcrum laterally and proximally to the ulnar styloid process of wrist and aligns the proximal arm parallel to the anterior midline of the humerus and the distal arm across the dorsal aspect of the forearm (just proximal to the styloid processes of the radius and ulna).
Movement	The clinician flexes the client's elbow to 90° and supports the forearm in a neutral position. The clinician passively moves the client's forearm to end range pronation. A normal end-feel is typically firm (to occasionally hard because of contact between the radius and ulna). This motion can be performed similarly actively by the client (without assistance from the clinician). Active range of motion should be performed prior to PROM to determine the client's willingness to move and so on.
Assessment	Clinician assesses for amount of ROM, end-feel, quality of the movement, client response, potential difference between AROM and PROM, and so on.

SUPINATION

Client Position	Sitting with arm at side
Clinician Position	Standing directly to the side of the client
Goniometer Alignment	The clinician positions the fulcrum medially and proximally to the client's ulnar styloid process, the proximal arm parallel to the anterior midline of the humerus, and the distal arm across the ventral surface of the forearm where the forearm is the most level. The distal arm should be parallel to the radial and ulnar styloid processes.
Movement	The clinician flexes the client's elbow to 90° and supports the forearm in a neutral position. The clinician passively moves the client's forearm to end range supination. A normal end-feel is typically firm (to occasionally hard because of contact between the radius and ulna). This motion can be performed similarly actively by the client (without assistance from the clinician). Active range of motion should be performed prior to PROM to determine the client's willingness to move and so on.
Assessment	Clinician assesses for amount of ROM, end-feel, quality of the movement, client response, potential difference between AROM and PROM, and so on.

Passive Accessories

Passive accessory motion assessment is essential in determination of the potential for joint-play dys-function in the joints being examined. The following section details distinct component assessments of passive joint mobility for the elbow joint.

HUMEROULNAR JOINT DISTRACTION

Client Position	Supine with arms relaxed at side, elbow resting on clinician's shoulder with forearm partially supinated
Clinician Position	Sitting at the client's elbow, facing the client
Stabilization	The rest of the client's body on the table serves as the stabilizing force. The clinician's stabilizing hand (left as shown) purchases the proximal humerus.
Movement and Direction of Force	The clinician's assessing hand (right as shown) purchases the proximal ulna, just distal to the elbow. The clinician uses their assessing hand to distract the ulna distally from the humerus at a 90° angle from the treatment plane, or an angle of 45° less flexion than the position of the ulnar shaft.
Assessment	Assessment is done for joint play/passive accessory motion, client response, and end-feel. Reproduction of concordant pain suggests dysfunction. Impaired joint mobility or end-feel may also suggest dysfunction if concordant pain is also reproduced.

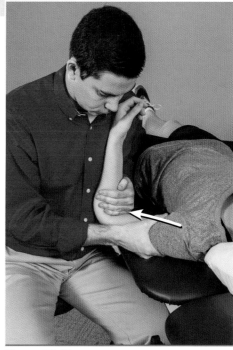

Figure 22.13

Critical Clinical Pearls

When performing humeroulnar joint distraction, keep the following in mind:

- Rule out any disruption to bony integrity.
- Ensure the shoulder joint and scapula are stabilized through your hand on the proximal humerus and the table.
- Watch for muscular guarding of client, which can give false information regarding the joint assessment.

HUMEROULNAR JOINT MEDIAL GLIDE

 Video 22.14 **in the web resource shows a demonstration of this test.**

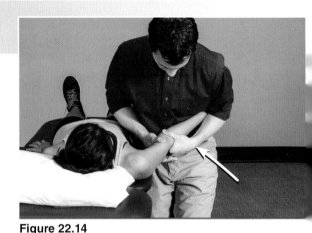

Figure 22.14

Client Position	Supine with arm relaxed at side
Clinician Position	Sitting or standing at the client's side with the client's arm braced between their side and mobilizing arm (left as shown). The clinician maintains the client's arm in a partially supinated position as they use their proximal hand (right as shown) to stabilize the medial distal humerus and their caudal hand (mobilizing hand; left as shown) to purchase the lateral aspect of the client's proximal forearm (radius).
Stabilization	The rest of the client's body on the table serves as a stabilizing force. The clinician's stabilizing hand purchases the distal humerus.
Movement and Direction of Force	The clinician's assessing hand purchases the proximal radius and ulna, just distal to the elbow. The clinician uses their assessing hand to glide the proximal ulna in a medial direction through the radius (assisting with their trunk).
Assessment	Assessment is done for joint play/passive accessory motion, client response, and end-feel. Reproduction of concordant pain suggests dysfunction. Impaired joint mobility or end-feel may also suggest dysfunction if concordant pain is also reproduced.

HUMEROULNAR JOINT LATERAL GLIDE

Client Position	Supine with arm relaxed at side
Clinician Position	Sitting or standing at the client's side with the client's arm braced between their side and mobilizing arm (left as shown). The clinician maintains the client's arm in a partially supinated position, using their cranial hand (right as shown) to stabilize the lateral distal humerus and their caudal hand (mobilizing hand; left as shown) to purchase the medial aspect of the proximal forearm (ulna).
Stabilization	The rest of the client's body on the table serves as a stabilizing force. The clinician's stabilizing hand purchases the distal humerus. They hold the rest of the client's arm between trunk and assessing arm.
Movement and Direction of Force	The clinician's assessing hand purchases the proximal ulna from the medial side, just distal to the elbow. The clinician uses their assessing hand to glide the proximal ulna in a lateral direction (assisting with their trunk).
Assessment	Assessment is done for joint play/passive accessory motion, client response, and end-feel. Reproduction of concordant pain suggests dysfunction. Impaired joint mobility or end-feel may also suggest dysfunction if concordant pain is also reproduced.

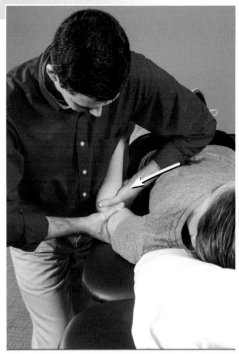

Figure 22.15

HUMERORADIAL JOINT DISTRACTION

Client Position	Supine with arms relaxed at side, forearm partially supinated and elbow slightly flexed
Clinician Position	Sitting or standing (as shown) at the client's elbow
Stabilization	The rest of the client's body on the table serves as a stabilizing force. The clinician's stabilizing hand (left as shown) purchases the distal humerus.
Movement and Direction of Force	The clinician's assessing hand (right) purchases the distal radius. The clinician uses their assessing hand to distract the radius distally from the humerus.
Assessment	Assessment is done for joint play/passive accessory motion, client response, and end-feel. Reproduction of concordant pain suggests dysfunction. Impaired joint mobility or end-feel may also suggest dysfunction if concordant pain is also reproduced.

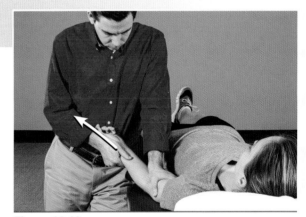

Figure 22.16

HUMERORADIAL JOINT POSTERIOR GLIDE

Client Position	Supine with arm relaxed at side, forearm fully supinated
Clinician Position	Standing at the client's elbow
Stabilization	The rest of the client's body on the table serves as a stabilizing force. The clinician's stabilizing hand (left as shown) purchases the distal humerus.
Movement and Direction of Force	The clinician's assessing hand (right as shown) purchases the proximal radius with the heel of their hand on the anterior surface. The clinician uses their assessing hand to glide the proximal radius in a posterior direction.
Assessment	Assessment is done for joint play/passive accessory motion, client response, and end-feel. Reproduction of concordant pain suggests dysfunction. Impaired joint mobility or end-feel may also suggest dysfunction if concordant pain is also reproduced.

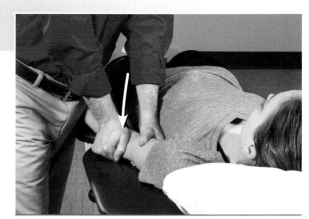

Figure 22.17

HUMERORADIAL JOINT ANTERIOR GLIDE

Client Position	Supine with arm relaxed at side, forearm in neutral with thumb facing up toward ceiling
Clinician Position	Sitting or standing at the client's elbow
Stabilization	The rest of the client's body on the table serves as a stabilizing force. The clinician's stabilizing hand (right as shown) purchases the distal humerus.
Movement and Direction of Force	The clinician's assessing hand (left as shown) purchases the proximal radius, with the heel of their hand on posterior or dorsal surface. The clinician uses their assessing hand to glide the proximal radius in an anterior direction.
Assessment	Assessment is done for joint play/passive accessory motion, client response, and end-feel. Reproduction of concordant pain suggests dysfunction. Impaired joint mobility or end-feel may also suggest dysfunction if concordant pain is also reproduced.

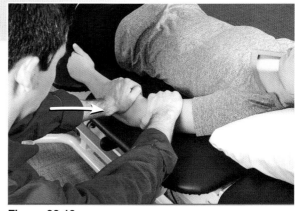

Figure 22.18

PROXIMAL RADIOULNAR JOINT POSTERIOR (DORSAL) GLIDE OF RADIAL HEAD

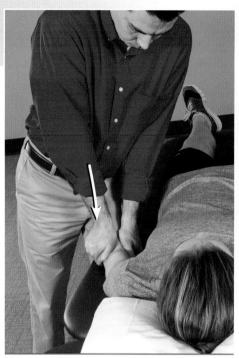

Client Position	Sitting with arm relaxed on table, elbow flexed to 70° and forearm in 35° supination
Clinician Position	Standing at the client's elbow
Stabilization	The rest of the client's body on the table serves as a stabilizing force. The clinician's stabilizing hand (left as shown) purchases the proximal ulna on posterior or dorsal side.
Movement and Direction of Force	The clinician's assessing hand (right as shown) purchases the proximal radius, with the heel of their hand purchasing the radial head on the anterior or volar side. The clinician uses their assessing hand to glide the proximal radius in a posterior or dorsal direction.
Assessment	Assessment is done for joint play/passive accessory motion, client response, and end-feel. Reproduction of concordant pain suggests dysfunction. Impaired joint mobility or end-feel may also suggest dysfunction if concordant pain is also reproduced.

Figure 22.19

PROXIMAL RADIOULNAR JOINT ANTERIOR (VOLAR) GLIDE OF RADIAL HEAD

 Video 22.20 **in the web resource shows a demonstration of this test.**

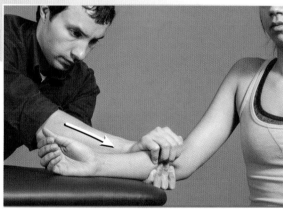

Figure 22.20

Client Position	Sitting with arm relaxed on table; elbow flexed to 70°, forearm in 35° supination
Clinician Position	Standing at the client's elbow
Stabilization	The rest of the client's body on the table serves as a stabilizing force. The clinician's stabilizing hand (left as shown) purchases the proximal ulna on the anterior or volar side.
Movement and Direction of Force	The clinician's assessing hand (right as shown) purchases the proximal radius, with the heel of their hand purchasing the radial head on the posterior or dorsal side. The clinician uses their assessing hand to glide the proximal radius in an anterior or volar direction.
Assessment	Assessment is done for joint play/passive accessory motion, client response, and end-feel. Reproduction of concordant pain suggests dysfunction. Impaired joint mobility or end-feel may also suggest dysfunction if concordant pain is also reproduced.

DISTAL RADIOULNAR JOINT POSTERIOR (DORSAL) GLIDE OF THE RADIUS

Client Position	Sitting with arm relaxed on table; elbow flexed with 10° supination
Clinician Position	Standing at the client's elbow
Stabilization	The rest of the client's body on the table serves as a stabilizing force. The clinician's stabilizing hand (left as shown) purchases the distal ulna on the posterior or dorsal side.
Movement and Direction of Force	The clinician's assessing hand (right as shown) purchases the distal radius, with the heel of their hand purchasing the radial head on the anterior or volar side. The clinician uses their assessing hand to glide the distal radius in a posterior or dorsal direction.
Assessment	Assessment is done for joint play/passive accessory motion, client response, and end-feel. Reproduction of concordant pain suggests dysfunction. Impaired joint mobility or end-feel may also suggest dysfunction if concordant pain is also reproduced.

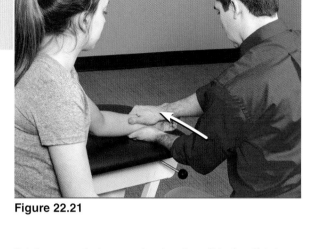

Figure 22.21

DISTAL RADIOULNAR JOINT ANTERIOR (VOLAR) GLIDE OF THE RADIUS

Client Position	Supine or sitting with arm resting on table; elbow flexed, 10° supination
Clinician Position	Standing at the client's elbow
Stabilization	The rest of the client's body on the table serves as a stabilizing force. The clinician's stabilizing hand (right as shown) purchases the distal ulna on the anterior or volar side.
Movement and Direction of Force	The clinician uses their assessing hand (left as shown) to purchase the distal radius, with the heel of their hand purchasing the radial head on the posterior or dorsal side. The clinician uses their assessing hand to glide the distal radius in an anterior or volar direction.
Assessment	Assessment is done for joint play/passive accessory motion, client response, and end-feel. Reproduction of concordant pain suggests dysfunction. Impaired joint mobility or end-feel may also suggest dysfunction if concordant pain is also reproduced.

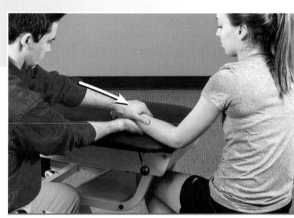

Figure 22.22

Flexibility

Refer to chapter 7 for relevant upper quarter flexibility assessments. As detailed in chapter 8, flexibility is the motion a particular joint is capable of.

Assessment of flexibility can assist the clinician in determining the potential presence of soft-tissue dysfunction. Each individual muscle can be evaluated based on the origin and insertion of the muscle (table 22.3).

TABLE 22.3　Elbow Muscles

Muscle	Origin	Insertion	Action	Innervation
FLEXION MUSCLES				
Biceps brachii (primary)	Long head: supraglenoid tubercle of scapula Short head: coracoid process of scapula	Radial tuberosity, fascia of forearm via aponeurosis	Flexion of elbow, supination at elbow, assists flexion at shoulder	Musculocutaneous nerve (C5, C6)
Brachialis (primary)	Distal half of anterior surface of humerus	Coronoid process and tuberosity of ulna	Flexion of elbow	Musculocutaneous nerve (C5, C6)
Brachioradialis (primary)	Proximal 2/3 of the lateral supracondylar ridge of distal humerus and intermuscular septum	Lateral aspect of distal radius just proximal to styloid process of radius	Flexion of elbow, assists with pronation and supination	Radial nerve (C5, C6)
Pronator teres	Humeral head: medial supracondylar ridge of humerus from the common flexor tendon, intermuscular septum, antebrachial fascia Ulnar head: medial side of the coronoid process of ulna	Midway along the lateral surface of the radius	Pronation, assists with flexion of elbow	Median nerve (C6, C7)
Flexor carpi radialis and ulnaris	Radialis: medial epicondyle of humerus and antebrachial fascia Ulnaris humeral head: medial epicondyle of humerus by common flexor tendon Ulnaris ulnar head: medial margin of olecranon and posterior border of ulna	Radialis: base of 2nd metacarpal bone and sends slip to base of 3rd metacarpal bone Ulnaris: pisiform bone with extensions attaching to hook of hamate, base of 5th metacarpal, and flexor retinaculum	Radialis: flexes hand at wrist, assists wrist abduction and flexion of elbow Ulnaris: flexes and adducts hand, assists flexion of elbow	Radialis: medial nerve (C6, C7) Ulnaris: ulnar nerve (C7, C8)
Extensor carpi radialis longus	Distal lateral supracondylar ridge of humerus	Base of 2nd metacarpal on dorsal aspect	Extends and abducts hand, assists with flexion of elbow	Radial nerve (C6, C7)
EXTENSION MUSCLES				
Triceps brachii (primary)	Long head: infraglenoid tubercle of scapula Medial head: distal 2/3 of medial and posterior humerus Lateral head: upper half of posterior humerus	Posterior surface of olecranon process of ulna	Extension of elbow; long head also assists with shoulder stabilization and adduction	Radial nerve (C6, C7, C8)
Anconeus	Lateral condyle of humerus	Lateral aspect of olecranon process and upper dorsal surface of ulna	Stabilize elbow, assist with extension of the elbow	Radial nerve (C7, C8)

(continued)

Table 22.3 *(continued)*

Muscle	Origin	Insertion	Action	Innervation
PRONATION MUSCLES				
Pronator teres (primary)	Humeral head: medial supracondylar ridge of humerus from the common flexor tendon, intermuscular septum, antebrachial fascia Ulnar head: medial side of the coronoid process of ulna	Midway along the lateral surface of the radius	Pronation, assists with flexion of elbow	Median nerve (C6, C7)
Pronator quadratus	Medial aspect of anterior surface of distal 1/4 of ulna	Distal 1/4 of the lateral border and anterior surface of the shaft of the radius	Pronation at forearm and wrist	Median nerve (C8, T1)
Flexor carpi radialis	Radialis: medial epicondyle of humerus and antebrachial fascia	Radialis: base of 2nd metacarpal bone and sends slip to base of 3rd metacarpal bone	Radialis: flexes hand at wrist, assists wrist abduction and flexion of elbow	Radialis: medial nerve (C6, C7)
SUPINATION MUSCLES				
Supinator	Lateral epicondyle of humerus, radial collateral ligament, annular ligament, supinator fossa, and crest of ulna	Lateral, posterior, and anterior surface of proximal third of radius	Supination	Radial nerve: deep branch (C5, C6, C7)
Biceps brachii (primary)	Long head: supraglenoid tubercle of scapula Short head: coracoid process of scapula	Radial tuberosity, fascia of forearm via aponeurosis	Flexion of elbow, supination at elbow, assists flexion at shoulder	Musculocutaneous nerve (C5, C6)

MUSCLE PERFORMANCE TESTING

Evaluating the integrity of each muscle can also provide additional information about the involvement of active structures around the joint and should be performed after assessment of motion testing.

ELBOW FLEXION

Client Position	Sitting, arms at side

- Forearm in supination to assess biceps
- Forearm in pronation to assess brachialis
- Forearm midway between supination and pronation to assess brachioradialis

Clinician Position	Standing directly in front of the client
Movement and Assessment	The clinician instructs the client to bend their elbow. The clinician provides resistance just proximal to the wrist with one hand and stabilizes the anterior shoulder with the other hand.

- Grade 5: completes motion against maximal resistance
- Grade 4: completes motion against strong resistance
- Grade 3: completes motion without resistance

The position for grades below 3 is as follows: The client sits with the arm abducted 90° and supported by the clinician. The clinician should position the forearm for the respective muscle group.

- Grade 2: completes full ROM
- Grade 1: muscle activity without movement
- Grade 0: no muscle activity

Primary Muscles	Biceps brachii
	Brachialis
	Brachioradialis
Secondary Muscles	Pronator teres
	Flexor carpi radialis and ulnaris
	Extensor carpi radialis longus
Primary Nerves	Musculocutaneous nerve (C5-6; biceps brachii and brachialis)
	Radial nerve (C5-6; brachioradialis)

ELBOW EXTENSION

Client Position	Prone on table, arm in 90° abduction, elbow flexed and forearm hanging vertically off edge of table
Clinician Position	Standing directly to the side of the client
Movement and Assessment	The clinician asks the client to straighten their elbow. The clinician provides resistance just proximal to the wrist with one hand and stabilizes the anterior shoulder with the other hand.

- Grade 5: completes motion against maximal resistance
- Grade 4: completes motion against strong resistance
- Grade 3: completes motion without resistance

The position to assess for grades below 3 is as follows: The client sits with the arm abducted 90° and supported by the clinician.

- Grade 2: completes full ROM in prone gravity minimized position
- Grade 1: muscle activity without movement
- Grade 0: no muscle activity

Primary Muscles	Triceps brachii
Secondary Muscles	Anconeus
Primary Nerve	Radial (C6-8)

FOREARM PRONATION

Client Position	Sitting on table, arm at side with elbow flexed 90° and forearm in supination
Clinician Position	Standing directly to the side of the client
Movement and Assessment	The clinician asks the client to pronate their forearm until the palm faces downward. The clinician provides resistance to the distal forearm or wrist with one hand and supports the client's elbow with the other hand.

- Grade 5: completes motion against maximal resistance
- Grade 4: completes motion against strong resistance
- Grade 3: completes motion without resistance

For the following grades, the client should sit with the shoulder flexed between 45° and 90°, the elbow flexed to 90°, and the forearm in neutral. The clinician supports the client's elbow.

- Grade 2: completes full ROM in position
- Grade 1: muscle activity without movement
- Grade 0: no muscle activity

Primary Muscles	Pronator teres
	Pronator quadratus
Secondary Muscles	Flexor carpi radialis
Primary Nerve	Median (C6-8)

FOREARM SUPINATION

Client Position	Sitting on table, arm at side and elbow in 90° flexion, forearm in pronation
Clinician Position	Standing directly to the side of the client
Movement and Assessment	The clinician asks the client to supinate their forearm until the palm faces the ceiling. The clinician provides resistance to the client's distal forearm or wrist with one hand and supports the client's elbow with their other hand.

- Grade 5: completes motion against maximal resistance
- Grade 4: completes motion against strong resistance
- Grade 3: completes motion without resistance

For the following grades, the client should sit with the shoulder flexed between 45° and 90°, the elbow flexed to 90°, and the forearm in neutral. The clinician supports the client's elbow.

- Grade 2: completes full ROM in position
- Grade 1: muscle activity without movement
- Grade 0: no muscle activity

Primary Muscles	Supinator
	Biceps brachii
Primary Nerve	Radial (C5-7)

SPECIAL TESTS

As mentioned in chapter 10 (Special Tests), in many cases the clinician is overly dependent on the performance and interpretation of special test findings with respect to differential diagnosis of the client's presenting pain. Utilization of special tests for ruling in (or helping to diagnose) a particular pathology should occur at this point in the examination process. It is also hoped that the clinician has a much clearer picture of the client's presentation prior to this point in the examination and will therefore depend minimally on special test findings with respect to diagnosis of the client's pain.

Ruling out other potential contributors to the client's pain is an essential part of the examination for the elbow joint. Refer to the Triage and Screening section of this chapter for more information. The following section includes specific special tests with detailed descriptions for the elbow joint and forearm to help rule in pathologies of this region. Similar to other body regions, clinicians should remember not to rely on special testing in isolation but instead to include it in the overall examination sequence.

Index of Special Tests

Alignment

Carrying Angle

Muscle Dysfunction

Lateral Epicondylopathy

Cozen's Test

Maudsley's Test

Medial Epicondylopathy

NA

Distal Biceps Tear or Rupture

Biceps Squeeze Test

Biceps Crease Interval (BCI)

Hook Test

Exam Cluster for Complete Tear

Passive Forearm Pronation

Bicipital Aponeurosis Flexion Test

Instability or Ligamentous Laxity

Medial Elbow or Ulnar Collateral Ligament

Moving Valgus Stress Test

Valgus Stress Test

Medial Elbow Instability Test

Lateral Elbow or Radial Lateral Collateral Ligament

Varus Stress Test

Posterolateral Rotatory Instability

Lateral Pivot Shift Test

Chair Push-Up Test

Posterolateral Rotatory Drawer Test

Tabletop Relocation Test

Prone Push-Up Test

Intra-Articular Pathology

Fracture

Elbow Extension Test (see Triage and Screening section of this chapter)

Elbow Pronation Test

Elbow Supination Test

Elbow Flexion Test

(continued)

Index of Special Tests *(continued)*

Nerve Entrapment

Cubital Tunnel or Ulnar Neuropathy

Pressure Provocation Test

Elbow Flexion Test for Cubital Tunnel

Tinel's Sign at the Elbow

Elbow Scratch Collapse Test

Elbow Flexion Test for Neuropathy

Elbow Osteoarthritis

NA

Case Studies

Go to www.HumanKinetics.com/OrthopedicClinicalExamination and complete these case studies for chapter 22:

- Case study 1 discusses a 19-year-old female water polo player with right elbow pain.
- Case study 2 discusses a 50-year-old male accountant and motocross racer with pain in his right shoulder and elbow when he rides.

Abstract Links

Go to www.HumanKinetics.com/OrthopedicClinicalExamination to access abstract links on these issues:

Arm squeeze test

Bony apprehension test

Elbow extension test

Hawkins-Kennedy test

Median nerve upper limb tension test

Olecranon-manubrium percussion test

Spurling's test

Tuning fork

ALIGNMENT

CARRYING ANGLE

Client Position	Standing with arms facing forward by sides in anatomical position
Clinician Position	Standing in front of and facing the client
Movement	None
Assessment	The clinician measures the elbow angle at the intersection of the bisected humerus and bisected axis of the forearm using a goniometer.

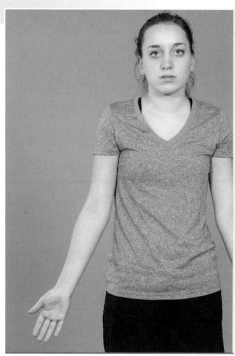

Figure 22.23

Statistics
- In a study of 1,275 healthy volunteers (mean age 22.9 ± 16 years, 644 women), elbow angle was measured with a goniometer. In both sexes the carrying angle in the dominant arm was significantly higher than in the nondominant arm, especially in age 14 and over. In the right-arm dominant group, the right angle was 11.3 ± 3.7° and the left angle was 10.6 ± 3.6°. In the left-arm dominant group, the right angle was 10.7 ± 4.0° and the left was 12.9 ± 4.2°.[89]

- In a study of 20 healthy volunteers (mean age 25 years, 50% women) using radiography as a reference standard, the mean carrying angle in extension of 11.6 ± 3.2° in men and 16.7 ± 3° in women was measured with a goniometer. With flexion, the carrying angles progressively decreased.[4]

- In a study of 51 healthy volunteers (mean age 31.7 ± 9 years, 31 women) with intratester reliability: ICC of 0.97 ± 0.003 (0.96–0.97) for goniometric measurements and intertester reliability for radiologic measurements: right side, ICC 0.99; left, ICC 0.99. The mean difference in goniometric measurement values when compared to radiography as a reference standard was –3.0° ± 3.2°.[90]

MUSCLE DYSFUNCTION: LATERAL EPICONDYLOPATHY

COZEN'S TEST

Client Position	Sitting or standing with elbow flexed at 90°, forearm pronation, hand in a fist, and fist in radial deviation
Clinician Position	Standing facing the client, palpating the lateral epicondyle with their thumb (left as shown)
Movement	The client extends the wrist against resistance applied by the clinician.
Assessment	A (+) test is reproduction of pain along the lateral epicondyle.
Statistics	NR[91]

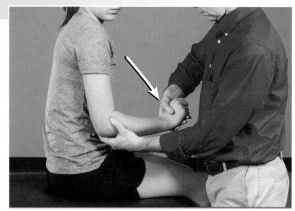

Figure 22.24

MAUDSLEY'S TEST

Client Position	Sitting with elbow flexed at 90°, fingers abducted and extended
Clinician Position	Facing the client and stabilizing the wrist
Movement	The clinician resists third digit extension.
Assessment	A (+) test is reproduction of pain.
Statistics	NR[92]

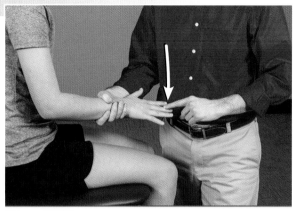

Figure 22.25

MUSCLE DYSFUNCTION: MEDIAL EPICONDYLOPATHY

There are no tests available for this condition.

MUSCLE DYSFUNCTION: DISTAL BICEPS TEAR OR RUPTURE

Critical Clinical Pearls

Regarding special tests for distal biceps tear or rupture, remember to do the following:

- Rule out instability or fractures of the bony joint structure.
- Ensure the client has normal pain-free PROM.
- Always examine the noninvolved side prior to the symptomatic side.

BICEPS SQUEEZE TEST

Client Position	Sitting with the forearm resting in their lap, elbow flexed at 60° to 80° and forearm in slight pronation
Clinician Position	Stands on the client's affected side and places one hand (right as shown) at the distal myotendinous junction and the other hand (left as shown) at the belly of the biceps brachii
Movement	The clinician squeezes the biceps firmly with both hands.
Assessment	A (+) test is lack of forearm supination as the biceps is squeezed.
Statistics	**SN 96 (NR), SP 100 (NR), +LR Inf, −LR 0.04,** QUADAS 9, in a study of 25 consecutive Navy corpsmen with presumptive distal biceps tendon ruptures (26 tendons, one had bilateral symptoms; mean age 42 years; all male; mean duration of symptoms NR), using arthroscopy as a reference standard (two clients had MRI as reference standard)[93]

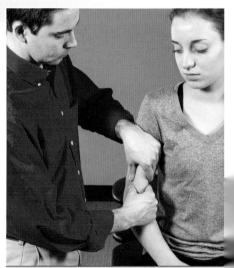

Figure 22.26

HOOK TEST

Client Position	Sitting or standing, with full forearm supination
Clinician Position	Facing client; for client's right elbow, clinician uses left index finger as shown.
Movement	The clinician uses their index finger from the lateral side to hook the tendon and pull it forward.
Assessment	A (+) test is if the clinician is not able to hook the tendon; there is no cordlike structure for the clinician to hook.

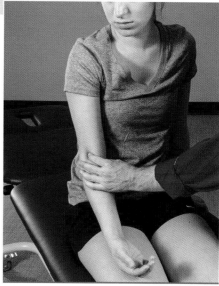

Figure 22.27

Statistics

- SN 100 (NR), SP 100 (NR), +LR Inf, –LR Inf, QUADAS 6, for complete tears in a study of 45 consecutive clients with a known or possible partial or complete avulsion of the distal biceps tendon (mean age 49; 1 woman; mean duration of symptoms: 31% acute [<10 days], 11% subacute [11-21 days], and 58% chronic [>21 days]), using arthroscopy or surgery as a reference standard (25 clients had MRIs: 13 complete tears, 12 partial tears). MRI for complete tears: SN 92 (NR), SP 85(NR), +LR 6.1, –LR 0.09.[56]

- Modified hook test for partial tears: pulling vigorously on biceps tendon after hooking it with index finger with a positive test of reproduction of pain. This modified test was performed in 9 out of 12 clients with partial tears; all were positive.[56]

- SN 81 (NR), SP 100 (NR), +LR Inf, –LR 0.19, QUADAS 7, diagnostic accuracy 94%, in a retrospective review of 17 clients who presented with suspected distal biceps tendon injury. All had physical maneuvers performed and had intraoperative data. Age greater than 18 years (mean age 47.2 years; 100% male; mean duration of symptoms: 9 acute <10 days after injury—mean 4.7 days, 8 chronic >90 days after injury—mean 165 days), using intraoperative examination as a reference standard.[94]

- **SN 81 (NR), SP 100 (NR), +LR Inf, –LR 0.19**, QUADAS 10, in a cohort study of 48 clients with suspected distal biceps tendon injuries (mean age 47 years; only 1 woman; mean duration of symptoms 76 days), using intraoperative examination or MRI as a reference standard.[95]

PASSIVE FOREARM PRONATION

Client Position	Sitting or standing, with arm in supination
Clinician Position	Facing the client and grasping their forearm
Movement	The clinician passively pronates the client's forearm.
Assessment	A (+) test is loss of visible and palpable proximal-to-distal movement of the biceps muscle belly.

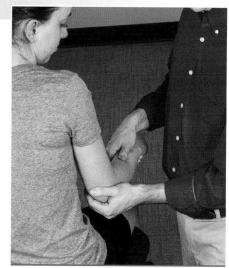

Figure 22.28

Statistics

- SN 87.5 (NR), SP 100 (NR), +LR Inf, –LR 0.12, QUADAS 7, diagnostic accuracy 94%, in a retrospective review of 17 clients who presented with suspected distal biceps tendon injury. All had physical maneuvers performed and had intraoperative data: age greater than 18 years (mean age 47.2 years), 100% male, mean duration of symptoms: 9 acute <10 days after injury—mean 4.7 days, 8 chronic >90 days after injury—mean 165 days, using intraoperative examination as a reference standard.[94]

(continued)

Passive Forearm Pronation *(continued)*

- **SN 95 (NR), SP 100 (NR), +LR Inf, –LR 0.05**, QUADAS 10, in a cohort study of 48 clients with suspected distal biceps tendon injuries (mean age 47 years; 1 woman; mean duration of symptoms 76 days), using intra-operative examination or MRI as a reference standard.[95] Movement of muscle belly is dependent on quantity and speed of movement into pronation.

BICEPS CREASE INTERVAL (BCI)

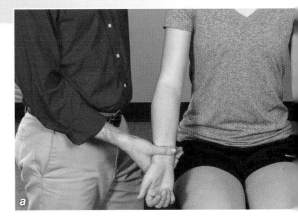

Client Position	Sitting or standing
Clinician Position	Facing client and grasping client's wrist
Movement	The clinician flexes the client's elbow to appreciate the main antecubital flexion crease, then passively extends and supinates the client's elbow *(a)*. Using a pen, the clinician traces the crease in the antecubital fossa and then strokes the distal biceps centrally parallel to the long axis (line might not be perpendicular to crease line; *b*). The clinician identifies the point where the distal biceps curve turns most sharply toward the antecubital fossa as the cusp of the distal descent, and marks a short transverse line at the cusp *(c)*. The clinician measures the distance between the biceps cusp and the antecubital crease in centimeters and repeats the process on the opposite arm.
Assessment	A (+) test for complete rupture is >6 cm for BCI. Biceps crease ratio (BCR) is calculated by BCI of injured side divided by BCI of unaffected side. BCR > 1.2 is a complete rupture.

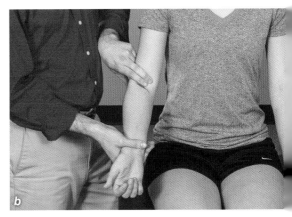

Statistics

- SN 92 (NR), SP 100 (NR), +LR Inf, –LR 0.08, QUADAS 5, diagnostic accuracy 93%, in a cohort study of 29 consecutive clients with suspected distal biceps tendon ruptures with confirmation by surgery or imaging (mean age 47 years; 100% male; mean duration of symptoms 49 days), using intraoperative examination or MRI as a reference standard. Reliability of >0.75.[96]

- SN 93 (NR), SP 100 (NR), +LR Inf, –LR 0.07, QUADAS 7, diagnostic accuracy 94%, in a retrospective review of 17 clients who presented with suspected distal biceps tendon injury. All had physical maneuvers performed and had intraoperative data: age greater than 18 years (mean age 47.2 years), 100% male, mean duration of symptoms: 9 acute <10 days after injury—mean 4.7 days, 8 chronic >90 days after injury—mean 165 days. Intraoperative examination was the reference standard.[94]

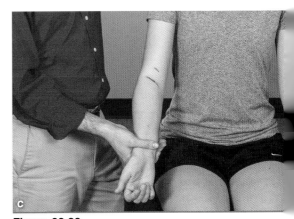

Figure 22.29

- **SN 88 (NR)**, SP 50 (NR), +LR 1.76, **–LR 0.24**, QUADAS 10, in a cohort study of 48 clients with suspected distal biceps tendon injuries (mean age 47 years; 1 woman; mean duration of symptoms 76 days), using intraoperative examination or MRI as a reference standard.[95]
- For BCR: SN 96 (NR), SP 80 (NR), +LR 4.8, –LR 0.08, QUADAS 5, diagnostic accuracy 93%, in a cohort study of 29 consecutive clients with suspected distal biceps tendon ruptures with confirmation by surgery or imaging (mean age 47 years; 100% male; mean duration of symptoms 49 days), using intraoperative examination or MRI. The BCI was measured on both arms and the BCR was calculated as the injured arm BCR divided by the uninjured arm BCI.[96] Calculations were also performed combining the BCI and BCR with a positive on either exam to indicate a complete rupture; values were exactly the same as BCR.[96]

EXAM CLUSTER FOR COMPLETE TEAR

The clinician performs the hook test, passive forearm pronation test, and BCI as described previously.

Assessment A (+) test occurs when all three tests are in agreement (either all [+] or all [–]). Conflicting results or equivocal findings suggest the need for soft-tissue imaging (MR or US).

Statistics **SN 100 (NR), SP 100 (NR), +LR Inf,, –LR 0**, QUADAS 10, in a cohort study of 48 clients with suspected distal biceps tendon injuries (mean age 47 years; 1 woman; mean duration of symptoms 76 days), using intraoperative examination or MRI as a reference standard.[95] The cluster will limit the need for imaging when all exam findings are in agreement. Follow-up with diagnostic imaging is only needed when conflicting examination findings are present.

BICIPITAL APONEUROSIS FLEXION TEST

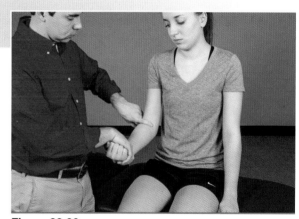

Figure 22.30

Client Position Sitting with arm in forearm supination

Clinician Position Facing client

Movement The clinician palpates the medial, lateral, and central parts of the antecubital fossa. The client makes a fist and flexes the wrist, then flexes the elbow and does an isometric hold at 75° of flexion. (The clinician can isometrically resist the forearm [with right arm as shown] as it moves into flexion and perform palpation [with left hand as shown] of the antecubital fossa.)

Assessment A (+) test is lack of sharp, thin edge of aponeurosis medially.

Statistics SN 100 (NR), SP 90 (NR), +LR 10, –LR 0, QUADAS 7, diagnostic accuracy 94%, in a retrospective review of 17 clients who presented with suspected distal biceps tendon injury. All had physical maneuvers performed and had intraoperative data: age greater than 18 years (mean age 47.2 years), 100% male, mean duration of symptoms: 9 acute <10 days after injury—mean 4.7 days, 8 chronic >90 days after injury—mean 165 days. Intraoperative examination was the reference standard.[94] This test can be used in triage and screening for biceps rupture earlier in the examination secondary to higher sensitivity of test.

INSTABILITY OR LIGAMENTOUS LAXITY: MEDIAL ELBOW OR ULNAR COLLATERAL LIGAMENT

MOVING VALGUS STRESS TEST

 Video 22.31 **in the web resource shows a demonstration of this test.**

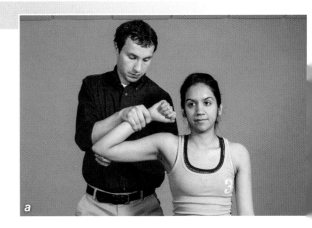

Client Position	Seated with arm abducted to 90°, elbow fully flexed
Clinician Position	Standing behind the client, supporting under the elbow and holding onto the wrist
Movement	The clinician provides a valgus stress at the client's elbow *(a)* until the shoulder reaches full ER and quickly extends the elbow to 30° *(b)*, while maintaining valgus torque.
Assessment	A (+) test is pain reproduction when the elbow is extended. The highest level of pain should be between 70° and 120° (shear angle).
Statistics	SN 100 (81-100), SP 75 (19-99), +LR 4.0, –LR 0, QUADAS 10, in a cohort study of 21 clients for suspected chronic ulnar collateral ligament (UCL) or medial collateral ligament (MCL) injuries (mean age 28 years; 2 women; mean duration of symptoms NR), using MRI and surgical assessment as reference standards[97]

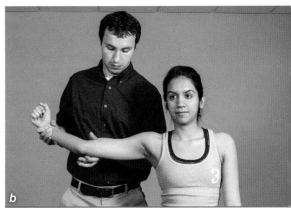

Figure 22.31

MEDIAL ELBOW INSTABILITY TEST

Client Position	Sitting or standing, with elbow extended
Clinician Position	Facing client and placing one hand at their elbow
Movement	The clinician palpates the client's ulnar nerve for tenderness or subluxation with flexion of the elbow. They examine the triceps mechanism for tenderness along the medial border and subluxation with resisted extension. They perform additional examination of the elbow for palpable ligamentous laxity.
Assessment	A (+) test is reproduction of pain medially at the joint line or laxity with palpation.
Statistics	SN 19 (4-46), SP 100 (40-100), +LR Inf, –LR 0.08, QUADAS 10, in a cohort study of 21 clients for suspected chronic UCL (MCL) injuries (mean age 28 years; 2 women; mean duration of symptoms NR), using MRI and surgical assessment as reference standards[97]

VALGUS STRESS TEST

Client Position	Sitting or standing, with elbow extended
Clinician Position	Facing client and placing one hand (left as shown) at their elbow and other hand (right as shown) at their wrist
Movement	The clinician applies an abduction or valgus force while palpating the ulnar or medial collateral ligament. The clinician applies the test again with the elbow at 20° to 30° of flexion.
Assessment	A (+) test is production of distraction pain medially and compression pain laterally at the joint line and laxity.

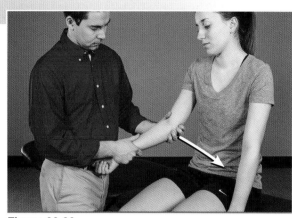

Figure 22.32

Statistics	SN 65 (38-86), SP 50 (7-93), +LR 1.3, –LR 0.7, QUADAS 10, in a cohort study of 21 clients for suspected chronic UCL (MCL) injuries (mean age 28 years; 2 women; mean duration of symptoms NR), using MRI and surgical assessment as reference standards.[97] This study also examined valgus stress at 30°, 60°, 70°, and 90° of flexion.

INSTABILITY AND LIGAMENTOUS LAXITY: LATERAL ELBOW OR RADIAL/LATERAL COLLATERAL LIGAMENT

VARUS STRESS TEST

Client Position	Sitting or standing, with elbow extended
Clinician Position	Facing the client and placing one hand (right as shown) at their elbow and other hand (left as shown) at their wrist
Movement	The clinician applies an adduction or varus force while palpating the radial (RCL) or lateral collateral ligament (LCL). They apply the test again with the elbow at 20° to 30° of flexion.
Assessment	A (+) test is production of distraction pain laterally and compression pain medially at the joint line and laxity.
Statistics	NR

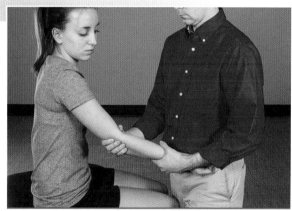

Figure 22.33

INSTABILITY OR LIGAMENTOUS LAXITY: POSTEROLATERAL ROTATORY INSTABILITY

LATERAL PIVOT SHIFT TEST

Client Position	Supine with arm over head in full shoulder ER and forearm supinated
Clinician Position	Standing at the client's head, with one hand (right as shown) blocking shoulder external rotation at the lateral elbow and other hand (left as shown) at the proximal wrist
Movement	The clinician flexes the client's elbow while applying a valgus, supinatory, and axial compressive force (maximal rotator displacement at 40° of flexion).
Assessment	A (+) test is apprehension, when performed in an awake client, and a palpable or visible clunk or dimple in the skin proximal to the radial head, when performed under anesthesia.
Statistics	• SN 38 (NR), SP (NR), +LR (NR), –LR (NR), QUADAS 8, in a cohort study of 8 clients for suspected elbow instability (mean age 44 years; 3 women; mean duration of symptoms 4.5 years), using surgical assessment as a reference. When under anesthesia, all 8 clients demonstrated a positive pivot shift, compared to only 3 when awake.[98]
	• NR[99]

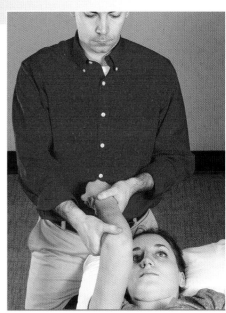

Figure 22.34

POSTEROLATERAL ROTATORY DRAWER TEST

Client Position	Sitting, arm resting in lap
Clinician Position	Standing at the client's side and providing stabilization at their humerus with one hand (right as shown)
Movement	The clinician pulls posteriorly on the lateral side of the proximal forearm.
Assessment	A (+) test is apprehension or a dimple of skin proximal to the radial head.
Statistics	NR[100]

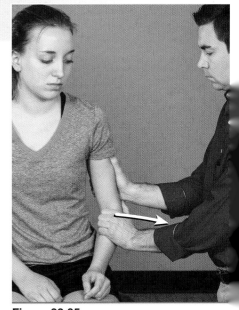

Figure 22.35

PRONE PUSH-UP TEST

Client Position	Prone on their stomach on the floor with elbows flexed at 90°, forearms supinated, and arms abducted to greater than shoulder width *(a)*
Clinician Position	NA
Movement	The client pushes up off the floor, extending the elbows *(b)*.
Assessment	A (+) test is apprehension occurring as the affected elbow is terminally extended from a flexed position, with voluntary or involuntary guarding. A complete dislocation is also considered (+).
Statistics	• SN 88 (NR), SP (NR), +LR (NR), –LR (NR), QUADAS 8, in a cohort study of 8 clients for suspected elbow instability (mean age 44 years; 3 women; mean duration of symptoms 4.5 years), using surgical assessment as a reference standard[98] • NR[101]

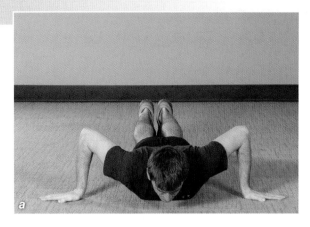

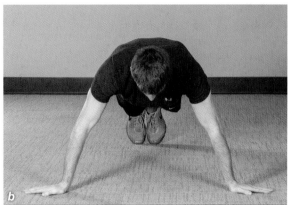

Figure 22.36

CHAIR PUSH-UP TEST

Client Position	Seated, with elbows flexed to 90°, forearms supinated, and arms abducted to greater than shoulder width
Clinician Position	NA
Movement	The client pushes down on the arms of the chair to rise, exclusively using upper extremity force.
Assessment	A (+) test is reluctance to extend the elbow fully as the client raises the body up from a chair as a result of apprehension or of complete dislocation.
Statistics	• SN 87 (NR), SP (NR), +LR (NR), –LR (NR), QUADAS 8, in a cohort study of 8 clients for suspected elbow instability (mean age 44 years; 3 women; mean duration of symptoms 4.5 years), using surgical assessment as a reference standard.[98] • SN 100 (NR), SP (NR), +LR (NR), –LR (NR), QUADAS 8, in a cohort study of 8 clients for suspected elbow instability (mean age 44 years; 3 women; mean duration of symptoms 4.5 years), using surgical assessment as a reference standard. When the push-up sign and chair sign were combined, SN increased.[98]

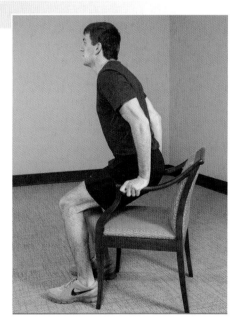

Figure 22.37

TABLETOP RELOCATION TEST

Client Position	Standing in front of the table with the hand of the symptomatic arm (or both arms) placed over the lateral edge of the table
Clinician Position	Standing next to the client and applying thumb pressure to the radial head, giving support and preventing posterior subluxation while the client performs the press-up the second time. Finally, the clinician removes their supporting thumb from the weight-bearing partially flexed elbow.

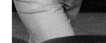

Figure 22.38

Movement	The client is asked to perform a press-up with the elbow pointing laterally (pressure is pushed down through the hand onto the table as the elbow is allowed to flex, bringing the chest toward the table). The maneuver is repeated, with the clinician using the thumb over the radial head to give support or prevent posterior subluxation while the client is performing the press-up.
Assessment	A (+) test is apprehension and pain as the elbow reaches 40° of flexion, or relief of pressure with the clinician applying pressure at the radial head. Clients with instability will report relief of pain and instability during the second press-up. The removal of the clinician's supporting thumb from the weight-bearing partially flexed elbow reproduces pain and apprehension again.
Statistics	• SN 100 (NR), SP (NR), +LR (NR), –LR (NR), QUADAS 6, in a cohort study of 8 clients for suspected elbow instability (mean age, gender, and mean duration of symptoms NR), using positive pivot shift test as a reference standard.[102] • NR[98, 101, 103]

INTRA-ARTICULAR PATHOLOGY

FRACTURE

Tuning fork and stethoscope (see Triage and Screening section)

Olecranon-manubrium percussion test (see Triage and Screening section)

Bony apprehension test (see Triage and Screening section)

Elbow extension test (see Triage and Screening section)

Overall AROM (see Triage and Screening section)

Overall AROM and tenderness to palpation (see Triage and Screening section)

ELBOW FLEXION TEST

Client Position	Lying supine
Clinician Position	NA
Movement	The client actively flexes the elbow. The clinician compares this movement to that of the unaffected side.
Assessment	A test is (+) when the client is unable to fully flex the elbow compared to the opposite side.
Statistics	SN 64 (50-69), **SP 100 (94-100)**, **+LR Inf**, –LR 0.36, QUADAS 11, in 115 consecutive clients (≥5 years of age) and subgrouped as adult (≥18 years) and children (<18 years) presenting to four emergency departments with acute elbow injury, <24 hours (mean age 29 years, 43% female; 71 adults: mean age 40.5 years, 45.5% female; 42 children: mean age 10.5 years, 41.5% female; mean duration of symptoms NR), using radiography as a reference standard[79]

ELBOW PRONATION TEST

Client Position	Lying supine
Clinician Position	NA
Movement	The client actively pronates the forearm. The clinician compares this movement to that of the unaffected side.
Assessment	A test is (+) when the client is unable to fully pronate the arm compared to the opposite side.
Statistics	SN 34 (22-48), **SP 100 (94-100)**, **+LR Inf**, –LR 0.66, QUADAS 11, in 115 consecutive clients (≥5 years of age) and subgrouped as adult (≥ 18 years) and children (<18 years) presenting to four emergency departments with acute elbow injury, <24 hours (mean age 29 years, 43% female; 71 adults: mean age 40.5 years, 45.5% female; 42 children: mean age 10.5 years, 41.5% female; mean duration of symptoms NR), using radiography as a reference standard[79]

ELBOW SUPINATION TEST

Client Position	Lying supine
Clinician Position	NA
Movement	The client actively supinates the forearm. The clinician compares the movement to that of the unaffected side.
Assessment	A test is (+) if the client is unable to fully supinate the arm compared to the opposite side.
Statistics	SN 43 (30-55), **SP 97 (88.5–100)**, **+LR 14.3**, –LR 0.58, QUADAS 11, in 115 consecutive clients (≥5 years of age) and subgrouped as adult (≥18 years) and children (<18 years) presenting to four emergency departments with acute elbow injury within 24 hours (mean age 29 years, 43% female; 71 adults: mean age 40.5 years, 45.5% female; 42 children: mean age 10.5 years, 59.5% male; mean duration of symptoms NR), using radiography as a reference standard[79]

NERVE ENTRAPMENT: CUBITAL TUNNEL AND ULNAR NEUROPATHY

PRESSURE PROVOCATION TEST

Client Position	Sitting
Clinician Position	Standing with two fingers over the client's ulnar nerve proximal to the cubital tunnel
Movement	The clinician moves the client's arm into 20° of flexion and forearm supination and maintains pressure over the ulnar nerve. The clinician holds this position for 60 seconds.
Assessment	A (+) test is reproduction of symptoms along the ulnar nerve.

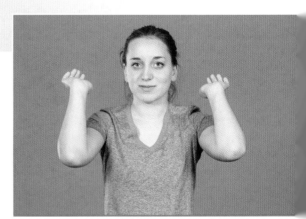

Figure 22.39

Statistics

- SN 46 (NR), SP 99 (NR), +LR 46, –LR 0.54, QUADAS 6, accuracy 81%, in 169 clients and 109 controls (mean age 52 years; 29 women; mean duration of symptoms 42 months) with 64 clients diagnosed with cubital tunnel by history, using examination and positive electrodiagnostic tests as reference standards[104]

- SN 60 (NR), SP (NR), +LR (NR), –LR (NR), QUADAS 12, accuracy 55%, in 192 clients including 55 controls (mean age, gender, and mean duration of symptoms NR), using sonography or electrodiagnostic tests as a reference standard[105]

- SN 89 (NR), SP 98 (NR), +LR 45, –LR 0.11, QUADAS 7, in 32 clients and 33 controls (mean age of clients 46, mean age of controls 41; gender NR; mean duration of symptoms NR), using electrodiagnostic tests as a reference standard[18]

ELBOW FLEXION TEST FOR CUBITAL TUNNEL

Client Position	Sitting in anatomical position
Clinician Position	NA
Movement	The client fully flexes the elbow and extends the wrist, then holds this position for 3 minutes while describing symptoms.
Assessment	A (+) test is reproduction of symptoms along the ulnar nerve distribution, including pain, tingling, and numbness.

Figure 22.40

Statistics

- SN 75 (NR), SP 99 (NR), +LR 75, –LR 0.25, QUADAS 7, in 32 clients and 33 controls (mean age of clients 46, mean age of controls 41; gender NR; mean duration of symptoms NR), using electrodiagnostic tests as a reference standard[18]

- SN 93 (NR), SP (NR), +LR NA, –LR NA, QUADAS 7, in 13 clients with cubital tunnel syndrome (mean age of clients 59 years; 100% males; mean duration of symptoms NR) as diagnosed, using electrophysiological tests as a reference standard[106]

TINEL'S SIGN AT THE ELBOW

Client Position	Sitting with elbow flexed at 90°
Clinician Position	Supporting client's elbow and forearm and placing finger just proximal to the medial cubital tunnel
Movement	The clinician taps over the ulnar nerve four to six times.
Assessment	A (+) test is reproduction of symptoms along the ulnar distribution.
Statistics	• SN 54 (NR), SP 99 (NR), +LR 54, –LR 0.46, QUADAS 6, accuracy 84%, in 169 clients and 109 controls (mean age 59 years; 29 females; mean duration of symptoms 42 months) with 64 diagnosed with cubital tunnel based on history, using examination and positive electrodiagnostic tests as reference standards.[104]

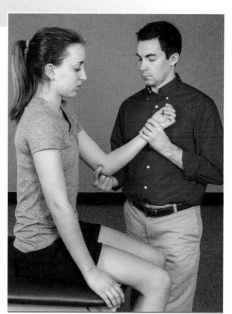

Figure 22.41

• SN 62 (NR), SP (NR), +LR (NR), –LR (NR), QUADAS 12, accuracy 59% in 192 clients including 55 controls (mean age, gender, and mean duration of symptoms NR), using sonography or electrodiagnostic tests as a reference standard.[105]
When Tinel's sign was combined with pressure provocation or flexion compression and nerve tenderness, SN 30 (NR), SP 84 (NR), +LR 1.84, –LR 0.83, QAUDAS 12.[105]

• SN 70 (NR), SP (NR), +LR 35, –LR 0.31, QUADAS 7, in 32 clients and 33 controls (mean age of clients 46, mean age of controls 41; gender and mean duration of symptoms NR), using electrodiagnostic tests as a reference standard.[18]

• Positive in 47 out of 204 asymptomatic clients; no diagnostic values available.[107]

ELBOW SCRATCH COLLAPSE TEST

Client Position	Sitting with elbows flexed to 90°
Clinician Position	Sitting or standing in front of the client
Movement	The clinician applies internal rotation force as the client resists with bilateral shoulder external rotation, then scratches or swipes their fingertips over the area of compressed ulnar nerve and repeats application of internal rotation force as the client resists with bilateral external rotation.
Assessment	A (+) test is weakness (unilaterally in affected area).

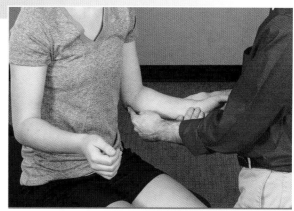

Figure 22.42

Statistics SN 69 (NR), SP 99 (NR), +LR 69, –LR 0.31, QUADAS 6, accuracy 89%, in 169 clients and 109 controls (mean age 52 years; 29 females; mean duration of symptoms 42 months) with 64 diagnosed with cubital tunnel based on history, using examination and positive electrodiagnostic tests as reference standards[104]

ELBOW FLEXION TEST FOR NEUROPATHY

Client Position	Sitting
Clinician Position	NA
Movement	The client fully flexes the elbows with neutral wrist and shoulder position *(a)*, then holds for 60 seconds. The client then moves to full flexion of elbows with neutral shoulder position and full wrist extension *(b)*, and holds this position for 60 seconds. The client then abducts the shoulders to 90°, places the elbows in full flexion and the wrists in full extension *(c)*, and holds this position for 90 seconds.
Assessment	A (+) test is reproduction of symptoms (in any of the positions) along the ulnar nerve distribution. The client does not move to the next position if they have symptoms in the preceding position.
Statistics	NR[107]

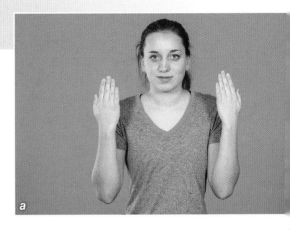

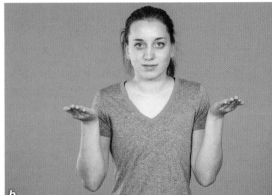

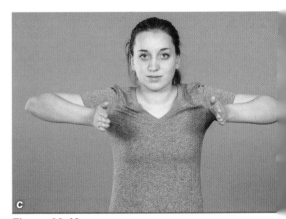

Figure 22.43

ELBOW OSTEOARTHRITIS

No special tests are described for osteoarthritis. As with all comprehensive examinations, screening out other competing diagnoses is paramount.

PALPATION

Thorough palpation of the affected joint and muscular structure can also help identify structures that are implicated. Palpation should be performed near the end of the examination after special tests to increase its utility (refer to chapter 11).

Elbow and Forearm

A complete examination sequence includes a thorough palpation of the area and is improved with a systematic approach to palpating all aspects of the elbow joint. During other parts of the sequence, the clinician should note if any of the structures are tender to the client during motion testing, muscle testing, and special tests. For more information, refer to chapter 11 (Palpation).

Anterior Aspect

Bony Structures

• **Coronoid fossa of humerus:** This is a small depression where the coronoid process of the ulna articulates during forearm flexion. It is located superior to the anterior trochlea and adjacent to the radial fossa of the humerus. This structure is hard to palpate because it is deep in the cubital fossa.

• **Coronoid process of ulna:** This projection from the upper and anterior aspect of the ulna is triangular in shape, and it articulates with the coronoid fossa during flexion. The ulnar collateral ligament attaches to the medial surfaces. The coronoid process is best felt by resisting the flexor digitorum superficialis and profundus muscles that attach to this structure. After resisting the muscles, the client should relax. Then the coronoid process can be felt deep under the muscular structures.

Soft-Tissue Structures

• **Cubital fossa:** Located in the anterior elbow joint, this triangular area is also called the antecubital fossa. The boundaries are formed medially by the pronator teres and laterally by the brachioradialis muscle. The proximal or superior boundary is formed by creating a horizontal line between the medial and lateral epicondyles of the humerus, resulting in an inferiorly directed apex of the triangle. The floor of the fossa is formed by the brachialis and supinator muscles and the roof is composed of skin, fascia, and bicipital aponeurosis. The following are contained within the cubital fossa, oriented medial to lateral:

- **Median nerve:** This is medial to the brachial artery. It crosses the cubital fossa deep to the pronator teres.

- **Brachial artery:** This is medial to the distal biceps tendon. It bifurcates into the radial and ulnar arteries at the apex of the fossa.

- **Biceps brachii tendon:** When resistance is applied to elbow flexion with forearm in supination, the distal tendon becomes more exposed. Moving more proximally, the muscle belly of the biceps can be appreciated.

Medial Aspect

Bony Structures

• **Medial epicondyle:** This is the most prominent projection on the medial aspect of the elbow. It serves as the attachment of the origin of the forearm flexors and common flexor tendon. Just proximal to the medial epicondyle is the medial supracondylar ridge, which can be palpated by moving in a superior direction from the largest prominence.

• **Trochlea of humerus:** This is the medial projection of the humerus that articulates with the trochlear notch on the ulna. After identification of the medial epicondyle, the trochlea can be palpated by moving in a posterolateral direction, just medial to the olecranon of the ulna. The trochlea can be palpated more easily with the elbow in a flexed position. Care should be taken to not irritate the ulnar nerve.

Soft-Tissue Structures

• **Ulnar nerve:** This is just posterior to the medial epicondyle and the intermuscular septum. It is very sensitive to palpation. The ulnar nerve can roll back and forth over the medial condyle. It is better appreciated with the arm in slight abduction, external rotation, and flexion between 20° and 70°. SN 31 (NR), SP (NR), +LR (NR), −LR (NR), QUADAS 12, accuracy 46% in 192 clients including 55 controls (mean age, gender, and mean symptoms NR), using sonography or electrodiagnostic tests as a reference for palpation of nerve tenderness in clients diagnosed with cubital tunnel symptoms.[105]

• **Forearm flexor mass:** As a unit, it becomes more palpable with resisted wrist flexion and adduction because it has a common origin off the medial epicondyle. Starting more proximally and moving distally, the muscles are the pronator teres, flexor carpi radialis, and palmaris longus.

Posterior Aspect

Bony Structures

• **Olecranon of ulna:** This is the midpoint of the straight line between the medial and lateral epicondyles when the elbow is extended. With ~30° elbow flexion, the triceps relaxes and the olecranon comes out of the fossa and moves inferiorly.

• **Olecranon fossa of humerus:** This is exposed with elbow flexion just proximally to olecranon on either side of the triceps tendon.

Soft-Tissue Structures

• **Triceps brachii tendon:** This inserts onto the olecranon process of the ulna and to the posterior wall of the elbow joint capsule. The clinician should resist elbow extension to increase the ability to palpate the borders of the triceps tendon.

• **Olecranon bursa:** This is only palpable if inflamed or thickened. The olecranon bursa is not attached to the synovial cavity. With extreme or chronic bursitis, inflammation of the bursa can be appreciated.

Lateral Aspect

Bony Structures

• **Lateral epicondyle:** This is the most prominent bony landmark laterally, and it continues proximally as the lateral supracondylar ridge.

• **Radial head:** This is located approximately 2 cm distal to the lateral epicondyle. It is best appreciated with one thumb on the lateral joint line and the other hand rotating the client's forearm into pronation and supination.

Soft-Tissue Structures

• **Forearm extensor mass:** Palpation of the common mass is made easier with the application of resistance to wrist extension because it has a common origin from the lateral epicondyle.

• **Brachioradialis:** With the forearm in neutral (midpoint of pronation and supination), the client is asked to clench the fist and flex the elbow.

• **Anconeus:** This is best palpated behind the radial head on the lateral aspect of the olecranon. It becomes more prominent when the elbow is extended against resistance.

PHYSICAL PERFORMANCE MEASURES

Unlike the lower extremity, less information is available about physical performance measures at the elbow. PPMs involving the entire upper extremity and utilizing the elbow can be used to provide objective data about the client's abilities, including strength, anaerobic power, endurance, speed, and fine dexterity. The clinician should start the client with measures that are appropriate but challenging and progress to more challenging activities as tolerated. Examples of tests are provided in table 22.4. The modified chair pick-up test was designed to reproduce symptoms in clients with lateral epicondylosis. Intrarater and interrater reliability were both high (ICC of 0.9–0.97 and 0.8–0.93, respectively) with low measurement error (5.8–7.2%).

TABLE 22.4 Physical Performance Measure Suggestions for the Elbow

Discrete physical parameter	Potential physical performance measurements for the lower-level client (if appropriate)	Potential physical performance measurements for the higher-level client (if appropriate)
Fundamental movement	Writing Modified chair pick-up	Any of the tests appropriate for the lower-level client Trunk stability push-up
Strength and power	Grip strength	Any of the tests appropriate for the lower-level client
Endurance	Grip endurance test Deep neck flexor test	Any of the tests appropriate for the lower-level client Repetitive box lifting task Periscapular endurance test Rotator cuff endurance test Repetitive push-up test

This results in strong negative correlation with peak or total force and pain with activities in clients with lateral epicondylosis.[108]

COMMON ORTHOPEDIC CONDITIONS OF THE ELBOW JOINT

While it is impossible to distinctly describe various pathological presentations of the elbow, there are evidence-based findings supportive of particular pathologies of this region of the body. Therefore, the intent of this section of the chapter is to present current evidence-supported findings suggestive of elbow pathologies. As previously described in chapter 4 (Evidence-Based Practice and Client Examination), not all examination findings are absolutely supported with clinical evidence, and the clinician should also rely on clinical experience and input from the client when performing differential diagnosis of a client's presentation of pain and dysfunction.

After completion of the examination, the clinician can start generating pathoanatomical hypotheses for the origin of the client's signs and symptoms. Some more frequently encountered orthopedic conditions of the elbow are discussed in the following sections with details of expected findings of each part of the orthopedic sequence.

Medial and Lateral Epicondylalgia

ICD-9: 726.31 (medial epicondylitis); 726.32 (lateral epicondylitis)

ICD-10: M 77.00 (medial epicondylitis, unspecified elbow); M77.10 (lateral epicondylitis, unspecified elbow)

Medial and lateral epicondylalgia are two of the most common pathologies at the elbow. They result from overuse repetitive activities. For lateral epicondylosis, the extensor carpi radialis brevis (ECRB) is the tendon most commonly involved, and shearing forces occur on the ECRB secondary to a more proximal origin than the axis for both flexion and extension movements.[108] Clients with lateral epicondylalgia, commonly called *tennis elbow*, report irritation on the lateral aspect of their elbow and forearm, which is increased with repetitive or gripping activities.[109]

Often medial epicondylalgia is called *golfer's elbow*. It results in symptoms similar to lateral epicondylalgia, only with irritation on the inside of the elbow or forearm. In young people, a variant of medial epicondylalgia is Little League elbow. This condition is a traction apophysitis of the medial epicondyle. As is implied by its name, it commonly occurs in youths who are baseball overhand pitchers. Repetitive valgus stress associated with pitches such as the curveball stress the growing bone to a greater extent than it can tolerate. It is generally believed that limited pitch counts and avoiding these types of throws until the pitcher is older are sound preventive measures.

I. Client Interview

Subjective History

- These pathologies are most common at the age of 40 to 60 years.[108, 110]
- They affect women more frequently than men.[110]
- The prevalence of lateral epicondylitis in the general populations is approximately 1.0% to 1.3% in men and 1.1% to 4.0% in women, and that of medial epicondylitis is nearly 0.3% to 0.6% in men and 0.3% to 1.1% in women.[110]
- Forceful activities, high force combined with high repetition or awkward posture, and awkward postures are associated with epicondylitis.[110]
- These conditions have a prevalence of up to 7.4% in engineering or labor occupations.[109]

Outcome Measures

- The DASH and QuickDASH have demonstrated clinical relevance for both medial and lateral epicondylalgia, although they are both regional measures.
- The Patient-Reported Tennis Elbow Evaluation (PRTEE) is a specific outcome measure for clients who have lateral epicondylalgia.

Diagnostic Imaging

- Imaging is not typically needed or performed except to rule out ligamentous instability.
- Ultrasound has been shown to demonstrate good to less than good ability to

help rule in (SP 77–90, +LR 3.2–9.2) and rule out (SN 77–92, –LR 0.09–0.31) lateral epicondylalgia.[51, 52]

- Ultrasound has been shown to demonstrate good ability to help **rule in** (SP 95, +LR 11.9) and **rule out** (SN 92, –LR 0.05) medial epicondylagia.[53]

II. Observation

- Client may have restricted grasping and might avoid shaking hands secondary to pain.

III. Triage and Screening

- All nonmusculoskeletal causes, as well as causes from related joints, should be ruled out.

- Olecranon-manubrium test: demonstrates good ability to help **rule out** (SN 84, –LR 0.3) and ideal ability to help **rule in** (SP 99, +LR 84) anterior shoulder dislocations, clavicle fractures, and humerus fractures.[75]

- The bony apprehension test: A (–) test has good ability to help **rule in** (SN 94, –LR 0.07) bony lesion.[77]

- Elbow extension test: A (–) test has ideal ability to help **rule in** (SN 95-100, –LR 0–0.06) fracture across three studies.[76, 78, 79]

- Elbow AROM: demonstrates ideal diagnostic accuracy to help both **rule out** (SN 100, –LR 0) and **rule in** (SP 97, +LR 33) fracture.[79]

- Clinicians should rule out cervical spine, shoulder, and neural tension from a more proximal cause.

IV. Motion Tests

- All motion and joint play assessments are recommended.

- For lateral epicondylalgia, all motions should be examined, but special attention should be paid to client response during active wrist extension and passive wrist flexion. Clients should perform wrist motions both with the elbow flexed and extended. The client will typically have maximum symptom reproduction with active wrist extension with the elbow in extension and the forearm pronated secondary to lengthened position of the lateral forearm extensor mass. Passive wrist flexion will reproduce pain when the elbow is extended and pronated.

- Conversely, active wrist flexion and passive wrist extension are more implicated with medial epicondylalgia, but all motions should be included in the physical examination. Clients should perform wrist motions both with the elbow flexed and extended. Maximum symptom reproduction typically occurs with active wrist flexion with the elbow in extension and the forearm supinated secondary to lengthened position of the medial forearm flexor mass. Passive wrist extension will reproduce pain when the elbow is extended and supinated.

V. Muscle Performance Testing

- Lateral epicondylalgia results in reduced strength and in pain with resisted wrist extension. Pain is greatest when the elbow is extended and the forearm is pronated.

- Pain and reduced strength might be appreciated with resisted wrist flexion and elbow extended for medial epicondylalgia.

VI. Special Tests

- Cozen's and Maudsley's tests have limited value because no diagnostic values are available.

VII. Palpation

- Palpation tends to elicit well-localized tenderness that is similar in quality and location to the pain experienced during activity.[111]

VIII. Physical Performance Measures

- Grip strength
- Modified chair pick-up test

POTENTIAL TREATMENT-BASED CLASSIFICATIONS

- Exercise and conditioning, pain control (if pain dominant), and mobility may be appropriate.

Distal Biceps Rupture ■ ■ ■ ■ ■ ■ ■

ICD-9: 841.8 (sprain or strains of other specified sites of elbow and forearm)

ICD-10: S53.499A (sprain of unspecified elbow)

Although 97% of all biceps ruptures occur at the proximal biceps, distal biceps injuries are typically a result of rapid loading to the arm. Typically the tear occurs at the biceps insertion to radial tuberosity, and delayed treatment can decrease positive prognosis, with complications and decreased outcome occurring as soon as 10 days after injury.[96] Distal biceps ruptures are often subcategorized as partial versus complete. If any fibers were present, then the tear is considered partial. Time needed to acquire imaging or a referral can negatively affect outcomes, which emphasizes the need for improved physical testing.[95]

I. Client Interview

Subjective History

- Distal biceps ruptures are most common at the age of 40 to 60 years.[96]

- The dominant arm is more commonly affected.[112]

- Acute traumatic load, typically eccentric force, results in sharp pain.

- Common activities that can result in eccentric force are starting a lawn mower, using overhead tennis serves, lifting weights overhead, and performing golf follow-throughs. Trying to control a fall on a flexed and supinated elbow can also cause great overload of the biceps.

- Degenerative tears can result from repetitive microtrauma, bony abnormalities, impingement, or hypovascularity.[113]

Outcome Measures

- The DASH and QuickDASH have demonstrated clinical relevance for distal biceps ruptures, although they are both regional measures.

Diagnostic Imaging

- US has growing support to increase reliability for diagnosis of partial tears and to decrease time from evaluation to treatment to improve outcomes. Current research shows that US demonstrates ideal ability to help **rule out** (SN 95-97, −LR 0.03-0.07) and good to less than good ability to help rule in (SP 71-100, +LR 3.28-Inf) distal biceps pathology.[55, 114]

- MRI has been considered a reference standard for diagnosis of distal biceps injuries, but it has better utility for detection of complete tears. MRI has ideal ability to help both **rule out** (SN 92, −LR 0.08) and **rule in** (SP 100, +LR Inf) distal biceps pathology.[54]

II. Observation

- For acute cases, the client might present with the arm guarded against the side of their body. Additionally, ecchymosis and swelling might be present, although an intact biceps aponeurosis might limit ecchymosis.[115]

- Palpable defect might be present and increased with biceps flexion.[116]

III. Triage and Screening

- All nonmusculoskeletal causes, as well as causes from related joints, should be ruled out.

- Olecranon-manubrium test: demonstrates good ability to help both **rule out** (SN 84, −LR 0.3) and ideal ability to help **rule in** (SP 99, +LR 84) anterior shoulder dislocations, clavicle fractures, and humerus fractures.[75]

- The bony apprehension test: A (−) test has good ability to help **rule in** (SN 94, −LR 0.07) bony lesion.[77]

- Elbow extension test: A (−) test has ideal ability to help **rule in** (SN 95-100, −LR 0–0.06) fracture across three studies.[76, 78, 79]

- Elbow AROM: demonstrates ideal ability to help both **rule out** (SN 100, −LR 0) and **rule in** (SP 97, +LR 33) fracture.[79]

- Clinicians should rule out cervical spine, shoulder, and neural tension from a more proximal cause.

IV. Motion Tests

- All motion and joint play assessments are recommended, especially those focused on active elbow flexion.

Clinicians should note decreased quality of movement and concordant pain.

V. Muscle Performance Testing

- Clients experience pain with active elbow flexion or supination and with reduced strength.[93, 117]

VI. Special Tests

- Exam cluster: For complete tear, a cluster of tests including the hook test, passive forearm pronation, and biceps crease interval, in that order, has demonstrated good ability to help **rule out** (SN 100, −LR 0) and **rule in** (SP 100, +LR NA) distal biceps injuries when all three tests were in agreement. Research suggests that if all three tests are in agreement imaging is not indicated, but further investigation by MRI or US is advised when conflicting or equivocal findings are present.[95]

- Hook test: A (+) test has ideal ability to help **rule in** (SP 100, +LR Inf) and good ability to help **rule out** (SN 81,−LR 0.19) suspected distal biceps tendon injuries in one low-bias study.[95]

- The biceps squeeze test: Both (−) and (+) tests have good ability to rule out or rule in the condition and demonstrate the greatest single-test abilities to help **rule out** (SN 96, −LR 0.04) and **rule in** (SP 100, +LR Inf) distal biceps ruptures.[93]

- Passive forearm pronation: Both (−) and (+) tests have ideal ability to help **rule out** (SN 95, −LR 0.05) and **rule in** (SP 100, +LR Inf) distal biceps ruptures.[95]

VII. Palpation

- Clients may experience tenderness to palpation at biceps muscle belly and distal insertion into radial tuberosity, with potential for palpable defect in musculature.

VIII. Physical Performance Measures

- Grip strength
- Biceps and supination endurance strength testing[117]

POTENTIAL TREATMENT-BASED CLASSIFICATIONS

- Protected mobility and pain control (if pain dominant) may be appropriate.

Ulnar Collateral Ligament (UCL) Sprain

ICD-9: 841.1 (ulnar collateral ligament sprain)

ICD-10: S53.449A (ulnar collateral ligament sprain of unspecified elbow)

The UCL is composed of three ligaments: transverse, anterior oblique, and posterior oblique ligaments. An injury to the UCL can be a progressive degeneration of the tissue due to repetitive overload or the less common acute rupture. The repetitive trauma overload injury is most likely due to repetitive throwing, such as pitching. The acute rupture most likely occurs as a result of a collision in sports like American football or wrestling where the elbow is in flexion.[24]

I. Client Interview

Subjective History

- History of repetitive sports or work activities
- Pain and tenderness on the inside of the elbow, especially during dynamic activities (throwing)
- Throwers: inability to achieve maximal velocity, decreased ball control
- Possible numbness and tingling into fourth and fifth digits
- Acute cases: pop, tearing, or pulling sensation at time of injury

Outcome Measures

- The DASH and QuickDASH have demonstrated clinical relevance for disorders related to medial elbow instability, although they are both regional measures.

Diagnostic Imaging

- MRI can be used to help visualize soft-tissue structures to help **rule in** (SP 100, +LR Inf) ulnar collateral ligament tears.[49]
- CT arthrograms can be used to help **rule out** (SN 86, −LR 0.15) and **rule**

in (SP 91, +LR 9.6) ulnar collateral ligament tears.[49]

- US can be used to visualize the soft-tissue structures of the elbow, and the use of contrast can increase ability to diagnose a small tear.[114]

II. Observation

- The client may have normal appearance unless injury is acute. The client might also present with arm in a guarded position against the front of their body. Swelling is also a possibility.

III. Triage and Screening

- All nonmusculoskeletal causes, as well as causes from related joints, should be ruled out.

- Olecranon-manubrium test: demonstrates good ability to help **rule out** (SN 84, −LR 0.3) and ideal ability to help **rule in** (SP 99, +LR 84) anterior shoulder dislocations, clavicle fractures, and humerus fractures.[75]

- The bony apprehension test: A (−) test has good ability to help **rule in** (SN 94, −LR 0.07) bony lesion.[77]

- Elbow extension test: A (−) test has ideal ability to help **rule in** (SN 95-100, −LR 0–0.06) fracture across three studies.[76, 78, 79]

- Elbow AROM: demonstrates ideal ability to help both **rule out** (SN 100, −LR 0) and **rule in** (SP 97, +LR 33) fracture.[79]

- Clinicians should rule out cervical spine, shoulder, and neural tension from a more proximal cause.

IV. Motion Tests

- Range of motion is variable in these clients. For acute injury, clinicians should anticipate slight restriction of motion with flexion, extension, and pronation, and greater limitations in supination. In chronic cases, range of motion can be within normal.

- Accessory glides that stress the medial ligamentous structures of the elbow can display hypermobility and possibly pain. Acutely injured clients might demonstrate muscular guarding for these motions.

V. Muscle Performance Testing

- Normal strength testing will be present in chronic instances, but clients may show reduced strength as well as associated pain of the forearm flexors and pronators in more acute situations.

VI. Special Tests

- Moving valgus stress test: A (−) test has ideal ability to help **rule out** (SN 100, +LR 4.0) suspected chronic UCL (MCL) injuries.[97]

- Valgus stress test: The test has less than good ability to help rule out (SN 66, +LR 1.65) and rule in (SP 60, −LR 0.56) UCL (MCL) tears.[48]

Differential Diagnosis of Medial Epicondylalgia and Chronic Ulnar Collateral Ligament Sprain

- Medial epicondylalgia affects more women than men.
- Symptoms of medial epicondylalgia are reproduced with active or resisted wrist flexion and pronation and passive wrist extension or supination.
- Chronic ulnar collateral ligament sprains commonly have pain-free motions within normal limits.
- Accessory glides of the elbow, especially with valgus force, will demonstrate hypermobility with a UCL sprain.
- The moving valgus stress test can be used to rule out a chronic UCL sprain, and the medial elbow instability test can be used to rule in a UCL sprain.

- Medial elbow instability test: A (+) test has ideal ability to help **rule in** (SP 100, +LR Inf) suspected chronic UCL (MCL) injuries.[97]

VII. Palpation

- Clients may have tenderness to palpation along the medial elbow joint and musculature.

- Tenderness to palpation: A (–) test has fair ability to help rule out (SN 81-94, –LR 0.2) UCL (MCL) tears.[48, 49]

VIII. Physical Performance Measures

- Grip strength

- For throwers, performance of athletic tasks and monitoring throwing or pitching velocity as well as accuracy can be an indicator for injury to the UCL (MCL).

POTENTIAL TREATMENT-BASED CLASSIFICATIONS

- Acute: pain modulation, modified immobility

- Chronic: activity modification, exercise and conditioning

Radial Head Subluxation or Dislocation

ICD-9: 841.1 (closed dislocation of elbow)

ICD-10: S53.096A (dislocation of unspecified radial head)

The acute subluxation or dislocation of the radial head typically occurs in the lateral direction; in pediatric clients, this is the most frequently dislocated joint.[118] Referred to as *nursemaid's elbow*, the radial head subluxes or dislocates as a result of a sudden pull on the upper limb with a forceful traction of the hand. If the arm is pronated and the elbow is extended (similar to the position used when swinging a child by their arms), the arm is more easily subluxed.

I. Client Interview

Subjective History

- Age < 6, most common under age of 4
- Pain occurs after fall or traction event

- Child avoids using arm
- Minimal swelling

Outcome Measures

- The DASH and QuickDASH have demonstrated clinical relevance for all upper extremity disorders, although both are regional measures. Since this condition is more common in pediatric clients, utility of this measure might be limited in the pediatric population.

Diagnostic Imaging

- Plain radiography, especially the lateral view, can help rule in a radial head dislocation. The radiocapitellar line is drawn through the center of the proximal radius at the intersection with the center of the capitellum. A radial head dislocation should be suspected if the line does not pass through the capitellum.[60]

- Radiographs should be performed to rule out additional fractures.

II. Observation

- Child with guarded position of arm
- Arm pronated and in slight flexion

III. Triage and Screening

- All nonmusculoskeletal causes, as well as causes from related joints, should be ruled out.

- Olecranon-manubrium test: demonstrates good ability to help **rule out** (SN 84, –LR 0.3) and ideal ability to help **rule in** (SP 99, +LR 84) anterior shoulder dislocations, clavicle fractures, and humerus fractures.[75]

- The bony apprehension test: A (–) test has good ability to help **rule in** (SN 94, –LR 0.07) bony lesion.[77]

- Elbow extension test: A (–) test has ideal ability to help **rule in** (SN 95-100, –LR 0–0.06) fracture across three studies.[76, 78, 79]

- Elbow AROM: demonstrates ideal ability to help both **rule out** (SN 100, –LR 0) and **rule in** (SP97, +LR 33) fracture.[79]

- Clinicians should rule out cervical spine, shoulder, and neural tension from a more proximal cause.

IV. Motion Tests

- Clinicians should watch for pain reproduced with extension and pronation of the elbow, both actively and passively.

V. Muscle Performance Testing

- Clients are typically unable to perform testing secondary to pain.

VI. Special Tests

- Chair push-up test: A (−) test has less than good ability to help rule out (SN 88-100, −LR NR) posterolateral instability or dislocation across two studies.[98, 102]

- Tabletop relocation test: A (−) test has less than good ability to help rule out (SN 100, −LR NR) posterolateral instability or dislocation in one study.[102]

- Lateral pivot shift and posterolateral rotator drawer tests might have implications, but research currently does not provide high values for SN, and SP was not reported.

VII. Palpation

- Clients experience tenderness laterally at the radial head.

VIII. Physical Performance Measures

- No physical performance measures are available for radial head subluxation or dislocation.

POTENTIAL TREATMENT-BASED CLASSIFICATIONS

- Immobility or protection and pain modulation may be appropriate.

Cubital Tunnel Syndrome

ICD-9: 354.2 (lesion of ulnar nerve)

ICD-10: G56.20 (lesion of ulnar nerve, unspecified upper limb)

Symptoms of cubital tunnel syndrome are a result of compression on the ulnar nerve as it travels on the medial aspect of the elbow in the cubital tunnel, which is formed by the two heads of the flexor carpi ulnaris muscle, the humeroulnar aponeurosis, and the medial ligaments of the elbow. The amount of angulation at the elbow, or the carrying angle, can also predispose the client's risk for ulnar nerve symptoms; a study of 36 clients with electrophysiologically confirmed diagnosis of ulnar neuropathy.[119]

I. Client Interview

Subjective History

- Medial elbow pain and paresthesia occur distally on the ulnar side of the forearm and hand.

- Sensation loss occurs in the hypothenar region; sensation typically occurs prior to weakness.

- Clients have weakness of ulnar innervated intrinsic hand muscles.

- Clients have a history of repetitive elbow flexion or extension or prolonged elbow flexion.[120]

Outcome Measures

- The DASH and QuickDASH have demonstrated clinical relevance for all upper extremity disorders, although both are regional measures.

Diagnostic Imaging

- Electromyography and nerve conduction velocity are typically used as gold standard, although a large range of sensitivities exist in the diagnosis of cubital tunnel (37–86%); thus a better reference standard might exist.[58]

- US can be used to measure ulnar nerve CSA on transverse scans, and swelling ratio can differentiate normal elbows from clients who have ulnar neuropathy at the elbow.[57, 68, 121]

- US maximum CSA >10 mm helps both rule out (SN 50, −LR 0.58) and rule in (SP 85, +LR 3.4) ulnar neuropathy at the elbow. US forearm swelling ratio > 2.9 mm helps both rule out (SN 42, −LR 0.66) and rule in (SP 87, +LR 3.2) ulnar neuropathy at the elbow.[57, 58]

- MR evaluation of nerve T2 signal increase helps **rule out** (SN 83, −LR 0.2) and **rule in** (SN 85, +LR 5.5) ulnar neuropathy at the elbow.[59]

II. Observation

- Typically clients have a normal appearing presentation, with no significant observational findings.

III. Triage and Screening

- All nonmusculoskeletal causes, as well as causes from related joints, should be ruled out.

- Olecranon-manubrium test: demonstrates good ability to help **rule out** (SN 84, −LR 0.3) and ideal ability to help **rule in** (SP 99, +LR 84) anterior shoulder dislocations, clavicle fractures, and humerus fractures.[75]

- The bony apprehension test: A (−) test has good ability to help **rule in** (SN 94, −LR 0.07) bony lesion.[77]

- Elbow extension test: A (−) test has ideal ability to help **rule in** (SN 95-100, −LR 0–0.06) fracture across three studies.[76, 78, 79]

- Elbow AROM: demonstrates strong diagnostic accuracy to both **rule out** (SN 100, −LR 0) and **rule in** (SP97, +LR 33) fracture.[79]

- Clinicians should rule out cervical spine, shoulder, and neural tension from a more proximal cause. It is especially important to rule out cervical radiculopathy (C7-8), brachial plexus injury, medial epicondylalgia, and thoracic outlet syndrome.

IV. Motion Tests

- Sustained elbow flexion reproduces symptoms.

V. Muscle Performance Testing

- Clients have potential for weak intrinsic forearm and hand muscles.

VI. Special Tests

- Pressure provocation test: A (+) test has fair ability to help rule in (SP 98-99, +LR 45-46) cubital tunnel syndrome across two studies with high risk of bias.[18, 104]

- Elbow flexion test for cubital tunnel: A (+) test has less than good ability to help rule in (SP 99, +LR 74) cubital tunnel syndrome in one study with high risk of bias.[18]

- Tinel's sign: A (+) test has less than good ability to help rule in (SP 98-99, +LR 35-54) cubital tunnel syndrome across three studies.[18, 104, 105]

- Elbow scratch test: A (+) test has less than good ability to help rule in (SP 99, +LR 69) cubital tunnel syndrome.[104]

VII. Palpation

- Clients may experience tenderness at medial elbow (maximum area of symptoms is 1 in. distal to epicondyle).

VIII. Physical Performance Measures

- Grip strength

POTENTIAL TREATMENT-BASED CLASSIFICATIONS

- Activity modification, exercise and conditioning, and potentially pain modulation (if pain dominant) may be appropriate.

Distal Humeral Fractures

ICD-9: 812.41 (closed supracondylar fracture of humerus)

ICD-10: S42.416A (nondisplaced supracondylar fracture)

Acute injury or trauma, including falling on an outstretched arm, impact to elbow, or twisting injury, can result in fractures of the elbow joint.[122] Classification systems have been created to describe the various types of fracture of the distal humerus, separating the extra-articular and intra-articular fractures. Further, intra-articular fractures are subdivided into transcondylar and bicondylar or intercondylar (Muller Classification of Distal Humerus Fractures). Accounting for 60% of all pediatric elbow fractures, supracondylar fractures can increase the risk of neurovascular compromise. Involvement of the growth plate occurs in 20% to 25% of pediatric fractures.[60]

I. Client Interview

Subjective History

- History of acute trauma or fall.

- Hearing a pop or crack during time of trauma.

- Pain at rest.
- Occurs more frequently in pediatric clients.
- If neurovascular compromise occurs, clients have loss of nerve function, typically with median nerve during posterolateral fracture displacement.

Outcome Measures

- The DASH and QuickDASH have demonstrated clinical relevance for all upper extremity disorders, although both are regional measures. Since falls and fractures are common in pediatric clients, utility of this measure might be limited in the pediatric population.

Diagnostic Imaging

- Radiographs are typically the first line for determining if a fracture has occurred following trauma, but newer research has used range of motion to decrease the need for radiographs in clients who have preservation of elbow range of motion.[76, 79, 123]

- Radiography: Standard views of anteroposterior and lateral images should be taken. A supracondylar fracture may cause the anterior humeral line to be anterior to the capitellum (or less than one-third of the capitellum is in front of the line).[60]

- CT is used when comminuted fractures are present to help with 3-D reconstruction for determining classification and assisting in surgical planning.[44, 124, 125]

II. Observation

- After a fall, the client will present with the arm guarded against their body and a decreased willingness to move. Swelling, bruising, and decreased willingness to move are also present after a fracture.

- Clients with an open fracture will present with a posterior wound proximal to the elbow joint.

III. Triage and Screening

- All nonmusculoskeletal causes, as well as causes from related joints, should be ruled out.

- Olecranon-manubrium test: demonstrates good ability to help **rule out** (SN 84, −LR 0.3) and ideal ability to help **rule in** (SP 99, +LR 84) anterior shoulder dislocations, clavicle fractures, and humerus fractures.[75]

- The bony apprehension test: A (−) test has good ability to help **rule in** (SN 94, −LR 0.07) bony lesion.[77]

- Elbow extension test: A (−) test has ideal ability to help **rule in** (SN 94.6–100, −LR 0–0.06) fracture across three studies.[76, 78, 79]

- Elbow AROM: demonstrates ideal ability to help both **rule out** (SN 100, −LR 0) and **rule in** (SP 97, +LR 33) fracture.[79]

- Clinicians should rule out cervical spine, shoulder, and neural tension from a more proximal cause.

IV. Motion Tests

- Clients may experience pain with flexion and extension more than in pronation and supination (depending on regions of fracture), both actively and passively.

- Clients may show hesitancy to move.

V. Muscle Performance Testing

- Clients are unable to perform testing secondary to pain.

VI. Special Tests

- Elbow flexion test: A (+) test has ideal ability to help **rule in** (SP 100, +LR Inf) a fracture in one high-quality study.[79]

- Elbow pronation test: A (+) test has ideal ability to help **rule in** (SP 100, +LR Inf) a fracture in one high-quality study.[79]

- Elbow supination test: A (+) test has ideal ability to help **rule in** (SP 97, +LR 14.3) a fracture in one high-quality study.[79]

- Olecranon-manubrium test and elbow AROM: See Triage and Screening section.

VII. Palpation

- Clients may experience tenderness at the elbow joint, typically throughout the entire joint, but more exquisite tenderness at the proximal joint.

VIII. Physical Performance Measures

- No physical performance measures are available for distal humeral fractures.

POTENTIAL TREATMENT-BASED CLASSIFICATIONS

- Immobility and pain modulation may be appropriate.

Radial Fractures

ICD-9: 813.00-813.93 (fractures of radius and ulna)

ICD-10: S52.90XA (unspecified closed fracture of forearm)

Acute injury or trauma, including falling on an outstretched arm, impact to elbow, or twisting injury, can cause fractures of the elbow joint that result in the radial head being driven into the capitellum. Radial head fractures are the most common elbow fracture in adults. Fat pad signs can assist with diagnosis. The *terrible triad* is associated defined as radial head fracture plus medial collateral ligament tear or dislocation and coronoid process fracture due to tension and compression forces, respectively, on the joint.[60]

I. Client Interview

Subjective History

- Occurs more frequently in adults than children
- History of acute trauma or fall
- Hearing a pop or crack during time of trauma
- Pain at rest and with movement
- Potential for mechanics block if fragment is displaced

Outcome Measures

- The DASH and QuickDASH have demonstrated clinical relevance for all upper extremity disorders, although both are regional measures. Since falls and fractures are common in pediatric clients, utility of this measure might be limited in the pediatric population.

Diagnostic Imaging

- Radiographs are typically the first line for determining if a fracture has occurred following trauma, but newer research has used range of motion to decrease the need for radiographs in clients who have preservation of elbow range of motion.[76, 79, 123]
- Radiography: Standard views of anteroposterior and lateral images should be taken. The lateral radiographs can indicate a positive fat pad sign or anterior sail sign. If a fracture is not seen on traditional views, an oblique view or radial head capitellar view (variation of lateral view) might visualize the radial head fracture better.[60]
- CT is used when comminuted fractures are present to help with 3-D reconstruction for determining classification and assisting in surgical planning.[44, 124, 125]

II. Observation

- After a fall, the client will present with the arm guarded against their body and with a decreased willingness to move. Swelling, bruising, and decreased willingness to move are also present after a fracture.
- Clients may have extensor weakness if the radial nerve is involved.

III. Triage and Screening

- All nonmusculoskeletal causes, as well as causes from related joints, should be ruled out.
- Olecranon-manubrium test: demonstrates good ability to help **rule out** (SN 84, −LR 0.3) and ideal ability to help **rule in** (SP 99, +LR 84) anterior shoulder dislocations, clavicle fractures, and humerus fractures.[75]
- The bony apprehension test: A (−) test has good ability to help **rule in** (SN 94, −LR 0.07) bony lesion.[77]
- Elbow extension test: A (−) test has ideal ability to help **rule in** (SN 94.6–

100, −LR 0–0.06) fracture across three studies.[76, 78, 79]

- Elbow AROM: demonstrates ideal ability to help both **rule out** (SN 100, −LR 0) and **rule in** (SP 97, +LR 33) fracture.[79]

- Clinicians should rule out cervical spine, shoulder, and neural tension from a more proximal cause.

IV. Motion Tests

- Pain with pronation and supination is greater than that with flexion and extension, but all movements are painful, both active and passive.

- Clients may have possible extensor weakness if the radial nerve is involved.

- Clients may show hesitancy to move.

V. Muscle Performance Testing

- Clients are unable to perform testing secondary to pain.

VI. Special Tests

- Elbow flexion test: A (+) test has ideal ability to help **rule in** (SP 100, +LR Inf) a fracture in one high-quality study.[79]

- Elbow pronation test: A (+) test has ideal ability to help **rule in** (SP 100, +LR Inf) a fracture in one high-quality study.[79]

- Elbow supination test: A (+) test has ideal ability to help **rule in** (SP 97, +LR 14.3) a fracture in one high-quality study.[79]

- The olecranon-manubrium test demonstrates good ability to help **rule out** (SN 84, −LR 0.3) and ideal ability to help **rule in** (SP 99, +LR 84) anterior shoulder dislocations, clavicle fractures, and humerus fractures.[75]

- Elbow AROM: demonstrates ideal ability to help both **rule out** (SN 100, −LR 0) and **rule in** (SP97, +LR 33) fracture.[79]

VII. Palpation

- Clients will experience tenderness at the elbow joint, typically throughout the entire joint, but more exquisite tenderness at the lateral joint.

VIII. Physical Performance Measures

- No physical performance measures are available for radial fractures.

POTENTIAL TREATMENT-BASED CLASSIFICATIONS

- Immobility and pain modulation may be appropriate.

Olecranon Fractures

ICD-9: 813.00-813.93 (fractures of radius and ulna)

ICD-10: ~ S52.90XA (unspecified closed fracture of forearm)

Two mechanisms result in fractures to the olecranon. A low-energy fracture results secondary to sudden concurrent pulling of triceps and brachialis muscles, usually in the elderly. High-energy fractures occur after a direct trauma to the olecranon process due to a high-energy force (concurrent comminuted ulnar shaft fracture may be present).[60]

I. Client Interview

Subjective History

- Occurs more frequently in adults than in children.

- History of acute trauma or direct blow to olecranon or fall onto flexed elbow.

- Hearing a pop or crack during time of trauma.

- Pain at rest.

- With throwers or pitchers, microtrauma can result in fracture over time.

Outcome Measures

- The DASH and QuickDASH have demonstrated clinical relevance for all upper extremity disorders, although both are regional measures. Since falls and fractures are common in pediatric clients, utility of this measure might be limited in the pediatric population.

Diagnostic Imaging

- Radiographs are typically the first line for determining if a fracture has occurred following trauma, but newer research has used range of motion to decrease the need for radiographs in clients who have preservation of elbow range of motion.[76, 79, 123]

- Radiography: Standard views of anteroposterior and lateral images should be taken. The lateral view best identifies olecranon fractures.[60]

- CT is used when comminuted fractures are present to help with 3-D reconstruction for determining classification and assisting in surgical planning.[124, 125]

II. Observation

- After a fall, the client will present with the arm guarded against their body and with a decreased willingness to move. Swelling, bruising, and decreased willingness to move are also present after a fracture.

III. Triage and Screening

- All nonmusculoskeletal causes, as well as causes from related joints, should be ruled out.

- Olecranon-manubrium test: demonstrates good ability to help **rule out** (SN 84, −LR 0.3) and ideal ability **rule in** (SP 99, +LR 84) anterior shoulder dislocations, clavicle fractures, and humerus fractures.[75]

- The bony apprehension test: A (−) test has good ability to help **rule in** (SN 94, −LR 0.07) bony lesion.[77]

- Elbow extension test: A (−) test has ideal ability to help **rule in** (SN 95-100, −LR 0–0.06) fracture across three studies.[76, 78, 79]

- Elbow AROM: demonstrates ideal ability to help both **rule out** (SN 100, −LR 0) and **rule in** (SP 97, +LR 33) fracture.[79]

- Clinicians should rule out cervical spine, shoulder, and neural tension from a more proximal cause.

IV. Motion Tests

- Pain with flexion and extension is greater than that with pronation and supination, but all movements are painful, both active and passive.

- Clients may show hesitancy to move.

V. Muscle Performance Testing

- Clients are unable to perform testing secondary to pain.

VI. Special Tests

- Elbow flexion test: A (+) test has ideal ability to help **rule in** (SP 100, +LR Inf) a fracture in one high-quality study.[79]

- Elbow pronation test: A (+) test has ideal ability to help **rule in** (SP 100, +LR Inf) a fracture in one high-quality study.[79]

- Elbow supination test: A (+) test has ideal ability to help **rule in** (SP 97, +LR 14.3) a fracture in one high-quality study.[79]

- The olecranon-manubrium test demonstrates good ability to help **rule out** (SN 84, −LR 0.3) and ideal ability to help **rule in** (SP 99, +LR 84) anterior shoulder dislocations, clavicle fractures, and humerus fractures.[75]

- Elbow AROM: demonstrates ideal ability to help both **rule out** (SN 100, −LR 0) and **rule in** (SP 97, +LR 33) fracture.[79]

VII. Palpation

- Clients may have tenderness at the elbow joint, typically throughout the entire joint, but more exquisite tenderness at the posterior joint.

VIII. Physical Performance Measures

- No physical performance measures are available for olecranon fractures.

POTENTIAL TREATMENT-BASED CLASSIFICATIONS

- Immobility and pain modulation may be appropriate.

Complex Elbow Instability: Fracture or Dislocation

ICD-9: 812.41 (closed supracondylar fracture of humerus); 813.00-813.93 (fractures of radius and ulna)

ICD-10: S42.416A (nondisplaced supracondylar fracture); ~ S52.90XA (unspecified closed fracture of forearm)

Acute injury or trauma including fall on an outstretched arm, impact to elbow, or twisting injury, can result in fractures of the elbow joint.[126] Elbow dislocations are fairly common, and only the shoulder is dislocated more often. Typically dislocations are described for the direction of radial or ulnar displacement, and complex dislocations have associated fractures (commonly the radial head and coronoid process) and the potential for neurovascular injuries.[118] The most common direction of dislocation is a combined posterior dislocation of the ulna and radius. Other possible directions of dislocation include anterior, lateral, or divergent.

A distal radioulnar dislocation with associated comminuted radial head fracture has been named the Essex-Lopresti fracture or dislocation; it also tears the interosseous membrane between the radius and ulna. Often a large amount of force or trauma produces this type of fracture or dislocation.[127] Another type of dislocation has been identified as the *terrible triad*, when a posterior elbow dislocation, radial head fracture, and coronoid fracture occur (possible MCL tear).[128] A Monteggia fracture or dislocation involves the presence of radial head dislocation in combination with an ulnar fracture. Several classification systems exist for Monteggia and other fractures or dislocations. Often a Monteggia fracture occurs with a direct blow to the forearm, which was held in a protective manner.[60, 129]

I. Client Interview

Subjective History

- Occurs more frequently in adults than children
- History of acute fall on outstretched arm with forced pronation, direct force when trying to protect self
- Hearing a pop or crack during time of trauma
- Pain at rest

Outcome Measures

- The DASH and QuickDASH have demonstrated clinical relevance for all upper extremity disorders, although both are regional measures. Since falls and fractures are common in pediatric clients, utility of this measure might be limited in the pediatric population.

Diagnostic Imaging

- Radiographs are typically the first line for determining if a fracture has occurred following trauma, but newer research has used range of motion to decrease the need for radiographs in clients who

have preservation of elbow range of motion.[76, 79, 123]

- Radiography: Standard views of anteroposterior and lateral images should be taken. Additional views including oblique views can help with diagnosis since radial head dislocation can be missed on radiographs.[60]
- CT is used when comminuted fractures are present to help with 3-D reconstruction for determining classification and assisting in surgical planning.[124, 125]

II. Observation

- After a fall, the client will present with the arm guarded against their body and with a decreased willingness to move. Swelling, bruising, and decreased willingness to move are also present after a fracture.
- The client may have extensor weakness if the radial nerve is involved.

III. Triage and Screening

- All nonmusculoskeletal causes, as well as causes from related joints, should be ruled out.
- Olecranon-manubrium test: demonstrates good ability to help **rule out** (SN 84, −LR 0.3) and ideal ability to help **rule in** (SP 99, +LR 84) anterior shoulder dislocations, clavicle fractures, and humerus fractures.[75]
- The bony apprehension test: A (−) test has good ability to help **rule in** (SN 94, −LR 0.07) bony lesion.[77]
- Elbow extension test: A (−) test has ideal ability to help **rule in** (SN 95-100, −LR 0–0.06) fracture across three studies.[76, 78, 79]
- Elbow AROM: demonstrates ideal ability to help both **rule out** (SN 100, −LR 0) and **rule in** (SP 97, +LR 33) fracture.[79]
- Clinicians should rule out cervical spine, shoulder, and neural tension from a more proximal cause.

IV. Motion Tests

- Clients experience pain with pronation, supination, flexion, and extension; all movements are painful, both active and passive.

- Clients may have possible extensor weakness if the radial nerve is involved.
- Clients may show hesitancy to move.

V. Muscle Performance Testing

- Clients are unable to perform testing secondary to pain.

VI. Special Tests

- Elbow flexion test: A (+) test has ideal ability to help **rule in** (SP 100, +LR Inf) a fracture in one high-quality study.[79]
- Elbow pronation test: A (+) test has ideal ability to help **rule in** (SP 100, +LR Inf) a fracture in one high-quality study.[79]
- Elbow supination test: A (+) test has ideal ability to help **rule in** (SP 97, +LR 14.3) a fracture in one high-quality study.[79]
- The olecranon-manubrium test demonstrates good ability to help **rule out** (SN 84, –LR 0.3) and ideal ability to help **rule in** (SP 99, +LR 84) anterior shoulder dislocations, clavicle fractures, and humerus fractures.[75]
- Elbow AROM: demonstrates ideal ability to help both **rule out** (SN 100, –LR 0) and **rule in** (SP 97, +LR 33) fracture.[79]

VII. Palpation

- Clients may experience tenderness at the elbow joint, typically throughout the entire joint, but more exquisite tenderness at the area of greatest joint disruption.

VIII. Physical Performance Measures

- No physical performance measures are available for complex elbow instability.

POTENTIAL TREATMENT-BASED CLASSIFICATIONS

- Immobility and pain modulation may be appropriate.

Elbow Osteoarthritis ▪ ▪ ▪ ▪ ▪ ▪ ▪

ICD-9: 715.12 (osteoarthrosis, localized, primary, upper arm)

ICD-10:M19.029 (primary osteoarthritis, unspecified elbow)

Elbow osteoarthritis (OA) is typically the result of idiopathic primary OA or of stiffness acquired post-traumatically.[130] Elbow OA is more common in men with a history of heavy upper extremity lifting or manual labor with initial findings at ends of motion, but as the disease progresses, pain is present throughout the entire range.[131] After any trauma to the elbow, post-traumatic arthritis may develop with pain and the possibility of associated impingement or nerve entrapment.[69] Clients with rheumatoid arthritis (RA) can develop elbow symptoms, complaining of pain throughout the arc of motion, with greater reports of pain laterally. The presence of RA should be ruled out.

I. Client Interview

Subjective History

- Gradual onset of pain and decreased ROM or function, with possible previous history of trauma
- Complaints of crepitus, grinding, or popping
- Character of pain: dull, ache
- Possible disruption of sleep
- Pain increases with activity and reduces with rest or heat
- Occurs more in men than in women[131]
- Age: middle to older age for primary, lower age with RA or previous trauma[61]
- Decreased strength

Outcome Measures

- The DASH and QuickDASH have demonstrated clinical relevance for all upper extremity disorders, although both are regional measures.

Diagnostic Imaging

- Radiographic findings include joint space narrowing, bone sclerosis, periarticular cysts, and osteophytes. Refer to chapter 6 for a definition of OA according to Kellgren and Lawrence.[132]
- AP, lateral with elbow at 90° flexion, and radiocapitellar radiographs are routinely performed even though no statically significant differences were present between normal elbows and those with primary OA.[61, 69]

- Development of classification system predictive of positive postoperative outcome is as follows:[61]
  - Class I: absence of degenerative changes in radiocapitellar joint but positive for degenerative changes in ulnotrochlear joint with presence of coronoid and olecranon spurring
  - Class II: mild joint space narrowing in radiocapitellar joint with marginal ulnotrochlear arthrosis
  - Class III: changes present in both classes I and II with radiocapitellar subluxation

II. Observation

- Clients may appear normal, with no significant observational findings. The client has potential of reduced functional ROM; if pain is dominant, the client might guard their arm against their body.

III. Triage and Screening

- All nonmusculoskeletal causes, as well as causes from related joints, should be ruled out.

- Olecranon-manubrium test: demonstrates good ability to help **rule out** (SN 84, −LR 0.3) and ideal ability to help **rule in** (SP 99, +LR 84) anterior shoulder dislocations, clavicle fractures, and humerus fractures.[75]

- The bony apprehension test: A (−) test has good ability to help **rule in** (SN 94, −LR 0.07) bony lesion.[77]

- Elbow extension test: A (−) test has ideal ability to help **rule in** (SN 95-100, −LR 0–0.06) fracture across three studies.[76, 78, 79]

- Elbow AROM: demonstrates ideal ability to help both **rule out** (SN 100, −LR 0) and **rule in** (SP 97, +LR 33) fracture.[79]

- Other types of arthritis should be ruled out, including rheumatoid arthritis and psoriatic arthritis, so a blood test might be indicated.

- Rare conditions of Lyme disease and acute infection can also manifest themselves in this joint and should be considered.[133]

IV. Motion Tests

- Clients might demonstrate reduction in motion in many directions. The location of symptoms will be influenced by previous trauma or repetitive activities and the location in the joint that was overstressed as a result of both of those.

- Primary limitations and pain will be present with forced flexion and extension of the elbow; less than 100° of total arc of motion will be possible.[61]

V. Muscle Performance Testing

- Clients show a slight reduction in strength globally but can display normal strength within pain-free ROM.

VI. Special Tests

- No special tests are described for osteoarthritis. As with all comprehensive examinations, screening out other competing diagnoses is paramount.

VII. Palpation

- Clients may experience possible (non-localized) tenderness around the elbow joint.

VIII. Physical Performance Measures

- Grip strength

POTENTIAL TREATMENT-BASED CLASSIFICATIONS

- Mobility and exercise and conditioning may be appropriate.

Osteochondritis Dissecans

ICD-9: 732.7 (osteochondritis dissecans)

ICD-10: M93.20 (osteochondritis dissecans of unspecified site)

Fragmentation of the articular cartilage of the elbow joint, or osteochondritis dissecans, can be a result of microtrauma to the elbow joint. Often the trauma creates an ischemic change or decreased blood flow in the area and compromises the cartilage integrity.

I. Client Interview

Subjective History

- Adolescence
- Pain increases with movement, especially extremes of motion
- Male–female ratio is 3:1
- History of significant trauma in >50%
- Poorly localized, possible deep pain
- Dominant arm
- Popping, clicking
- History of racquetball, baseball, gymnastics, or heavy weightlifting

Outcome Measures

- The DASH and QuickDASH have demonstrated clinical relevance for all upper extremity disorders, although both are regional measures.

Diagnostic Imaging

- Radiographs are typically the first line for determining if a fracture has occurred following trauma, but newer research has used range of motion to decrease the need for radiographs in clients who have preservation of elbow range of motion.[76, 79, 123]
- MRI is used to determine amount and location of cartilage damage and to augment radiographs.[50]

II. Observation

- If injury is acute, swelling and ecchymosis might be present.
- Clients may exhibit signs of distress during active movement and potential catching during motion.

III. Triage and Screening

- All nonmusculoskeletal causes, as well as causes from related joints, should be ruled out.
- Olecranon-manubrium test: demonstrates good ability to help **rule out** (SN 84, −LR 0.3) and ideal ability to help **rule in** (SP 99, +LR 84) anterior shoulder dislocations, clavicle fractures, and humerus fractures.[75]
- The bony apprehension test: A (−) test has good ability to help **rule in** (SN 94, −LR 0.07) bony lesion.[77]
- Elbow extension test: A (−) test has ideal ability to help **rule in** (SN 94.6–100, −LR 0–0.06) fracture across three studies.[76, 78, 79]
- Elbow AROM: demonstrates ideal ability to help both **rule out** (SN 100, −LR 0) and **rule in** (SP 97, +LR 33) fracture.[79]
- Clinicians should rule out cervical spine, shoulder, and neural tension from a more proximal cause.

IV. Motion Tests

- Clients exhibit decreased motion and pain with end-range extension and flexion.

V. Muscle Performance Testing

- Testing should be within normal limits.

VI. Special Tests

- Active radiocapitellar compression test: The client pronates and supinates their forearm while flexing and extending the elbow.

VII. Palpation

- Typically no specific tenderness occurs secondary to deep palpation; potential for tenderness at muscular structures secondary to irritation to those structures has developed.

VIII. Physical Performance Measures

- Grip strength
- Functional activity or performance

POTENTIAL TREATMENT-BASED CLASSIFICATIONS

- Mobility, pain modulation, and exercise and conditioning may be appropriate.

CONCLUSION

A structured orthopedic evaluation and examination sequence assists clinicians in determining the origin of the client's symptoms and generating both a treatment-based classification and pathoanatomical diagnosis. The client interview consisting of subjective findings, outcome measures, results from diagnostic imaging, and observation provides sig-

nificant information to the clinician. After the client interview, the clinician should use the examination to first rule out serious pathology through triage and then use the remainder of the sequence (motion testing, muscle performance, special tests, palpation, and physical performance measures) to confirm the involved structures. Synthesis of the information gathered during the examination provides the clinician with impairments and treatment interventions for creating a client-centered rehabilitation program.

23

WRIST AND HAND

Jonathan Sylvain, PT, DPT, OCS, FAAOMPT
Michael P. Reiman, PT, DPT, OCS, SCS, ATC, FAAOMPT, CSCS
Gary P. Austin, PT, PhD, OCS, FAFS, FAAOMPT

The wrist and hand (WH) complex is composed of many static and dynamic components. The interplay and intricate balance of these structures allows for incredible power, dexterity, and precision. Disruption of any of these components significantly affects each client's ability to perform activities of daily living and occupational or recreational tasks. The WH is an extremely active portion of the upper extremity but is tremendously vulnerable to injury.[1,][2] The challenge during the examination of the wrist and hand lies in accurately revealing the causative component in order to ascertain the most effective treatment approach. Often times diagnosis is vague and uninformative; therefore, during each client interaction, including clients with WH-region pain, components of the clinical examination (including, but not limited to, the subjective history, outcome measures, diagnostic imaging, objective examination, and special testing) should involve assessments with their own ability to shift the probability of a particular diagnosis. This chapter presents an evidence-based approach in the examination of the WH complex.

CLINICALLY APPLIED ANATOMY

The distal radioulnar joint is in very close proximity to the wrist (see chapter 22 for greater detail). Some detail is given here due to its relationship with the wrist and hand. This joint is a pivot joint that unites the distal radius and ulna with the articular disc, or triangular fibrocartilage complex (TFCC). The TFCC assists in adjoining the radius, and it is the primary stabilizer of the distal radioulnar joint. The TFCC also transmits an axial load from the hand to the forearm and cushions weight-bearing forces, and it is an attachment site for ligaments (figure 23.1).

The wrist is made up of eight carpal bones arranged in two rows, proximal and distal. The scaphoid, lunate, triquetrum, and pisiform carpal bones make up the proximal row, while the trapezium, trapezoid, capitate, and hamate carpal bones make up the distal row (figure 23.2). Collectively, the carpal bones of the proximal row have a convex shape proximally and concave shape distally. Distally from the carpal bones are the metacarpals and then the phalanges. The metacarpal bones make up the dorsum (dorsal surface) and palm (volar

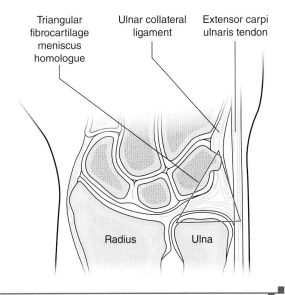

Figure 23.1 Articular disc as part of the triangular fibrocartilage complex (TFCC).

surface) of the hand. These bones have little movement on each other. The phalanges, on the other hand, must have a significant amount of movement in order to allow the hand to manipulate objects.

Due to several variables (multiple small bones, the presence of several joints, and the amount of movement necessary for the hand to manipulate objects), proper stability in the hand requires an

intricate working relationship of the multiple muscles used to move the hand and the ligaments that stabilize the multiple joints (figure 23.3). Proper stability of the hand is necessary for the muscles to perform their tasks.

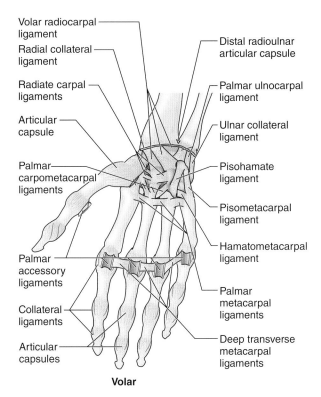

Volar

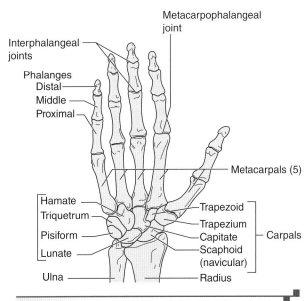

Figure 23.2 Bones of the wrist and hand.

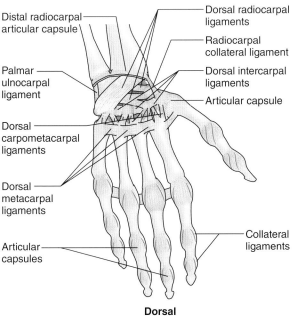

Dorsal

Figure 23.3 Volar (palmar) and dorsal ligaments of the wrist and hand.

Several of these carpal bones have characteristics important to the clinician. The scaphoid bone makes up the floor of the anatomical snuffbox (figure 23.4). The scaphoid is also the most commonly fractured carpal bone. The commonly described mechanism for such a fracture is a fall on an outstretched hand (FOOSH) injury. The lunate is also susceptible to FOOSH injury, with the potential for subluxation or dislocation. The capitate is the most central and largest of the carpal bones. Distally it articulates with the third metacarpal bone. It is considered the keystone of the proximal transverse arch of the hand. The hook of the hamate is attached to the flexor retinaculum.

The extensor and flexor retinacula of the wrist prevent bowstringing of the extensor and flexor tendons, respectively. This allows for mechanical efficiency of wrist and hand movements. The flexor retinaculum (transverse carpal ligament) is commonly described as a contributor to the pathology of carpal tunnel syndrome due to its compression of the median nerve in the carpal tunnel (figure 23.5). Surgical correction of this pathology often involves partially releasing this retinaculum to decrease the pressure on the median nerve.

The anatomical structure of the fingers involves a complex interaction of tendons and ligamentous support. At the level of the metacarpophalangeal (MCP) joint, the tendon of the extensor digitorum fans out to cover the posterior aspect of the joint, much like a hood. A complex tendon covering the posterior (dorsal) aspect of the digits is formed by

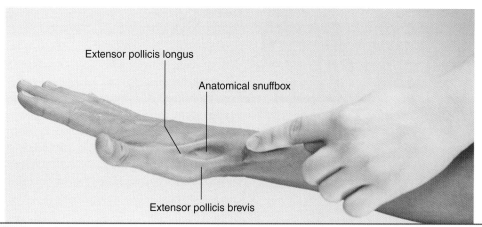

Figure 23.4 Anatomical snuffbox.

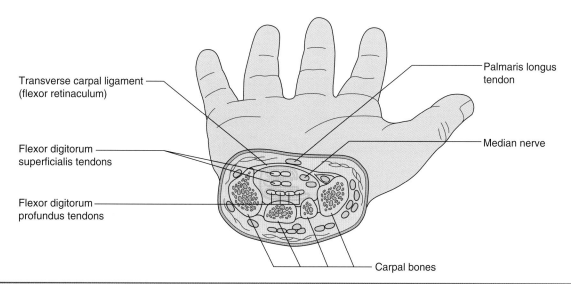

Figure 23.5 Transverse view of the carpal tunnel, showing the median nerve and flexor tendons.

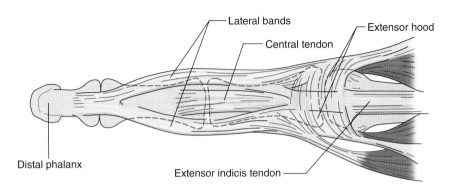

Figure 23.6 Extensor hood and tendons.

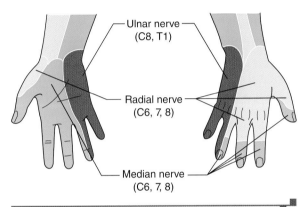

Figure 23.7 Innervations for the volar and dorsal aspects of the hand.

a combination of tendons and insertion from the extensor digitorum, extensor indicis, and the extensor digiti minimi (figure 23.6).

The innervation of the hand is complex. As demonstrated in figure 23.7, the three primary nerves of the arm (ulnar, radial, and median) all provide innervation to the hand. Understanding the complexity of nerve innervation here can assist the clinician with differential diagnosis of nerve-related symptoms.

CLIENT INTERVIEW

This interview is typically the first encounter the clinician has with the client. As previously discussed in chapter 5 (Client Interview and Observation), this component of the examination can provide the clinician with a significant amount of information relevant to the probability of the client's presenting diagnosis. For purposes of this text, the interview is described relative to each body part or section but generally includes subjective reports by the client, as well as findings from their outcome measures. Also included in this section is radiographic imaging. While clinicians should avoid biasing their examination by interpreting findings of radiographic imaging prior to seeing clients (in most cases without concerns for red flags and major medical-related issues), this point in the examination is most likely where clinicians will encounter radiographic imaging. Additionally, in some instances, clinicians must interpret radiographic imaging early in the examination to rule out serious pathology prior to continuing with other components of the examination sequence.

Subjective

Most injuries of the wrist and hand are obvious, but often it can be difficult to detect subtle injuries. Therefore, a systematic examination is vital. Furthermore, when examining the distal upper extremities, the clinician should screen proximal structures to determine if they are involved in the client's presentation. The subjective examination will provide relevant clues beneficial for differential diagnosis and will assist in determining the scope of the physical examination.

As with all areas of the body, when examining the client with musculoskeletal pain, early in the examination the clinician must clearly understand the nature of the condition, the mechanism of injury, if present, and the concordant sign. Details of the nature of the condition and mechanism of injury can be extremely helpful in determining the potential pain generator. Falling on an outstretched hand, for example, has been shown to be a common mechanism for wrist and hand trauma[3] resulting in fractures of the distal radius[4] and scaphoid bones.[5] Also, repetitive microtrauma is particularly common in the wrist and hand, leading to carpal tunnel and various tenosynovitis pathologies.[6-9] The reason for the repetitive nature of the pain onset must also be determined (e.g., occupation, recreational activities, hobbies).

The wrist and hand region is a vital component with activities of daily living, recreational activities, hobbies, and work-related activities. Therefore, the effect of the client's pain on their daily function must be determined. The clinician must clearly understand the specific tasks, whether they are daily, work, or hobby tasks, most commonly affected by the injury in order to determine the extent of the impairment to the client. For example, if the greatest disability is with an infrequent activity, it is much less likely to affect the client's function than a task that the client is required to do frequently on a daily basis, such as typing for an administrative assistant.

Clinicians must inquire about the client's age and occupation, the location and longevity of the symptoms, when the symptoms are at their worse and when they are relieved, the functional tasks that aggravate or relieve the symptoms, previous treatment, and any diagnostic test or imaging performed as well as what the results were.

The clinician should also be concerned with the presence and location of altered sensation, such as numbness and tingling. For example, nocturnal paresthesia is considered a classic symptom of carpal tunnel syndrome. However, its presence in isolation does not appear to have significant diagnostic accuracy (sensitivity [SN] 77, specificity [SP] 27, +LR 1.1, −LR 0.9).[10] The wrist and hand neurovascular system is quite complex and proficient. Decreased sensation to the touch described by the client should alert the clinician to potential neurovascular compromise. The presence of altered sensation in the median nerve, although suggestive of carpal tunnel or median nerve compromise, has been shown to only minimally assist in the potential to rule in (SP 67, +LR 1.2) such pathology.[11]

Outcome Measures

Outcome assessment has become important in evaluating the efficacy and effectiveness of treatment procedures. Commonly used outcome measures specifically utilized for the wrist and hand are the Disabilities of the Arm, Shoulder, and Hand (DASH) question-

naire, QuickDASH, Patient-Specific Functional Scale (PSFS), Patient-Rated Wrist Evaluation questionnaire (PRWE), Patient-Rated Wrist/Hand Evaluation questionnaire (PRWHE), the Brigham and Women's carpal tunnel questionnaire (CTQ), and the Gartland and Werley score. These outcome measures for the wrist and hand typically include measures common to the rest of the upper extremity (namely the DASH and QuickDASH), common overall measures (such as the PSFS), and those more exclusive to the wrist and hand (such as PRWE, CTQ, and Gartland and Werley score). The complexity of the wrist and hand, in several aspects, exceeds that of many other areas of the body. Outcome measures are such an area. Therefore, greater detail on the respective outcome measures is given for the wrist and hand measures here than in most of the other chapters.

The DASH[12] and QuickDASH[13] are measures commonly used with clients presenting with limitation throughout the upper extremity that assess symptoms and function, as discussed in chapters 21 (Shoulder) and 22 (Elbow and Forearm). Within the wrist and hand, the DASH has demonstrated very good validity,[13-15] good reliability,[13-17] and very good responsiveness.[13-15, 18, 19] Minimal detectable change (MDC) and minimal clinical important difference (MCID) are 13.7[16, 20] and 10.0 to 10.83 (SN 82, SP 74)[16, 21, 22] The QuickDASH has demonstrated good validity,[13, 17] reliability,[13, 17] and responsiveness.[13, 23] MDC and MCID are 11.0[23] and 8.0 to 15.91 (SN 79-80, SP 75-77).[22, 24, 25]

The PSFS is a generic outcome measure that assesses function. It is completed by the client. Clients rate their ability to complete up to three activities on an 11-point scale.[26] The PSFS has demonstrated good validity (construct and concurrent),[27] reliability,[27] and responsiveness[27] in clients with upper extremity musculoskeletal problems. MDC and MCID have been found to be 3.0[27] and 1.16 (SN 88, SP 79).[27]

The CTQ is a diagnosis-specific measure that assesses client's symptoms and function. It consists of a 19-item questionnaire in which clients rate the severity of their symptoms (symptom severity score, known as SSS) and functional status with carpal tunnel syndrome.[28] The CTQ has demonstrated fair validity,[14, 28] good reliability[14, 28] and responsiveness.[29] MCID in clients post injection in the SSS component of the CTQ is 1.04.[30] In postoperative clients, MCID is 0.92 overall, and 1.14 in SSS and 0.74 in FSS.[31]

The PRWE is a 15-item questionnaire, completed by the client, that rates wrist-related pain and disability in functional activities and specific tasks.[32] The PRWE has demonstrated fair validity[14, 32] and good reliability[14, 32] and responsiveness.[14, 18] MDC and MCID have been found to be 12.2[20] and 14.[22] The PRWE was modified to include the hand and the wrist, becoming the PRWHE.[19] The PRWHE is similar to the PRWE. It is a 15-item questionnaire, completed by the client, that rates wrist- and hand-related pain and disability in functional activities and specific tasks. The PRWHE has demonstrated good validity,[33] reliability,[14, 33] and responsiveness.[19] MDC and MCID are currently not available.

The Gartland and Werley measures function and is region specific to the wrist and hand. Unlike the previously mentioned measures, the clinician completes scoring after the client has been examined.

This system is based on a demerit point system, which involves an objective evaluation of wrist function.[34] No validity or reliability studies have been carried out to date. It is one of the few outcome measures that provides an objective evaluation of outcome, and it is popular among orthopedic surgeons.[14]

Diagnostic Imaging

Different imaging techniques used for the WH are likely dependent on the pathology. The specific diagnostic accuracy of the most commonly used imaging modalities for the WH is listed in table 23.1.

TABLE 23.1 **Diagnostic Accuracy of Imaging Modalities for the Wrist and Hand**

Pathology	Diagnostic test	Reference standard	SN/SP
Osteoarthritis	MRI	Variable	61/82[35]#
		Histology	74/76[35]#
		Radiographs	61/81[35]#
Carpal tunnel	EMG	Clinical findings	**91/81**[36]
	MRI		43-88/40-100*[36]
	CT		Pooled analysis: 68-97/48-87*[36]
	US		Pooled analysis: 77-88/46-79*[36]
		Clinical or electrodiagnostic testing	Pooled analysis: **87/83**[37]
		Electrodiagnostic testing	Pooled analysis: **78/87**[38]
			Pooled analysis: **84/78**[39]
Extensor tendon rupture	CT	Arthroscopy	33-95/82-99^[40]
Distal radius fracture	Radiography	CT	75/68[41]
TFCC injury	MRI	Arthroscopy	Pooled analysis: 75/81[42]
			Pooled results: **83/80**[43]
			100/90[44]
	MRA		Pooled analysis: **84/95**[42]
	X-ray arthrography	Variable	Pooled analysis: 76/93[45]
Scaphoid fracture	Bone scintigraphy	Variable	Pooled analysis: **97/89**[46]
			94-100[47]/60-95[48]
	MRI	Clinical testing	Pooled analysis: **96/99**[46]
			100/100[49]
	CT	Arthroscopy	77/86[50]
		Clinical testing/radiographs	**89-97/85-91**[51]
			94/100[52]
	Radiographs	Arthroscopy	45/95[50]

= The Menashe study[35] investigated osteoarthritis in multiple joints (hip, knee, and hand). The majority of studies were performed on knee osteoarthritis. * = diagnostic accuracy dependent on location modality utilized; ^ = diagnostic accuracy dependent on tendon involved; EMG = electromyography; MRI = magnetic resonance imaging; MRA = magnetic resonance arthrography; CT = computed tomography; TFCC = triangular fibrocartilaginous complex; US = ultrasound

The color coding for suggestion of **good** and **ideal** diagnostic accuracy values reported in this table are without quality scoring (QUADAS), a very important aspect of determination of the clinical utility of such values. Therefore, it is suggested that the reader keep this in mind when interpreting such values.

Routine radiographic imaging can often serve as the primary imaging modality, especially with fractures. Advanced imaging techniques such as radionuclide bone imaging, computed tomography (CT), or magnetic resonance imaging (MRI) should not be first choice modalities in clients with distal radius fractures (figure 23.8) or scaphoid fractures (figure 23.9), and should be used only when conventional radiographs are inconclusive. Scintigraphy can be helpful for diagnosing occult fractures and for documenting fracture healing and ligamentous or cartilaginous post-traumatic disorders, as well as for diagnosis and follow-up of reflex sympathetic dystrophy. A disadvantage of scintigraphy is its poor localization of pathology. Indications for CT include the confirmation of occult fractures suspected on the basis of the findings of physical examination and focally hot bone scintigrams when plain films are normal or inconclusive. In comparison with conventional radiography, CT is superior for the preoperative evaluation of complex comminuted distal radius fractures, depicting the distal radial articular surface and size and position of fracture fragments, as well as for the assessment of fracture healing. Additionally, CT is the imaging technique of choice for the correct diagnosis of subluxations of the distal radioulnar joint. MRI is an important diagnostic technique for the evaluation of suspected injuries of soft tissues related to distal radius fractures, such as to the flexor and extensor tendons or the median nerve, and for the early diagnosis of necrosis of the scaphoid or lunate (figure 23.10). Other indications include identification of triangular fibrocartilage complex perforations (figure 23.11), ruptures of carpal ligaments, and demonstration of contents of the carpal tunnel.[53]

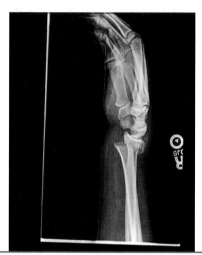

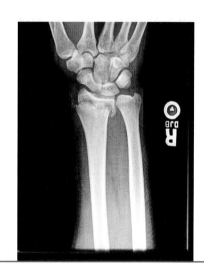

Figure 23.8   Radiograph: distal radius fracture.
© MedPix

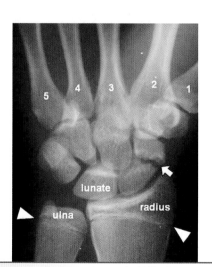

Figure 23.9   Radiograph: scaphoid fracture.
© MedPix

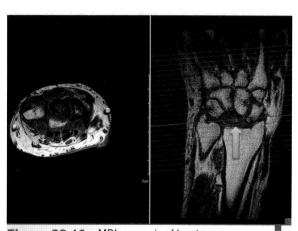

Figure 23.10   MRI: necrosis of lunate.
© MedPix

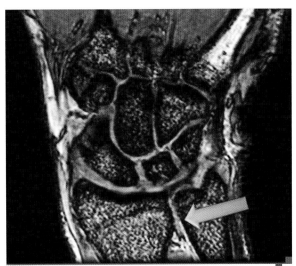

Figure 23.11   MRI: triangular fibrocartilage complex perforations.

© MedPix

Radiographs

As with imaging of all other areas of the body, radiographs are typically the most readily available imaging modality to the clinician investigating wrist and hand dysfunction. As noted previously, radiographs are often the first choice imaging modality with fracture pathologies of the WH.

Magnetic Resonance Imaging

MRI diffusion-weighted imaging of peripheral nerves might prove to be the most useful imaging sequence for the detection of early nerve dysfunction. Electrodiagnostic studies are likely to remain the pivotal diagnostic examination in clients with suspected carpal tunnel syndrome (CTS) for the foreseeable future. With advances in both software and hardware, however, high-resolution MRI imaging of peripheral nerves will become faster, cheaper, and likely more accurate, possibly paving the way for an expanded role in the diagnosis of this common syndrome.[54]

Ultrasound

In sonographically accessible regions, US is the preferred initial imaging modality for anatomic evaluation of suspected peripheral nervous system lesions. Imaging frequently detects peripheral nerve pathology and contributes to the differential diagnosis in clients with mononeuropathies and brachial plexopathies. Ultrasound is more SN than MRI (93% vs. 67%), and it has equivalent SP (86%) and better identifies multifocal lesions than MRI.[55]

Ultrasound (US) is more frequently being utilized for several pathologies, including carpal tunnel. The clinical value of it is still being determined. Currently, US using cross-sectional area of the median nerve is not an acceptable alternative to electrodiagnostic testing for diagnosis of carpal tunnel syndrome, but it could give complementary results.[39, 56] High-frequency diagnostic ultrasound of the hand, wrist, and elbow has significant potential to improve the quality of diagnosis and care provided by neuromuscular and musculoskeletal specialists. In clients referred for weakness, pain, and numbness of the hand, wrist, or elbow, diagnostic ultrasound can be an adjunct to electrodiagnosis and can help in identifying ruptured tendons and treating conditions such as carpal tunnel syndrome or trigger finger. Clinicians should use a small high-frequency (>10 MHz) transducer, an instrument with a blunt-pointed tip to enhance sonopalpation, and a model of the hand, wrist, and elbow to enhance visualization of small anatomical structures and complex bony contours. A range of conditions, including tendon and ligament ruptures, trigger finger, de Quervain tenosynovitis, intersection syndrome, lateral epicondylitis, and osteoarthritis, can be assessed with US.[57]

Review of Systems

Refer to chapter 6 (Triage and Differential Diagnosis) for detail on review of systems relevant to the wrist and hand.

OBSERVATION

A general observable event occurs during the initial contact and introduction with the client. When greeting the client, the clinician may observe the client's subsequent refusal or willingness to move, apprehension, or hand substitution, which can possibly indicate the significance of pain with such tasks as handshaking and therefore the client's reluctance to use the injured hand. Observation of the hand in the resting position can be useful in identifying hand dysfunction. Clinicians should observe the wrists and hands from both the anterior and posterior aspects. Loss of normal posturing may be caused by pathology. For example, a client presenting with a flexed finger may have a disrupted extensor tendon; conversely, a client with an extended finger may have a disrupted flexor tendon.

Clinicians should also assess hand textures and contours of the skin of bilateral upper extremities, specifically looking for changes in skin color or ability to sweat, which may indicate a digital nerve injury; capillary refill insufficiencies, which may indicate microvascular compromise; two-point discrimination difficulties, which may indicate neurologic compromise;[58] edema, which may be related to soft-tissue injuries or fracture; or significant atrophy, which may be associated with an upper motor neuron lesion[59] or peripheral nerve, or nerve root, injury. Assessment of edema or significant atrophy typically will occur during the observation component of the exam. Most often it is useful to obtain an objective measure to assess for change during subsequent visits. Assessment of swelling with the use of the figure-eight method or obtaining volumetric measurements has demonstrated good validity ($r = 0.92$–0.94) and reliability (ICC = 0.98–0.99).[60]

Typically the resting position of the hand is slight wrist flexion involving the metacarpophalangeal, proximal interphalangeal, and distal interphalangeal joints. Clients presenting with various nerve palsies may display muscle wasting or altered resting positions of the wrist and hand. Radial nerve palsy results in the inability to extend the wrist; thus the client may present with flexed wrist posturing. Median nerve palsy results in the inability to appropriately perform pinching tasks due to weakness in the flexor pollicis longus and flexor digitorum profundus. During pinching, the client will exhibit pad-to-pad pinching with the inability to flex the interphalangeal joint.

TRIAGE AND SCREENING

Triage and screening is a necessary component of the examination process that must be completed prior to continuing with the examination. As with all specific body part examinations, at this point the clinician must decide whether or not to continue with the examination. Specifically, they should determine whether to continue examining the client or refer them to a physician. Ruling out serious pathology (refer to chapter 6, Triage and Differential Diagnosis) and pain generation from other related (or close-proximity) structures assists the clinician with more accurately determining the necessity of continuing with the other examination components to identify the actual source of the client's pain. Additionally, clinicians should implement strong screening tests (tests of high SN and low –LR) at this point in the examination to narrow down the competing diagnoses of the respective body region (cervical spine and more proximal upper extremity in this case) when this is applicable.

The clinician must be aware of disorders affecting the wrist and hand that require the need for medical intervention, such as fractures or dislocations that occur due to trauma. Refer to chapters 4 and 6 for additional detail on differential diagnosis.

Ruling Out Serious Pathology: Red Flags

Special testing for potential red flags related to fracture or dislocation of the forearm, wrist, and hand should utilize the use of a tuning fork, active and passive range of motion assessments, palpation, and a gripping assessment.

TUNING FORK

Client Position	Supine or sitting with upper extremity relaxed
Clinician Position	Standing at the side of the upper extremity to be assessed, directly facing the client
Movement	The clinician places a stethoscope on the proximal aspect of the respective phalange, metacarpal, radius, or ulna. The clinician taps and places the tuning fork on the distal aspect of the respective phalange, metacarpal, radius, or ulna.
Assessment	A (+) test is a muffled or absent sound.
Statistics	• Placement over bony landmark: SN 83, SP 80, +LR 4.2, –LR 0.21, QUADAS 6, in a study of 37 clients (ages 7-60 years, 18 females) with various locations and types of fractures, using a criterion reference of radiography[61] • Placement over swelling area: SN 83, SP 92, +LR 10.4, –LR 0.2, in the same study[61]

Physical Findings for Wrist Fracture Following Acute Trauma

Physical findings found most useful in screening for wrist fracture for clients with acute wrist trauma are the following:[62]

- Localized tenderness (SN 94)
- Pain on active motion (SN 97)
- Pain on passive motion (SN 94)
- Pain on grip (SN 71)
- Pain on supination (SN 68)

A client presenting with any of the preceding findings who has a history of trauma should be sent for radiographs.

Clinical Prediction Rule for Acute Pediatric Wrist Injuries

A clinical prediction rule was developed to attempt to identify clinical variables that are most likely to be associated with acute pediatric wrist injuries. Significant variables included the following:

- Reduction in grip strength ≥ 20% compared to contralateral side
- Distal radius point tenderness
- Statistics: SN 79, SP 63, +LR 2.14, −LR 0.33[63]

Ruling Out Pain Generation From Other Related Structures

As with all joints, clinicians should screen the joints above and below the injury for potential contribution to pain generation. Ruling out the cervical spine is of particular importance due not only to its close proximity to the shoulder, but its potential for referral into the shoulder and the entire upper extremity.[64] Once red flags have been ruled out, an efficient way to begin to differentiate the many potential pain referral sources is through the upper quarter screening examination. The traditional upper quarter screen consists of testing of dermatomes, myotomes, deep tendon reflexes, and possible upper motor involvement. A systematic approach to ruling out these other areas is suggested. The key points of this approach are listed in the following section. Refer to chapters 17 (Cervical Spine), 21 (Shoulder), and 22 (Elbow and Forearm) for greater detail regarding these examination procedures.

Rule Out Cervical Spine

The upper quarter screen will determine cervical spine range of motion (ROM) and the potential for the cervical spine as a pain generator to the client's complaints of wrist and hand pain.

Radiculopathy and Discogenic-Related Pathology

These can be ruled out with a combination of Spurling's compression test and the upper limb tension test (median nerve bias):

- Spurling's test: **SN 93 (77-99), SP 95 (76-100), +LR 19.6, −LR 0.07**, QUADAS 9[65]
- Median nerve upper limb tension test: **SN 97 (85-99)**, SP 22 (12-33), +LR 1.3, −**LR 0.12**, QUADAS 10[66]
- Arm squeeze test (described for cervical nerve root compression): SN 95 (85-99), SP 96 (87-99), +LR 24, −LR 0.05, QUADAS 8[67]

Facet Joint Dysfunction

As noted in chapter 17 (Cervical Spine), facet joint dysfunction can be ruled in with reproduction of concordant pain with posterior–anterior spinal joint play assessment or facet joint block.

Rule Out Shoulder and Elbow Joints

The upper quarter screen will determine shoulder and elbow ROM and the potential for these joints as pain generators to the client's complaints of wrist and hand pain. Full active range of motion (AROM) and the application of overpressure for each motion at those joints (if pain-free) will help eliminate those motions and joints as contributors to the client's symptoms. Additionally, as with any joint, clearing AROM with or without overpressure is necessary. AROM of all motions as per the upper quarter screen described in chapter 7 should be implemented. In order to fully clear the cervical spine, full AROM (with overpressure if pain-free) must be present.

Rule Out Shoulder: Impingement

- Hawkins-Kennedy test
  - Pooled analysis: SN 74 (57-85), SP 57 (46-67), +LR 1.7, −LR 0.5, in six studies with 1,029 clients[68]
  - Pooled analysis: SN 80 (72-86), SP 56 (45-67), +LR 1.84, −LR 0.35, in seven studies with 944 clients[69]

Rule Out Elbow: Fracture

- Elbow extension test
  - **SN 97 (85-100)**, SP 69 (57-80), +LR 3.1, **−LR 0.04**, QUADAS 10[70]
  - **SN 100, SP 100, +LR Inf, −LR 0**, QUADAS 11[71]
- Overall active ROM: **SN 100 (93-100), SP 97 (88-100), +LR 33, −LR 0**, QUADAS 11[71]
- Tenderness to palpation: **SN 100 (93-100)**, SP 67 (53-78), +LR 3, **−LR 0**, QUADAS 11[71]

Additionally, as with any joint, clearing AROM with or without overpressure is necessary. AROM of all motions as per the lower quarter screen described in chapter 7 should be implemented. In order to fully clear the above stated joints, full AROM (with overpressure if pain-free) must be present. In order to fully clear the wrist and hand, full AROM (with overpressure if pain-free) must be present. Detail in this regard is described in the following section.

Critical Clinical Pearls

When performing the subjective examination, keep the following in mind:

- The subjective examination provides insight to the possible source of the client's symptoms and helps guide the clinician in prioritizing the objective examination.
- The clinician should develop a clear understanding of the nature of the condition; the mechanism of injury, if present; the behavior of the symptoms; and the concordant sign.
- The clinician should screen proximal neuromusculoskeletal structures of the cervical spine, shoulder, and elbow to determine their involvement in the client's presentation.
- Outcome measure assessment at the initial evaluation is valuable in evaluating the effectiveness of selected interventions.

MOTION TESTS

Motion assessment is a very important aspect of the examination for the orthopedic client. Motion dysfunction can be used to differentiate contractile versus noncontractile tissue (see chapter 9). Assessment of end-feel, potential capsular patterns, and ROM norm values can give the clinician an appreciation of the potential impairments for the orthopedic client they are assessing. Active ROM, passive ROM (PROM), and joint-play assessments are necessary to determine not only the presence or absence of joint , but also the precise aspects of the motion that are dysfunctional. The close-packed position, resting position, capsular pattern, ROM norms, and end-feel for the joints of the wrist and hand are displayed in table 23.2.

Passive and Active Range of Motion

Range of motion (ROM) at the wrist and hand may be limited due to a number of pathological reasons. Furthermore, the anatomical complexities of the wrist and hand deem it necessary to view for significant and subtle deviations during objective movement assessment. ROM measurements at the wrist and hand include active range of motion (AROM) and passive range of motion (PROM) assessments.

Typically clinicians perform these measurements with the use of a goniometer or inclinometer, but more often than not, many rely on obtaining visual measurements. Current literature calls for the use of goniometers and inclinometers in order to make reliable decisions due to motion restrictions.[72]These

TABLE 23.2 Wrist and Hand Arthrology

Joint	Close-packed position	Resting position	Capsular pattern	ROM norms	End-feel
Wrist	Extension with radial deviation	10° flexion and slight UD	Equal limitation of flexion and extension, slight limitations of RD and UD	85° flexion 70° extension 20° RD 30° UD	Firm for flexion, extension, and UD Hard for RD
MCP (2-5)	Full flexion	Slight flexion	Equal limitation of flexion and extension	Up to 90° for flexion 45° and greater for extension	Hard for flexion (firm also described) Firm for extension and abduction Soft for adduction
PIP	Full extension	Slight flexion	Equal restriction of flexion and extension	100° for digits 2-5 Extension is a return to 0°	Hard for flexion Firm for extension
DIP	Full extension	Slight flexion	Equal restriction flexion and extension	90° flexion for digits 2-5 Extension is a return to 0°	Firm for both motions
1st CMC	Full opposition	Midrange of motion	Limitation of abduction and slight limitation in extension	0–15° flexion 20–80° since thumb may start in some flexion Thumb and 5th finger touch for opposition	Soft or firm for flexion Firm for extension and abduction Soft for adduction and opposition
1st MCP	Full flexion	Slight flexion	Greater restriction in flexion than extension	50° flexion Extension to neutral	Firm or hard for flexion Firm for extension
1st IP	Full extension	Slight flexion	Equal restriction in flexion and extension	80° flexion 20° past neutral for extension	Firm for both flexion and extension

RD = radial deviation; UD = ulnar deviation; MCP = metacarpal phalangeal; PIP = proximal interphalangeal; DIP = distal interphalangeal; CMC = carpometacarpal; IP = interphalangeal

measurements are used to assess for ROM impairments or restrictions, with the ultimate goal of making clinical decisions with clients. It is essential that clinical measures be valid and reliable so that they can be used to discriminate between clients. Values involving goniometric measurement at the WH have demonstrated good reliability.[72-78]

ROM measurements taken for the wrist and hand typically occur in single planes of motion, and they are not representative of normal functional ranges of movement that occur on a daily basis. However, decreased motion assessed during planar movements has been associated with a decline in the client's perceived function.[79] The motions of pronation and supination are listed in chapter 22 (Elbow and Forearm). Refer to that chapter for details of these measurements.

WRIST FLEXION

Client Position	Sitting with the distal arm off the edge of the table, hand in neutral
Clinician Position	Standing or sitting directly to the side of the client
Goniometer Alignment	The clinician should place the fulcrum on the lateral aspect of the client's wrist over the triquetrum and align the proximal arm with the lateral midline of the ulna using the olecranon as a reference and the distal arm with the lateral midline of the fifth metacarpal.
Movement	The clinician stabilizes the client's radius and ulna with their proximal hand and grasps the client's hand with their distal hand. The clinician then passively moves the hand into wrist flexion to end range (end-feel is firm). Similarly, the client can perform this motion actively (without assistance from the clinician). AROM should be performed prior to PROM to determine the client's willingness to move and so on.
Assessment	Clinician assesses for amount of ROM, end-feel, quality of the movement, client response, potential difference between AROM and PROM, and so on.

EXTENSION

Client Position	Sitting with the distal arm off the edge of the table, hand in neutral
Clinician Position	Standing or sitting directly to the side of the client
Goniometer Alignment	The clinician positions the fulcrum on the lateral aspect of the client's wrist over the triquetrum and aligns the proximal arm with the lateral midline of the ulna using the olecranon as a reference and the distal arm with the lateral midline of the fifth metacarpal.
Movement	The clinician stabilizes the client's radius and ulna with their proximal hand and grasps the client's hand with their distal hand. The clinician then passively moves the client's hand into wrist extension to end range (end-feel is firm). Similarly, the client can perform this motion actively (without assistance from the clinician). AROM should be performed prior to PROM to determine the client's willingness to move and so on.
Assessment	Clinician assesses for amount of ROM, end-feel, quality of the movement, client response, potential difference between AROM and PROM, and so on.

RADIAL DEVIATION

Client Position	Sitting with the distal arm supported on table, hand in neutral
Clinician Position	Standing or sitting directly to the side of the client
Goniometer Alignment	The clinician positions the fulcrum on the dorsal aspect of the client's wrist over the capitate and aligns the proximal arm with the dorsal midline of the forearm and the distal arm with the dorsal midline of the third metacarpal.
Movement	The clinician stabilizes the client's radius and ulna with their proximal hand and grasps the client's hand with their distal hand. The clinician then passively moves the client's hand into radial deviation to end range (end-feel is hard). Similarly, the client can perform this motion actively (without assistance from the clinician). Active range of motion should be performed prior to PROM to determine the client's willingness to move and so on.
Assessment	Clinician assesses for amount of ROM, end-feel, quality of the movement, client response, potential difference between AROM and PROM, and so on.

ULNAR DEVIATION

Client Position	Sitting with the distal arm supported on table, hand in neutral
Clinician Position	Standing or sitting directly to the side of the client
Goniometer Alignment	The clinician positions the fulcrum on the dorsal aspect of the client's wrist over the capitate and aligns the proximal arm with the dorsal midline of the forearm and the distal arm with the dorsal midline of the third metacarpal.
Movement	The clinician stabilizes the client's radius and ulna with their proximal hand and grasps the client's hand with their distal hand. The clinician then passively moves the client's hand into ulnar deviation to end range (end-feel is hard). Similarly, the client can perform this motion actively (without assistance from the clinician). AROM should be performed prior to PROM to determine the client's willingness to move and so on.
Assessment	Clinician assesses for amount of ROM, end-feel, quality of the movement, client response, potential difference between AROM and PROM, and so on.

HAND METACARPOPHALANGEAL (MCP) JOINT FLEXION

Client Position	Sitting with the distal arm supported on table, forearm and hand in neutral
Clinician Position	Standing or sitting directly to the side of the client
Goniometer Alignment	The clinician positions the fulcrum on the dorsal aspect of the client's metacarpophalangeal joint and aligns the proximal arm with the dorsal midline of the metacarpal and the distal arm with the dorsal midline of the proximal phalanx.
Movement	The clinician stabilizes the client's metacarpal with their proximal hand and grasps the client's dorsal surface of the proximal phalanx with their distal hand. The clinician then passively moves the finger toward the palm to end range (end-feel is hard). A small finger goniometer is necessary for this measurement. Similarly, the client can perform this motion actively (without assistance from the clinician). AROM should be performed prior to PROM to determine the client's willingness to move and so on.
Assessment	Clinician assesses for amount of ROM, end-feel, quality of the movement, client response, potential difference between AROM and PROM, and so on.

MCP JOINT EXTENSION

Client Position	Sitting with the distal arm supported on table, forearm and hand in neutral
Clinician Position	Standing or sitting directly to the side of the client
Goniometer Alignment	The clinician positions the fulcrum on the dorsal aspect of the client's metacarpophalangeal joint and aligns the proximal arm with the dorsal midline of the metacarpal and the distal arm with the dorsal midline of the proximal phalanx.
Movement	The clinician stabilizes the client's metacarpal with their proximal hand and grasps the client's dorsal surface of the proximal phalanx with their distal hand. The clinician then passively moves the finger away from the palm to end range (end-feel is firm). A small finger goniometer is necessary for this measurement. Similarly, the client can perform this motion actively (without assistance from the clinician). AROM should be performed prior to PROM to determine the client's willingness to move and so on.
Assessment	Clinician assesses for amount of ROM, end-feel, quality of the movement, client response, potential difference between AROM and PROM, and so on.

MCP JOINT ABDUCTION AND ADDUCTION

Client Position	Sitting with the distal arm supported on table, forearm pronated and hand in neutral
Clinician Position	Standing or sitting directly to the side of the client
Goniometer Alignment	The clinician positions the fulcrum on the dorsal aspect of the client's metacarpophalangeal joint and aligns the proximal arm with the dorsal midline of the metacarpal and the distal arm with the dorsal midline of the proximal phalanx.
Movement	The clinician stabilizes the client's metacarpal with their proximal hand and grasps the client's dorsal surface of the proximal phalanx with their distal hand. The clinician then passively moves the finger away from the midline of the hand to end range (end-feel is firm). A small finger goniometer is necessary for this measurement. Adduction of this joint is recorded as the return from full abduction with same set-up. Similarly, the client can perform this motion actively (without assistance from the clinician). AROM should be performed prior to PROM to determine the client's willingness to move and so on.
Assessment	Clinician assesses for amount of ROM, end-feel, quality of the movement, client response, potential difference between AROM and PROM, and so on.

PROXIMAL INTERPHALANGEAL (PIP) AND DISTAL INTERPHALANGEAL (DIP) JOINT FLEXION

Client Position	Sitting with the distal arm supported on table, forearm and hand in neutral
Clinician Position	Standing or sitting directly to the side of the client
Goniometer Alignment	The clinician positions the fulcrum on the dorsal aspect of the PIP joint or DIP joint and aligns the proximal arm with the dorsal midline of the proximal phalanx (PIP) or the dorsal midline of the middle phalanx (DIP) and the distal arm with the dorsal midline of the middle phalanx (PIP) or the dorsal midline of the distal phalanx.
Movement	The clinician stabilizes the client's proximal phalanx (PIP joint) or middle phalanx (DIP) with their proximal hand and grasps the client's dorsal surface of the middle phalanx (PIP) or dorsal surface of the distal phalanx (DIP) with their distal hand. The clinician then passively moves the finger toward the palm of the hand to end range (end-feel is hard [PIP] or firm [DIP]). A small finger goniometer is necessary for this measurement. Similarly, the client can perform this motion actively without assistance from the clinician. AROM should be performed prior to PROM to determine the client's willingness to move and so on. • PIP extension: stabilization and goniometer alignment same as for PIP flexion; end-feel is firm. • DIP extension: stabilization and goniometer alignment same as for DIP flexion; end-feel is firm.
Assessment	Clinician assesses for amount of ROM, end-feel, quality of the movement, client response, potential difference between AROM and PROM, and so on.

THUMB CARPOMETACARPAL (CMC) JOINT FLEXION

Client Position	Sitting with the distal arm supported on table, forearm and hand in neutral
Clinician Position	Standing or sitting directly to the side of the client
Goniometer Alignment	The clinician positions the fulcrum over the palmar aspect of the client's first CMC joint and aligns the proximal arm with the ventral midline of the radius using the radial styloid process as a reference and aligns the distal arm with the ventral midline of the first metacarpal.

(continued)

Thumb Carpometacarpal (CMC) Joint Flexion *(continued)*

Movement	The clinician stabilizes the client's carpals, radius, and ulna with their proximal hand and grasps the dorsal surface of the client's metacarpal (thumb) with their distal hand. The clinician then passively moves the thumb toward the ulnar aspect of the hand to end range (end-feel is soft or firm). A small finger goniometer is necessary for this measurement. Similarly, the client can perform this motion actively (without assistance from the clinician). AROM should be performed prior to PROM to determine the client's willingness to move and so on.
Assessment	Clinician assesses for amount of ROM, end-feel, quality of the movement, client response, potential difference between AROM and PROM, and so on.

THUMB CMC JOINT EXTENSION

Client Position	Sitting with the distal arm supported on table, forearm and hand in neutral
Clinician Position	Standing or sitting directly to the side of the client
Goniometer Alignment	The clinician positions the fulcrum over the palmar aspect of the client's first CMC joint and aligns the proximal arm with the ventral midline of the radius using the radial styloid process as a reference and aligns the distal arm with the ventral midline of the first metacarpal.
Movement	The clinician stabilizes the client's carpals, radius, and ulna with their proximal hand and grasps the dorsal surface of the client's metacarpal (thumb) with their distal hand. The clinician then passively moves the thumb toward the radial aspect of the hand to end range (end-feel is firm). A small finger goniometer is necessary for this measurement. Similarly, the client can perform this motion actively (without assistance from the clinician). AROM should be performed prior to PROM to determine the client's willingness to move and so on.
Assessment	Clinician assesses for amount of ROM, end-feel, quality of the movement, client response, potential difference between AROM and PROM, and so on.

THUMB CMC JOINT ABDUCTION

Client Position	Sitting with the distal arm supported on table, forearm midway between pronation and supination and hand in neutral
Clinician Position	Standing or sitting directly to the side of the client
Goniometer Alignment	The clinician positions the fulcrum over the lateral aspect of the radial styloid process, aligns the proximal arm with the lateral midline of the client's second metacarpal using the center of the MCP joint for reference, and aligns the distal arm with the lateral midline of the first metacarpal using the center of MCP joint for reference.
Movement	The clinician stabilizes the client's carpals and second metacarpal with their proximal hand and grasps the medial and lateral surface of the client's metacarpal (thumb) with their distal hand. The clinician then passively moves the thumb away from the palm of the hand to end range (end-feel is firm). A small finger goniometer is necessary for this measurement. Similarly, the client can perform this motion actively (without assistance from the clinician). AROM should be performed prior to PROM to determine the client's willingness to move and so on.

- CMC joint adduction: recorded as the return from full abduction.
- CMC joint opposition: The clinician should move the first and fifth metacarpals toward each other. The distance between the fingers is measured. The normal end-feel is soft.

Assessment	Clinician assesses for amount of ROM, end-feel, quality of the movement, client response, potential difference between AROM and PROM, and so on.

THUMB MCP JOINT FLEXION

Client Position	Sitting with the distal arm supported on table, forearm in full supination and hand in neutral
Clinician Position	Standing or sitting directly to the side of the client
Goniometer Alignment	The clinician positions the fulcrum over the dorsal aspect of the MCP joint and aligns the proximal arm with the dorsal midline of the metacarpal and the distal arm with the dorsal midline of the proximal phalanx.
Movement	The clinician stabilizes the client's first metacarpal with their proximal hand and grasps the client's dorsal aspect of proximal phalanx with their distal hand. The clinician then passively moves the thumb toward the ulnar aspect of the hand to end range (end-feel is hard). A small finger goniometer is necessary for this measurement. Similarly, the client can perform this motion actively (without assistance from the clinician). AROM should be performed prior to PROM to determine the client's willingness to move and so on.
Assessment	Clinician assesses for amount of ROM, end-feel, quality of the movement, client response, potential difference between AROM and PROM, and so on.

THUMB MCP JOINT EXTENSION

Client Position	Sitting with the distal arm supported on table, forearm in full supination and hand in neutral
Clinician Position	Standing or sitting directly to the side of the client
Goniometer Alignment	The clinician positions the fulcrum over the dorsal aspect of the client's MCP joint and aligns the proximal arm with the dorsal midline of the metacarpal and the distal arm with the dorsal midline of the proximal phalanx.
Movement	The clinician stabilizes the client's first metacarpal with their proximal hand and grasps the client's dorsal aspect of the proximal phalanx with their distal hand. The clinician then passively moves the thumb toward the radial aspect of hand to end range (end-feel is firm). A small finger goniometer is necessary for this measurement. Similarly, the client can perform this motion actively (without assistance from the clinician). AROM should be performed prior to PROM to determine the client's willingness to move and so on.
Assessment	Clinician assesses for amount of ROM, end-feel, quality of the movement, client response, potential difference between AROM and PROM, and so on.

THUMB INTERPHALANGEAL (IP) JOINT FLEXION

Client Position	Sitting with the distal arm supported on table, forearm in full supination and hand in neutral
Clinician Position	Standing or sitting directly to the side of the client
Goniometer Alignment	The clinician positions the fulcrum over the dorsal aspect of the IP joint and aligns the proximal arm with the dorsal midline of the proximal phalanx and the distal arm with the dorsal midline of the distal phalanx.
Movement	The clinician stabilizes the client's first proximal phalanx with their proximal hand and grasps the client's dorsal aspect of the distal phalanx with their distal hand. The clinician then passively moves the tip of the thumb toward the ulnar aspect of the hand to end range (end-feel is firm). A small finger goniometer is necessary for this measurement. Similarly, the client can perform this motion actively (without assistance from the clinician). AROM should be performed prior to PROM to determine the client's willingness to move and so on. IP joint extension: moving palmar aspect of distal phalanx toward radial aspect of hand; end-feel is firm.
Assessment	Clinician assesses for amount of ROM, end-feel, quality of the movement, client response, potential difference between AROM and PROM, and so on.

Passive Accessories

Mobility testing of the wrist and hand has multiple components. Passive accessory movements can be useful in identifying each client's concordant sign that relates to the numerous joints of the wrist and hand. If a concordant sign is identified during examination, the clinician must determine the effect of the movement during sustained or oscillatory movements. The clinician should find out if the concordant sign becomes better or worse, or does not change at all. This information will prove useful when developing a treatment plan of care. Assessing the relationship of the carpal joints and their relationship to the client's symptoms is assessed as normal, hypermobile, or hypomobile. In a group of clients with similar symptoms, the percent of agreement between two different skilled clinicians ranged from 60% to 100%.[80]

WRIST (RADIOCARPAL AND ULNOCARPAL) POSTERIOR (DORSAL) GLIDE

Client Position	Sitting with the wrist in neutral, with the forearm supported on the table and the thumb facing the ceiling
Clinician Position	Standing or sitting (as shown) at the client's side to be assessed
Stabilization	The rest of the client's body on the table serves as a stabilizing force. The clinician's stabilizing hand (right as shown) purchases the distal radius and ulna against the table.
Movement and Direction of Force	The clinician's assessing hand (left as shown) purchases the proximal row of carpal bones. The clinician's assessing hand glides the proximal row of carpal bones in a posterior (dorsal) direction (away from clinician).
Assessment	Assessment is done for joint play/passive accessory motion, client response, and end-feel. Reproduction of concordant pain suggests dysfunction. Impaired joint mobility or end-feel may also suggest dysfunction if concordant pain is also reproduced.

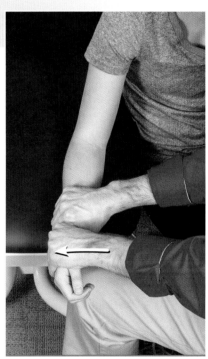

Figure 23.12

Notes
- This technique can also be performed with the client's forearm fully supinated and with the clinician standing and gliding the carpal bones posteriorly (dorsally) toward the floor.
- The midcarpal joint posterior (dorsal) glide can be performed the same way, with the clinician using the stabilizing hand to purchase the proximal row of carpal bones and the wrist and the assessing hand to purchase the distal row of carpal bones, and performing the posterior (dorsal) glide as described.

WRIST ANTERIOR (VOLAR/PALMAR) GLIDE

Client Position	Sitting with the wrist in neutral, with the forearm on the table and the thumb facing the ceiling
Clinician Position	Standing or sitting (as shown) at the client's side to be assessed
Stabilization	The rest of the client's body on the table serves as a stabilizing force. The clinician's stabilizing hand (left as shown) purchases the distal radius and ulna against the table.
Movement and Direction of Force	The clinician's assessing hand (right as shown) purchases the proximal row of carpal bones. The clinician uses their assessing hand to glide the proximal row of carpal bones in an anterior (volar/palmar) direction (away from clinician).
Assessment	Assessment is done for joint play/passive accessory motion, client response, and end-feel. Reproduction of concordant pain suggests dysfunction. Impaired joint mobility or end-feel may also suggest dysfunction if concordant pain is also reproduced.
Notes	• This technique can also be performed with the client's forearm fully pronated. The clinician stands and glides the carpal bones anteriorly (volar/palmar direction) toward the floor.
	• The midcarpal joint anterior (volar/palmar) glide can be performed the same way. The clinician uses the stabilizing hand to purchase the proximal row of carpal bones and wrist and the assessing hand to purchase the distal row of carpal bones, and then performs the anterior (volar/palmar) glide as described.

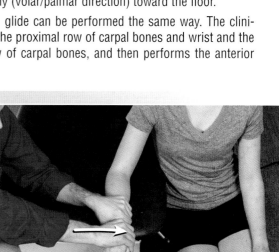

Figure 23.13

WRIST RADIAL GLIDE

Client Position	Sitting with the wrist in neutral, with the forearm supported on the table and fully pronated
Clinician Position	Standing or sitting (as shown) at the client's side to be assessed
Stabilization	The rest of the client's body on the table serves as a stabilizing force. The clinician's stabilizing hand (left as shown) purchases the distal radius and ulna against the table.
Movement and Direction of Force	The clinician's assessing hand (right as shown) purchases the proximal row of carpal bones. The clinician uses the assessing hand to glide the proximal row of carpal bones in a radial direction (away from clinician).
Assessment	Assessment is done for joint play/passive accessory motion, client response, and end-feel. Reproduction of concordant pain suggests dysfunction. Impaired joint mobility or end-feel may also suggest dysfunction if concordant pain is also reproduced.
Note	The midcarpal joint radial glide can be performed the same way. The clinician uses the stabilizing hand to purchase the proximal row of carpal bones and the wrist and the assessing hand to purchase the distal row of carpal bones, then performs the radial glide as described.

Figure 23.14

WRIST ULNAR GLIDE

Client Position	Sitting with the wrist in neutral, with the forearm supported on the table and fully supinated
Clinician Position	Standing or sitting (as shown) at the client's side to be assessed
Stabilization	The rest of the client's body on the table serves as a stabilizing force. The clinician's stabilizing hand (left as shown) purchases the distal radius and ulna against the table.
Movement and Direction of Force	The clinician's assessing hand (right as shown) purchases the proximal row of carpal bones. The clinician uses the assessing hand to glide the proximal row of carpal bones in an ulnar direction (away from clinician).

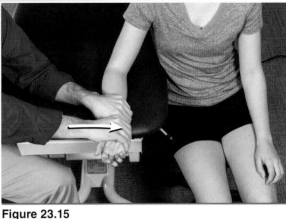

Figure 23.15

Assessment	Assessment is done for joint play/passive accessory motion, client response, and end-feel. Reproduction of concordant pain suggests dysfunction. Impaired joint mobility or end-feel may also suggest dysfunction if concordant pain is also reproduced.
Note	The midcarpal joint ulnar glide can be performed the same way. The clinician uses the stabilizing hand to purchase the proximal row of carpal bones and the wrist and the assessing hand to purchase the distal row of carpal bones, then performs the ulnar glide as described.

SPECIFIC CARPAL BONE POSTERIOR (DORSAL) GLIDE

Client Position	Sitting with the wrist in neutral, with the forearm supported on the table and fully supinated
Clinician Position	Standing at the client's side to be assessed
Stabilization	The rest of the client's body on the table serves as a stabilizing force. The clinician's stabilizing hand (right as shown) purchases the distal radius and ulna against the table.
Movement and Direction of Force	The clinician's assessing hand (left as shown) purchases the given proximal carpal bone. The clinician uses the assessing hand to glide the given carpal bone in a posterior (dorsal) direction (away from clinician and toward the floor).

Figure 23.16

Assessment	Assessment is done for joint play/passive accessory motion, client response, and end-feel. Reproduction of concordant pain suggests dysfunction. Impaired joint mobility or end-feel may also suggest dysfunction if concordant pain is also reproduced.
Note	• Scaphoid posterior glide on radius. • Lunate posterior (dorsal) glide on radius. • Triquetrum posterior (dorsal) glide on disc. • Each carpal bone can be posteriorly (dorsally) glided on the neighboring carpal bone. • Midcarpal joint posterior (dorsal) glide (specific carpals)

- Trapezium and trapezoid posterior (dorsal) glide on scaphoid.
- Capitate posterior (dorsal) glide on lunate.
- Hamate posterior (dorsal) glide on triquetrum.

SPECIFIC CARPAL BONE ANTERIOR (VOLAR/PALMAR) GLIDE

Client Position	Sitting with the wrist in neutral, with the forearm supported on the table and fully pronated
Clinician Position	Standing at the client's side to be assessed
Stabilization	The rest of the client's body on the table serves as a stabilizing force. The clinician's stabilizing hand purchases the distal radius and ulna against the table.
Movement and Direction of Force	The clinician's assessing hand purchases the given proximal carpal bone. The clinician uses the assessing hand to glide the given carpal bone in an anterior (volar/palmar) direction (away from clinician and toward floor).
Assessment	Assessment is done for joint play/passive accessory motion, client response, and end-feel. Reproduction of concordant pain suggests dysfunction. Impaired joint mobility or end-feel may also suggest dysfunction if concordant pain is also reproduced.
Note	• Scaphoid anterior (volar/palmar) glide on radius.

- • Lunate anterior (volar/palmar) glide on radius.
- • Triquetrum anterior (volar/palmar) glide on disc.
- • Each carpal bone can be anteriorly (volar/palmar direction) glided on the neighboring carpal bone.
- • Midcarpal joint anterior (volar/palmar) glide (specific carpals).
    - Trapezium and trapezoid anterior (volar/palmar) glide on scaphoid
    - Capitate anterior (volar/palmar) glide on lunate
    - Hamate anterior (volar/palmar) glide on triquetrum

TRAPEZIOMETACARPAL JOINT (THUMB) POSTERIOR (DORSAL) GLIDE

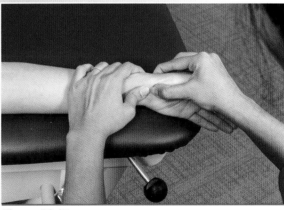

Figure 23.17

Client Position	Sitting with the wrist in neutral, with the forearm supported on the table and the thumb facing the ceiling
Clinician Position	Sitting at the client's side to be assessed
Stabilization	The rest of the client's body on the table serves as a stabilizing force. The clinician's stabilizing hand (left as shown) purchases the trapezium and wrist against the table.
Movement and Direction of Force	The clinician uses their assessing hand (right as shown) to purchase the proximal metacarpal, with their thumb on the anterior (volar/palmar) surface and their index finger on the posterior (dorsal) surface. The clinician uses the assessing hand to glide the proximal metacarpal in a posterior (dorsal) direction (away from clinician).
Assessment	Assessment is done for joint play/passive accessory motion, client response, and end-feel. Reproduction of concordant pain suggests dysfunction. Impaired joint mobility or end-feel may also suggest dysfunction if concordant pain is also reproduced.

TRAPEZIOMETACARPAL JOINT (THUMB) ANTERIOR (VOLAR/PALMAR) GLIDE

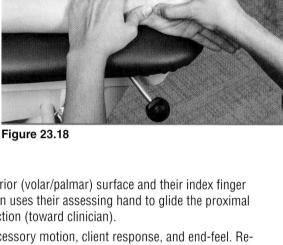

Figure 23.18

Client Position — Sitting with the wrist in neutral, with the forearm supported on the table and the thumb facing the ceiling

Clinician Position — Sitting at the client's side to be assessed

Stabilization — The rest of the client's body on the table serves as a stabilizing force. The clinician's stabilizing hand (left as shown) purchases the trapezium and wrist against the table.

Movement and Direction of Force — The clinician uses their assessing hand (right as shown) to purchase the proximal metacarpal, with their thumb on the anterior (volar/palmar) surface and their index finger on the posterior (dorsal) surface. The clinician uses their assessing hand to glide the proximal metacarpal in an anterior (volar/palmar) direction (toward clinician).

Assessment — Assessment is done for joint play/passive accessory motion, client response, and end-feel. Reproduction of concordant pain suggests dysfunction. Impaired joint mobility or end-feel may also suggest dysfunction if concordant pain is also reproduced.

TRAPEZIOMETACARPAL JOINT (THUMB) RADIAL GLIDE

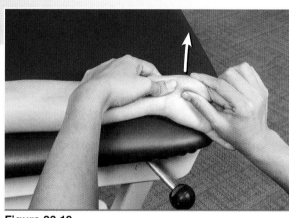

Figure 23.19

Client Position — Sitting with the wrist in neutral, with the forearm supported on the table and the thumb facing the ceiling

Clinician Position — Sitting at the client's side to be assessed

Stabilization — The rest of the client's body on the table serves as a stabilizing force. The clinician's stabilizing hand (left as shown) purchases the trapezium and wrist against the table.

Movement and Direction of Force — The clinician uses their assessing hand (right as shown) to purchase the proximal metacarpal, with their thumb on the ulnar surface and their index finger on the radial surface. The clinician uses their assessing hand to glide the proximal metacarpal in a radial direction (toward the ceiling).

Assessment — Assessment is done for joint play/passive accessory motion, client response, and end-feel. Reproduction of concordant pain suggests dysfunction. Impaired joint mobility or end-feel may also suggest dysfunction if concordant pain is also reproduced.

TRAPEZIOMETACARPAL JOINT (THUMB) ULNAR GLIDE

Client Position	Sitting with the wrist in neutral, with the forearm supported on the table and the thumb facing the ceiling
Clinician Position	Sitting at the client's side to be assessed
Stabilization	The rest of the client's body on the table serves as a stabilizing force. The clinician's stabilizing hand (left as shown) purchases the trapezium and wrist against the table.
Movement and Direction of Force	The clinician uses their assessing hand (right as shown) to purchase the proximal metacarpal, with their thumb on the ulnar surface and their index finger on the radial surface. The clinician uses their assessing hand to glide the proximal metacarpal in an ulnar direction (toward the floor).
Assessment	Assessment is done for joint play/passive accessory motion, client response, and end-feel. Reproduction of concordant pain suggests dysfunction. Impaired joint mobility or end-feel may also suggest dysfunction if concordant pain is also reproduced.

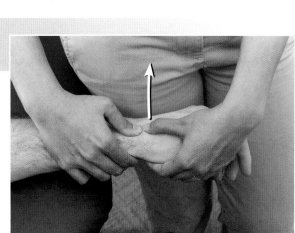

Figure 23.20

CARPOMETACARPAL JOINTS 2-5 POSTERIOR (DORSAL) GLIDE

Client Position	Sitting with the wrist in neutral, with the forearm fully pronated
Clinician Position	Standing at the client's side to be assessed
Stabilization	The rest of the client's body on the table serves as a stabilizing force. The clinician's stabilizing hand (right as shown) purchases the carpal bones and wrist against the table.
Movement and Direction of Force	The clinician uses their assessing hand (left as shown) to purchase the proximal metacarpal, with their thumb on the posterior (dorsal) surface and their index finger on the anterior (volar/palmar) surface. The clinician uses their assessing hand to glide the proximal metacarpal in a posterior (dorsal) direction (toward the ceiling).
Assessment	Assessment is done for joint play/passive accessory motion, client response, and end-feel. Reproduction of concordant pain suggests dysfunction. Impaired joint mobility or end-feel may also suggest dysfunction if concordant pain is also reproduced.

Figure 23.21

CARPOMETACARPAL JOINTS 2-5 VOLAR/PALMAR GLIDE

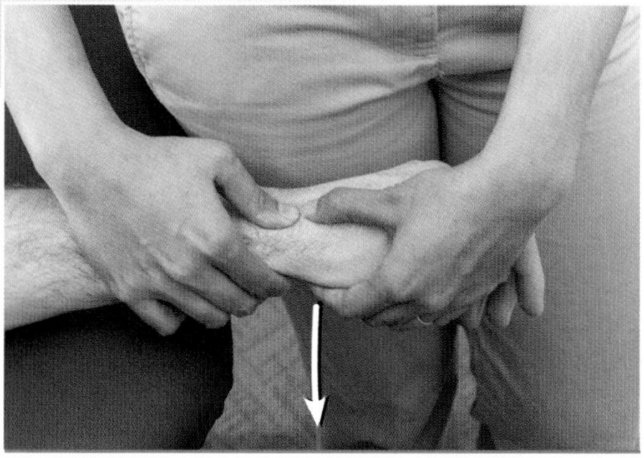

Client Position	Sitting with the wrist in neutral, with the forearm fully pronated
Clinician Position	Standing at the client's side to be assessed
Stabilization	The rest of the client's body on the table serves as a stabilizing force. The clinician's stabilizing hand (right as shown) purchases the carpal bones and wrist against the table.
Movement and Direction of Force	The clinician uses their assessing hand (left as shown) to purchase the proximal metacarpal, with their thumb on the posterior (dorsal) surface and their index finger on the anterior (volar/palmar) surface. The clinician uses their assessing hand to glide the proximal metacarpal in an anterior (volar/palmar) direction (toward the floor).
Assessment	Assessment is done for joint play/passive accessory motion, client response, and end-feel. Reproduction of concordant pain suggests dysfunction. Impaired joint mobility or end-feel may also suggest dysfunction if concordant pain is also reproduced.

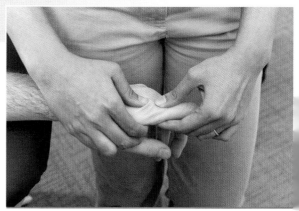

Figure 23.22

METACARPOPHALANGEAL JOINTS 1-5 GLIDES

Client Position	Sitting with the wrist in neutral, with the forearm fully pronated
Clinician Position	Standing at the client's side to be assessed
Stabilization	The rest of the client's body on the table serves as a stabilizing force. The clinician's stabilizing hand (right as shown) purchases the metacarpal bone and hand.
Movement and Direction of Force	The clinician's assessing hand (left as shown) purchases the proximal phalanx. The clinician uses the assessing hand to glide the proximal phalanx in the respective direction.
Assessment	Assessment is done for joint play/passive accessory motion, client response, and end-feel. Reproduction of concordant pain suggests dysfunction. Impaired joint mobility or end-feel may also suggest dysfunction if concordant pain is also reproduced.
Note	• Posterior glide (proximal phalanx toward the clinician and ceiling)
	• Anterior glide (proximal phalanx away from clinician and toward the floor)
	• Radial glide (proximal phalanx toward the radius)
	• Ulnar glide (proximal phalanx toward the ulna)

Figure 23.23

INTERPHALANGEAL JOINTS 1-5 GLIDES

Client Position	Sitting with the wrist in neutral, with the forearm fully pronated
Clinician Position	Standing at the client's side to be assessed
Stabilization	The rest of the client's body on the table serves as a stabilizing force. The clinician's stabilizing hand (right as shown) purchases the client's proximal phalanx and hand.
Movement and Direction of Force	The clinician's assessing hand (left as shown) purchases the distal phalanx. The clinician uses the assessing hand to glide the distal phalanx in the respective direction.

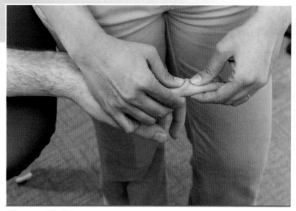

Figure 23.24

Assessment	Assessment is done for joint play/passive accessory motion, client response, and end-feel. Reproduction of concordant pain suggests dysfunction. Impaired joint mobility or end-feel may also suggest dysfunction if concordant pain is also reproduced.
Note	• Posterior glide (distal phalanx toward the clinician and ceiling)
	• Anterior glide (distal phalanx away from the clinician and toward the floor)

Flexibility

See chapter 21 (Shoulder) for appropriate flexibility assessments.

MUSCLE PERFORMANCE TESTING

Manual muscle testing and handheld dynamometric testing are accurate, valid, and reliable methods for assessing and measuring muscle strength.[81-85] Common manual muscle tests of the wrist and hand are outlined here.

WRIST FLEXION

Client Position	Sitting, with forearm supinated and wrist in neutral
Clinician Position	Standing directly to the side of the client
Movement and Assessment	The clinician stabilizes the client's forearm under the wrist and uses the other hand to give resistance to the entire palm of the hand as the client attempts to flex the wrist (for the flexor carpi radialis, force is focused over the radial side of the palm; for the flexor carpi ulnaris, the force is focused over the ulnar side of the palm).

- Grade 5: completes full range with maximal resistance
- Grade 4: completes full range with strong resistance
- Grade 3: completes full range without resistance
- Grade 2: completes only partial range with forearm in neutral supination or pronation
- Grade 1: muscle activity without movement
- Grade 0: no muscle activity

Primary Muscles	Flexor carpi radialis
	Flexor carpi ulnaris

(continued)

Wrist Flexion *(continued)*

Secondary Muscles	Palmaris longus
	Flexor digitorum superficialis
	Flexor digitorum profundus
	Abductor pollicis longus
	Flexor pollicis longus
Primary Nerves	Median (C6-7; flexor carpi radialis)
	Ulnar (C7-T1; flexor carpi ulnaris)

WRIST EXTENSION

Client Position	Sitting, with forearm pronated and wrist in neutral
Clinician Position	Standing directly to the side of the client
Movement and Assessment	The clinician stabilizes the client's forearm under the wrist and uses their other hand to give resistance to the entire dorsum of the hand as the client attempts to extend the wrist (for the extensor carpi radialis longus and brevis, force is focused over the radial side of the dorsum; for extensor carpi ulnaris, force is focused over the ulnar side of the dorsum).

- Grade 5: completes full range with maximal resistance
- Grade 4: completes full range with strong resistance
- Grade 3: completes full range without resistance
- Grade 2: completes only partial range with forearm in neutral supination or pronation
- Grade 1: muscle activity without movement
- Grade 0: no muscle activity

Primary Muscles	Extensor carpi radialis longus and brevis
	Extensor carpi ulnaris
Secondary Muscles	Extensor digitorum
	Extensor digiti minimi
	Extensor indicis
Primary Nerve	Radial (C6-8)

FINGER METACARPOPHALANGEAL (MCP) FLEXION

Client Position	Sitting with forearm supinated, wrist in neutral, and MCP extended
Clinician Position	Standing directly to the side of the client
Movement and Assessment	The clinician stabilizes the client's metacarpals proximal to the MCP joint and uses their other hand to give resistance to the proximal row of phalanges on the volar/palmar surface. Meanwhile, the client attempts to flex the MCP joint. Fingers may also be tested separately.

- Grade 5: completes full range with strong resistance
- Grade 4: completes full range with some resistance
- Grade 3: completes full range without resistance
- Grade 2: completes only partial range with forearm in neutral supination or pronation
- Grade 1: muscle activity without movement
- Grade 0: no muscle activity

Primary Muscles	Lumbricals
	Dorsal interossei
	Palmar interossei
Secondary Muscles	Flexor digitorum superficialis
	Flexor digitorum profundus
	Flexor digiti minimi
Primary Nerves	Median (C8-T1; lumbricals 1 and 2)
	Ulnar (C8-T1; lumbricals 3 and 4)

FINGER MCP EXTENSION

Client Position	Sitting with forearm pronated, wrist in neutral, and MCP relaxed
Clinician Position	Standing directly to the side of the client
Movement and Assessment	The clinician stabilizes the client's metacarpals proximal to the MCP joint and uses their other hand to give resistance to the proximal row of phalanges on the dorsal surface. Meanwhile, the client attempts to extend the MCP joint. Fingers may also be tested separately (extensor indicis for index finger, extensor digiti minimi for 5th digit).

- Grade 5: completes full range with strong resistance
- Grade 4: completes full range with some resistance
- Grade 3: completes full range without resistance
- Grade 2: completes only partial range with forearm in neutral supination or pronation
- Grade 1: muscle activity without movement
- Grade 0: no muscle activity

Primary Muscles	Extensor digitorum
	Extensor indicis
	Extensor digiti minimi
Primary Nerve	Radial (C7-8)

FINGER PROXIMAL INTERPHALANGEAL (PIP) AND DISTAL INTERPHALANGEAL (DIP) FLEXION

Client Position	Sitting with forearm supinated, wrist in neutral, and MCP relaxed
Clinician Position	Standing directly to the side of the client
Movement and Assessment	The clinician stabilizes all fingers (except the one to be tested) into extension with one hand and uses their other hand to give resistance to the volar/palmar aspect of the distal end of the middle phalanx of the finger being tested. Meanwhile, the client attempts to flex the respective joint.

- Grade 5: completes full range with strong resistance
- Grade 4: completes full range with some resistance
- Grade 3: completes full range without resistance

Forearm is in the mid-position of supination or pronation for all grades below grade 3.

- Grade 2: completes only partial range with forearm in neutral supination or pronation
- Grade 1: muscle activity without movement
- Grade 0: no muscle activity

(continued)

Finger Proximal Interphalangeal (PIP) and Distal Interphalangeal (DIP) Flexion *(continued)*

Primary Muscles	Flexor digitorum superficialis
	Flexor digitorum profundus
Primary Nerves	Median (C8-T1; flexor digitorum superficialis and profundus fingers 2 and 3)
	Ulnar (C8-T1; flexor digitorum profundus fingers 4 and 5)

FINGER ABDUCTION

Client Position	Sitting with forearm pronated, wrist in neutral, and MCP relaxed
Clinician Position	Standing directly to the side of the client
Movement and Assessment	The clinician stabilizes the client's wrist with one hand and uses their other hand to give resistance to the radial and ulnar aspects of the two corresponding fingers. Meanwhile the client attempts to abduct the two fingers away from each other.

- Grades 5 and 4 are subjective.
- Grade 3: can abduct any given finger without resistance
- Grade 2: completes only partial range of any given finger
- Grade 1: muscle activity without movement
- Grade 0: no muscle activity

Primary Muscles	Dorsal interossei
	Abductor digiti minimi
Secondary Muscles	Extensor digitorum
	Extensor digiti minimi
Primary Nerve	Ulnar (C8-T1)

FINGER ADDUCTION

Client Position	Sitting with forearm pronated, wrist in neutral, and MCP relaxed
Clinician Position	Standing directly to the side of the client
Movement and Assessment	The clinician stabilizes the client's wrist with one hand and uses their other hand to give resistance to pull the fingers apart. Meanwhile, the client attempts to adduct the fingers and keep them in contact with each other.

- Grades 5 and 4 are subjective: fingers are very weak with this motion
- Grade 3: can adduct any given finger without resistance
- Grade 2: completes only partial range of any given finger
- Grade 1: muscle activity without movement
- Grade 0: no muscle activity

Primary Muscle	Palmar interossei
Secondary Muscle	Extensor indicis
Primary Nerve	Ulnar (C8-T1)

THUMB MCP AND IP FLEXION

Client Position	Sitting with forearm supinated, wrist and thumb in neutral
Clinician Position	Standing directly to the side of the client
Movement and Assessment	The clinician stabilizes the client's respective proximal bone (1st metacarpal or phalanx) and uses their other hand to give one-finger resistance to the palmar aspect of distal bone. Meanwhile, the client attempts to flex the respective joint (MCP or IP).

- Grade 5: completes full range with maximal resistance
- Grade 4: completes full range with moderate resistance
- Grade 3: completes full range without resistance
- Grade 2: completes only partial range
- Grade 1: muscle activity without movement
- Grade 0: no muscle activity

Primary Muscles	Flexor pollicis brevis for MCP flexion
	Flexor pollicis longus for IP flexion
Primary Nerves	Median (C8-T1; flexor pollicis longus and brevis superficial head)
	Ulnar (C8-T1; flexor pollicis brevis deep head)

THUMB MCP AND IP EXTENSION

Client Position	Sitting with forearm in neutral supination or pronation, wrist in neutral, and thumb in neutral
Clinician Position	Standing directly to the side of the client
Movement and Assessment	The clinician stabilizes the client's respective proximal bone (1st metacarpal or phalanx) and uses their other hand to give one-finger resistance to the dorsal aspect of the distal bone. Meanwhile, the client attempts to extend the respective joint (MCP or IP).

- Grades 5 and 4 are subjective: fingers are very weak with this motion
- Grade 3: completes full range some resistance
- Grade 2: completes only partial range
- Grade 1: muscle activity without movement
- Grade 0: no muscle activity

Primary Muscles	Extensor pollicis brevis for MCP extension
	Extensor pollicis longus for IP extension
Primary Nerve	Radial (C7-8)

THUMB ABDUCTION

Client Position	Sitting with forearm supinated, wrist in neutral, and thumb adducted
Clinician Position	Standing directly to the side of the client
Movement and Assessment	The clinician stabilizes the client's hand and uses their other hand to give resistance distal to the ulnar aspect of the thumb CMC joint. Meanwhile, the client attempts to abduct the thumb (lifting it up toward the ceiling or directly off the palm and index finger).

- Grade 5: completes full range with strong resistance
- Grade 4: completes full range with moderate resistance
- Grade 3: completes full range with some resistance

Forearm in mid supination or pronation for the following grades:

- Grade 2: completes only partial range
- Grade 1: muscle activity without movement
- Grade 0: no muscle activity

Primary Muscles	Abductor pollicis longus
	Abductor pollicis brevis
Secondary Muscles	Palmaris longus
	Extensor pollicis brevis
	Opponens pollicis
Primary Nerves	Median (C8-T1; abductor pollicis brevis)
	Ulnar (C7-8; abductor pollicis longus)

THUMB ADDUCTION

Client Position	Sitting with forearm pronated, wrist in neutral, and thumb abducted
Clinician Position	Standing directly to the side of the client
Movement and Assessment	The clinician stabilizes the client's hand with one hand and uses the other hand to give resistance distal to the radial aspect of thumb's CMC joint. Meanwhile, the client attempts to adduct the thumb (lifting it up to the palm and index finger).

- Grade 5: completes full range with strong resistance
- Grade 4: completes full range with moderate resistance
- Grade 3: completes full range with some resistance

Forearm in mid supination or pronation for the following grades:

- Grade 2: completes only partial range
- Grade 1: muscle activity without movement
- Grade 0: no muscle activity

Primary Muscle	Adductor pollicis
Secondary Muscle	1st dorsal interosseus
Primary Nerve	Ulnar (C8-T1)

OPPOSITION (THUMB TO FIFTH FINGER)

Client Position	Sitting with forearm supinated, wrist in neutral, and thumb relaxed
Clinician Position	Standing directly to the side of the client
Movement and Assessment	The clinician stabilizes client's hand while giving resistance distal to the head of the 1st metacarpal of the thumb and the 5th finger simultaneously. Meanwhile, the client attempts to touch these two fingers.

- Grade 5: completes full range with maximal resistance
- Grade 4: completes full range with moderate resistance
- Grade 3: completes full range with some resistance
- Grade 2: completes only partial range
- Grade 1: muscle activity without movement
- Grade 0: no muscle activity

Primary Muscles	Opponens pollicis
	Opponens digiti minimi
Secondary Muscles	Abductor pollicis brevis
	Flexor pollicis brevis
Primary Nerves	Median (C8-T1; opponens pollicis)
	Ulnar (C8-T1; both muscles)

SPECIAL TESTS

As mentioned in chapter 10 (Special Tests), in many cases the clinician is overly dependent on the performance and interpretation of special test findings with respect to differential diagnosis of the client's presenting pain. Utilization of special tests for ruling in (or helping to diagnose) a particular pathology should occur at this point in the examination process. It is also hoped that the clinician has a much clearer picture of the client's presentation prior to this point in the examination and will therefore depend minimally on special test findings with respect to diagnosis of the client's pain.

Specific testing to rule in or out the wrist and hand for various pathologies is listed in the following section with detailed test descriptions. Remember that special tests are a very minor component of the overall examination; therefore, depending on findings from special testing alone is inadequate clinical practice.

Index of Special Tests

Carpal Tunnel Syndrome

Upper Limb Neurodynamic Test (Median Nerve)

Upper Limb Neurodynamic Test (Radial Nerve)

Wainner's Clinical Prediction Rule for Carpal Tunnel Syndrome

Phalen's Test

Reverse Phalen's Test

Modified Phalen's Test

Tinel's Sign

Flick Sign

Hand Elevation Test

Tethered Median Nerve Stress Test

Closed-Fist or Lumbrical Provocation Test

Wrist-Ratio Index

Katz Hand Diagram

Median Nerve Digit Score

(continued)

Case Studies

Go to www.HumanKinetics.com/OrthopedicClinicalExamination and complete these case studies for chapter 23:

- Case study 1 discusses a 22-year-old male hockey player with right wrist pain.
- Case study 2 discusses a 47-year-old female secretary with pain in her right and left wrists and hands.

Abstract Links

Go to www.HumanKinetics.com/OrthopedicClinicalExamination to access abstract links on these issues:

Anatomical snuffbox tenderness

Clinical stress test (distal radial fracture)

Closed fist test (lumbrical provocation test)

Elbow extension test

Extensor carpi ulnaris (ECU) synergy test

Finkelstein's test

Flick sign

Garcia-Elias test

Gilliat tourniquet test

Hand elevation test

Hawkins-Kennedy test

Hem's questionnaire for carpal tunnel syndrome

Katz hand diagram

Modified carpal compression test

Modified Phalen's test

Phalen's test

Press test (TFCC)

Pronation with ulnar deviation of the wrist

Reverse Phalen's test

Scaphoid compression test

Spurling's test

Tethered median nerve stress test

Thenar atrophy

Ulnar collateral ligament test

Upper limb tension test (median nerve)

Watson scaphoid test

Wrist flexion and median nerve compression

Wrist-radio index

CARPAL TUNNEL SYNDROME

UPPER LIMB NEURODYNAMIC TEST (MEDIAN NERVE)

Refer to chapter 7 (Orthopedic Screening and Nervous System Examination) for the performance and diagnostic accuracy of this test.

UPPER LIMB NEURODYNAMIC TEST (RADIAL NERVE)

Refer to chapter 7 (Orthopedic Screening and Nervous System Examination) for the performance and diagnostic accuracy of this test.

WAINNER'S CLINICAL PREDICTION RULE FOR CARPAL TUNNEL SYNDROME

Five test variables are used to predict the presence of carpal tunnel syndrome: (1) moving, shaking, or positioning the wrist or hands improves symptoms, (2) wrist ratio index > 0.67, (3) Brigham and Women's Hospital Hand Symptom Severity Scale score > 1.9, (4) diminished sensation in the median sensory field of thumb, or (5) age > 45 years.

Assessment A (+) test is meeting two or more of the five variables.

Statistics
- Two variables or greater: **SN 98 (14-100)**, SP 14 (13-23), +LR 1.1, **–LR 0.14**, QUADAS 10, in a study of 82 clients with carpal tunnel syndrome (mean age 45 ± 12 years; 41 women; mean duration of symptoms 183 days), using electrodiagnostic testing as a reference standard[86]
- Three variables or greater: **SN 98 (14-100)**, SP 54 (40-67), +LR 2.1, **–LR 0.04**, QUADAS 10[86]
- Four variables or greater: SN 77 (61-93), **SP 83 (73-93)**, +LR 4.6, –LR 0.28, QUADAS 10[86]
- All five variables positive: SN 18 (3-31), **SP 99 (97-100)**, **+LR 18.3**, –LR 0.83, QUADAS 10[86]

Critical Clinical Pearls

When performing the upper limb tension test for carpal tunnel syndrome, keep the following in mind:

- It is not uncommon for asymptomatic clients to experience limitations or discomfort.
- The clinician should perform the examination on the uninvolved side first.
- The clinician should perform the movements in a sequential order on both upper extremities each time the testing procedure is performed.
- A positive finding requires the following:
  - A reproduction of the client's concordant sign.
  - Test responses that are altered by the movement of a distant component.
  - A difference between the uninvolved side and involved side. The differences may be found in range, resistance during movement, and symptom response.

PHALEN'S TEST

Client Position	Sitting with arm relaxed and elbows and forearm horizontal
Clinician Position	Sitting next to the client
Movement	The client relaxes the wrists and allows them to fall into a gravity-assisted wrist flexion, then holds them there for up to 60 seconds. The clinician questions the client with regard to symptoms at 15-second intervals during the 60-second period. A variation of this test is for the client to approximate the dorsum of both hands to introduce bilateral wrist flexion.
Assessment	A (+) test is reproduction or exacerbation of paresthesias or anesthesia in the cutaneous distribution of the median nerve in the hand.

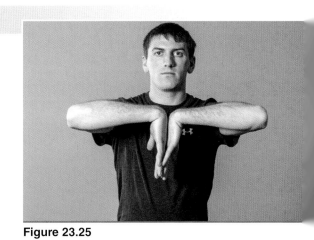

Figure 23.25

Statistics
- Overall estimate: SN 68 (not reported, or NR), SP 73 (NR), +LR 2.3, –LR 0.44, over 31 studies and 3,218 clients with pathology and 1,637 control clients[87]
- SN 77 (61-93), SP 40 (26-53), +LR 1.3, –LR 0.58, QUADAS 10, in a study of 82 clients with carpal tunnel syndrome (mean age 45 ± 12 years; 41 women; mean duration of symptoms 183 days), using electrodiagnostic testing as a reference standard[86]
- SN 75 (62-82), **SP 95 (85-100), +LR 15**, –LR 0.3, QUADAS 10, in a study of 100 consecutive clients/157 hands all using electrodiagnostic testing as an inclusion criterion and 50 healthy volunteers/100 hands (age range of all clients 18-73 years; 111 women; duration of symptoms ranged from 2 weeks to 20 years), using hand, wrist, and forearm problems and surgery as reference standards[88]
- SN 34 (24-43), SP 74 (62-87), +LR 1.3, –LR 0.9, QUADAS 11, in a study of 142 clients with suggestion of carpal tunnel (mean age 46.6 years; 82 women; duration of symptoms NR), using electrodiagnostic testing as a reference standard[89]
- Modification with 2.83 unit Semmes-Weinstein monofilament testing: **SN 82 (NR), SP 86 (NR),+LR 5.9, –LR 0.21**, QUADAS 11, in a study of 21 clients (33 hands) with suggestion of carpal tunnel (mean age 60 years [range 28-85 years]; 18 women; duration of symptoms 3 weeks to 10 years), using electrodiagnostic testing as a reference standard[90]
- **SN 80 (NR), SP 100 (NR), +LR Inf, –LR 0.20**, QUADAS 9, in a study of 37 clients (66 hands) with carpal tunnel syndrome (ages 27-88 years; 26 women; duration of symptoms NR) confirmed with electrodiagnostic testing as a reference standard[91]
- SN 61 (53-69), SP 83 (77-89), +LR 3.6, –LR 0.47, QUADAS 8, in a study of 83 clients/90 hands with carpal tunnel syndrome (mean age 56.9 [range 48-64 years]; 76 women; mean duration of symptoms NR), using electrodiagnostic testing as a reference standard[92]

REVERSE PHALEN'S TEST

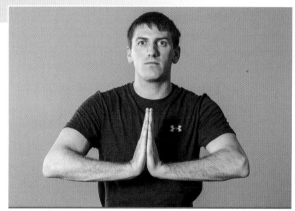

Figure 23.26

Client Position	Sitting with arm relaxed
Clinician Position	Sitting next to the client
Movement	The clinician instructs the client to place the wrists of both hands in complete dorsal extension for 60 seconds.
Assessment	A (+) test is reproduction of numbness and tingling along the distribution of the median nerves within 60 seconds.

Statistics
- SN 41 (NR), SP 55 (NR), +LR 0.9, –LR 1.1, QUADAS 10, in a study of 50 clients with CTS (mean age NR; 43 women; duration of symptoms NR), using nerve conduction studies as a reference standard[93]
- SN 42 (36-49), SP 35 (29-42), +LR 0.65, –LR 1.7, QUADAS 9, in a study of 232 clients with CTS (mean age NR [range 20-91 years]; 163 women; duration of symptoms NR), using the American Academy of Neurology clinical diagnostic criteria,[94] US, and electrodiagnostic studies as reference standards[95]
- SN 55 (NR), SP 96 (NR), +LR 14, –LR 0.5, QUADAS 8, in a study of 179 clients with CTS (mean age 53 years; 142 women; duration of symptoms NR), using clinical history, physical examination, and abnormalities of median nerve sensory and motor conduction velocities as reference standards[96]

MODIFIED PHALEN'S TEST

Client Position	Sitting with arm relaxed, resting on a pillow or arm holders with the hands floating at the end
Clinician Position	Sitting or standing next to the client
Movement	The clinician passively flexes the client's hands up to 90°.
Assessment	A (+) test is reproduction of symptoms along the distribution of the median nerve in the hand.
Statistics	No diagnostic accuracy studies determining SN and SP have been performed to date for this clinical test. The test differs from Phalen's test by having the forearms vertical in a relaxed position and having the clinician perform the passive wrist flexion.[97]

TINEL'S SIGN

Client Position	Sitting with the arm relaxed
Clinician Position	Sitting next to the client
Movement	The clinician flexes the client's elbow from 0° to 30° and places the forearm in a supinated position while supporting the client's wrist and hand in a neutral position. The clinician positions a tendon reflex hammer about 6 in. (15 cm) above the wrist and allows it to fall four to six times over the median nerve located between the tendons of the flexor carpi radialis and the palmaris longus at the proximal wrist crease.

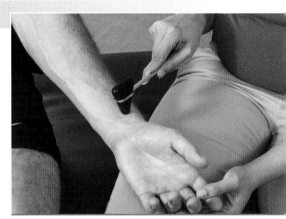

Figure 23.27

Assessment	A (+) test has been described as either nonpainful tingling sensation radiating distally along the course of the nerve or discomfort or pain that is related to the client's condition occurring at the wrist or radiating distally along the course of the nerve.
Statistics	These statistics are for nonpainful tingling sensation radiating distally along the course of the nerve:

- Overall estimate: SN 50 (NR), SP 77 (NR), +LR 2.3, –LR 0.44, over 28 studies and 2,640 clients with pathology and 1,614 control clients[87]
- SN 41 (22-59), SP 58 (45-72), +LR 0.98, –LR 1.0, QUADAS 10, in a study of 82 clients with carpal tunnel syndrome (mean age 45 ± 12 years; 41 women; mean duration of symptoms 183 days), using electrophysiologic examination as a reference standard[86]
- SN 64 (53-75), **SP 99 (96-100)**, **+LR 64**, –LR 0.4, QUADAS 10, in a study of 100 consecutive clients/157 hands all with electrodiagnostic testing as an inclusion criterion and 50 healthy volunteers/100 hands (age range of all clients 18-73 years; 111 women; duration of symptoms ranged from 2 weeks to 20 years), using hand, wrist, and forearm problems and surgery as a reference standard[88]
- SN 27 (18-36), SP 91 (62-87), +LR 3.0, –LR 0.8, QUADAS 11, in a study of 142 clients with suggestion of carpal tunnel (mean age 46.6 years; 82 women; duration of symptoms NR), using electrodiagnostic testing as a reference standard[89]
- SN 74 (66-81), **SP 91 (86-95)**, **+LR 8.2**, –LR 0.29, QUADAS 9, in a study of 83 clients/90 hands with carpal tunnel syndrome (mean age 56.9 [range 48-64 years]; 76 women; mean duration of symptoms NR), using electrodiagnostic testing as a reference standard[92]

These statistics are for discomfort or pain at the wrist or radiating distally along the course of the nerve that is related to the client's condition:

- SN 48 (29-67), SP 67 (54-79), +LR 1.4, –LR 0.78, QUADAS 10, in a study of 82 clients with carpal tunnel syndrome (mean age 45 ± 12 years; 41 women; mean duration of symptoms 183 days), using electrophysiologic examination as a reference standard[86]

FLICK SIGN

Client Position	Sitting with arms relaxed
Clinician Position	Standing, monitoring client
Movement	The clinician instructs the client to vigorously shake or flick their hands.
Assessment	A (+) test is resolution of symptoms of paresthesia during or following the test.
Statistics	

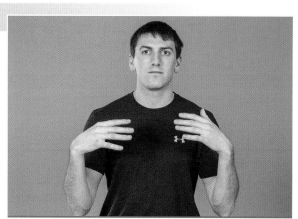

Figure 23.28

- Overall estimate: SN 47 (NR), SP 62 (NR), +LR 2.3, –LR 0.44, over four studies and 5,036 clients with pathology and 3,854 control clients[87]
- SN 37 (27-46), SP 74 (62-87), +LR 1.4, –LR 0.9, QUADAS 11, in a study of 142 clients with suggestion of carpal tunnel syndrome (mean age 47 years; 82 women; duration of symptoms NR), using electrodiagnostic testing as a reference standard[89]
- SN 50 (NR), SP 61 (NR), +LR 1.3, –LR 0.8, QUADAS 10, in a study of 50 clients with carpal tunnel syndrome symptoms (mean age NR; 43 women; duration of symptoms NR), using electrodiagnostic testing as a reference standard[93]
- **SN 90 (80-96)**, SP 30 (20-42), +LR 1.3, **–LR 0.3**, QUADAS 13, in a study of 59 clients/75 hands with carpal tunnel syndrome (mean age 47 years [range 15-82 years]; 43 women; duration of symptoms NR), using clinical and neurophysiological testing as a reference standard[11]

HAND ELEVATION TEST

Client Position	Sitting or standing comfortably
Clinician Position	Seated or standing at the client's side
Movement	The client actively raises both arms overhead and maintains the position for up to 2 minutes or until symptoms are provoked.
Assessment	A (+) test is provocation of paresthesia or numbness in the median nerve distribution.
Statistics	

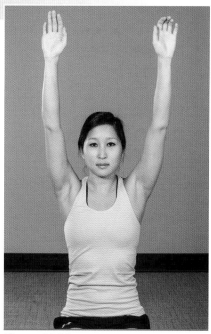

Figure 23.29

- SN 76 (NR), SP 99 (NR), +LR 50.3, –LR 0.25, QUADAS 8, in a study of 118 clients (200 symptomatic hands) with carpal tunnel syndrome (mean age 55.3 years [range 44-75 years]; 118 women; mean duration of symptoms greater than 6 months) confirmed with electrodiagnostic testing as a reference standard[98]
- **SN 87 (NR)**, **SP 89 (NR)**, +LR 7.8, –LR 0.15, QUADAS 9, in a study of 83 clients/90 hands with carpal tunnel syndrome (mean age 57 [range 48-64 years]; 76 women; duration of symptoms NR), using electrodiagnostic testing as a reference standard[92]

(continued)

Hand Elevation Test *(continued)*

- SN 99, SP 91, +LR 11.5, –LR 0.02, QUADAS 7, in a study of 70 clients with carpal tunnel syndrome (mean age 58 [range 26-87 years]; 51 women; duration of symptoms NR), using electrodiagnostic testing as a reference standard[99]
- SN 88 (81-94), SP 98 (95-100), +LR 44, –LR 0.12, QUADAS 7, in a study of 48 clients (60 hands) with carpal tunnel syndrome (mean age 56 [range 27-92 years]; 32 women; duration of symptoms NR), using electrodiagnostic testing as a reference standard[100]

TETHERED MEDIAN NERVE STRESS TEST

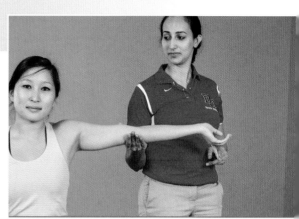

Client Position	Comfortably positioned, either sitting down or lying supine
Clinician Position	Positioned comfortably next to the client
Movement	With the client's forearm in supination, the clinician passively hyperextends the wrist while passively extending the distal interphalangeal joint of the index finger. This position is maintained for 15 seconds.
Assessment	A (+) test is provocation of pain in the proximal volar aspect of the forearm.

Figure 23.30

Statistics	SN 50 (NR), SP 59 (NR), +LR 1.22, –LR 0.59, QUADAS 11, in a study of 102 clients with carpal tunnel syndrome (mean age 53 years; 5 women; duration of symptoms 3-12 months), using electrodiagnostic testing as a reference standard[101]

CLOSED-FIST OR LUMBRICAL PROVOCATION TEST

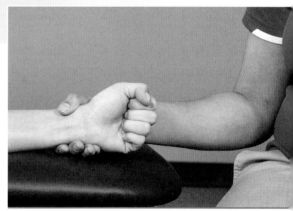

Client Position	Comfortably positioned, either sitting down or lying in supine
Clinician Position	Positioned comfortably next to the client
Movement	The client moves the fingers into a fully flexed position and maintains a fist for up to 60 seconds or until the onset of symptoms. The clinician holds the client's wrist.
Assessment	A (+) test is the provocation of paresthesia or numbness in the median nerve distribution.

Figure 23.31

Statistics	• Pooled synthesis: SN 48, SP 81, +LR 2.5, –LR 0.64 in a systematic review of two studies including 159 clients[102] • SN 37 (NR), SP 71 (NR), +LR 1.28, –LR 0.89, QUADAS 8, in a study of 96 clients with carpal tunnel syndrome (mean age 53 years; 6 women; duration of symptoms 3-12 months), using electrodiagnostic testing as a reference standard[103]

WRIST-RATIO INDEX

Client Position	Seated with the arm resting on the table
Clinician Position	Seated next to the client
Measurement	Using a standard sliding caliper, the clinician measures the dorsal-ventral and radial-ulnar dimensions of the wrist at the level of the distal palmar wrist crease.
Assessment	A (+) test occurs if the wrist ratio (D-V/R-U) is $\geq$ 0.70.
Statistics	SN 69 (NR), SP 73 (NR), +LR 2.6, –LR 0.42, QUADAS 10, in a study of 143 clients (228 hands) clients with carpal tunnel syndrome (mean age, number of females, and duration of symptoms NR), using electrodiagnostic testing as a reference standard[104]

KATZ HAND DIAGRAM

Client Position	The client fills out a self-administered hand diagram using a key of numbness, tingling, and decreased sensation.
Assessment	The Katz hand diagram divides clients into the categories of classic, probable, possible, and unlikely carpal tunnel syndrome.

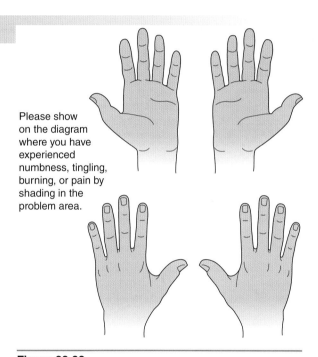

Please show on the diagram where you have experienced numbness, tingling, burning, or pain by shading in the problem area.

Figure 23.32

Statistics

- Pooled synthesis: SN 75, SP 72, +LR 2.7, –LR 0.35 in a systematic review of six studies including 293 clients.[102]

- **SN 80 (NR)**, SP 90 (NR), +LR 3.6, **–LR 0.1**, QUADAS 11, in a study of 63 clients (83 hands) with carpal tunnel syndrome (mean age, gender, and duration of symptoms NR), using objective clinical criteria including electrodiagnostic testing as a reference standard[105]

- SN 33-40 (20-52), SP 76-81 (69-87), +LR 1.38–2.11, –LR 0.89–0.74, QUADAS NR, in a study of 221 workers with carpal tunnel syndrome (mean age 32 years; 65 women; duration of symptoms NR), using electrodiagnostic testing as a reference standard[106]

MEDIAN NERVE DIGIT SCORE

Client Position	The client fills out a self-administered hand diagram using a key of numbness, tingling, and decreased sensation.
Assessment	The clinician scores the diagrams according to the number of digits indicated by the client (thumb, index, and long finger) with shading. Each digit is scored separately as involved or uninvolved.

Statistics

- Overall SN 54-58 (40-69), SP 70-76 (62-83), +LR 1.8–2.4, –LR 0.66–0.55, QUADAS 9, in a study of 221 workers with carpal tunnel syndrome (mean age 32 years; 65 women; duration of symptoms NR), using electrodiagnostic testing as a reference standard[106]
- Long finger: SN 67 (52-79), SP 65-73 (57-80), +LR 1.9–2.5, –LR 0.45–0.51[106]
- Index finger: SN 54-59 (40-70), SP 67-73 (60-80), +LR 1.6–2.2, –LR 0.69–0.56[106]
- Thumb: SN 31-35 (21-50), SP 77-79 (70-85), +LR 1.4–1.7, –LR 0.89–0.82[106]

THENAR ATROPHY

Client Position	Sitting with arms relaxed on the table
Clinician Position	Sitting next to the client
Assessment	The clinician visually inspects the thenar eminence for loss of bulk in the abductor pollicis brevis muscle. A (+) test is the presence of observable atrophy.
Statistics	• Pooled synthesis: SN 12, SP 94, +LR 2.0, –LR 0.94, in a systematic review of two studies including 107 clients[102]
	• SN 18 (NR), **SP 96 (NR)**, +LR 4.5, –LR 0.85, QUADAS 9, in a study of 88 clients diagnosed with carpal tunnel syndrome (mean age 56 [range 21-85 years]; 55 women; mean duration of symptoms NR), using electrodiagnostic testing as a reference standard[107]

WRIST FLEXION AND MEDIAN NERVE COMPRESSION

 Video 23.33 **in the web resource shows a demonstration of this test.**

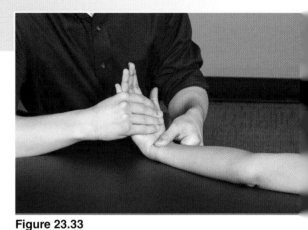

Client Position	Sitting with the elbows fully extended, forearm supinated, and wrist flexed to 60°
Clinician Position	Sitting next to the client
Movement	The clinician applies even and constant pressure over the median nerve at the carpal tunnel.

Figure 23.33

Assessment	A (+) test is the reproduction of the client's symptoms along the median nerve distribution within either 20 or 30 seconds.
Statistics	• Pooled synthesis: SN 80, SP 92, +LR 10, –LR 0.22, in a systematic review of three studies including 190 clients[102]
	• 30-second cutoff: **SN 86 (80-92), SP 95 (91-99)**, +LR 17.2, **–LR 0.15**, QUADAS 9, in a study of 114 clients/191 hands with CTS (mean age NR; 32% females; mean duration of symptoms NR), using electrodiagnostic testing as a reference standard[108]
	• 20-second cutoff: **SN 82 (76-89), SP 99 (97-100)**, +LR 82, **–LR 0.18**, QUADAS 9, in a study of 114 clients/191 hands (mean age NR; 32% females; mean duration of symptoms NR) with CTS, using electrodiagnostic testing as a reference standard[108]

MEDIAN NERVE COMPRESSION TEST

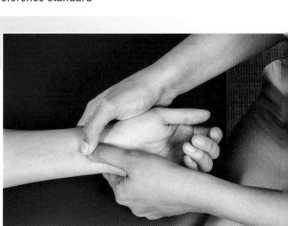

Client Position	Sitting with arms relaxed on the table
Clinician Position	Sitting opposite the client, with their thumbs placed directly over the median nerve as it passes under the flexor retinaculum between the flexor carpi radialis and the palmaris longus
Movement	The clinician applies even and constant pressure with the thumbs for 15 seconds to 2 minutes. Afterward, the clinician removes their thumbs and questions the client on the relief of symptoms.

Figure 23.34

Assessment	A (+) test is the reproduction of the client's symptoms (pain, paresthesia, or numbness) distal to the site of compression along the median nerve distribution.
Statistics	Pooled synthesis: SN 64, SP 83, +LR 3.8, –LR 0.43, in a systematic review of 17 studies including 1,985 clients[102]

CARPAL COMPRESSION TEST (DURKAN'S TEST)

Client Position	Sitting with arms relaxed on the table
Clinician Position	Sitting opposite to the client and placing their thumbs directly over the client's median nerve
Movement	The clinician applies even and constant pressure over the proximal edge of the carpal ligament (proximal wrist crease) with their thumbs for 30 seconds.
Assessment	A (+) test is the reproduction of the client's symptoms (pain, paresthesia, or numbness) distal to the site of compression along the median nerve distribution.
Statistics	• Pooled synthesis: SN 64, SP 83, +LR 3.8, –LR 0.43, in a systematic review of 17 studies including 1,985 clients[102]
	• SN 75 (67-82), **SP 93 (88-97)**, **+LR 10.7**, –LR 0.27, QUADAS 9, in a study of 83 clients/90 hands with carpal tunnel syndrome (mean age 56.9 [range 48-64 years]; 76 women; mean duration of symptoms NR), using electrodiagnostic testing as a reference standard[92]
	• SN 77 (NR), SP 18 (NR), +LR 0.9, –LR 1.29, QUADAS 9, in a study of 88 clients diagnosed with carpal tunnel syndrome (mean age 56 [range 21-85 years]; 55 women; mean duration of symptoms NR), using electrodiagnostic testing as a reference[107]

MODIFIED CARPAL COMPRESSION TEST

Client Position	Sitting with forearms in supination on a table, with wrists in neutral alignment
Clinician Position	Sitting opposite to the client, with their thumbs placed directly over the palmar aspect of the carpal tunnel with adjacent thumbs
Movement	The clinician applies an oscillatory pressure over the palmar aspect of the carpal tunnel.
Assessment	A (+) test is reproduction of the client's symptoms in the median nerve distribution of the volar/palmar aspect within 5 seconds.
Statistics	SN 14 (8-24), SP 96 (72-100), +LR 3.5, –LR 0.89, QUADAS 9, in a study of 43 clients/86 hands with the diagnosis of carpal tunnel syndrome (mean female age: 47 years, mean male age: 52; 32 women; mean duration of symptoms NR), using electrodiagnostic testing as a reference standard[109]

TWO-POINT DISCRIMINATION

Client Position	Sitting with arms relaxed on the table
Clinician Position	Sitting next to the client
Movement	The clinician uses a two-point esthesiometer applied to the pulp of the index finger until the skin just blanches. The client distinguishes between the touch of the prongs (either one or two). The clinician records, in millimeters, the smallest distance perceived as two separate points.
Assessment	A (+) test is the client's inability to detect a distance of 6 mm or more.
Statistics	Pooled synthesis: SN 24, SP 93, +LR 4.8, –LR 0.80, in a systematic review of six studies including 381 clients[102]

SEMMES-WEINSTEIN MONOFILAMENT TEST

Client Position	Sitting with the arms relaxed on the table
Clinician Position	Sitting next to the client
Movement	The clinician applies the monofilament perpendicular to the palmar digital surface of the digital pulp of digits 1, 2, and 3 on the affected hand. The clinician applies pressure until the monofilament begins to bend. They repeat this process three times.
Assessment	A (+) test is occurs when the client, with their eyes closed, can verbally report which digit is receiving pressure at 2.83 mg.
Statistics	Pooled synthesis: SN 72, SP 62, +LR 1.9, –LR 0.45, in a systematic review of 11 studies including 811 clients[102]

HYPOESTHESIA

Client Position	Sitting with the arms relaxed on the table
Clinician Position	Sitting or standing next to the client
Movement	The clinician rolls a pinwheel across the client's hand in the distribution of the median nerve.
Assessment	A (+) test is the client's ability to report a decrease in their capability to detect pain in the hand along the distribution of the median nerve.
Statistics	SN 51 (NR), SP 85 (NR), +LR 3.4, –LR 0.6, QUADAS 10, in a study of 143 clients (228 hands) with carpal tunnel syndrome (mean age, number of females, and duration of symptoms NR), using electrodiagnostic testing as a reference standard[104]

GILLIAT TOURNIQUET TEST

Client Position	Sitting with the arms relaxed on the table
Clinician Position	Sitting or standing next to the client
Movement	The clinician places a blood pressure cuff over the client's arm proximal to the elbow and inflates it to either a suprasystolic pressure (above the client's systolic pressure) or an infrasystolic pressure (70 mmHg) for 60 seconds.
Assessment	A (+) test is either the reproduction or exacerbation of paresthesia or numbness in the client's thumb or index finger within 60 seconds.
Statistics	• Pooled synthesis (suprasystolic): SN 59, SP 61, +LR 1.5, –LR 0.67, in a systematic review of six studies including 306 clients[102] • Suprasystolic: SN 67 (53-80), SP 33 (1-91), +LR 1, –LR 1, QUADAS 8, in a study of 49 clients/52 hands with carpal tunnel syndrome (mean age 52 years; 40 women; mean duration of symptoms NR), using electrodiagnostic testing as a reference standard[110] • Infrasystolic: SN 55 (40-69), SP 100 (29-100), +LR 55, –LR 0.46, QUADAS 8, in a study of 49 clients/52 hands (mean age 52 years; 40 women; mean duration of symptoms NR) with carpal tunnel syndrome, using electrodiagnostic testing as a reference standard[110]

ABNORMAL VIBRATION

Client Position	Sitting with the arms relaxed on the table
Clinician Position	Sitting or standing next to the client
Movement	The clinician will use a tuning fork with 256 cycles per second. The clinician strikes the tuning fork against a firm object and then places it against the fingertip of each digit on the client's hand. They then compare the testing to the contralateral upper extremity.
Assessment	A (+) test occurs when the client reports that the perception of the stimulus was altered and that they could qualify the difference as being lesser, being greater, or similar.
Statistics	Pooled synthesis: SN 55, SP 81, +LR 2.9, –LR 0.56, in a systematic review of six studies including 343 clients[102]

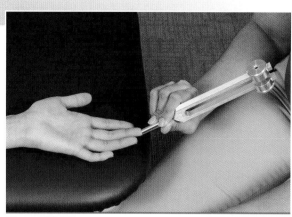

Figure 23.35

ABDUCTOR POLLICIS BREVIS WEAKNESS

Client Position	Sitting with the arms relaxed on the table and the thumb positioned in neutral
Clinician Position	Sitting or standing next to the client
Movement	The clinician instructs the client to move the thumb into abduction as they apply a force directed toward the palm.
Assessment	A (+) test is weakness of thumb abduction.
Statistics	• Pooled synthesis: SN 29, SP 80, +LR 1.5, –LR 0.89, in a systematic review of two studies including 107 clients[102]

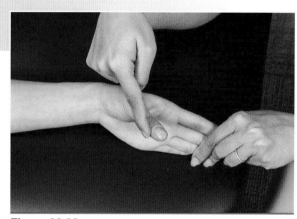

Figure 23.36

• SN 37 (NR), SP 73 (NR), +LR 1.4, –LR 0.86, QUADAS 9, in a study of 88 clients diagnosed with carpal tunnel syndrome (mean age 56 [range 21-85 years]; 55 women; mean duration of symptoms NR), using electrodiagnostic testing as a reference[107]

HEMS' QUESTIONNAIRE FOR CARPAL TUNNEL SYNDROME

The questionnaire has two sections. The client completes the first section and the clinician completes the second section. The questionnaire is scored according to the following system:

- Age: below 60 years (2 points), above 60 years (0 points)
- Symptoms: night pain (2 points), paresthesia median nerve distribution (2 points), relief pain by shaking (2 points), relief pain by splint (1 point), clumsiness (1 point)
- Signs: Tinel's sign (2 points), Phalen's test (1 point), alteration in sensation in distribution of median nerve (2 points), wasting of thenar eminence (2 points)
- Total: (17 points)

Statistics
- Score ≥ 6: SN 92 (83-97), SP 61 (36-83), +LR 2.4, –LR 0.13, QUADAS 7, in a study of 91 clients/52 hands with carpal tunnel syndrome (mean age 55 years; 108 women; symptom duration ranged from 3 months to more than 1 year), using nerve conduction studies as a reference standard[111]

- Score ≥ 7: SN 82 (72-90), SP 67 (41-87), +LR 2.5, –LR 0.27, QUADAS 7, in a study of 91 clients/52 hands with carpal tunnel syndrome (mean age 55 years; 108 women; symptom duration ranged from 3 months to more than 1 year), using nerve conduction studies as a reference standard[111]

- Score ≥ 8: SN 70 (58-80), SP 72 (47-90), +LR 2.5, –LR 0.42, QUADAS 7, in a study of 91 clients/52 hands with carpal tunnel syndrome (mean age 55 years; 108 women; symptom duration ranged from 3 months to more than 1 year), using nerve conduction studies as a reference standard[111]

THUMB INSTABILITY

ULNAR COLLATERAL LIGAMENT TEST (GAMEKEEPER'S OR SKIER'S THUMB)

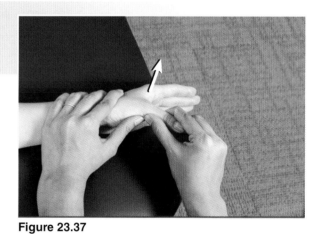

Figure 23.37

Client Position Sitting with the arms relaxed

Clinician Position Sitting next to the client

Movement The clinician stabilizes the client's hand or fingers with their cranial hand and takes the client's thumb into extension with their caudal hand. Maintaining thumb extension, the clinician applies a valgus stress to the metacarpophalangeal joint of the thumb.

Assessment A (+) test has been described as valgus movement greater than 30°.

Statistics SN 94 (NR), SP (NR), +LR (NR), –LR (NR), QUADAS 8, in a prospective study of 23 clients with acute ulnar collateral ligament injuries (mean age NR; number of women NR; mean duration of symptoms 7 days), using surgery as a reference standard[112]

THUMB TENOSYNOVITIS

FINKELSTEIN'S TEST

Client Position	Sitting with the arms relaxed
Clinician Position	Sitting next to the client
Movement	The client makes a fist with the thumb placed inside the fingers. The clinician stabilizes the proximal forearm and deviates the client's wrist in an ulnar direction.
Assessment	A (+) test has been described as pain over the abductor pollicis longus (APL) and extensor pollicis brevis (EPB) tendons.

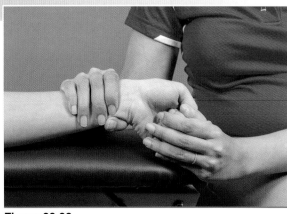

Figure 23.38

Statistics

- NR

- The extensor pollicis brevis test has been performed to determine if a septum was present between the EPB and APL. The test consists of two parts: (1) The clinician resists thumb metacarpophalangeal joint extension and then (2) resists thumb palmar abduction. A (+) test occurs when the pain produced by part (1) is greater than that in (2).

- **SN 81 (NR)**, SP 50 (NR), +LR 1.62, **–LR 0.38**, QUADAS 9, in a study of 178 clients with de Quervain's (mean age 46 years; 138 women; mean duration of symptoms NR), using surgery as a reference standard.[113]

EXTENSOR CARPI ULNARIS TENDINOSIS

EXTENSOR CARPI ULNARIS (ECU) SYNERGY TEST

Client Position	Sitting with arms relaxed with the arm to be assessed on the table with the elbow flexed at 90°, forearm in full supination, wrist in neutral, and fingers fully extended
Clinician Position	Sitting next to the client, the clinician grasps the client's thumb and middle finger with one hand and palpates the ECU tendon with the other hand.
Movement	The client radially abducts the thumb against resistance.
Assessment	A (+) test has been described as reproduction of pain along the dorsal aspect of the wrist.
Statistics	• NR

- Part of a clinical algorithm in a prospective study of 55 clients with dorsal-ulnar-sided wrist pain, using MRI or wrist arthroscopy as a reference standard. Authors suggest that the ECU synergy test compose part of a clinical algorithm that may help to differentiate between intra-articular and extra-articular pathology, and it may minimize the need for wrist MRI and diagnostic arthroscopy.[114]

SCAPHOID FRACTURE

SCAPHOID COMPRESSION TEST

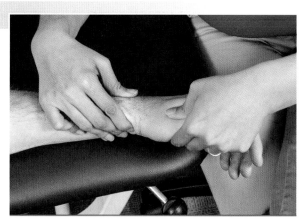

Figure 23.39

Client Position	Sitting with the arms relaxed
Clinician Position	Sitting next to the client
Movement	The clinician provides longitudinal pressure through the thumb, producing compression on the scaphoid.
Assessment	A (+) test is a reproduction of the client's pain at the wrist.
Statistics	• SN 70 (NR), SP 22 (NR), +LR 0.90, −LR 1.4, QUADAS 9, in a prospective study of 99 clients with scaphoid fracture (mean age NR [range 10-74 years]; 44 females with acute wrist injuries, duration of symptoms NR), using initial X-rays or repeat X-ray or bone scan 2 weeks after injury as a reference standard[115]
	• **SN 100 (94-100)**, SP 48 (40-60), +LR 1.92, **−LR 0**, QUADAS 9, in a prospective study of 215 clients with scaphoid fracture (median age 36 years; 48% women; duration of symptoms within 24 hours), using initial X-rays or repeat X-ray or bone scan 2 weeks after injury as a reference standard[116]

ANATOMICAL SNUFFBOX TENDERNESS

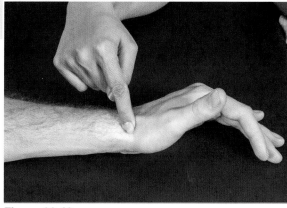

Figure 23.40

Client Position	Sitting with the arms relaxed
Clinician Position	Sitting next to the client
Movement	The clinician palpates and provides pressure on the anatomical snuffbox.
Assessment	A (+) test is pain or tenderness during palpation with pressure.
Statistics	• SN 90 (80-100), SP 40 (33-47), +LR 2.37, −LR 2.25, QUADAS 8, in a study of 246 clients with a suspected scaphoid injury (mean age, number of females, and mean duration of symptoms NR), using initial X-rays or repeat X-rays 14 days later as a reference standard[117]
	• **SN 100 (94-100)**, SP 19 (13-26), +LR 1.23, **−LR 0**, QUADAS 9, in a prospective study of 215 clients with scaphoid fracture (median age 36 years; 48% females; duration of symptoms within 24 hours), using initial X-rays or repeat X-ray or bone scan 2 weeks after injury as a reference standard[116]

SCAPHOID TUBERCLE TENDERNESS

Client Position	Sitting with the arms relaxed
Clinician Position	Sitting next to the client
Movement	The clinician extends the client's wrist with one hand and then palpates and provides pressure to the tuberosity at the proximal wrist with the other hand.
Assessment	A (+) test is pain or tenderness during palpation with pressure.

Statistics
- SN 87 (75-99), SP 57 (50-64), +LR 1.55, –LR 1.51, QUADAS 8, in a study of 246 clients with a suspected scaphoid injury (mean age, number of females, and mean duration of symptoms NR), using initial X-rays or repeat X-rays 14 days later as a reference standard[117]
- **SN 100 (94-100)**, SP 30 (23-38), +LR 1.43, **–LR 0**, QUADAS 9, in a prospective study of 215 clients with scaphoid fracture (median age 36 years; 48% females; duration of symptoms within 24 hours), using initial X-rays or repeat X-ray or bone scan 2 weeks after injury as a reference standard[116]

PRONATION WITH ULNAR DEVIATION OF THE WRIST

Client Position	Sitting with the arms relaxed
Clinician Position	Sitting next to the client
Movement	The clinician instructs the client to pronate their wrist to end range, followed by ulnar deviation.
Assessment	A (+) test is described as pain in the anatomical snuffbox.
Statistics	• NR
	• Powell and colleagues demonstrated that the test gave a 52% positive predictive value and a 100% negative predictive value in a prospective study of 73 clients.[118]

The next 10 tests for scaphoid fracture were examined and performed on 41 clients after a fall on an outstretched hand. MRI was used as a reference standard. Three orthopedic surgeons who had 10 years of clinical experience in treating trauma reviewed the MRIs. The orthopedists were provided the results of the clinical tests prior to interpreting each MRI. The clinical tests were performed in the following order, which may have had an effect on pain tolerance; this could have adversely affected the outcomes.[119]

ABDUCTION OF THE THUMB

Client Position	Sitting with the arms relaxed
Clinician Position	Sitting next to the client
Movement	The clinician asks the client to actively abduct their thumb.
Assessment	A (+) test is a reproduction of pain during thumb abduction.
Statistics	SN 73 (NR), SP 50 (NR), +LR 1.45, –LR 0.55, QUADAS 11, in a study of 41 clients with clinically suspected occult scaphoid fractures (median age 29 years; 12 females; duration of symptoms NR), using MRI as a reference standard[119]

RADIAL DEVIATION OF THE WRIST

Client Position	Sitting with the arms relaxed
Clinician Position	Sitting next to the client
Movement	The clinician asks the client to actively deviate their wrist radially.
Assessment	A (+) test is a reproduction of pain during radial deviation.
Statistics	SN 68 (NR), SP 33 (NR), +LR 1.03, –LR 0.95, QUADAS 11, in a study of 41 clients with clinically suspected occult scaphoid fractures (median age 29 years; 12 females; duration of symptoms NR), using MRI as a reference standard[119]

AXIAL LOADING OF THE THUMB

Client Position	Sitting with the arms relaxed
Clinician Position	Sitting next to the client
Movement	The clinician produces a compressive load through the client's thumb.
Assessment	A (+) test is a reproduction of the client's pain during the compressive loading.
Statistics	SN 71 (NR), SP 35 (NR), +LR 1.10, –LR 0.82, QUADAS 11, in a study of 41 clients with clinically suspected occult scaphoid fractures (median age 29 years; 12 females; duration of symptoms NR), using MRI as a reference standard[119]

FLEXION OF THE WRIST

Client Position	Sitting with the arms relaxed
Clinician Position	Sitting next to the client
Movement	The clinician instructs the client to actively flex their wrist.
Assessment	A (+) test is a reproduction of the client's pain during wrist flexion.
Statistics	SN 71 (NR), SP 50 (NR), +LR 1.43, –LR 0.57, QUADAS 11, in a study of 41 clients with clinically suspected occult scaphoid fractures (median age 29 years; 12 females; duration of symptoms NR), using MRI as a reference standard[119]

EXTENSION OF THE WRIST

Client Position	Sitting with the arms relaxed
Clinician Position	Sitting next to the client
Movement	The clinician instructs the client to actively extend their wrist.
Assessment	A (+) test is a reproduction of the client's pain during wrist extension.
Statistics	SN 72 (NR), SP 60 (NR), +LR 1.81, –LR 0.46, QUADAS 11, in a study of 41 clients with clinically suspected occult scaphoid fractures (median age 29 years; 12 females; duration of symptoms NR), using MRI as a reference standard[119]

POWER GRIP OF THE HAND

Client Position	Sitting with the arms relaxed
Clinician Position	Sitting next to the client
Movement	The clinician and client set up in a handshake position. The clinician instructs the client to squeeze their hand.
Assessment	A (+) test is a reproduction of pain while the client squeezes the clinician's hand.
Statistics	SN 67 (NR), SP 20 (NR), +LR 0.83, –LR 1.67, QUADAS 11, in a study of 41 clients with clinically suspected occult scaphoid fractures (median age 29 years; 12 females; duration of symptoms NR), using MRI as a reference standard[119]

ULNAR DEVIATION OF THE WRIST

Client Position	Sitting with the arms relaxed
Clinician Position	Sitting next to the client
Movement	The clinician instructs the client to actively perform ulnar deviation of their wrist.
Assessment	A (+) test is a reproduction of the client's pain during ulnar deviation.
Statistics	SN 70 (NR), SP 36 (NR), +LR 1.10, –LR 0.83, QUADAS 11, in a study of 41 clients with clinically suspected occult scaphoid fractures (median age 29 years; 12 females; duration of symptoms NR), using MRI as a reference standard[119]

PRONATION OF THE FOREARM

Client Position	Sitting with the arms relaxed
Clinician Position	Sitting next to the client
Movement	The clinician instructs the client to actively pronate their forearm.
Assessment	A (+) test is a reproduction of the client's pain during pronation.
Statistics	SN 79 (NR), SP 58 (NR), +LR 1.90, –LR 0.35, QUADAS 11, in a study of 41 clients with clinically suspected occult scaphoid fractures (median age 29 years; 12 females; duration of symptoms NR), using MRI as a reference standard[119]

SUPINATION OF THE FOREARM

Client Position	Sitting with the arms relaxed
Clinician Position	Sitting next to the client
Movement	The clinician instructs the client to actively supinate their forearm.
Assessment	A (+) test is a reproduction of the client's pain during supination.
Statistics	SN 76 (NR), SP 50 (NR), +LR 1.52, –LR 0.48, QUADAS 11, in a study of 41 clients with clinically suspected occult scaphoid fractures (median age 29 years; 12 females; duration of symptoms NR), using MRI as a reference standard[119]

THUMB-INDEX FINGER PINCH

Client Position	Sitting with the arms relaxed
Clinician Position	Sitting next to the client
Movement	The clinician instructs the client to actively pinch their thumb and index finger together.
Assessment	A (+) test is a reproduction of pain while pinching.
Statistics	SN 73 (NR), SP 75 (NR), +LR 2.92, –LR 0.36, QUADAS 11, in a study of 41 clients with clinically suspected occult scaphoid fractures (median age 29 years; 12 females; duration of symptoms NR), using MRI as a reference standard[119]

WRIST LAXITY

GARCIA-ELIAS TEST

Wrist laxity is evaluated using four clinical tests. Each test is given a score of 1 to 50 points, with a score of 1 point indicating the greatest stiffness and a score of 50 indicating the highest joint laxity. All four test scores are added together for a range of 4 to 200. Clients are ranked based on their laxity score. A (+) test is a rank in the top 25% of total clients. The four clinical tests are the following:

- Measurement in millimeters of the shortest perpendicular distance between the center of the thumbnail and the forearm when the client was asked to move the thumb maximally toward the forearm while extending the wrist
- Measurement of the angle of the wrist when the client was asked to extend the wrist maximally
- Measurement in millimeters of the shortest perpendicular distance between the center of the thumbnail and the forearm when the client was asked to move the wrist in maximal flexion
- Measurement of the angle of the wrist when the client was asked to flex the wrist maximally

Statistics   SN 20 (NR), SP 55 (NR), +LR 0.44, −LR 1.46, QUADAS 8, in a study of 50 healthy premenopausal female clients, using clinical evaluations from two expert surgeons that resulted in a final score on a Likert scale as a reference standard[120]

BEIGHTON METHOD

The Beighton method of assessment of generalized ligamentous laxity is described in detail in chapter 8 (Range of Motion Assessment).

AROM METHOD

A measurement device was created, based on a validated clinical goniometer, to measure the AROM of the wrist. The forearm and hand were fixed so that the movement was localized to the wrist, although researchers stated that minor carpal motion could not be prevented.

Statistics   SN 54 (NR), SP 67 (NR), +LR 1.61, −LR 0.69, QUADAS 8, in a study of 50 healthy premenopausal female clients, using clinical evaluations from two expert surgeons that resulted in a final score on a Likert scale as a reference standard[120]

WRIST INSTABILITY

WATSON SCAPHOID TEST (SCAPHOID INSTABILITY)

Client Position	Sitting with the arm slightly pronated
Clinician Position	Sitting or standing next to the client. The clinician grasps the client's wrist from the radial side with their thumb over the scaphoid tubercle. With the other hand, the clinician grasps the client's metacarpals.
Movement	The clinician moves the client's hand from ulnar deviation and slight extension to radial deviation and slight flexion. The clinician uses their thumb to push the scaphoid out of its normal

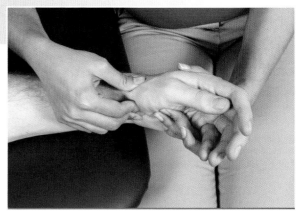

Figure 23.41

alignment when laxity is present. When the thumb is released, a thunk is heard as the scaphoid returns to its normal alignment.

Assessment   A (+) test occurs when there is a subluxation or clunk at the clinician's thumb and a reproduction of pain reported by the client.

Statistics   SN 69 (NR), SP 66 (NR), +LR 2.0, –LR 0.47, QUADAS 12, in a retrospective study of 50 clients with wrist pain (median age 38 years; 24 women; duration of symptoms of at least 4 weeks), using arthroscopy as a reference standard[121]

ULNOMENISCOTRIQUETRAL DORSAL GLIDE OR PIANO KEY TEST (TFCC TEAR OR TRIQUETRAL INSTABILITY)

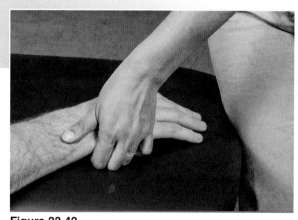

Client Position   Sitting with the arms relaxed

Clinician Position   Sitting or standing at the client's side. The clinician places their thumb dorsally over the client's ulna and places the proximal interphalangeal joint of their index finger over the pisotriquetral complex.

Movement   The clinician produces a dorsal glide of the pisotriquetral complex by squeezing their thumb and index finger together.

Figure 23.42

Assessment   A (+) test is described as a reproduction of pain or laxity in the ulnomeniscotriquetral region.

Statistics   SN 66 (NR), SP 64 (NR), +LR 1.8, –LR 0.5, QUADAS 12, in a retrospective study of 50 clients with wrist pain (median age 38 years; 24 women; duration of symptoms of at least 4 weeks), using arthroscopy as a reference standard[121]

BALLOTTEMENT TEST (LUNOTRIQUETRAL LIGAMENT INTEGRITY)

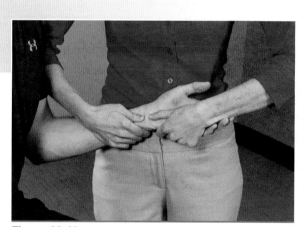

Client Position   Sitting with the arms relaxed

Clinician Position   Sitting or standing next to the client. The clinician grasps the triquetrum with the thumb and index finger of one hand and uses the other thumb and index finger of the other hand to grasp the lunate.

Movement   The clinician moves the lunate in a palmar and dorsal direction in regard to the triquetrum.

Figure 23.43

Assessment   A (+) test is laxity, crepitus, or reproduction of the client's pain during movement.

Statistics   SN 64 (NR), SP 44 (NR), +LR 1.14, –LR 0.82, QUADAS 12, in a retrospective study of 50 clients with wrist pain (median age 38 years; 24 women; duration of symptoms of at least 4 weeks), using arthroscopy as a reference standard[121]

WRIST FLEXION AND FINGER EXTENSION TEST (SCAPHOLUNATE PATHOLOGY)

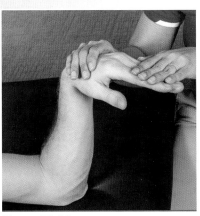

Client Position	Sitting with the elbow placed on the table
Clinician Position	Sitting or standing next to the client
Movement	The clinician places and holds the client's wrist in flexion and instructs the client to extend their fingers against resistance.
Assessment	A (+) test is a reproduction of pain over the scaphoid.
Statistics	• NR
	• Truong and colleagues[122] described this test as a component of five clinical exam tests used in determining scapholunate pathology.

Figure 23.44

DORSAL CAPITATE DISPLACEMENT APPREHENSION TEST (STABILITY OF THE CAPITATE BONE)

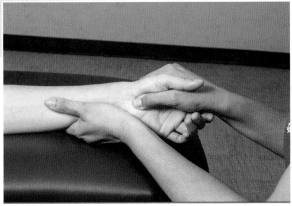

Client Position	Sitting facing the clinician
Clinician Position	Sitting or standing next to the client. The clinician uses one hand to hold the client's hand in neutral. With the other hand, the clinician places their thumb over the palmar aspect of the capitate and their fingers on the dorsal surface.
Movement	The clinician pushes the capitate posterior and applies a counterpressure with the fingers on the dorsal surface.
Assessment	A (+) test is a reproduction of the client's pain, apprehension, or if half of the proximal pole of the capitate is displaced past the lunate fossa.
Statistics	• NR
	• Truong and colleagues[122] described a similar test, called the capitolunate instability pattern wrist maneuver, as a component of five clinical exam tests used in determining scapholunate pathology.

Figure 23.45

CLINICAL STRESS TEST (DISTAL RADIUS FRACTURE)

Client Position	Sitting with the arms relaxed
Clinician Position	Sitting or standing next to the client. The clinician grasps the client's radius with the forearm in a neutral position.
Movement	The clinician fixes the distal ulna between their thumb and index finger and then tries to force the distal ulna in a dorsal and palmar direction in regard to the radius.
Assessment	A (+) test occurs when the ulna is displaced relatively to the contralateral side with the existence of pain or apprehension.

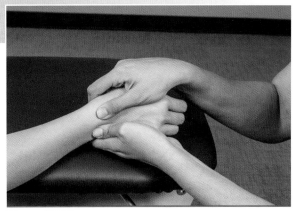

Figure 23.46

Statistics
- NR
- Kim and colleagues[123] determined the kappa values for agreement of the results regarding distal radial ulnar joint instability by comparing CT measurements and the clinical stress test. Reliability values are as follows: 0.33 for the modified radioulnar line, 0.56 for the epicenter, and 0.41 for the radioulnar ratio method. A limitation with this study was that a second clinician did not retest the reliability of the clinical stress test.

ULNOCARPAL STRESS TEST

Client Position	Sitting with the elbow fully flexed, forearm supinated, and wrist in full ulnar deviation
Clinician Position	Sitting or standing next to the client, supporting their elbow and grasping the palm of the hand
Movement	The clinician maintains ulnar deviation while moving the wrist in supination and pronation.
Assessment	A (+) test is a click and pain along the medial aspect of the wrist within the ulnocarpal region.
Statistics	• NR

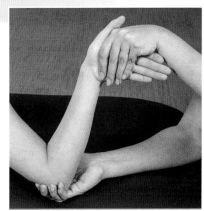

Figure 23.47

- Moriya and colleagues[124] evaluated this test on 11 fresh and frozen cadaver specimens. Investigators released the triangular ligament to simulate instability of the distal radial ulnar joint.

GRIND TEST (TFCC)

Client Position	Sitting with the arms relaxed
Clinician Position	Sitting or standing next to the client
Movement	The clinician compresses and rotates the client's first metacarpal bone and trapezium.
Assessment	A (+) test is reproduction of pain and crepitus due to the test movement.
Statistics	NR

PRESS TEST (TFCC)

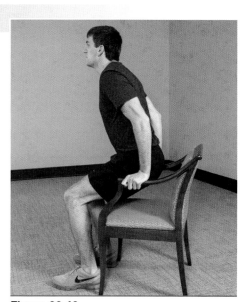

Figure 23.48

Client Position	Sitting in a stable chair with both hands and arms on the armrests
Clinician Position	Sitting or standing next to the client
Movement	The client pushes off the armrests to suspend their body only using the hands.
Assessment	A (+) test is a reproduction of the wrist pain while the client is pressing up their body weight.
Statistics	• SN 100, QUADAS 7, in a prospective study of 27 clients with a working diagnosis of a triangular fibrocartilage complex tear (median age 31 years; 9 women; duration of symptoms NR), using arthroscopic surgery as a reference standard.[125] Due to methodology of the test design, SP could not be determined.
	• SN 79, QUADAS 7, in a prospective study of 27 clients with a working diagnosis of a triangular fibrocartilage complex tear (median age 31 years; 9 females; duration of symptoms NR), using MRI arthrogram as a reference standard.[125] Due to methzzodology of the test design, SP could not be determined.

SUPINATION LIFT TEST (TFCC)

Client Position	Sitting with the elbows flexed to 90° and the forearms supinated. The client lays their hands flat on the undersurface of a heavy stable table or against the clinician's hands.
Clinician Position	Sitting or standing next to the client
Movement	The client is instructed to lift the table or to push up against the clinician's hands.
Assessment	A (+) test is pain localized to the ulnar side of the wrist or if the client has difficulty applying the force.
Statistics	NR

PALPATION

Palpation of the WH will include bony and soft-tissue structures. Soft-tissue and bony palpation will begin proximally at the elbow at the epicondyles and continue distally into the structures of the hand. Specific bony structures to be assessed are the epicondyles of the humerus, the olecranon of the humerus, the shafts of the distal radius and ulna, the radial head and styloid process of the radius, the carpal and metacarpal bones, and the phalanges. Soft-tissue palpation should include the musculature, ligamentous, tendinous, and neural structures of the elbow and forearm, specifically assessing structures identified as areas of concern from previously exposed subjective and objective findings. Specific palpatory findings have been shown to be useful in assisting with diagnosis:

- The lack of a palpable mass proximal to the metacarpophalangeal joint can be used to rule out a complete tear of the UCL of the thumb (SN 100).[112]

- Physical findings found most useful in screening for wrist fracture for clients with acute wrist trauma included localized tenderness (SN 94).[62]

- Tenderness with palpation of the distal radius was found in children following acute trauma in the absence of obvious deformity: SN 79, SP 63.[63]

Here are the main anatomical landmarks commonly assessed during palpatory assessment of the wrist and hand (refer to figures 23.2 and 23.3).

- **Radial styloid process:** This is located on the distal most and lateral portion of the radius that attaches to the first row of carpal bones. The clinician should palpate the distal end of the radius, just proximal to the scaphoid.

- **Ulnar styloid process:** This is located on the distal most and dorsal surface of the ulna. The clinician should palpate the distal end of the ulna.

- **Anatomical snuffbox:** This is bordered medially by the extensor pollicis longus and laterally by the extensor pollicis brevis and the abductor pollicis longus (see figure 23.4). It can be seen best by having the client actively extend the thumb. The scaphoid can be palpated inside the snuffbox.

- **Scaphoid (navicular):** This bone represents the floor of the snuffbox. It is the largest bone of the proximal carpal row. With ulnar deviation, the scaphoid slides out from under the radial styloid process so that it can become more palpable.

- **Lunate:** This is located just lateral to scaphoid, distal to radius, and directly proximal to capitate. As the wrist is flexed, the lunate becomes prominent on the dorsal aspect of the wrist.

- **Triquetrum:** This is located just distal to the ulnar styloid process, in the proximal row of carpal bones. This carpal bone is difficult to palpate, even with radial wrist deviation.

- **Pisiform:** The sesamoid bone formed within the flexor carpi ulnaris. It is easily moveable with palpation.

- **Hook of hamate:** This is located slightly distal and radial to pisiform. With the interphalangeal joint of the palpating thumb on the pisiform, the clinician should point the tip of the thumb into the client's palm, palpating the hook of the hamate. It forms the lateral border of the tunnel of Guyon (ulnar nerve and artery of hand pass through here).

- **Trapezium:** This is located on the radial side of the carpals, and it articulates with the 1st metacarpal. The clinician should ask the client to flex and extend their thumb, and then palpate just proximal to scaphoid and just distal to the 1st metacarpal.

- **Capitate:** This lies between the 3rd metacarpal and the radius. With the wrist in neutral, a small depression is noted in the area of the capitate. Flexing the wrist causes the capitate to slide out from under the lunate, creating a fullness (or prominence) where the depression was located.

- **Metacarpophalangeal joints:** The clinician should move distal from metacarpals to the knuckles of the hand. Palpating along the side, the clinician can palpate the joint line.

- **Flexor carpi ulnaris (FCU):** The FCU is most easily palpated just proximal to the pisiform bone. It is more easily palpated with active wrist flexion or ulnar deviation.

- **Palmaris longus:** See figure 23.49. The clinician can have the client flex their wrist and touch the tips of their thumb and 5th finger together in opposition. If present (it is absent in 7–10% of population), it will be prominent with this movement because it lies anterior to the flexor retinaculum.

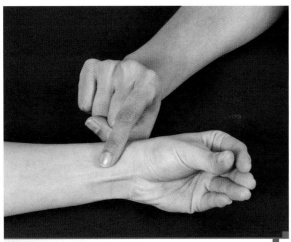

Figure 23.49 Palmaris longus.

• **Radial artery:** This is palpable just proximal to the radial styloid and radial to the flexor carpi radialis.

• **Ulnar artery:** This is palpable just proximal to the pisiform bone and radial to the FCU.

PHYSICAL PERFORMANCE MEASURES

Physical performance measures of the upper extremity are applicable for use in clients presenting with wrist and hand dysfunction. For more information, refer to chapter 21 (Shoulder). Specifically, the most commonly used measures for the wrist and hand are grip strength and measures of fine motor control of the wrist and hand. Gross wrist or hand strength assessments are the following:

• Maximum grip strength
• Tip pinch strength
• Key pinch strength
• Tripod pinch strength

Selection and utilization of these tests will be individualistic to each client dependent on their functional status and goals. As mentioned in previous chapters, selection and utilization of these measures should move from least challenging to most.

Grip strength is one of the most commonly used physical performance measures. It is typically used with clients with dysfunction in the wrist and hand. Grip strength is often considered an index of the power that the hand can exert during activities. Maximum grip strength has been shown as an important predictor of hand function, and is used to evaluate change over time following intervention.[126] Grip testing is commonly used in clinical settings to evaluate hand and upper extremity function, level of impairment, and physical performance.[18, 127-130] Grip strength has also been proposed as a possible predictor of mortality,[131] and a loss of grip strength may imply a loss of independence.[132]

Test–retest reliability of grip strength has demonstrated good reliability in asymptomatic[133-137] and symptomatic clients.[129, 130, 135, 138] Furthermore, several studies have demonstrated the reliability of grip strength testing in children,[139] adolescents,[140, 141] and adults[134-136] Grip strength reference values have been determined for healthy adults of both genders across a wide age range, and are essential in aiding clinical decisions about the normality of a client's status compared to the general population.[142-144]

Fine motor control, commonly referred to as *dexterity*, is an important skill that is required in order to perform activities of daily living and occupational-related tasks, and is frequently affected in clients presenting with wrist and hand dysfunction. Dexterity is defined as "fine, voluntary movements used to manipulate small objects during a specific task."[145] Dexterity assessments provide objective information for clients presenting with wrist and hand impairments, and they can demonstrate functional recovery after injury or lack thereof. Dexterity has been described by two related terms: *manual dexterity* and *fine motor dexterity*. Manual dexterity is the ability to coordinate movements and handle objects skillfully with the hand and fine motor dexterity refers to in-hand skillful manipulations of a tool or object with the fingers.[21, 145] Dexterity performance measures are used to quantify abilities by evaluating a client's speed and quality of movement as the hand controls and works with objects and tools related to activities of daily living and occupational or recreational tasks. Numerous dexterity performance measures have been found to be reliable and valid tools to evaluate a client's manual and fine motor dexterity.[146] Yancosek and colleagues recommend the use of the box and block test for manual dexterity and the Purdue peg board for fine motor dexterity. Table 23.3 provides an outline of the most commonly used dexterity testing performance measures.

TABLE 23.3 Summary of Frequently Used Dexterity Tests

Dexterity testing	Initially described	Bilateral or unilateral	Manual or fine dexterity	Reliability
Functional dexterity test	Aaron et al., 2003[147]	Unilateral	Manual	**Aaron et al.**[147] N = 339 based on 5 different combined studies Population: students, workers, uninjured and injured hands of hand therapy clients Interrater reliability ICC = 0.82–0.93 Intrarater reliability ICC = 0.91 **Sartorio et al.**[21] N = 324 subjects Population: clinically and functionally asymptomatic clients Test–retest reliability ICC $\geq$ 0.90
Purdue pegboard test	Tiffin et al., 1948[148]	Unilateral	Fine	**Gallus et al.**[149] N = 25 total; 22 female, 3 male Population: clients with multiple sclerosis Test–retest reliability for 1 trial ICC 0.85–0.90 Test–retest reliability for 3 trial ICC 0.92–0.96 **Buddenberg et al.**[150] N = 47 total; 33 female, 14 male Population: college students Test–retest reliability for 1 trial ICC 0.37–0.70 Test–retest reliability for 3 trial ICC 0.81–0.89
Nine hole peg test	Kellor et al., 1971[151]	Unilateral	Fine	**Svensson et al.**[152] N = 20 total; 11 female, 9 male Population: Swedish adults with Charcot-Marie-Tooth disease Test–retest ICC for right hand = 0.99 Test–retest ICC for left hand = 0.80 **Grice et al.**[153] N = 25 for reliability tests Population: college students/community volunteers Interrater reliability: Pearson r coefficient: right: $r = 0.984$, left: $r = 0.993$ Test–retest reliability: Pearson r coefficient: right: $r = 0.459$, left: $r = 0.442$ **Mathiowetz et al.**[154] N = 644 Population: 26 female occupational therapy students and 618 volunteers Interrater reliability: Pearson r coefficient: right: $r = 0.97$, left: $r = 0.99$ Test–retest reliability: Pearson r coefficient: right: $r = 0.69$, left: $r = 0.43$

(continued)

Table 23.3 *(continued)*

Dexterity testing	Initially described	Bilateral or unilateral	Manual or fine dexterity	Reliability
Jebsen-Taylor hand function test	Jebsen et al., 1969[155]	Unilateral	Manual and fine	**Jebsen et al.**[155] N = 300 total; 30 female, 30 male in age (y.o.) categories 20-29, 30-39, 40-49, 50-59, and 60-94 Population: 300 healthy adults and 60 clients Test–retest reliability: Pearson *r* coefficient = 0.60–0.99
Box and block test	Mathiowetz et al., 1985[156]	Unilateral	Manual	**Svensson et al.**[152] N = 20 total; 11 female, 9 male Population: Swedish adults with Charcot-Marie-Tooth disease Test–retest ICC for right hand = 0.95 Test–retest ICC for left hand = 0.96 **Platz et al.**[157] N = 56 total Population: neurologically impaired adults Interrater reliability and test–retest reliability ICCs and Spearman rho all > 0.95 **Desrosiers et al.**[158] N = 35 healthy adults, 34 impaired adults, 104 (for the construct validity test), and N = 360 (for the norming) Population: clients older than 60 y.o. with and without UE impairment Reliability: ICC = 0.89 and 0.97 **Mathiowetz et al.**[156] N = 628; 318 female, 310 male Population: volunteers from 7 different counties in Milwaukee area Interrater reliability: Pearson *r* coefficient: right: *r* = 1.00, left: *r* = 0.999

N = number of clients; ICC = interclass correlation coefficient; y.o. = years old; UE = upper extremity

COMMON ORTHOPEDIC CONDITIONS OF THE WRIST AND HAND

While it is impossible to distinctly describe various pathological presentations of the wrist and hand, there are evidence-based findings supportive of particular pathologies of this region of the body. Therefore, the intent of this section of the chapter is to present current evidence-supported findings suggestive of wrist and hand pathologies. As previously described in chapter 4 (Evidence-Based Practice and Client Examination), though, not all examination findings are absolutely supported with clinical evidence, and the clinician should also rely on clinical experience and input from the client when performing differential diagnosis of a client's presentation of pain and dysfunction.

The following section discusses and provides an evidence-based examination template for common orthopedic conditions of the wrist and hand. The section highlights current evidence for each particular diagnosis including each section of the examination template: the subjective history, outcome measures, diagnostic imaging, observation, triage, motion tests, muscle performance testing, special tests, palpation, and physical performance measures. Finally, potential treatment-based classifications are proposed for each condition.

Carpal Tunnel Syndrome (CTS) ▪▪▪▪▪▪▪▪▪▪▪▪▪▪▪▪▪▪▪

ICD-9: 354.0 (carpal tunnel syndrome)

ICD-10: G56.0 (carpal tunnel syndrome, unspecified upper limb)

The carpal tunnel is bordered volarly by the extensor retinaculum. Carpal tunnel syndrome is compression of the median nerve in this tunnel, eliciting pain, paresthesia, numbness, and other associated median nerve symptoms. It is the most common compressive neuropathy in the upper extremity. The diagnosis of CTS continues to generate some controversy.[159]

I. Client Interview

Subjective History

- The most bothersome symptoms being pain, numbness, and tingling versus loss of feeling helps **rule in** (SP 91, +LR 0.42) carpal tunnel syndrome.[86]

- Not having paresthesia along the median nerve distribution that awakens the client at night helps **rule out** (SN 96, −LR 0.04;[88] SN 84, −LR 0.5[160]) and **rule in** (SP 100, +LR Inf)[88] carpal tunnel syndrome.

- Not having paresthesia in the thumb, index, and long finger helps **rule out** (SN 95, −LR 0.19) carpal tunnel syndrome.[11]

- Symptom behavior being intermittent and variable, not constant, helps rule in (SP 89, +LR 2.1) carpal tunnel syndrome.[86]

- If hand shaking does not improve symptoms, it helps **rule out** (SN 81, −LR 0.34) carpal tunnel syndrome.[86]

- A variety of factors have been described to lead to CTS: heredity, size of carpal tunnel, associated local and systemic diseases, and certain habits involving repetitive or sustained wrist flexion.[88, 161]

- The subjective report of swelling in the region of the carpal tunnel does little to rule out (SN 49, −LR 1.3) or rule in (SP 32, +LR 0.8) the presence of CTS.[162]

- General risk factors:[163]

- Female gender [odds ratio, or OR = 3.7 (2.6–5.2)]

- Middle age (40-60 years old) [OR = 2.2 (0.9–4.9)]

- Overweight or obesity [OR = 1.5 (1.1–1.9)]

- Diabetes mellitus [OR = 5.3 (1.6–16.8)]

- Excessive alcohol abuse [OR = 2.3 (0.7–2.3)]

- Occupational risk factors:[164]

- Repetition [OR = 2.7 (1.8–39)]

- Chronic wrist flexion [OR = 1.7 (1.0–0.6)]

- Powerful grip [OR = 4.4 (1.4–13.6)]

- Chronic vibration load [OR = 2.6 (1.7–4.0)]

Outcome Measures

- Brigham and Women's Hospital Hand Symptom Severity Scale > 1.9 helps rule out carpal tunnel syndrome.[86]

- A possible rating on the Katz hand diagram provided good (**SP 98, +LR 38**)[88] to less than good (SP 90, +LR 3.6[105]) ability to help rule in carpal tunnel syndrome.

- An unlikely rating on the Katz hand diagram provided some assistance to **rule out** (SN 90, −LR 0.1[105]) carpal tunnel syndrome.

- Using the clinical diagnosis of CTS as criterion standard, the Katz hand diagram had favorable diagnostics to help rule out (SN 90) CTS among a population-based sample of people with numbness and tingling in the hand.[165]

- The Katz hand diagram also demonstrated that the drawing of an expanded area of symptoms prior to surgery was correlative with poorer outcomes.[166]

Diagnostic Imaging

- EMG compared to clinical findings provided moderate assistance to help **rule out** (SN 91) and **rule in** (SP 81) CTS.[36] EMG is typically the first choice because it has the highest specificity and sensitivity compared to other imaging modalities.

- CT compared to clinical findings provided some assistance to help rule out (SN 68-97) and rule in (SP 48-87) CTS. However, diagnostic accuracy was dependent on the location where the modality was utilized.[36]

- MRI compared to clinical findings provided some assistance to help rule out (SN 43-88) and rule in (SP 40-100) CTS. However, diagnostic accuracy was dependent on the location where the modality was utilized.[36]

- US may provide some assistance to help rule out (SN 77-88) and rule in (SP 46-87) CTS.[36-39] However, diagnostic accuracy was dependent on the location where the modality was utilized. The advantages of US compared to electrodiagnostic testing are that it takes less time to perform, causes less discomfort to the client, and is less expensive.

- Nerve conduction testing provided some assistance to help rule out (SN 70) and rule in (SP 82) population-based CTS. However, this study demonstrated a relatively high level of false-positive test results (18%).[165]

II. Observation

- The client may shake their hands in an attempt to relieve symptoms.
  - This flick sign, when (+), provides ideal ability to help **rule out** (SN 90, −LR 0.3) carpal tunnel syndrome, although in only one study.[11]

- Long-standing carpal tunnel syndrome may lead to atrophy of the thenar eminence musculature.

- Thenar atrophy, when present, provides good ability to help **rule in** (SP 96, +LR 4.5) carpal tunnel syndrome.[107]

III. Triage and Screening

- All nonmusculoskeletal causes, as well as neuromusculoskeletal causes from proximal joints, should be ruled out.[64]

- A lack of localized tenderness (SN 94), pain on active motion (SN 97), and pain on passive motion (SN 94) help **rule out** fracture of the wrist.[62]

- CTS is characterized by motor, sensory, and autonomic nerve impairment resulting in numbness and tingling in the median nerve distribution of the hand, hypotrophy of the thenar musculature, dropping of items and decreased sweat function in the hand, with symptom exacerbation at night and after frequent or repetitive use of the wrist and hand.[167]

- Abnormal vibration sense: A (−) test has less than good ability to help rule out (SN 87)[88] CTS and a (+) test has less than good ability to help rule in (SP 80, +LR 3.1;[168] SP 85, +LR 1.4[169]) carpal tunnel syndrome.

- Having reduced sensation to touch in the thumb, index finger, and long fingers has less than good ability to help rule in (SP 67, +LR 1.2) carpal tunnel syndrome.[11]

- Having the appearance of white fingers in the thumb, index finger, and long fingers has less than good ability to help rule in (SP 83, +LR 1.4) carpal tunnel syndrome.[11]

IV. Motion Tests

- Client may possibly have limited and painful wrist active and passive ROM.

V. Muscle Performance Testing

- Abductor pollicis brevis weakness has less than good ability to help rule in (SP 80-89, +LR 1.5–1.7) carpal tunnel syndrome.[86, 87]

- Long-standing carpal tunnel syndrome may lead to weakness of opposition and grip or pincer strength.[161]

- Grip, key pinch, three-jaw pinch, and tip-pinch weakness or pain provided little help in ruling in or out carpal tunnel syndrome.[88]

VI. Special Tests

- Clinical prediction rule is as follows:[86]
  - 2 or more variables present: limited ability to rule in or rule out carpal tunnel syndrome
  - All 5 variables present: has ideal ability to help **rule in** (SP 95, +LR 18.3) carpal tunnel syndrome

- Variables: (1) hand shaking improves symptoms, (2) wrist–ratio index > 0.67, (3) Brigham and Women's Hospital Hand Symptom Severity Scale score > 1.9, (4) diminished sensation in median sensory field of thumb, and (5) age > 45 years

- CTS-6 diagnostic clinical criteria for CTS are as follows:[170]

  - Numbness and tingling in the median nerve distribution

  - Nocturnal numbness

  - Weakness or atrophy of the thenar musculature

  - Tinel's sign

  - Phalen's test

  - Loss of two-point discrimination

- Phalen's test: provides less than good ability to help rule in or out carpal tunnel syndrome in pooled analysis[87] and several other studies.[86, 89, 92]

- Phalen's test: A (+) test has good (**SP 86-100, +LR 5.9-Inf**)[90, 91] to ideal ability (**SP 95, +LR 15**)[88] to help rule in carpal tunnel syndrome.

- Phalen's test: A (−) test had good ability to help **rule out** (SN 82, −LR 0.21) in one high-quality study.[90]

- Reverse Phalen's and modified Phalen's tests have less than good ability to rule out or rule in carpal tunnel syndrome.

- Tinel's test provides less than good ability to help rule in or out carpal tunnel syndrome in pooled analysis[87] and two other studies.[86, 89]

- Tinel's test: A (+) test has good (**SP 91, +LR 8.2**)[92] to ideal ability (**SP 99, +LR 64**)[88] to help rule in carpal tunnel syndrome.

- Tinel's, Phalen's, reverse Phalen's, and carpal tunnel compression tests are more SN; they are SP for the diagnosis of tenosynovitis of the flexor muscles of the hand, rather than being specific tests for carpal tunnel syndrome and can be used as an indicator for medical management of the condition.[95]

- Flick sign: provides less than good ability to rule in or out carpal tunnel syndrome in pooled analysis[87] and two other studies.[89, 93]

- Flick sign: A (−) test had ideal ability to help **rule out** (SN 90, −LR 0.3) carpal tunnel syndrome in one high-quality study.[11]

- Hand elevation test: A (−) test had good ability to help **rule out** (SN 87, −LR 0.15) and **rule in** (SP 89, +LR 7.8) carpal tunnel in one high-quality study,[92] while other studies of lesser quality demonstrated less than good ability for ruling in or out carpal tunnel.

- Upper limb tension test (median nerve bias): A (−) test had good ability to help **rule out** (SN 92, −LR 0.56) carpal tunnel syndrome in one study,[171] but not in another high-quality study (SN 75, −LR 1.9).[86]

- Upper limb tension test (radial nerve bias), tethered median nerve stress test, closed-fist or lumbrical provocation test, modified carpal compression, wrist-ratio index, median nerve digit score, Semmes-Weinstein monofilament test, hypoesthesia, Gilliat tourniquet test, abnormal vibration, abductor pollicis brevis weakness, and Hems' questionnaire all provide less than good ability to rule in or out carpal tunnel syndrome.

- Thenar atrophy (SP 96, +LR 4.5),[107] carpal compression test (SP 83-93, +LR 3.8–10.7),[87, 92] and two-point discrimination (SP 93, +LR 4.8),[87] when (+), all provided good ability to **rule in** carpal tunnel syndrome.

- Katz hand diagram: See information under prior Outcome Measures section.

- Physical examination tests have a low yield for the diagnosis of carpal tunnel in workplace surveillance and pre-placement screening programs, with only the Semmes-Weinstein sensory test scoring above SN of 31 (actual value: SN 58).[172]

- Other studies also suggest that physical examination is minimally useful as a screening mechanism for carpal tunnel in working populations.[165, 173]

VII. Palpation

- The median nerve and corresponding area are likely to be tender to palpation, and palpation may produce paresthesia.

VIII. Physical Performance Measures

- Grip strength and measures of fine motor control of the wrist and hand may be used. Selection and utilization of these tests will be individual to each client and dependent on their functional status and goals.

POTENTIAL TREATMENT-BASED CLASSIFICATIONS

- Neurodynamics, mobility, and exercise and conditioning may be used.

Triangular Fibrocartilaginous Complex (TFCC) Injury

ICD-9: 842.01 (sprain of carpal [joint] of wrist); 842.09 (other sprains and strains of wrist)

ICD-10: M24.139 (other articular cartilage disorders, unspecified wrist)

The TFCC is a cartilaginous disc at the distal ulna that is triangular in shape and serves several important functions: It dissipates compressive loads with ulnar weight bearing, serves as a connection with the radius, covers the head of the ulna, allows for forearm rotation, and serves as a stabilizing force in the distal radioulnar joint. A TFCC injury is caused by acute trauma (type 1), or can be due to degenerative (type 2) changes at the wrist related to previous injuries, distal radial ulnar joint conditions, or inflammatory conditions.[174, 175]

I. Client Interview

Subjective History

Differential Diagnosis of Carpal Tunnel Syndrome and Cervical Radiculopathy (C6-7)

- CTS is characterized by paresthesias or pain in the distribution of the median nerve along the thumb, index, and middle fingers, and along the medial half of the ring finger on the palmar aspect.
- CTS symptoms are often reported as worse at night, causing the client to wake up.
- Untreated CTS results in atrophy and weakness within the thenar muscles, resulting in difficulty with handgrip and opposition of the thumb.
- Cervical radiculopathy may be identified by the occurrence of cervical spine pain, reproduction of UE pain with cervical spine active range of motion, muscle weakness along a myotomal pattern, reflex impairment or loss, or motor or sensory disturbances, not within the distribution of median nerve.
  - C6 radiculopathy is associated with pain along the superior lateral aspect of the arm into the thumb and index fingers, a diminished biceps and brachioradialis reflex, and weakness with elbow flexion and wrist extension.
  - C7 radiculopathy is associated with pain along the dorsal aspect of the arm and the posterolateral aspect of the forearm into the third digit, a diminished triceps reflex, and weakness of elbow extension and wrist flexion.
- Spurling's compression test may exacerbate (have positive findings) C6-C7 radicular pain, but not median nerve entrapment.
- Selected special tests may be useful in ruling in or out carpal tunnel syndrome. (See Carpal Tunnel Syndrome.)
- Diagnostic imaging can be a helpful adjunct during differential diagnosis.

- Clients report wrist pain of a mechanical nature (with possible clicking and joint crepitus), localized swelling, weakness of the wrist or forearm, and instability.[176]

- Clients with the following experiences are at risk for type 1 traumatic TFCC injuries:[176, 177]

  - They have sustained a fall onto an outstretched hand.

  - They participate in repetitive, forceful twisting or pulling movements with palmar rotation such as with the use of heavy tools or equipment or when participating in sports that involve the use of a racket, a bat, or a club (tennis, baseball, golf) or that involve direct pressure on the hands (gymnastics, wrestling).

- The following clients are at risk for type 2 degenerative TFCC injuries: [176, 177]

  - Clients with a previous history of fracture at the distal radius or ulna, or a history of a wrist fracture during childhood.

  - Clients with congenital abnormalities presenting with positive ulnar variance, in which the ulna is anatomically longer than the radius. Research demonstrates that in people with neutral variance, the TFCC accepts around 20% of the loading forces, whereas in those with positive variance, loading forces can exceed 40%.[178]

  - Clients of advancing age.

    - Degenerative TFCC tears were present in 7.6% of wrists by age 30, 18.1% of wrists by age 40, 40% of wrists by age 50, 42.8% of wrists by age 60, and 53.1% of wrists in clients after 60 years of age.[177]

    - Osteoporosis, which is characterized by low bone mass and microarchitectural deterioration, is a major risk factor for fractures of the hip, vertebrae, and distal forearm.[179]

Outcome Measures

- The DASH, QuickDASH, PRWHE, and PSFS are appropriate for this client population. All have demonstrated clinical applicability in clients with upper extremity dysfunction.

Diagnostic Imaging

- The TFCC is not visible on radiographs, but radiographs are helpful for ruling out possible scaphoid or distal radius fractures, positive ulnar variance, avulsion of the ulnar styloid, or carpal instability (specifically, volar intercalated segment instability [VISI deformity]).

- X-ray arthrography, with a triple compartment injection, helps **rule in** (SP 93) a complete tear of the TFCC and provides little help to rule out (SN 76) the injury.[45]

- Magnetic resonance imaging (MRI) and magnetic resonance arthrography (MRA) have better capability to help **rule in** and **rule out** a TFCC injury and aid in ascertaining the location of the tear.

  - MRA detection of tear:

    - SN 84, SP 95[42]

  - MRI detection of tear:

    - Pooled results: SN 83, SP 80[43]

    - SN 75, SP 81[42]

    - SN 100, SP 90[44]

  - MRI location of tear:

    - SP 75, SN 100[44]

II. Observation

- The clinician may observe excessive dorsal prominence of the distal ulna relative to the adjacent radius and carpal bones.

III. Triage and Screening

- All nonmusculoskeletal causes, as well as neuromusculoskeletal causes from proximal joints, should be ruled out.[64]

- No localized tenderness (SN 94), pain on active motion (SN 97), and pain on passive motion (SN 94) help **rule out** fracture of the wrist.[62]

IV. Motion Tests

- Clients may demonstrate limitations and pain with forearm pronation or supination and ulnar deviation of the wrist.[176]
- Clients may have pain with passive accessory assessment during movement of the carpals against the head of the ulna.

V. Muscle Performance Testing

- Clients may have possible difficulty and pain during resisted wrist radial deviation and thumb extension.

VI. Special Tests

- Ulnomeniscotriquetral dorsal glide or piano key test: provides less than good ability to help rule out (SN 66, −LR 0.5) or rule in (SP 64, +LR 1.8) a TFCC injury.
- Press test, supination lift test, and grind test: All should be used with caution due to poor methodology. They provide less than good ability to either rule in or rule out TFCC.
- Watson scaphoid test (scaphoid instability), ballottement test (lunotriquetral ligament integrity), wrist-flexion and finger extension test (scapholunate pathology), dorsal capitate displacement apprehension test (capitate stability), clinical stress test (distal radius fracture), and ulnocarpal stress test all provide less than good ability to rule in or rule out their respective pathologies.

VII. Palpation

- The TFCC is best palpated in the soft spot between the ulnar styloid, flexor carpi ulnaris, volar surface of the ulnar head, and pisiform. A reproduction of pain in this area may be indicative of a foveal disruption of the TFCC or ulnotriquetral ligament. This test is termed the *ulna fovea sign* and has less than good ability to help rule out (SN 95) and rule in (SP 87) a TFCC injury.[180]
- Peritriquetral tenderness may be noted.[181]

VIII. Physical Performance Measures

- Grip strength and measures of fine motor control of the wrist and hand may be used. Selection and utilization of these tests will be individual to each client, dependent on their functional status and goals.

POTENTIAL TREATMENT-BASED CLASSIFICATIONS

- Bracing, stabilization, mobility, pain control, and exercise and conditioning may be used.

De Quervain's Tenosynovitis

ICD-9: 727.04 (radial styloid tenosynovitis)

ICD-10: M65.4 (radial styloid tenosynovitis [de Quervain])

De Quervain's tenosynovitis is a stenosing tenosynovitis of the sheath surrounding the tendons of the extensor pollicis brevis (EPB) and abductor pollicis longus (APL) at the styloid process of the radius. These muscles are directly next to each other with a common function of thumb extension.

I. Client Interview

Subjective History

- Risk factors include female gender, age greater than 40, and black race.[182]
- Onset is gradual and is not associated with trauma.[183]
- The symptoms are similar to those with other types of tenosynovitis, which commonly include pain, swelling, and difficulty moving the involved joint (thumb in this case).
- Clients have difficulty with repetitive gripping, lifting, and twisting motions.
- Dorsolateral radial-sided wrist pain may radiate proximally into the forearm with gripping and thumb extension.
- Pain has been described as a "constant aching, burning, pulling sensation."[184]
- This condition is common in pregnant or postpartum women.[185-188]

Outcome Measures

- The DASH, QuickDASH, PRWHE, and PSFS are appropriate for this client population. All have demonstrated clinical applicability in clients with upper extremity dysfunction.

Diagnostic Imaging

- Radiographs may be beneficial for differential diagnosis purposes to assess the carpometacarpal joint for arthrosis.
- Ultrasound was found to be a cost-effective and advantageous method for evaluating the tendon and surrounding sheaths, assessing for pathologic modifications,[189] and detecting anatomic abnormalities.[190]
- A retrospective review of wrist MR images revealed increased thickness of the EPB, APL, and peritendinous edema. The findings were found to be reliable and clinically correlated.[191]

II. Observation

- The clinician should assess the resting position of the wrist and hand, specifically evaluating the thumb.
- The clinician should assess for inflammation at the dorsal lateral aspect of the thumb or in close proximity to the radial styloid process.

III. Triage and Screening

- All nonmusculoskeletal causes, as well as neuromusculoskeletal causes from proximal joints, should be ruled out.[64]
- No localized tenderness (SN 94), pain on active motion (SN 97), and pain on passive motion (SN 94) help **rule out** fracture of the wrist.[62]

IV. Motion Tests

- Pain may increase with abduction of the thumb and ulnar deviation of the wrist.[183]
- Increased tensile loads in the APL and EPB during passive stretching may reproduce concordant pain.[183]

V. Muscle Performance Testing

- Grip testing may be diminished secondary to pain.[183]
- An increased tensile load in the APL and EPB during manual muscle testing may reproduce concordant pain.[183]

VI. Special Tests

- Finkelstein test: This is a commonly used test, but to date no diagnostic accuracy studies have been performed to determine the SN and SP.
- Extensor pollicis brevis test: This is used to determine if a septum was present between the EPB and APL; it provided good ability to help **rule out** (SN 81, −LR 0.38) de Quervain's tenosynovitis when test was (−).[113]

VII. Palpation

- Palpation at the radial styloid tends to elicit well-localized tenderness that is similar in quality and location to the pain experienced during activity.[192]
- The clinician should look for tenderness at the radial styloid process, palpable thickening of the extensor sheaths of the first dorsal compartment, and crepitus of the tendons moving within the extensor sheath.[193]

VIII. Physical Performance Measures

- Grip strength and measures of fine motor control of the wrist and hand may be used. Selection and utilization of these tests will be individual to each client, dependent on their functional status and goals.

POTENTIAL TREATMENT-BASED CLASSIFICATIONS

- Bracing, mobility, pain or inflammation control, and exercise and conditioning may be used.

Osteoarthritis

ICD-9: 715.14 (osteoarthrosis, localized, primary, hand)

ICD-10: M19.039 (primary osteoarthritis, wrist); M19.049 (primary osteoarthritis, unspecified hand)

Osteoarthritis (OA), also known as degenerative joint disease, is the degeneration of articular cartilage and subchondral bone. Osteoarthritis is the most common joint disorder in the United States.[194] It is a group of overlapping and distinct diseases that will affect one out of three adults over the age of 55.[195] Wrist and hand OA will include any of the multiple joints in bilateral extremities. Symptomatic hand OA is most prevalent in the DIP joint, followed by the first carpometacarpal, PIP, and MCP joints.[196] Ninety-five percent of degenerative wrist arthritis occurs as periscaphoid area problems, commonly secondary to trauma.[197] Primary OA is a multifactorial, heterogeneous, and complex disease. Secondary OA is caused by comorbidities, infection, trauma, and joint laxity.

I. Client Interview

Subjective History

- Occurs most often in fifth or seventh decades of life[198]
- Report of pain, aching, and stiffness[199]
- Risk factors for hand OA include the following:[196]
  - Age over 40 years
  - Female gender
  - Positive family history
  - History of occupational usage
  - Obesity
  - History of finger joint injury

Outcome Measures

- A number of validated and reliable outcome measures are available to specifically assess function in clients with hand OA. These measures include the Health Assessment Questionnaire (HAQ),[200] the Arthritis Hand Function Test (AHFT),[201] the Arthritis Impact Measurement Scale 2 (AIMS2),[202] the Score for Assessment and quantification of Chronic Rheumatic Affections of the Hands (SACRAH),[203, 204] the Functional Index for Hand Osteoarthritis (FIHOA),[205, 206] the Cochin scale,[207, 208] and the Australian/Canadian Osteoarthritis Hand Index (AUSCAN).[209]
- A systematic review of a selection of these measures has been completed with the goal to provide an overall review of the literature but not to provide a recommendation on any one measure. The results of the review demonstrated that the AIMS2, HAQ, AUSCAN, Cochin, and FIHOA performed well and are useful with clients presenting with hand OA.[210]

Diagnostic Imaging

- Plain radiographs are the initial primary diagnostic imagining tool utilized to assess for osteoarthritic changes of the wrist and hand that demonstrated high intra-observer reliability.[211, 212] Radiographic findings include joint space narrowing, bone sclerosis, periarticular cysts, and osteophytes. Refer to chapter 6 for a definition of OA according to Kellgren and Lawrence.[213]
- Plain radiographs have also demonstrated sensitivity to change over time (1 year).[211]
- Radiographic signs of hand OA, osteophytes, or joint space narrowing are prevalent in up to 81% of the elderly population.[214]
- MRI can provide some assistance to help rule out or rule in the presence of OA. Menashe and colleagues[35] investigated osteoarthritis in multiple joints (hip, knee, and hand). The majority of studies were performed on knee osteoarthritis.
  - SN 61, SP 82 with variable reference standard
  - SN 74, SP 76 with histology used as reference standard
  - SN 61, SP 81 with radiographs used as a reference standard

II. Observation

- Heberden's and Bouchard's nodes can be clinically assessed by observation with a high percentage of agreement between assessors.[215]
  - Heberden's nodes are cystic swellings containing gelatinous hyaluronic acid that appear on the dorsolateral aspects of DIP joints.[216, 217]
  - Bouchard's nodes are cystic swellings containing gelatinous hyaluronic acid that appear on the dorsolateral aspects of PIP joints.[216, 217]

III. Triage and Screening

- All nonmusculoskeletal causes, as well as neuromusculoskeletal causes from proximal joints, should be ruled out.[64]

- No localized tenderness (SN 94), pain on active motion (SN 97), and pain on passive motion (SN 94) help **rule out** fracture of the wrist.[62]

IV. Motion Tests

- Clients may have limited and painful active and passive ROM of the affected joint.

V. Muscle Performance Testing

- Clients may have limitation of muscular performance in the region of the affected joint due to pain.

- Clients may have difficulty with gripping and twisting.

VI. Special Tests

- Clinical prediction rule for osteoarthritis of the hand,[218] hand pain, aching, or stiffness, *and* 3 or 4 of the following:

  - Enlargement of ≥2 joints of 10 selected joints*

  - Swelling of ≤3 MCP joints

  - Enlargement of ≥2 DIPs

  - Deformity of 1 of 10 selected joints*

    - *2nd and 3rd DIP, 2nd and 3rd PIP, and 1st CMC of each hand

  - Good ability to help **rule in** (SP 87, +LR 7.2) and limited ability to help rule out (SN 94, −LR 0.7) OA of the hand.

VII. Palpation

- Heberden's and Bouchard's nodes and joint line tenderness can be clinically assessed by palpation with a high percentage of agreement between assessors.[215]

VIII. Physical Performance Measures

- Grip strength and measures of fine motor control of the wrist and hand may be used. Selection and utilization of these tests will be individual to each client, dependent on their functional status and goals.

POTENTIAL TREATMENT-BASED CLASSIFICATIONS

- Mobility, pain or inflammation control, exercise and conditioning, and bracing may be used.

Rheumatoid Arthritis

ICD-9: 714.0 (rheumatoid arthritis)

ICD-10: M06.9 (rheumatoid arthritis, unspecified); M05.40 (rheumatoid myopathy with rheumatoid arthritis of unspecified site); M05.449 (rheumatoid myopathy with rheumatoid arthritis of unspecified hand); M05.439 (rheumatoid myopathy with rheumatoid arthritis of unspecified wrist)

Rheumatoid arthritis (RA) is a complex disease to diagnose and treat. RA is a chronic and progressive autoimmune condition that affects the organs and joints, particularly of the wrist, hands, and feet. It is considered a lifelong disease, although patients can go into remission. The prevalence range in North America is 0.9 to 1.1 in the general adult population.[219] RA is characterized by persistent synovitis, systemic inflammation, autoantibodies, and a wide array of multisystem comorbidities. Proper diagnosis and treatment are required to decrease the progression of joint deformity, which leads to limitations with daily functional activities. Delayed diagnosis can result in long-term joint injury.[220] Laboratory studies and imaging are useful in confirming the diagnosis and tracking disease progression, but diagnosis is primarily based on clinical findings. Researchers have reported that several environmental and genetic factors contribute to having an increased risk of developing RA, which are listed in the following section. Currently, there is no treatment to cure RA. Current treatments include physical therapy, occupational therapy, corticosteroids or nonsteroidal anti-inflammatory drugs (NSAIDs), and biologic or nonbiologic disease-modifying antirheumatic drugs (DMARDs).[221] These treatments are aimed at decreasing pain, maintaining mobility and function, and slowing down the progression of the disease. Poor prognosis has been correlated to low functional scores early in the disease progression, lower socioeconomic status, lower education level, strong family history of the disease, and early involvement of many joints.[222]

I. Client Interview

Subjective History

- Age of onset between 30 and 50 years of age[222]

- Complaints of pain and stiffness in multiple joints[222]

- Complaints of puffy hands secondary to increased blood flow to affected areas[222]
- Insidious onset of morning stiffness or diffuse aching that lasts 1 hour or longer[221]
- Symptoms may begin after a trigger event, such as a viral illness.[222]
- Environmental risk factors for RA include the following:[222,223]
  - Hormonal exposure
  - Tobacco use
  - Microbial exposure
  - Smoking
  - Consumption of more than 3 cups of decaffeinated coffee per day
  - Silicate exposure
- Genetic risk factors for RA include the following:[222, 223]
  - Female gender
  - Positive family history
  - Older age
  - HLA genotype

Outcome Measures

- The American College of Rheumatology convened a working group to conduct a systematic review of the literature to identify RA disease activity measures. The working group recommended the following activity measures: Clinical Disease Activity Index, Disease Activity Score with 28-joint counts (erythrocyte sedimentation rate (ESR) or C-reactive protein (CRP)), Patient Activity Scale (PAS), PAS-II, routine assessment of patient index data with three measures, and the Simplified Disease Activity Index.[224]
- These activity measures have been validated and have demonstrated accurate reflections of disease activity. They are sensitive to change and practical to use in the clinical settings. They discriminate between low, moderate, and high disease activity states and discuss remission criteria.[224]

Diagnostic Imaging

- Conventional radiography is the imaging modality of choice. Radiography can detect bone erosions, joint space narrowing, juxta-articular osteoporosis, cysts, joint subluxations, malalignment, or ankylosis. However, limitations exist with its use for early detection of RA due to limitations in detecting soft-tissue changes and the early stages of bone erosion.[225]
- Conventional radiograph is helpful in monitoring disease progression. Validated scoring methods assessing radiologic damage are available, including the Larsen method, the Sharp method, and their modifications.[225]
- MRI and ultrasound allow for direct visualization of early inflammatory and destructive joint changes in affected regions. Current evidence evaluating the use of MRI for the diagnosis and prognosis of early RA is inadequate. Literature demonstrates that sensitivity and specificity ranged from 20% to 100% and 0% to 100%, depending on MRI criteria used.[226]

II. Observation

- Clients may have symmetric joint swelling.[221]
- Clients may have atrophy of musculature in proximity of involved joints.[221]
- Affected joints will be held in flexion by clients to decrease painful distention of the joint capsules.[221]
- 25% of clients will present with rheumatoid nodules of varying size. The common location will be the extensor area of the forearm.[221]

III. Triage and Screening

- All nonmusculoskeletal causes, as well as neuromusculoskeletal causes from proximal joints, should be ruled out.[64]
- No localized tenderness (SN 94), pain on active motion (SN 97), and pain on passive motion (SN 94) help **rule out** fracture of the wrist.[62]

IV. Motion Tests

- Clients may have limited and painful active and passive ROM of the affected joint.

V. Muscle Performance Testing

- Clients may have limitation of muscular performance in the region of the affected joint due to pain.
- Clients may have difficulty with gripping and twisting.

VI. Special Tests

- The American College of Rheumatology and European League Against Rheumatism classification criteria for rheumatoid arthritis are as follows:[227]
  - Joint involvement (0–5)
    - 1 medium-to-large joint (0)
    - 2 to 10 medium-to-large joints (1)
    - 1 to 3 small joints (large joints not counted) (2)
    - 4 to 10 small joints (large joints not counted) (3)
    - More than 10 joints (at least one small joint) (5)
  - Serology (0-3)
    - Negative rheumatoid factor (RF) and negative anticitrullinated protein antibody (ACPA) (0)
    - Low positive RF or low positive ACPA (2)
    - High positive RF or high positive ACPA (3)
  - Acute-phase reactants (0-1)
    - Normal CRP and normal ESR (0)
    - Abnormal CRP or abnormal ESR (1)
  - Duration of symptoms (0-1)
    - Less than 6 weeks (0)
    - 6 weeks or more (1)

VII. Palpation

- Affected joints may be warm, tender, and boggy to palpation.[221]

VIII. Physical Performance Measures

- Grip strength and measures of fine motor control of the wrist and hand may be used. Selection and utilization of these tests will be individual to each client, dependent on their functional status and goals.

POTENTIAL TREATMENT-BASED CLASSIFICATIONS

- Mobility, pain or inflammation control, exercise and conditioning, and bracing may be used.

Differential Diagnosis of Osteoarthritis and Rheumatoid Arthritis

- Symptomatic OA of the fingers is most prevalent in the DIP joints and is frequently associated with Heberden's nodes. In contrast, RA is most prevalent in MCP and PIP joints. It is not associated with Heberden's nodes but with symmetrical joint swelling.
- RA age of onset is typically between 30-50 years old compared to OA age of onset, which occurs after the fifth decade of life.
- Palpation of joint enlargement in clients with OA is hard and bony. In contrast, soft, warm, boggy, and tender joints are typical of RA.
- Insidious onset of morning stiffness or diffuse aching that lasts at least 1 hour is present with RA. Morning stiffness in OA, when present, is usually transient and is decreased with movement.
- Radiographs can assist in distinguishing RA from OA. OA radiographs are characterized by narrowing of the joint space due to cartilage loss or osteophytes. In contrast, RA radiographs demonstrate erosions or cysts.

Colles' Fracture

ICD-9: 813.41 (closed Colles' fracture)

ICD-10: S52.539 (Colles' fracture of unspecified radius)

Fractures of the radius or ulna account for 44% of all hand and forearm fractures.[228] A Colles' fracture is an extra-articular fracture of the distal radius. The fracture typically occurs following a fall on an outstretched hand with the wrist extended. The fracture is usually associated with a dorsal and radial displacement of the distal fragment and disturbance of the radial-ulnar articulation. Associated injuries, which include an ulnar styloid fracture, TFCC tear, and scapholunate dissociation, may occur and can lead to difficulties with differential diagnosis.

I. Client Interview

Subjective History

- This injury occurs in more women than men (6:1), and increased risk of injury is correlated with age. There is a bimodal age distribution with an increased risk in young men and elderly women.[4, 229, 230]

- This injury is typically secondary to a trauma with a fall on an outstretched hand with the forearm pronated and the wrist extended.

- Clients report decreased range of motion of the wrist.

- Clients have complaints of dorsal and radial wrist pain.

Outcome Measures

- The DASH, QuickDASH, PRWE, PRWHE, and PSFS are appropriate for this client population. All have demonstrated clinical applicability in clients with upper extremity dysfunction.

- According to one study, the normal course of recovery, with the use of the PRWE, is for pain and functional limitations to become mild within 3 months.[231]

Diagnostic Imaging

- Plain radiographs, with PA and lateral views, are the initial primary diagnostic imagining tool utilized to assess for the presence of a Colles' fracture.[232]

- A CT scan can help assess for intra-articular fractures, the extent of articular surface depression, and comminution.[233]

- MRI is useful in identifying fractures and concomitant soft-tissue injury.[232]

II. Observation

- Possible increased angulation of the distal radius

- Dorsal wrist effusion

III. Triage and Screening

- All nonmusculoskeletal causes, as well as neuromusculoskeletal causes from proximal joints, should be ruled out.[64]

- No localized tenderness (SN 94), pain on active motion (SN 97), and pain on passive motion (SN 94) help **rule out** fracture of the wrist.[62]

IV. Motion Tests

- Clients may have pain with wrist flexion, extension, and ulnar or radial deviation in AROM and PROM.

V. Muscle Performance Testing

- Clients may have pain and difficulty with gripping.

VI. Special Tests

- No tests have been currently investigated that are particular to Colles' fracture. Refer to other fracture tests to help rule out the possibility of their presence.

VII. Palpation

- Clients may have pain or tenderness to palpation at the distal radius.

VIII. Physical Performance Measures

- Grip strength and measures of fine motor control of the wrist and hand may be used. Selection and utilization of these tests will be individualistic to each client dependent on their functional status and goals.

POTENTIAL TREATMENT-BASED CLASSIFICATIONS

- Immobilization and pain or inflammation control may be used.

Scaphoid Fracture ▪ ▪ ▪ ▪ ▪ ▪ ▪ ▪

ICD-9: 814.01 (closed fracture of navicular [scaphoid] bone of wrist); 814.11 (open fracture of navicular [scaphoid] bone of wrist)

ICD-10: S62.009A (unspecified fracture of navicular [scaphoid] bone of unspecified wrist, initial encounter for closed fracture); S62.009B (unspecified fracture of navicular [scaphoid] bone of unspecified wrist, initial encounter for open fracture)

Fractures of the hand account for 14% to 19% of all hand and forearm fractures[228, 234] and 8% are of the carpal bones. The scaphoid carpal bone is located in the anatomical snuffbox (ASB) of the hand, and it is the most commonly fractured carpal bone, accounting for almost 90%.[235, 236] These fractures are most commonly the result of the client falling and reaching out to catch themselves during their fall, commonly referred to as *falling on an outstretched hand*, or FOOSH.[237] A FOOSH is characterized by forceful wrist hyperextension and radial deviation. During radial deviation and extension of the wrist, the scaphoid approximates to the radius, resulting in limiting further motion.

Early and accurate diagnosis is essential due to the poor blood supply of the scaphoid. The clinician should be cognizant of detecting the potential for these fractures to minimize insufficient treatment, which would risk future complications, including avascular necrosis, nonunion, carpal instability, and osteoarthritis.[238] On the other hand, overtreatment must also be avoided due to the increased costs of health care and the potential for the client to miss days of work due to immobilization or work restrictions.

The majority of scaphoid fractures occur at the transverse waist, but they may also occur at the proximal pole, distal pole, and tubercle.[48, 237] Fracture to the proximal pole may be manifested by avascular necrosis due to associated injury to the arterial blood supply.

I. Client Interview

Subjective History

- Typically young males between 10 and 29 years of age are at the highest risk,[237, 239] with the median age of injury in men at 25 years old, according to one recent epidemiologic study.[237]

- Pain is described as a "deep, dull ache" in the radial wrist.[5]

- The most common mechanism of injury is described as a FOOSH. Less common mechanisms are wrist hyperextension injuries associated with deceleration (such as against the steering wheel of a car), machinery kickback injuries, falls onto the dorsum of the hand (i.e., hyperflexion injuries), forced ulnar deviation, direct loading of the scaphoid, and stress-related fractures in athletes.[235, 237, 240]

- Clients may complain of painful wrist movements, specifically wrist extension, flexion, and radial deviation.

- Clients report pain with gripping activities.[5]

Outcome Measures

- The DASH, QuickDASH, PRWHE, and PSFS are appropriate for this client population. All have demonstrated clinical applicability in clients with upper extremity dysfunction.

Diagnostic Imaging

- Plain radiographs, with four standard views (posteroanterior [PA], PA ulnar deviation, lateral and semipronated oblique), are the initial primary diagnostic imaging tool utilized to assess scaphoid fracture. However, there is a great deal of variability in the sensitivities found in the literature (SN 35-86).[48, 50, 241-243] Specificity has been found to be as high as (SP 92-95).[50, 243]

- Bone scintigraphy can be used to help **rule out** (SN 94-100;[47] SN 97, −LR 0.03[46]) and help **rule in** (SP 89, +LR 8.8) scaphoid fractures.[46] However, a recent review found that scintigraphy has a high false positive rate (up to 25%) and low specificity (SP 60-95). Therefore, a positive scan will require further imaging.[48]

- MRI is typically not recommended during the initial evaluation, but it can be helpful for **ruling in** (SP 100;[49] SP 99, +LR 96;[46] SP 86[50]) and **ruling out** (SN 100;[49] SN 96, −LR 0.04[46]) scaphoid fractures if the initial plain radiograph is negative. The cost of MRI is higher; therefore, it is typically not utilized in the acute stage. However, a recent study demonstrates that MRI may be cost-effective in the overall management of clients with scaphoid fractures since it may prevent unnecessary cast immobilization and the use of health care dollars.[238]

- CT scans can be used to help **rule out** (SN 89-97;[51] SN 94[52]) and **rule in** (SP 85-91;[51] SP 100[52]) scaphoid fractures. CT is useful in assessing the morphology of the fracture and bony architecture of the scaphoid.[52]

II. Observation

- Mild swelling and bruising of the dorsal wrist and fullness of the ASB[5]

III. Triage and Screening

- All nonmusculoskeletal causes, as well as neuromusculoskeletal causes from proximal joints, should be ruled out.[64]
- No localized tenderness (SN 94), pain on active motion (SN 97), and pain on passive motion (SN 94) help **rule out** fracture of the wrist.[62]

IV. Motion Tests

- Clients may have limited and painful wrist active and passive ROM, specifically wrist extension, flexion, and radial deviation.
- Range of thumb movement does little to help rule in or out a scaphoid fracture (SN 69, SP 66).[116]

V. Muscle Performance Testing

- Clients may have pain in the ASB with resisted forearm supination.[244]
- Clients may have pain with gripping.[5]

VI. Special Tests

- Thumb-index finger pinch (SN 73, SP 75, +LR 2.92, −LR 0.36) and pain during pronation of the forearm (SN 79, SP 58, +LR 1.90, −LR 0.35) were found to be more valuable than other physical examination maneuvers in detecting scaphoid bone injuries, but they provide less than good ability to help rule out or rule in their existence.[119]

- Scaphoid compression test: A (−) test has less than good ability to help rule out a scaphoid fracture (SN 70, +LR 0.90;[115] SN 100, +LR 1.92[116]).
- A combination of clinical signs (ASB tenderness, scaphoid tubercle tenderness, and longitudinal compression), used within the first 24 hours of injury, has less than good ability to help rule in or rule out a scaphoid fracture (SN 100, SP 74).[116]

VII. Palpation

- Negative tenderness to palpation at the ASB (SN 90, −LR 2.25) or scaphoid tubercle (SN 87, −LR 1.51) has less than good ability to help rule out scaphoid fracture.[117]

VIII. Physical Performance Measures

- Grip strength and measures of fine motor control of the wrist and hand may be used. Selection and utilization of these tests will be individual to each client, dependent on their functional status and goals.

POTENTIAL TREATMENT-BASED CLASSIFICATIONS

- Immobilization and pain or inflammation control may be used.

Kienböck's Disease

ICD-9: 732.3 (juvenile osteochondrosis of upper extremity)

ICD-10: M87.9 (osteonecrosis, unspecified)

Kienböck's disease is an avascular necrosis of the lunate in the proximal carpal row of wrist. The lunate bone is most frequently involved in dislocations, fracture dislocations, and perilunate dislocations, accounting for about 10% of all wrist injuries.[245, 246] The exact etiology is unknown, but clients will commonly report trauma, with a FOOSH being the most common such mechanism. The lunate, similar to the scaphoid, has a limited blood supply, making avascular necrosis a significant possibility following trauma. Morphologic variations such as negative ulnar variance,[247] abnormal radial inclination, trapezoidal shape of the lunate, and variations in the vascularity to the lunate may be predisposing factors.[248]

Clients in the early stage of the disease process rarely seek medical attention; therefore, the true incidence and natural history of the disease are unknown.[249] Progression of the disease leads to collapse of the lunate, with subsequent carpal destabilization and wrist joint osteoarthritis. Early diagnosis and treatment are essential to stop the progression and minimize complications.

I. Client Interview

Subjective History

- Most common in young men aged 18-40.[250, 251]
- Typically unilateral.[250]
- Activity-related dorsal wrist pain may radiate into the forearm.[251]
- Stiffness, tenderness, and swelling are reported.
- Reported history of wrist trauma.[249]
- The client's complaint of symptoms may have begun several months to years earlier.[249]

Outcome Measures

- Progression of the disease can be monitored clinically by the DASH and the loss of flexion of the wrist.[252]
- The DASH, QuickDASH, PRWHE, and PSFS are appropriate for this client population. All have demonstrated clinical applicability in clients with upper extremity dysfunction.

Diagnostic Imaging

- Negative ulnar variance, which can be detected with plain radiographs, has been associated with Kienböck's disease.[247]
- Plain radiographs are the primary diagnostic imagining tool utilized for diagnosis and staging of Kienböck's disease. The modified Stahl's classification and Lichtman's radiographic classification are the primary staging systems used.
- MRI is useful in the earlier stages of the disease, particularly when findings are absent on plain films. MRI enables for an earlier and more extensive detection of changes.[250, 253]

- Osteonecrosis of the carpal bones shows correlation of MRI findings with histological examination of bone biopsies.
    - Pooled results: accuracy 0.98 (95% confidence interval [CI] 90-100), SN 97, and SP 100.[43]
- CT is useful for determining the stage and extent of the disease.[251, 253]

II. Observation

- In later stages, dorsal swelling around the location of the lunate may be present due to synovitis of the radiocarpal joint.[251]

III. Triage and Screening

- All nonmusculoskeletal causes, as well as neuromusculoskeletal causes from proximal joints, should be ruled out.[64]
- No localized tenderness (SN 94), pain on active motion (SN 97), and pain on passive motion (SN 94) help **rule out** fracture of the wrist.[62]

IV. Motion Tests

- Clients may have painful and limited wrist flexion and extension.[249-251]

V. Muscle Performance Testing

- Clients may have weakness and pain with grip assessment.[249-251]

VI. Special Tests

- No tests are particular to Kienböck's disease.

VII. Palpation

- Clients may have localized dorsal wrist pain at the lunate.[250]

VIII. Physical Performance Measures

- Grip strength and measures of fine motor control of the wrist and hand may be used. Selection and utilization of these tests will be individual to each client, dependent on their functional status and goals.

POTENTIAL TREATMENT-BASED CLASSIFICATIONS

- Immobilization and pain or inflammation control may be used.

Ulnar Collateral Ligament Tear of the Thumb (Gamekeeper's Thumb or Skier's Thumb)

ICD-9: Stener lesion: 719.94 (unspecified disorder of joint, hand)

ICD-10: Stener lesion: M25.9 (joint disorder, unspecified)

Ulnar collateral ligament tear of the thumb is an injury that is described as an insufficiency of the ulnar collateral ligament (UCL) of the metacarpophalangeal (MCP) joint of the thumb. The injury is a result of a sudden valgus force placed onto the abducted MCP joint or due to repetitive abduction strain, and it has been previously described as gamekeeper's thumb (a chronic injury) and skier's thumb (an acute injury).[254, 255] Other underlying pathologies that may cause a UCL tear include rheumatoid arthritis and generalized ligamentous laxity.

Injuries to the UCL can be partial or complete tears. Complete tears can further be divided into displaced and undisplaced. A Stener lesion, a displaced tear, occurs when the adductor aponeurosis becomes interposed between the ruptured UCL and its site of insertion at the base of the proximal phalanx. The distal portion of the ligament therefore retracts and points superficially and proximally. The UCL no longer contacts its area of insertion and cannot heal. This lesion can also be associated with a gamekeeper's fracture. The incidence of a Stener lesion associated with rupture of the UCL has been reported as high as 45% based on operative findings.[256] An untreated UCL tear of the MCP joint may lead to significant functional limitations and chronic pain due to instability of the joint.[257]

I. Client Interview

Subjective History

- Clients will complain of pain and weakness with any activity requiring adduction or flexion of the thumb's MCP joint, including prehension grip.[258]
- Clients experience pain, swelling, and stiffness.[258, 259]
- Clients are likely to describe limited ability to abduct and possibly extend the thumb without pain.[258, 260]
- This injury may also be as the result of nonacute, repetitive tasks stressing the MCP of the thumb into abduction.[258, 260]

- Clients have subjective report of trauma or repeated strain.[259]

Outcome Measures

- The DASH, QuickDASH, PRWHE, and PSFS are appropriate for this client population. All have demonstrated clinical applicability in clients with upper extremity dysfunction.

Diagnostic Imaging

- Stress radiographs (radiographs obtained with the thumb in the flexed and extended positions and with valgus stress at the MCP joint) can help determine the degree of instability of partial tears of the UCL.[257]
- Arthrography, ultrasound, and MRI have been used to identify complete tears; however, these tests are not particularly cost-effective and are not 100% accurate.[257, 261, 262]

II. Observation

- Ecchymosis or bruising is commonly seen in the acutely injured client.[257-260]

III. Triage and Screening

- All nonmusculoskeletal causes, as well as neuromusculoskeletal causes from proximal joints, should be ruled out.[64]
- No localized tenderness (SN 94), pain on active motion (SN 97), and pain on passive motion (SN 94) help **rule out** fracture of the wrist.[62]

IV. Motion Tests

- Accessory testing of the MCP joint of the thumb will be excessive or painful with a valgus stress.[258, 263]
- Clients may have limited ability to abduct and possibly extend thumb without pain.[258, 260]

V. Muscle Performance Testing

- Weakness of maximum grip strength and pincer grip[257, 259]

VI. Special Tests

- Stress testing at 30°: The lack of a definite end point on stress testing at 30° flexion is likely to indicate a complete rupture of the ulnar collateral ligament.[263]

- Ulnar collateral ligament test: A (−) test has less than good ability to help rule out (SN 94) ulnar collateral ligament injuries.[112] This test should be used with caution due to poor methodology.

VII. Palpation

- The lack of a palpable mass proximal to the metacarpophalangeal joint can be used to help rule out (SN 100) a complete tear of the UCL of the thumb.[112]
- Clients may have tenderness to palpation over the UCL at the MCP of the thumb.[258, 259, 263]
- In the instance of a Stener lesion, there may also be a palpable mass proximal to the adductor aponeurosis.[259, 264]

VIII. Physical Performance Measures

- Grip strength and measures of fine motor control of the wrist and hand may be used. Selection and utilization of these tests will be individual to each client, dependent on their functional status and goals.

POTENTIAL TREATMENT-BASED CLASSIFICATIONS

- Bracing and pain or inflammation control may be used.

Boxer's Fracture

ICD-9: 815 (fracture of metacarpal bone)

ICD-10: S62 (fracture at the wrist and hand level)

A boxer's fracture occurs as a result of axial loading of the 4th or 5th transverse neck of the metacarpal bone secondary to an indirect force such as striking an object with a closed fist. Boxer's fractures represent over half of all metacarpal fractures.[265]

I. Client Interview

Subjective History

- This injury is most likely to be aggression related, such as punching an object with a closed fist.[265, 266]
- Clients report having had a cracking, snapping, or popping sensation.[266]
- Pain description is most likely isolated to the region of the hand.

- Males are nearly 50% more likely to sustain a fracture from a punch mechanism than females.[265]
- Aggression-related fractures occurred at a median age of 22 (7-51) years old.[266]
- Accident-related fracture occurred at a median age of 34 (2-90) years old.[266]

Outcome Measures

- The DASH, QuickDASH, PRWHE, and PSFS are appropriate for this client population. All have demonstrated clinical applicability in clients with upper extremity dysfunction.

Diagnostic Imaging

- Standard views of anteroposterior and lateral views are typically sufficient for diagnosis.[267, 268]
- Sonographic examination has been shown to be an effective diagnostic tool in clients with fifth metacarpal fractures: SN 97 (84-99), SP 92 (79-98), +LR 14 (4.6–41), −LR 0.03.[269]
- Aggression-related fractures are typically located in the neck of the metacarpal bone.[266]
- Accident-related fractures are located approximately equally in the subcapital, diaphyseal, and basal parts of the metacarpal bone.[266]

II. Observation

- If presenting acutely, the client likely will have swelling, ecchymosis, and guarded movement of involved upper extremity.[265, 268, 270, 271]
- The client may also present with abrasions or cuts and demonstrable displacement of the involved metacarpal.[265, 268, 270, 271]

III. Triage and Screening

- All nonmusculoskeletal causes, as well as neuromusculoskeletal causes from proximal joints, should be ruled out.[64]
- No localized tenderness (SN 94), pain on active motion (SN 97), and pain on passive motion (SN 94) help **rule out** fracture of the wrist.[62]

IV. Motion Tests

- Clients may have limited ROM of MCP and more distal motions; possible wrist ROM limitation is also likely.[265, 271]

V. Muscle Performance Testing

- Clients may have limited strength of MCP and more distal joints; possible wrist weakness is also likely.[265, 271]

VI. Special Tests

- No tests are particular to Boxer's fracture.

VII. Palpation

- Tenderness description is most likely isolated to the region of the hand.[265, 268, 271]

VIII. Physical Performance Measures

- Grip strength and measures of fine motor control of the wrist and hand may be used. Selection and utilization of these tests will be individual to each client, dependent on their functional status and goals.

POTENTIAL TREATMENT-BASED CLASSIFICATIONS

- Immobilization and pain or inflammation control may be used.

Boutonniere Deformity

ICD-9: 736.21 (Boutonniere deformity)

ICD-10: M20.029 (Boutonniere deformity of unspecified finger)

A boutonniere deformity (BD) is a deformity of one of the digits where the proximal interphalangeal (PIP) joint is flexed and the distal interphalangeal (DIP) joint is hyperextended. This occurs due to deformity or disruption of the central slip, a key component of the extensor mechanism of the PIP joint. Weakening or disruption of the central slip with compromise of the triangular ligament subjects the lateral bands to migrate volar to the axis of rotation of the PIP joint. As the deformity progresses, the now-dominant flexor superficialis creates constant flexion at the PIP joint. Over time, BDs may become fixed as the surrounding volar plate and ligaments become contracted.

While this injury is traditionally believed to be the result of jamming the involved finger, only 5% of clients who jammed their finger and up to 50% of clients with rheumatoid arthritis were estimated to develop BD.[270] The main etiologies described in the literature are rheumatoid arthritis, mechanical trauma, burns, and infections.

Dorsal avulsion fractures or any fractures involving the base of the middle phalanx are at high risk for developing BD. Open or closed fractures appear to have the same incidence of subsequent BD formation.

I. Client Interview

Subjective History

- Clients may describe an acute mechanical trauma, such as jamming the involved finger.
- A history of rheumatoid arthritis, burns, or infections has also been described as predisposing a factor.

Outcome Measures

- The DASH, QuickDASH, PRWHE, and PSFS are appropriate for this client population. All have demonstrated clinical applicability in clients with upper extremity dysfunction.

Diagnostic Imaging

- Standard radiographs of the hand and digit, including posterior–anterior, oblique, and lateral views, are typically sufficient. If these are negative and a high suspicion of fracture or deformity exists, stress views and or fluoroscopic examination may be warranted.[270]

II. Observation

- The clinician should observe flexion of the PIP and hyperextension of the DIP joint of the involved digit.
- The PIP joint may appear swollen and painful.
- The deformity may not appear immediately after injury; several weeks may pass before the muscle imbalance around the PIP joint occurs.[272]

III. Triage and Screening

- Standard radiographs can be used to rule out fracture. See prior Diagnostic Imaging section.

IV. Motion Tests

- A loss of active extension of the PIP joint of ≥20°, with the wrist and MCP fully flexed, is helpful in diagnosing BD.[270]

- Clients will have difficulty with active PIP joint extension but will be able to actively hold the digit in extension if placed in the position passively.

V. Muscle Performance Testing

- Clients will have difficulty with active PIP joint extension.

VI. Special Tests

- Haines-Zancolli test:
  - A test is (−) if passive flexion of the DIP is still possible with the PIP maintained in extension.
  - A test is (+) if flexion of the DIP is not possible with PIP in extension.
  - No diagnostic accuracy studies, determining SN and SP, have been performed to date for this clinical test.

VII. Palpation

- Clients may have possible tenderness to palpation at the affected digit.

VIII. Physical Performance Measures

- Grip strength and measures of fine motor control of the wrist and hand may be used. Selection and utilization of these tests will be individual to each client, dependent on their functional status and goals.

POTENTIAL TREATMENT-BASED CLASSIFICATIONS

- Upper extremity orthotics and pain or inflammation control may be used.

Swan-Neck Deformity

ICD-9: 736.22 (swan-neck deformity)

ICD-10: M20.039 (swan-neck deformity of unspecified finger)

Swan-neck deformity (SND) is a deformity of the digits in which the PIP is hyperextended and the DIP is flexed (figure 23.50). The deformity may start

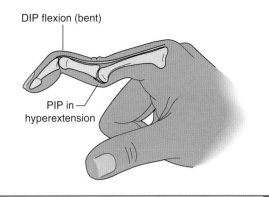

DIP flexion (bent)

PIP in hyperextension

Figure 23.50   Swan neck deformity.

at either the DIP or PIP. SND has been associated with rheumatologic diseases (rheumatoid arthritis), neurologic disorders (cerebral palsy), hypermobility syndromes (Ehlers-Danlos syndrome), and trauma.[273] The primary lesion is laxity in the volar plate that allows hyperextension of the PIP joint. Causes include trauma, generalized ligament laxity, and rheumatoid arthritis. Secondary lesions occur due to an imbalance of forces on the PIP joint. Causes include MCP joint volar subluxation, mallet injury, flexor digitorum superficialis laceration, rupture, or excision, and intrinsic contracture.

Clients will present with an observable deformity in the affected digit and may report snapping or locking of the digit. Diagnosis is typically evident from the physical exam. Physicians may order X-rays to assess the condition of the affected joint surfaces. Recognition of the underlying clinical diagnosis that is responsible for the SND is vital. Conservative treatment will include client education, activity modification, and splinting. Splinting will permit active PIP flexion and limit hyperextension of the joint. In client cases where balance cannot be restored, surgical intervention may be necessary.

Mallet Finger

ICD-9: 736.1 (mallet finger)

ICD-10: M20.019 (mallet finger of unspecified fingers)

The deformity is produced by disruption of the terminal extensor mechanism at the distal interphalangeal (DIP) joint (figure 23.51). Mallet finger is a common closed tendon injury that is seen in

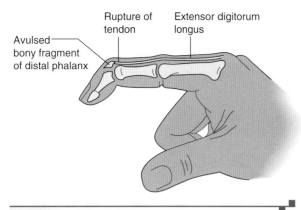

Figure 23.51   Mallet finger.

athletes; this injury is also common in nonathletes after minor trauma.[274] Injury occurs from forcible flexion of the extended DIP joint, which results in unopposed flexion from the flexor digitorum profundus.

Mallet finger has also been referred to as drop, hammer, or baseball finger (although baseball accounts for only a small percentage of such injuries). Clients will report pain in the DIP region and display difficulty in extending the injured digit. The 3rd, 4th, and 5th digits of the dominant hand are the most frequently involved.[274] Often times the client will need radiographs to rule out an avulsion fracture or fracture to the articular surface.[274]

Nonsurgical management is the standard of care for mallet injuries. Treatment consists of putting the finger in a mallet splint for 6 to 8 weeks, which allows the tendon to return to its normal resting length. The involved digit is placed in extension or slight hyperextension at the DIP joint. Although splint management is simple with minimal complications, client education with specific attention to detail is vitally necessary to ensure a successful outcome. Long-term follow-up status post splinting has demonstrated favorable results,[275] and researchers have demonstrated high client satisfaction following splinting despite the possibility of residual deformity.[276]

Surgical intervention is recommended when clients present with an open fracture or if the intra-articular fracture comprises more than 30% of the joint surface.[274] An untreated mallet finger is painful. If left untreated, the digit will eventually develop a swan neck deformity due to compensatory hyperextension at the proximal interphalangeal joint.[274, 277]

Flexor Tenosynovitis

ICD-9: 727.0 (synovitis and tenosynovitis)

ICD-10: M65 (synovitis and tenosynovitis)

Tendon sheaths are lined by paratenon and synovium; therefore, the same disease process affects the tendons as the joints. Symptoms of tenosynovitis may occur before those of intra-articular disease. The affected sites are the dorsal and volar aspects of the wrist, because the tendons are covered by synovium as they pass under the flexor and extensor retinaculum and under the wrist, and the volar aspect of the digits, because the tendons are covered by synovium in the fibro-osseous canals in the finger. Synovitis of the tendons can cause pain, dysfunction, and eventual rupture of tendons.

When the condition causes the respective finger to get stuck in a flexed position, the condition is called *stenosing tenosynovitis*, more commonly referred to as *trigger finger* (figure 23.52). This condition often coexists with tendinitis. Trigger finger results from a difference in the diameter of the flexor tendon and the retinacular sheath due to thickening and narrowing of the sheath. Narrowing of the A1 pulley at the metacarpal head occurs most often due to its location leading to high forces during normal and forceful gripping.[278] Thus abnormalities of the gliding mechanism of the tendon will occur resulting in inflammation, which causes nodular enlargement of the tendon distal to the pulley.

Proposed causes include repetitive finger movements and trauma.[279, 280] In certain circumstances,

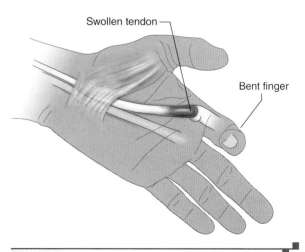

Figure 23.52   Trigger finger.

occupational-related tasks (i.e., extensive gripping or shearing), could be predisposing factors.[281, 282] However, the relationship is questionable, and research displays that trigger finger is not related to occupation.[283, 284] Therefore, clinicians should consider the cause as multifactorial in nature.

Trigger finger occurs most commonly in clients between 50 and 60 years old and is six times more likely to occur in women than men.[285] The lifetime risk is 2.6% in the general population[286] and increases to 10% in the diabetic population.[287] The reason is not glycemic but is related to the duration of the disease. Trigger finger can concomitantly occur with carpal tunnel syndrome, de Quervain's disease, hypothyroidism, rheumatoid arthritis, renal disease, and amyloidosis.[288-291]

The client will report initial gradual painless popping, snapping, clicking, locking, stiffness, or difficulty extending a flexed digit at the DIP or PIP joints, with pain developing as the condition progresses. Trigger finger most often occurs in the thumb followed by the third and fourth digits.[292] A painful palpable nodule may be found in the palmar aspect of the hand in the region of the MCP joint. As the disease progresses, the client may avoid use of the hand due to pain and popping or clicking, resulting in secondary contractures of the PIP joint.[289] There are no objective confirmatory tests. Imaging tests are generally not done; if completed, they are usually normal. Laboratory tests may be useful for detecting the presence of related conditions such as diabetes, hypothyroidism, or rheumatoid arthritis.[293]

Due to the chronic nature of the symptoms associated with trigger finger, conservative treatment is often not successful and is often frustrating for clients. However, conservative management, consisting of client education, activity modification, MCP joint mobilization, nonsteroidal anti-inflammatory drugs, splinting, or corticosteroid injection, is typically recommended prior to surgical intervention.[294]

The aim of splinting is to reduce tendon excursion through the A1 pulley in order to allow the inflammation to resolve.[278, 295] Splinting consists of wearing a custom-made splint to hold the MCP joint at 10° to 15° of flexion, with the PIP and DIP joints left free. Research has demonstrated that splinting can be effective for certain clients; however, for those with more severe disease and a longer duration of symptoms, it can yield lower success rates.[295, 296]

Corticosteroid injections have been demonstrated to provide a resolution or improvement of symptoms in up to 93% of clients.[297] The shot is injected into the affected tendon; if symptoms do not resolve or recur, a second injection has been demonstrated to be half as efficacious as the initial.[298]

Operative treatment is considered the gold standard of treatment if unsuccessful with conservative management. Common surgical techniques include an open procedure, endoscopy, or percutaneous release. Complication can include long-term scar tenderness, inadequate release, nerve damage, and flexor sheath infection.[299]

Bennett's Fracture

ICD-9: 815 (fracture of metacarpal bone)

ICD-10: S62 (fracture at wrist and hand level)

Bennett's fracture is a fracture of the base of the first metacarpal bone, which extends into the CMC joint (figure 23.53). This intra-articular fracture is the most common type of fracture of the first metacarpal. Its prevalence accounts for about one-third of all fractures of the first metacarpal,[300] and it is nearly always accompanied by some degree of subluxation or frank dislocation of the carpometacarpal joint. On radiographs, the fracture line runs obliquely and involves the first carpometacarpal joint.[301] A Bennett's fracture occurs from axial force directed against a partially flexed metacarpal. The injury typically occurs in young males[301, 302] in their dominant hand[302] due to a blow on a partially closed fist, which may occur during a fall or when

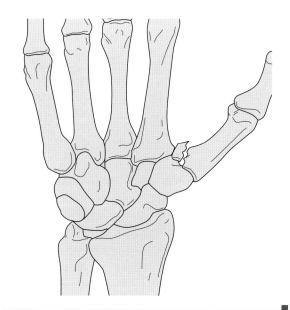

Figure 23.53 Bennett's fracture.

involved in athletic activities (i.e. boxing, martial arts).[301] Clients will present with complaints of pain, loss of function of the first carpometacarpal joint, acute edema, tenderness to palpation at the first metacarpal, decreased AROM, difficulty with grip, and weakness with pincer grip.[303]

Treatment of this fracture can be difficult. Prognostic factors include the location and displacement of the fracture, the extent of impaction at the metacarpal, and the presence or absence of articular damage to the trapezium. Due to the fracture being unstable, concern exists that inadequate fixation may lead to long-term consequences, such as osteoarthritis, weakness of the hand, or decreased function in the first carpometacarpal joint.[303, 304] Bennett fractures can be treated conservatively with closed reduction and casting, closed reduction and percutaneous Kirschner wire fixation, or open reduction and internal fixation (ORIF). Studies offer conflicting evidence for the best results and most reliable reduction of the fracture and subluxation[302, 305-307]

Irrespective of treatment selection for optimal post injury recovery, it is recommended that a reduction of less than 1 mm of displacement be achieved.[308, 309] After immobilization or surgical intervention, the goal of rehabilitation will be to decrease pain and edema and increase strength and AROM to restore functional capabilities.

Dupuytren's Contracture

ICD-9: 728.6 (contracture of palmar fascia)

ICD-10: M72.0 (palmar fascial fibromatosis [Dupuytren])

Dupuytren's contracture is characterized as a progressive disorder of the palmar fascia that results in shortening, thickening, and fibrosis of the fascia and aponeurosis (figure 23.54). Dupuytren's contracture affects the palmar hand, causing progressive, permanent, and symptomatic flexion contractures of the metacarpals. Incidence is highest in male[310-312] Caucasian clients of northern European descent.[310] The average age of onset is 60, with the incidence increasing with age.[312]

Risk factors for Dupuytren's contracture include a history of smoking,[313, 314] alcohol consumption,[314, 315] adhesive capsulitis,[316] epilepsy,[317] diabetes mellitus,[314, 318] history of manual labor,[173] hand trauma,[319] and genetics.[315] However, further research is needed due to the fact that current evidence is weak in nature.

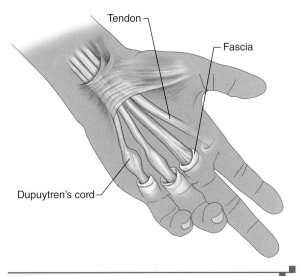

Figure 23.54 Dupuytren's contracture.

The physical examination is the mainstay for diagnosis of Dupuytren's disease. Clients will present with nodules or thickening of the skin on the volar/palmar aspect of the hand, skin pitting and dimples, palmar digital contractures of the MCP joint, and bands of fibrotic tissue.[312] Dupuytren's contracture typically occurs bilaterally and most often in the fourth and fifth digits.[320] The Hueston tabletop test can aid in diagnosis. The client is instructed to lay their palm flat on a tabletop; if they cannot do so, the test is considered positive. No diagnostic accuracy studies have been performed to date.

Surgical intervention is the mainstay of treatment for Dupuytren's contracture. Due to this fact, the clinician's main role occurs postoperatively, which includes client education, splinting, therapeutic exercise, and edema and scar management.

CONCLUSION

The wrist and hand are some of the most complex anatomical structures in the body. They have many static and dynamic components, making them vulnerable to injury. The interplay and balance of these structures allows for a wide range of daily functional activities that allow for power, dexterity, and precision. Injury to any of the components of the WH complex will lead to client difficulties with occupational and recreational tasks. During the examination of the WH complex, the challenge lies in ascertaining the causative component. This chapter provides a comprehensive overview of the structural and biomechanical basis of the WH complex, an evidence-based examination outline, and an evidence-based discussion of common orthopedic conditions of the wrist and hand. Clinicians must keep in mind that the components of the clinical examination, including (but not limited to) the subjective history, outcome measures, diagnostic imaging, objective examination, and special testing, are assessments with their own ability to shift the probability of a particular diagnosis.

24

HIP

Michael P. Reiman, PT, DPT, OCS, SCS, ATC, FAAOMPT, CSCS

Differential diagnosis of the hip joint poses a diagnostic dilemma, particularly given that pain in the hip region is often difficult to localize to a specific pathological structure. With the evolution of improved diagnostic imaging and advanced surgical techniques, examination of the coxofemoral (hip) joint and periarticular structures as a primary pain source for hip-related pain and dysfunction has received a significant increase in attention.[1-3] Although limited information exists in support of diagnostic utility, emphasis on patient history, clinical examination findings, magnetic resonance imaging (MRI), arthrogram, and anesthetic intra-articular injection pain response are currently advocated for determining the presence of intra-articular hip joint pathology.[4] Combined use of these examination processes by health care practitioners has been only marginally effective. Authors have reported that clients visit, on average, 3.3 health care providers over a period of 21 months before being correctly diagnosed with a hip labral tear.[5] Confounding the diagnostic process of the hip joint is a lack of consensus regarding the actual examination.[6] Additionally confounding variables for the differential diagnosis of hip joint labral tear are the variability in reported prevalence of acetabular labral tears in clients with hip or groin pain and the complex interaction among the lumbar spine, pelvis, and hip.[7-12] Reports of the prevalence of labral tear pathology range anywhere from 22% to 55%.[13-16] The extent to which various pathologies in the hip—such as femoroacetabular impingement (FAI), labral tear, and osteoarthritis—coexist is also not clearly defined.

CLINICALLY APPLIED ANATOMY

The hip joint is a large synovial joint that attaches the trunk to the lower leg. Like the shoulder, it is a ball-and-socket joint. Unlike the shoulder, it is a primary weight-bearing joint. With a convex femoral head articulating with the concave acetabulum, the mechanics of the hip joint are similar to that of the shoulder. Therefore, the hip does have a fair amount of mobility. It is also an inherently very stable joint due to its architectural structure, ligamentous support, and load-bearing function.

The acetabular labrum deepens the acetabulum to increase hip joint stability (figure 24.1). The orientation of the femur and the ligamentous strength also contribute to hip joint stability. Biomechanical analyses suggest that the labrum is stressed by compressive loads and extremes of hip joint motion.[17-19] Therefore, a tear of the labrum likely alters physiological functions, such as enhancing joint stability and load distribution.[17]

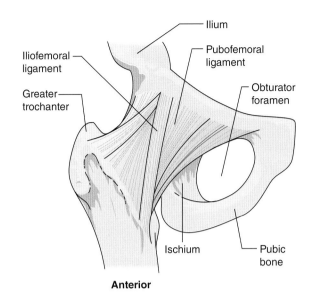

Figure 24.1 Acetabular labrum.

The femur is slightly anteverted, slightly anterior to the frontal plane relative to the shaft of the femur (figure 24.2). The acetabulum is typically slightly anteverted as well. Therefore, when a client has a limitation or pain with the combined motions of flexion, adduction and internal rotation, the clinician should be suspicious of a mechanical impingement due to either a retroverted acetabulum or bony abnormality of the femoral head.

Ligamentous support is an important variable for hip stability (figure 24.3). The three primary ligaments of the hip (iliofemoral, ischiofemoral, and pubofemoral) all have a primary function of stability for the hip joint. All three ligaments are taut with hip extension, although some findings suggest that

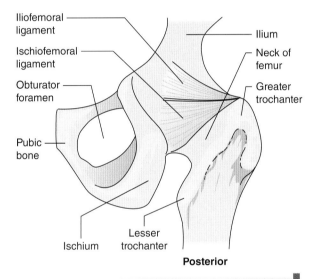

Figure 24.3 Primary ligaments around the hip.

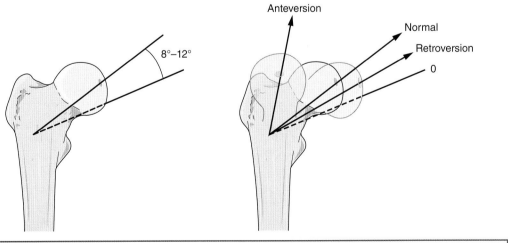

Figure 24.2 Angle of torsion: normal, anteversion, and retroversion.

the ischiofemoral ligament tightens during flexion. Additional motions stressing combinations of these ligaments are primarily hip abduction and external rotation. Clients with ligamentous laxity likely will have excessive hip external rotation.[20, 21]

The loads on the hip joint can be variable.[22] Standing exerts 0.3 times the client's body weight, walking exerts between 1.3 times and 5.8 times body weight, walking up stairs exerts 3 times body weight, and running exerts over 4.5 times body weight on the hip joint.

CLIENT INTERVIEW

This interview is typically the first encounter the clinician will have with the client. As previously discussed in chapter 5 (Client Interview and Observation), this component of the examination can provide the clinician with a significant amount of information relevant to the probability of the client's presenting diagnosis. For purposes of this text, the interview is described relative to each body part or section but generally includes subjective reports by the client, as well as findings from their outcome measures. Also included in this section is radiographic imaging. While clinicians should avoid biasing their examinations by interpreting findings of radiographic imaging prior to seeing clients (in most cases without concerns for red flags and major medical-related issues), this point in the examination is most likely where clinicians will encounter radiographic imaging. Additionally, in some instances, clinicians must interpret radiographic imaging early in the examination to rule out serious pathology prior to continuing with other components of the examination sequence.

Subjective

The client should be encouraged to describe in detail the specific location of their concordant pain. As previously described, differential diagnosis of the lumbar spine, pelvis, and hip is often difficult. A few variables have been shown to demonstrate a strong predilection to hip pain. The presence of a limp, groin pain, or limited internal rotation (IR) of the hip significantly predicted diagnosis of disorder as originating primarily from hip opposed to the spine. Patients with a limp were 7 times more likely to have hip disorder than spine disorder, while those with groin pain were 7 times more likely to have hip disorder alone or hip and spine disorder versus spine disorder alone. Limited IR in a patient was 14 times more likely to suggest a hip disorder only or hip and spine disorder versus spine disorder only.[23] Additionally complicating the differential diagnosis of the pain generator in the hip joint region are the multiple potential causes of pain in this area. Clearly delineating the specific cause requires deliberate questioning. Details about specific pain location, level of irritability, pain duration, and onset (all information discussed in chapters 4 through 6) are paramount.

Potential Causes of Various Hip Pathologies

Trauma or Repeated Microtrauma

Hip dislocation

Hip subluxation with or without acetabulum or labral injury

Fracture or stress fracture of acetabulum, femur, or pelvis

Avulsion injury of iliac spine, hip, or pelvic girdle

Contusion of iliac spine (hip pointer)

Muscle strain (most likely adductors or hamstrings)

Ligament sprain

Loose bodies in joint

Acetabular labral tears

Athletic pubalgia or sports hernia

Femoral or inguinal hernia

Soft-tissue contusion injuries

Myositis ossificans

Tendinitis or tendinopathy

Pubic symphysis dysfunction

Sacroiliac joint dysfunction

Femoroacetabular impingement

(continued)

Infectious

Osteomyelitis

Hip pyarthrosis

Urinary tract infection

Septic arthritis

Inflamed lymph nodes

Neurologic

Herniated nucleus pulposus

Nerve entrapment

- Femoral
- Obturator
- Piriformis

- Lateral femoral cutaneous (meralgia paresthetica)
- Genitofemoral
- Ilioinguinal

Neurovascular injury

Degenerative

Osteoarthritis

- Spine
- Femoroacetabular joint

- Sacroiliac joint
- Pubic symphysis

Osteolysis

Inflammatory

Rheumatoid arthritis

Juvenile rheumatoid arthritis

Ankylosing spondylitis

Bursitis

- Trochanteric or subtrochanteric
- Iliopectineal
- Ischiogluteal
- Iliopsoas

Osteitis pubis

Tendinitis

Pelvic inflammatory disease

Crohn's disease

Reiter's syndrome

Systemic lupus erythematosus

Prostatitis

Gynecologic

Epididymitis

Hydrocele

Varicocele

Renal lithiasis

Referred visceral pain

Inflamed lymph nodes

Transient synovitis

Metabolic

Gout

Metabolic bone disease

Vascular

Osteonecrosis or avascular necrosis (e.g., osteochondritis dissecans)

Chondrolysis

Sickle-cell disease

Neurovascular injury

Thrombosis

Neoplastic

Pelvic

Acetabulum

Femur

Testicular

Gynecologic

Some specific questions (besides those listed in chapters 4 through 6) are relevant to the hip joint. Age of the client will assist with differential diagnosis of hip pain. Pediatric and adolescent pathologies, such as Legg-Calvé-Perthes (typical age of onset is 3 to 12 years old) and slipped capital femoral epiphysis (average age of 12.1 years for girls and 14.4 years for boys), will significantly differ in client age compared to acetabular labral tear (adolescents to older adults) and hip osteoarthritis, osteoporotic femoral neck fractures, or gluteal tendinopathy (older adults).

Mechanism of onset can assist with differential diagnosis of hip pathology. Acetabular labral tears, for example, have four primary mechanisms of onset or contributing factors: traumatic, dysplasia, femoroacetabular impingement (FAI), and laxity and hypermobility.[24] Soft-tissue injuries should be suspected in athletes who while sprinting felt a pop, either posteriorly (hamstring)[25, 26] or in the medial thigh (adductors).[27, 28] Careful questioning of the client can be extremely helpful in determining the potential primary structures involved.

Groin pain is a common location for multiple hip pathologies (as well as lumbar spine and pelvic girdle pathologies). Groin and thigh pain were found in 55% and 57% of hip joint pain clients, respectively. However, pain referral was also seen in the buttock and lower extremity distal to the knee in 71% and 22%, respectively.[29] The most common locations of pain for clients with labral tear were the central groin and lateral peritrochanteric area.[30] The clinician should therefore systematically differentially diagnose the commonly reported groin pain presentation. Paresthesia in the anterior groin and thigh is more suggestive of femoral nerve versus obturator peripheral nerve involvement (medial thigh) once the lumbar spine is ruled out.

Complaints of clicking, catching, and snapping should include labral tear, intra-articular pathology, and snapping hip on the differential diagnosis.[16, 31-33] Carefully delineating the source (and relevance) of such symptoms is imperative to properly diagnosing the client. For example, 91% of ballet dancers reported snapping hip; 60% of them could volitionally produce this snapping, yet only 7% were not able to continue dancing due to the snapping.[34]

Thus, the question of whether the condition is worsening, staying the same, or improving is relevant, as is the degree to which their current symptoms affect their daily and recreational activities. Diagnosis such as hip osteoarthritis will likely continue to progress in terms of pathology, but the client may just limit their daily activities. Younger clients may report a greater effect on their activities due to unwillingness to limit such activities. Therefore, as with all other regions of assessment, the clinician should have a clear understanding of the client's symptoms, how they affect their functional status, where the symptoms are located, aggravating and relieving factors, and so on.

Outcome Measures

Clinicians can use multiple outcome measures. Outcome measures formulated, implemented in research studies, and utilized in daily clinical practice are multiple for the hip joint. The specific outcome measure utilized is also sometimes dependent on the hip pathology. No conclusive evidence supports a single patient-reported outcome measure questionnaire for the evaluation of patients undergoing hip arthroscopy. Investigation of the most efficacious hip outcome measure for hip arthroscopy patients suggests that the Nonarthritic Hip Score (NAHS) was the best-quality questionnaire among it, the Hip Outcome Score (HOS), and the Modified Harris Hip Score (MHHS).[35] The NAHS demonstrated the highest content validity, while the HOS scored best on agreement, internal consistency, and responsiveness.[35]

For the evaluation of treatment goals in patients with hip osteoarthritis, the following measurement instruments were recommended: Lequesne index, Western Ontario and McMaster Universities (WOMAC) osteoarthritis index, Hip disability and Osteoarthritis Outcome Score, Knee injury and Osteoarthritis Outcome Score, patient-specific complaint list, Visual Analogue Scale for pain, Intermittent and Constant Osteoarthritis Pain questionnaire, goniometry, Medical Research Council for strength, and the handheld dynamometer.[36] The fact that multiple measures were recommended underlies the importance of a comprehensive assessment approach, as discussed in chapter 4 of this text. Function is a multifactorial variable that requires a comprehensive approach to assessment.

As part of the comprehensive assessment of function, a proposal for the development of a standardized battery of physical performance outcome measures to complement self-report measures when capturing the construct of function in patients with hip osteoarthritis (OA) has been suggested.[37] Part of the reasoning for such a proposal is the evidence questioning the construct validity and longitudinal validity of the WOMAC-PF for assessing physical function, a previously recommended leading self-report measure for the assessment of function in these patients. Recommendations for the use of both self-report measures and physical performance measures of physical function are needed for a more comprehensive assessment of function in patients with hip OA.[37]

A recent systematic review investigated utilization of 12 different outcome measures. They concluded that the Hip dysfunction and Osteoarthritis Outcome Score (HOOS) contains adequate measurement qualities for evaluating patients with hip OA or total hip replacement (THR). The HOS is the best available questionnaire for evaluating hip arthroscopy, but the Inguinal Pain Questionnaire, the only identified questionnaire for evaluating groin disability, does not contain adequate measurement qualities.

The HOOS was recommended for evaluating patients with hip OA undergoing nonsurgical treatment and surgical interventions such as THR. The HOS is recommended for evaluating patients undergoing hip arthroscopy. The authors concluded that these questionnaires should also be evaluated in younger patients (age < 50) with hip or groin disability, including surgical and nonsurgical patients.[38]

A newly developed tool, the 33-item International Hip Outcome Tool (iHOT-33) has been suggested as a primary outcome measure for acetabular labral tear (ALT) clients due to its development following large sample sizes and the most rigorous methodology. This questionnaire uses a visual analogue scale response format designed for computer self-administration by young, active patients with hip pathology. The iHOT-33 has been shown to be reliable and highly responsive to clinical change, and it has demonstrated face, content, and construct validity.[39] A short version of the International Hip Outcome Tool (iHOT-12) has been developed. It has very similar characteristics to the original rigorously validated 33-item questionnaire, losing very little information despite being only one-third the length. It is valid, reliable, and responsive to change. It can be used for initial assessment and postoperative follow-up in routine clinical practice.[40]

The Copenhagen Hip and Groin Outcome Score (HAGOS) has also been suggested for the assessment of symptoms, activity limitations, participation restrictions, and quality of life in physically active, young to middle-aged patients with long-standing hip or groin pain. The HAGOS consists of six separate subscales assessing pain, symptoms, physical function in daily living, physical function in sport and recreation, participation in physical activities, and hip- or groin-related quality of life. It is also valid, reliable, and responsive to change. This measure is suggested for use in interventions where the client's perspective and health-related quality of life are of primary interest.[41]

The Short Musculoskeletal Function Assessment (SMFA) had good overall responsiveness in clients with hip fractures and has been recommended for use as one of the measures to evaluate the outcome after a hip fracture.[42]

The Children's Hospital Oakland Hip Evaluation Scale (CHOHES) is a modification of the Harris Hip Score (HHS). It does appear to be an easy-to-use, valid, and reliable assessment tool and should be considered for use in the routine clinical evaluation of sickle-cell disease patients with avascular necrosis (AVN).[43]

Diagnostic Imaging

Radiographic examination of the hip joint, as of other regions of the body, is dependent on the type of pathology. Diagnostic imaging, like clinical examination techniques, continues to be refined. Some types of imaging have been utilized in the same type of pathology with comparison studies to determine the best diagnostic or screening procedure. Diagnostic imaging, like each component of the examination for potential hip joint pathology, provides relevant and valuable information for the clinician in order to make the best clinical decisions regarding the client's diagnosis and potential treatments. Not unlike other portions of the examination of the hip joint, diagnostic imaging requires careful interpretation on part of the clinician. Several studies have found hip pathological changes in asymptomatic people.[44-47] Therefore, diagnosis made solely on diagnostic imaging interpretation is not sensible clinical practice.

While there are many different imaging methods, and sometimes choices of method, for a particular pathology (table 24.1), the value of diagnostic imaging should be carefully weighted for some diagnoses, such as developmental hip dysplasia and FAI.[48] For imaging of intra-articular hip pathology, MRI represents the best technique because it enables clinicians to directly visualize cartilage, it provides superior soft-tissue contrast, and it offers the prospect of multidimensional imaging. However, opinions differ on the diagnostic efficacy of MRI

TABLE 24.1   Diagnostic Accuracy of Various Imaging Modalities for the Hip

Pathology	Diagnostic test	Reference standard	SN/SP
Osteoarthritis	Radiographs: various criteria (e.g., joint space width, ostephyte presence, and so on)	Surgery	Not investigated
	MRI	Variable	Pooled analysis: 61/82[54]#
		Histology	Pooled analysis: 74/76[54]#
		Radiographs	Pooled analysis: 61/81[54]#
Intra-articular pathology	Intra-articular injection	Surgery	90% accuracy[1]
Labral tear	CT	Surgery	**97/87**[55]
			92/100[56]
	MRI		Pooled analysis: 66/79[57]
			91/80[58]
	MRA		Pooled analysis: 87/64[57]
	US		82/60[58]
Articular cartilage lesion	MRA	Surgery	58-81/69-100[59]
			50-79/77-84[60]
			49-67/76-89[61]
			Pooled analysis: 62/**86**[62]
	CT		70-79/**93-94**[61]
			88/82[55]
	MRI		Pooled analysis: 59/**94**[62]
Impingement	MRA	Surgery	87/64[57]
	CT scan		**92-97/87-100**[55, 56]
	MRI		66/79[57]
	Bone scan	Hip pain, (+) impingement test, and (+) radiographs	**85/63**[63]
Proximal femur fracture (e.g., neck, intertrochanteric)	Radiograph	Surgery	**90-95/68-100**[64]
	Bone scan		**91/100**[65]
	MRI		**100/100**[65]
	CT		NR
Femoral shaft stress fracture	Bone scan	Surgery	**91/100**[65]
	Radiograph		**90-95/68-100**[64]
	MRI		**100/100**[65]
AVN/osteonecrosis of femoral head	MRI	Surgery	**99/99**[66]
			SN 100[67]
	Bone scan		SN 81[67]
Gluteal tendon tear	MRI	Surgery	33-100/**92-100**[68]
			93/92[69]
	US		SN 79-100[68]
			PPV 95-100[68]
		Surgery/histopathological findings	61/100[70]
Sport-related chronic groin pain	MRI	Comprehensive clinical exam	78/**88**[71]

= the Menashe study[54] investigated osteoarthritis in multiple joints (hip, knee, and hand). The majority of studies were performed on knee osteoarthritis. CT = computed tomography; MRI = magnetic resonance imaging; MRA = magnetic resonance arthrography; US = ultrasonography; NR = not reported

The color coding for suggestion of **good** and **ideal** diagnostic accuracy values reported in this table are without quality scoring (QUADAS), a very important aspect of determination of the clinical utility of such values. Therefore, it is suggested that the reader keep this in mind when interpreting such values.

and on the question of which MRI technique is most appropriate.[49] A large-field-of-view MRI survey of the pelvis, combined with high-resolution MRI of the pubic symphysis, is an excellent means of assessing various causes of athletic pubalgia, providing information about the location of injury, and delineating the severity of disease.[50] Due to the fact that various findings have been discovered in subjects with groin pain,[50-52] such an approach is suggested.

Groin pain, arising from injuries to the hip and pelvis, accounts for 5% to 6% of athletic injuries in adults and 10% to 24% of these injuries in children.[51] Diagnostic imaging of clinical value is necessary for differentially diagnosing what has been termed as "the Bermuda triangle of sports medicine."[53]

Radiographs

Anteroposterior (AP) and lateral (axial "frog leg") views are the standard views utilized in plain film radiographs. As with all extremity joints, comparison between sides is necessary. Assessment of particular aspects on the AP view includes the following:

- Hip dislocations and most fractures are often seen on AP and lateral views.

- An AP view with the hip internally rotated provides a necessary view of the femoral neck with those patients in whom femoral neck fractures are suspected but standard radiographic findings are negative.

- Neck-shaft angle: An abnormal head neck offset (or pistol grip deformity) can be seen on these views.

- Alpha angle: The alpha angle is a parameter used to quantify the degree of femoral deformity that reflects the insufficient anterolateral head-neck offset and femoral head aspheric-

ity.[72] Alpha angles greater than 60° have been suggested to be associated with symptomatic impingement[72, 73] (figure 24.4), although other findings have suggested much higher values to discriminate between subjects with pathology and controls.[74] Cam impingement is associated with a larger than normal alpha angle.

- Crossover sign: A crossover sign on the AP view is where a portion of the anterior wall of the acetabulum projects farther laterally, or crosses over the posterior wall (figure 24.5). This sign is associated with pincer-type impingement of the hip. The three different types of femoroacetabular impingement are depicted in figure 24.6.

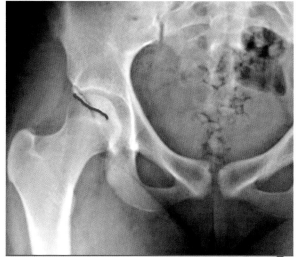

Figure 24.5 Crossover sign of the hip joint. Posterior wall of acetabulum (red line) crosses over anterior wall of acetabulum (blue line).

© Michael Reiman

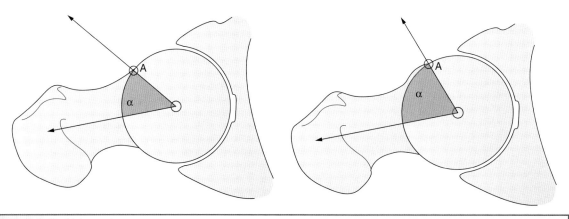

Figure 24.4 Alpha angle.

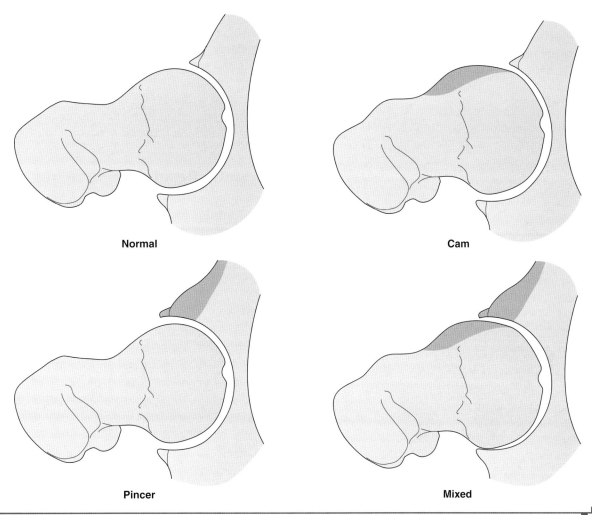

Figure 24.6 Femoroacetabular impingement types.

- Contour of femoral head.
- Femoral head and acetabulum orientation: assessment for acetabular dysplasia and acetabular protrusio (acetabular overcoverage; coxa profunda). Acetabular protrusio is diagnosed on the AP view demonstrating a center-edge angle (figure 24.7; angle between red [line from midpoint of femoral head to lateral edge of acetabular rim] and blue [line from midpoint of femoral head straight vertical] lines) greater than 40° (figure 24.8) and medialization of the medial wall of the acetabulum (red arrow in figure 24.9) past the ilioischial line (blue arrow in figure 24.9).
- Neck-shaft angle: assessment for coxa vara or coxa valga.

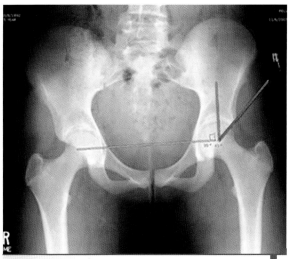

Figure 24.7 Center-edge angle.

© Michael Reiman

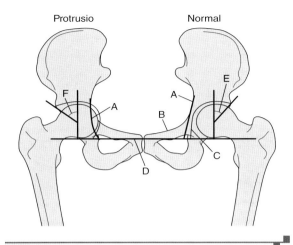

Figure 24.8 Excessive center-edge angle demonstrating protrusio.

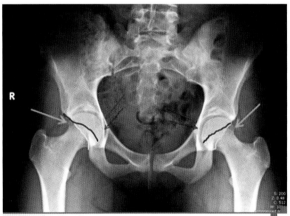

Figure 24.9 Acetabular protrusio (red arrow pointing to acetabular line) projecting medial to the ilioischial line (blue arrow). The green arrows show cam deformity.

© Michael Reiman

- Joint space width and osteophytes for assessment of osteoarthritis.
- Bone disease such as bony cysts (suggestive of OA), tumors, Legg-Calvé-Perthes disease.

Lateral view radiographs are performed with the client's hip flexed, abducted, and externally rotated while they are lying supine. This view allows clinicians the capability to view for any possible pelvic obliquity or slipped capital femoral epiphysis (SCFE). Children with suggestive groin symptoms should have hip AP and frog-leg lateral radiographs to rule out SCFE.[75]

Measures of joint space, the maximum thickness of subchondral sclerosis, and the size of the largest osteophyte have been utilized to diagnose hip OA with radiographs. Minimal joint space (i.e., the shortest distance between the femoral head margin and the acetabulum) was the index most strongly associated with other radiologic features of OA. Mild to moderate hip OA was defined as ≥2 mm of joint space available, while severe OA was defined as ≤1.5 mm of minimum joint space on radiographs.[76]

Magnetic Resonance Imaging

Magnetic resonance imaging is increasingly being utilized for the assessment of hip pathology presence. Both soft tissue (e.g., tendon, labral, and bursal lesions) and osseous tissue (e.g., stress fractures and osteonecrosis) can reliably be assessed with MRI. Since MRI is more sensitive to bone marrow edema, it is often used to assess subtle occult fractures and diagnoses such as sport-related chronic groin pain, osteitis pubis, or bone stress injuries of the pubis bone.[77] Combining arthrography (magnetic resonance arthrography) has recently been shown to be both more sensitive and specific for the diagnoses of hip pathological lesions such as labral tears than MRI,[57] although less sensitive and specific for diagnosis such as gluteal tendinopathy.[68] Magnetic resonance imaging with arthrogram (MRA) has also been used for many of the same types of pathologies that MRI is used for. Abnormal findings on MRI and MRA for various pathologies should caution the clinician regarding interpretation of such findings and diagnosis.[44, 78]

Computed Tomography

Computed tomography scans are traditionally utilized for acetabular wall and femoral head fractures, as well as the more subtle hip dislocations. The assessment of osseous abnormalities, such as shape and size of the femoral head (as in a bony exostosis for cam impingement; figure 24.10) and acetabulum, anteversion, and retroversion measurements are important uses of CT scan. As with radiographs and MRI or MRA, findings of abnormalities in asymptomatic clients[45] require caution in diagnostic interpretation of CT findings in the hip joint.

Ultrasound

Ultrasound, or ultrasonography, is an imaging technique that does not involve radiation. It is typically used for the assessment of tendon pathology in the hip,[68] although it has also been suggested for various other soft-tissue hip and lower extremity pathol-

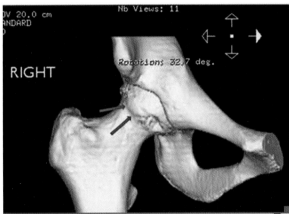

Figure 24.10 Three-dimensional CT scan demonstrating pistol grip deformity associated with cam-type impingement in the hip joint.

© Michael Reiman

ogies.[79] Ultrasonography has even been suggested for the use of screening for developmental hip dysplasia,[80] although a recent systematic review cautions its use in this manner due to weak evidential support for the clinical utility of ultrasonography.[81]

Bone Scan (Scintigraphy)

Bone scans are typically utilized to help diagnosis tumors, necrosis, and stress fractures of the hip. This is particularly the case with proximal femoral (femoral neck and intertrochanteric) fractures.

Review of Systems

Refer to chapter 6 (Triage and Differential Diagnosis) for detail on review of systems relevant to the hip joint.

OBSERVATION

Observation of the client presenting with hip pain should (as with all portions of the body) include general postural assessment (both statically and dynamically), gait, transfers, and potential limitations in strength and mobility with daily tasks. Static posture assessment should be viewed from both the anteroposterior view as well as laterally. Looking for asymmetry from side to side can alert the clinician to structural abnormalities. Iliac crest height, greater trochanter height, and anterior and posterior superior iliac spine levels (as also observed for the lumbar spine and pelvis) can alert the clinician to some potential structural dysfunctions that may be contributing to the client's hip pain. Postural

dysfunctions, such as lower crossed syndrome and scoliosis (see chapter 14) can have significant effects on the hip joint.

While more detail regarding posture is given in chapter 14, some additional things are worth mentioning here. From all views, the clinician should assess for scars, skin discoloration, changes in texture, and so on. From both the lateral and posterior views, the clinician can assess for gluteal atrophy, which is strongly correlated with hip osteoarthritis.[82, 83]

Several hip muscles are active during gait. Principal among them are the gluteal muscles. The gluteus medius (GMed) is a broad, fan-shaped muscle with attachments to the superior and flared portion of the ilium, as well as distally attaching to the lateral and superior–posterior aspect of the greater trochanter.[84] The GMed has been anatomically divided into three parts (anterior, middle, and posterior), each performing specific functions. As an entire muscle, the GMed stabilizes the femur and pelvis during weight-bearing activities. The greatest GMed activation has been observed during the stance phase of gait.[85, 86] The gravitational torque about the hip during single leg stance is counteracted by an abduction torque on the stance hip, stabilizing the pelvis relative to the femur. Additionally, these muscles are required to rotate the pelvis in the same direction as the advancing contralateral swinging leg.[87] Therefore, dysfunction of these muscles (primarily the gluteus medius and gluteus minimus) is depicted in an excessive contralateral (or non-weight-bearing swinging) side of the pelvis, or Trendelenburg gait pattern. A compensated gait pattern would present when the client excessively shifts their upper body mass toward the involved side to decrease the length of the lever arm acting on the weight-bearing hip joint and therefore prevent the non-weight-bearing side of the pelvis from dropping. The clinician should be cognizant of these different compensatory gait patterns for dysfunction in the hip abductor muscle group when examining hip dysfunction clients. Clients with hip osteoarthritis[88] and slipped capital femoral epiphysis,[89] for example, have demonstrated this type of gait dysfunction. The Trendelenburg test is discussed later in the Special Tests section regarding specific diagnostic and clinical relevance.

The hip extensor muscles, as a group, produce the greatest torque across the hip joint compared to any other muscle group.[90] This torque is utilized to propel the upper body of a person upward and forward from a position of hip flexion.[87, 91] Such examples during gait movements would include standing up out of a chair, climbing a steep hill or incline, and pushing off into a sprint. If the gluteus maximus is paralyzed, the client's trunk must be thrown posterior at heel strike to prevent the trunk from falling forward with the flexion moment at the hip. The typical orthopedic or sports client with hip dysfunction involving the gluteus maximus is more likely to present with deficits in stairs, step-ups, and sit-to-stand maneuvers due to the torque production discussed previously.

Therefore, deficits detected with sit-to-stand and stand-to-sit transfers may be indicative of dysfunction in the gluteal muscles. Additionally the clinician should be cognizant of joint changes, such as labral tear, impingement, dysplasia, and osteoarthritis. Each of these conditions could lead to muscle performance or joint mobility dysfunction contributing to limitations in these activities.

The client with joint changes may have complaints with some combination of hip joint positions involving flexion, adduction, or internal rotation.[16] Pain may therefore be detected in the groin region or described as a *C-sign pattern* (because the client uses their hand in the shape of the letter

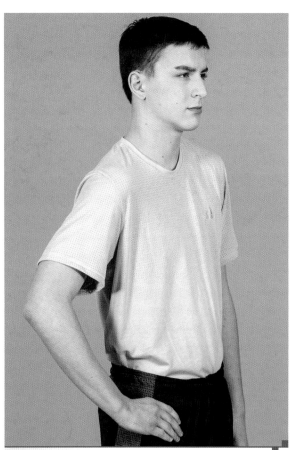

Figure 24.11 C-sign.

C to demonstrate pain location; see figure 24.11), indicative of potential intra-articular involvement.[92] Pain posturing on part of the client may be seen when sitting in chairs (especially lower level chairs), stepping up with the involved leg, squatting, and so forth, since these motions will replicate the combinations of these movements in the hip.

Range of motion of the hip can also be observed without formal assessment. In the supine position, the clinician can assess generally for anterior capsular laxity. The client lying supine with relaxed legs and demonstrating enough external rotation for the lateral border of that foot to touch the table likely has laxity of the anterior capsule or excessive femoral anterior torsion. Alternatively, the client presenting with very little to no external rotation in this position should heighten the clinician's concern for limited anterior capsular mobility or femoral retrotorsion.

Limitations in hip range of motion (ROM) can be assessed with daily activities. Gait on level surfaces requires only 30° to 44° of hip flexion, while ascending and descending stairs requires 45° to 66° of hip flexion.[93, 94] Sitting in a chair of an average seat height requires 112° of hip flexion. Putting on socks requires 120° of flexion, 20° of abduction, and 20° of external rotation.[95] Clients with FAI cannot squat as deeply as those without FAI.[96] Difficulty performing such daily tasks can alert the clinician as to which particular motions to more closely examine.

TRIAGE AND SCREENING

Triage and screening is a necessary component of the examination process that should be done prior to continuing with the examination. As with all specific body part examinations, at this point the clinician must decide whether or not to continue with the examination. Specifically, they should determine whether to continue examining the client or refer them to a physician. Ruling out serious pathology (refer to chapter 6, Triage and Differential Diagnosis) and pain generation from other related (or close-proximity) structures helps the clinician more accurately determine the necessity of continuing with the other examination components to identify the actual source of the client's pain. Additionally, implementing strong screening tests (tests of high SN and low −LR) at this point in the examination is suggested for narrowing down the competing diagnoses of the respective body regions (lumbar spine, pelvis and knee in this case) when this is applicable.

Ruling Out Serious Pathology: Red Flags

A careful subjective history and observation of the client will help the clinician triage the client. The clinician must be aware of disorders affecting the abdominal and pelvic organs that can also refer pain to the hip region, mimicking a musculoskeletal dysfunction. Previous history of cancer, such as prostate cancer in men or any reproductive cancer or breast cancer in a woman, is a red flag since these cancers may be associated with metastases to the hip joint.[97]

In a study of women with groin pain, multiple sources of pathology were discovered, further suggesting the need for a detailed screen as part of the clinical examination.[98] Other red flags include a history of trauma, fever, unexplained weight loss, burning with urination, night pain, and prolonged corticosteroid use.[99-101] The clinician should also be aware of other variables, such as previous history of surgeries to the hip or proximal lower extremity, previous abdominal or pelvic organ surgery, insidious onset of pain, symptoms unchanged by position or movement, symptoms related to a woman's menstrual cycle, neurological or vascular diseases that the client may have, acute hip pain with fever, malaise, night sweats, unexplained weight loss, intravenous drug use, night pain unrelieved by position change, compromised immune system, a history of corticosteroid exposure or alcohol abuse (risk for avascular necrosis), and previous history of cancer, as mentioned before. Awareness of these potential red flag concerns can alert the clinician of the need for medical intervention. Refer to chapter 6 for additional details on differential diagnosis.

During special testing for potential red flags from non-musculoskeletal causes related to the hip, clinicians should utilize the resisted straight leg raise and the heel strike tests. The details of these tests are listed here.

RESISTED STRAIGHT-LEG RAISE TEST

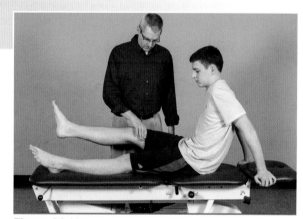

Figure 24.12

Client Position	Sitting and leaning back on the hands or lying supine
Clinician Position	Standing at the side of lower extremity to be assessed
Movement	The client raises the lower extremity 30 cm off the table. The client resists as the clinician applies a downward pressure at the distal thigh.
Assessment	A (+) test is indicated if pain is reproduced in the lower quadrant, indicating possible peritoneal inflammation, appendicitis, or inflammation of the iliopsoas muscle. A test is (+) for labral tear with reproduction of concordant pain or clicking or catching in the anterior hip, not the lower quadrant of abdomen.
Statistics Regarding Appendicitis	SN 16 (not reported, or NR), SP 95 (NR), +LR 2.4, –LR 0.90, in a study reporting summary estimates for the diagnosis of acute appendicitis[102]
Statistics Regarding Intra-Articular Hip Pathology	• SN 59 (57-96), SP 32 (9-48), +LR 0.9, –LR 1.3, QUADAS 7, in a study of 50 clients with signs or symptoms suggestive of hip pathology (mean age 60.2 years; 30 women; symptom duration NR), using ≥80% improvement in pain after intra-articular hip joint injection as a reference standard.[103]
	• SN 56 (NR), SP not tested, QUADAS 9, in a study of 51 clients (52 hips). Of these clients the average age was 35 years, 22 were female, and the symptom duration ranged from 3 months to 15 years. Symptomatic FAI and radiography (all subjects) or surgery (43 subjects) were used as a reference standard.[104]

HEEL STRIKE TEST[105]

Client Position	Supine on the table, arms relaxed
Clinician Position	Standing at the client's feet, directly facing the client
Movement	Clinician lifts the lower extremity to be assessed. Keeping the client's knee straight, the clinician uses their hand (right as shown) to strike the client's heel.
Assessment	A (+) test is indicated by the production of pain or the reproduction of the client's symptoms, specifically deep hip pain.
Statistics	NR

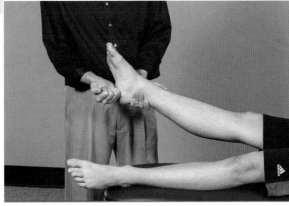

Figure 24.13

Rule Out Fracture

A particular concern of triage involving the hip joint is the ruling out of a fracture. Osteoporosis, which is characterized by low bone mass and microarchitectural deterioration, is a major risk factor for fractures of the hip, vertebrae, and distal forearm. Hip fracture is the most detrimental fracture, being associated with 20% mortality and 50% permanent loss in function.[106] Presence of a hip fracture warrants referral to a physician. Testing to rule in or rule out the presence of a fracture or stress fracture of the hip region includes the patellar-pubic percussion test and the fulcrum test. Details of these tests are listed here.

STRESS FRACTURE TEST (FULCRUM TEST)

Client Position	Relaxed sitting position on the end of the table, with bilateral feet over the edge
Clinician Position	Sitting at the end of the table, directly the facing client
Movement	The clinician places one forearm (left as shown) under the client's thigh to be tested. With their other hand (right as shown), the clinician applies a downward pressure to the proximal knee. This test can be repeated in successively more proximal areas on the femur assuming the test is negative with testing of previous location.
Assessment	A test is considered (+) for stress fractures if the client reports pain with the maneuver.
Statistics	• SN 93 (NR), SP 75 (NR), +LR 3.7, –LR 0.09, QUADAS 5, in a study of 7 clients with proximal femur stress fractures (mean age 19.8 years; 4 were female; mean symptom duration NR), using bone scan or radiography as a reference standard.[107]
	• SN 88 (NR), SP 13 (NR), +LR 1.0, –LR 0.92, QUADAS 7, in a study of 6 clients with proximal femur stress fractures (age range 19-23 years; all were female; mean symptom duration NR), using radiography, bone scan, or MRI as a reference standard.[108]
	• Confirmation of a stress fracture requires a bone scan; therefore, a positive finding warrants physician referral.

Figure 24.14

PATELLAR-PUBIC PERCUSSION TEST

 Video 24.15 **in the web resource shows a demonstration of this test.**

Client Position	Relaxed supine position with bilateral lower extremities straight
Clinician Position	Standing at the side of the lower extremity to be tested, directly facing the client
Movement	The clinician places a stethoscope over the pubic tubercle on the ipsilateral side of the lower extremity being tested (right as shown). The clinician listens through the stethoscope as they tap the ipsilateral patella. Tapping and placing a tuning fork over the patella can also be used in place of tapping the patella directly.
Assessment	A (+) test is a diminished percussion noted on the side of pain indicating a potential femur fracture.
Statistics	• Pooled analysis: **SN 95 (92-97)**, **SP 86 (78-92)**, **+LR 6.11**, **–LR 0.07**, across three studies with 782 clients[109]
	• **SN 94 (NR)**, **SP 95 (NR)**, **+LR 20.4**, **–LR 0.06**, QUADAS 9, in a study of 41 consecutive clients (mean age, gender, and symptom duration NR) presenting to emergency department with a history of hip trauma necessitating radiographic examination, using radiography as a reference standard[110]
	• SN 91 (NR), SP 82 (NR), +LR 5.1, –LR 0.11, QUADAS 8, in a study of 100 consecutive clients with suspected femoral neck fracture (mean age 78.6 years; 82 women; mean symptom duration NR), using radiography as a reference standard[111]
	• **SN 96 (87-99)**, **SP 86 (49-98)**, **+LR 6.7**, **–LR 0.75**, QUADAS 10, in a study of 290 consecutive clients with suspected occult femoral neck fracture (mean age 72 ± 6.8 years; 236 women; mean duration of symptoms NR), using radiography, bone scan, MRI, or CT as a reference standard[112]

Figure 24.15

Ruling Out Pain Generation From Other Related Structures

Once red flags are ruled out, an efficient way to begin to differentiate the many potential pain referral sources is through the lower quarter screening examination. The traditional lower quarter screen consists of testing of dermatomes, myotomes, deep tendon reflexes, and possible upper motor involvement. The clinician should differentially diagnose the potential contribution of the sacroiliac joint or pelvic girdle and lumbar spine as the primary pain generator for the client's hip pain. Screening tests for these areas are employed to limit the extent of the differential diagnosis for pathology contributing to the client's hip pain. A systematic approach

to ruling out these other areas is suggested. The key points of this approach are listed here. Refer to chapters 19 (Lumbar Spine) and 20 (Sacroiliac Joint and Pelvic Girdle) for greater detail regarding these examination procedures.

Rule Out Lumbar Spine

The following section lists suggested special tests for ruling out the lumbar spine as a potential pain generator for the client with presentation of hip pain. The details of each of these tests can be found in chapter 19.

Radiculopathy or Discogenic-Related Pathology
This is ruled out with a combination of ROM and special tests assessments.

Repeated Motions (ROM)

- Centralization and peripheralization: 5-20 reps

    - **SN 92 (NR)**, SP 64 (NR), +LR 2.6, **−LR 0.12**, QUADAS 12[113]

    - SN 40 (28-54), **SP 94 (73-99), +LR 6.7**, −LR 0.63, QUADAS 13[114]

Special Tests

- Straight leg raise test

    - **SN 97 (NR)**, SP 57 (NR), +LR 2.2, **−LR 0.05**, QUADAS 10[115]

    - Pooled analysis: **SN 92 (87-95)**, SP 28 (18-40), +LR 2.9, **−LR 0.29**[116]

    - **SN 91 (82-94)**, SP 26 (16-38), +LR 2.7, **−LR 0.35**[117]

- Slump test

    - **SN 83 (NR)**, SP 55 (NR), +LR 1.8, **−LR 0.32**, QUADAS 11[118]

    - SN 84 (NR), SP 83 (NR), +LR 4.9, −LR 0.19, QUADAS 7[119]

Facet Joint Dysfunction This is ruled out with the seated extension–rotation test. As noted in chapter 19 (Lumbar Spine), facet joint dysfunction is ruled in with posterior-to-anterior spinal joint-play assessments eliciting stiffness and concordant pain.

Seated Extension–Rotation

- **SN 100 (NR)**, SP 22 (NR), +LR 1.3, **−LR 0.0**, QUADAS 11[120]

- **SN 100 (NR)**, SP 12 (NR), +LR 1.1, **−LR 0.0**, QUADAS 10[121]

Rule Out SIJ Dysfunction

The following section lists suggested special tests for ruling out the SI joint as a potential pain generator for the client with presentation of hip pain. The details of each of these tests can be found in chapter 20.

Pain provocation cluster testing:[122] **SN 91 (62-98), SP 83 (68-96), +LR 6.97, −LR 0.11, QUADAS 13**

- Thigh thrust test: **SN 88 (64-97)**, SP 69 (47-82), +LR 2.80, **−LR 0.18**; QUADAS 12[123]

- Gaenslen's test: SN 50-53, SP 71-77, +LR 1.8–2.2, −LR 0.66, QUADAS 12[123]

- Distraction test: SN 60 (36-80), SP 81 (65-91), +LR 3.20, −LR 0.49; QUADAS 12[123]

- Compression test: SN 69 (44-86), SP 69 (51-79), +LR 2.20, −LR 0.46; QUADAS 12[123]

- Sacral thrust test: SN 63 (39-82), SP 75 (58-87), +LR 2.50, −LR 0.50; QUADAS 12[123]

Laslett and colleagues assessed the diagnostic utility of the McKenzie method of mechanical assessment combined with the following sacroiliac tests: distraction, thigh thrust, Gaenslen, sacral thrust, and compression. The McKenzie assessment consisted of flexion in standing, extension in standing, right and left side gliding, flexion in lying, and extension in lying. The movements were repeated in sets of 10, and centralization and peripheralization were recorded. If it was determined that repeated movements resulted in centralization, the client was considered to present with pain of discogenic origin. If discogenic origin of pain was ruled out, the cluster of tests exhibited the following (3 out of 5 required to be positive): SN 94 (72-99), SP 78 (61-89), +LR 4.29, −LR 0.80, QUADAS 12.[123]

The test with the strongest diagnostic capability of ruling out SIJ-related dysfunction is the thigh thrust test: **SN 88 (64-97)**, SP 69 (47-82), +LR 2.80, **−LR 0.18**, QUADAS 12.[123]

Additionally, as with any joint, clearing AROM with or without overpressure is necessary. AROM of all motions as per the lower quarter screen described in chapter 7 should be implemented. In order to fully clear the lumbar spine and peripheral joints, full AROM (with overpressure if pain-free) must be present.

Sensitive Tests for the Hip

Ruling out particular pathologies in the hip joint can be complicated. Once competing pain-generating joints have been ruled out as outlined previously, it is suggested that SN tests of the hip joint be implemented to narrow down the potential diagnoses. The use of special tests can be of assistance (as well as all other components of the funnel examination approach). These tests, along with their correlation with pathology, are presented here. Additionally, the diagnostic accuracy of these tests relative to the pathology investigated is also presented.

Ruling out hip osteoarthritis is described. To assist in ruling out hip impingement, labral tear, or intra-articular pathology, clinicians should implement the flexion-adduction-internal rotation (FADDIR) and flexion-internal rotation tests.

- The gold standard clinical diagnosis for hip osteoarthritis is as follows: Clients with hip pain and hip internal rotation (IR) range of motion (ROM) $\geq 15°$ who experienced pain with IR, had morning stiffness ≤ 60 minutes, and were 50 years old or older could be identified as having hip OA (SN 86).[124]

- Hip impingement or labral tear and potential intra-articular involvement: FADDIR test.
  - Pooled analysis: **SN 94 (88-97)**, SP 8 (2-20), **+LR 1.02, −LR 0.48**, across four studies with 128 clients (MRA reference standard)[109]
  - Pooled analysis: **SN 99 (95-100)**, SP 7 (0-34), **+LR 1.06, −LR 0.15**, across two studies with 157 clients (arthroscopy reference standard)[109]

- Flexion-internal rotation test.
  - Pooled analysis: **SN 96 (82-100)**, SP 17 (12-54), **+LR 1.12, −LR 0.27**, across three studies with 42 clients[109]

The use of fluoroscopically guided intra-articular hip injection has been suggested to differentiate the pain source in clients with concomitant hip and lumbar spine arthritis. This technique demonstrated an **SN 100, SP 81, +LR 11.1, −LR 0**.[125]

Additionally, as with any joint, clearing AROM with or without overpressure is necessary. In order to fully clear the hip joint, full AROM (with overpressure if pain-free) must be present. Details in this regard are described in the following section.

MOTION TESTS

Motion assessment is a very important aspect of the examination for the orthopedic client. Motion dysfunction can be used to differentiate contractile versus non-contractile tissue (see chapter 9). Assessment of end-feel, potential capsular patterns, and ROM norm values can give the clinician an appreciation of the potential impairments for the orthopedic client they are assessing (table 24.2). Active range of motion (AROM), passive range of motion (PROM), and joint-play assessments are necessary to determine not only the presence or absence of joint dysfunction but also the precise aspects of the motion that are dysfunctional.

Passive and Active ROMs

Intrarater reliability of hip ROM was shown to be moderate to excellent (intraclass correlation coefficient or ICC = 0.50–0.97) in clients with and without hip OA.[126-128] Specific hip ROM measures have shown excellent interrater reliability, ranging from ICC of 0.76 to 0.97.[129] When assessing passive and active ROM, the clinician should consider the potential pathology. Clients with hip FAI and osteoarthritis, for example, have been shown to have limited hip IR, while clients with FAI and labral tear alone exhibited reduced motions in hip flexion, internal rotation, and adduction.[5, 11, 104, 124, 130-132] Therefore, the clinician can expect to find such limitations when assessing clients suspected of having these pathologies.

TABLE 24.2   Hip Joint Arthrology

Joint	Close-packed position	Resting position	Capsular pattern	ROM norms	End-feel
Femoral-acetabular	Full extension, abduction, internal rotation	30° flexion, 30° abduction, slight external rotation	Flexion, abduction, internal rotation	Flexion: 140° with knee flexed Extension: 20° Internal rotation: 45° External rotation: 45° Abduction: 40° Adduction: 25°	Firm for all motions

HIP FLEXION

Client Position	Supine with the leg to be assessed lying straight on the table
Clinician Position	Standing directly to the side of the client
Goniometer Alignment	The clinician positions the fulcrum over the lateral aspect of the greater trochanter and aligns the proximal arm with the lateral midline of the trunk and the distal arm with the lateral midline of the femur, using the lateral epicondyle of the knee as a reference.
Movement	The clinician stabilizes the client's pelvis with their proximal hand and grasps the client's distal lower extremity with their distal hand. The clinician then passively raises the lower extremity until a firm end-feel (due to stretching of hamstrings) is felt. Bending the knee will allow for increased hip flexion due to putting the hamstrings on slack. The clinician passively moves the hip to end range flexion (end-feel is soft due to approximation of the quadriceps muscle group approximating the abdomen). Assessment in this position is a more accurate measure of hip joint passive ROM. These motions can be performed similarly actively by the client (without assistance from the clinician). Active range of motion should be performed prior to PROM to determine the client's willingness to move and so on.
Assessment	Clinician assesses for amount of ROM, end-feel, quality of the movement, client response, potential difference between AROM and PROM, and so on.

HIP EXTENSION

Client Position	Prone with the leg to be assessed lying straight on the table
Clinician Position	Standing directly to the side of the client
Goniometer Alignment	The clinician positions the fulcrum over the lateral aspect of the greater trochanter and aligns the proximal arm with the lateral midline of the trunk and the distal arm with the lateral midline of the femur, using the lateral epicondyle of the knee as a reference.
Movement	The clinician's proximal hand stabilizes the pelvis while the distal hand grasps the lower extremity to be assessed just above the knee and passively lifts the lower extremity to end range extension (end-feel is firm due to stretching of the anterior joint capsule and ligaments). If the knee is flexed, the end-feel is firm due to the tension on the rectus femoris muscle. These motions can be performed similarly actively by the client (without assistance from the clinician). Active range of motion should be performed prior to PROM to determine the client's willingness to move and so on.
Assessment	Clinician assesses for amount of ROM, end-feel, quality of the movement, client response, potential difference between AROM and PROM, and so on.

HIP INTERNAL ROTATION

Client Position	Supine with the lower extremity to be assessed at 90° of hip and knee flexion
Clinician Position	Standing directly to the side of the client
Goniometer Alignment	The clinician positions the fulcrum over the anterior aspect of patella and aligns the proximal arm perpendicular to the client's body or parallel to a line bisecting the anterior superior iliac spine (ASIS) on both sides and the distal arm with the midline of the tibia to a point midway between the medial and lateral malleoli.
Movement	The clinician's proximal hand stabilizes the femur and their distal hand grasps the client's foot or heel. The clinician passively rotates the lower extremity into end range internal rotation by pulling the heel laterally while maintaining the femur in neutral adduction or abduction. The end-feel is

firm due to tension in the posterior joint capsule and external hip rotators. This motion can be performed similarly actively by the client (without assistance from the clinician). Active range of motion can be performed in same position but should be performed in the sitting position if there is compensation of hip adduction/abduction and done prior to PROM to determine the client's willingness to move and so on.

Assessment	Clinician assesses for amount of ROM, end-feel, quality of the movement, client response, potential difference between AROM and PROM, and so on.

HIP EXTERNAL ROTATION

Client Position	Supine with the lower extremity to be assessed in 90° of hip and knee flexion
Clinician Position	Standing directly to the side of the client
Goniometer Alignment	The clinician positions the fulcrum over the anterior aspect of patella, aligns the proximal arm perpendicular to the client's body or parallel to a line bisecting the ASIS on both sides, and aligns the distal arm with the midline of the tibia to a point midway between the medial and lateral malleoli.
Movement	The clinician's proximal hand stabilizes the femur and their distal hand grasps the client's foot or heel. The clinician passively rotates the lower extremity into end range external rotation by pushing the heel medially while maintaining the femur in neutral adduction or abduction. The end-feel is firm due to tension in the anterior joint capsule and the iliofemoral and pubofemoral ligaments. This motion can be performed similarly actively by the client (without assistance from the clinician). Active range of motion can be performed in the same position but should be performed in the sitting position if there is compensation of hip adduction/abduction and done prior to PROM to determine the client's willingness to move and so on.
Assessment	Clinician assesses for amount of ROM, end-feel, quality of the movement, client response, potential difference between AROM and PROM, and so on.

HIP ABDUCTION

Client Position	Supine with the leg to be assessed lying straight on the table
Clinician Position	Standing directly to the side of the client
Goniometer Alignment	The clinician positions the fulcrum over the ipsilateral ASIS and aligns the proximal arm along a line bisecting the ASIS on each side and the distal arm along the length of the ipsilateral femur, using the patella for a reference.
Movement	The clinician's proximal hand stabilizes the pelvis and their distal hand grasps the lower extremity to be assessed just above the knee. The clinician passively moves the lower extremity to end range abduction (end-feel is firm due to tension in the adductor muscle group, medial joint capsule and ligaments). This motion can be performed similarly actively by the client (without assistance from the clinician). Active range of motion should be done prior to PROM to determine the client's willingness to move and so on.
Assessment	Clinician assesses for amount of ROM, end-feel, quality of the movement, client response, potential difference between AROM and PROM, and so on.

HIP ADDUCTION

Client Position	Supine with the lower extremity to be assessed lying straight on table. The leg not being assessed is abducted, allowing for end range assessment on the lower extremity being assessed.
Clinician Position	Standing directly to the side of the client
Goniometer Alignment	The clinician positions the fulcrum over the ipsilateral ASIS and aligns the proximal arm along a line bisecting the ASIS on each side and the distal arm along the length of the ipsilateral femur using the patella for reference.
Movement	The clinician's proximal hand stabilizes the pelvis and their distal hand grasps the lower extremity to be assessed just above the knee. The clinician passively moves the lower extremity to end range adduction (end-feel is firm due to tension in the lateral joint capsule, IT band, and the gluteus medius muscle). This motion can be performed similarly actively by the client (without assistance from the clinician). Active range of motion should be done prior to PROM to determine the client's willingness to move and so on.
Assessment	Clinician assesses for amount of ROM, end-feel, quality of the movement, client response, potential difference between AROM and PROM, and so on.

Passive Accessories

Passive accessory motion assessment is essential for determining the potential for joint-play dysfunction in the joints being examined. The following section details distinct component assessments of passive joint mobility for the hip joint.

INDIRECT DISTRACTION

Client Position	Supine with bilateral legs relaxed
Clinician Position	Standing at the client's foot, facing the client's hip
Stabilization	The rest of the client's body on the table serves as a stabilizing force, especially with the lumbar spine side-bent away from the clinician. A belt may be wrapped around the client's pelvis and the treatment table to help stabilize the pelvis.
Movement and Direction of Force	The clinician grabs the client's leg proximal to the knee (supracondylar ridges of femur) with both hands. Additionally,

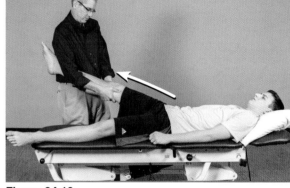

Figure 24.16

the clinician can place the client's leg between their arm and trunk as shown for improved purchase and ability to provide force. The clinician places the hip in the resting position (30° flexion, 30° abduction, and slight external rotation). Distraction force in caudal direction is imposed through both hands. The clinician can also lean back and use their entire body to utilize more force during the assessment. The direction of force is directly inferior and along longitudinal axis from hip joint, imparted through the clinician's body leaning back.

Assessment	Assessment is done for joint play/passive accessory motion, client response, and end-feel. Reproduction of concordant pain suggests dysfunction. Impaired joint mobility or end-feel may also suggest dysfunction if concordant pain is also reproduced.

ANTERIOR GLIDE

Client Position	Prone with bilateral legs relaxed
Clinician Position	Standing directly to the side of the client's hip to be assessed. The clinician should support the client's leg between their trunk and stabilizing hand.
Stabilization	The client's body resting on the table serves as a stabilizing force. A belt may be wrapped around the client's pelvis and the treatment table to help stabilize the pelvis. The clinician's stabilizing hand (right as shown) is positioned on the anterior surface of the distal thigh/knee. This hand controls the position of the femur.
Movement and Direction of Force	The clinician's assessing hand (left as shown) purchases the posterior surface of the most proximal portion of the client's thigh (just below the buttock) with a broad hand placement (force across the entire hand). The clinician should be careful not to extend the hip to the close-packed position (end range hip extension, abduction, and internal rotation). The clinician's assessing hand glides the femur in an anterior direction.
Assessment	Assessment is done for joint play/passive accessory motion, client response, and end-feel. Reproduction of concordant pain suggests dysfunction. Impaired joint mobility or end-feel may also suggest dysfunction if concordant pain is also reproduced.

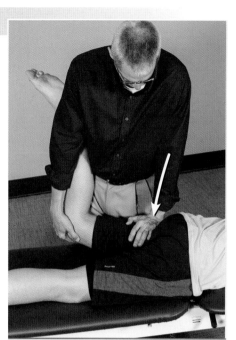

Figure 24.17

POSTERIOR GLIDE I

Client Position	Supine with bilateral legs relaxed
Clinician Position	Standing at the side of the client's hip or leg to be assessed, directly facing the client
Stabilization	The client's body resting on the table serves as a stabilizing force. A belt may be wrapped around the client's pelvis and the treatment table to help stabilize the pelvis. The clinician's stabilizing hand (right as shown) holds the client's thigh just proximal to the knee. The amount of internal or external rotation can be varied to find the position that most effectively stretches the hip.
Movement and Direction of Force	The clinician's assessing hand (left as shown) purchases the anterior surface of the proximal thigh (just distal to the groin). This hand contact should be broad and should glide the femur in a posterior to posterior inferior direction along the plane of the joint from a resting position of the hip initially.
Assessment	Assessment is done for joint play/passive accessory motion, client response, and end-feel. Reproduction of concordant pain suggests dysfunction. Impaired joint mobility or end-feel may also suggest dysfunction if concordant pain is also reproduced.

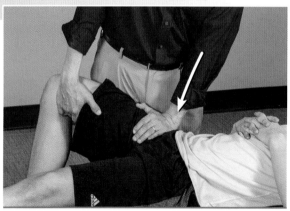

Figure 24.18

POSTERIOR GLIDE II

 Video 24.19 in the web resource shows a demonstration of this test.

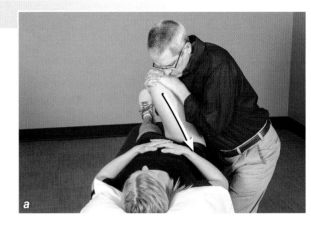

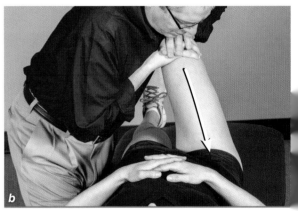

Figure 24.19

Client Position	Supine with bilateral legs relaxed
Clinician Position	Standing next to the client's hip to be assessed *(a)* or on opposite side of hip to be assessed *(b)*, directly facing the client
Stabilization	The client's body resting on the table serves as a stabilizing force.
Movement and Direction of Force	Both of the clinician's hands purchase the client's knee, with the hip in combined flexion and slight adduction (approximating the joint restricted position as tolerated). The clinician uses both hands and their body to provide a force longitudinally through the femur and directed in a posterior and lateral direction. Utilizing the technique standing on the side opposite of leg to be assessed *(b)*, the clinician can also grab the edge of the table on the opposite side pelvis (same side of leg to be assessed) with the most cranial hand (right as shown) for additional stabilization and force generation in cases of very stiff hips.
Assessment	Assessment is done for joint play/passive accessory motion, client response, and end-feel. Reproduction of concordant pain suggests dysfunction. Impaired joint mobility or end-feel may also suggest dysfunction if concordant pain is also reproduced.

Critical Clinical Pearls

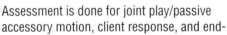

When performing joint-play assessment, the clinician should keep the following in mind:

- The hip joint is a very large joint that likely will require more force to assess joint play than most other extremity joints.
- As always when assessing joint play in any joint, the clinician should take up the soft tissue slack and glide the joint in the direction required, assessing for joint mobility, end-feel, and client response.
- The clinician is referred to table 24.2 for resting position, close-packed position, and end-feel of the hip joint.

Flexibility

As detailed in chapter 7, flexibility is the motion that a particular joint is capable of. Assessment of flexibility can assist the clinician in determining the potential presence of soft-tissue dysfunction of various soft tissues listed in table 24.3.

- Thomas Test: see Special Tests section.
- Ober's Test: see Special Tests section.

TABLE 24.3 Hip Muscles

Muscle	Origin	Insertion	Action	Innervation
HIP FLEXORS				
Iliacus (primary)	Iliac fossa	Lesser trochanter (with psoas major) of femur	Flexion of thigh, slight adduction of the thigh of free limb	Femoral nerve L1-L4
Psoas (primary)	Bodies and transverse processes of lumbar vertebrae	Lesser trochanter of femur	Flexion of thigh, slight adduction of the thigh of free limb	L1-L4
Rectus femoris	Anterior inferior iliac spine, ilium, and above the acetabulum	Patella and through patellar ligament to tibial tuberosity	Extension of leg, flexion of thigh	Femoral nerve L1-L4
Tensor fasciae latae	Iliac crest posterior to anterior superior iliac spine (ASIS)	Iliotibial tract	Flexion, medial rotation, and abduction of thigh	Superior gluteal nerve L4-S1
Sartorius	ASIS	Medial surface, proximal end of tibia just distal to tibial tuberosity	Flexion, abduction, and lateral rotation of thigh; flexion of leg	Femoral nerve
Pectineus	Superior ramus of pubis	Femur just distal to lesser trochanter	Flexion and adduction of thigh	Femoral nerve, possibly obturator or accessory obturator nerve or both
Adductor brevis	Body and inferior ramus of pubis	Pectineal line, proximal part of linea aspera of femur	Adduction and flexion of thigh	Obturator nerve
Adductor longus	Pubic tubercle	Medial lip of linea aspera of femur	Adduction and flexion of thigh	Obturator nerve
Adductor magnus (superior fibers)	Inferior ramus of pubis, ramus of ischium, ischial tuberosity	Linea aspera (anterior fibers), adductor tubercle of femur (posterior fibers)	Adduction, flexion (anterior fibers), and extension (posterior fibers) of thigh	Obturator nerve (anterior fibers), sciatic nerve (posterior fibers)
Gluteus medius (anterior)	Lateral surface of ilium between anterior and posterior gluteal line	Greater trochanter	Abduction, medial rotation and flexion (anterior fibers), and lateral rotation and extension (posterior fibers) of thigh	Superior gluteal nerves L5-S1
Piriformis	Sacrum (pelvic surface)	Greater trochanter of femur	Lateral rotation of thigh of extended hip, abduction of thigh when thigh is flexed	Ventral rami S1 and S2
HIP ADDUCTOR MUSCLES				
Pectineus	Superior ramus of pubis	Femur just distal to lesser trochanter	Flexion and adduction of thigh	Femoral nerve L2-L3

(continued)

Table 24.3 *(continued)*

Muscle	Origin	Insertion	Action	Innervation
HIP ADDUCTOR MUSCLES				
Adductor longus	Pubic tubercle	Medial lip of linea aspera of femur	Adduction and flexion of thigh	Obturator nerve L2-4
Gracilis	Inferior ramus of pubis, ramus of ischium	Medial surface, proximal end of tibia just distal to medial condyle	Adduction of thigh, flexion of leg, medial rotation of flexed leg	Obturator nerve L3-L4
Adductor brevis	Body and inferior ramus of pubis	Pectineal line, proximal part of linea aspera of femur	Adduction and flexion of thigh	Obturator nerve L2-4
Adductor magnus	Inferior ramus of pubis, ramus of ischium, ischial tuberosity	Linea aspera (anterior fibers), adductor tubercle of femur (posterior fibers)	Adduction, flexion (anterior fibers), and extension (posterior fibers) of thigh	Obturator nerve (anterior fibers), sciatic nerve (posterior fibers) L2-4
HAMSTRING MUSCLES				
Semitendinosus	Ischial tuberosity	Medial surface of proximal end of tibia	Extension of thigh, flexion of leg, medial rotation of flexed leg	Sciatic nerve: tibial branch L4-S2
Semimembranosus	Ischial tuberosity	Medial condyle of tibia	Extension of thigh, flexion of leg, medial rotation of flexed leg	Sciatic nerve: tibial branch L4-S2
Biceps femoris	Long head: ischial tuberosity Short head: linea aspera of femur and lateral intermuscular septum	Lateral head of fibula and lateral tibial condyle	Extension of thigh (long head), flexion of leg, lateral rotation of flexed leg	Sciatic nerve: tibial branch to long head (L5-S3), common fibular branch to short head (L5-S2)

PSOAS ASSESSMENT I[133]

Client Position	Prone with upper trunk relaxed
Clinician Position	Standing directly to the side of the leg to be assessed
Movement	The clinician lifts the client's leg with the knee flexed while preventing pelvic motion at the ischial tuberosity until engaging the barrier.
Assessment	Normally the knee can be lifted 6 in. (15 cm) off the table. If this distance is less than 6 in., tightness and shortness of the psoas are present. Shortness and tightness are present if the ROM is asymmetric.
Statistics	NR

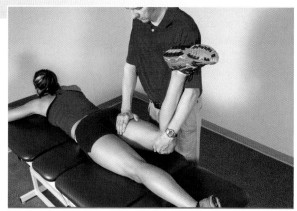

Figure 24.20

PSOAS ASSESSMENT II[133]

Client Position	Supine at the end of the table
Clinician Position	Standing or kneeling at the side of the leg to be assessed
Movement	The client holds the non-test leg in a flexed position while the clinician passively lowers the leg to be tested into end-range hip extension. The stationary arm of the goniometer is lined up parallel with the trunk; the axis is at the middle of the hip joint and the moving arm runs parallel to the thigh, using the lateral epicondyle of the knee as a reference point.

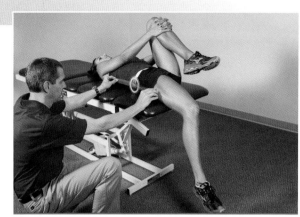

Figure 24.21

Assessment	If the back of the thigh does not contact the table, psoas shortness is present.[133] If a hip flexion angle of at least 7° below horizontal is not achieved, the iliopsoas is considered tight.[134]
Statistics	NR; see Special Tests section for diagnostic accuracy of this test for hip labral tear pathology.

RECTUS FEMORIS ASSESSMENT[133, 135]

Client Position	Supine with buttocks on the end of the table
Clinician Position	Standing or kneeling at the side of the leg to be assessed
Movement	The client holds the non-test leg in a flexed position while the clinician passively lowers the leg to be tested into end-range hip extension. The stationary arm of the goniometer is parallel to the thigh and femur and lined up with the middle of the hip joint. The clinician aligns the axis at mid-knee and the moving arm at the lateral malleolus of the ankle as it runs parallel to the mid-tibia.

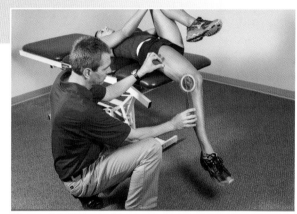

Figure 24.22

Assessment	The following are guidelines to use in order to determine which specific structure is at fault:

- Less than 10° to 15° of hip extension indicates a tight iliopsoas. Simultaneous extension of the knee during this maneuver indicates tightness of the rectus femoris.[133]
- Knee flexion: If less than 100° to 105° is available, the rectus femoris is tight.[133]
- With low back and sacrum flat on the table, the posterior thigh touches the table and the knee flexes approximately 80°.[135]
- Shortness in the tensor fasciae latae is indicated by abduction of the thigh as the hip extends, by extension of the knee if the thigh is prevented from abducting or is passively adducted as the hip is extended, or by internal rotation of the thigh.[135]

Statistics	NR

HIP ADDUCTOR ASSESSMENT (LONG VERSUS SHORT)[133]

Client Position	Supine with the leg to be tested close to the edge of the table
Clinician Position	Standing directly next to the leg to be assessed
Movement	The client's non-test leg is fully flexed at the hip.
Assessment	Maintaining the leg to be assessed in full extension, the clinician passively abducts it (normal range is 40°). When the full ROM is reached, the clinician passively flexes the knee of the test leg and attempts to abduct the leg further.

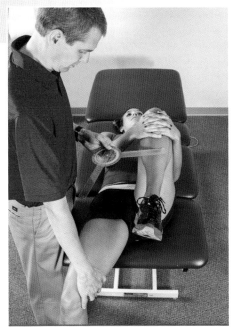

Goniometric measurement is as with standard hip abduction technique.

- Hip abduction: If less than 15° to 20° is available, the short hip adductors are tight.
- If the maximum hip abduction range does not increase when the knee is flexed, the single joint adductors (pectineus, adductor magnus, adductor longus, and adductor brevis) are shortened.

Figure 24.23

- If the hip abduction range does increase with the knee passively flexed, the double joint adductors (gracilis, semimembranosus, and semitendinosus) are shortened.

Statistics NR

HAMSTRING LENGTH: PASSIVE SUPINE 90/90 POSITION ASSESSMENT[136]

Client Position	Supine, with hip flexed to 90°
Clinician Position	Standing next to the leg to be assessed, directly facing the client
Movement	The clinician places the contralateral lower extremity on the support surface with knee fully extended. They extend the client's knee through full available ROM passively until firm muscular resistance is felt, while maintaining the hip in 90° of flexion. The clinician aligns the goniometer *(a)* with the stationary arm along the femur or the inclinometer *(b)* along the mid-shin, with the greater trochanter of the femur as the reference point. The axis of movement is the lateral epicondyle at the knee, and the moving arm is aligned with the lateral malleolus.
Assessment	The clinician should use the angle measured as the score. Youdas and colleagues[137] have assessed hamstring muscle length in both males and females, and have determined normative data for those in the age range of 20 to 80 years.

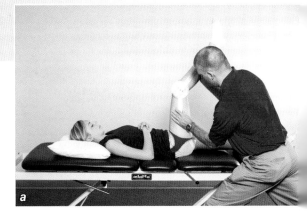

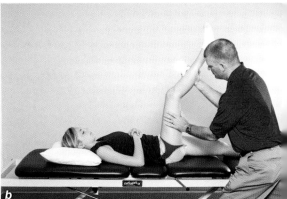

Figure 24.24

Results indicate that males have a popliteal angle ranging from 138.1° to 142.8°, with an average of 141.4°. Women of the same age have popliteal angles that range from 148.7° to 154.8°, with an average of 152.0°. These data seem to indicate that women have greater hamstring length at all ages than their male counterparts.

Statistics NR

MUSCLE PERFORMANCE TESTING

Manual muscle testing (MMT) of the hip can implicate soft-tissue dysfunction, muscle weakness, and so on, but it is also a good reminder that many clients with other pathology may also have weaknesses demonstrated with MMT. Hip MMT in subjects with and without OA has shown moderate to excellent reliability.[128]

HIP FLEXION

Client Position	Seated with bilateral knees flexed over the edge of the table
Clinician Position	Standing directly to the side of the client
Movement and Assessment	The clinician stabilizes the client's pelvis with their proximal hand and provides resistance on the anterior aspect of the distal femur

- Grade 5: completes motion against maximum resistance
- Grade 4: completes motion against strong resistance
- Grade 3: completes motion without resistance
- Grade 2: completes motion in side-lying position without resistance
- Grade 1: muscle activity without movement
- Grade 0: no muscle activity

Primary Muscles	Psoas major
	Iliacus
Secondary Muscles	Rectus femoris
	Sartorius
	Tensor fasciae latae
	Pectineus
	Adductor longus, brevis, and magnus
	Anterior gluteus medius
Primary Nerves	L2-4 (psoas)
	Femoral nerve (L2-3; iliacus)

HIP EXTENSION

Client Position	Prone with the leg to be assessed lying straight on the table
Clinician Position	Standing directly to the side of the client
Movement and Assessment	The clinician's proximal hand stabilizes the pelvis, while their distal hand provides resistance on the posterior aspect of the distal femur, with lower extremity either straight or with knee bent (to isolate gluteus maximus).

- Grade 5: completes motion against maximum resistance
- Grade 4: completes motion against strong resistance
- Grade 3: completes motion without resistance
- Grade 2: completes motion in side-lying position without resistance
- Grade 1: muscle activity without movement
- Grade 0: no muscle activity

Primary Muscles	Gluteus maximus
	Hamstring group

- Semitendinosus
- Semimembranosus
- Biceps femoris

Secondary Muscles	Adductor magnus
	Posterior gluteus medius
Primary Nerves	Inferior gluteal nerve (L5-S2; gluteus maximus)
	Tibial portion of sciatic nerve (L5-S2; hamstrings)

HIP INTERNAL ROTATION

Client Position	Sitting with lower extremity to be assessed at 90° of hip and knee flexion, legs off the end of the table
Clinician Position	Standing directly in front of the client
Movement and Assessment	The clinician's proximal hand stabilizes the femur, and their distal hand provides resistance on the lateral aspect of the distal lower extremity (just above the lateral malleolus), trying to externally rotate the client's lower extremity.

- Grade 5: completes motion against maximum resistance
- Grade 4: completes motion against strong resistance
- Grade 3: completes motion without resistance
- Grade 2: completes motion in supine with legs extended position without resistance
- Grade 1: muscle activity without movement
- Grade 0: no muscle activity

Primary Muscles	Anterior gluteus minimus
	Anterior gluteus medius
	Tensor fasciae latae
Secondary Muscles	Semitendinosus
	Semimembranosus
Primary Nerve	Superior gluteal nerve (L4-S1)

HIP EXTERNAL ROTATION

Client Position	Supine with lower extremity to be assessed in 90° of hip and knee flexion
Clinician Position	Standing directly to the side of the client
Movement and Assessment	The clinician's proximal hand stabilizes the femur, and their distal hand provides resistance on the medial aspect of the distal lower extremity (just above the medial malleolus), trying to internally rotate the client's lower extremity.

- Grade 5: completes motion against maximum resistance
- Grade 4: completes motion against strong resistance
- Grade 3: completes motion without resistance
- Grade 2: completes motion in supine with legs extended position without resistance
- Grade 1: muscle activity without movement
- Grade 0: no muscle activity

Primary Muscles	Gluteus maximus
	Superior and inferior gemellus
	Obturator internus and externus
	Quadratus femoris
	Piriformis
Secondary Muscles	Sartorius
	Biceps femoris
	Posterior gluteus medius
	Psoas major
	Adductor longus
Primary Nerves	Inferior gluteal nerve (L4-S1; gluteus maximus)
	Nerve to quadratus femoris (L5-S1; quadratus femoris and inferior gemellus)
	Nerve to obturator internus (L5-S1; obturator internus and superior gemellus)
	Nerve to piriformis (S1-2; piriformis)
	Obturator nerve (L3-4; obturator externus)

HIP ABDUCTION

Client Position	Side lying with the lower extremity to be assessed on top of the non-testing lower extremity
Clinician Position	Standing directly behind the client
Movement and Assessment	The clinician's proximal hand stabilizes the pelvis and their distal hand provides resistance over the lateral femoral condyle.

- Grade 5: completes motion against maximum resistance
- Grade 4: completes motion against strong resistance
- Grade 3: completes motion without resistance
- Grade 2: completes motion in supine with legs extended position without resistance. The clinician can hold the leg at the heel just off table to avoid friction with the table.
- Grade 1: muscle activity without movement
- Grade 0: no muscle activity

(continued)

Hip Abduction *(continued)*

Primary Muscles	Gluteus medius
	Gluteus minimus
Secondary Muscles	Cranial fibers of gluteus maximus
	Tensor fasciae latae
	Sartorius
Primary Nerve	Superior gluteal nerve (L4-S1)

HIP ADDUCTION

Client Position	Side lying with the lower extremity to be assessed below the non-testing lower extremity
Clinician Position	Standing directly behind the client
Movement and Assessment	The clinician's proximal hand holds the non-testing lower extremity while their distal hand provides resistance over the medial femoral condyle.

- Grade 5: completes motion against maximum resistance
- Grade 4: completes motion against strong resistance
- Grade 3: completes motion without resistance
- Grade 2: completes motion in supine with the legs extended without resistance. The clinician can hold the leg at the heel just off the table to avoid friction.
- Grade 1: muscle activity without movement
- Grade 0: no muscle activity

Primary Muscles	Adductor magnus
	Adductor longus
	Adductor brevis
	Gracilis
	Pectineus
Secondary Muscles	Obturator externus
	Caudal fibers of gluteus maximus
Primary Nerves	Obturator nerve (L2-4)
	Femoral nerve (L2-3; pectineus)

SPECIAL TESTS

As mentioned in chapter 10 (Special Tests), in many cases the clinician is overly dependent on the performance and interpretation of special test findings with respect to differential diagnosis of the client's presenting pain. Utilization of special tests for ruling in (or helping to diagnose) a particular pathology should occur at this point in the examination process. It is also hoped that the clinician has a much clearer picture of the client's presentation prior to this point in the examination and will therefore depend minimally on special test findings with respect to diagnosis of the client's pain.

When examining the hip joint, the clinician should rule out the potential contribution of the client's pain coming from related structures, most notably the lumbar spine and SIJ or pelvic girdle. Refer to the section on triage and screening for this. Specific testing for ruling in the hip joint's various pathologies is listed in the following section with test descriptions. The clinician is cautioned regarding study findings suggesting limitations in the clinical applicability of many hip special tests.[109, 138, 139] Remember that special tests are a very small component of the overall examination. Reliance of findings on special testing alone is inadequate clinical practice.

Index of Special Tests

Alignment

Test for True Leg Length
Apparent Leg Length Discrepancy

Craig's Test

Muscle Dysfunction

Gluteal Tendinopathy
Trendelenburg's Sign
Resisted External Derotation Test

Resisted Hip Abduction Test
FABER Test

Piriformis Syndrome
Piriformis Syndrome (FAIR Test)

Sport-Related Chronic Groin Pain
Single Adductor Test
Squeeze Test

Bilateral Adductor Test

Hamstring Injury
Puranen-Orava Test
Bent Knee Stretch Test

Modified Bent Knee Stretch Test
Taking Off the Shoe Test

Muscle Length Testing

Thomas Test

Ober's Test: Iliotibial Band

Ligamentous Laxity

Dial Test
Log Roll Test

Long-Axis Femoral Distraction Test
Abduction-Extension-External Rotation Test

Intra-Articular Pathology

Flexion-Adduction Test (detecting pathologic changes)
Hip Scour Test

FABER Test (Patrick's Test, Figure-Four Test)
Ligamentum Teres Test (detection of torn ligamentum teres)

Hip Osteoarthritis

Trendelenburg's Sign
FABER Test

Resisted Hip Abduction

Impingement or Labral Tear

Femoral Acetabular Impingement Test (Flexion-Adduction-IR Test, FADDIR Test)
Flexion-IR Test

Flexion-Adduction-Axial Compression Test
Internal Rotation-Flexion-Axial Compression Test

Hip Dysplasia

Passive Hip Abduction Test

Case Studies

Go to www.HumanKinetics.com/OrthopedicClinicalExamination and complete these case studies for chapter 24:

- Case study 1 discusses a 27-year-old female with left buttock pain into the posterior thigh and lateral hip that is worse with walking, standing, ambulating stairs, sitting, and standing from a chair.
- Case study 2 discusses a 24-year-old female with right hip and groin pain that is worse with running, yoga, and low squatting and sitting.

Abstract Links

Go to www.HumanKinetics.com/OrthopedicClinicalExamination to access abstract links on these issues:

Craig's test

FABER's test

Femoral acetabular impingement test

Flexion-adduction-internal rotation test (FADDIR)

Flexion-IR test

Hip scour test

Internal rotation-flexion-axial compression test

Ligamentum teres test

Log roll test

Ober's test

Passive hip abduction test

Patellar-pubic percussion test

Piriformis syndrome (FAIR test)

Puranen-Orava test

Repeated motions, centralization and peripheralization

Resisted straight leg raise test

Seated extension-rotation

Sensitive tests for the hip

Single adductor test

Slump test

Straight leg raise test

Stress fracture test (fulcrum test)

Taking off the shoe test

Test for true leg length

Thomas test

Trendelenburg's sign

ALIGNMENT

TEST FOR TRUE LEG LENGTH

Client Position	Supine with bilateral legs extended and arms relaxed. Both legs should be in the same degree of abduction or adduction and internal or external rotation for reliability. The client should also be lying straight on the table.
Clinician Position	Standing at the side of the leg to be measured
Movement	Measurement is taken from the ASIS to the distal medial malleolus on the same side.

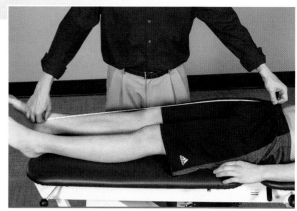

Figure 24.25

Assessment The clinician performs a comparison from side to side. True leg length discrepancy is further assessed in supine with bilateral knees flexed and feet flat on table. In this position, the clinician should observe whether the knees are at the same height. If the knee extends farther (cranial to caudal) on the long side, then shortening is suggested to be due to a difference in femoral length. If the knee is lower (vertically) on the short side, then the difference in leg length is suggested to be due to a shortened tibia.

Statistics Reliability has been shown to be good to excellent across different studies and statistical analysis,[140-142] although correlation to pathology is tenuous at best.[143-146]

Note A difference of 1 to 1.5 cm is considered normal, but can still be a cause of symptoms.

APPARENT LEG LENGTH DISCREPANCY

Client Position Supine with bilateral legs extended and arms relaxed. Both legs should be in the same degree of abduction or adduction and internal or external rotation for reliability. The client should also be lying straight on the table.

Clinician Position Standing at the side of the leg to be measured

Movement The clinician takes a measurement from the umbilicus to the medial malleolus on both sides.

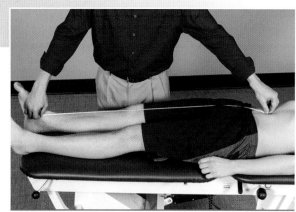

Figure 24.26

Assessment A difference in measurement signifies a difference of apparent leg length.

Statistics NR

Note This test is performed after true leg length discrepancy is ruled out.

CRAIG'S TEST

Client Position Prone with the knee flexed to 90°

Clinician Position Standing or sitting on the side of the hip to be assessed

Movement The clinician palpates the posterior aspect of the greater trochanter of the femur. The hip is then passively rotated internally and externally until the greater trochanter is parallel with the examining table or it reaches its most lateral position. The angle is measured with a goniometer.

Assessment The degree of antetorsion can be assessed by measuring the angle of internal/external rotation at the femur with the stationary arm parallel to the table (horizontally) and the moving arm of the goniometer along the tibia through the midpoint of the anterior ankle. The normal range of anterior torsion is 10° to 15° of external rotation. Antetorsion is any angle greater than the normal range and retrotorsion is any angle below this normal range.

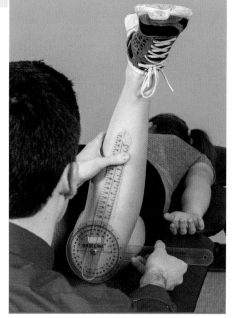

Figure 24.27

(continued)

Craig's Test *(continued)*

Statistics   Reliability: $ICC_{(2,1)}$ = 0.45 (0.10; 0.70)[147]

This measure also correlated with MRI only moderately. It had wide confidence intervals (CIs), and its clinical utility is questioned.[148]

MUSCLE DYSFUNCTION: GLUTEAL TENDINOPATHY OR GREATER TROCHANTERIC PAIN SYNDROME (GTPS)

TRENDELENBURG'S SIGN

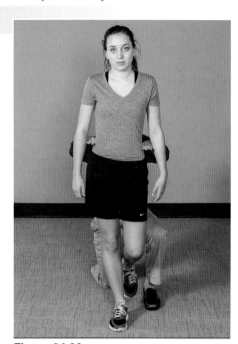

Figure 24.28

Client Position	Standing on both lower extremities
Clinician Position	Standing directly behind the client to observe posture
Movement	The client is asked to stand on one lower limb (right as shown). The clinician monitors for dropping of pelvis.
Assessment	A positive test is indicated if the pelvis on the opposite side (nonstance side) drops (left pelvis dropping as shown) when the client stands on the affected leg.

Statistics

- Pooled analysis: SN 61 (46-75), **SP 92 (83-97)**,**+LR 6.83**, –LR 0.25, across three studies with 78 subjects[109]

- SN 73 (NR), SP 77 (NR), +LR 3.2, –LR 0.4, QUADAS 10, in a study of 24 clients with clinical features consistent with GTPS (age range 36-75 years; 24 women; mean duration of symptoms NR), and MRI as a reference standard[149]

- SN 24 (5-57), **SP 94 (53-100)**, **+LR 3.6**, –LR 0.82, QUADAS 12, in a study of 40 clients with unilateral hip pain (mean age 54.4 ± 9.5 years; 37 were female; symptom duration variable: less than 1 year to greater than 5 years), and MRI as a reference standard[150]

- **SN 97 (NR), SP 96 (NR), +LR 24.3, –LR 0.03**, QUADAS 10, in a study of 17 clients with refractory GTPS (mean age 68.1 ± 10.8 years; 16 were female; mean duration of symptoms 13 ± 10.5 months), and MRI or surgery as a reference standard[151]

- SN 55 (NR), SP 70 (NR), +LR 1.83, –LR 0.82, QUADAS 10, in a study of 20 healthy adults and 20 adults with radiographically documented hip OA (mean age 50.4 to 53.4 years; 10 females in each group; mean symptom duration NR), and radiography as a reference standard[88]

RESISTED EXTERNAL DEROTATION TEST

Client Position	Supine, hip flexed 90° and in external rotation
Clinician Position	Standing just to the side of the client's leg being tested, slightly decreases external rotation just enough to relieve pain (if any was present)
Movement	The client actively returns the leg to neutral position (placing the leg along the axis of the bed) against resistance. If the test result is (–), the test is repeated with the client lying prone, with the hip extended, the knee flexed to 90°.

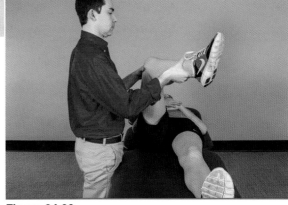

Figure 24.29

Assessment	A (+) test is spontaneous reproduction of client's concordant pain.
Statistics	**SN 88 (NR)**, **SP 97 (NR)**, **+LR 32.6**, **–LR 0.12,** QUADAS 10, in a study of 17 clients with refractory GTPS (mean age 68.1 ± 10.8 years; 16 were female; mean duration of symptoms NR), and a reference standard of MRI[151]

RESISTED HIP ABDUCTION TEST

See description under hip osteoarthritis.

FABER TEST

See description under intra-articular pathology.

MUSCLE DYSFUNCTION: PIRIFORMIS SYNDROME

PIRIFORMIS SYNDROME (FAIR TEST)

Client Position	Side lying on contralateral side with the hip and knee slightly bent for stability. Trunk is in normal postural alignment.
Clinician Position	Standing directly behind the client at the level of the hips
Movement	The clinician grasps the client's shin and brings the leg to be tested into a position of flexion, adduction, and internal rotation (FAIR). Fishman and colleagues (2002) later described the addition of simultaneous downward pressure at the flexed knee and passive superolateral movement of the shin.[152]

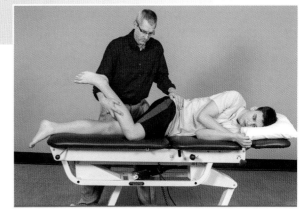

Figure 24.30

Assessment	A (+) test is reproduction of client's concordant pain.
Statistics	SN 88 (NR), SP 83 (NR), +LR 5.2, –LR 0.14, QUADAS 8, in a sample of 918 consecutive clients (1,014 legs) with follow-up on 733 legs (mean age, gender, and symptom duration NR), and a reference standard of H reflex testing[152, 153]

MUSCLE DYSFUNCTION: SPORT-RELATED CHRONIC GROIN PAIN

SINGLE ADDUCTOR TEST

Client Position	Supine with bilateral legs extended
Clinician Position	Standing at client's foot to be assessed
Movement	The clinician passively flexes the leg to be assessed to 30°. The client resists the clinician's attempt to abduct the leg to be tested, effectively contracting their adductor muscles on that side.
Assessment	A (+) test is reproduction of client's concordant pain.
Statistics	SN 30 (NR), SP 91 (NR), +LR 3.3, –LR 0.66, QUADAS 7, in a study of 89 Australian rules football players with chronic groin pain (mean age and symptom duration NR; all were male), and a reference standard of MRI[27]

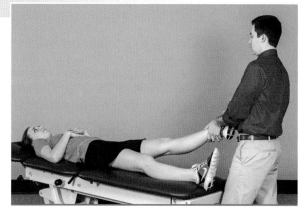

Figure 24.31

SQUEEZE TEST

Client Position	Supine with bilateral hips flexed 45° and knees flexed 90° so that bilateral feet are flat on table
Clinician Position	Standing at the client's bilateral knees, placing a fist between knees
Movement	The client is asked to maximally contract both adductor muscles simultaneously to squeeze the fist effectively.
Assessment	A (+) test is reproduction of client's concordant pain.
Statistics	SN 43 (NR), SP 91 (NR), +LR 4.8, –LR 0.63, QUADAS 7, in a study of 89 Australian Rules football players with chronic groin pain (mean age and symptom duration NR; all were male), and a reference standard of MRI[27]

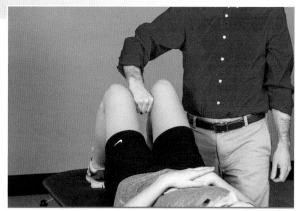

Figure 24.32

BILATERAL ADDUCTOR TEST

Client Position	Supine with bilateral legs extended
Clinician Position	Standing at the client's bilateral feet, directly facing the client
Movement	The clinician passively flexes the client's leg to be assessed to 30°. The client is asked to maximally contract both adductor muscles simultaneously, thereby attempting to bring bilateral legs together.

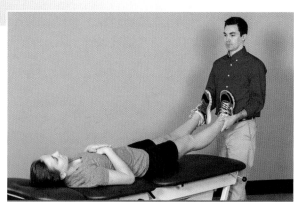

Figure 24.33

Assessment A (+) test is reproduction of client's concordant pain.
Statistics SN 54 (NR), SP 93 (NR), +LR 7.7, –LR 0.49, QUADAS 7, in a study of 89 Australian rules football players with chronic groin pain (mean age and symptom duration NR; all were male), and a reference standard of MRI[27]

MUSCLE DYSFUNCTION: HAMSTRING INJURY

PURANEN-ORAVA TEST

Client Position Standing
Clinician Position Standing at the client's side to be assessed
Movement The client actively stretches the hamstring muscles in the standing position with the hip flexed at about 90°, the knee fully extended, and the foot on a solid support surface.
Assessment A (+) test is reproduction of client's concordant pain.
Statistics SN 76 (61-87), SP 82 (68-92), +LR 4.2, –LR 0.29, QUADAS 8, in a study of 46 symptomatic and 46 asymptomatic athletes with a 15-month average duration of symptoms (mean age 22.8 ± 2.3 years; 12 were females; mean duration of symptoms 15.0 ± 7.2 months), and a reference standard of MRI[154]

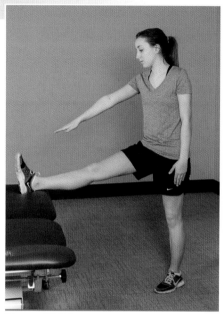

Figure 24.34

BENT KNEE STRETCH TEST

Client Position Supine with legs relaxed
Clinician Position Standing at the client's side to be assessed, directly facing the client
Movement The clinician grasps the symptomatic leg behind the heel with one hand (left as shown) and at the knee with the other hand (right as shown). The clinician maximally flexes the hip and knee, and then *slowly* straightens the knee.
Assessment A (+) test is reproduction of client's concordant pain.

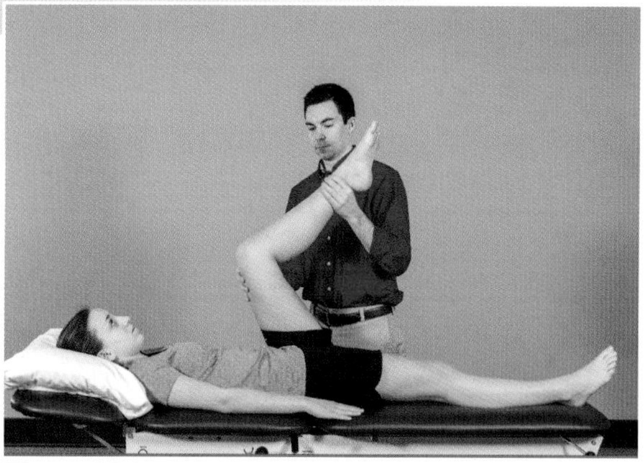

Figure 24.35

Statistics SN 84 (71-93), SP 87 (73-95), +LR 6.5, –LR 0.18, QUADAS 8, in a study of 46 symptomatic and 46 asymptomatic athletes with a 15-month average duration of symptoms (mean age 22.8 ± 2.3 years; 12 were females; mean duration of symptoms 15.0 ± 7.2 months), and a reference standard of MRI[154]

MODIFIED BENT KNEE STRETCH TEST

Client Position	Supine with legs relaxed
Clinician Position	Standing at client's side to be assessed, directly facing the client
Movement	The clinician grasps the symptomatic leg behind the heel with one hand and at the knee with the other hand. The clinician maximally flexes the hip and knee, and then *rapidly* straightens the knee. This test is similar to prior test, except the movement is *rapid*.
Assessment	A (+) test is reproduction of client's concordant pain.
Statistics	SN 89 (76-96), SP 91 (79-97), +LR 9.9, –LR 0.12, QUADAS 8, in a study of 46 symptomatic and 46 asymptomatic athletes with a 15-month average duration of symptoms (mean age 22.8 ± 2.3 years; 12 were females; mean duration of symptoms 15.0 ± 7.2 months), and a reference standard of MRI[154]

TAKING OFF THE SHOE TEST

Client Position	Standing
Clinician Position	Standing at client's side to be assessed
Movement	The client is asked to take their affected side shoe off with the help of their other shoe. The affected leg during this maneuver has approximately 90° of external rotation at the hip and 20° to 25° of flexion at the knee.
Assessment	A (+) test is reproduction of client's concordant pain.
Statistics	SN 100 (97-100), SP 100 (97-100), +LR 280, –LR 0.0, QUADAS 6, in a study of 140 symptomatic professional soccer players (age range 17-33 years; all were male; duration of symptoms was between 0 and 42 days from injury), and a reference standard of US[155]

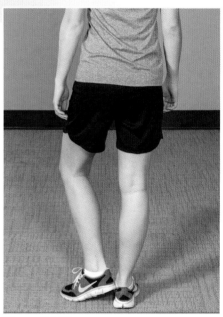

Figure 24.36

MUSCLE LENGTH TESTING

THOMAS TEST

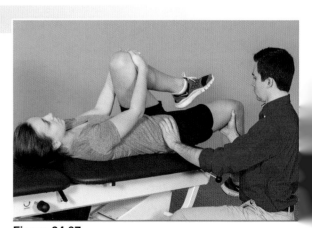

Figure 24.37

Client Position	Supine at end of table, holding the leg not being tested (left as shown) in a flexed position
Clinician Position	Standing or kneeling to the side of the leg to be assessed
Movement	The clinician passively extends the leg being tested (right as shown).
Assessment	The back of the thigh should contact the table. If not, psoas shortness is present. The goniometer's stationary arm is lined up parallel with trunk, the axis with the mid-hip joint, and the moving arm runs parallel with thigh, using a reference point of lateral epicondyle of knee. For a labral tear, a (+) test is reproduction of painful clicking during testing.

Statistics
(for labral tear
pathology only)

SN 89 (NR), SP 92 (NR), +LR 11.1, −LR 0.12, QUADAS 10, in a study of 59 clients with refractory hip pain (35 clients with labral tear; mean age 37 years; 32 were female; mean duration of symptoms NR), and arthroscopy as a reference standard[14]

Note

The clinician can use the proximal hand to monitor lumbar spine position. The lumbar spine should maintain contact with table. The client can compensate with increased lumbar lordosis or anterior pelvic tilt.

- To determine which specific structures are at fault: If less than 0° of hip extension is achieved, this indicates a tight iliopsoas. Simultaneous extension of the knee during this maneuver indicates tightness of the rectus femoris.
- Lumbar extension can alter position of pelvis.[156]
- Modified approach of having the client perform a volitional posterior pelvic tilt during test to ensure lumbar stability is advocated.[134]

OBER'S TEST: ILIOTIBIAL BAND

Client Position

Side lying with the side to be tested on top. The bottom leg should be bent to allow for a more stable base to prevent trunk and total body rotation. Alignment should be in the frontal plane throughout the body, not allowing for rotation or hip flexion compensation.

Clinician Position

Standing directly behind the client. Their cranial hand (right as shown) stabilizes the pelvis to prevent tilting in frontal plane or rotation. Their caudal hand (left as shown) grasps under the knee.

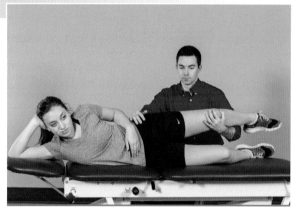

Figure 24.38

Movement

The clinician maintains the client in frontal plane alignment, not allowing the client to rotate at the trunk. They stabilize the ipsilateral hip and hold the client's leg just under the knee. The client's knee should be flexed approximately 20° and the hip slightly externally rotated. The clinician should extend the client's leg and gradually lower it while maintaining hip stabilization.

Assessment

The clinician can measure the distance from the medial epicondyle of the knee to the table for objective measurement. Comparison is made from side to side. Kendall interprets normal measurement as when the thigh drops to 10° below the horizontal. Anything above this level is indicative of IT band tightness.

Statistics

- Restricted and painful finding: SN 41 (26-58), SP 95 (75-100), +LR 8.2, −LR 0.62, QUADAS 10, in a study of 84 clients including controls, those with osteoarthritis, and those with GTPS (67% of clients; 41 had GTPS; mean age 53.8 years; 38 were female; mean duration of symptoms 3-24+ months), and using GTPS definition, radiographs to rule out hip OA and subsequent US guided local anesthetic injection as a reference standard[157]
- Reliability
  - ICC (goniometer) = 0.82–0.92[158]
  - (inclinometer) = 0.94[159]
  - (inclinometer) = 0.91[160]

LIGAMENTOUS LAXITY

DIAL TEST

Client Position	Supine in relaxed position with bilateral lower extremities extended and arms relaxed
Clinician Position	Standing at side of leg to be tested, facing the client
Movement	With the hip in a neutral flexion–extension and abduction–adduction position, the clinician grasps the client's leg at the femur and tibia and passively rolls it into full IR. The leg is released and allowed to ER.

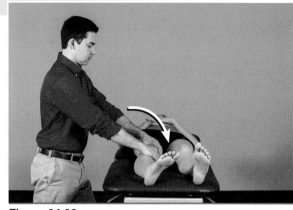

Figure 24.39

Assessment	The clinician should evaluate side-to-side ROM differences and clicking. A (−) dial test constitutes ER of the lower limb less than 45°, as measured vertically, with a firm endpoint. Clients with passive ER greater than 45° are considered to have a (+) dial test. This test is repeated for the contralateral leg, and comparisons are made as to the degree of rotation and bilateral endpoints. A relationship between the dial test and capsular laxity has been suggested.[21]
Statistics	NR
Note	The potential for muscle guarding and possible false-negative results must be recognized with this test.

LOG ROLL TEST

Client Position	Supine in relaxed position with bilateral legs relaxed
Clinician Position	Standing at side of leg to be tested, facing the client
Movement	With the hip in a neutral flexion–extension and abduction–adduction position, the client's lower extremity is passively rolled into full IR and ER (as shown).

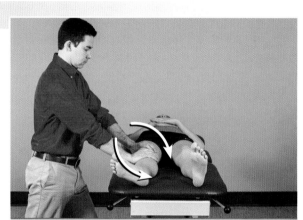

Figure 24.40

Assessment	The clinician should evaluate side-to-side ROM differences and clicking. A click reproduced during the test is suggestive of labral tear, while increased ER ROM may indicate iliofemoral ligament laxity.
Statistics	• Interrater reliability: ICC = 0.63;[161] (κ) = 0.61.[162] • The potential for muscle guarding and possible false-negative results must be recognized with this test.

LONG-AXIS FEMORAL DISTRACTION TEST

Client Position	Supine, bilateral legs extended with arms relaxed at the sides
Clinician Position	Standing at the foot of the table, directly facing the client
Movement	The clinician grasps the client's leg to be distracted just above the medial malleoli with the hip in 30° flexion, 30° abduction, and 10° to 15° ER. Distraction is provided by clinician leaning backward while holding the lower extremity.

Figure 24.41

Assessment	A client with capsular laxity may have increased motion and a feeling of apprehension with this maneuver. Comparatively, a client with hypomobility may have decreased motion and relief of pain.[161]
Statistics	• NR
	• The potential for muscle guarding and possible false-negative results must be recognized with this test.

ABDUCTION-EXTENSION-EXTERNAL ROTATION TEST

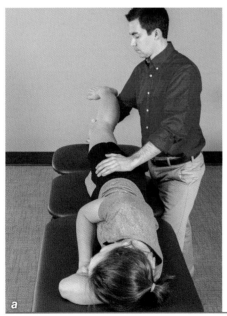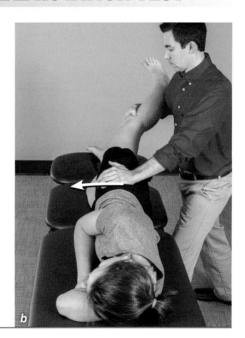

Figure 24.42

Client Position	Side lying with involved side on top, noninvolved lower extremity flexed at hip and knee for trunk stabilization
Clinician Position	Standing behind client at the level of the hips. The clinician grasps the client's leg to be tested under the knee with the caudal hand (right as shown). The cranial hand (left as shown) is placed just posterior to the greater trochanter.
Movement	The knee is kept straight, with the hip abducted at 30° and neutral rotation, and brought from 10° flexion *(a)* to terminal extension, externally rotating the straight leg while pushing forward on the greater trochanter *(b)* to reproduce any complaint of pain or discomfort.

(continued)

Abduction-Extension-External Rotation Test *(continued)*

Assessment   A (+) test is reproduction of concordant pain or increased laxity or ROM compared to the other side. A (+) test can be associated with microinstability, hyperlaxity, strain of the ilio-femoral ligament, or combined anterior antetorsion and acetabular anteversion summation.

Statistics   • NR

• This test is comparable to the apprehension test in the shoulder.

Critical Clinical Pearls

The clinician is reminded of the limitations in alignment and laxity joint testing:

• These tests have extremely limited investigation regarding their diagnostic accuracy.

• Discrepancies in leg length, for example, may or may not have clinical relevance, and findings should be interpreted with this in mind.

• Laxity, especially anterior capsular laxity, may be a result of alignment of the hip joint (e.g., femoral retrotorsion would increase hip ER ROM and limit hip IR ROM).

INTRA-ARTICULAR PATHOLOGY

FLEXION-ADDUCTION TEST (DETECTING PATHOLOGIC CHANGES)

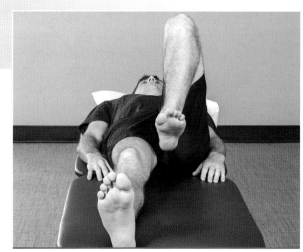

Figure 24.43

Client Position   Supine with bilateral legs extended, arms relaxed

Clinician Position   Standing at client's bilateral feet, directly facing the client

Movement   Hip is flexed to 90° and placed in neutral rotation. The hip is then allowed to adduct as far as possible.

Assessment   In the normal population, the knee should adduct to their opposite shoulder (right as shown). Pathologic changes allow adduction to only the other leg (right as shown) or less.

Statistics   NR

HIP SCOUR TEST

Video 24.44 in the web resource shows a demonstration of this test.

Client Position	Supine with arms relaxed, positioned close to the edge of the table
Clinician Position	Standing at the client's side to be assessed, directly facing the client
Movement	The clinician flexes and adducts *(a)* the hip until resistance to the movement is detected or the client's pelvis begins to lift on the table (assesses inner quadrant). The clinician then maintains flexion into resistance and moves the hip into abduction and external rotation *(b)* (outer quadrant), and then brings the hip through two full arcs of motion. If the client reports no pain, the clinician then repeats the test while applying long-axis compression through the femur.
Assessment	A (+) test is reproduction of clicking or catching with concordant pain.
Statistics	• SN 50 (26-74), SP 29 (12-51), +LR 0.70, –LR 1.72, QUADAS 7, in a study of 50 clients with variable hip pathologies (mean age 62 years; 30 were female; mean symptom duration NR), and intra-articular hip injection as a reference standard.[103]
	• The reliability of the Scour test is good (ICC of 0.87, 0.96, and 0.96) for rating of hip pain.[163]

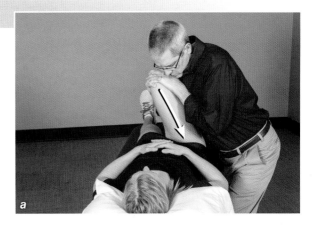

Figure 24.44

FABER TEST (PATRICK'S TEST, FIGURE-FOUR TEST)

Client Position	Supine with arms relaxed
Clinician Position	Standing at client's side, directly facing the client
Movement	The clinician places the client's heel of the leg to be tested (left as shown) over the opposite knee (right as shown). They passively externally rotate and abduct the hip joint by placing pressure over the ipsilateral knee, while stabilizing the contralateral innominate.
Assessment	The clinician should look for quantity and quality of motion, as well as for concordant pain (dependent on pathology) as a (+) test.
Statistics	• SN 81 (57-96), SP 25 (9-48), +LR 1.1, –LR 0.72, QUADAS 7, in a study of 50 clients with variable hip pathologies (mean age 60.2 years; 30 were female; mean duration of symptoms from 3-24+ months), and intra-articular hip injection as a reference standard[103]

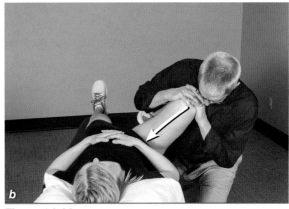

Figure 24.45

(continued)

FABER Test (Patrick's Test, Figure-Four Test) *(continued)*

- SN 60 (41-77), SP 18 (7-39), +LR 0.73, –LR 2.2, QUADAS 9, in a study of 105 clients with hip pain (mean age 42 ± 15 years; 24 were female; mean duration of symptoms 1.9 years), and MRA and intra-articular injection as a reference standard[4]
- SN 42 (NR), SP 75 (NR), +LR 1.7, –LR 0.8, QUADAS 9, in a study of 18 clients with previous periacetabular osteotomy (17 had labral tear; age range 32-56 years; 16 were female; mean duration of symptoms NR), and MRA as a reference standard[164]

Greater Trochanteric Pain Syndrome (GTPS)
SN 83 (68-93), SP 90 (68-99), +LR 8.3, –LR 0.19, QUADAS 10, in a study of 84 clients including controls, those with osteoarthritis, and those with GTPS (67% of clients; 41 had GTPS; mean age 53.8 years; 38 were female; mean duration of symptoms 3-24+ months), and using GTPS definition, radiographs to rule out hip OA, and subsequent US guided local anesthetic injection as a reference standard[157]

GTPS Versus Hip OA
- A (+) restricted and painful (lateral hip pain) FABER test is strongly associated with GTPS and not hip OA (**SN 81, SP 82, +LR 4.5, –LR 0.23**).[157]
- Reliability:
  - (κ) = 0.63 (interrater), % agreement = 84%[162]
  - ICC = 0.87 (interrater)[163]
  - ICC = 0.93 (intratester)[165]
  - ICC for motion assessment = 0.90; (κ) for end-feel = 0.47 (intertester)[166]
  - ICC = 0.66 and 0.74 (interrater)[167]
- The MDC for the FABER test for range of motion is 8° difference in motion, while the MDC for pain is a change of more than 1.6 points of the NPRS.[168]

LIGAMENTUM TERES TEST (DETECTION OF TORN LIGAMENTUM TERES)

 Video 24.46 in the web resource shows a demonstration of this test.

Client Position	Supine with leg relaxed to start
Clinician Position	Standing directly on the side of the client's leg to be assessed
Movement	The clinician passively flexes the hip fully, then extends it 30°, leaving the hip at about 70° flexion (knee is flexed 90°). The hip is then abducted fully and then adducted 30°, typically leaving it at about 30° abduction. The leg is then passively externally *(a)* and internally *(b)* rotated to available end-range.
Assessment	A (+) test is reproduction of concordant pain with either external or internal rotation.
Statistics	**SN 90 (81-96), SP 85 (75-92), +LR 6.5, –LR 0.11,** QUADAS 10, in a study of 75 consecutive clients (mean age 34.2 years; 29 females; mean duration of symptoms all over 3 months), and surgery as a reference standard[169]

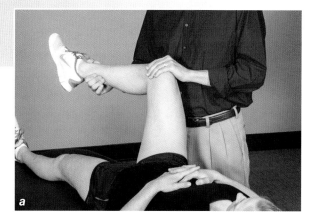

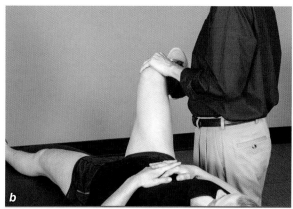

Figure 24.46

HIP OSTEOARTHRITIS

TRENDELENBURG'S SIGN

See the section on Muscle Dysfunction: Gluteal Tendinopathy or Greater Trochanteric Pain Syndrome (GTPS).

FABER TEST

See the section on Intra-Articular Pathology.

RESISTED HIP ABDUCTION

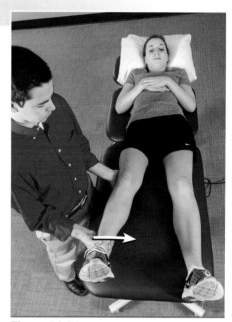

Client Position	Supine with leg relaxed to start
Clinician Position	Standing directly on the side of the client's leg to be assessed holding a handheld dynamometer (if available; not shown here)
Movement	The clinician applies a force to the leg with the handheld dynamometer, resisting hip abduction. A "make" manual muscle test is utilized when assessing for hip osteoarthritis.[88]
Assessment	Weakness is noted with a test using 30% client body-weight resistance criteria.
Statistics	• SN 35 (NR), SP 90 (NR), +LR 3.5, –LR 0.72, QUADAS 10, in a study of 20 healthy adults and 20 adults (mean age 50.4–53.4 years; 10 females in each group; mean duration of symptoms NR), and radiographically documented hip OA[88]
	• Gluteal tendinopathy or GTPS assessment (without dynamometer): SN 71 (51-87), **SP 84 (71-93)**, **+LR 5.5**, –LR 0.37, across two studies with 79 subjects[109]

Figure 24.47

IMPINGEMENT OR LABRAL TEAR

FEMORAL ACETABULAR IMPINGEMENT TEST (FLEXION-ADDUCTION-IR TEST, FADDIR TEST)

 Video 24.48 **in the web resource shows a demonstration of this test.**

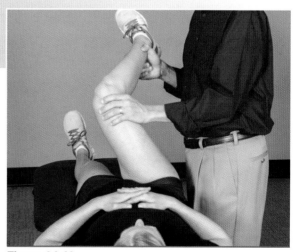

Client Position	Supine with bilateral legs lying extended and arms relaxed at side
Clinician Position	Standing next to leg to be assessed, directly facing the client
Movement	The combined motions of flexion (typically about 90°) and adduction to end range are initially performed as shown.

Figure 24.48

(continued)

Femoral Acetabular Impingement Test (Flexion-Adduction-IR Test, FADDIR Test) *(continued)*

The clinician then maintains adduction with overpressure while performing IR of the hip with overpressure to that motion as well.

Assessment Reproduction of the client's concordant groin pain and/or clicking or popping with concordant pain is suggestive of hip impingement or labral tear. This combined movement engages the femoral head–neck junction into the anterior superior labrum and acetabular rim.[170] It is suggested that this combined motion causes a mechanical abutment of the femoral head on the acetabulum and/or shearing force on the labrum.

Statistics
- Pooled analysis: **SN 94 (88-97)**, SP 8 (2-20), +LR 1.02, **–LR 0.48**, across four studies with 128 clients (MRA reference standard)[109]
- Pooled analysis: **SN 99 (95-100)**, SP 7 (0-34), +LR 1.06, **–LR 0.15**, across two studies with 157 clients (arthroscopy reference standard)[109]
- **SN 99 (NR)**, SP 25 (NR), +LR 1.3, **–LR 0.04**, QUADAS 9, in a study of 30 clients with FAI or labral tear (mean age 40.7 years; 13 were female; mean duration of symptoms > 3 months), using MRA or CT scan as a reference standard[171]
- SN 99 (NR), SP 5 (NR), +LR 1.0, –LR 0.2, QUADAS 8, in a study of 101 clients with labral tear and concurrent pathology (mean age 37.6 years; 71 were female; mean duration of symptoms 21.6 months), and MRA and arthroscopy as a reference standard[172]
- SN 97 (NR), SP 13 (NR), +LR 1.1, –LR 0.23, QUADAS 7, in a study of 23 clients with labral tear (mean age 40.2 years; 14 were female; mean duration of symptoms 3.5 years), and surgery as a reference standard[173]
- SN 78 (59-89), SP 10 (3-29), +LR 0.9, –LR 2.2, QUADAS 9, in a study of 105 clients with various intra-articular pathology (mean age 42 ± 15 years; 24 were female; mean duration of symptoms 1.9 years), and MRA or intra-articular injection as a reference standard[4]
- SN 97 (NR), SP 4 (NR), +LR 1.0, –LR 0.75, QUADAS 10, in a study of 35 adolescent clients with FAI or labral tear (mean age 16 years; 30 were female; duration of symptoms ranged between 3 months to 3 years), and MRI or MRA as a reference standard[174]
- SN 59 (NR), SP 75 (NR), +LR 2.4, –LR 0.55, QUADAS 9, in a study of 18 clients with labral tear (age range 32-56 years; 16 were female; mean duration of symptoms NR), and MRA as a reference standard[164]

FLEXION-IR TEST

Client Position Supine with bilateral legs lying extended and arms relaxed at side

Clinician Position Standing next to leg to be assessed, directly facing the client

Movement The clinician grasps the client's ankle and supports the client's knee if necessary. Combined motions of flexion to 90° and end range IR (with overpressure) are performed.

Assessment A (+) test is reproduction of concordant pain and/or clicking with concordant pain. As with the impingement test, pain in the groin is indicative of labral degeneration, fraying, or tearing.

Statistics
- Pooled analysis: **SN 96 (82-100)**, SP 17 (12-54), +LR 1.12, **–LR 0.27**, across three studies with 42 clients[109]
- **SN 98 (NR)**, SP 8 (NR), +LR 1.1, **–LR 0.25**, QUADAS 11, in a study of 30 clients with labral tear (mean age 41 years; 13 females; mean duration of symptoms NR), and MRA as a reference standard[175]

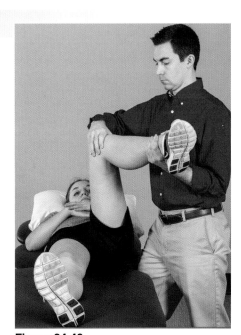

Figure 24.49

- **SN 97 (NR)**, SP 25 (NR), +LR 1.3, **–LR 0.12**, QUADAS 11, in a study of 30 clients with labral tear (mean age 41 years; 13 were female; mean duration of symptoms NR), and arthroscopy as a reference standard[175]
- **SN 94 (NR)**, SP 13 (NR), +LR 1.1, **–LR 0.46**, QUADAS 8, in a study of 10 clients with labral tear (mean age 28.7 years; 7 were female; mean duration of symptoms 2.9 years), and arthroscopy as a reference standard[176]
- **SN 94 (NR)**, SP 17 (NR), +LR 1.1, **–LR 0.35**, QUADAS 9, in a study of 10 clients with labral tear (mean age 38.4 years; 5 were female; mean duration of symptoms NR), and arthroscopy as a reference standard[177]

FLEXION-ADDUCTION-AXIAL COMPRESSION TEST

Client Position	Supine with bilateral legs lying extended and arms relaxed at side or resting on the stomach
Clinician Position	Standing next to the leg to be assessed, directly facing the client. The clinician clasps the patellofemoral joint with bilateral hands.
Movement	Combined motions of flexion to 90°, IR to end range, and adduction are performed as shown.
Assessment	The clinician should look for reproduction of the client's concordant pain with or without clicking or catching as a (+) test.
Statistics	SN 100 (NR), SP not tested, QUADAS 8, in a study of 10 clients with labral tear (mean age 28.7 years; 7 were female; mean duration of symptoms 2.9 years), and arthroscopy as a reference standard[176]

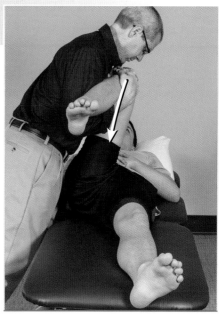

Figure 24.50

INTERNAL ROTATION-FLEXION-AXIAL COMPRESSION TEST

Client Position	Supine with bilateral legs lying extended and arms relaxed at side or resting on their stomach
Clinician Position	Standing next to leg to be assessed, directly facing the client. Bilateral hands are clasped over the patello-femoral joint.
Movement	The clinician supports the client's leg as shown. Combined motions of flexion to 90° and IR to end range with axial compression are performed.
Assessment	Reproduction of pain indicates a (+) test.
Statistics	SN 75 (19-99), SP 43 (18-72), +LR 1.3, –LR 0.58, QUADAS 8, in a study of 18 athletic clients with complaints of groin pain (mean age 30.5 ± 8.5 years; 5 were female; mean duration of symptoms NR), and MRA as a reference standard[16]

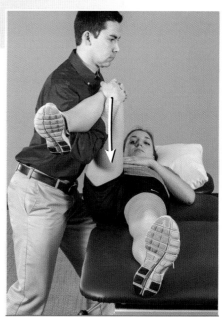

Figure 24.51

HIP DYSPLASIA

PASSIVE HIP ABDUCTION TEST

This test is specific to neonates.

Client Position	Supine on table
Clinician Position	Standing facing the client
Movement	The clinician passively flexes the client's bilateral hips to 90°. The clinician then passively abducts both hips to end ROM.
Assessment	A (+) test is indicated by a restriction in abduction ROM as compared to the opposite side.
Statistics	• SN 70 (NR), SP 90 (NR), +LR 7.0, −LR 0.33, QUADAS 7, in a study of 1,107 neonates considered to be at risk of hip dysplasia (gender not reported), and ultrasonography as a reference standard.[178]
	• Unilateral limitation of hip abduction was considered to be an important clinical sign, and its presence in an infant over the age of 4 months makes further investigation essential.

PALPATION

The clinician should potentially palpate the entire lumbopelvic and hip complex when assessing the hip joint, dependent on the particular client presentation. Refer to chapters 19 (Lumbar Spine) and 20 (Sacroiliac Joint and Pelvic Girdle) to review palpation of these structures.

Anterior Aspect

Bony Structures

• **Iliac crest:** This structure is very easy to locate and is prominent for palpation. The clinician can place their hands along the side of the client at the level of the pelvic girdle, and then slide bilateral hands up and down until they feel the ridge of the iliac crest. The clinician can compare side to side to ascertain if the crests are level.

• **Iliac tubercle:** This is the widest portion of the iliac crest.

• **ASIS:** See chapter 19 for a description of performance.

• **Pubic tubercles:** See chapter 19 for a description of performance.

• **Greater trochanters:** The clinician can start on the iliac crest and palpate distally along the lateral midline until they reach a small plateau. The clinician can put extended hands to rest on top of the greater trochanters bilaterally to determine the symmetry of height and so on. They should have the client internally and externally rotate the thigh to determine the most prominent portion of the trochanter to determine angle of torsion (figure 24.52).

• **Posterior approach to the femoral head:** With the client in a prone position, the clinician can mobilize the hip by rotating it medially to push the femoral head posteriorly. The head is accessible through the muscular mass of the gluteus maximus between the greater trochanter and the lateral surface of the iliac bone.

• **Anterior approach to the femoral head:** With the client side lying, the clinician can stabilize the client's pelvis with their hip. The clinician can place their proximal hand on the anteromedial aspect of the hip and grip its anterior aspect, using their finger and thumb. Their distal hand supports

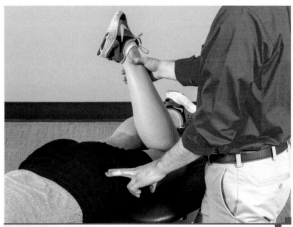

Figure 24.52 Palpation of the greater trochanter.

the anteromedial aspect of the thigh as the clinician slowly brings the limb into extension (stabilizing the pelvis with their hip). The fingers of their proximal hand will gradually feel the femoral head. The clinician will be able to feel the pulse of the femoral artery, which is pushed forward by the femoral head. Palpation of femoral pulse is appropriate for differential diagnosis of potential lower-extremity vascular compromise.

Soft-Tissue Structures

• **Inguinal ligament:** This structure attaches from the ASIS to the pubic tubercle. It can be palpated using transverse palpation. An inguinal hernia may be present if a bulge is found. Typically, it is not tender (perhaps due to peripheral nerve entrapment).

• **Femoral triangle:** This is located in the area directly distal to the crease of the groin (figure 24.53). The base of the triangle is formed by the inguinal ligament. The lateral border is the medial aspect of the sartorius and the medial border is the adductor longus. The floor is comprised of the iliacus, psoas major, adductor longus, and pectineus. The femoral vessels are superficial. They consist of (from lateral to medial) the femoral nerve, artery, and vein. The triangle and its components are most easily palpable in the FABER position. Swollen lymph nodes can be palpated in the superior aspect of the triangle. The psoas bursa may also be palpated within the triangle, but only if it is swollen.

• **Femoral nerve, artery, and vein:** The femoral vein and nerve are not easily palpable normally. The femoral pulse (femoral artery) can most easily be detected at the midway point between the pubic tubercle and the ASIS. This is a normally strong

pulse. Occlusion of the aorta or the iliac arteries should be a consideration with a weak pulse.

• **Sartorius:** In the same FABER position, it is most easily palpable at the proximal anteromedial aspect of the thigh.

• **Adductor longus:** It is palpable at the proximal medial aspect of the thigh inferior to the pubic symphysis. It can be more easily palpated by having the client resist adduction.

• **Pectineus:** This is found in the depression just lateral to the adductor longus muscle. It forms the medial aspect of the floor of Scarpa's triangle.

• **Rectus femoris:** Its origin is at the anterior inferior iliac spine (AIIS) (just distal to ASIS) between the tensor fasciae latae (TFL) and the sartorius.

• **Iliopsoas muscle at the distal aspect:** The clinician can place their grip medial to the proximal course of the sartorius, close to its origin at the ASIS. It is lined medially by the pectineus muscle. When it is placed under tension (the clinician resists hip flexion with their distal hand), the clinician can palpate this muscle's contracting fibers at the level of the iliopectineal process.

Posterior Aspect

Bony Structures

Please refer to chapter 19 for details on palpation of these structures.

• Posterior superior iliac spines (PSIS)
• Sacroiliac joint
• Ischial tuberosity

Side-Lying Position

Soft-Tissue Structures

• **Piriformis muscle and sciatic nerve:** See chapter 19 for details on performance.

• **Gluteus maximus:** The client lies prone with the knee flexed. The clinician can resist hip extension and palpate the mid-posterior buttock. The clinician should remember the borders: the iliac crest, sacrum, and lateral trochanter or gluteal tuberosity on the femur.

• **Gluteus medius:** Bony landmarks are the anterior part of the iliac crest and superior border of the greater trochanter. The clinician should ask the client to abduct the leg (from side lying) in the frontal plane. Internal rotation will mobilize the anterior fibers, as well as the gluteus minimus.

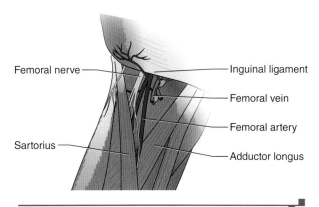

Femoral nerve

Sartorius

Inguinal ligament

Femoral vein

Femoral artery

Adductor longus

Figure 24.53 Femoral triangle.

- **Tensor fasciae latae:** In side-lying position, the client flexes their hip slightly. Abduction in this plane will make the TFL more prominent.

PHYSICAL PERFORMANCE MEASURES

Physical performance measures of the hip joint are applicable to the lumbar spine or pelvis and lower extremities. As with PPMs in other areas of the body, selection and utilization of these tests should go from least to most challenging to the client. Since the hip is a lower-extremity weight-bearing joint, the parameters of interest to assess with PPMs could potentially include strength, anaerobic power, endurance, balance, trunk endurance, speed, agility, and quickness, depending on the pathology, the client's functional level, and so on. Examples of potentially appropriate tests are given in table 24.4.

A systematic review[179] supports the use of the single-leg stance, single-leg squat, and star excursion balance tests (SEBT) for hip pathology clients. Clients with FAI had decreased mean peak squat depth compared to controls, suggesting that maxi-

TABLE 24.4 Physical Performance Measure Suggestions for the Hip Joint

Discrete physical parameter	Potential physical performance measurements for the lower-level client (if appropriate)	Potential physical performance measurements for the higher-level client (if appropriate)
Balance	Single-leg stance test Romberg test Four square step test Functional reach test Sidestep test Tandem walking Tinetti test	Any of the tests appropriate for the lower-level client Star excursion balance test Multiple single-leg hop stabilization test
Fundamental movement	Deep squat test Sock test Sit-to-stand test Self-paced walking test Timed up and go test	Any of the tests appropriate for the lower-level client Rotational stability Trunk stability push-up
Strength and power	1RM leg press Lunge test Knee bending in 30 s	Any of the tests appropriate for the lower-level client Jump and hop tests
Lower extremity anaerobic power	Only if appropriate and necessary	Any of the tests appropriate for the lower-level client Wingate anaerobic power test Lower extremity functional test
SAQ	Only if appropriate and necessary	Any of the tests appropriate for the lower-level client Edgren sidestep test Illinois Agility test Pro agility test Zigzag run test
Trunk endurance	Supine bridge test	Trunk flexion, extension, and lateral flexion bilaterally Repetitive box lifting task

SAQ = speed, agility, and quickness

mal squat depth is a valid measure of assessment for FAI.[96] The SEBT, a purported measure of balance, range of motion, and muscle performance,[180-182] recruited the gluteus medius at 49% of maximal volitional isometric contraction with a medial reach.[183] The single-leg squat also demonstrated a relationship to hip abductor function.[184] Dysfunction in any of these PPMs should alert the clinician to perform measures previously discussed (motion tests, muscle performance tests, and so on).

Normative and discriminatory values for involved to noninvolved lower extremities on various hop, speed, and agility tests have been reported.[185] Most of these tests are reported for either normative values or on knee and ankle pathologies. The reliability of these measures specifically for hip dysfunction has not been established. The sport test has been advocated to objectively assess a client's readiness to return to sport following hip arthroscopy. Rather than measuring isolated movements, it analyzes a client's coordinated movement patterns and power of an involved extremity. The sport test includes single-knee bends, side-to-side lateral movement, diagonal side-to-side movement, and forward box lunges. Clients must score 17/20 or higher to pass each of the four components of the test.[186] Although the application of this test to those with ALT has not been investigated, this test could ideally function as an advanced assessment of sport-related ability for those clients with ALT since it replicates most components of sporting activity. Again, though, it is worth noting that a limitation is lack of diagnostic accuracy or ability to predict return to sport.

COMMON ORTHOPEDIC CONDITIONS OF THE HIP JOINT

While it is impossible to distinctly describe various pathological presentations of the hip joint, there are evidence-based findings supportive of particular pathologies of this region of the body. Therefore, the intent of this section of the chapter is to present current evidence-supported findings that are suggestive of hip pathologies. As previously described in chapter 4 (Evidence-Based Practice and Client Examination), though, not all examination findings are absolutely supported with clinical evidence. Clinicians should also rely on clinical experience and input from the client when performing differential diagnosis of a client's presentation of pain and dysfunction.

Hip joint dysfunction and pathology, much like other joint pathology, can have variable presentations. These pathological presentations can also have similarities in their presentation. Differentiating among their clinical findings is helpful for the clinician to determine not only the appropriate clinical intervention but also the necessity of referral to other potentially more appropriate health care clinicians.

Differential Diagnosis of Pain Related to the Hip Joint and Lumbar Spine

- Clients who limp were shown to be 7 times more likely to have a hip disorder than a spine disorder.
- Clients who had groin pain were 7 times more likely to have a hip disorder alone versus a hip and spine disorder or a spine disorder alone.
- Clients with limited hip IR were 14 times more likely to have a hip disorder alone versus a hip and spine disorder or a spine disorder alone.
- Painful joint mobility assessment of the respective body section (hip or lumbar spine) can assist with implicating that body part as the pain generator, especially if joint motion is restricted and joint motion or pain improves with repeated joint-mobility treatment.
- Intra-articular hip joint pathology often presents with deep groin pain that is not palpable.

Hip Osteoarthritis

ICD-9: 721.5 (degenerative joint disease; hip arthritis)

ICD-10: M16.0 (hip osteoarthritis)

Hip osteoarthritis is a common type of osteoarthritis (OA). Since the hip is a weight-bearing joint, OA can cause significant problems. Hip OA is caused by deterioration of articular cartilage and breakdown of the joint surfaces. According to the American College of Rheumatology classification criteria, osteoarthritis of the hip must involve hip pain and at least two of the following three criteria:

- Erythrocyte sedimentation rate < 20 mm per hour
- Femoral or acetabular osteophytes seen on radiograph
- Joint space narrowing seen on radiograph

I. Client Interview

Subjective History

- Stiffness first thing in morning for ≤ 60 minutes.[187]
- Gradual, insidious onset of pain.[131, 187]
- Pain that progressively worsens with activity and exercise is common. Pain may be prolonged after activity as well.
- The more common locations of pain reported were in the ischial tuberosity and anterior thigh.[30]
- Previous hip injury was associated with unilateral hip OA.[188]
- Obesity is associated with hip OA.[188-190]
- There is a negative association between cigarette smoking and OA among men.[188, 190]
- A weak positive association exists between prolonged regular sporting activity and hip OA.[188]
- Lifting of heavy loads and occupation-related risk factors are present for OA.[189, 190]
- More women than men have OA.[190]
- Older age, previous knee trauma, hand OA, and presence of Heberden's nodes have also been described as risk factors.[188, 190]

- Groin and thigh pain were found in 55% and 57% of hip joint–pain clients, respectively. However, pain referral was also seen in the buttock and lower extremity distal to the knee in 71% and 22%, respectively.[29]
- Composite of signs and symptoms:
  - Hip pain and hip IR < 15° and hip flexion ≤ 115° *or*
  - Hip IR ≥ 15° and pain with IR and morning stiffness ≤ 60 minutes and age > 50 years
  - Helps **rule out** (SN 86, −LR 0.2) and rule in (SP 75, +LR 3.4) hip OA in a study of 201 clients who experienced hip pain for most days of the prior month[124]

Outcome Measures

- The WOMAC, Physical Function Subscale, and LEFS have demonstrated clinical applicability in these clients, although they are highly influenced by client pain levels.[191-194]
- Findings caution against the isolated use of self-report assessments of physical function, since change in the pain level significantly affected change in self-report measures of physical function.[191-193]

Diagnostic Imaging

- Radiographic findings include joint space narrowing, bone sclerosis, periarticular cysts, and osteophytes. Refer to chapter 6 for a definition of OA according to Kellgren and Lawrence.[195]
- Minimal joint space was the index most strongly associated with other radiologic features of OA.[76]
- Clients meeting the previously discussed clinical signs and symptoms criteria from Altman and colleagues[124] demonstrated hip OA on radiography.
- Radiographs help rule out (SN 61, −LR 0.6) and rule in (SP 81, +LR 3.2) hip osteoarthritis.[54]
- MRI helps rule out (SN 61, −LR 0.6) and rule in (SP 82, +LR 3.4) hip osteoarthritis.

II. Observation

- Gluteal atrophy has been observed in clients with hip OA.[82, 83]

- Trendelenburg's sign is present in clients with gluteal tendinopathy or hip OA;[150, 166] therefore, clinicians should observe for compensated or uncompensated gluteus medius gait pattern.

- Soft-tissue and sacrolumbar joint ROM restrictions have been suggested to limit frontal plane pelvic ROM during normal gait.[196]

- The hip being held in resting position (hip flexion, slight abduction, and external rotation) generally indicates the presence of hip effusion.

III. Triage and Screening

- All non-musculoskeletal causes, as well as causes from related joints, should be ruled out.

- The patellar-pubic percussion test helps **rule out** (pooled SN 95, −LR 0.07) and **rule in** (pooled SP 86, +LR 6.1) femoral fracture.[109]

- Prostate cancer in men or any reproductive cancer or breast cancer in a woman is a red flag since these cancers may be associated with metastases to the lumbar spine or hip joint.[97]

- Rule out lumbar spine and SIJ or pelvic girdle dysfunction when suspecting hip pathology.

IV. Motion Tests

- All motions and joint-play assessments are recommended, especially IR and flexion ROM;[131, 150, 187] therefore, posterior and inferior joint-play glides are recommended due to their correlation with these motions.

- Impaired range of joint motion resulted in reduced functional status.[197, 198]

- Having no motions of restricted mobility helped **rule out** (SN 100) hip OA in a study of 195 subjects presenting with new episodes of hip pain to various general practitioners.[131]

- Having two planes of motion that were restricted in movement helped rule in (SP 77, +LR 2.5) mild to moderate and severe hip OA (SP 69, +LR 2.6).[131]

- Having three planes of motion that were restricted in movement helped **rule in** (SP 93, +LR 4.7) mild to moderate and severe hip OA (SP 88, +LR 4.5).[131]

- Decreased passive hip IR (SP 86, +LR 3.0), pain with passive hip IR (SP 86, +LR 3.7), and pain with active hip IR (SP 86, +LR 2.2) all helped rule in hip OA or gluteal tendinopathy in 40 clients with unilateral hip pain.[150]

- The clinical prediction rule for predicting hip OA is as follows:

  - Self-report of squatting as aggravating factor

  - Scour test with adduction causing groin or lateral hip pain

  - Active hip flexion causing lateral hip pain

  - Passive hip IR ≤ 25°

  - Active hip extension causing pain:

    - CPR helps **rule out** hip OA when ≥1 predictor (SN 95, −LR 0.27) or ≥2 predictors (SN 81, −LR 0.31) are present; helps **rule in** hip OA when 5 predictors (SP 98, +LR 7.3) or ≥4 predictors (SP 98, +LR 24.3) are present, or **rule in** hip OA when ≥3 predictors (SP 86, +LR 5.2) are present.[166]

- More recent findings suggest that in clients with hip symptoms, hip internal rotation <24° and flexion <114° were found to be the cutoffs with the highest discriminative ability to distinguish between clients with and without radiographic features.[132]

- Intrarater reliability is generally moderate to good for clients with hip intra-articular pathology.[126, 127, 199]

V. Muscle Performance Testing

- Greater muscle strength, aerobic capacity, and standing balance were protective factors for preventing deterioration of functional status.[197, 198]

- Gluteus medius and maximus weakness and atrophy are correlated with hip osteoarthritis.[82, 83, 200]

VI. Special Tests

- Trendelenburg test: has poor ability to help rule out (SN 55, −LR 0.8) and rule in (SP 70, +LR 1.83) hip OA when utilized in a study of 20 healthy adults and 20 adults with radiographically documented hip OA.[88]

- Resisted hip abduction test: A (+) test has less than good ability to help rule in (SP 90, +LR 3.5) hip OA.[88]

- A (+) restricted and painful (lateral hip pain) FABER test is strongly associated with GTPS and not OA (**SN 81, SP 82, +LR 4.5, −LR 0.23**).[157]

- FABER test: A (+) test helps rule in (SP 71, +LR 1.9) hip OA.[166]

- The scour test, although limited on diagnostic investigation, is likely a (+) test in these clients.

VII. Palpation

- Palpation of the anterior hip joint and gluteal muscles is especially appropriate.

VIII. Physical Performance Measures[201]

- 6-meter walk test
- Timed up and go test
- Sit-to-stand test
- Self-paced walk tests
- Stair climbing
- Sock test
- Pain and functional status seem to deteriorate slowly.[198]
- The self-paced walk, stair test, timed up and go, and 6-minute walk have been suggested as more complete measures of physical function for these clients.[191-194]
- Terwee and colleagues identified 26 performance-based tests; many represent variations on the same theme. The most useful test was unable to be determined because consensus is lacking on what activities and functional parameters should be included.[202]

- Mobility, pain control (if pain dominant), and exercise and conditioning may be used.

Hip Impingement or Labral Tear

ICD-9: 719.45; 719.95; 718.85

ICD-10: S76 (other specified injury of hip and thigh)

Femoroacetabular impingement (FAI) is a mechanical abutment between the femoral head and acetabulum, typically in the superior-anterior portion of the acetabulum. FAI generally has two primary types: cam and pincer impingement. The cam type describes the femoral head and neck relationship as aspherical, or not perfectly round. This aspherical shape contributes to abnormal contact between the head and socket. The pincer type describes the situation where the socket or acetabulum has too much coverage of the ball or femoral head. This overcoverage typically results in the labral cartilage being pinched between the rim of the socket and the anterior femoral head–neck junction. The pincer form of the impingement is typically secondary to *retroversion*, a turning back of the socket, *profunda*, a socket that is too deep, or *protrusio*, a situation where the femoral head extends into the pelvis. Most of the time, the cam and pincer forms exist together, i.e., *mixed impingement*. Femoroacetabular impingement is one of the primary causes (along with hip dysplasia, trauma, and hip joint laxity) of hip labral tear.

I. Client Interview

Subjective History

- C-sign pain description.[92]
- Groin pain is predominant. Clients may complain of sharp or dull pain, and pain is likely to be activity related.[5]
- The most common locations of pain were the central groin and lateral peritrochanteric area.[30]
- Groin pain 96%[172] and 100%[14] SN to help **rule out** labral tear.
- Anterior groin pain worsens with prolonged periods of standing, sitting, or walking.[203]

- Inguinal clicking and giving way correlated ($r = 0.79$) with labral tear.[14]

- Sharp pain, especially with clicking for labral tear, helps to **rule out** (SN 100, −LR 0) and **rule in** (SP 85, +LR 6.7)[16] labral tear.

- More recently, the most commonly reported locations of pain were the central groin and the lateral peritrochanteric area. The least common were the ischial tuberosity and the anterior thigh.[30]

- FAI is more common in those with decreased hip IR[204] and increased body mass.[74]

- 90% of clients with labral tears had FAI morphology.[205]

- Recent findings suggest increased prevalence of FAI in those participating in sports, particularly American football,[206] hockey,[44] and soccer.[46]

- Clients may have pain with squatting.[96, 207]

Outcome Measures

- Hip Outcome Score[208]
- International Hip Outcome Tool[39, 40]

Diagnostic Imaging

- Increased alpha angle in cam-type impingement.[204]

- Alpha angle measurement (with cutoff of 55°) on MRA provides some assistance to **rule in** impingement due to excessive alpha angle (SP 70).[209]

- Magnetic resonance imaging helps **rule in** hip impingement (SP 79, −LR 0.43).[57]

- Ischial spine projection assessing for retroversion on radiographs helps **rule in** (SP 91, +LR 45.5) and **rule out** (SN 98, −LR 0.09) hip impingement.[210]

- Computed tomography scan for assessment provides much greater ability to **rule out** (SN 92-97, −LR 0.03–0.08) and **rule in** (SP 87-100, +LR 7.5) hip impingement.[55]

- Computed tomography helps **rule out** (SN 92-97, −LR 0.03–0.08) and **rule in** (SP 87-100, +LR 7.5) labral tear.[55, 56]

- Magnetic resonance imaging arthrogram is more helpful for **ruling out** (pooled SN 87, −LR 0.20) labral tear versus MRI (pooled SN 66, −LR 0.34), while MRI is more helpful for **ruling in** (pooled SP 79, +LR 3.1) labral tear than MRA (pooled SP 64, +LR 2.4).[57]

II. Observation

- Clients avoid deep squatting motions, sitting in low chairs, and adduction and IR combined motions.[18] Squatting with the hips internally rotated causes increased pain versus squatting with legs externally rotated.

- Decreased gluteal muscle performance and labral tear[15] suggest that functional limitations may also be found in the propulsion phase of gait, standing up out of a chair, climbing a steep hill or incline, and pushing off into a sprint.

- The hip being held in the resting position (hip flexion, slight abduction, and external rotation) generally indicates the presence of hip effusion.

- During normal gait, clients with FAI have demonstrated less hip abduction, frontal pelvic ROM, and overall frontal plane ROM.[196]

- 37% of athletic clients undergoing hip arthroscopy had generalized ligamentous laxity,[211] which could present with increased external rotation on that hip during gait, standing, and/or relaxed supine postures.

III. Triage and Screening

- All non-musculoskeletal causes, as well as causes from related joints, should be ruled out.

- The patellar-pubic percussion test helps **rule out** (pooled SN 95, −LR 0.07) and **rule in** (pooled SP 86, +LR 6.1) femoral fracture.[109]

- Prostate cancer in men or any reproductive cancer or breast cancer in a woman is a red flag since these cancers may be associated with metastases to the lumbar spine or hip joint.[97]

- Rule out lumbar spine and SIJ or pelvic girdle dysfunction.

- Soft-tissue and sacroiliac and lumbar joint ROM restrictions have been suggested to limit frontal-plane pelvic ROM during normal gait.[196]

IV. Motion Tests

- Soft-tissue restrictions are suggested to limit frontal-plane pelvic ROM during normal gait.[196]

- Clients with FAI and labral tear exhibited reduced motions in hip flexion, internal rotation, and adduction.[5, 11, 104, 130]

- Using 3-D CT kinematic analysis, hips with FAI had decreased flexion, internal rotation, and abduction. Internal rotation decreased with increasing flexion and adduction.[212]

- Internal rotation ROM decreased in clients with FAI.[204, 213-216]

- Intrarater reliability is generally moderate to good for clients with hip intra-articular pathology.[126, 127, 199]

V. Muscle Performance Testing

- Hip flexor weakness and endurance deficits were noted in clients with FAI.[217, 218]

- Labral tear clients have decreased gluteal muscle performance.[15]

- Gluteus medius and maximus weakness and atrophy are correlated with hip osteoarthritis.[82, 83, 200]

VI. Special Tests

- Hip impingement and labral tear tests are generally better at **ruling out** versus **ruling in** pathology.[109]

- FADDIR: A (−) test has good ability to help **rule out** (SN 94-99, −LR 0.15–0.48) FAI or labral tear across a pooled analysis of six studies.[109]

- Flexion IR: A (−) test has good ability to help **rule out** (SN 96, −LR 0.27) FAI or labral tear across a pooled analysis of four studies.[109]

- The FADDIR test position allows for testing the widest zone of the acetabulum and is not localized to abutment in the anterolateral acetabulum.[219]

- Thomas test: A (−) test is helpful for **ruling out** (SN 89, −LR 0.12) hip labral tear and a (+) test is helpful for **ruling it in** (SP 92, +LR 11.1).[14] The greatest tensile strains on the hip were found on the anterior–superior portion of the capsule or labrum,[15] likely the mechanism for a (+) Thomas test.

- The scour test, although limited on diagnostic investigation, is likely a (+) test in these clients.

- The flexion-adduction-axial compression and internal rotation-axial compression tests have poor ability to rule out or in FAI or labral tear.

VII. Palpation

- Although pain referral for these clients is typically to the groin and, to a lesser degree, the buttock and lateral trochanter,[220] these areas of the hip are typically not tender to palpation unless there is also extra-articular involvement.

- Because of recent findings implicating the psoas major as a potential contributor to ALT pathology,[220-222] palpation of this structure for concordant pain is merited.

VIII. Physical Performance Measures

- Clients with FAI are not able to squat as low as those without FAI due to decreased sagittal pelvic ROM.[96]

- Squat performance improved post-surgically for clients with FAI despite overall pelvic ROM not improving, suggesting that squat improvement is likely due to increased knee and ankle angles, as well as increased posterior pelvic tilt during descent of squat. Therefore, posterior glide mobilizations are important to the femoral head.[207]

- Clinicians can perform occupation- and sport-specific testing as warranted.

POTENTIAL TREATMENT-BASED CLASSIFICATIONS

- Mobility, pain control (if pain dominant), exercise and conditioning, and possibly stability may be used.

Differential Diagnosis
of Hip FAI or Labral Tear and OA

- Pathology related to FAI or labral tear is more likely in younger to middle-aged adults versus middle-aged to older adults for hip OA.

- Pathology related to FAI or labral tear typically has a consistent mechanical-type pain (locking, clicking, catching) presentation versus hip OA, which can have these symptoms but also more likely has consistent weight-bearing pain than FAI or labral tear.

- Both FAI or labral tear and hip OA clients have been suggested to have limited hip flexion and IR.

- More advanced hip OA is suggested to have multiplanar ROM restrictions.

- Radiographic imaging of joint space narrowing, osteophytes, and subchondral sclerosis is more likely suggestive of hip OA versus findings of cam and pincer morphology on FAI client radiographs.

- Clients with both pathologies have been suggested to have pain with squatting, as well as with tests such as the scour and FADDIR.

- Some literature suggests that FAI or labral tear pathology is a precursor to hip OA pathology, although this is yet to be conclusively proven.

Femoral Stress Fracture

ICD-9: 820.0 (femoral neck fracture); 821.0 (fracture of shaft or unspecified part of femur closed)

ICD-10: S72 (fracture of neck of femur)

A femoral stress fracture is an incomplete fracture of the femur. Typically the highest prevalence of these stress fractures occurs in the femoral neck or femoral shaft.

I. Client Interview

Subjective History[223-229]

- These fractures are more common in women than in men. Caucasian women are 1.5 to 4 times more likely than African-American women to have a hip fracture after the age of 40.

- Pain is often described as aching or deep hip or groin pain.

- Pain location: proximal anterior or lateral hip or groin region.

- Pain increases with activity and is often relieved with rest.

- Night pain is not uncommon.

- A history of osteoporosis is a risk factor for hip fracture.

- Hip fracture is the most detrimental fracture, being associated with 20% mortality and 50% permanent loss in function.

Outcome Measures

- Any appropriate hip measure can be used.

Diagnostic Imaging

- Bone scan (**SN 91, SP 100, +LR Inf, − R Infa**),[65] radiographs (**SN 90-95, SP 68-100, +LR 2.1-Inf, − R 2.1-In**),[64] and MRI (**SN 100, SP 100**)[65] have all shown the capability to rule in and rule out femoral stress fractures.

II. Observation

- Clients have decreased weight bearing on the involved leg.[224, 225, 227]

- Antalgic gait with decreased step length was noted.[224, 225, 227]

- Trendelenburg's sign is present in clients with gluteal tendinopathy or hip OA;[150, 166] therefore, clinicians should observe for a compensated or uncompensated gluteus medius gait pattern.[225]

- The hip being held in a resting position (hip flexion, slight abduction, and external rotation) generally indicates the presence of hip effusion.

III. Triage and Screening

- All non-musculoskeletal causes, as well as causes from related joints, should be ruled out.

- Rule out complete fracture: clients who are not able to bear weight on the involved leg, leg giving out, pain with active or passive movement, sign of the buttock, and so on.

- Prostate cancer in men or any reproductive cancer or breast cancer in a woman is a red flag since these cancers may be associated with metastases to the lumbar spine or hip joint.[97]

- Clinicians should rule out lumbar spine and SIJ or pelvic girdle dysfunction.

- Soft-tissue and sacroiliac and lumbar joint ROM restrictions have been suggested to limit frontal-plane pelvic ROM during normal gait.[196]

- The scour test, although limited on diagnostic investigation, is likely a good test for ruling out intra-articular involvement.

IV. Motion Tests

- Intrarater reliability of hip ROM was shown to be moderate to excellent (ICC = 0.50–0.97) in clients with and without hip OA.[126-128] Specific hip ROM measures have shown excellent interrater reliability, ranging from ICC of 0.76 to 0.97.[129]

V. Muscle Performance Testing

- Hip weakness, especially with abduction, is likely.[225]

VI. Special Tests

- Patellar-pubic percussion test: A (−) test helps **rule out** (pooled SN 95, −LR 0.07) and a (+) test helps **rule in** (pooled SP 86, +LR 6.1) femoral fracture in pooled analysis.[109]

- Fulcrum test: helps rule out (SN 88-93, −LR 0.09–0.92) stress fracture in studies of high bias.[107, 108]

- Clients will likely have pain with resisted SLR test.

VII. Palpation

- Palpation is especially appropriate for the proximal anterior and lateral thigh or groin, or around a suspected fracture location.

VIII. Physical Performance Measures

- This type of testing is most likely not appropriate for these clients. Only lower-level testing is suggested, if this type of testing is appropriate at all, in the acute assessment of this pathology.

POTENTIAL TREATMENT-BASED CLASSIFICATIONS

- If detected acutely, the clinician will likely refer the client out to a physician (definitely should in the case of a fracture).

- Stability

- Mobility, pain control (if pain dominant), exercise and conditioning

Avascular Necrosis

ICD-9: 733.40 (aseptic necrosis of bone, site unspecified)

ICD-10: M87.9 (osteonecrosis, unspecified)

Avascular necrosis (AVN, also osteonecrosis, bone infarction, aseptic necrosis, and ischemic bone necrosis) is a disease resulting from cellular death (necrosis) of bone components due to interruption of the blood supply. The bone tissue therefore dies and the bone collapses. Avascular necrosis involving the bones of a joint often leads to destruction of the joint articular surfaces.

I. Client Interview

Subjective History

- Association with various conditions, including corticosteroid use, alcoholism, and sickle-cell anemia.[230]

- Clients often report groin pain that is exacerbated by weight bearing. The pain may initially be mild, but it progressively worsens over time and with use. Eventually, the pain is present at rest and may be present at night.

- Groin and thigh pain were found in 55% and 57% of hip joint–pain clients, respectively. However, pain referral was also seen in the buttock and lower extremity distal to the knee in 71% and 22%, respectively.[29]

Outcome Measures

- Any appropriate hip outcome measure can be used.

Diagnostic Imaging

- Bone scan has some ability to **rule out** (SN 81)[67] avascular necrosis, while MRI is more helpful for **ruling out** (SN 99[66] and 100[67]) and **ruling in** (SP 99, +LR 99)[66] avascular necrosis.

II. Observation

- Trendelenburg's sign is present in clients with gluteal tendinopathy or hip OA;[150, 166] therefore, clinicians should observe for a compensated or uncompensated gluteus medius gait pattern.
- The hip being held in a resting position (hip flexion, slight abduction, and external rotation) generally indicates the presence of hip effusion.

III. Triage and Screening

- All non-musculoskeletal causes, as well as causes from related joints, should be ruled out.
- The patellar-pubic percussion test helps **rule out** (pooled SN 95, −LR 0.07) and **rule in** (pooled SP 86, +LR 6.1) femoral fracture.[109]
- Prostate cancer in men or any reproductive cancer or breast cancer in a woman is a red flag since these cancers may be associated with metastases to the lumbar spine or hip joint.[97]
- Clinicians should rule out lumbar spine and SIJ or pelvic girdle dysfunction.
- The scour test, although limited on diagnostic investigation, is likely a good test for ruling out intra-articular hip joint involvement.
- Soft-tissue and sacroiliac and lumbar joint ROM restrictions have been suggested to limit frontal-plane pelvic ROM during normal gait.[196]

IV. Motion Tests

- Limitations in hip motion are common.
- Intrarater reliability is generally moderate to good for clients with hip intra-articular pathology.[126, 127, 199]

V. Muscle Performance Testing

- Hip muscle weakness is often general.

VI. Special Tests

- Extension < 15° is the most helpful limitation in motion to help rule in (SP 92, +LR 2.4) avascular necrosis.
- External rotation < 60° (SP 73, +LR 0.48) and pain with internal rotation (SP 86, +LR 0.93) are less helpful for ruling in avascular necrosis.[231]

VII. Palpation

- Due to the location of the pathology, the clinician should palpate the anterior and lateral hip.

VIII. Physical Performance Measures

- None is appropriate for the acutely diagnosed client.

POTENTIAL TREATMENT-BASED CLASSIFICATIONS

- If detected acutely, refer the client out to a physician.
- Stability
- Mobility, pain control (if pain dominant), exercise and conditioning

Snapping Hip Syndrome

ICD-9: 719.65 (other symptoms referable to joint, pelvic region and thigh)

ICD-10: M76.1 (psoas tendinitis)

In this syndrome, a snapping sensation in the lateral or deep anterior hip is associated with sudden, sharp pain in the area of the greater trochanter or anterior hip. The snapping sensation and pain are the result of the iliopsoas tendon subluxing over the greater trochanter or iliopectineal eminence. Three types of snapping hip syndrome exist: external (iliotibial band snapping over the greater trochanter), internal (iliopsoas snapping over the iliopectineal eminence or femoral head), and intra-articular (hip intra-articular involvement eliciting the snapping sensation).

I. Client Interview

Three types:[31, 33, 232-234]

- External: IT band snapping over greater trochanter
- Internal: iliopsoas tendon snapping over iliopectineal eminence or femoral head
- Intra-articular: labral tear, loose bodies, and articular cartilage defects

Subjective History

- Audible snapping when hip is brought from flexion to extension; or around greater trochanter with hip flexed, adducted, and rotated.
- Common in dancers.[34, 235-237]
- Variable disability, often snapping is not of significance.[31, 237]
- Groin and thigh pain was found in 55% and 57% of hip joint pain clients, respectively. However, pain referral was also seen in the buttock and lower extremity distal to the knee in 71% and 22%, respectively.[29]

Outcome Measures

- Any appropriate hip measure can be used.

Diagnostic Imaging

- None specific

II. Observation

- Clients may have coxa vara.[31]
- Dancers will often stand with bilateral legs externally rotated.[34, 235-237]
- The hip being held in a resting position (hip flexion, slight abduction, and external rotation) generally indicates the presence of hip effusion.
- Clients may avoid transitional movements or complain of pain with them.

III. Triage and Screening

- All non-musculoskeletal causes, as well as causes from related joints, should be ruled out.
- The patellar-pubic percussion test helps **rule out** (pooled SN 95, −LR 0.07) and **rule in** (pooled SP 86, +LR 6.1) femoral fracture.[109]

- The scour test, although limited on diagnostic investigation, is likely a good test for ruling out intra-articular involvement.
- Prostate cancer in men or any reproductive cancer or breast cancer in a woman is a red flag since these cancers may be associated with metastases to the lumbar spine or hip joint.[97]
- Clinicians should rule out lumbar spine and SIJ or pelvic girdle dysfunction.
- Soft-tissue and sacroiliac and lumbar joint ROM restrictions have been suggested to limit frontal-plane pelvic ROM during normal gait.[196]

IV. Motion Tests

- Clients will often have increased hip abduction, extension, or external rotation (especially dancers).[34, 235-237]
- Intrarater reliability is generally moderate to good for clients with hip intra-articular pathology.[126, 127, 199]

V. Muscle Performance Testing

- Weakness of hip abductors, external rotators, and flexors can be common in dancers.[34, 235-237]

VI. Special Tests

- Tests involving dynamic movement of the hip (e.g., scour, ligamentum teres tear test) are often (+).
- Reproduction of clicking or popping are likely reproduced with many special tests and ROM movements involving triplanar movement in large amplitude movements. Differential diagnosis of clicking or popping generation should be determined.

VII. Palpation

- The lateral trochanter (external) and anterior hip, especially the psoas major (internal), will be tender to palpation.

VIII. Physical Performance Measures

- Appropriate hip measures are dependent on the client's status and function.

- Stability
- Pain control (if pain dominant), exercise and conditioning, and possibly mobility

Slipped Capital Femoral Epiphysis

ICD-9: 732.2 (nontraumatic slipped upper femoral epiphysis)

ICD-10: S76 (other specified injury of hip and thigh)

A slipped capital femoral epiphysis (SCFE) is a separation of the femoral head of the hip joint from the femur at the upper growth plate of the bone. The failure of the epiphyseal plate occurs as a result of the shear forces applied parallel to the growth plate. It is actually the neck that comes upward and outward while the head remains in the acetabulum. A SCFE can be stable or unstable. Adverse complications include avascular necrosis and chondrolysis (both are rare). The cause is relatively unknown, but it is thought to be related to growth hormone or endocrine abnormalities.

I. Client Interview

Subjective History[238-243]

- Occurs from age 8 to 17 years; the average age for girls is 12.1 ± 1 years and for boys is 14.4 ± 1.3 years.
- Clients generally report pain in the hip, groin, thigh, or knee; pain is often vague in nature.
- Approximately 15% of those with SCFE will have medial knee pain and distal thigh pain. Of these, 46% will have initial symptoms of medial knee or distal thigh pain.
- Clients with SCFE usually report symptoms to be dull, vague, and intermittent.
- Groin and thigh pain were found in 55% and 57% of hip joint–pain clients, respectively. However, pain referral was also seen in the buttock and lower extremity distal to the knee in 71% and 22%, respectively.[29]

- 95% of clients with SCFE are obese or overweight.
- In 60% of cases, the clients are male.
- The onset is generally insidious.
- Acute onset is usually trauma related.
- African-American clients are affected more often than Caucasian.
- Clients have vague thigh or knee pain.

Outcome Measures

- Any appropriate hip measure can be used.

Diagnostic Imaging

- AP and frog-leg lateral radiographs of the pelvis confirm a diagnosis of SCFE since the slip is always posterior.

II. Observation

- Clients may have Trendelenburg gait, excessive trunk lean to the involved side, or an antalgic gait pattern.[238, 239]
- Clients may have difficulty bearing weight on the externally rotated leg.[243]
- The hip being held in resting position (hip flexion, slight abduction, and external rotation) generally indicates the presence of hip effusion.
- Quadriceps atrophy is present in some clients.[244]

III. Triage and Screening

- All non-musculoskeletal causes, as well as causes from related joints, should be ruled out.
- The patellar-pubic percussion test helps **rule out** (pooled SN 95, –LR 0.07) and **rule in** (pooled SP 86, +LR 6.1) femoral fracture.[109]
- The scour test, although limited on diagnostic investigation, is likely a good test for ruling out intra-articular involvement.
- Prostate cancer in men or any reproductive cancer or breast cancer in a woman is a red flag since these cancers may be associated with metastases to the lumbar spine or hip joint.[97]
- Clinicians should rule out lumbar spine and SIJ or pelvic girdle dysfunction.

- Soft-tissue and sacroiliac and lumbar joint ROM restrictions have been suggested to limit frontal-plane pelvic ROM during normal gait.[196]

IV. Motion Tests

- Clients may have limited hip IR or full pain-free range of motion in the lumbar spine and knee.[238, 239]
- Other findings report limited hip motions in a capsular pattern (IR, abduction, and flexion).[243]
- Intrarater reliability is generally moderate to good for clients with hip intra-articular pathology.[126, 127, 199]

V. Muscle Performance Testing

- Hip abductor weakness is described in these clients.[243]

VI. Special Tests

- Assessing hip IR with hip flexed to 90° is an often employed screening maneuver.[245]

VII. Palpation

- Clients may have generalized tenderness in the anterior and lateral hip.[245]

VIII. Physical Performance Measures

- None is appropriate for the acutely diagnosed client.

POTENTIAL TREATMENT-BASED CLASSIFICATIONS

- If detected acutely, refer the client out to a physician.
- Stability
- Mobility, pain control (if pain dominant), and exercise and conditioning

Legg-Calvé-Perthes Disease

ICD-9: 732.1 (juvenile osteochondrosis of hip and pelvis)

ICD-10: M91.1 (juvenile osteochondrosis of head of femur)

This disease is an osteochondritis dissecans of the femoral head. A definitive cause remains unknown, and onset is typically insidious.

I. Client Interview

Subjective History

- Unilateral in 90% of cases.
- 4 times more common in boys than girls.
- Clients have complaints of vague, aching pain in groin that can radiate to medial thigh and knee.
- Groin and thigh pain were found in 55% and 57% of hip joint–pain clients, respectively. However, pain referral was also seen in the buttock and lower extremity distal to the knee in 71% and 22%, respectively.[29]
- Muscle spasm is a common complaint.

Outcome Measures

- Any appropriate hip measure can be used.

Diagnostic Imaging

- Conventional radiography was less sensitive in identifying the degree of lateral subluxation and the extent of the necrosis in the femoral head than MRI.[246, 247]
- MRI may show proximal femoral abnormalities before radiography.[247]

II. Observation

- Clients may have Trendelenburg gait, excessive trunk lean to the involved side, or an antalgic gait pattern.[238, 239]
- Limp is usually an initial sign; the client may drag the leg slightly, and the leg is often externally rotated during gait.
- Clients may have atrophy of the thigh.
- The hip being held in the resting position (hip flexion, slight abduction, and external rotation) generally indicates the presence of hip effusion.

III. Triage and Screening

- All non-musculoskeletal causes, as well as causes from related joints, should be ruled out.
- The patellar-pubic percussion test helps **rule out** (pooled SN 95, −LR 0.07) and **rule in** (pooled SP 86, +LR 6.1) femoral fracture.[109]
- The scour test, although limited on diagnostic investigation, is likely a good test for ruling out intra-articular involvement.

- Prostate cancer in men or any reproductive cancer or breast cancer in a woman is a red flag since these cancers may be associated with metastases to the lumbar spine or hip joint.[97]
- Clinicians should rule out lumbar spine and SIJ or pelvic girdle dysfunction.
- Soft-tissue and sacroiliac and lumbar joint ROM restrictions have been suggested to limit frontal-plane pelvic ROM during normal gait.[196]

IV. Motion Tests

- Clients usually have limitations in hip abduction and internal rotation ROM.
- Intrarater reliability is generally moderate to good for clients with hip intra-articular pathology.[126, 127, 199]

V. Muscle Performance Testing

- Clients are likely to have general hip weakness.[245]

VI. Special Tests

- No tests are specifically designated for this pathology.

VII. Palpation

- The anterior hip may be tender to palpation.[245]

VIII. Physical Performance Measures

- None is appropriate for the acutely diagnosed client.

POTENTIAL TREATMENT-BASED CLASSIFICATIONS

- If detected acutely, refer the client out to a physician.
- Stability
- Mobility, pain control (if pain dominant), and exercise and conditioning

Adductor Tendinopathy or Sport-Related Chronic Groin Pain

ICD-9: 762.5; 843.9 (sprains and strains of hip and thigh)

ICD-10: S76.2 (injury of adductor muscle and tendon of thigh)

This is a tendinopathy of the adductor muscle group. Sport-related chronic groin pain itself is a broad terminology potentially encompassing a multifactorial etiology of chronic groin pain in athletes.

I. Client Interview

Subjective History

- Pubic-related pain is most significant in soccer players[248, 249] and in hockey players.[250, 251]
- Pain occurs predominantly in the groin.[77, 248-252]
- Acutely injured athletes report a distinctive mechanism of injury with immediate pain and possibly hearing a pop.
- Several studies suggest a correlation between FAI and adductor tendinopathy, with prevalence as high as 94%,[253] although recent findings suggest this potential correlation does not prevent successful rehabilitation with long-term follow-up.[254]

Outcome Measures

- The Inguinal Pain Questionnaire is the only questionnaire investigating groin pain, but it is in need of further validation.[38]

Diagnostic Imaging

- Pubic edema is noted on MRI,[77, 255] although correlation to pathology is unknown.
- Magnetic resonance imaging is better at ruling in (**SP 88**, **+LR 4.0**) than ruling out (SN 78) sport-related chronic groin pain.[71]

II. Observation

- Acutely injured clients will have difficulty with adduction movements (e.g., supine to sit, getting in and out of car, and so on).
- Acutely injured clients may present with swelling or bruising of involved musculature.
- The hip being held in a resting position (hip flexion, slight abduction, and external rotation) generally indicates the presence of hip effusion.

III. Triage and Screening

- All non-musculoskeletal causes, as well as causes from related joints, should be ruled out.

- Clinicians should rule out urological, gynecological, rheumatologic, oncologic, and inflammatory sources of groin pain.[256]

- The patellar-pubic percussion test helps **rule out** (pooled SN 95, −LR 0.07) and **rule in** (pooled SP 86, +LR 6.1) femoral fracture.[109]

- The scour test, although limited on diagnostic investigation, is likely a good test for ruling out intra-articular involvement.

- Prostate cancer in men or any reproductive cancer or breast cancer in a woman is a red flag since these cancers may be associated with metastases to the lumbar spine or hip joint.[97]

- Clinicians should rule out lumbar spine and SIJ or pelvic girdle dysfunction.

- Soft-tissue and sacroiliac and lumbar joint ROM restrictions have been suggested to limit frontal-plane pelvic ROM during normal gait.[196]

IV. Motion Tests

- Restricted adductor flexibility is moderately associated with groin pain in athletes.[250]

- Limited hip IR and ER,[255] as well as total hip ROM, were noted in athletes with sport-related chronic groin pain.[252]

V. Muscle Performance Testing

- Evidence suggests a correlation between adductor muscle weakness and groin pain in hockey players[250, 251] and soccer players.[248, 249]

VI. Special Tests

- The single adductor (SP 91, +LR 3.3), squeeze test (SP 91, +LR 4.8), and bilateral adductor (SP 93, +LR 7.7) tests, when (+), all help rule in sport-related chronic groin pain.[27]

VII. Palpation

- Tenderness over adductors, especially proximally (and can be on pubis), is significant in these athletes.[27, 257, 258]

VIII. Physical Performance Measures

- Since these clients are most frequently athletes, the specific lower extremity functional components of the athlete's sport should be assessed.

- Speed and agility and quickness testing are likely most appropriate for most of these athletes.

POTENTIAL TREATMENT-BASED CLASSIFICATIONS

- Mobility, pain control (if pain dominant), and exercise and conditioning can be used.

Hamstring Strain

ICD-9: 843.9 (sprains and strains of hip and thigh)

ICD-10: S76.3 (injury of muscle and tendons of the posterior muscle group at thigh level)

A hamstring strain or injury is an excessive stretch or tearing of the muscle fibers of the hamstring muscles and related tissues. Hamstring strains can occur at one of the attachment sites or at any point along the length of the muscle. They are classified as first, second, or third degree depending on the severity.

- First degree: excessive stretching or minor tearing of a few muscle fibers. The pain can often be localized with one finger. Some stiffness and weakness will also be present. If exercise is attempted, the pain and stiffness may decrease during the activity but return after, often with much greater intensity.

- Second degree: moderate tearing of muscle fibers with pain generally covering a larger area than the first-degree strain. Stiffness and weakness will be felt, and the painful area may appear black and blue due to bleeding within the injured muscle. Significant limping may also occur when walking.

- Third degree: a complete tear of the muscle. Widespread bruising will be present. The clinician may see or feel a balling up of the muscle. Third-degree strains are a rare occurrence.

I. Client Interview

Subjective History

- More likely in athletes.[25, 26, 259-262]

- Acutely injured athletes report a distinctive mechanism of injury with immediate pain and possibly hearing a pop.

- Pain is located is the posterior thigh, often close to the buttock.

- Pain gets worse with activity involving resisted hip extension or resisted knee flexion (such as stairs).

- Hamstring injuries (HI) are one of the most common soft-tissue injuries in athletes.[25, 259, 263-267]

- In athletes, two proposed injury mechanisms include high-speed running and slow-speed overstretching (as in dancers).[25, 262] The role of the hamstrings is to brake knee extension (up to ~85% of running cycle—elongation stress).[268]

- Injury can also result from falling forward over a fixed foot and therefore from flexion at the hip with the knee relatively straight. This mechanism is also possible in waterskiers.[269]

- Clients complain of immediate pain with later presentation of ecchymosis and potential inflammation.[259, 269]

Outcome Measures

- Any appropriate hip measure can be used.

Diagnostic Imaging

- Magnetic resonance imaging and US are considered the criterion reference standards for diagnosis of hamstring injury,[270-272] although both MRI[273, 274] and US[275] continue to show (+) findings on clients returning to sport and should not be used as the sole criterion of a client's ability to return to sport.

II. Observation

- Acutely injured clients will likely present with limited weight bearing, decreased stride length during gait, and possible inflammation.[259, 269]

- The hip being held in a resting position (hip flexion, slight abduction, and external rotation) generally indicates the presence of hip effusion.

III. Triage and Screening

- All non-musculoskeletal causes, as well as causes from related joints, should be ruled out.

- The patellar-pubic percussion test helps **rule out** (pooled SN 95, −LR 0.07) and **rule in** (pooled SP 86, +LR 6.1) femoral fracture.[109]

- The scour test, although limited on diagnostic investigation, is likely a good test for ruling out hip intra-articular involvement.

- Prostate cancer in men or any reproductive cancer or breast cancer in a woman is a red flag since these cancers may be associated with metastases to the lumbar spine or hip joint.[97]

- Clinicians should rule out lumbar spine and SIJ or pelvic girdle dysfunction.

- Soft-tissue and sacroiliac and lumbar joint ROM restrictions have been suggested to limit frontal-plane pelvic ROM during normal gait.[196]

IV. Motion Tests

- Clients may have restricted hip flexion and combined hip flexion and knee extension ROM.[28, 269, 276, 277]

V. Muscle Performance Testing

- Clients have weakness in hip extension and in combined hip extension and knee flexion ROM.[28, 269, 276, 277]

- Eccentric hamstring weakness is most significant.[278]

VI. Special Tests

- The Puranen-Orava test, bent knee stretch, and modified bent knee stretch tests when (−) have less than good ability to help rule out (SN range of 76-89, −LR 0.12–0.29) and when (+) help rule in (SP range of 82-91, +LR 4.2–9.9) hamstring injury.[154]

- The taking off the shoe test, active ROM, passive ROM, and resisted ROM tests all have less than good ability to help rule out (SN range of 55-100, −LR 0.0–0.5) and rule in (SP 100) hamstring injury due to being performed in a study of high bias.[155]

- 57% of rugby players with grade I hamstring strain had adverse neural tension with the slump test.[279]

VII. Palpation

- Area is likely tender at the location of the tear.[26, 276, 280]

- The more distal the tenderness is to the ischial tuberosity, the longer the return to sport.[280]

VIII. Physical Performance Measures

- Since these clients are most frequently athletes, the specific lower extremity functional components of the athlete's sport should be assessed.

- Speed and agility and quickness testing are likely most appropriate for most of these athletes.

POTENTIAL TREATMENT-BASED CLASSIFICATIONS

- Pain (if pain dominant), mobility, and exercise and conditioning may be used.

Gluteus Medius Tendinopathy and Tear or Greater Trochanteric Pain Syndrome

ICD-9: 843.9 (sprains and strains of hip and thigh); GTPS: 726.5 (enthesopathy of hip region)

ICD-10: S76 (injury of muscle and tendon of hip); GTPS: M70.6 (trochanteric bursitis)

This involves tendinopathy, dysfunction, or altered muscle control of the gluteus medius muscle compared to an actual tear of the muscle itself. Greater trochanteric pain syndrome (GTPS) is defined as a history of lateral hip pain (LHP; 7 cm proximal and distal, and 3 cm anterior and posterior of the greater trochanter) and experiencing LHP with one or more of the following:

- When lying on the ipsilateral side
- During weight-bearing activities
- During sitting

I. Client Interview

Subjective History

- Gluteal tendinopathy most frequently occurs in late-middle-aged women.[281]

- Commonly presents with dull pain in the lateral hip.[281]

- Much of the subjective is similar to that described by clients with hip osteoarthritis: weakness, pain, functional limitation, and stiffness.

- Pain in lateral hip is worse with resisted hip abduction activities.[151, 281]

- GTPS is suggested to be defined as a history of LHP in the absence of difficulty with putting shoes and socks on.[157]

Outcome Measures

- The WOMAC, Physical Function Subscale, and LEFS have demonstrated clinical applicability in these clients, although they are highly influenced by client pain levels.[191-194]

Diagnostic Imaging

- Magnetic resonance imaging and US both appear to have capability to assist with **ruling in** and **ruling out** gluteal tendon tears across multiple studies.[68-70]

- Sclerotic bone reaction on radiography underlies gluteus medius tear in 55% of all clients with tears and 100% of all clients with large tears.[282]

- Of clients with trochanteric symptoms, 50% had gluteal tendinosis, 0.5% had gluteal tendon tears, and 29% had thickened IT band. 80% did not have bursitis on US.[283]

- 88% of hips with trochanteric symptoms had gluteal tendinopathy.[284]

- US findings demonstrate tendinopathy and bursal pathology coexist in GTPS.[70]

II. Observation

- Trendelenburg's sign is present in clients with gluteal tendinopathy or hip OA;[150, 166] therefore, clinicians should observe for a compensated or uncompensated gluteus medius gait pattern.

- Atrophy of gluteal muscles is suggestive of gluteal tendon or OA pathology.[82, 83]
- The hip being held in a resting position (hip flexion, slight abduction, and external rotation) generally indicates the presence of hip effusion.

III. Triage and Screening

- All non-musculoskeletal causes, as well as causes from related joints, should be ruled out.
- The patellar-pubic percussion test helps **rule out** (pooled SN 95, −LR 0.07) and **rule in** (pooled SP 86, +LR 6.1) femoral fracture.[109]
- Prostate cancer in men or any reproductive cancer or breast cancer in a woman is a red flag since these cancers may be associated with metastases to the lumbar spine or hip joint.[97]
- Clinicians should rule out lumbar spine and SIJ or pelvic girdle dysfunction.
- Soft-tissue and sacrolumbar joint ROM restrictions have been suggested to limit frontal-plane pelvic ROM during normal gait.[196]

IV. Motion Tests

- Decreased passive IR (SP 86, +LR 3.0) and pain with passive hip IR (SP 86, +LR 3.7) helps rule in gluteal tendinopathy.[150]
- Passive hip abduction test: A (+) test has good ability to help **rule in** (SP 93, +LR 8.3) gluteal tendinopathy.
- Intrarater reliability is generally moderate to good for clients with hip intra-articular pathology.[126, 127, 199]

V. Muscle Performance Testing

- Greater muscle strength, aerobic capacity, and standing balance were protective factors for preventing deterioration of functional status.[197, 198]
- Clients have gluteus medius and maximus weakness and atrophy.[82, 83, 150, 200, 281]
- Pain with resisted muscle testing of both gluteus medius and minimus helps **rule in** (SP 86, +LR 3.3) gluteal tendinopathy.[150]

VI. Special Tests

- A (+) restricted and painful (lateral hip pain) FABER test is strongly associated with GTPS and not OA (**SN 81, SP 82, +LR 4.5, −LR 0.23**).[157]
- FABER test: A (+) test has ideal ability to help **rule in** (SP 90, +LR 8.3) GTPS and a (−) test has good ability to help **rule out** (SN 83, −LR 0.19) GTPS.[157]
- Trendelenburg's sign: A (+) test has ideal ability (**SP 92, +LR 6.8**) in pooled analysis, and good (**SP 94, +LR 3.6**) to ideal ability (**SP 96, +LR 24.3**) in single studies to help rule in gluteal tendinopathy or GTPS.[109]
- Resisted external derotation test: A (+) test has ideal ability to help **rule in** (SP 97, +LR 32.6) and a (−) test has good ability to help **rule out** (SN 88, −LR 0.12) GTPS.[151]

VII. Palpation

- Gluteal musculature is most clinically applicable because the area is often focally tender.[281]

VIII. Physical Performance Measures

- Lower-level balance, fundamental movement, and such tests are most clinically applicable, if any tests at all are appropriate for the specific client.

POTENTIAL TREATMENT-BASED CLASSIFICATIONS

- Pain (if pain dominant), mobility, exercise and conditioning
- Possibly stability

Bursitis

ICD-9: 726.5 (enthesopathy of hip region); 727.3 (other bursitis)

ICD-10: (other specified injuries of hip and thigh)

Bursitis is the swelling and irritation of a bursa. A bursa is a fluid-filled sac that acts as a cushion between muscles, tendons, and joints. Trochanteric bursitis is inflammation of the trochanteric bursa, which is situated over the lateral trochanter. The bursa provides lubrication and cushioning to allow the muscles to flex and extend over the trochanter

Differential Diagnosis of Hip Osteoarthritis and Greater Trochanteric Pain Syndrome or Gluteus Medius Tendinopathy

- A (+) restricted *and* painful (lateral hip pain) FABER test is strongly associated with GTPS and not hip OA.
- Hip OA has a characteristic restricted ROM limitation (limited hip flexion and IR) with a characteristic hard end-feel.
- These pathologies, along with their findings, often coexist.
- Radiographic findings for hip OA are more significant (e.g., joint space narrowing, articular cartilage damage, potential osteophytes) than findings for GTPS.
- Subjective history of weakness, pain, functional limitations, and stiffness, as well as a (+) Trendelenburg sign can help rule in both pathologies.

without damaging the muscles. It also cushions the tendon before the attachment of the gluteus medius and minimus muscles. Other common bursae of the hip include the iliopsoas bursa and iliopectineal bursa. Bursitis, especially as an isolated pathology, must be questioned due to findings of low prevalence on imaging[283] and lack of bursal inflammation on histology, suggesting there is no etiologic role of bursal inflammation in the trochanteric pain syndrome.[285]

I. Client Interview

Subjective History

- Iliopsoas bursitis
  - Deep snapping sensation[286, 287]
  - Tenderness in the femoral triangle[286, 287]
  - Anterior hip pain with activity[286, 287]
  - Associated with trauma, overuse, athletic activity, osteoarthritis, and rheumatoid arthritis[286]
- Trochanteric bursitis
  - Associated with athletic activity, especially running and overuse[286, 288]
  - Can be associated with falls[286, 288]

Outcome Measures

- Any appropriate hip measures are applicable.

Diagnostic Imaging

- Of clients with trochanteric symptoms, 50% had gluteal tendinosis, 0.5% had gluteal tendon tears, and 29% had

thickened IT band. 80% did not have bursitis on US.[283]
- 88% of hips with trochanteric symptoms had gluteal tendinopathy.[284]

II. Observation

- Clients may have pain with transitional movements, especially those involving hip flexion to or from extension.[227]
- The hip being held in a resting position (hip flexion, slight abduction, and external rotation) generally indicates the presence of hip effusion.

III. Triage and Screening

- All non-musculoskeletal causes, as well as causes from related joints, should be ruled out.
- The patellar-pubic percussion test helps **rule out** (pooled SN 95, −LR 0.07) and **rule in** (pooled SP 86, +LR 6.1) femoral fracture.[109]
- Prostate cancer in men or any reproductive cancer or breast cancer in a woman is a red flag since these cancers may be associated with metastases to the lumbar spine or hip joint.[97]
- Clinicians should rule out lumbar spine and SIJ or pelvic girdle dysfunction.
- Soft-tissue and sacroiliac and lumbar joint ROM restrictions have been suggested to limit frontal-plane pelvic ROM during normal gait.[196]

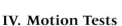

IV. Motion Tests

- Intrarater reliability is generally moderate to good for clients with hip intra-articular pathology.[126, 127, 199]
- Pain is reproduced with hip rotation, abduction, and adduction of hip.[286, 289]
- Clients have limited hip extension.[227]

V. Muscle Performance Testing

- Clients have pain and weakness with resisted hip flexion (especially iliopsoas), often with snapping.[286]

VI. Special Tests

- Pain may be elicited with resisted external derotation and FAIR tests (trochanteric bursitis).[151-153, 288]
- Pain may be elicited with hip impingement or labral tear testing involving flexion, adduction, or internal rotation movements.[216]
- Clients are likely to have (+) Thomas test for limited iliopsoas flexibility.[227, 287]

VII. Palpation

- Tenderness in femoral triangle (iliopsoas bursitis)[286, 287]
- Tenderness over lateral trochanter (trochanteric bursitis)[286, 288]

VIII. Physical Performance Measures

- Appropriate measures depend on the client's functional level, impairments, and occupation or hobbies.

POTENTIAL TREATMENT-BASED CLASSIFICATIONS

- Pain control may be used (if pain dominant); otherwise most likely treatments will be mobility or exercise and conditioning.

Piriformis Syndrome

ICD-9: 843.9 (sprains and strains of hip and thigh)

ICD-10: S76 (injury of muscle and tendon of hip)

Piriformis syndrome is often described similarly to other muscle and tendon dysfunctions (pain with resistance and with muscle elongation). It has also been described in presentation similarly to sciatica due its close anatomical proximity to the sciatic nerve and the view that dysfunction in this muscle can produce similar symptoms. Evidence findings supporting the clinical presentation of piriformis syndrome are described as follows.

I. Client Interview

Subjective History

- Pain is often described in the gluteal or buttock region, although the client may also have pain radiating down the involved leg.
- Clients may have a history of trauma, including a fall or twisting mechanism.
- Clients often have difficulty and pain with walking.
- Acute pain is often noted with squatting, bending, and stooping.

Differential Diagnosis of Age-Related Pathologies

The age of the client can assist with differential diagnosis of various hip pathologies:

- Pediatric age (typically aged 3 to 12 years) is more indicative of Legg-Calvé-Perthes disease.
- Adolescent age (typically 12 to 14.5 years) is more indicative of slipped capital femoral epiphysis.
- Adolescent to middle age is more likely indicative of femoroacetabular impingement or labral tear.
- Older adult age is more likely indicative of hip osteoarthritis and/or GTPS.
- Some pathologies, like AVN and FAI or labral tear, can exist across multiple age categories (adolescents through older adult).

Outcome Measures

- Any hip or lumbar spine measure can be applicable.

Diagnostic Imaging

- This syndrome typically requires a diagnosis of exclusion.

II. Observation

- The client may be reluctant to sit or shift weight onto the involved side.
- Clients may present with an antalgic gait pattern.
- Clients often have difficulty or pain posturing with squatting, standing up out of chair, stooping, and lifting activities.
- The hip being held in a resting position (hip flexion, slight abduction, and external rotation) generally indicates the presence of hip effusion.

III. Triage and Screening

- All non-musculoskeletal causes, as well as causes from related joints, should be ruled out.
- Clinicians should rule out sign of the buttock (see chapter 20, Sacroiliac Joint and Pelvic Girdle).
- The patellar-pubic percussion test helps **rule out** (pooled SN 95, −LR 0.07) and **rule in** (pooled SP 86, +LR 6.1) femoral fracture.[109]
- The scour test, although limited on diagnostic investigation, is likely a good test for ruling out intra-articular involvement.
- Prostate cancer in men or any reproductive cancer or breast cancer in a woman is a red flag since these cancers may be associated with metastases to the lumbar spine or hip joint.[97]
- Clinicians should rule out lumbar spine and SIJ or pelvic girdle dysfunction.
- Soft-tissue and sacroiliac and lumbar joint ROM restrictions have been suggested to limit frontal-plane pelvic ROM during normal gait.[196]

IV. Motion Tests

- Pain is often noted with passive internal rotation due to stretch of the piriformis.
- It is not common for clients to have accessory motion restrictions unless coexisting joint dysfunction is also present.

V. Muscle Performance Testing

- Clients have weakness in the hip, most notably with external and (to a lesser degree) internal rotation.
- Weakness may be present in gluteal muscles.
- Clients have pain with resisted hip external rotation.

VI. Special Tests

- FAIR test: A (−) test has less than good ability to help rule out (SN 88, −LR 0.14) and a (+) test helps rule in (SP 83, +LR 5.2) piriformis syndrome.[152, 153]
- Clinicians should always be cognizant of the fact that this position is similar to the FADDIR test for intra-articular hip pathology and should clearly discern where the client's pain reproduction is.

VII. Palpation

- The area will often be tender to palpation, generally in the involved side buttock, but more notably over the piriformis.

VIII. Physical Performance Measures

- Depend on the client's functional level
- Hip or lumbar spine assessments as appropriate for client

POTENTIAL TREATMENT-BASED CLASSIFICATIONS

- Pain control (if pain dominant), mobility (especially if related to joint dysfunction), and exercise and conditioning may be used.

CONCLUSION

The hip joint has an interdependent mechanical and pain-generation relationship with the lumbar spine, pelvis, and the knee joint. Differential diagnosis of this joint requires careful interpretation of the client's clinical presentation. Integration of best evidence as suggested here in this chapter, as well as the systematic examination approach, should be used to minimize further complicating the differential diagnosis of this region of the body. A systematic, evidence-based funnel approach suggests to the practicing clinician the importance of using all components of the examination process. Additionally, it suggests that the clinician focus on ruling out or screening for potential competing pathologies early in the examination process and attempting to rule in or diagnose particular pathologies later in the examination process. Utilization of a systematic screening process early in the examination funnels or narrows down potential competing diagnoses that can then be more likely ruled in with more SP findings or testing.

KNEE

David Logerstedt, PT, PhD, MPT, SCS
Michael P. Reiman, PT, DPT, OCS, SCS, ATC, FAAOMPT, CSCS

A primary goal of diagnosis is to match the client's clinical presentation with the most efficacious treatment approach.[1] Diagnosis of ligamentous injuries of the tibiofemoral joint can be made with a reasonable level of certainty with certain clinical findings.[2] For meniscal injuries, only a fair level of certainty can be made; for articular cartilage injuries, certainty is reduced to a low level.[3] In a small percentage of clients, trauma to the thigh and knee may be some-thing more serious than the commonly occurring injuries.[4, 5]

CLINICALLY APPLIED ANATOMY

The knee joint (figure 25.1) is actually comprised of two joints: the tibiofemoral joint and the

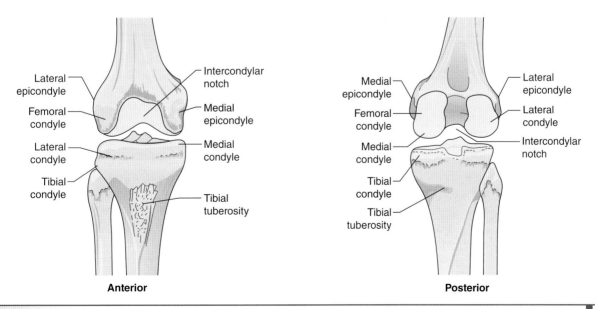

Figure 25.1 Knee joint.

patellofemoral joint. The tibiofemoral joint is the largest synovial joint in the body, connecting the two longest lever arms (femur and tibia). It is a modified hinge joint with two articulations (medial and lateral compartments), allowing flexion and extension with accessory rotation. It is a major weight-bearing joint, supporting two to five times body weight during functional activities. The functional stability of the tibiofemoral joint is derived from the passive restraint of the ligaments, the active support of muscles, the joint geometry, and the compressive forces between the tibia and femur.

The patellofemoral joint is comprised of the patella articulating with the trochlear groove. The patella is a large sesamoid bone embedded in the quadriceps mechanism. The role of the patella is to increase the torque of the quadriceps muscles by increasing the distance from the axis of motion. Additionally, it provides bony protection to the distal joint surfaces of the femoral condyles when the knee is flexed and prevents damaging compressive forces on the quadriceps tendon with resisted knee extension.

The ligamentous support provides passive stability to the knee joint (figure 25.2). Four primary ligaments (anterior cruciate ligament [ACL], posterior cruciate ligament [PCL], medial (tibial) collateral ligament [MCL], and lateral (fibular) collateral ligament [LCL]) provide the primary passive stability to the tibiofemoral joint. The ACL is the primary restraint to anterior translation of the tibia relative to the femur[6] and a major secondary restraint to internal rotation, particularly when the joint is near full extension.[7] The PCL is the primary restraint to posterior tibial translation, contributing about 90%

of the resistance across the knee flexion arc,[8] and is the secondary restraint to external rotation of the tibia on the femur.[9] The superficial MCL provides 57% of the restraining knee valgus moment at 5° of knee flexion and 78% of the restraining moment at 25° of knee flexion, due to decreased contribution from the posterior capsule.[10] The LCL is the main structure responsible for resisting varus moments, particularly in the initial 0° to 30° of knee flexion, and has a role in limiting external rotation of a flexed knee.[10]

The medial and lateral menisci cover the superior aspect of the tibia (figure 25.3).[11] Each meniscus is comprised of fibrocartilage. Although both are wedge shaped, the lateral meniscus is more circular, whereas the medial meniscus is more crescent shaped. The lateral meniscus is more mobile than the medial meniscus. The menisci function to distribute stress across the knee during weight bearing, provide shock absorption, serve as secondary joint stabilizers, facilitate joint gliding, prevent hyperextension, and protect the joint margins.[11]

The loads on the knee joint vary depending on the activity. Using an instrumented knee implant, average peak resultant forces range from 107% of body weight during double-leg stance to 346% of body weight during stair descent.[12]

CLIENT INTERVIEW

This interview is typically the first encounter the clinician will have with the client. As previously discussed in chapter 5 (Client Interview and Observation), this component of the examination can provide the clinician with a significant amount of information relevant to the probability of the client's presenting diagnosis. For purposes of this text, the interview is described relative to each body part or section but generally includes subjective reports by the client, as well as findings from their outcome measures. Also included in this section is radiographic imaging. While clinicians should avoid biasing their examination by interpreting findings of radiographic imaging prior to seeing the client (in most cases without concerns for red flags and major medical-related issues), this point in the examination is most likely where clinicians will encounter radiographic imaging. Additionally, in some instances, clinicians must interpret radiographic imaging early in the examination to rule out serious pathology prior to continuing with other components of the examination sequence.

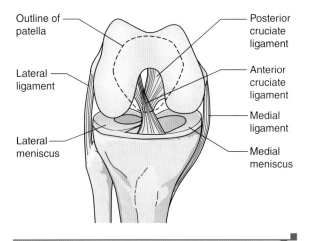

Figure 25.2 Ligaments of the tibiofemoral joint.

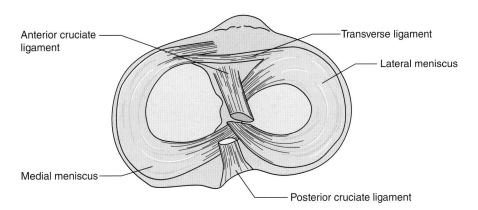

Figure 25.3 Menisci of the knee.

The examination process of the knee begins with the client interview. It allows the clinician to gather information from the client about the chief complaint, the mechanism of injury, and the location and irritability of pain associated with the injury. The clinician uses data gathered from the client interview to generate an initial set of hypotheses concerning the underlying cause of impairments and functional deficits[13] and the structures that are injured.[14] From this, the clinician can generate client-identified problem lists that can be used to guide and formulate an examination strategy.

Subjective

The client should be encouraged to describe in detail the specific location of their concordant pain. This is especially relevant in the location about the knee. Differential diagnosis of the knee provides some challenges to the clinician. A primary goal of diagnosis is to match the client's clinical presentation with the most efficacious treatment approach, as well as to determine whether physical therapy management is appropriate.[1] Complicating the differential diagnosis of the pain generator in the knee joint region are the multiple potential causes of pain in this area. Clearly delineating the specific cause requires deliberate questioning. Gathering details on the specific pain location, level of irritability, pain duration, and onset (all information discussed in chapter 5) is paramount.

Some specific questions are relevant to the knee joint. Knowing the age of the client will assist with differential diagnosis of knee pain. Pediatric and adolescent pathologies, such as Osgood-Schlatter lesion and Sinding-Larsen-Johansson lesion, will significantly differ in client age compared to patella tendinopathy (adolescents to older adults).

Mechanism of onset can assist with differential diagnosis of knee pathology. Careful questioning of the client can be extremely helpful in determining the potential primary structures involved. Deceleration and acceleration motions with noncontact valgus load at or near full extension are indicative of an ACL tear.[16, 17] A twisting injury may indicate a ligament or meniscal tear. Acute trauma with hemarthrosis within 2 hours is associated with intra-articular knee injuries (ACL tear, meniscus tear, or an osteochondral fracture).[18-20]

The clinician should therefore systematically differentially diagnose the commonly reported knee pain presentation. Paresthesia in the medial knee is more suggestive of saphenous nerve versus femoral peripheral nerve involvement (medial knee) once the lumbar spine is ruled out. Complaints of clicking, catching, snapping, or locking should include meniscal tear, intra-articular pathology, and osteochondral injury on the differential diagnosis.[20, 21] Carefully delineating the source (and relevance) of such symptoms is imperative to properly diagnosing the client. Thus, the question of whether the condition is worsening, staying the same, or improving is relevant, as is the degree to which the client's current symptoms affect their daily and recreational activities. Diagnosis such as knee osteoarthritis will likely continue to progress in terms of pathology, but the client may just limit their daily activities. Younger clients may report a greater influence on their activities due to unwillingness to limit such activities. Therefore, as with all other regions of assessment, the clinician should have a clear understanding of the client's symptoms, how they affect

Potential Causes of Knee Pain by Location

Anterior Knee Pain

Patellar subluxation or dislocation

Patellar apophysitis (Sinding-Larsen-
Johansson lesion)

Tibial apophysitis (Osgood-Schlatter lesion)

Patellar tendinitis (jumper's knee)

Patellofemoral pain syndrome

Medial Knee Pain

Tibial (medial) collateral ligament sprain

Medial meniscal tear

Pes anserine bursitis

Medial plica syndrome

Medial articular cartilage lesion

Slipped capital femoral epiphysis (referred from the
hip)

Lateral Knee Pain

Fibular (lateral) collateral ligament sprain

Lateral meniscal tear

Iliotibial band syndrome

Lateral articular cartilage lesion

Posterior Knee Pain

Popliteal cyst (Baker's cyst)

Posterior cruciate ligament injury

Posterolateral corner injury

Distal hamstring injury

Proximal gastrocnemius injury

Nonspecific Knee and Thigh or Leg Symptoms

Arthrofibrosis

Deep vein thrombosis

Dislocation

Fracture

Neurovascular compromise

Osteoarthritis

Rheumatoid arthritis

Septic arthritis

Referred pain from hip pathology

Peripheral nerve entrapment

Lumbar radiculopathy

Adapted from Calmbach and Hutchens 2003.[15]

their functional status, where the symptoms are located, aggravating and relieving factors, and so on.

Outcome Measures

Multiple outcome measures exist for the knee joint that are formulated, implemented in research studies, and utilized in daily clinical practice. The specific outcome measure utilized is sometimes dependent on the knee pathology. Investigation of the most efficacious knee outcome measure for ACL patients suggested that the IKDC 2000 subjective knee form was a more useful questionnaire than the KOOS;

however, the KOOS outperformed the IKDC 2000 for sports and recreation and quality of life subscales.[22] For the evaluation of treatment goals in clients with knee disorders, the following types of measurement instruments were recommended: validated patient-reported outcome measure, general health questionnaire, validated activity scale, physical performance measures, goniometry, and muscle strength testing.[2] The fact that multiple measures were recommended underlies the importance of a comprehensive assessment approach, as discussed in chapter 4 of this text. Function is a multifactorial variable that requires a comprehensive approach to assessment.

Caution against the isolated use of self-report assessments of physical function has been advocated since change in pain level significantly affected change in self-report measures of physical function.[23, 24] Physical performance measures, along with these self-report outcome measures, have been advocated as a more accurate measure of a client's function.[23, 24] As part of the comprehensive assessment of function, it has been suggested that clinicians develop a standardized battery of physical performance outcome measures to complement client-reported measures when capturing the construct of function in clients with knee injuries.[25, 26] Performance-based measures are important indicators of knee function after knee surgery,[27] and they capture different aspects of overall knee performance and function from physical impairments[25] and client-reported outcomes.[28-30] Both self-report measures and physical performance measures of physical function are needed for a more comprehensive assessment of function in clients with knee pathology.

Diagnostic Imaging

The knee is one of the most frequently injured joints in the body.[31] Radiographic examination of the knee is highly dependent on the type of pathology. Diagnostic imaging continues to be improved and refined. The use of diagnostic imaging can provide key information detailing soft tissue, articular surface, and bone injury and morphology, enhancing the clinician's ability to make informed clinical decisions. It can greatly help the clinician detect knee disorders and direct targeted treatment interventions. Diagnostic imaging requires appropriate interpretation; clinical decision making based solely on diagnostic imaging is not advised. Studies have found knee abnormalities in asymptomatic clients.[32-34] Therefore, it is recommended that clinical signs and symptoms match the findings from diagnostic imaging to provide clinicians with the best treatment options and with a more accurate prognosis.[19, 34, 35] Table 25.1 presents the diagnostic accuracy of different imaging modalities for specific conditions of the knee joint.

TABLE 25.1 Diagnostic Accuracy of Imaging Modalities for the Knee Joint

Pathology	Diagnostic test	Gold standard	SN/SP
Osteoarthritis	MRI	Variable	61/82[36]#
		Histology	74/76[36]#
		Radiographs	61/81[36]#
		Arthroscopy	0-86/48-95[37]
Articular cartilage abnormalities	MRI	Arthroscopy	26-96/50-100[37]
			83/94[38]
Meniscus tear	MRI	Arthroscopy	Pooled analysis: MM
			91/81[39]
			93/88[40]
			Pooled analysis: LM
			76/93[39]
			79/96[40]
ACL	MRI	Arthroscopy	Pooled analysis:
			87/95[39]
			94/94[40]
	Stress radiograph		81/82[41]
PCL	MRI	Arthroscopy	100/100[42]

\# = The Menashe study[36] investigated osteoarthritis in multiple joints (hip, knee and hand). The majority of studies were performed on knee osteoarthritis.
ACL = anterior cruciate ligament; PCL = posterior cruciate ligament; MM = medial meniscus; LM = lateral meniscus

The color coding for suggestion of **good** and **ideal** diagnostic accuracy values reported in this table are without quality scoring (QUADAS), a very important aspect of determination of the clinical utility of such values. Therefore, it is suggested that the reader keep this in mind when interpreting such values.

Radiographs

Plain film radiography is typically the first imaging step in the evaluation of knee disorders. Supine anteroposterior (AP) and cross-table lateral projections of the knee and patella, and the tangential projection (sunrise or Merchant methods) are recommended routine views for plain film radiography. Additionally, a posteroanterior axial view of the intercondylar fossa may be included. Limb-to-limb comparisons should be made. Standing series may be obtained in nontraumatic injuries and can best evaluate joint space and alignment.

The use of plain radiographs can reveal fractures, osteochondral lesions, bony malalignment and abnormalities, joint effusion, and joint space narrowing. Particular aspects of AP and lateral views include the following:

- Fractures of the distal femur and proximal tibia are likely visualized on AP and lateral views. Acute knee injuries should be assessed using the Ottawa Knee Rules.[43]

- Alignment of long axes of the femur and tibia, such as genu varum and genu valgum, can be seen.

- Kellgren-Lawrence grading is the accepted standard for radiographic osteoarthritis (OA) diagnosis (figure 25.4).[44]

  - Grade 0: No radiographic features of OA

  - Grade 1: Doubtful joint space narrowing, possible osteophyte formation

  - Grade 2: Possible joint space narrowing, defined osteophytes

  - Grade 3: Definite joint space narrowing, multiple osteophytes, possible bony malalignment

  - Grade 4: Large osteophyte formation, marked joint space narrowing, bony malalignment, bone sclerosis

- Marrow fat can be released into the joint if a fracture has extended into the joint, resulting in a lipohemarthrosis. It is best viewed from a lateral radiograph.

Tangential projection provides an axial view of the patellofemoral joint space and the articular cartilage of the patella and femur. Particular aspects of tangential views include the following:

- Patella disorders (fracture, subtle patella instability)

- Sulcus angle (figure 25.5): angle between the lines drawn from the highest points of the femoral condyles to the deepest point of the trochlear groove (142.4° ± 6.9° is considered normal)[45]

- Patella axis (figure 25.6): angle between the midline axial section of the patella and the line drawn parallel to the posterior femoral condyles[45]

- Lateral patellofemoral length (figure 25.7): distance between the most lateral part of the patella and the line drawn parallel to the lateral side of the femur condyle[45]

- Lateral patellofemoral angle (figure 25.8): angle between the line parallel to the tip of the anterior condyles and the lateral patellar facet[45]

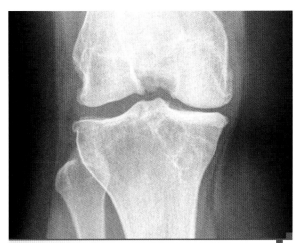

Figure 25.4 Radiography of osteoarthritic knee.

Courtesy of David Logerstedt

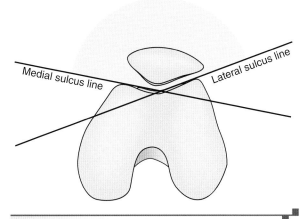

Figure 25.5 Sulcus angle.

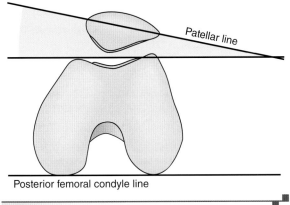

Figure 25.6 Patella axis.

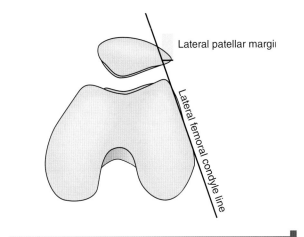

Figure 25.7 Lateral patellofemoral length.

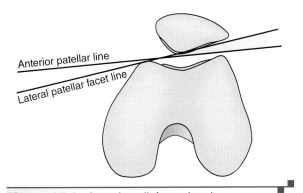

Figure 25.8 Lateral patellofemoral angle.

Ottawa Knee Rules A knee radiograph is required only for acute knee-injury clients with one or more of these findings related to age, tenderness, or function: [43]

- Age 55 years or older
- Tenderness at head of fibula
- Isolated tenderness of patella
- Inability to flex to 90°
- Inability to bear weight both immediately and in the emergency department (four steps)

The presence of one or more of these findings would have identified the 68 fractures in the study population with a sensitivity (SN) of 100 (95% confidence interval [CI], 95-100) and a specificity (SP) of 54 (51-57). Application of the rule would have led to a 28% relative reduction in the use of radiography from 68.6% to 49.4% in the study population.

Additional studies have supported the use of this rule. Prospective validation has shown the Ottawa Knee Rules to be 100% SN for identifying fractures of the knee and to have the potential to allow physicians to reduce the use of radiography in clients with acute knee injuries. [46] Additionally, a systematic review of six studies involving 4,249 adult clients determined a pooled SN of 98.5, –LR of 0.05, and a pooled SP of 49. [47]

Pittsburg Decision Rule This decision rule states that a knee radiograph is required only for an acute fall or blunt trauma and with clients who have either the inability to ambulate or an age younger than 12 or older than 50 years. [48] This decision rule has been validated with good results, SN ranging from 77 to 100, and SP ranging from 57 to 79. [48-50] A study also suggested that it had better pooled SP (51) than the Ottawa Knee Rules (27) when compared directly. [51]

Magnetic Resonance Imaging

Clinical examination by well-trained clinicians may be as accurate as magnetic resonance imaging (MRI) in regard to the diagnosis of ligamentous and meniscal lesions (figure 25.9) of the knee joint. [19, 35, 52] For articular cartilage pathology, clinical examination is frequently inconclusive because clients present with nonspecific symptoms of joint pain or swelling that may not develop until late in the course of the disease. [53, 54] MRI may be reserved for clients with persistent symptoms of pain and swelling that may indicate occult cartilage or meniscal pathology. [35] Limited diagnostic accuracy of MRI accuracy has been undertaken with respect to articular cartilage degeneration or arthritic changes in the knee joint. Extensive variability regarding diagnostic accuracy has been shown currently. [37] There is evidence in some MRI protocols that MRI is a relatively valid, SN, SP, accurate, and reliable clinical tool for

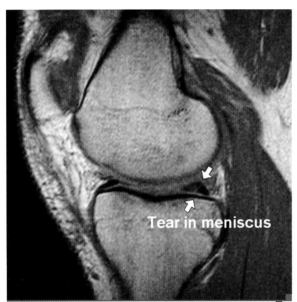

Figure 25.9 MRI of knee with meniscal tear.
© MedPix

identifying articular cartilage degeneration. Unfortunately, due to the heterogeneity of MRI sequences, it is not possible to make definitive conclusions regarding its global clinical utility for guiding diagnosis and treatment strategies.[37]

Computed Tomography

Computed tomography (CT) can be helpful in the diagnosis of subtle fractures following knee trauma when radiographs are negative. CT arthrography has the most accuracy for evaluating cartilage thickness.[55] It is more reliable for delineating focal cartilage lesions[56] and visualizing subchondral bone sclerosis and osteophyte formation.[55, 57]

Review of Systems

Refer to chapter 6 (Triage and Differential Diagnosis) for detail on review of systems relevant to the knee.

OBSERVATION

Observation of the client presenting with knee pain should (as with all portions of the body) include general postural assessment (static and dynamic), gait, transfers, and potential limitations in strength and mobility with daily tasks. Static posture assessment should be viewed from both the anteropos-

terior and lateral views. Looking for asymmetry from side to side can alert the clinician to structural abnormalities. Iliac crest height, greater trochanter height, anterior and posterior superior iliac spine levels (as also observed for the lumbar spine and pelvis), leg length discrepancy, genu valgus and varus, and knee flexion can alert the clinician to some potential structural dysfunctions that may be contributing to the client's knee pain.

While more detail regarding posture is given in chapter 14, some additional things are worth mentioning here. From all views, the clinician should assess for scars, skin discoloration, changes in texture, and so on. From both the lateral and anterior views, the clinician can assess for quadriceps atrophy, which is strongly correlated with quadriceps weakness.[58]

After a knee injury, clients typically demonstrate an antalgic gait pattern. A knee stiffening strategy (decreased knee flexion with increased co-contraction of the quadriceps and hamstrings muscles) during stance phase of gait can be seen after an ACL injury.[59] In those with dynamic knee instability or pain, a reduced knee extension moment and stance time on the injured limb may develop. Changes in hip excursion may also be present after ACL injury.[60] Many clients with medial knee OA exhibit an increase in external knee adduction moment, which predicts the presence,[61] severity,[62] and rate of progression of the disease.[63] Similarly to other knee disorders, clients with knee OA ambulate with knee stiffening strategy.

Limitations in knee range of motion (ROM) can influence activities of daily living. Stance phase of gait on level surfaces requires 20° of knee flexion, while swing phase requires 70° of knee flexion.[64] Ascending and descending stairs require 80° to 110° of knee flexion, respectively. Sitting in or rising from a chair requires 85° of knee flexion, while donning a sock or tying a shoelace requires 120° of knee flexion. Difficulty performing such daily tasks can alert the clinician as to which particular motions to more closely examine.

TRIAGE AND SCREENING

Triage and screening is a necessary component of the examination process that must be completed prior to continuing with the examination. As with all specific body part examinations, at this point the clinician must decide whether or not to continue with the examination. Specifically, they should determine whether to continue examining the client or refer them to a physician. Ruling out serious pathology (refer to chapter 6, Triage and Differential Diagnosis) and pain generation from other related (or close-proximity) structures assists the clinician with more accurately determining the necessity of continuing with the other examination components to identify the actual source of the client's pain. Additionally, clinicians should implement strong screening tests (tests of high SN and low –LR) at this point in the examination to narrow down the competing diagnoses of the respective body region(s) (lumbar spine, pelvis, and hip in this case) when this is applicable.

Ruling Out Serious Pathology: Red Flags

Clinicians must be able to recognize clients with serious pathology and refer them to the appropriate health care professional.[65] Red flag findings can be indicators of serious pathology. Red flag concerns for the knee and distal lower extremity include fractures, peripheral arterial disease, deep venous thrombosis, compartment syndrome, septic arthritis, and cellulitis. Fractures have been well investigated with respect to the knee. The Ottawa Knee Rules,[43] as previously described, should be implemented in any case with suspicion of fracture. Once red flag concerns are alleviated, the clinician should rule out pain referral from another region of the body as listed in the following section.

Rule Out Fracture

The report of any knee trauma should alert the clinician to the possibility of fracture. Properly identifying when to obtain radiographs can eliminate unnecessary radiographs and can be cost-effective.[47]

- Ottawa Knee Rules for screening or diagnosing knee fracture
  - Pooled analysis: **SN 99 (93-100)**, SP 49 (43-51), +LR 1.9, **–LR 0.02**, across six studies with 4,249 adult clients (radiography reference standard)[47]
  - **SN 100 (96-100)**, SP 52 (49-55), +LR 2.1, **–LR 0.01** for identifying fractures of the knee and allowing physicians to reduce the use of radiography in clients with acute knee injuries[46]

- Pittsburg Decision Rule
  - Pooled analysis: **SN 86 (57-96)**, SP 51 (44-59), +LR 1.8, **–LR 0.27**, across 90 injured clients (radiography reference standard)[51]

Ruling Out Pain Generation From Other Related Structures

Once red flags are ruled out, an efficient way to begin to differentiate the many potential pain referral sources is through the lower quarter screening examination. The traditional lower quarter screen consists of testing of dermatomes, myotomes, deep tendon reflexes, and possible upper motor involvement. The clinician should differentially diagnose the potential contribution of the sacroiliac joint or pelvic girdle, lumbar spine, and hip as the primary pain generator for the client's knee pain. Screening tests for these areas are employed to limit the extent of the differential diagnosis for pathology contributing to the client's knee pain. A systematic approach to ruling out these other areas is suggested. The key points of this approach are listed here. Refer to chapters 19 (Lumbar Spine) and 20 (Sacroiliac Joint and Pelvic Girdle) for greater detail regarding these examination procedures.

Rule Out Lumbar Spine

The following section lists suggested special tests for ruling out the lumbar spine as a potential pain generator for the client with presentation of knee pain. The details of each of these tests can be found in chapter 19.

Radiculopathy or Discogenic-Related Pathology   This is ruled out with a combination of ROM and special tests assessments.

Repeated Motions (ROM)

Centralization and peripheralization: 5-20 reps

- **SN 92 (not reported, or NR)**, SP 64 (NR), +LR 2.6, **–LR 0.12**, QUADAS 12[66]
- SN 40 (28-54), **SP 94 (73-99)**, **+LR 6.7**, –LR 0.64, QUADAS 13[67]

Special Tests

- Straight leg raise test
  - **SN 97 (NR)**, SP 57 (NR), +LR 2.3, **–LR 0.05**, QUADAS 10[68]
  - Pooled analysis: **SN 92 (87-95)**, SP 28 (18-40), +LR 2.9, **–LR 0.29**[69]

- Slump test
  - **SN 83 (NR)**, SP 55 (NR), +LR 1.8, **−LR 0.32**, QUADAS 11[70]

Facet Joint Dysfunction   This is ruled out with the seated extension–rotation test. As noted in the lumbar spine chapter, facet joint dysfunction is ruled in with posterior-to-anterior spinal joint-play assessments eliciting stiffness and concordant pain.

- Seated extension–rotation: **SN 100 (NR)**, SP 22 (NR), +LR 1.3, **−LR 0.0**, QUADAS 11[71]

Rule Out SI Joint Dysfunction

Sacroiliac joint (SIJ) dysfunction is ruled out with pain provocation cluster testing and the thigh thrust test.

- Pain provocation cluster testing:[72] **SN 91 (62-98)**, **SP 83 (68-96)**, **+LR 6.97**, **−LR 0.11**, QUADAS 13
- Thigh thrust test: **SN 88 (64-97)**, SP 69 (47-82), +LR 2.80, **−LR 0.18**; QUADAS 12[73]

Rule Out Hip Joint Dysfunction

Hip ROM limitations should be ruled out in all planes (see chapter 24). Intra-articular hip joint involvement is ruled out with the flexion-adduction-internal rotation (FADDIR) test:

- Pooled **SN 94 (88-97)**, SP 8 (2-20), +LR 1.02, **−LR 0.48**, across four studies with 128 clients (MRA reference standard)[74]
- Pooled **SN 99 (95-100)**, SP 7 (0-34), +LR 1.06, **−LR 0.15**, across two studies with 157 clients (arthroscopy reference standard)[74]

As with any joint, clearing AROM with or without overpressure is necessary. AROM of all motions as per the lower quarter screen described in chapter 7 should be implemented. In order to fully clear the hip joint, full AROM (with overpressure if pain-free) must be present.

Additionally, as with any joint, clearing AROM with or without overpressure is necessary. In order to fully clear the knee joint, full AROM (with overpressure if pain-free) must be present. Detail in this regard is described in the following section.

MOTION TESTS

Motion assessment is a very important aspect of the examination for the orthopedic client. Motion dysfunction can be used to differentiate contractile versus non-contractile tissue (see chapter 9). Assessment of end-feel, potential capsular patterns, and ROM norm values can give the clinician an appreciation of the potential impairments for the orthopedic client they are assessing (table 25.2).

TABLE 25.2   Knee Joint Arthrology

Joint	Close-packed position	Resting position	Capsular pattern	ROM norms	End-feel
Tibiofemoral	Full extension and external rotation of tibia	25–30° flexion	Flexion > extension	0–150°	Flexion = soft-tissue approximation Extension = firm
Tibiofibular	Ankle dorsiflexion	0° of ankle plantar flexion	Pain with contraction of the biceps femoris		Firm
Patellofemoral	Full knee flexion	Hyperextension to 5° of knee flexion		Moves 8-10 mm from full flexion to extension	
Motions of the patellofemoral joint include flexion and extension, medial and lateral glides, medial and lateral tilts, medial and lateral rotation, and anterior and posterior tilts. With knee flexion, the patella will inferiorly glide and vice versa with knee extension. The patella also goes through medial and lateral gliding motions. During lateral glide, the lateral edge of the patella moves closer to the lateral side of the knee. During medial glide, the medial side moves toward the medial edge of the knee.					

Active ROM, PROM, and joint-play assessments are necessary to determine not only the presence or absence of joint dysfunction but also the precise aspects of the motion that are dysfunctional.

Loss of range of motion after a knee injury is a common impairment, but it can be devastating to the functional recovery of the client. Active motion testing of the knee can indicate a client's ability and willingness to perform the motion, the amount of range of motion available, and muscle function. Passive motion testing provides the clinician with information regarding joint end-feel and irritability of the joint.

Passive and Active ROMs

Intrarater reliability of knee passive ROM was shown to be good to excellent (intraclass correlation coefficient or ICC = 0.85–0.99) and interrater reliability of knee passive ROM was moderate to excellent (ICC = 0.62–0.99).[75] Intrarater reliability of knee active knee extension was good ($ICC_{2,1}$ = 0.85) and knee active flexion was excellent ($ICC_{2,1}$ = 0.95).[76] When assessing passive and active ROM, the clinician should consider the potential pathology. Clients with ACL injury or reconstruction, meniscus or articular cartilage surgery, and knee osteoarthritis, for example, have limited knee extension and flexion,[77, 78] while clients with patellofemoral pain syndrome and patella tendinopathy infrequently exhibit reduced ROM. Therefore, the clinician can expect to find such impairments when assessing clients suspected of having these pathologies.

KNEE FLEXION

Client Position	Supine with the leg to be assessed lying straight on the table
Clinician Position	Seated directly to the side of the client
Goniometer Alignment	The fulcrum is centered over the lateral epicondyle, the proximal arm is aligned with the midline of the femur (greater trochanter as a reference), and the distal arm is aligned with the midline of the fibula (using the lateral malleolus and fibular head for reference).
Movement	The clinician passively flexes the client's hip to 90° and stabilizes the thigh with their proximal hand and passively flexes the heel toward the buttock to end range flexion (normal end-feel is soft in most clients due to soft tissue approximation). This motion can be performed similarly actively by the client (without assistance from the clinician). Active range of motion should be performed prior to PROM to determine the client's willingness to move and so on.
Assessment	Clinician assesses for amount of ROM, end-feel, quality of the movement, client response, potential difference between AROM and PROM, and so on.

KNEE EXTENSION

Client Position	Supine with heel of the leg to be assessed placed on a bolster
Clinician Position	Seated directly to the side of the client
Goniometer Alignment	The fulcrum is centered over the lateral epicondyle, the proximal arm is aligned with the midline of the femur (greater trochanter as a reference), and the distal arm is aligned with the midline of the fibula (using the lateral malleolus and fibular head for reference).
Movement	The clinician passively extends the client's knee to end range extension (normal end-feel is firm). This motion can be performed similarly actively by the client (without assistance from the clinician). Active range of motion should be performed prior to PROM to determine the client's willingness to move and so on.
Assessment	The clinician assesses for amount of ROM, end-feel, quality of the movement, client response, potential difference between AROM and PROM, and so on.

Passive Accessories

Passive accessory motion is the movement that occurs between one articulating joint surface relative to another. These motions are also referred to as *joint arthrokinematics*. Passive accessory motion assessment is essential for determining the potential for joint-play dysfunction in the joints being examined. The following section details distinct component assessments of passive joint mobility for the knee and patellofemoral joint.

Little to no reliability or validity testing for passive accessory motion for the knee or patellofemoral joints has been published. A few unpublished dissertations have reported poor to fair reliability of passive accessory motion testing in the knee.[79-81]

TIBIOFEMORAL JOINT DISTRACTION

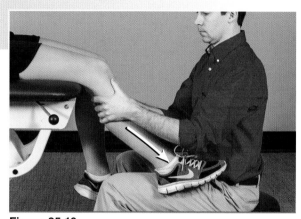
Figure 25.10

Client Position	Sitting with the leg to be assessed hanging over the edge of the table, with the knee bent to approximately 25°
Clinician Position	Sitting, directly facing the client's knee to be assessed.
Stabilization	The rest of the client's body on the table serves as a stabilizing force.
Movement and Direction of Force	With both hands, the clinician purchases the proximal tibia on the medial and lateral sides. They can also perform the assessment with the client in supine and the femur stabilized under a solid towel roll or small bolster. The clinician uses both hands to simultaneously distract the tibia distally in a direction parallel to the long axis of the tibia.
Assessment	Assessment is done for joint play/passive accessory motion, client response, and end-feel. Reproduction of concordant pain suggests dysfunction. Impaired joint mobility or end-feel may also suggest dysfunction if concordant pain is also reproduced.

TIBIOFEMORAL JOINT POSTERIOR GLIDE

Figure 25.11

Client Position	Sitting with the leg to be assessed hanging over the edge of the table, and the knee bent approximately 25°
Clinician Position	Sitting, directly facing the client's knee to be assessed
Stabilization	The client's body resting on the table serves as a stabilizing force. The clinician's stabilizing hand (right as shown) purchases the distal femur and holds it against the table.
Movement and Direction of Force	The clinician's assessing hand (left as shown) purchases the proximal tibia on the anterior surface (primary purchase with web space of hand). Assessment can also be performed with the client in supine and the femur stabilized under a solid towel roll or small bolster. The clinician uses their assessing hand to glide the tibia in a posterior direction.

Assessment Assessment is done for joint play/passive accessory motion, client response, and end-feel. Reproduction of concordant pain suggests dysfunction. Impaired joint mobility or end-feel may also suggest dysfunction if concordant pain is also reproduced.

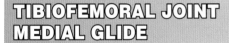

TIBIOFEMORAL JOINT ANTERIOR GLIDE

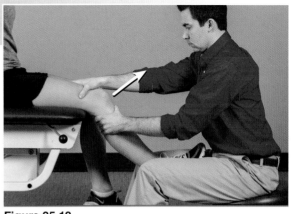

Figure 25.12

Client Position	Sitting with the leg to be assessed hanging over the edge of the table and the knee bent approximately 25°
Clinician Position	Sitting, directly facing the client's knee to be assessed
Stabilization	The client's body resting on the table serves as a stabilizing force. The clinician's stabilizing hand (right as shown) purchases the distal femur and holds it against the table.
Movement and Direction of Force	The clinician's assessing hand (left as shown) purchases the proximal tibia on the posterior surface (primary purchase with fingers). Assessment can also be performed with the client in supine and the femur stabilized under a solid towel roll or small bolster. The clinician uses their assessing hand to glide the tibia in an anterior direction.
Assessment	Assessment is done for joint play/passive accessory motion, client response, and end-feel. Reproduction of concordant pain suggests dysfunction. Impaired joint mobility or end-feel may also suggest dysfunction if concordant pain is also reproduced.

TIBIOFEMORAL JOINT MEDIAL GLIDE

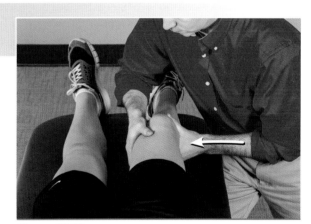

Figure 25.13

Client Position	Supine on a table
Clinician Position	Standing at the side of client's leg to be assessed
Stabilization	The client's body resting on the table serves as a stabilizing force. The client's knee is flexed approximately 25°. The clinician's stabilizing hand (right as shown) purchases the distal femur from the medial side.
Movement and Direction of Force	The clinician's assessing hand (left as shown) is parallel to the stabilizing hand. This hand purchases the lateral proximal aspect of the tibia primarily with the web space. The clinician uses their assessing hand to glide the proximal tibia in a medial direction.
Assessment	Assessment is done for joint play/passive accessory motion, client response, and end-feel. Reproduction of concordant pain suggests dysfunction. Impaired joint mobility or end-feel may also suggest dysfunction if concordant pain is also reproduced.

TIBIOFEMORAL JOINT LATERAL GLIDE

Client Position	Supine on a table
Clinician Position	Standing at the side of the client's leg to be assessed
Stabilization	The client's body resting on the table serves as a stabilizing force. The client's knee is flexed approximately 25°. The clinician's stabilizing hand (left hand as shown) purchases the distal femur from the lateral side.
Movement and Direction of Force	The clinician's assessing hand (right as shown) is parallel to the stabilizing hand. This hand purchases the medial proximal aspect of the tibia primarily with the web space. The clinician uses their assessing hand to glide the proximal tibia in a lateral direction.
Assessment	Assessment is done for joint play/accessory motion, client response, and end-feel. Reproduction of concordant pain suggests dysfunction. Impaired joint mobility or end-feel may also suggest dysfunction if concordant pain is also reproduced.

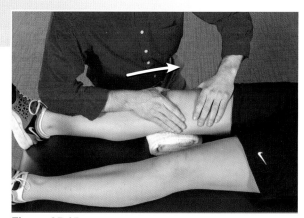

Figure 25.14

PATELLOFEMORAL JOINT SUPERIOR GLIDE

Client Position	Supine on a table
Clinician Position	Sitting at the side of the client's leg to be assessed
Stabilization	The client's body resting on the table serves as a stabilizing force. The client's knee is flexed approximately 5° to 10°. The clinician's stabilizing hand (left as shown) purchases the distal femur.
Movement and Direction of Force	The clinician's assessing hand (right as shown) is placed along the tibia. It purchases the distal patella with the web space between the thumb and index finger (broad, comfortable purchase). The clinician uses their assessing hand to glide the patella along the plane of the joint in a superior direction.
Assessment	Assessment is done for joint play/passive accessory motion, client response, and end-feel. Reproduction of concordant pain suggests dysfunction. Impaired joint mobility or end-feel may also suggest dysfunction if concordant pain is also reproduced.

Figure 25.15

PATELLOFEMORAL JOINT INFERIOR GLIDE

Client Position	Supine on a table
Clinician Position	Sitting at the side of their client's leg to be assessed
Stabilization	The client's body resting on the table serves as a stabilizing force. The client's knee is flexed approximately 5° to 10°. The clinician's stabilizing hand (right as shown) purchases the proximal tibia.
Movement and Direction of Force	The clinician's assessing hand (left as shown) is placed along femur. It purchases the proximal patella with the web space between the thumb and index finger (broad, comfortable purchase). The clinician uses their assessing hand to glide the patella along the plane of the joint in an inferior direction.
Assessment	Assessment is done for joint play/passive accessory motion, client response, and end-feel. Reproduction of concordant pain suggests dysfunction. Impaired joint mobility or end-feel may also suggest dysfunction if concordant pain is also reproduced.

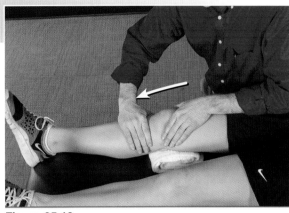

Figure 25.16

PATELLOFEMORAL JOINT MEDIAL GLIDE

Client Position	Supine on a table
Clinician Position	Sitting at the side of the client's leg to be assessed
Stabilization	The client's body resting on the table serves as a stabilizing force. The client's knee is flexed approximately 5° to 10°.
Movement and Direction of Force	The clinician purchases bilateral thumbs (or the heel of one hand) on the lateral border of the patella (broad, comfortable purchase) (as shown). The clinician uses bilateral thumbs (or the heel of one hand) to glide the patella in a medial direction.
Assessment	Assessment is done for joint play/passive accessory motion, client response, and end-feel. Reproduction of concordant pain suggests dysfunction. Impaired joint mobility or end-feel may also suggest dysfunction if concordant pain is also reproduced.

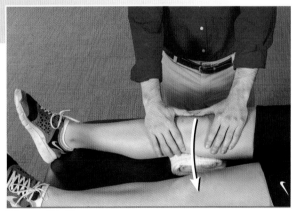

Figure 25.17

PATELLOFEMORAL JOINT LATERAL GLIDE

Client Position	Supine on a table
Clinician Position	Sitting at the side of the client's leg to be assessed
Stabilization	The client's body resting on the table serves as a stabilizing force. The client's knee is flexed approximately 5° to 10°.
Movement and Direction of Force	The clinician purchases bilateral thumbs (or the heel of one hand) on the medial border of the patella (broad, comfortable purchase) (as shown). The clinician uses bilateral thumbs (or the heel of one hand) to glide the patella in a lateral direction.

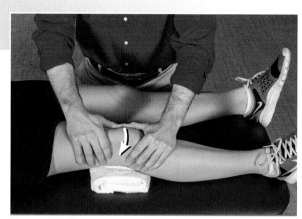

Figure 25.18

Assessment	Assessment is done for joint play/passive accessory motion, client response, and end-feel. Reproduction of concordant pain suggests dysfunction. Impaired joint mobility or end-feel may also suggest dysfunction if concordant pain is also reproduced.

PATELLOFEMORAL JOINT MEDIAL TILT

Client Position	Supine on a table
Clinician Position	Sitting at the side of the client's leg to be assessed
Stabilization	The client's body resting on the table serves as a stabilizing force. The client's knee is flexed approximately 5° to 10°.
Movement and Direction of Force	The clinician purchases bilateral thumbs on the lateral border of the patella, just under the inferior lateral edge (broad, comfortable purchase) (as shown). The clinician uses bilateral thumbs to lift the lateral border of the patella in an anterior direction (tilting the medial border posteriorly into the trochlear groove).

Figure 25.19

Assessment	Assessment is done for joint play/passive accessory motion, client response, and end-feel. Reproduction of concordant pain suggests dysfunction. Impaired joint mobility or end-feel may also suggest dysfunction if concordant pain is also reproduced.

PATELLOFEMORAL JOINT LATERAL TILT

This is not commonly a necessary assessment due to patella lateral tilt orientation. If it is necessary to assess, the purchase would be on the medial border of the patella, and the patella would be tilted laterally.

Flexibility

Refer to chapter 24 (Hip) for flexibility assessments appropriate for the knee.

MUSCLE PERFORMANCE TESTING

The diagnostic accuracy of manual muscle testing for knee extension is limited as a screening tool for strength impairments.[82] Muscle imbalances and asymmetries are modifiable risk factors that can contribute to injury or reinjury in the knee. Athletes are more likely to sustain more lower-extremity injuries if knee flexor and hip extensor strength asymmetries are present.[83, 84] Athletes with eccentric hamstring strength asymmetries were at greater risk of sustaining a hamstring muscle injury than those without asymmetries.[85] Athletes in field sports had an increased risk with ankle strength imbalances,[86] and had an increased risk of trauma with low hamstring-to-quadriceps ratio and increased risk of overuse with high hamstring-to-quadriceps ratio.[87] Asymmetries in the lower extremity exist after injury[88] and can persist for years.[89]

KNEE FLEXION

Client Position	Prone, leg straight and foot off end of table
Clinician Position	Standing directly to the side of the client
Movement and Assessment	The client is instructed to flex the knee to less than 90° as the clinician resists just proximal to ankle. The clinician can place their other hand over the hamstring tendons. With the leg in internal rotation, the clinician can assess the medial hamstrings. With the leg in external rotation, they can assess the lateral hamstrings.

- Grade 5: completes motion against maximal resistance
- Grade 4: completes motion against strong resistance
- Grade 3: completes motion without resistance

The position to assess for grade 2 is side lying with the non-testing leg on table and the leg to be assessed straight and supported by the clinician.

- Grade 2: completes full ROM in side-lying gravity-minimized position

For the following grades, the client is in a prone position, as with grades 5, 4, and 3:

- Grade 1: tendons become prominent without movement
- Grade 0: no muscle activity

Primary Muscles	Hamstrings

- Biceps femoris
- Semitendinosus
- Semimembranosus

Secondary Muscles	Sartorius
	Gracilis
	Gastrocnemius
	Popliteus
	Plantaris
Primary Nerves	Common peroneal nerve (sciatic; L5-S2; biceps femoris)
	Tibial (sciatic; L5-S2; all 3 muscles)

KNEE EXTENSION

Client Position	Sitting, with a towel under the distal thigh and tibia hanging vertically off the edge of the table
Clinician Position	Standing directly to the side of the client
Movement and Direction of Force	The client is instructed to extend their knee as the clinician resists on the dorsum of the distal tibia, just proximal to the ankle. Slightly flexing the knee is suggested to avoid locking the knee out.

- Grade 5: completes motion against maximal resistance
- Grade 4: completes motion against strong resistance
- Grade 3: completes motion without resistance

The position to assess for grades below 3 is side lying with the non-testing leg on the table and the leg to be assessed held in about 90° flexion and supported by the clinician.

- Grade 2: completes full ROM in prone gravity-minimized position
- Grade 1: muscle activity without movement
- Grade 0: no muscle activity

Primary Muscles	Quadriceps femoris

- Rectus femoris
- Vastus medialis longus and oblique
- Vastus lateralis
- Vastus intermedius

Primary Nerve	Femoral nerve (L2-4; entire quadriceps femoris)

SPECIAL TESTS

As mentioned in chapter 10 (Special Tests), in many cases the clinician is overly dependent on the performance and interpretation of special test findings with respect to differential diagnosis of the client's presenting pain. Utilization of special tests for ruling in (or helping to diagnose) a particular pathology should occur at this point in the examination process. It is also hoped that the clinician has a much clearer picture of the client's presentation prior to this point in the examination and will therefore depend minimally on special test findings with respect to diagnosis of the client's pain.

A significant number of pathologies and special tests are relevant to the knee. The knee has also had a fair amount of investigation undertaken regarding the diagnostic accuracy of the special tests for each relevant pathology. As with each of the other chapters in parts III and IV of this text, the reader is advised to look at systematic reviews and meta-analysis (when available). The tests with the strongest diagnostic accuracy and clinical applicability are highlighted as appropriate.

Index of Special Tests

Fracture of Knee

Ottawa Knee Rules (see Diagnostic Imaging section for full description)

Meniscal Tear

Composite Physical Examination

McMurray's Test

Thessaly Test

Ege's Test

Apley's Test

Joint Line Tenderness

Steinmann Sign I

Steinmann Sign II

Axial Pivot-Shift Test

Dynamic Knee Test

Medial-Lateral Grind Test

Bounce-Home Test

Squat or Duck Waddle Test

Forced Flexion

Effusion

Payr Sign

Anterior Cruciate Ligament Tear and Anterior Rotary Instability

Composite Physical Examination

Lachman's Test

Anterior Drawer Test

Pivot Shift Test

Anterior Drawer in External Rotation (ACL and Anterior-Medial Instability)

Anterior Drawer in Internal Rotation (ACL and Anterior-Lateral Instability)

Active Lachman's Test

Posterior Cruciate Ligament Tear and Posterior Rotary Instability

Composite Physical Examination

Posterior Sag Sign (Godfrey's Test)

Quadriceps Active Drawer

Reverse Pivot-Shift Test (posterolateral instability tear)

Reverse Lachman's Test (Trillet's Test)

Posterior Drawer Test

Medial Collateral Ligament Tear

Valgus Stress Test at 30° Knee Flexion

Lateral Collateral Ligament Tear

Varus Stress Test

Composite Physical Examination

Patellofemoral Pain Syndrome

Q-Angle Measurement

Patellar Tilt Test

Patellar Apprehension Test

Pain With Squatting

Pain With Stair Climbing

Pain With Kneeling

Resisted Knee Extension

Compression Test

Waldron's Test Phase 1 (supine)

Waldron's Test Phase 2 (standing)

Clarke's Sign or Patellar Grind Test

Lateral Pull Test

Eccentric Step-Down Test

Palpation for Tendinopathy

Plica Syndrome

Composite Physical Examination

Proximal Tibiofibular Joint Instability

Fibular Head Translation Test

Radulescu Sign

Knee Effusion

Modified Stroke Test

Ballottement Test

Self-Noticed Swelling

Cluster of Test Findings

Knee Osteoarthritis

Composite Examination for Osteoarthritis

Osteochondral Lesion

Composite Examination for Loose Bodies

Composite Examination for Chondral Fracture

Case Studies

Go to www.HumanKinetics.com/OrthopedicClinicalExamination and complete these case studies for chapter 25:

- Case study 1 discusses a 48-year-old male with complaints of catching and pain in his right medial knee.
- Case study 2 discusses a 16-year-old female who injured her knee while playing soccer.

Abstract Links

Go to www.HumanKinetics.com/OrthopedicClinicalExamination to access abstract links on these issues:

Anterior cruciate ligament tear, composite physical exam

Apley's test

Bounce-home test

Dynamic knee test

Ege's test

Forced flexion

Knee effusion

Lachman test

McMurray's test

Medial-lateral grind test

Meniscal tear, composite physical exam

Pain provocation cluster testing

Patellar tendinopathy

Patellofemoral pain syndrome

Payr sign

Pivot shift test

Posterior cruciate ligament tear, composite physical exam

Posterior drawer test

Proximal tibiofibular joint instability

Repeated motions, centralization and peripheralization

Slump test

Steinmann sign I

Straight leg raise test

Thessaly test

MENISCAL TEAR

COMPOSITE PHYSICAL EXAMINATION

Multiple studies have included different clusters of findings to establish a composite physical exam:

- Pooled analysis: **SN 86 (79-92)**, SP 72 (61-83), +LR 3.1, **–LR 0.19**, in a study of 274 clients with medial meniscus injuries across five studies, using arthroscopy and MRI as reference standards[18]
- Pooled analysis: **SN 88 (77-99)**, **SP 92 (89-95)**, **+LR 11**, **–LR 0.13**, in a study of 274 clients with lateral meniscus injuries across five studies, using arthroscopy and MRI as reference standards[18]
- **SN 87 (NR)**, SP 68 (NR), +LR 2.7, **–LR 0.19**, QUADAS 10, in a study of medial meniscal tears in 50 clients with differential diagnosis of meniscal tear (mean age 22 years; 13 women; mean duration of symptoms NR), using joint-line tenderness and McMurray, Steinmann, and modified Apley's tests as the physical exam and MRI as a reference standard[35]
- SN 75 (NR), **SP 95 (NR)**, **+LR 15**, –LR 0.26, QUADAS 10, in a study of lateral meniscal tears in 50 clients with differential diagnosis of meniscal tear (mean age 22 years, 13 women, mean duration of symptoms NR) using joint-line tenderness, and McMurray, Steinmann, and modified Apley's tests as the physical exam and MRI as a reference standard[35]

- SN 87 (NR), **SP 93 (NR)**, **+LR 12.4**, –LR 0.14, QUADAS 9, in a study of 290 clients with medial meniscus injuries (mean age 38 years; 97 women; mean duration of symptoms NR), using arthroscopy as a reference standard[90]
- **SN 81 (NR)**, **SP 93 (NR)**, **+LR 11.6**, **–LR 0.10**, QUADAS 9, in a study of 290 clients with lateral meniscus injuries (mean age 38 years; 97 women; mean duration of symptoms NR), using arthroscopy as a reference standard[90]
- **SN 87 (NR)**, **SP 93 (NR)**, **+LR 12.4**, **–LR 0.14**, QUADAS 9, in a study of 195 clients with intra-articular lesions (medial meniscus injuries; mean age 36 years; 73 women; mean duration of symptoms NR), using arthroscopy as a reference standard[91]
- **SN 81 (NR)**, **SP 93 (NR)**, **+LR 11.6**, **–LR 0.2**, QUADAS 9, in a study of 195 clients with intra-articular lesions (lateral meniscus injuries; mean age 36 years; 73 women; mean duration of symptoms NR), using arthroscopy as a reference standard[91]

MCMURRAY'S TEST

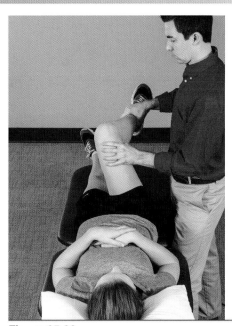 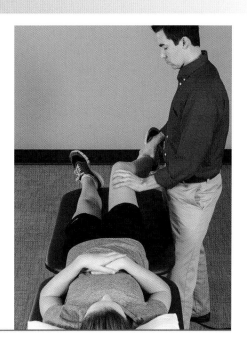

Figure 25.20

Client Position	Supine on a table
Clinician Position	Standing directly next to the limb being tested. The clinician grasps the ankle of the tested limb with their distal hand (right as shown) and places their proximal hand (right as shown) on the lateral aspect of the distal femur (as shown) or on anterior aspect of the tested knee. The thumb of the proximal hand can be placed over the lateral joint line and the middle finger is placed over the medial joint line if purchase is on the anterior knee and clinician can adequately control the knee with this purchase.
Movement	To assess the integrity of the medial meniscus, the clinician maximally flexes and externally rotates the tested knee, and slowly extends the knee. To assess the integrity of the lateral meniscus, the clinician maximally flexes and internally rotates the tested knee, and slowly extends the knee. A varus or valgus stress may be applied during the McMurray test.
Assessment	A (+) test is indicated if a palpable or audible thud or click is appreciated. Isolated re-creation of pain constitutes a (+) test.
Statistics	• Pooled analysis: SN 75 (71-79), SP 67 (64-69), +LR 2.3, –LR 0.37, across six studies with QUADAS score > 10 with 931 clients[92]
	• Pooled analysis: SN 55 (50-60), SP 77 (62-87), +LR 2.4, –LR 0.58, across four studies with 1,232 clients[93]

(continued)

McMurray's Test *(continued)*

- SN 50 (38-62), SP 77 (57-90), +LR 2, −LR 0.6, QUADAS 8, in a study of medial meniscal tears in 109 clients with differential diagnosis of meniscal tear (mean age 39 ± 12; 29 women; mean duration of symptoms NR), and arthroscopy as a reference standard[94]
- SN 21 (9-43), SP 94 (85-98), +LR 3, −LR 0.8, QUADAS 8, in a study of lateral meniscal tears in 109 clients with differential diagnosis of meniscal tear (mean age 39 ± 12; 29 women; mean duration of symptoms NR), and arthroscopy as a reference standard[94]
- SN 28 (NR), **SP 92 (NR)**, **+LR 3.5**, −LR 0.8, QUADAS 11, in a study of 63 clients with knee injury (mean age, gender, and mean duration of symptoms NR), and MRI as a reference standard[95]
- SN 50 (NR), SP 78 (NR), +LR 2.3, −LR 0.6, QUADAS 11, in a study of 32 clients with medial meniscus tear (mean age 27 years; 2 women; mean duration of symptoms NR), and arthroscopy as a reference standard[96]
- SN 79 (NR), SP 40 (NR), +LR 1.3, −LR 0.5, QUADAS 10, for meniscal tears in a study of 80 clients with an ACL injury (mean age 26.6; 4 women; mean duration of symptoms NR), and arthroscopy as the reference standard[97]
- SN 16 (NR), **SP 98 (NR)**, **+LR 8**, −LR 0.9, QUADAS 10, in a study of medial meniscal tears in 104 clients with differential diagnosis of meniscal tear (mean age, gender, and mean duration of symptoms NR), and arthroscopy as a reference standard[98]

Note Many authors suggest the described rotation biases as described above are not particular to either the medial or lateral meniscus as both are potentially being stressed.

THESSALY TEST

 Video 25.21 **in the web resource shows a demonstration of this test.**

Client Position	Standing on the tested lower extremity with the tested knee flexed to 5° and then 20°
Clinician Position	Standing directly in front of the client as shown to permit the client to use the clinician's hands as upper extremity support
Movement	The client is asked to internally and externally rotate their knee and body three times (rotate their body).
Assessment	A (+) test is indicated if discomfort or a sense of locking or catching in the knee over the medial or lateral joint line occurs.

Statistics

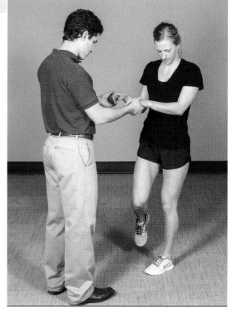

Figure 25.21

- SN 41 (30-54), SP 68 (47-84), +LR 1, −LR 0.9, QUADAS 8, for Thessaly test at 5° in a study of medial meniscal tears in 109 clients with differential diagnosis of meniscal tear (mean age 39 ± 12; 29 women; mean duration of symptoms NR), and arthroscopy as a reference standard[94]
- SN 66 (NR), **SP 96 (NR)**, **+LR 16**, −LR 0.35, QUADAS 9, for Thessaly test at 5° in a study of medial meniscal tears in 213 clients with a knee injury with an initial diagnosis of meniscal tear (mean age 29.4 years; 56 women; mean duration of symptoms NR), and MRI as a reference standard[99]
- SN 59 (47-71), SP 67 (45-83), +LR 2, −LR 0.6, QUADAS 8, for Thessaly test at 20° in a study of medial meniscal tears in 109 clients with differential diagnosis of meniscal tear (mean age 39 ± 12; 29 women; mean duration of symptoms NR), and arthroscopy as a reference standard[94]

- **SN 89 (NR), SP 97 (NR), +LR 29, −LR 0.11**, QUADAS 9, for Thessaly test at 20° in a study of medial meniscal tears in a study of medial meniscal tears in 213 clients with a knee injury with an initial diagnosis of meniscal tear (mean age 29.4 years; 56 women; mean duration of symptoms NR), and MRI as a reference standard[99]
- SN 16 (6-38), SP 89 (78-94), +LR 1, −LR 0.9, QUADAS 8, for Thessaly test at 5° in a study of lateral meniscal tears in 109 clients with differential diagnosis of meniscal tear (mean age 39 ± 12; 29 women; mean duration of symptoms NR), and arthroscopy as a reference standard[94]
- **SN 81 (NR), SP 91 (NR), +LR 9, −LR 0.21**, QUADAS 9, for Thessaly test at 5° in a study of lateral meniscal tears in 213 clients with a knee injury with an initial diagnosis of meniscal tear (mean age 29.4 years; 56 women; mean duration of symptoms NR), and MRI as a reference standard[99]
- SN 31 (15-54), SP 95 (87-98), +LR 6, −LR 0.7, QUADAS 8 for Thessaly test at 20° in a study of lateral meniscal tears in 109 clients with differential diagnosis of meniscal tear (mean age 39 ± 12; 29 women; mean duration of symptoms NR), and arthroscopy as a reference standard[94]
- **SN 92 (NR), SP 96 (NR), +LR 23, −LR 0.08**, QUADAS 9, for Thessaly test at 20° in a study of lateral meniscal tears in 213 clients with a knee injury with an initial diagnosis of meniscal tear (mean age 29.4 years; 56 women; mean duration of symptoms NR), and MRI as a reference standard[99]

EGE'S TEST

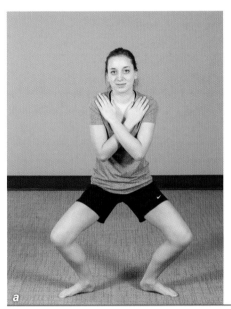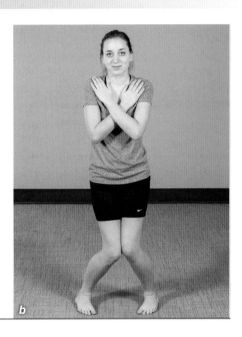

Figure 25.22

Client Position	Standing with bilateral knees in full extension and feet 30 to 40 cm apart
Clinician Position	Standing in front of the client
Movement	For detecting a medial meniscus, the client maximally externally rotates both lower extremities and then squats *(a)* and returns to full erect standing slowly. For detecting a lateral meniscus, the client maximally internally rotates both lower extremities and then squats *(b)* and returns to full erect standing slowly.
Assessment	A pain or a click on the corresponding joint line is considered a (+) test.
Statistics	• SN 67 (NR), SP 81 (NR), +LR 3.5, −LR 0.4, QUADAS 11, for detecting medial meniscal tears in a study of 150 clients with meniscal tears (mean age 35.7 years; 40 women; mean duration of symptoms NR), and arthroscopy as a reference standard[100] • SN 64 (NR), **SP 90 (NR)**, **+LR 6.4**, −LR 0.4, QUADAS 11, for detecting lateral meniscal tears in a study of 150 clients with meniscal tears (mean age 35.7 years; 40 women; mean duration of symptoms NR), and arthroscopy as a reference standard[100]

APLEY'S TEST

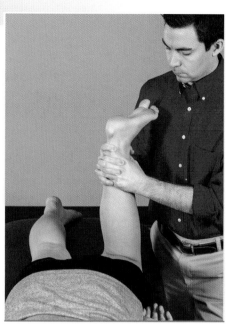

Figure 25.23

Client Position	Prone on a table
Clinician Position	Standing directly next to the limb being tested. The clinician grasps the ankle of the tested limb and flexes the knee to 90°.
Movement	With the client's knee flexed to 90°, the clinician distracts and rotates the tibia. The clinician then compresses and rotates the tibia.
Assessment	Worsening pain with distraction and rotation is considered a (+) test for a soft-tissue sprain. Worsening pain with compression and rotation is considered a (+) test for meniscal tear.
Statistics	• SN 41 (NR), **SP 93 (NR)**, **+LR 5.9**, –LR 0.6, QUADAS 9, in a study of 213 clients with medial meniscus tear (mean age 29.4 years; 56 women; mean duration of symptoms NR), and MRI as a reference standard[99]
	• **SN 81 (NR)**, SP 56 (NR), +LR 1.8, **–LR 0.3**, QUADAS 11, in a study of 32 clients with medial meniscus tear (mean age 27 years; 2 women; mean duration of symptoms NR), and arthroscopy as a reference standard[96]

• SN 41 (NR), SP 86 (NR), +LR 2.9, –LR 0.7, QUADAS 9, in a study of 213 clients with lateral meniscus tear (mean age 29.4 years; 56 women; mean duration of symptoms NR), and MRI as a reference standard[99]

• SN 13 (NR), SP 90 (NR), +LR 1.3, –LR 1.0, QUADAS 10, in a study of 156 clients with meniscus tear (mean age 23 years; 73 women; mean duration of symptoms NR), and arthroscopy as a reference standard[101]

• SN 16 (NR), SP 80 (NR), +LR 0.8, –LR 1.1, QUADAS 10, in a study of 161 clients with meniscus tear (mean age 33 years; 55 women; mean duration of symptoms NR), and arthroscopy as a reference standard[102]

JOINT LINE TENDERNESS

Client Position	Supine on a table
Clinician Position	Standing next to the testing leg
Movement	The clinician palpates the medial and lateral joint lines of the knee.
Assessment	The presence of tenderness along the medial or lateral joint line of the knee indicates a (+) finding.
Statistics	• Pooled analysis: SN 76 (73-80), SP 77 (64-87), +LR 3.3, –LR 0.31, across four studies with 1,354 subjects[93]
	• SN 83 (71-90), SP 76 (55-86), +LR 3, –LR 0.2, QUADAS 8, in a study of medial meniscal tears in 109 clients with differential diagnosis of meniscal tear (mean age 39 ± 12 years; 29 women; mean duration of symptoms NR), and arthroscopy as a reference standard[94]
	• SN 68 (46-85), SP 97 (89-99), +LR 22, –LR 0.3, QUADAS 8, in a study of lateral meniscal tears in 109 clients with differential diagnosis of meniscal tear (mean age 39 ± 12 years; 29 women; mean duration of symptoms NR), and arthroscopy as a reference standard[94]

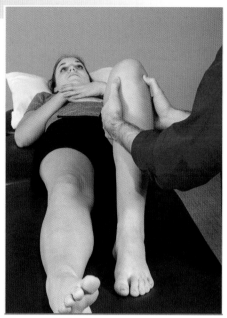

Figure 25.24

STEINMANN SIGN I

Client Position	Supine on a table
Clinician Position	Standing next to the testing leg
Movement	The clinician grasps the heel of the tested limb with their distal hand and places their contralateral hand (proximal) on the anterior aspect of the tested knee. The thumb of the proximal hand is placed over the lateral joint line and the middle finger is placed over the medial joint line. The clinician flexes the knee and hip to varying degrees and then internally and externally rotates the tibia without flexing or extending the knee.
Assessment	Joint-line pain is considered a (+) test for meniscal tear.
Statistics	• SN 29 (NR), **SP 100 (NR), +LR Inf**, –LR 0.7, QUADAS 11, in a study of 63 clients with knee injury (mean age, sex, and mean duration of symptoms NR), and MRI as a reference standard[95]
	• SN 66 (NR), **SP 83 (NR), +LR 3.9**, –LR 0.4, QUADAS 11, in a study of 32 clients with medial meniscus tear (mean age 27 years; 2 women; mean duration of symptoms NR), and arthroscopy as a reference standard[96]
	• **SN 86 (NR), SP 88 (NR), +LR 7.2, –LR 0.2**, QUADAS 9, in a study of 68 clients with meniscal tear (mean age, sex, and mean duration of symptoms NR), and arthroscopy as a reference standard[103]

STEINMANN SIGN II

Client Position	Supine on a table
Clinician Position	Standing next to the testing leg
Movement	The clinician grasps the heel of the tested limb with their distal hand and places their contralateral hand (proximal) on the anterior aspect of the tested knee. The thumb of the proximal hand is placed over the lateral joint line and the middle finger is placed over the medial joint line. The clinician flexes the knee and hip to varying degrees.
Assessment	Joint-line pain that moves in posterior direction during knee flexion is considered a (+) test for meniscal tear.
Statistics	NR

AXIAL PIVOT-SHIFT TEST

Client Position	Supine with bilateral legs and arms relaxed
Clinician Position	Standing directly to the side of the client on the side of the leg to be assessed
Movement	The clinician applies a valgus and internal rotational torque at the proximal tibia. The clinician applies an axial load through the foot while flexing the knee to 30° to 45° of knee flexion. The combined valgus, internal rotation, and axial load is continually applied while the knee is extended to the starting position.
Assessment	Joint-line pain or click felt by the clinician indicates a (+) test for meniscal tear.
Statistics	SN 71 (NR), **SP 83 (NR)**, **+LR 4.2**, –LR 0.4, QUADAS 10, study of 156 clients with meniscus tear (mean age 23 years; 73 women; mean duration of symptoms NR), and arthroscopy as a reference standard[101]

DYNAMIC KNEE TEST

Client Position	Supine on a table, with the knee flexed to 90° and the hip abducted to 60°, flexed to 45°, and externally rotated
Clinician Position	Standing next to the testing leg, palpating the lateral joint line
Movement	The clinician adducts the hip while the knee maintains 90° flexion.
Assessment	Sharp pain at end range of hip adduction or an increase in pain at the lateral joint line is considered a (+) test for lateral meniscus injury.
Statistics	SN 85 (NR), **SP 90 (NR)**, **+LR 8.5**, –LR 0.2, QUADAS 9, in a study of 421 (knees) clients with lateral meniscus tear (mean age, sex, mean duration of symptoms NR), and arthroscopy as a reference standard[104]

MEDIAL-LATERAL GRIND TEST

Client Position Supine on a table

Clinician Position Standing next to the testing leg

Movement The clinician grasps the heel of the tested limb with their distal hand and places their contralateral hand (proximal) on the anterior aspect of the tested knee. The thumb of the proximal hand is placed over the lateral joint line and the middle finger is placed over the medial joint line. The clinician applies a valgus torque to the knee as the knee is flexed to 45°. The clinician applies a varus torque to the knee as the knee is extended. The combined motion is circumduction of the knee.

Assessment A grinding sensation felt by the clinician indicates a (+) test for a meniscus tear.

Statistics SN 70 (NR), SP 67 (NR), +LR 2.1, –LR 0.45, QUADAS 9, in a study of 93 clients (100 knees) with meniscal tear (mean age 31 years; 24 women; mean duration of symptoms NR), and arthroscopy as a reference standard[105]

BOUNCE-HOME TEST

Client Position Supine on a table

Clinician Position Standing at the end of the testing leg

Movement The clinician extends the test knee to end-range extension.

Assessment A mechanical block that limits full knee extension or pain at extension end-range indicates (+) test for a meniscus tear.

Statistics
- SN 47 (NR), SP 67 (NR), +LR 1.4, –LR 0.8, QUADAS 10, study of 156 clients with meniscus tear (mean age 23 years; 73 women; mean duration of symptoms NR), and arthroscopy as a reference standard[101]
- SN 38 (NR), SP 67 (NR), +LR 1.2, –LR 0.9, QUADAS 9, in a study of 200 clients with meniscus tear (mean age, sex, and mean duration of symptoms NR), and arthroscopy as a reference standard[106]
- SN 44 (NR), SP 85 (NR), +LR 2.9, –LR 0.7, QUADAS 10, in a study of 161 clients with meniscus tear (mean age 33 years; 55 women; mean duration of symptoms NR), and arthroscopy as a reference standard[102]

SQUAT OR DUCK WADDLE TEST

Client Position Standing

Clinician Position Standing in front of the client

Movement The client squats; if no pain is reproduced, the client walks like a duck.

Assessment A mechanical block that limits full knee flexion or pain at flexion end-range indicates (+) test for a meniscus tear.

Statistics
- SN 55 (NR), SP 67 (NR), +LR 1.7, –LR 0.7, QUADAS 9, in a study of 200 clients with meniscus tear (mean age, sex, and mean duration of symptoms NR), and arthroscopy as a reference standard[106]
- SN 68 (NR), SP 60 (NR), +LR 1.7, –LR 0.5, QUADAS 11, in a study of 100 clients with knee injury (mean age 27.9 years; 5 women; mean duration of symptoms NR), and MRI as a reference standard[95]

FORCED FLEXION

Client Position	Supine on a table
Clinician Position	Standing at the end of the testing leg
Movement	The clinician flexes the test knee to end-range extension.
Assessment	A mechanical block that limits full knee flexion or pain at flexion end-range indicates (+) test for a meniscus tear.
Statistics	• SN 44 (NR), SP 57 (NR), +LR 1.0, –LR 1.0, QUADAS 9, in a study of 200 clients with meniscus tear (mean age, sex, and duration of symptoms NR), and arthroscopy as a reference standard[106]
	• SN 50 (NR), SP 68 (NR), +LR 1.6, –LR 0.7, QUADAS 10, in a study of 161 clients with meniscus tear (mean age 33 years; 55 women; mean duration of symptoms NR), and arthroscopy as a reference standard[102]
	• SN 77 (NR), SP 41 (NR), +LR 1.3, –LR 0.6, QUADAS 11, in a study of 134 clients with meniscus tear (mean age 40.2 ± 12.2 years; 70 women; mean duration of symptoms NR), and MRI as a reference standard[107]

EFFUSION

Client Position	Supine on a table
Clinician Position	Standing next to the client
Movement	The clinician measures the amount of swelling about the knee.
Assessment	More swelling present on the test knee compared to the contralateral knee indicates (+) test for a meniscus tear.
Statistics	SN 53 (NR), SP 54 (NR), +LR 1.2, –LR 0.9, QUADAS 9, in a study of 200 clients with meniscus tear (mean age, sex, and duration of symptoms NR), and arthroscopy as a reference standard[106]

PAYR SIGN

Client Position	Seated on a table with the foot of the test leg on the contralateral knee, forming a figure-four position
Clinician Position	Standing next to the client's test leg
Movement	The clinician pushes the affected knee downward toward the floor.
Assessment	Pain over the medial joint line indicates a (+) test for a posterior horn tear of the medial meniscus.
Statistics	SN 54 (NR), SP 44 (NR), +LR 1.0, –LR 1.1, QUADAS 11, in a study of 64 clients with meniscus tear (mean 38.5 years; 22 women; mean duration of symptoms NR), and arthroscopy as a reference standard[108]

Critical Clinical Pearls

When performing tests to assess the integrity of a ligament, a positive test is indicated from the following:

- Increase in excursion compared to the contralateral knee
- Abnormal end-feel compared to the contralateral knee
- Pain in the ligament when force is applied

ANTERIOR CRUCIATE LIGAMENT TEAR

COMPOSITE PHYSICAL EXAMINATION

- SN 62 (NR), SP 75 (NR), +LR 2.5, –LR 0.5, QUADAS 12, in a study of 118 clients with acute knee injury (mean age, sex, and duration of symptoms NR), using Lachman's test and the anterior drawer test as the physical exam for ACL tear and examination under anesthesia as a reference standard for an ACL tear. The diagnostic accuracy of composite physical exam is limited due to the sample size and injury rate.[109]

- **SN 100 (75-100), SP 99 (94-100), +LR 100, –LR 0**, QUADAS 10, in 100 clients with ACL tears (mean age, sex, and mean duration of symptoms NR), using Lachman's test, the anterior drawer test, and the pivot shift test as the physical exam for ACL tear and MRI as the reference standard.[110]

- **SN 100 (NR), SP 100 (NR), +LR Inf, –LR Inf**, QUADAS 10, in a study of 50 clients with differential diagnosis of ACL tear (mean age 22 years; 13 women; mean duration of symptoms NR), using Lachman's test, the anterior drawer test, and the pivot shift test as the physical exam and MRI as the reference standard.[35]

- **SN 81 (NR), SP 91 (NR), +LR 9, –LR 0.2**, QUADAS 11, in a study of 32 children and adolescents (mean age 12.6 ± 2.1 years; 18 women; mean duration of symptoms NR), using a clinical examination and MRI as a reference standard.[111]

- SN 18 (0-36), **SP 98 (96-100), +LR 9.8**, –LR 0.8, QUADAS 11, in a study of 134 clients with an acute knee injury (mean age 40.2 ± 12.2; 60 women; mean duration of symptoms NR), using a history of effusion, popping, and episodes of giving way and MRI as the reference standard.[112]

- SN 19 (0-38), **SP 99 (98-100), +LR 19.9**, –LR 0.8, QUADAS 11, in a study of 134 clients with an acute knee injury (mean age 40.2 ± 12.2; 60 women; mean duration of symptoms NR), using an anterior drawer test and a history of effusion, popping, and episodes of giving way and MRI as the reference standard.[112]

LACHMAN'S TEST

 Video 25.25 in the web resource shows a demonstration of this test.

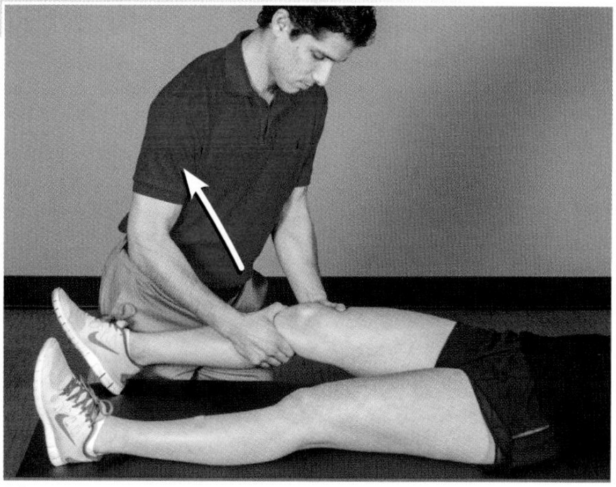

Client Position	Supine on a table with the involved knee in 20° to 30° knee flexion
Clinician Position	Standing directly next to the limb being tested
Movement	The clinician stabilizes the femur with one hand (left as shown) and places the other hand (right as shown) on the posteromedial aspect of the proximal tibia with the thumb placed over the anteromedial aspect of the proximal tibia. A force is applied anteriorly to displace the tibia.

Figure 25.25

Assessment	Increased anterior tibial excursion relative to the femur with a soft end-feel compared to the contralateral knee indicates a (+) test.
Statistics	• Pooled **SN 85 (83-87), SP 94 (92-95), +LR 10.2, –LR 0.2**, in a meta-analysis of 1,729 clients with both acute and chronic ACL tears[113]
	• Pooled **SN 94 (91-96), SP 97 (93-99), +LR 9.4, –LR 0.1**, in a meta-analysis of 377 clients with acute ACL tears[113]

(continued)

Lachman's Test *(continued)*

- Pooled **SN 95 (91-97)**, **SP 90 (87-94)**, **+LR 7.1**, **–LR 0.2**, in a meta-analysis of 375 clients with chronic ACL tears[113]
- Pooled **SN 87 (76-98)**, **SP 93 (89-96)**, **+LR 12.4**, **–LR 0.14**, in a study of 274 clients with knee injuries and arthroscopy for ACL tears and MRI as reference standards[18]

ANTERIOR DRAWER TEST

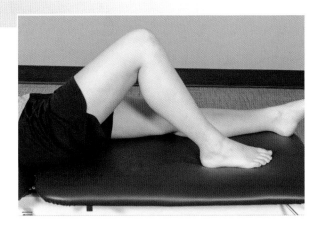

Client Position	Supine hook lying with knee flexed 90° and foot on table
Clinician Position	Sitting on client's foot to stabilize leg
Movement	The clinician places bilateral hands on the posterior aspect of the tibia and their thumbs on each respective joint line. The clinician translates the proximal tibia anteriorly and assesses motion.
Assessment	Increased anterior tibial excursion relative to the femur with a soft end-feel compared to the contralateral knee indicates a (+) test.

Statistics

- Pooled SN 55 (52-58), **SP 92 (90-94)**, **+LR 7.3**, –LR 0.5, in a meta-analysis of 1,420 clients with both acute and chronic ACL tears[113]
- Pooled SN 49 (43-55), SP 58 (39-76), +LR 1.4, –LR 0.7, in a meta-analysis of 77 clients with acute ACL tears[113]
- Pooled **SN 92 (88-95)**, **SP 91 (87-94)**, **+LR 8.9**, **–LR 0.1**, in a meta-analysis of 375 clients with chronic ACL tears[113]
- Pooled SN 48 (38-59), **SP 87 (83-91)**, **+LR 3.7**, –LR 0.6, in a study of 274 clients with knee injuries and arthroscopy for ACL tears and MRI as a reference standards[18]

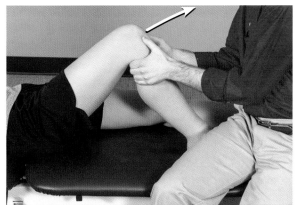

Figure 25.26

PIVOT SHIFT TEST

Video 25.27 in the web resource shows a demonstration of this test.

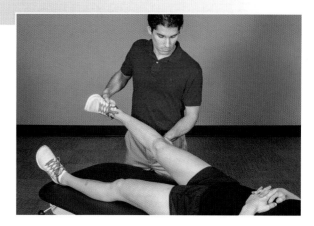

lient Position — Supine with bilateral legs and arms relaxed

Clinician Position — Standing directly to the side of the client on the side of the leg to be assessed

Movement — The clinician flexes the knee to 20° to 30° of flexion and places torque on the tibia while rotating it internally (with right hand as shown). At the same time, the clinician applies a valgus stress with the heel of the hand (left as shown) behind the proximal fibula and flexes the knee. The clinician then returns the leg to the starting position with continued valgus stress.

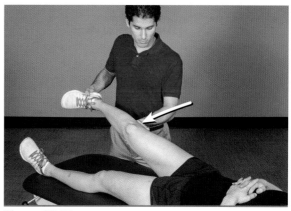

Assessment — A (+) test is an anterior subluxation of the lateral tibial plateau with flexion that reduces with bringing the leg back to the starting position.

Figure 25.27

Statistics

- Pooled SN 24 (21-27), **SP 98 (96-99)**, **+LR 8.5**, –LR 0.9, in a meta-analysis of 1,073 clients with both acute and chronic ACL tears[113]

- Pooled SN 32 (25-38), **SP 100 (98-100)**, **+LR Inf**, –LR 0.68, in a meta-analysis of 27 clients with acute ACL tears[113]

- Pooled SN 40 (29-52), **SP 97 (95-99)**, **+LR 7.7**, –LR 0.8, in a meta-analysis of 395 clients with chronic ACL tears[113]

- Pooled SN 61 (40-82), **SP 97 (93-99)**, **+LR 20.3**, –LR 0.4, in a study of 274 clients with knee injuries and arthroscopy for ACL tears and MRI as reference standards[18]

- SN 56 (NR), **SP 92 (NR)**, **+LR 7.0**, –LR 0.47, QUADAS 9, in a study of 300 clients with partial ACL tears (mean age 29.5 ± 11.3 years; 141 women; mean duration of injury range from 6.5 months to 19 months), and a side-to-side difference of anterior tibial displacement from 4 to 9 mm with stress radiographs as a reference standard[114]

- **SN 88 (NR)**, **SP 96 (NR)**, **+LR 22**, **–LR 0.13**, QUADAS 9, in a study of 300 clients with complete ACL tears (mean age 29.5 ± 11.3 years; 141 women; mean duration of injury range from 6.5 months to 19 months), and a side-to-side difference of anterior tibial displacement from 4 to 9 mm with stress radiographs as a reference standard[114]

- **SN 82 (NR)**, **SP 87 (NR)**, **+LR 6.3**, **–LR 0.21**, in a study of 171 clients with acute complete ACL tears (mean age 30.2 ± 11.0 years; 64 women; mean time from injury to surgery 21.5 weeks), and arthroscopy as a reference standard[41]

ANTERIOR DRAWER IN EXTERNAL ROTATION (ACL AND ANTERIOR-MEDIAL INSTABILITY)

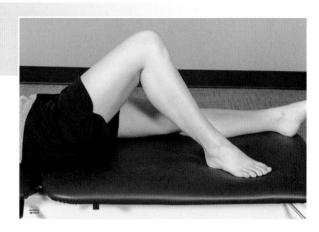

Client Position	Supine hook lying with knee flexed 90°, tibia externally rotated 15°, and foot on table
Clinician Position	Sitting on client's foot to stabilize leg
Movement	The clinician places bilateral hands on the posterior aspect of tibia and their thumbs on each respective joint line. The clinician translates the proximal tibia anteriorly and assesses motion.
Assessment	Increased anterior tibial excursion relative to the femur with a soft end-feel compared to the contralateral knee indicates a (+) test.
Statistics	NR

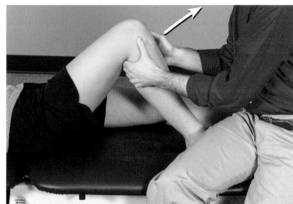

Figure 25.28

ANTERIOR DRAWER IN INTERNAL ROTATION (ACL AND ANTERIOR-LATERAL INSTABILITY)

Client Position	Supine hook lying with knee flexed 90°, tibia internally rotated 30°, and foot on table
Clinician Position	Sitting on client's foot to stabilize leg
Movement	The clinician places bilateral hands on the posterior aspect of tibia and their thumbs on each respective joint line. The clinician translates the proximal tibia anteriorly and assesses motion.
Assessment	Increased anterior tibial excursion relative to the femur with a soft end-feel compared to the contralateral knee indicates a (+) test.
Statistics	NR

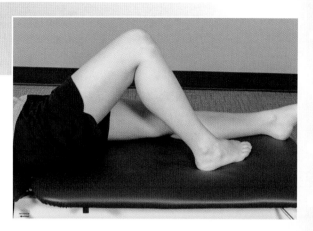

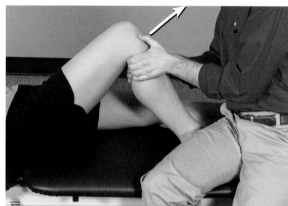

Figure 25.29

ACTIVE LACHMAN'S TEST

Client Position	Supine with a bolster behind the affected knee (30–40° knee flexion)
Clinician Position	Standing next to the client
Movement	The client actively extends the leg and returns the leg to the starting position.
Assessment	An anterior glide of the proximal tibia indicates a (+) test.
Statistics	NR

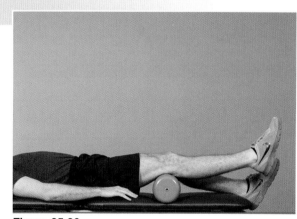

Figure 25.30

POSTERIOR CRUCIATE LIGAMENT TEAR

COMPOSITE PHYSICAL EXAMINATION

Pooled **SN 81 (63-98)**, **SP 95 (81-100)**, **+LR 16.2**, **–LR 0.2**, in a study of 274 clients with knee injuries, using arthroscopy and MRI as a reference standards[18]

Composite Physical Examination	• Reverse Lachman's test, reverse Lachman's endpoint, reverse pivot shift, posterior drawer, posterior sagittal sign, external rotation recurvatum, quadriceps active drawer, and dynamic posterior shift test
	• Pooled **SN 90 (84-94)**, **SP 99 (96-100)**, **+LR 90**, **–LR 0.10**, QUADAS 9, in a study of 18 clients (mean age, sex, and mean duration of symptoms NR), with chronic PCL tears and arthroscopy as a reference standard[115]

POSTERIOR DRAWER TEST

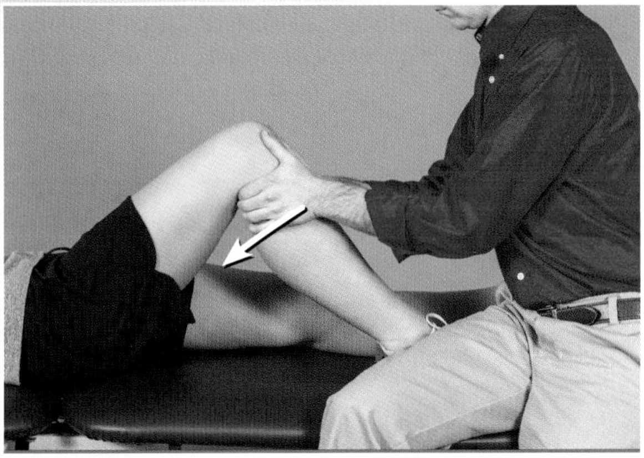

Client Position	Supine hook lying with knee flexed 90° and foot on table
Clinician Position	Sitting on client's foot to stabilize leg
Movement	The clinician places bilateral hands on the anterior surface of tibia and their thumbs on each respective joint line. The clinician translates the proximal tibia posteriorly and assesses motion. Internal and external rotation of foot can also be utilized for directional assessment.
Assessment	A (+) test is increased posterior tibial translation: Grade I+ (0-5 mm), grade II+ (6-10 mm), grade III+ (11+ mm).
Statistics	**SN 90 (NR)**, **SP 99 (NR)**, **+LR 90**, **–LR 0.1**, QUADAS 9, in a study of 18 clients (mean age, sex, and mean duration of symptoms NR), with chronic PCL tears and arthroscopy as a reference standard[115]

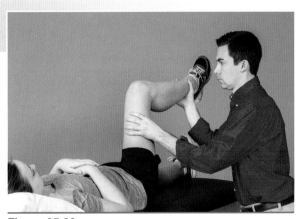

Figure 25.31

POSTERIOR SAG SIG (GODFREY'S TEST)

Client Position	Supine with hip and knee flexed 90°
Clinician Position	Standing directly to side of leg to be tested
Movement	The clinician supports the leg at the ankle and heel, suspending it in the air.
Assessment	A (+) test is posterior sagging of the tibia secondary to gravitational pull.
Statistics	SN 79 (54-94), **SP 100 (95-100)**, **+LR 88.4**, –LR 0.28, QUADAS 9, in a study of 18 clients (mean age, sex, and mean duration of symptoms NR), with chronic PCL tears and arthroscopy as a reference standard[115]

Figure 25.32

QUADRICEPS ACTIVE DRAWER

Client Position	Supine hook lying with knee flexed 90° and foot on table
Clinician Position	Standing at client's feet, directly facing them
Movement	The clinician supports the client's thigh and proximal tibia (medial-lateral without anterior-posterior stabilization of tibia). While stabilizing the foot, they ensure that the client's thigh is relaxed. The clinician asks the client to slide the foot gently down the table.
Assessment	A (+) test is anterior tibial displacement due to quadriceps contraction.
Statistics	SN 53 (29-76), **SP 96 (88-100)**, **+LR 12.0**, –LR 0.50, QUADAS 9, in a study of 18 clients (mean age, sex, and duration of symptoms NR), with chronic PCL tears and arthroscopy as a reference standard[115]

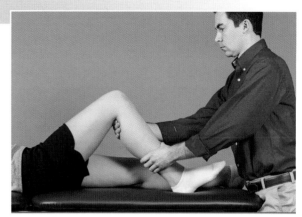

Figure 25.33

REVERSE PIVOT-SHIFT TEST (POSTEROLATERAL INSTABILITY TEAR)

Client Position	Supine with knee flexed to 70° to 80°. External rotation is applied to the lower leg with distal hand (left as shown).
Clinician Position	Standing directly to the side of the leg to be assessed
Movement	The clinician lets the weight of the leg straighten the knee. A slight axial load is then applied through the leg with distal hand (left as shown) and a valgus stress is applied at the knee with proximal hand (right as shown). As the knee approaches 20° of flexion, the clinician feels and observes for the lateral tibial plateau moving anteriorly with a jerk-like movement from a position of posterior subluxation and external rotation to a position of reduction and neutral rotation.
Assessment	A (+) test is the change to the reduction and neutral rotation position.
Statistics	• Reverse pivot shift: SN 26 (12-49), **SP 95 (85-98)**, **+LR 4.9**, –LR 0.78, QUADAS 9, in a study of 18 clients (mean age, sex, and mean duration of symptoms NR), with chronic PCL tears and arthroscopy as a reference standard[115]
	• Dynamic pivot shift: SN 58 (36-77), **SP 95 (85-98)**, **+LR 10.8**, –LR 0.45, QUADAS 9, in a study of 18 clients (mean age, sex, and mean duration of symptoms NR), with chronic PCL tears and arthroscopy as a reference standard[115]

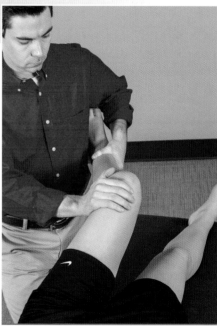

Figure 25.34

REVERSE LACHMAN'S TEST (TRILLET'S TEST)

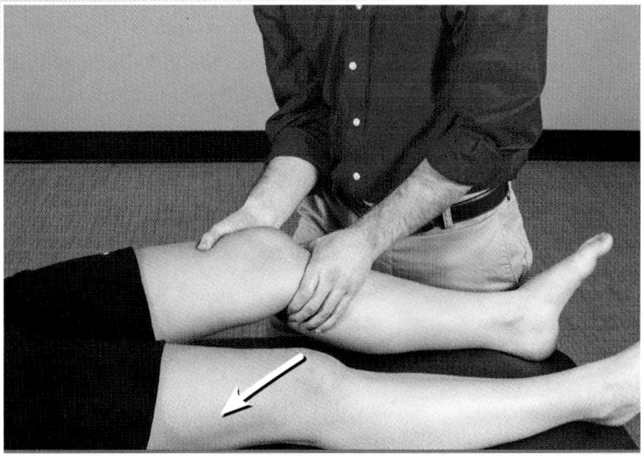

Client Position	Supine with knee flexed 20° to 30°
Clinician Position	Standing directly to the side of leg to be assessed
Movement	The clinician stabilizes the distal femur with one hand (right as shown) and grasps the posterior proximal tibia with the other (left as shown). The clinician applies an anterior tibial force followed by a posterior tibial force to the proximal tibia with the distal hand (left as shown).
Assessment	A (+) test is an increased posterior tibial translation or absent endpoint in the posterior direction.
Statistics	SN 63 (41-81), **SP 89 (79-95)**, **+LR 5.6**, –LR 0.43, QUADAS 9, in a study of 18 clients (mean age, sex, and mean duration of symptoms NR), with chronic PCL tears and arthroscopy as a reference standard[115]

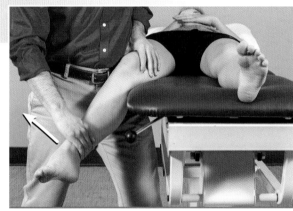
Figure 25.35

MEDIAL COLLATERAL LIGAMENT TEAR

VALGUS STRESS TEST AT 30° KNEE FLEXION

Client Position	Supine on a table with the testing limb over the edge of the table and the knee flexed to 30°
Clinician Position	Standing next to the testing leg and facing toward the client's feet
Movement	The clinician grasps the ankle of the test limb with the outside hand (right as shown). The clinician places their outer thigh against the thigh of the test limb. The contralateral hand of the clinician (left as shown) is over the medial joint line of the test limb. A valgus force is applied by abducting the ankle with the thigh stabilized.
Assessment	Pain at the MCL or increased excursion between the femur and tibia are suggestive of MCL disruption.
Statistics	• SN 78 (64-92), SP 67 (57-76), +LR 2.3, –LR 0.3, QUADAS 11, for pain in a study of 134 clients (mean age 40.2 ± 12.2 years; 60 women; 36 days [9-81]), with acute traumatic knee injury and MRI as a reference standard[116]
	• **SN 91 (81-100)**, SP 49 (39-59), +LR 1.8, **–LR 0.2**, QUADAS 11, for laxity in a study of 134 clients with acute traumatic knee injury (mean age 40.2 ± 12.2 years; 60 women; 36 days [9-81]), and MRI as a reference standard[116]

Figure 25.36

LATERAL COLLATERAL LIGAMENT TEAR

VARUS STRESS TEST

Client Position	Supine on a table with the testing limb over the edge of the table and the knee flexed to 30°
Clinician Position	Standing next to the testing leg and facing the client's feet
Movement	The clinician grasps the ankle of the testing limb with their outside hand (right as shown). The clinician places their outer thigh against the thigh of the testing limb. The contralateral hand of the clinician (left as shown) is over the lateral joint line of the testing limb. A varus force is applied by adducting the ankle with the thigh stabilized.
Assessment	Pain at the LCL or increased excursion between the femur and tibia is suggestive of LCL disruption.
Statistics	NR

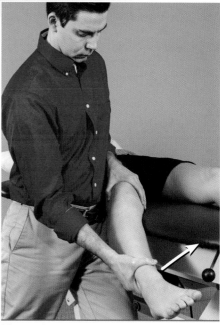

Figure 25.37

COMPOSITE PHYSICAL EXAMINATION

Clinical examination in combination with ACL, PCL, and LM lesions.

- **SN 100 (NR)**, SP 20 (NR), +LR 1.3, **–LR 0.0**, QUADAS 12, in a study of 118 clients with acute knee injury (mean age, sex, and mean duration of symptoms NR) and examination under anesthesia as a reference standard. The diagnostic accuracy of composite physical exam is limited due to the sample size and injury rate.[109]

PATELLOFEMORAL PAIN SYNDROME

Q-ANGLE MEASUREMENT

Client Position	Supine with test knee in full extension
Clinician Position	Standing next to the testing leg
Movement	The fulcrum of the large goniometer is placed over the mid-patella. The stationary arm is aligned along the anterior thigh toward the anterior superior iliac spine of the pelvis. The moving arm is aligned along the anterior shank over the tibial tubercle.
Assessment	An angle greater than 10° for men and greater than 15° for women is considered a (+) test.
Statistics	SN 76 (NR), SP 63 (NR), +LR 2.1, –LR 0.4, QUADAS 11, in a study of 29 clients with PFPS (mean age, sex, and mean duration of symptoms NR), and 17 healthy controls as a reference standard[117]

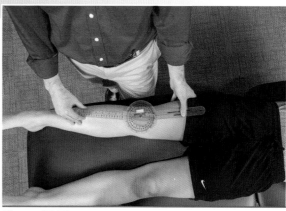

Figure 25.38

PATELLAR TILT TEST

Client Position	Supine on a table with knees extended and relaxed
Clinician Position	Sitting next to the test knee
Movement	The clinician tilts the lateral aspect of the patella using the thumbs (lifting lateral border of patella anterior out of the groove) and index fingers (pushing medial portion of patella posteriorly into the groove).
Assessment	The patella moving out of the trochlear groove and subluxing laterally indicates (+) test of patellofemoral joint instability.

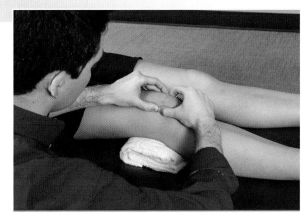

Figure 25.39

Statistics
- SN 19 (13-22), SP 83 (68-93), +LR 1.1, –LR 0.9, QUADAS 8, in a study of 59 clients with PFPS (mean age, sex, and mean duration of symptoms NR), and 23 healthy controls as a reference standard[118]
- SN 43 (31-55), SP 92 (75-98), +LR 5.4, –LR 0.6, QUADAS 10, in a study of 61 clients with PFPS (mean age, sex, and mean duration of symptoms NR), and 25 healthy controls as a reference standard[119]

PATELLAR APPREHENSION TEST

Client Position	Supine with the test knee flexed to 30°
Clinician Position	Standing next to the testing leg
Movement	With one hand (right as shown), the clinician places a maximal lateral glide to the patella. With the other hand (left as shown), the clinician grasps the ankle and slowly flexes the knee and hip from full extension, or from 90° flexion (as shown), to 30° flexion with a sustained lateral glide to the patella.
Assessment	Reproduction of the client's pain or apprehension presented by the client is considered a (+) test.

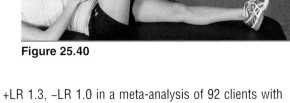

Figure 25.40

Statistics
- Pooled SN 15 (9-24), SP 89 (77-95), +LR 1.3, –LR 1.0 in a meta-analysis of 92 clients with PFPS (mean age, sex, and mean duration of symptoms NR), and 53 healthy controls as a reference standard[120]
- SN 32 (NR), SP 86 (NR), +LR 2.3, –LR 0.8, QUADAS 11, in a study of 31 clients with PFPS (mean age 31.0 ± 15.2; 9 women; mean duration of symptoms [pain] 45.1 ± 55.2 months), and 28 healthy controls as a reference standard[121]
- SN 7 (NR), SP 92 (NR), +LR 0.9, –LR 1.0, QUADAS 10, in a study of 61 clients with PFPS (mean age, sex, and mean duration of symptoms NR), and 25 healthy controls as a reference standard[119]

PAIN WITH SQUATTING

Movement The client performs a squatting motion that feels normal to them.

Assessment Reports of pain by the client or reproduction of pain during test activities indicates (+) test for patellofemoral pain syndrome.

Statistics
- **SN 91 (NR)**, SP 50 (NR), +LR 1.8, **–LR 0.2**, QUADAS 10, in a study of 52 clients with PFPS (mean age 49.3 ± 13.5 years; 17 women; mean duration of symptoms [pain] 34.3 ± 55.6 months), and physician's diagnosis as a reference standard[122]
- **SN 94 (NR)**, SP 46 (NR), +LR 1.7, **–LR 0.1**, QUADAS 11, in a study of 29 clients with PFPS (mean age, sex, and mean duration of symptoms NR), and 17 healthy controls as a reference standard[117]

PAIN WITH STAIR CLIMBING

Movement The client climbs stair in their normal way.

Assessment Reports of pain by the client or reproduction of pain during test activities indicates (+) test for patellofemoral pain syndrome.

Statistics
- SN 75 (NR), SP 43 (NR), +LR 1.3 (1.0–1.9), –LR 0.6 (0.03–1.1), QUADAS 10, in a study of 52 clients with PFPS (mean age 49.3 ± 13.5 years; 17 women; mean duration of symptoms [pain] 34.3 ± 55.6 months), and physician's diagnosis as a reference standard[122]
- **SN 94 (NR)**, SP 45 (NR), +LR 1.7, **–LR 0.1**, QUADAS 11, in a study of 29 clients with PFPS (mean age, sex, and mean duration of symptoms NR), and 17 healthy controls as a reference standard[117]

PAIN WITH KNEELING

Movement The client kneels as they normally would.

Assessment Reports of pain by the client or reproduction of pain during test activities indicates (+) test for patellofemoral pain syndrome.

Statistics **SN 84 (NR)**, SP 50 (NR), +LR 1.7, **–LR 0.3**, QUADAS 10, in a study of 52 clients with PFPS (mean age 49.3 ± 13.5 years; 17 women; mean duration of symptoms [pain] 34.3 ± 55.6 months), and physician's diagnosis as a reference standard[122]

RESISTED KNEE EXTENSION

Client Position Seated on the end of a table with feet off the ground and knees in a flexed position

Clinician Position Next to the client's test leg

Movement The client extends the knee while the clinician resists knee extension.

Assessment Reproduction of pain during test activities indicates (+) test for patellofemoral pain syndrome.

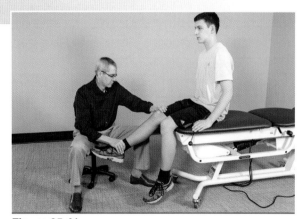

Figure 25.41

Statistics
- SN 39 (NR), SP 82 (NR), +LR 2.2, –LR 0.8, QUADAS 10, in a study of 52 clients with PFPS (mean age 49.3 ± 13.5 years; 17 women; mean duration of symptoms [pain] 34.3 ± 55.6 months), and physician's diagnosis as a reference standard[122]
- SN 21 (NR), **SP 95 (NR)**, **+LR 4.2**, –LR 0.8, QUADAS 9, in a study of 20 clients with patellofemoral pain (mean age 41 ± 12 years; 6 women; mean duration of symptoms NR), and a healthy group as a reference standard[123]

COMPRESSION TEST

Client Position	Long-sitting on a table
Clinician Position	Next to the client's test leg
Movement	The clinician pushes the patella directly into the femoral trochlea.
Assessment	A reproduction of the client's pain is considered a (+) test.
Statistics	• SN 83 (66-92), SP 18 (6-41), +LR 1.0, –LR 1.0, QUADAS 11, in a study of 29 clients with PFPS (mean age, sex, and mean duration of symptoms NR), and 17 healthy controls as a reference standard[117]

Figure 25.42

• SN 68 (NR), SP 54 (NR), +LR 1.5, –LR 0.6, QUADAS 10, in a study of 52 clients with PFPS (mean age 49.3 ± 13.5 years; 17 women; mean duration of symptoms [pain] 34.3 ± 55.6 months), and physician's diagnosis as a reference standard[122]

WALDRON'S TEST PHASE 1 (SUPINE)

Client Position	Supine with test knee in full extension
Clinician Position	Standing next to the test leg
Movement	The clinician compresses the patella against the femur with one hand while passively flexing the knee with the other hand.
Assessment	Crepitus and reproduction of pain is considered a (+) test.
Statistics	SN 45 (28-64), SP 68 (48-83), +LR 1.4, –LR 0.8, QUADAS 11, in a study of 31 clients with PFPS (mean age 31.0 ± 15.2; 9 women; mean duration of symptoms [pain] 45.1 ± 55.2 months) and 28 healthy controls as a reference standard[121]

WALDRON'S TEST PHASE 2 (STANDING)

Client Position	Standing
Clinician Position	Standing next to the client
Movement	The client slowly performs a full squat while the clinician gently compresses the patella against the femur.
Assessment	Crepitus and reproduction of pain is considered a (+) test.
Statistics	SN 23 (10-42), SP 79 (59-91), +LR 1.1, –LR 1.0, QUADAS 11, in a study of 31 clients with PFPS (mean age 31.0 ± 15.2; 9 women; mean duration of symptoms [pain] 45.1 ± 55.2 months), and 28 healthy controls as a reference standard[121]

CLARKE'S SIGN OR PATELLAR GRIND TEST

Client Position	Supine with the test knee in slight flexion
Clinician Position	Standing next to the testing leg with one hand on the superior aspect of the patella
Movement	The clinician glides the patella inferiorly (as with an inferior patella glide mobility assessment) and the client contracts the quadriceps muscles.
Assessment	Reproduction of the client's pain is considered a (+) test.
Statistics	SN 48 (31-67), SP 75 (55-89), +LR 1.9, –LR 0.7, QUADAS 11, in a study of 31 clients with PFPS (mean age 31.0 ± 15.2; 9 women; mean duration of symptoms [pain] 45.1 ± 55.2 months), and 28 healthy controls as a reference standard[121]

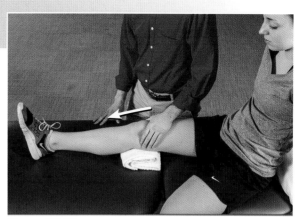

Figure 25.43

LATERAL PULL TEST

Client Position	Supine with test knee in full extension
Clinician Position	Standing next to the client, stabilizing the lower extremity in neutral rotation
Movement	The client performs an isometric quadriceps muscle contraction. The clinician observes the movement of the patella with and without slight pressure to the superior aspect of the patella.
Assessment	The patella tracking more laterally than superiorly is considered a (+) test.
Statistics	SN 25 (NR), **SP 100 (NR), +LR 249**, –LR 0.8, QUADAS 10, in a study of 61 clients with PFPS (mean age, sex, and mean duration of symptoms NR), and 25 healthy controls as a reference standard[119]

ECCENTRIC STEP-DOWN TEST

Client Position	Hands on hips, standing on an elevated platform
Clinician Position	Standing in front of and facing the client
Movement	The client steps down anteriorly with one leg from the platform as slowly and with as much control as possible.
Assessment	Reproduction of pain is considered a (+) test.
Statistics	SN 42 (NR), SP 82 (NR), +LR 2.3, –LR 0.7, QUADAS 11, in a study of 31 clients with PFPS (mean age 31.0 ± 15.2; 9 women; mean duration of symptoms [pain] 45.1 ± 55.2 months), and 28 healthy controls as a reference standard[121]

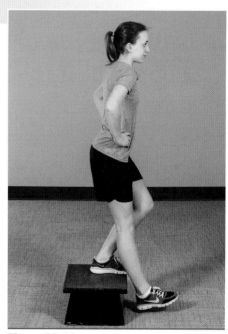

Figure 25.44

PATELLAR TENDINOPATHY

PALPATION FOR TENDINOPATHY

Client Position	Supine with test knee in full extension
Clinician Position	Standing next to the client
Movement	The clinician anteriorly tilts the inferior pole of the patella and then palpates the inferior pole of the patella.
Assessment	Reproduction of pain is considered a (+) test.
Statistics	SN 56 (NR), SP 47 (NR), +LR 1.0, −LR 0.9, QUADAS 12, in a study of 163 clients with patella tendinopathy (mean age 16.4 ± 1.0 years; 83 women; mean duration of symptoms NR), and ultrasonography as a reference standard[124]

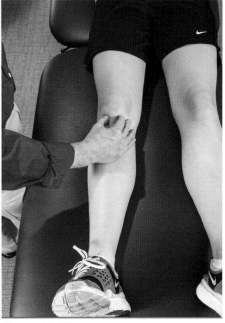

Figure 25.45

PLICA SYNDROME

Plica syndrome has several tests used to assess the findings; however, the diagnostic accuracy of these tests has not been investigated.

Composite Physical Examination	Performance of the physical examination is not described.
Statistics	SN 70 (NR), **SP 99 (NR)**, **+LR 70**, −LR 0.3, QUADAS 9, in a study of 195 clients with intra-articular lesions (mean age 36 years; 73 women; mean duration of symptoms NR), and arthroscopy as a reference standard[91]

PROXIMAL TIBIOFIBULAR JOINT INSTABILITY

FIBULAR HEAD TRANSLATION TEST

Client Position	Supine on a table
Clinician Position	Standing next to the client with one hand on the fibular head and the other on the proximal tibia
Movement	The clinician anteriorly and posteriorly translates the fibular head.
Assessment	Reproduction of the client's pain or apprehension presented by the client is considered a (+) test.
Statistics	NR[125]

RADULESCU SIGN

Client Position   Prone on a table with knee flexed at 90°

Clinician Position   Standing next to the client with one hand on the posterior thigh and the other on the distal tibia

Movement   The clinician internally rotates the tibia.

Assessment   Reproduction of the client's pain, fibular subluxation, or apprehension presented by the client is considered a (+) test.

Statistics   NR[126]

KNEE EFFUSION

MODIFIED STROKE TEST

Client Position   Supine on a table

Clinician Position   Standing next to the client

Movement   The clinician begins by stroking any fluid proximally at the medial tibiofemoral joint line multiple times *(a)*. If the fluid does not immediately return, the clinician then strokes distally along the distal lateral thigh *(b)* and observes for any return of fluid at the medial sulcus.

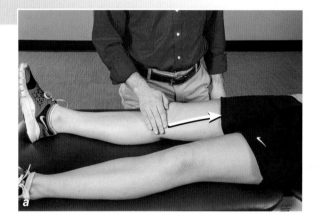

Assessment   The test is graded:

- No wave was produced with the downward stroke (0)

- Small wave of fluid returns at the medial sulcus with the downward stroke (trace)

- Larger return wave of fluid was produced at the medial knee (1+)

- Swelling returns without the downward stroke (2+)

- Inability to move the effusion out of the medial sulcus (3+)

Statistics   NR[127]

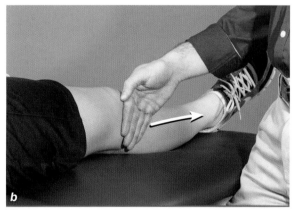

Figure 25.46

BALLOTTEMENT TEST

Client Position	Long-sitting on a table
Clinician Position	Standing next to the client with one hand superior to the patella and the other hand inferior to the patella
Movement	The clinician approximates the hands toward the patella. Then the clinician pushes the patella directly into the femoral trochlea and observes the return of the patella to the start position.
Assessment	The sense of the patella floating back to the start position is indicative of a (+) test.

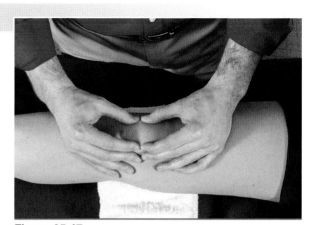
Figure 25.47

Statistics SN 83 (71-94), SP 49 (39-59), +LR 1.6, –LR 0.3, QUADAS 13, in a study of 134 clients with traumatic knee complaints (mean age 40.2 ± 12.2 years; 60 women; mean duration of symptoms 36 days [9-81]), and MRI as a reference standard[128]

SELF-NOTICED SWELLING

Assessment	The client reports knee swelling.
Statistics	SN 80 (68-92), SP 45 (35-59), +LR 1.5, –LR 0.4, QUADAS 13, in a study of 134 clients with traumatic knee complaints (mean age 40.2 ± 12.2 years; 60 women; mean duration of symptoms 36 days), and MRI as a reference standard[128]

CLUSTER OF TEST FINDINGS

Ballottement test, self-noticed swelling

Statistics SN 67 (52-81), SP 82 (73-90), +LR 3.6, –LR 0.4, QUADAS 13, in a study of 134 clients with traumatic knee complaints (mean age 40.2 ± 12.2 years; 60 women; mean duration of symptoms 36 days), and MRI as a reference standard[128]

KNEE OSTEOARTHRITIS

Composite Examination for Osteoarthritis	Performance of the physical examination is not described.
Statistics	• SN 94 (NR), SP 94 (NR), +LR 15., –LR 0.06, QUADAS 9, in a study of 195 clients with intra-articular lesions (mean age 36 years; 73 women; mean duration of symptoms NR), and arthroscopy as a reference standard[91]
	• SN 94 (NR), SP 100 (NR), +LR Inf, –LR 0.06, QUADAS 9, in a study of 290 clients with intra-articular lesions (mean age 38 years; 97 women; mean duration of symptoms NR), and arthroscopy as a reference standard[90]

OSTEOCHONDRAL LESION

Composite Examination for Loose Bodies	Performance of the physical examination is not described.
Statistics	• SN 67 (NR), **SP 98 (NR)**, **+LR 33.5**, −LR 0.3, QUADAS 9, in a study of 195 clients with intra-articular lesions (mean age 36 years; 73 women; mean duration of symptoms NR), and arthroscopy as a reference standard[91] • SN 65 (NR), **SP 99 (NR)**, **+LR 65**, −LR 0.4, QUADAS 9, in a study of 290 clients with intra-articular lesions (mean age 38 years; 97 women; mean duration of symptoms NR), and arthroscopy as a reference standard[90]
Composite Examination for Chondral Fracture	Performance of the physical examination is not described.
Statistics	• SN 14 (NR), **SP 99 (NR)**, **+LR 14**, −LR 0.9, QUADAS 9, in a study of 195 clients (mean age 36 years; 73 women; mean duration of symptoms NR), with intra-articular lesions and arthroscopy as a reference standard[91] • SN 15 (NR), **SP 98 (NR)**, **+LR 7.5**, −LR 0.9, QUADAS 9, in a study of 290 clients (mean age 38 years; 97 women; mean duration of symptoms NR), with intra-articular lesions and arthroscopy as a reference standard[90]

PALPATION

The clinician should potentially palpate the knee, as well as the hip complex and lower leg, when assessing the knee joint, dependent on the particular client's presentation. The clinician is referred to the hip and lower leg chapters to review palpation of these structures.

Anterior Aspect

Bony Structures (see figure 25.48)

• **Patella:** This is the prominent sesamoid bone on the anterior aspect of the knee.

• **Tibial tubercle:** This large prominence of bone is directly below the tibial plateaus.

• **Tibial plateaus:** These are the smooth bony surfaces of the proximal tibia condyles. The clinician can place their fingers in the indentation medial and lateral to the patella ligament. The edge of the plateau is palpable.

• **Femoral condyles:** These are two large bony projections of the distal femur, lined with articular cartilage. With the knee flexed, the condyles are palpable directly medial and lateral to the patella.

• **Trochlear groove:** This concave surface on the femur articulates with the retropatellar surface.

• **Gerdy's tubercle:** This is a small tubercle of the anterolateral aspect of the proximal tibia.

Soft-Tissue Structures

• **Quadriceps tendon:** This is the tendon that attaches the distal quadriceps to the superior aspect of the patella.

• **Patella ligament and tendon:** This ligament attaches the inferior pole of the patella to the tibial tubercle.

• **Pes anserine tendon:** This conjoined tendon of the sartorius, gracilis, and semitendinosus attaches to the anteromedial aspect of the proximal tibia at the inferior portion of the medial tibial plateau.

• **Medial and lateral patella retinaculum:** These are extensions of the aponeuroses of the quadriceps muscles. They attach the medial and lateral borders of the patella to the distal femur and proximal tibia.

• **Infrapatellar fat pad:** This is a cylindrical piece of fat situated retro to the patella ligament. It is palpable with the knee fully extended as the patella ligament pushes portions of the fat pad medial and lateral to the ligament.

Medial Aspect

Bony Structures

• **Medial epicondyle:** This is a large bony protrusion located on the medial aspect of the distal end of the femur.

• **Adductor tubercle:** This is a small protrusion at the summit of the medial condyle that affords

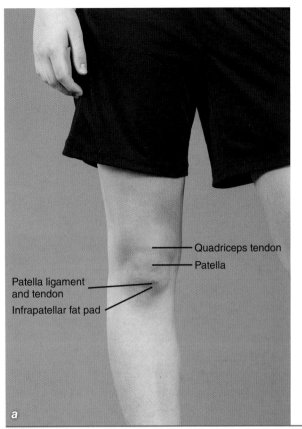
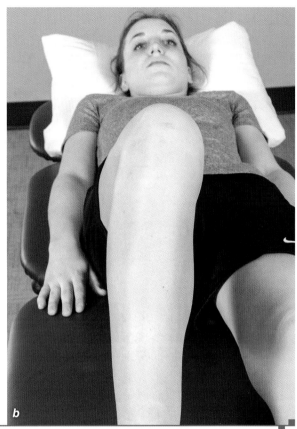

Quadriceps tendon
Patella
Patella ligament and tendon
Infrapatellar fat pad

Figure 25.48   *(a)* Anterior knee; *(b)* anterior knee with knee flexed.

attachment of the adductor magnus tendon. It can be best palpated by moving a hand distally over the adductor muscles until a ridge is felt just proximal to the medial epicondyle.

Soft-Tissue Structures

• **Medial collateral ligament:** This ligament attaches from the medial epicondyle of the femur to the medial condyle and shaft of the tibia. The deep fibers have direct attachment to the medial meniscus. Palpating along the medial joint line, the MCL becomes apparent as the joint line disappears under the ligament.

• **Medial joint line:** The medial joint line is the space between the medial femoral condyle and the medial tibial plateau. It is best appreciated with the knee flexed.

• **Gracilis tendon:** This tendon passes posterior to the medial femoral condyle, coursing around the medial tibial condyle, forming a conjoined tendon with the sartorius and semitendinosus muscles (pes anserinus), and attaching to the anteromedial aspect of the proximal tibia.

• **Sartorius tendon:** This tendon courses anteriorly and medially across the anterior aspect of the femur, forming a conjoined tendon with the gracilis and semitendinosus muscles (pes anserinus), and attaching to the anteromedial aspect of the proximal tibia.

Lateral Aspect

Bony Structures

• **Lateral epicondyle:** This is a bony protrusion located on the lateral aspect of the distal end of the femur, sometimes obscured by the iliotibial band.

• **Fibular head:** This is the proximal end of the fibula, just distal to the lateral tibial plateau, providing attachment for the biceps femoris muscle, lateral collateral ligament, and other soft-tissue structures.

Soft-Tissue Structures

• **Lateral collateral ligament:** The ligament attaches the lateral femur condyle to the fibular head. It is best palpated with the knee flexed to 90° and the hip externally rotated.

- **Iliotibial band:** This thick fibrous band of connective tissue attaches distally at Gerdy's tubercle on the proximal aspect of the anterolateral tibia.

- **Lateral joint line:** The lateral joint line is the space between the lateral femoral condyle and the lateral tibial plateau. It is best appreciated with the knee flexed.

- **Common peroneal nerve:** This nerve descends along the lateral aspect of the popliteal fossa and winds around the head of the fibula, where it is palpable.

Posterior Aspect

Bony Structures

- No bony structures are prominent for palpation here.

Soft-Tissue Structures (see figure 25.49)

- **Biceps femoris tendon:** The distal tendon is a conjoined tendon of the long and short heads of the biceps femoris that attaches to the lateral aspect of the head of the fibula and to a small portion to the lateral tibial condyle.

- **Semimembranosus tendon:** The distal tendon primarily attaches to the posteromedial aspect of the medial tibial condyle.

- **Semitendinosus tendon:** The distal tendon courses along the medial aspect of the popliteal fossa and around the medial tibial condyle, forming

a conjoined tendon with the gracilis and sartorius (pes anserinus), and attaching to the anteromedial aspect of the proximal tibia.

- **Popliteal fossa:** This is a shallow depression on the posterior aspect of the knee, bordered superiorly and medially by the semitendinosus and semimembranosus muscles, superiorly and laterally by the biceps femoris muscle, inferiorly and medially by the medial head of the gastrocnemius muscle, and inferiorly and laterally by the lateral head of the gastrocnemius muscle. It contains the popliteal artery, popliteal vein, and the posterior tibial nerve.

PHYSICAL PERFORMANCE MEASURES

It was found that collectively the walk test, the timed up and go test, and the 6-minute walk test yielded two factors consistent with the health concepts of pain and function. The application of these tests may provide clinicians and clinical researchers with more distinct impressions of pain and function that complement information from self-report measures.[23, 24, 129] Table 25.3 provides suggestions of physical performance measures for lower-level and higher-level clients.

COMMON ORTHOPEDIC CONDITIONS OF THE KNEE

While it is impossible to distinctly describe various pathological presentations of the knee, there are evidence-based findings supportive of particular pathologies of this region of the body. Therefore, the intent of this section of the chapter is to present current evidence-supported findings suggestive of knee pathologies. As previously described in chapter 4 (Evidence-Based Practice and Client Examination), though, not all examination findings are absolutely supported with clinical evidence, and the clinician should also rely on clinical experience and input from the client when performing differential diagnosis of a client's presentation of pain and dysfunction.

The knee is one of the most frequently injured joints in physically active people.[130-132] Injuries of the knee can be the result of repetitive microtrauma from overuse, an acute traumatic event, or

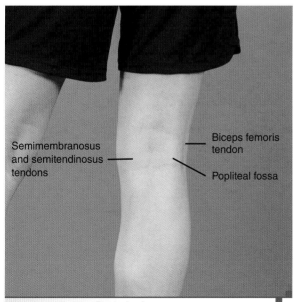

Figure 25.49   Posterior knee.

TABLE 25.3 Physical Performance Measure Suggestions for the Knee Joint

Discrete physical parameter	Potential physical performance measurements for the lower-level client (if appropriate)	Potential physical performance measurements for the higher-level client (if appropriate)
Balance	Single-leg stance test Romberg test Four square step test Functional reach test Sidestep test Tandem walking Tinetti test	Any of the tests appropriate for the lower-level client Star excursion balance test Y balance test Multiple single-leg hop Stabilization test
Fundamental movement	Deep squat test Sock test Sit-to-stand test 30 s chair stand test Self-paced walking test Timed up and go test Stair climbing test	Any of the tests appropriate for the lower-level client Rotational stability Trunk stability push-up
Strength and power	1RM leg press Lunge test Knee bending in 30 s	Any of the tests appropriate for the lower-level client Jump and hop tests Vail Sport Test
Lower extremity anaerobic power	Only if appropriate and necessary	Any of the tests appropriate for the lower-level client Wingate anaerobic power test Lower extremity functional test
SAQ	Only if appropriate and necessary	Any of the tests appropriate for the lower-level client Edgren sidestep test Illinois agility test Pro agility test Zigzag run test
Trunk endurance	Supine bridge test	Trunk flexion, extension, and lateral flexion bilaterally Repetitive box lifting task

SAQ = speed, agility, and quickness

Critical Clinical Pearls

When administering potential physical performance measurements for the higher-level client, the client should have the following:

- Trace to no joint effusion
- Full, passive ROM
- Injured knee's quadriceps strength greater than 80% compared to the contralateral knee's quadriceps strength
- Ability to ambulate with normal gait pattern and run with normal gait pattern for higher-level tests
- Ability to hop in place on the injured limb without joint pain

a combination of acute or chronic injury. Overuse injuries to the knee, such as patellofemoral pain and patella tendinopathy, typically occur as a result of microtrauma, abnormal joint alignment, or poor training strategies or techniques that do not allow adequate healing to take place.[133] Many of these injuries, such as intra-articular fractures, ligamentous ruptures, and meniscal and articular cartilage injuries,[134] are traumatic in nature and occur during sports involving jumping, cutting, and pivoting.[135] Traumatic knee injuries place people at high risk for the development of post-traumatic osteoarthritis (PTOA). PTOA is a major contributor to the prevalence of knee OA because people with a previous knee injury have an over 50% lifetime risk of developing symptomatic knee OA.[136] These injuries can lead to short-term disability and long-term morbidity, resulting in impaired function and reduced quality of life.

ACL Injury

ICD-9: 844.2 (sprain of cruciate ligament of knee)

ICD-10: S83.5 (sprain and strain involving anterior cruciate ligament of knee)

Injury to the ACL is most likely traumatic and related to sports activity. The mechanism is frequently a plant and cut or twisting type of activity. There is frequently significant swelling, pain, and limited ROM immediately after surgery. Since the ACL is a major stabilizer of the knee, the client may have complaints of instability in their knee.

I. Client Interview

Subjective History

- Decelerating or accelerating with non-contact dynamic valgus load near full extension[17]
- Feeling or hearing a pop at the time of injury[18]
- Swelling in the knee within 2 hours after the injury[18]
- History of knee giving way or buckling[137, 138]

Outcome Measures

- Knee Outcome Survey-Activities of Daily Living Scale (KOS-ADLS)[139]
- International Knee Documentation Committee 2000 (IKDC 2000) subjective knee form[140, 141]

- Knee Injury and Osteoarthritis Outcome Score (KOOS)[142]
- Lysholm Knee Scale[143]
- Sports Activity Level[137]
- Marx Activity Level Scale[144]
- Tegner Activity Level Scale[145]
- Shortened version of Tampa Scale of Kinesiophobia-11 (TSK-11)[146, 147]
- ACL-Return to Sports After Injury (ACL-RSI)[148, 149]

Diagnostic Imaging

- MRI is helpful for **ruling out** (pooled SN 87-94) and **ruling in** (pooled SP 94-95) ACL injury.[39, 40]

II. Observation

- Quadriceps atrophy[58, 150]
- Client ambulates with stiff knee gait with flexed knee.[151]

III. Triage and Screening

- All non-musculoskeletal causes, as well as causes from related joints, should be ruled out.
- If necessary, the Ottawa Knee Rules can help to **rule out** (SN 100) fractures of the knee.[43]
- A classification system can determine which active clients with an ACL tear will likely return to high functioning levels without surgery for a short period of time (i.e., to finish a sports season or work opportunity). Clients must meet all the following criteria to be classified as a potential coper:[138, 152]
  - Number of giving-way episodes of the knee ≤ 1
  - Single-leg 6 m timed hop symmetry index ≥ 80%
  - KOS-ADLS ≥ 80%
  - GRS ≥ 60%

IV. Motion Tests

- Loss of full knee ROM after ACL injury influences knee ROM loss after surgery.[153-155]
- 25 % of clients had greater than 5° differences in passive knee extension 4 weeks after ACL reconstruction.[78]

- Clinicians should look for patella mobility.[154, 156]

V. Muscle Performance Testing

- Quadriceps and hamstrings muscle strength deficits are present after ACL injury.[29, 157-162] One year after ACL injury, greater limb-to-limb asymmetries in quadriceps muscles are reported, whereas symmetry in hamstrings muscles is restored.[162]
- Preoperative quadriceps strength predicts knee function after ACL reconstruction.[158, 163-165]

VI Special Tests

- Composite physical examination: has better ability to help **rule in** (range SP 75-100, range +LR 2.5-Inf) than to help **rule out** (range SN 18-100, range −LR 0.8–0.0) ACL injury across multiple high-quality studies.[35, 109-112]
- Lachman's test: has ideal ability to help **rule in** (SP 94, +LR 10.2) and good ability to help **rule out** (SN 85, −LR 0.2) both acute and chronic injuries.[113, 166]
- Lachman's test: has ideal ability to help **rule out** (SN 94, −LR 0.1) and **rule in** (SP 97, +LR 9.4) acute injuries.[113]
- Lachman's test: has ideal ability to help **rule out** (SN 95, −LR 0.2) and **rule in** (SP 90, +LR 12.4) chronic injuries.[113]
- The pivot shift test is the best test to help **rule in** (SP 98 , +LR 8.5) ACL injury, but it has poor ability to help rule out (SN 24, −LR 0.9) ACL injury.[113]
- Pivot shift test: in pooled analyses has ideal ability to help **rule in** (SP 97-100, +LR 7.7-Inf) acute and chronic injuries.[18, 113]
- Pivot shift test: In two separate studies it shows good ability to help **rule out** (SN 82-88, −LR 0.21–0.13) and good to ideal ability to help **rule in** (SP 87-96, +LR 6.3–22) complete chronic injuries.[41, 114]
- Anterior drawer test: has a poor ability to help rule out (SN 49, −LR 0.88) or rule in (SP 58, +LR 1.17) acute injuries.[113]

- Anterior drawer test: has ideal ability to help **rule out** (SN 92, −LR 0.1) and **rule in** (SP 91, +LR 8.9) chronic injuries.[113]
- Anterior drawer test: has poor ability to help rule out (SN 55, −LR 0.5) but ideal ability to **rule in** (SP 92, +LR 7.3) combined acute and chronic injuries.[113]
- Composite physical examination: only helps **rule in** (SP 98, +LR 33.5) the potential for an osteochondral lesion to exist.[91]

VII. Palpation

- Tibial plateau to evaluate possible associated fracture
- Joint line to evaluate possible associated meniscus injury
- MCL and LCL to evaluate possible associated concomitant ligament injury

VIII. Physical Performance Measures

- Single-leg hops can predict self-reported knee function after ACL injury and reconstruction. A cutoff score greater than 88% on the single-hop for distance after ACL injury can be used to identify with high probability that the client will have normal knee function 1 year later.[167] Single-leg hop tests conducted 6 months after ACL reconstruction can predict the likelihood of successful and unsuccessful outcome 1 year after ACL reconstruction. Clients demonstrating less than the 88% cutoff score on the 6 m timed hop test at 6 months may benefit from targeted training to improve limb symmetry in an attempt to normalize function. Clients with minimal side-to-side differences on the crossover hop test at 6 months will possibly have good knee function at 1 year if they continue with their current training regimen. Preoperative single-leg hop tests are not able to predict postoperative outcomes.[168]

POTENTIAL TREATMENT-BASED CLASSIFICATIONS

- Acute: immobilization and pain control (most likely)
- Post-operative: pain control and mobility

- Rehabilitation: mobility and exercise and conditioning during the majority of the time (whether postoperatively or nonoperatively)
- Stability when managed nonoperatively

PCL Injury

ICD-9: 844.2 (sprain of cruciate ligament of knee)

ICD-10: S83.5 (sprain and strain involving posterior cruciate ligament of knee)

Injury to the PCL, similar to the ACL, is most likely traumatic and related to sports activity. The mechanism is frequently directly landing on the proximal tibia of a flexed knee with the foot in plantar flexion or sudden forceful knee hyperextension. There is frequently significant swelling, pain, and limited ROM immediately after surgery. While the PCL is a significant stabilizer of the knee, clients may have complaints of instability in their knee similar to an ACL injury. PCL injuries are less frequent than ACL injuries.

I. Client Interview

Subjective History

- Typically, clients report a fall on a flexed knee with the foot in plantar flexion.
- In an automobile accident, clients may report that the proximal tibia hit the dashboard (posterior directed force on the proximal tibia).
- Abrasions or ecchymosis may be present on the anterior aspect of the proximal tibia.
- Clients may complain of localized posterior pain in the knee with kneeling or decelerating.

Outcome Measures

- Knee Outcome Survey-Activities of Daily Living Scale (KOS-ADLS)[139]
- International Knee Documentation Committee 2000 (IKDC 2000) subjective knee form[140, 141]
- Knee Injury and Osteoarthritis Outcome Score (KOOS)[142]
- Lysholm Knee Scale[143]

- Sports Activity Level[137]
- Marx Activity Level Scale[144]
- Tegner Activity Level Scale[145]

Diagnostic Imaging

- The literature reporting on diagnostic imaging for PCL tears is limited.[169]

II. Observation

- The clinician should look for abrasions or ecchymosis on the anterior aspect of the proximal tibia in an acute setting.

III. Triage and Screening

- All non-musculoskeletal causes, as well as causes from related joints, should be ruled out.
- If necessary, the Ottawa Knee Rules can help to **rule out** (SN 100) fractures of the knee.[43]

IV. Motion Tests

- ROM in the involved knee may be restricted due to effusion. Long-term outcomes have noted no differences between the PCL injured knee and the uninvolved knee.[170]

V. Muscle Performance Testing

- Inconsistent findings for quadriceps muscle strength deficits after PCL injury have been reported.[171] Hamstring muscle weakness has been reported 6 months after PCL injury.[172]

VI. Special Tests

- Composite clinical examination: has good ability to help **rule out** (pooled SN 81-90, −LR 0.2–0.1) and good to ideal ability to help **rule in** (pooled SP 95-99, +LR 16-90) PCL injuries.[18, 115]
- Posterior drawer test: has good ability to help **rule in** (SP 99, +LR 90) and **rule out** (SN 90, +LR 0.1) chronic injuries.[115]
- Posterior sag sign (SP 100, +LR 88), quadriceps active drawer (SP 96, +LR 12), reverse pivot shift (SP 95, +LR 4.9), dynamic posterior shift (SP 95, +LR 10.8), and the reverse Lachman's (SP 89, +LR 5.6) tests all have good ability to help **rule in** PCL injuries.[115]

- Composite physical examination: only helps **rule in** (SP 98, +LR 33.5) the potential for an osteochondral lesion to exist.[91]

VII. Palpation

- Tibial plateau to evaluate possible associated fracture
- Joint line to evaluate possible associated meniscus injury
- MCL and LCL to evaluate possible associated concomitant ligament injury
- Posterolateral corner of the knee to evaluate possible associated posterolateral involvement

VIII. Physical Performance Measures

- Physical performance measures that are easily reproducible can be used to assess clients with activity limitations and participation restrictions associated with PCL injuries. Single-leg hops may assess functional recovery, rehabilitation progress, and readiness to return to sport.

POTENTIAL TREATMENT-BASED CLASSIFICATIONS

- Acute: immobilization and pain control (most likely)
- Postoperative: pain control and mobility
- Rehabilitation: mobility and exercise and conditioning during the majority of the time (whether postoperatively or nonoperatively)
- Stability when managed nonoperatively

Patellofemoral Pain Syndrome

ICD-9: 719.46 (pain in joint, lower leg)

ICD-10: M22.2 (patellofemoral disorders)

Patellofemoral pain syndrome (PFPS) is a broad term for various pathologies of the patellofemoral joint. This syndrome encompasses pathologies attributed to excessive movement of the patella, excessive compression of the patella in the femoral groove, as well as various other potential pathologies. The clinician is advised to perform a compre-hensive examination to determine the pathological process attributed to the client's pain.

I. Client Interview

Subjective History

- Clients report an insidious onset of poorly defined pain localized to the anterior aspect of the knee. The onset of symptoms can be slowly or acutely developed with a worsening of pain with prolonged sitting, squatting, ascending or descending stairs, or running, especially with hills.[173]

Outcome Measures

- Lower Extremity Functional Scale (LEFS)[174]
- KOS-ADLS
- Anterior Knee Pain Scale (AKPS)
- IKDC 2000
- PFPS severity scale (PSS)[175]

II. Observation

- Q-angle in standing and supine
- Leg length
- Patellar tracking
- Patella alta

III. Triage and Screening

- All non-musculoskeletal causes, as well as causes from related joints, should be ruled out.
- If necessary, the Ottawa Knee Rules can help **rule out** (SN 100) fractures of the knee.[43]

IV. Motion Tests

- Joint mobility of the patella is necessary in order to permit full and pain-free tibiofemoral range of motion. Clients with hypomobility of the patella may have difficulty with activities that require full knee ROM, whereas hypermobility of the patella may be an indication of ligamentous laxity or instability of the patella. Several motion tests are appropriate for determining joint play mobility:
  - Passive gliding patella
  - Patellar translation superiorly–inferiorly

- Patellar translation medially–laterally
- Patella inferior pole test

V. Muscle Performance Testing

- Resisted isometric quadriceps contraction
- Vastus medialis coordination test

VI. Special Tests

- Patellar tilt test: has poor ability to help rule out PFPS (SN 19, −LR 0.9;[118] SN 43, −LR 0.6);[119] however, it has ideal ability to help **rule in** the syndrome (SP 92, +LR 5.4) in studies with low bias for PFPS.[119]

- Patellar apprehension test: has poor ability to help rule out PFPS in studies of low bias (SN 32, −LR 0.8;[121] SN 7, −LR 1.0[119]) and in pooled analyses (SN 15, −LR 1.0).[120] It has poor to fair ability to help rule in PFPS in studies of low bias (SN 86, +LR 2.3;[121] SN 92, +LR 0.9[119]) and in pooled analyses (SP 89, +LR 1.3).[120]

- Compression test: has poor ability to help rule out (SN 83, −LR 1.0;[117] SN 68, −LR 0.6[122]) and rule in PFPS (SP 18, +LR 1.0[117] SP 54, +LR 1.5[122]) in studies of low bias.

- Clarke sign: has poor ability to help rule out PFPS (SN 48, −LR 0.7) and rule in (SP 75, +LR 1.9) in one study with low bias.[121]

- Waldron's test (phase 1 and phase 2): has poor ability to help rule out (SN 45, −LR 0.8; SN 23, −LR 1.0) and rule in PFPS (SP 68, +LR 1.4; SP 79, +LR 1.1) in one study with low bias.[121]

- Pain with squatting (**SN 91-94, −LR 0.2–0.1**)[117, 122] and pain with stair climbing (**SN 94, −LR 0.1**)[122] have ideal ability to help rule out PFPS, while pain with kneeling (SN 84, −LR 0.3)[122] has good ability to help **rule out** PFPS.

- Resisted knee extension: has good ability to help **rule in** (SP 95, +LR 4.2) PFPS.[123]

- Composite physical examination: only helps **rule in** (SP 98, +LR 33.5) the potential for an osteochondral lesion to exist.[91]

VII. Palpation

- Medial facet
- Lateral facet
- Inferior pole of the patella
- Superior pole of the patella

VIII. Physical Performance Measures

- Activities and tasks, such as kneeling, prolonged sitting, squatting, and stair climbing[176] can exacerbate pain symptoms in clients with PFPS. Pain during squatting and stair climbing are associated with an increase in patellofemoral joint reaction force. Several functional tests have been used to assess reliability and changes in pain; however, the validity of these tests has not been determined.

  - Bilateral squat
  - Eccentric step test or step-down
  - Anteromedial lunge
  - Single-leg press
  - Balance and reach

POTENTIAL TREATMENT-BASED CLASSIFICATIONS

- Pain control
- Exercise (strengthening, neuromuscular control) and conditioning
- Mobility and flexibility

Meniscus Tear

ICD-9: 836.0 (tear of medial cartilage or meniscus of knee); 836.2 (other tear of cartilage or meniscus of knee)

ICD-10: S83.2 (tear of meniscus); M23.2 (derangement of meniscus due to old tear or injury)

The menisci are cartilage structures between the femur and tibia serving stabilizing and compressive-loading functions in the knee. The mechanism of meniscal tear is similar to the ACL injury (plant and cut or rotational twisting with the foot on the ground). The client may also complain of symptoms similar to the ACL injury (locking and catching), although much less frequent symptoms of the knee giving out are noted for meniscal tears compared to ACL injury.

Differential Diagnosis of a Meniscus Tear

- Delayed effusion compared to cruciate ligament tears (more immediate effucsion)
- Reported catching or locking of the knee similar to cruciate ligament tear but less frequent and lack of distinct instability complaints as with a cruciate ligament tear
- Catching sensation with meniscal tear is more distinct and deep in joint compared to PFPS catching
- Pain with
  - Forced hyperextension
  - Maximum flexion
  - McMurray's test or similar movements (both weight-bearing and nonweight-bearing)
- Discomfort or sense of catching or locking over either joint line during any Thessaly test position

I. Client Interview

Subjective History

- Feeling tearing sensation or hearing a pop at the time of injury, accompanied by severe pain[18]
- Swelling in the knee delayed (6-24 hours) after the injury[18]
- Knee pain with twisting maneuver in full weight bearing[11, 18]
- History of catching or locking of the knee[177]

Outcome Measures

- Knee Outcome Survey-Activities of Daily Living Scale (KOS-ADLS)[139]
- International Knee Documentation Committee 2000 (IKDC 2000) subjective knee form[140, 141]
- Knee Injury and Osteoarthritis Outcome Score (KOOS)[142, 178]
- Lysholm Knee Scale[179]
- Sports Activity Level[137]
- Marx Activity Level Scale[144]
- Tegner Activity Level Scale[179]

Diagnostic Imaging

- MRI is more helpful for **ruling out** (pooled SN 91-93) than **ruling in** (pooled SP 81-88) medial meniscus tear.[39, 40]
- MRI is less helpful for ruling out (pooled SN 76-79) than **ruling in** (pooled SP 93-95) lateral meniscus tear.[39, 40]

II. Observation

- Quadriceps atrophy[58, 150]
- Client ambulates with stiff knee gait with flexed knee.[151]

III. Triage and Screening

- All non-musculoskeletal causes, as well as causes from related joints, should be ruled out.
- If necessary, the Ottawa Knee Rules can help **rule out** (SN 100) fractures of the knee.[43]

IV. Motion Tests

- Pain with hyperextension of the knee can help **rule in** (SP 86.3) a meniscal tear.
- Pain with forced knee flexion has low SN (47.7) and SP (58.8) for a meniscal tear.

V. Muscle Performance Testing

- Quadriceps strength deficits have been reported to persist up to 4 years after arthroscopic partial meniscetomy.[180]

VI. Special Tests

- Pooled analysis of clustered testing: has good ability to help **rule out** medial (SN 86, −LR 0.19) and lateral (SN 88, −LR 0.13) meniscal tears, with ideal ability to help **rule in** (SP 92, +LR 11) lateral meniscal tears.[18]
- McMurray's test: has shown only fair ability to help rule in (SP 67-77, +LR 2.4) and rule out (SN 55-75, −LR

0.58–0.37) meniscal tears in pooled analysis.[92, 93]

- In low-bias single studies, McMurray's test is poor at helping rule out and poor (SP 40, +LR 1.3),[97] good (**SP 92, +LR 3.5**),[95] and ideal (**SP 98, +LR 8**)[98] at helping rule in meniscal tear.

- McMurray's test: has low to moderate ability to help **rule out** (SN 75, −LR 0.70) meniscal tear in studies of low bias[92] and pooled analysis (SN 55, −LR 0.6),[93] as well as to help **rule in** (SP 67, +LR 3.6)[92] meniscal tear in studies of low bias and in pooled analysis (SP 77, +LR 2.4).

- Thessaly's test: has poor (SN 66, −LR 0.35) to good ability (**SN 81-92, +LR 0.21–0.08**)[99] when performed at different degrees of knee flexion in a single low-bias study to help rule out meniscal tear, and a good ability to help **rule in** (SP 91-97, +LR 9-29) meniscal tear.[99]

- Thessaly's test: has good ability to help **rule in** (SP 91-97, +LR 9-29) various types of meniscal tears.[99]

- Ege's test: has good (**SP 81, +LR 3.5**; medial meniscus) to ideal (**SP 90, +LR 6.4**; lateral meniscus) ability to help rule in meniscal tear.[100]

- Apley's test: has poor ability to help rule out meniscal tear (SN 61, −LR 0.6) in studies of low bias[92] and pooled analysis (SN 22, −LR 1.0),[93] as well as to help rule in meniscal tear (SP 64, +LR 1.9) in studies of low bias[92] and in pooled analysis (SP 88, +LR 1.0).[93]

- Apley's test: in separate isolated studies, demonstrated good ability to help rule out (SN 81, −LR 0.3)[96] and rule in (SP 93, +LR 5.9)[99] meniscal tear.

- Steinman sign I: has poor to good (**SN 86, −LR 0.2**)[103] ability to help rule out and good (**SP 83-88, +LR 3.9–7.2**)[96] to ideal (**SP 100, +LR Inf**)[95] ability to help rule in meniscal tear.

- Dynamic knee test: has good ability to help **rule in** (SP 90, +LR 8.5) meniscal tear.[104]

- Axial pivot-shift test: has good ability to help **rule in** (SP 83, +LR 4.2) meniscal tear.[101]

- Joint line tenderness, Payr's sign, presence of joint effusion, forced knee flexion, squat test, bounce-home test, Steinmann sign II, and medial–lateral grind tests: have poor ability to help rule in or rule out meniscal tears in low-bias studies.

- Composite score: consisting of McMurray's test, pain with knee hyperextension, history of mechanical symptoms, joint line tenderness, and pain with forced knee flexion. Positive findings on all five tests had ideal ability to help **rule in** (SP 99, +LR 11.45) meniscal tears. Positive findings on three or more tests had good ability to help **rule in** (SP 90, +LR 3.15) meniscal tears.[177]

- Composite physical examination: only helps **rule in** (SP 98, +LR 33.5) the potential for an osteochondral lesion to exist.[91]

VII. Palpation

- Joint line tenderness has some moderate ability to help **rule out** meniscal tear in studies of low bias (SN 61, −LR 0.72)[92] and in pooled analysis (SN 76, −LR 0.3),[93] as well as to help **rule in** meniscal tear in studies of low bias (SP 77, +LR 4.1)[92] and in pooled analysis (SP 77, +LR 3.3).

VII. Physical Performance Measures

- Physical performance measures that are easily reproducible can be used to assess clients with activity limitations and participation restrictions associated with meniscal injuries.

POTENTIAL TREATMENT-BASED CLASSIFICATIONS

- Acute: immobilization and pain control (most likely)

- Postoperative: pain control and mobility

- Rehabilitation: mobility and exercise and conditioning during the majority of the time (whether postoperative or nonoperative)

MCL or LCL Tear

ICD-9: 844.0 (sprain of lateral collateral ligament of knee)

ICD-10: S83.429A (sprain of lateral collateral ligament of unspecified knee)

Injuries to the MCL are typically the result of contact to the lateral knee and occur most frequently in collision and contact sports.[2] LCL injuries are the least common of knee ligament injuries and usually occur as part of more extensive injuries involving the posterolateral corner of the knee.[181]

I. Client Interview

Subjective History

- For MCL tears, clients typically report a direct hit to the lateral aspect of the knee while in a weight-bearing position,[182] resulting in a sudden application of a valgus torque to the knee.[183] Noncontact valgus external rotation can occur in alpine skiing[184] or in other types of cutting or pivoting sports.

- Pain is worse in partial tears compared to complete tears.[185]

Outcome Measures

- Knee Outcome Survey-Activities of Daily Living Scale (KOS-ADLS)[139]

- International Knee Documentation Committee 2000 (IKDC 2000) subjective knee form[140, 141]

- Knee Injury and Osteoarthritis Outcome Score (KOOS)[142]

- Lysholm Knee Scale[143]

- Sports Activity Level[137]

- Marx Activity Level Scale[144]

- Tegner Activity Level Scale[145]

II. Observation

- More than three-fourths of clients with complete ruptures can ambulate without support.[185]

III. Triage and Screening

- All non-musculoskeletal causes, as well as causes from related joints, should be ruled out.

- If necessary, the Ottawa Knee Rules can help **rule out** (SN 100) fractures of the knee.[43]

IV. Motion Tests

- With incomplete tears of the MCL, end-range knee extension and flexion may be limited due to pain.

V. Muscle Performance Testing

- The long-term outcomes for isolated complete tears of the MCL were much worse than for incomplete tears, with a higher rate of medial instability, muscle weakness, and poor functional outcomes.[186]

VI. Special Tests

- Valgus stress test performed at 30° of knee flexion: This test is performed to isolate the integrity of the MCL. Limited diagnostic accuracy on valgus stress testing is available. SN 86-86 has been reported in two studies, but methodological flaws limit their findings.[187] More recent work reported good ability of assessing laxity with valgus stress at 30° to help **rule out** an MCL injury (SN 91, −LR 0.2), but poor ability to help rule in an MCL injury (SP 49, +LR 1.8).[116] Additionally, pain with valgus stress test at 30° has moderate to fair ability to help rule out (SN 78, −LR 0.3) and rule in (SP 67, +LR 2.3) an MCL injury.[116]

- Varus stress testing for LCL injury does not have reported diagnostic accuracy.

- Composite physical examination: only helps **rule in** (SP 98, +LR 33.5) the potential for an osteochondral lesion to exist.[91]

VII. Palpation

- Tenderness with palpation of the medial femoral epicondyle, joint line, or proximal tibia should be noted.[188]

- Palpatory provocation of MCL reproduces familiar pain.[2]

VIII. Physical Performance Measures

- Since these clients are most frequently athletes, the specific lower extremity functional components of the athlete's sport should be assessed.

- Speed, agility, and quickness testing is likely most appropriate for most of these athletes.

POTENTIAL TREATMENT-BASED CLASSIFICATIONS

- Acute: immobilization and pain control (most likely)
- Postoperative: pain control and mobility
- Rehabilitation: mobility and exercise and conditioning for the majority of the time (whether postoperatively or nonoperatively)
- Stability when managed nonoperatively

Patellar Tendinopathy

ICD-9: 726.9 (enthesopathy of unspecified site)

ICD-10: M77.9 (enthesopathy, unspecified)

Patellar tendinopathy is a broad term encompassing tendinitis, tendinosis, and peritendinitis. Several authors have suggested the term *patellar tendinopathy* as a clinical condition that encompasses all overuse conditions involving the patellar tendon from the proximal attachment on the inferior pole of the patella to the distal attachment on the tibial tubercle.[189-192]

I. Client Interview

Subjective History

- Clients complain of anteriorly well-localized pain, typically at the proximal attachment of the patella ligament to the inferior pole of the patella exacerbated by physical activity or prolonged knee flexion.[189] Pain may be present at the initiation of or throughout activities, affecting performance.

Outcome Measures

- Victorian Institute of Sport Assessment-patellar tendinopathy (VISA-P)[193, 194]

II. Observation

- Increased body mass index may be a risk factor for patellar tendinopathy.[195]

III. Triage and Screening

- All non-musculoskeletal causes, as well as causes from related joints, should be ruled out.

- If necessary, the Ottawa Knee Rules can help **rule out** (SN 100) fractures of the knee, as determined in a study of 1,047 adults with acute knee injuries.[43]

IV. Motion Tests

- Decreased quadriceps and hamstrings flexibility may be associated with patellar tendinopathy.[195]
- Limited ankle dorsiflexion (<36.5°) increases the risk of developing patellar tendinopathy within 1 year.[196]

V. Muscle Performance Testing

- Quadriceps strength deficits may increase the risk for patellar tendinopathy.[195]

VI. Special Tests

- Palpation for tendinopathy: has poor ability to help rule in or rule out the pathology.[124]
- Performing single-legged squat on a decline has been suggested as a special test or functional test for patellar tendinopathy;[197] however, the validity of this test has not be established.

VII. Palpation

- Palpation tends to elicit well-localized tenderness that is similar in quality and location to the pain experienced during activity.[198]

VIII. Physical Performance Measures

- Vertical jumping performance may be higher in athletes with patella tendinopathy.[195]

POTENTIAL TREATMENT-BASED CLASSIFICATIONS

- Pain control
- Exercise (strengthening, neuromuscular control) and conditioning
- Mobility and flexibility

Knee Osteoarthritis

ICD-9: 715.16 (osteoarthrosis, localized, primary, lower leg)

ICD-10: M17.10 (unilateral primary osteoarthritis, unspecified knee)

Differential Diagnosis of PFPS and Patella Tendinopathy

- Although palpation diagnostic accuracy is limited in both cases, the client with PFPS is more likely to have pain on the medial or lateral patella facets versus the client with patella tendinopathy (more likely to have tenderness on patella tendon, inferior patella pole, or tendon insertion into tibial tubercle).
- Both conditions are likely to have relatively insidious onset of poorly localized pain on the anterior aspect of the knee, pain with squatting, and pain with resisted knee extension.
- PFPS is more likely to have pain with prolonged sitting than is tendinopathy.
- Special testing, in general, is of poor diagnostic ability to differentiate these conditions.
- The client with patella tendinopathy is more likely to have pain with isometric contraction at full knee extension with initial contraction, but pain will likely improve with repetition.
- The client with PFPS is more likely to have pain with isometric contraction in knee flexion at or greater than 30° knee flexion (where the patella contacts the trochlear groove).

Osteoarthritis (OA) of the knee is characterized by degeneration of the articular cartilage, morphologic changes to the subchondral bone, and damage to the surrounding soft tissue.[199] These structural changes lead to joint pain, muscle weakness, reduced range of motion, and joint instability.[200, 201] As a result, most people with symptomatic knee OA report difficulty with walking, stair climbing, rising from a car, or carrying heavy loads.[202]

I. Client Interview

Subjective History

- More likely in a client over the age of 50 years old.[203, 204]
- Women over the age of 65 are twice as likely to have knee OA than men over the same age.[205]
- Female gender,[206, 207] previous knee trauma,[207] and older age[207] were strong risk factors for knee OA.
- Body mass index is positively associated with knee OA.[206, 207]
- Clients may have diffuse tenderness and morning stiffness for <30 minutes.[208]
- Clients may complain of clicking and catching in knee, especially with activity.[208]
- Mechanism of onset is typically insidious, unless client has a previous history of trauma.[208]

- Criteria for classification of osteoarthritis of the knee:[203]
  - Age > 50 years
  - Knee crepitus
  - Palpable bony enlargement
  - Bony tenderness to palpation
  - Morning stiffness that improves in less than 30 minutes
  - No palpable warmth of the synovium
    - If the client does not have three of these variables, this helps **rule out** (SN 95, −LR 0.07) the likelihood of knee OA.
    - >3 variables present in a client is less impressive for helping **rule in** (SP 69, +LR 3.1) knee OA.

Outcome Measures

- The WOMAC, Physical Function subscale, and LEFS have demonstrated clinical applicability in these clients, although they are highly influenced by client pain levels.[23, 24, 209, 210]
- Findings caution against the isolated use of self-report assessments of physical function since change in pain level significantly affected change in self-report measures of physical function.[23, 24, 209]

Diagnostic Imaging

- Bone marrow lesions on MRI for clients with osteoarthritis have been associated with pre-existing and future cartilage loss.[211]

- Radiographic findings include joint space narrowing, bone sclerosis, periarticular cysts, and osteophytes. Refer to chapter 6 for definition of OA according to Kellgren and Lawrence.[212]

- MRI is less helpful for **ruling out** (SN 83) than **ruling in** (SP 94) articular cartilage damage.[38]

II. Observation

- Clients may ambulate with antalgic gait and have loss of ROM and general joint effusion.[3, 204]

- The knee may have a redness in appearance.[204]

III. Triage and Screening

- All non-musculoskeletal causes, as well as causes from related joints, should be ruled out.

- If necessary, the Ottawa Knee Rules can help **rule out** (SN 100) fractures of the knee.[43]

IV. Motion Tests

- Clients have loss of ROM, typically in a capsular pattern.[204, 213]

- Clients have limited joint mobility, especially with anterior and posterior glides of the tibiofemoral joint.[3, 208, 213]

- Clicking or catching may be noted with passive joint mobility testing.[208]

- Impaired range of joint motion resulted in reduced functional status.[214, 215]

V. Muscle Performance Testing

- Greater muscle strength, aerobic capacity, and standing balance were protective factors for preventing deterioration of functional status.[214, 215]

VI. Special Tests

- Diagnosis of knee OA is based predominantly on history, physical examination, and diagnostic imaging.[213]

- Composite physical examination: helps **rule out** (SN 94, −LR 0.06) and **rule in** (SP 94, +LR 15.7) OA.[91]

- Composite physical examination: only helps **rule in** (SP 98, +LR 33.5) the potential for an osteochondral lesion to exist.[91]

- The clinician will want to rule out potential for meniscal or ligamentous tears associated with knee OA.

VII. Palpation

- Clients may have palpable bony enlargement, bony tenderness to palpation, and no palpable warmth of the synovium.[203]

- Clients may have diffuse tenderness around knee.[3, 208]

- The knee may be warm to palpation.[204]

VIII. Physical Performance Measures

- Pain and functional status seem to deteriorate slowly.[215]

- Self-paced walk, stair test, timed up-and-go, and the 6 min walk have been suggested as more complete measures of physical function for these clients.[23, 24, 209, 210]

- Terwee and colleagues identified 26 performance-based tests; many represent variations on the same theme. The most useful test was unable to be determined because consensus is lacking on what activities and functional parameters should be included.[216]

POTENTIAL TREATMENT-BASED CLASSIFICATIONS

- Mobility for pain and limited motion, pain control, and exercise and conditioning may be used.

CONCLUSION

The knee joint has an interdependent mechanical and pain-generation relationship with the entire lower extremity and trunk. Differential diagnosis of this joint requires careful interpretation of the client's clinical presentation. Clinicians should integrate best evidence as suggested in this chapter as well as the systematic examination approach to minimize further complicating the differential diagnosis of this region of the body. A systematic, evidence-based funnel approach suggests to the practicing clinician the importance of all components of the examination process. Additionally, it suggests that the clinician focus on ruling out or screening for potential competing pathologies early in the examination process and attempting to rule in or diagnose particular pathologies later in the examination process. Utilization of a systematic screening process early in the examination funnels or narrows down potential competing diagnoses that can then be more likely ruled in with more SP findings or testing.

LOWER LEG, ANKLE, AND FOOT

Shefali Christopher, PT, DPT, SCS, LAT, ATC
Michael P. Reiman, PT, DPT, OCS, SCS, ATC, FAAOMPT, CSCS

The lower leg, ankle, and foot are the most distal joints in the body and are important to evaluate because they can influence the knee, hip, and other proximal structures, and vice versa. The foot and ankle have the unique function of being both stable and flexible to assist with function. The functions of the foot and ankle include adapting to uneven terrain, absorbing ground reaction force, providing a stable base of support, and being rigid enough for push-off. The lower leg, foot, and ankle are defined in this chapter as the tibia, fibula, talus, calcaneus, cuneiforms, cuboid, navicular, metatarsals, phalanges, and their joint articulations.

A systematic, evidence-based funnel approach suggests to the practicing clinician the importance of all components of the examination process. This chapter provides information on client interview, observation, triage and screening, motion tests, muscle performance tests, special tests, palpation, and physical performance tests as well as common orthopedic conditions specific to the lower leg, foot, and ankle. With the help of this funnel, clinicians can collect pertinent information that will help them put their clients in an appropriate treatment-based classification group and address impairments.

CLINICALLY APPLIED ANATOMY

The lower leg, ankle, and foot involve a complex relationship of multiple bones and joints. This complexity is further compounded by the fact that the entire lower leg is a continuation, functionally, of the pelvic girdle, hip, and knee (figure 26.1). Movements at the proximal and distal lower extremities have been suggested to contribute to dysfunction at the other area. Pain and osteoarthritis at the knee and foot have been linked to problems with foot structure.[1, 2]

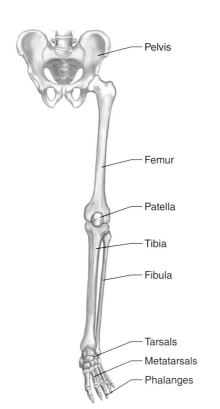

Figure 26.1 Relationship of pelvic girdle and distal lower extremity.

The lower leg consists of two primary bones, the tibia and fibula. The tibia is the second largest bone and is a weight-bearing bone. The fibula is used mostly in stability and muscle attachments. These two bones articulate proximally at the proximal tibiofibular joint and distally at the distal tibiofibular joints. Distally these bones are connected via

the dense syndesmotic tissue between them, and are called the syndesmotic joint. The stability of the syndesmosis is provided by the fibula, since it sits in the anterior and posterior tibial processes.[3] The anteroinferior tibiofibular ligament, the posteroinferior tibiofibular ligament, the inferior transverse ligament, the interosseous ligament, and the deep portion of the deltoid ligament add to the stability of the joint.[3] There is limited movement at both of these joints; however, the fibula moves during gait to accommodate the talus.

The ankle joint consists of three primary joints (figure 26.2). The joint traditionally thought of as the ankle joint is the talocrural joint. This joint is an articulation of the distal tibia (concave) and the superior portion of the talus (convex). This is a uniaxial synovial hinge joint whose primary motions are plantarflexion and dorsiflexion. The joint is surrounded by the strong deltoid ligament medially and the weaker lateral ligaments (anterior talofibular ligaments [ATFL], posterior talofibular ligaments [PTFL] and calcaneofibular ligament [CFL]; figure 26.3) on the lateral portion of the ankle. The anterior talofibular ligament requires the lowest maximal load to produce failure to the lateral ligaments, although it has the highest strain to failure of the group.[4] The joint congruency also provides stability to the joint. The two primary reasons medial ankle sprains are infrequent are the strength of the deltoid ligament as well as how the fibula extends farther than the tibia distally. The ankle joint sustains the greatest load per surface area of any joint in the body.[5]

The subtalar joint is a diarthrodial joint consisting of the calcaneus and talus. This joint produces the triplanar motions of pronation and supination (figure 26.4). Open kinetic chain pronation at the subtalar

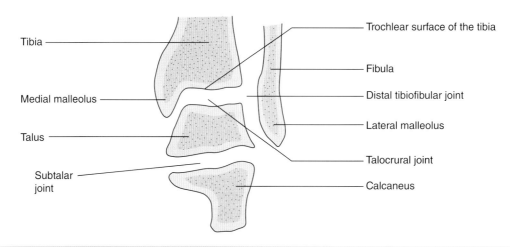

Figure 26.2 Distal tibiofibular, talocrural, and subtalar joints.

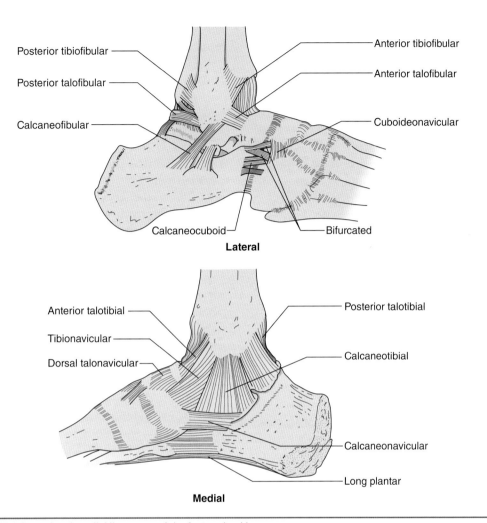

Figure 26.3 Lateral and medial ligaments of the foot and ankle.

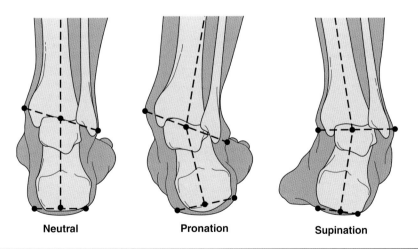

Figure 26.4 Motions of the subtalar joint: neutral, pronation, and supination.

joint consists of calcaneal eversion in the frontal plane, abduction in the transverse plane, and dorsiflexion in the sagittal plane. Open kinetic chain supination at the subtalar joint consists of calcaneal inversion in the frontal plane, adduction in the transverse plane, and plantarflexion in the sagittal plane. Closed chain pronation at the subtalar joint consists of calcaneal eversion, talar plantarflexion and adduction, and tibial internal rotation. Closed chain supination at the subtalar joint consists of calcaneal inversion, talar dorsiflexion and abduction, and tibial external rotation.

The ankle and foot region includes multiple bones, joint articulations, and complex movements. The foot (figure 26.5) is typically functionally divided into the rearfoot, midfoot, and forefoot. The rearfoot consists of the subtalar joint, the midfoot is made up of the tarsal bones (navicular, cuboid, and the three cuneiforms), and the forefoot consists of the five metatarsals and their phalanges. The commonly described first ray is the first metatarsal, which articulates with the first cuneiform. The fifth ray is the fifth metatarsal.

The primary function of the rearfoot is to convert the torque of the lower limb, influence the functioning of the foot and forefoot, as well as convert transverse rotation of the lower extremity to sagittal, frontal, and transverse plane movements. The midfoot transfers motion from the rearfoot to the forefoot and provides stability as the forefoot manipulates terrain, even or uneven.[6] The long bones of the foot are the metatarsals. Their articulations are in the forefoot. These joints are the tarsometatarsal and metatarsophalangeal joints.

The arches of the foot consist of the medial longitudinal arch, the lateral longitudinal arch, and the transverse arch (figure 26.6). The medial longitudinal arch's apex is the navicular, and its height is often measured to determine pathology locally and globally. The lateral longitudinal arch is on the lateral side, with the apex being the cuboid. The transverse arch runs transversely.

CLIENT INTERVIEW

This interview is typically the first encounter the clinician will have with the client. As previously discussed in chapter 5, this component of the examination can provide the clinician with a significant amount of information relevant to the probability of the client's presenting diagnosis. For purposes of this text, the interview is described relative to each body part or section, but it generally includes subjective reports by the client, as well as findings from their outcome measures. Also included in this section is radiographic imaging. While clinicians should avoid biasing their examination by interpreting findings of radiographic imaging prior to seeing the client (in most cases without concerns for red flags and major medical-related issues), this point in the examination is most likely where clinicians will encounter radiographic imaging. Additionally, in some instances, clinicians must interpret radiographic imaging early in the examination to rule out serious pathology prior to continuing with other components of the examination sequence.

Subjective

The subjective history should be initiated with broad, open-ended questions that help the clinician gather pertinent information. The client should be encouraged to describe the concordant pain with a history of where the pain started and what the mechanism of injury was. As stated in chapter 5, the clinician should ask questions that encourage

Critical Clinical Pearls

The medial longitudinal arch is important for the following reasons:

- A high or low arch may indicate pathology, such as with plantar fasciitis.
- Arch is elevated during terminal stance to enable windlass mechanism.
- Measurement of arch height using navicular height, navicular position test, or arch ratio can provide the clinician with objective information that can help with evaluation and treatment of a variety of pathologies.

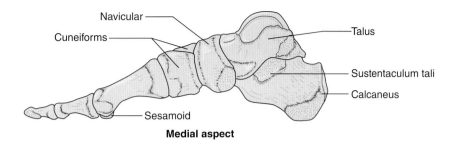

Medial aspect

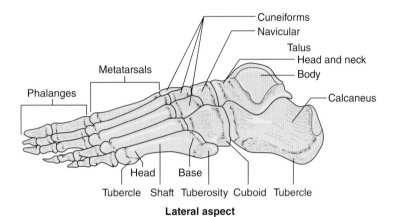

Lateral aspect

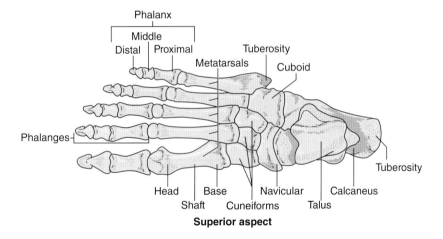

Superior aspect

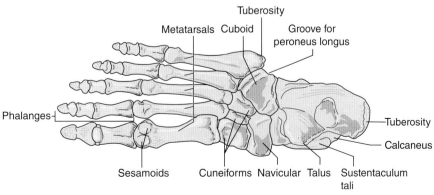

Plantar aspect

Figure 26.5 Bones of the foot and ankle.

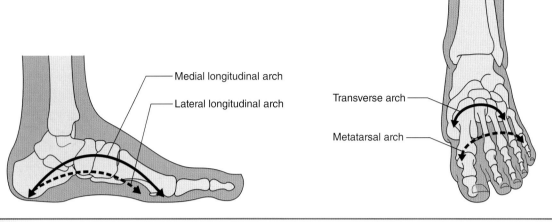

Figure 26.6 Medial, lateral, and transverse arches of the foot.

the client to provide information about whether the concordant pain has gotten progressively better or worse, which activities and times of day influence the pain (worse and better), as well as what kind of pain the client is experiencing (e.g., dull, achy, sharp, stabbing). When looking at the lower leg, ankle, or foot, clinicians should include questions regarding pertinent past medical history such as diabetes, rheumatoid arthritis, gout, osteoarthritis, past pregnancies, and menstrual cycle, as well as musculoskeletal impairments and problems, especially those pertaining to trunk, hip, and knee injuries.[1] At times childhood pathologies, such as clubfoot, may contribute to current impairments and thus must not be missed during subjective history review.

When looking at the foot and ankle, the clinician should learn about the client's footwear preference because wearing poor footwear may significantly contribute to the client's pain and development of impairment.[7, 8, 9] Further questioning should include shoe type for daily use and whether the client wears inserts or any other orthotics or brace. The age of and amount of mileage on the shoes and the orthotics may be pertinent because many patients wear their orthotics and shoes too long. This results in breakdown of the supportive capabilities, which is individualized depending on the forces put through it as well as materials used. The footwear assessment form (figure 26.7) could also be a helpful tool in collecting this information.[10] Questions about the client's occupation may be pertinent if they stand for long periods of time, as well as what shoes they wear to work and what kind of surface they stand on at work.[6]

For the athletic population, other considerations include history of weight loss or weight gain, what athletic activities they perform and the shoe they perform them in, how long they have been performing the athletic activity and on what surface, what their workouts typically consist of (distance vs. speed), if they participate in any dynamic warm-up before or static stretching after, as well as whether they are training for any race in the near future. Understanding the client's goal for coming to physical therapy is of utmost importance, since it could be an area of motivation or lack of compliance with the prescribed home exercise program.[6]

Outcome Measures

A variety of outcome measures are used for the lower leg, foot, and ankle. This section lists some available outcome measures and the pathologies that they have been utilized for.

The Foot and Ankle Ability Measure (FAAM) is the only outcome measure validated in a physical therapy setting for plantar fasciitis clients. It consists of a 21-item activity of daily living (ADL) subscale and an 8-item sports subscale. The test–retest reliability was 0.89 and 0.87 for the ADL and sports subscales, respectively. The minimally clinically important difference for the FAAM was 8 points for the ADL subscale and 9 points for the sports subscale.[11]

The Foot and Ankle Disability Index (FADI) assesses activities of daily living, and the FADI Sport assesses sport-related tasks that are more difficult. Hale and Hertel[12] tested the reliability and sensitivity of the FADI and FADI Sport in young adults with

1. FIT

Foot length [____]   **Thumb width** [____]

Fit of shoe (length) – rule of thumb (wearer's thumb)

Palpation: Good [ ]   Too short (< ½ thumb) [ ]   Too long (> 1 ½) [ ]
Straw =   Good [ ]   Too short (< ½ thumb) [ ]   Too long (> 1 ½) [ ]

Fit of shoe (width) – grasp test   Good [ ]   Too narrow [ ]   Too wide [ ]
Fit of shoe (depth)   Good [ ]   Too shallow [ ]

2. GENERAL

Age of shoe   0 - 6 months [ ]   6 - 12 months [ ]   > 12 months [ ]

Footwear style

Walking shoe [ ]	Athletic shoe [ ]	Oxford shoe [ ]	Moccasin [ ]
Boot [ ]	UGG boot [ ]	High heel [ ]	Thong/Flip-flop [ ]
Slipper [ ]	Backless slipper [ ]	Court shoe [ ]	Mule [ ]
Sandal [ ]	Surgical/Bespoke [ ]	Other (specify) [_____]	

Materials (upper)   Leather [ ]   Synthetic [ ]   Mesh [ ]   Other [_____]
Materials (outsole)   Rubber [ ]   Plastic [ ]   Leather [ ] Other [_____]

Weight [_____]   **Length** [_____]   **Weight/Length** [_____]

3. GENERAL STRUCTURE

Heel height =

0 - 2.5 cm [ ]   2.6 - 5.0 cm [ ]   > 5.0 cm [ ]

Forefoot height (measured at point of the 1st and MTPJs) =

0 - 0.9 cm [ ]   1.0 - 2.0 cm [ ]   > 2.0 cm [ ]

Longitudinal profile (heel – forefoot difference) =

Flat (0 - 0.9 cm) [ ]   Small heel rise (1 - 3 cm) [ ]   Large heel rise (> 3 cm) [ ]

Last (center goniometer at 50% shoe length) =

Straight (< 5°) [ ]   Semicurved (5 - 15°) [ ]   Curved (> 15°) [ ]

Fixation of upper to sole

Board [ ]   Combination [ ]   Slip-lasted [ ]

Forefoot sole flexion point

At level of MTPJs [ ]   Proximal to 1st MTPJ [ ]   Distal to 1st MTPJ [ ]

Figure 26.7 Comprehensive footwear assessment tool.

Reprinted from C.J. Barton, D. Bonanno, and H.B. Menz, 2009, "Development and evaluation of a tool for the assessment of footwear characteristics," *Journal of Foot Ankle Research* 23: 2:10. doi: 10.1186/1757-1146-2-10

(continued)

4. MOTION CONTROL PROPERTIES

Density   Single ☐   Dual ☐

Fixation   None ☐   Laces ☐   Straps/Buckles ☐   Velcro ☐   Zips ☐
                Number of eyelets ☐

Heel counter stiffness (20 mm above bottom or upper)

No heel counter ☐   Minimal (> 45°) ☐   Moderate (< 45°) ☐   Rigid (0-10°) ☐

Midfoot sole sagittal stability

Minimal (> 45°) ☐   Moderate (< 45°) ☐   Rigid (0-10°) ☐

Midfoot sole frontal stability (torsional)

Minimal (> 45°) ☐   Moderate (< 45°) ☐   Rigid (0-10°) ☐

5. CUSHIONING

Presence   None ☐   Heel ☐   Heel/Forefoot ☐

Lateral midsole hardness   Soft ☐   Firm ☐   Hard ☐

Durometer readings   1st ☐   2nd ☐   3rd ☐   Mean ☐

Medial midsole hardness   Soft ☐   Firm ☐   Hard ☐

Durometer readings   1st ☐   2nd ☐   3rd ☐   Mean ☐

Heel sole hardness (center of inside heel shoe interface)   Soft ☐   Firm ☐   Hard ☐

Durometer readings   1st ☐   2nd ☐   3rd ☐   Mean ☐

6. WEAR PATTERNS

Upper   Medial tilt (> 10°) ☐   Neutral ☐   Lateral tilt (> 10°) ☐

Midsole   Medial compression signs ☐   Neutral ☐   Lateral compression signs ☐

Tread pattern   **A**   Textured ☐   Smooth (i.e., no pattern) ☐
                     B   Not worn ☐   Partly worn ☐   Fully worn ☐

Outsole wear pattern   None ☐   Normal ☐   Lateral ☐   Medial ☐

L 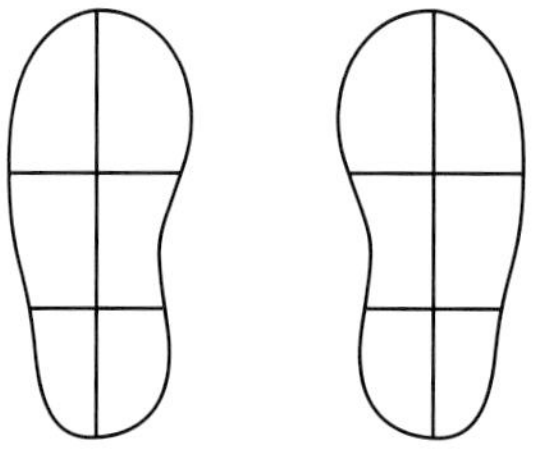   R

Figure 26.7   *(continued)*

chronic ankle instability (CAI) and concluded that the FADI and FADI Sport tools were reliable in detecting the functional limitations of subjects with CAI (intraclass correlation coefficient [ICC] after 1 week was 0.89 and 0.84). The tools were sensitive to differences between healthy subjects and subjects with CAI as well as to improvements after rehabilitation of subjects. After 4 weeks of rehabilitation, they saw significant score increase, showing the responsiveness of the scale.

The Foot Function Index (FFI) has 23 items that measure pain, disability, and activity restriction. The score is based on a visual analogue scale.[13, 14] It is a validated and reliable instrument for people with rheumatoid arthritis and has been seen to be sensitive to change.[13, 15] The FFI was also a reliable tool for measuring outcomes of foot and ankle surgery. Landorf and Radford[16] reported that the minimal important difference for the FFI for pain was an improvement of 12 points and for disability was an improvement of 7 points. Minimal detectable difference of the total score was 7.

The Ankle Osteoarthritis Scale was modified from the FFI and was seen to be a valid and reliable tool for measuring symptoms and disability in patients with ankle osteoarthritis (OA).[17]

Despite the fact that the Lower Extremity Functional Scale (LEFS) is not foot specific, it is often used in practice due to its reliability, validity, and 90% confidence interval of minimal detectable change.[18, 19] It is comprised of 20 items and is scored on a 0 to 4 scale, with 0 being unable to perform and 4 being not difficult.

Diagnostic Imaging

An accurate diagnosis is important because it initiates a treatment plan that will get a person back to 100% function or back to playing sport. Correct use of imaging modalities may be critical to this process. Table 26.1 highlights the diagnostic accuracy of several imaging modalities for different foot and ankle pathologies.

TABLE 26.1   Diagnostic Accuracy of Imaging Modalities for the Lower Leg, Ankle, and Foot

Pathology	Diagnostic test	Gold standard	SN/SP
Syndesmotic ankle injury	US	Uninjured ankle comparison	100/100[20]
	MRI	Surgery	SN 73[21]
Osteomyelitis of foot and ankle	MRI	Variable	Pooled analysis: 77-100/40-100[22]
Bone marrow lesions	CT	MRI	90/81[23]
Achilles tendon tear	MRI	Surgery	SN 91[24]
			94/6[21]
Achilles tendon tear (partial)	US	Surgery	94/100[25]
Posterior tibial tendon tear	MRI	Surgery	94/6[21]
Ankle collateral ligament injury	MRI	Surgery	SN 73[21]
Peroneus longus and brevis tendon tear	MRI	Surgery	SN 57[21]
			83/75[26] (brevis)
			55/89[27]
Peroneal tendinopathy	MRI	Surgery	84/75[27]
Peroneal tendon dislocation	MRI	Surgery	75/99[27]

US = ultrasound; MRI = magnetic resonance imaging; CT = computed tomography; SN = sensitivity; SP = specificity

The color coding for suggestion of **good** and **ideal** diagnostic accuracy values reported in this table are without quality scoring (QUADAS), a very important aspect of determination of the clinical utility of such values. Therefore, it is suggested that the reader keep this in mind when interpreting such values.

Radiographs

Sesamoiditis, spiral fibular fractures (figure 26.8), turf toe, stress fractures (initially shows no injury but pain and symptoms; figure 26.9), Lisfranc fracture (figure 26.10), or midfoot injuries and ankle sprains (if indicated by the Ottawa Ankle Rules) are some common foot and ankle pathologies where radiographs are used.[28]

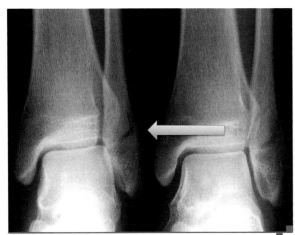

Figure 26.8 Spiral fibular fractures, occurring at the level of the syndesmosis. There may be an associated injury to the deltoid-medial malleolus complex.

© MedPix

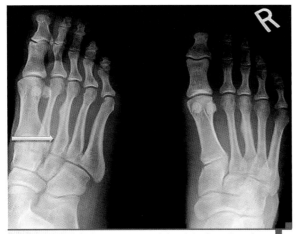

Figure 26.9 Radiographs of the right foot that show focal periosteal reaction and callous formation about the right third metatarsal diaphysis, helping to show the exact location of this stress fracture.

© MedPix

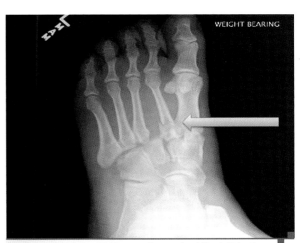

Figure 26.10 Oblique radiograph of the left foot shows a fracture of the base of the 2nd metatarsal and dislocation of bases of the 3rd to 5th metatarsals at the tarsometatarsal joints consistent with fracture or dislocation at the Lisfranc joint.

© MedPix

- **Ottawa Ankle Rules:** The Ottawa Ankle Rules (OAR; figure 26.11) were prospectively derived (N = 750 patients), refined, and validated (N = 1,485). They incorporate simple historical and physical findings that are well defined to determine if clients require radiography of their ankle or foot following a traumatic injury.[29] Radiographs are required only if the client has pain near the malleolus *and* one or more of the following:[29]
  - Bone tenderness along the distal 6 cm of the posterior edge of the tibia or tip of the medial malleolus
  - Bone tenderness along the distal 6 cm of the posterior edge of the fibula or tip of the lateral malleolus
  - Inability to bear weight for four steps, both immediately after the injury and in the emergency department
- **Ottawa Foot Rules:** Radiographs are required only if the client has pain in the midfoot *and* one or more of the following:[29]
  - Bone tenderness at the base of the fifth metatarsal
  - Bone tenderness at the navicular bone
  - Inability to bear weight for four steps, both immediately after the injury and in the emergency department

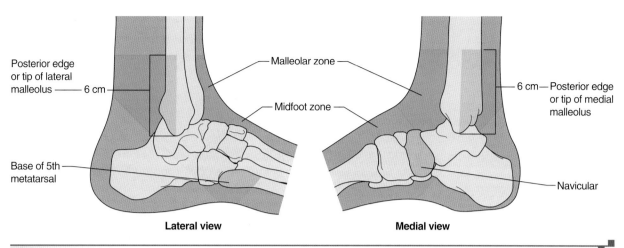

Figure 26.11 Landmarks for Ottawa Ankle and Foot Rules.

An intervention study[30] demonstrated a 27% relative reduction in radiography rates in the intervention hospital versus a 2% increase at the control hospital. For foot injuries, the difference was a 14% relative reduction at the intervention hospital versus a 13% increase at the control hospital. The study also found that clients spent approximately 36 minutes less time in the emergency department without radiography and had similar levels of patient satisfaction. Most importantly, there were no missed fractures using the rule, and similar radiography rates remained at the intervention hospital 12 months after the study concluded.

Bachmann and colleagues[31] did a systematic review on the accuracy of the OAR and concluded the pooled negative likelihood ratios (−LRs) for the ankle and midfoot were 0.08 and 0.08, respectively. The pooled sensitivity (SN) was 99.6 to 96.4 (combined assessment), whereas the specificity (SP) was 26.3 (combined assessment). For children, the pooled −LR was 0.07. The pooled SN was 99.6 when the rule was applied within 48 hours of injury and SN was 96.4 when combining studies that included both foot and ankle.

Dowling and colleagues[32] performed a meta-analysis looking at the accuracy of the OAR for excluding fractures of the ankle and midfoot in children. The study concluded that in children older than 5 years presenting with ankle and midfoot injuries, the OAR was a reliable tool. The pooled SN was 98.5 with the pool estimate of X-ray reduction at 24.8%.

The Bernese Ankle Rules were developed to improve SP of the Ottawa Ankle Rules in identifying fracture after midfoot trauma or low energy malleolar trauma. The exam is three steps: indirect pressure 10 cm proximal to the fibular tip, direct medial malleolar stress, and simultaneous compression of midfoot and hindfoot.[33] The study was done in 354 patients who presented to the ER with the chief complaint of acute varus stress with the foot extended. The SN was 100 and SP was 91, using radiographs as the reference standard.[34]

Magnetic Resonance Imaging

Magnetic resonance imaging (MRI) is often used as a standard procedure for evaluating and diagnosing morphologic changes in the ankle. Both ultrasound (US) and MRI were equally sensitive in detecting the presence (or absence) of the muscle, tendon, and ligament ankle injury, whereas US was less specific than MRI in detecting grade 3 or complete tear injury.[35] Thickening of the plantar fascia insertion more than 5 mm either on US or MRI is suggestive of plantar fasciopathy.[36] If a client complains of pain, instability, crepitus, catching, or locking with little to no improvement after 4 to 6 weeks of nonsurgical treatment for ankle sprain, an MRI is recommended for further diagnosing the presence of osteochondral lesions.[37]

Computed Tomography

For tendon dislocation, entrapment, rupture or injury, and bone chip intercalation, Yu and colleagues[38] found an accuracy of 98.4 (SN 88.8, SP 98.1; 27 patients: 24 men and 8 women [5 subjects were lost to follow up in the study] with an average age of 43 years and surgery as the reference standard) when using computed tomography (CT). Singh and colleagues[39] reported high diagnostic accuracy of using SPECT-CT for ankle and foot pathology when a definitive clinical diagnosis could not be reached with exam and radiography. They reported SN 95.5, SP 83, +LR 5.59, and –LR 0.06 (50 patients: 35 women and 15 men; average age 51.6 years). Guggenberger and colleagues[23] compared MRI to CT when looking at distinct traumatic bone marrow lesions of the ankle joint and concluded that images constructed from CT had high SN and excellent negative predictive value but moderate SP and low positive predictive value.

Ultrasound

Ultrasound is superior to MRI for diagnosis of plantar fibroma because small low-signal lesions on MRI are similar to the normal plantar fascia signal. Ultrasound demonstrates low echogenicity compared with the echogenic plantar fascia.[36]

Review of Systems

Refer to chapter 6 (Triage and Differential Diagnosis) for details on review of systems relevant to the ankle and foot.

OBSERVATION

Observation of the lower leg, foot, and ankle (LLFA) should include both weight-bearing (WB) and non-weight-bearing (NWB) positions. With both positions, the clinician should observe the client in their normal stance or posture without correction to ascertain their most typical presentation. In the WB position, the clinician should observe for LLFA posture statically and during gait due to the relationship between static foot posture and mobility.[40] Gait assessment is one of the most important parts of the LLFA exam, and it can often give the clinician a sense of the client's functional ability in WB.[41] Clients may have an altered heel toe progression to decrease weight bearing or painful dorsiflexion and may adopt different compensations either in the foot or up the kinetic chain.[42] More information on gait assessment can be found in chapter 13.

The clinician should observe shoulder and pelvic height, spinal curvature, pelvic rotation, femoral anteversion or retroversion (refer to chapter 14), amount of knee flexion or extension, degree of valgus and varus of the knee and tibia, foot position, and navicular drop in standing (refer to Special Tests section for methodology).[42] Other things that are important to observe are the following: subtalar pronation; tibial torsion; distal tibiofemoral joint; rearfoot to leg orientation; forefoot to rearfoot orientation; degrees of pronation and supination, both weight-bearing and non-weight-bearing; foot deviations such as pes planus, pes cavus, talipes equinus or talipes equinovarus, and hallux valgus; degree of toe out; forefoot equinus; talar bulge; condition of nails and toes; edema, bruising, or swelling; calluses; vasomotor or circulatory changes; shoes and shoe wear; and skin health (dryness, sweating, or perfusion).[1]

Observing the foot and ankle mechanics during functional tasks such as walking, stair climbing, and performing a single-leg squat and step-down can provide valuable information for the clinician. Plantar load distribution during these functional tasks is an important observational measurement as increased pain has been seen to correlate with increased plantar loading.[1] These functional tests can also be used to evaluate balance and proprioception.[43, 44]

Here are some common deformities, deviations, and injuries to the LLFA. For common observation tests and measures, refer to the Special Tests section.

- **Hammer toe:** flexion contracture of the plantar surface of the proximal interphalangeal (PIP) with a mild associated contracture of the metatarsophalangeal (MTP) joint (figure 26.12).[6]
- **Mallet toe:** flexion deformity of the distal interphalangeal joint with plantar contracture.[6]
- **Claw toe:** hyperextension of the MTP joints and flexion of the PIP and distal interphalangeal (DIP) joints (figure 26.13). This is a more advance contracture of the intrinsic muscles

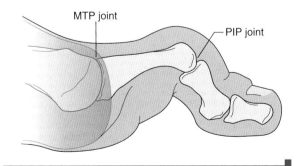

Figure 26.12 Hammer toe.

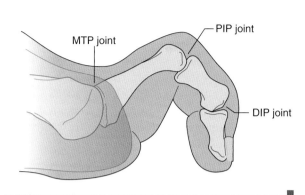

Figure 26.13   Claw toe.

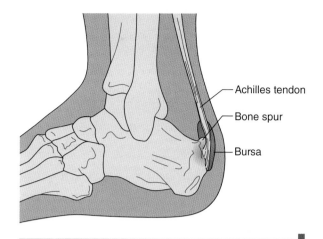

Figure 26.14   Haglund's deformity.

and capsules, which can be associated with pes cavus, muscle pathology to lumbricales or interosseous muscles, or neurologic pathology.[6]

- **Bunion:** Hallux valgus formed by the first metatarsal bone and the proximal phalanx of the hallux.[265]

- **Bunionette (tailor's bunion):** painful prominence on the lateral aspect of the fifth metatarsal head due to bony enlargement of the head itself; increased intermetatarsal angle; bowing of the fifth metatarsal; or posttraumatic, iatrogenic, or inflammatory arthropathy; or due to extrinsic factors such as footwear or working position. Depending on the symptoms, the client could conservatively treat this deformity; however, if that fails, surgical treatment should be performed.[45]

- **Pes planus:** flat footedness, can be flexible or rigid.

- **Helbing's sign:** a curving inward of the Achilles tendon that happens most often with flat footedness.

- **Pes cavus:** foot has a high arch, which results in limited weight bearing on the plantar aspect of the foot and, in turn, pressure placed on the heel and metatarsal heads.[46]

- **Pump bump:** Haglund's deformity (figure 26.14) is the bony enlargement on the back of the heel, which can develop bursitis.

- **Equinus deformity (talipes equinus):** limited dorsiflexion (lack of 10°); may be due to

contracture of gastrocnemius or soleus muscle groups or due to trauma, inflammatory disease, or spasticity structural bone deformities. Clients with this deformity may have symptoms of medial arch pain, posterior leg pain, plantar heel pain, talonavicular pain, lateral ankle sprains, or metatarsalgia.[47]

- **Clubfoot:** includes a wide range of deformities, most of which involve the heel (figure 26.15). Talipes equinovarus is the most common. Two categories are present: flexible or resistant form. The flexible form can be treated conservatively with orthotics and footwear modifications. The resistant form requires surgery due to the presence of stiffness.[6] (Refer to chapter 29, Pediatric Examination, for more detail on clubfoot.)

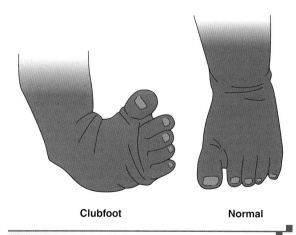

Clubfoot   Normal

Figure 26.15   Clubfoot.

- **Hindfoot varus (subtalar varus):** most common abnormality. Inversion of the calcaneus when subtalar joint is neutral.

- **Hindfoot valgus:** eversion of the calcaneus when subtalar joint is neutral.[6]

- **Forefoot valgus:** when the plane of the metatarsal head is in an everted or valgus position. All of the metatarsal heads may be everted, or the first metatarsal head may be plantar flexed while the second to fifth lie in the correct plane.[6]

- **Forefoot varus:** inversion of the forefoot on the rearfoot when the subtalar joint is neutral.[48] Garbalosa and colleagues found a mean of 8° of forefoot varus in studies of 120 healthy subjects, showing that a certain amount of varus may be characteristic of a healthy population.[49]

- **Metatarsus adductus (hooked forefoot):** adduction of the five metatarsals at the tarsometatarsal joints, in the transverse plane.

- **Morton's metatarsalgia (interdigital neuroma):** Entrapment of the interdigital nerve occurs as the nerve passes on the plantar aspect of the transverse intermetatarsal ligament where it is vulnerable to a traction injury and compression during repetitive toe-rise or toe-off phase in running. The third interdigital nerve is most commonly involved and can be found between the third and fourth metatarsal heads. Clients will often report forefoot burning, cramping, numbness in the toes of the involved interspace, and tingling; they may also report proximal radiation into the foot. Diagnosis can be made through physical exam; however, ultrasound and MRI can aid this. With footwear modifications, orthosis, injections, sclerosing and steroids, this can be treated nonoperatively; however, if these methods fail, conservative treatment nerve decompression or a neurectomy may surgically help symptoms.[50]

- **Hallux rigidus:** Decreased dorsiflexion of the first MTP joint and pain and swelling in the posterior aspect of the joint[51] are usually due to osteochondritis dissecans (OCD) or localized articular disorder in adolescents and generalized degenerative arthritis in adults.[6]

- **Morton's foot:** This short first metatarsal with long second metatarsal leads to increased loading of second metatarsal head and callus formation.

- **Tarsal coalition:** This is a connection of two bones of the mid- or rearfoot, either a fibrous, cartilaginous, or bony connection (figure 26.16). Plane radiographs assist with diagnosing it, since it is difficult to diagnose such malformations during the physical exam.[6] Clients may complain of vague pain with insidious onset in the rearfoot or midfoot or of frequent ankle sprains.[52]

- **Os trigonum:** This separation of the secondary center of the lateral tubercle from the remainder of the posterior talus (figure 26.17) is due to either repeated microtrauma during development or a fracture that has not united. The client will report pain during passive plantarflexion between the Achilles tendon and the lateral malleolus.[53]

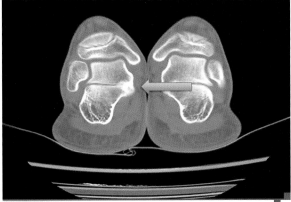

Figure 26.16 Tarsal coalition.
© MedPix

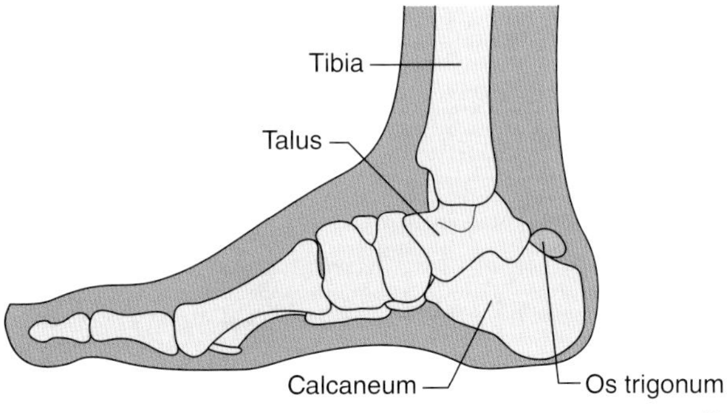

Tibia

Talus

Calcaneum — Os trigonum

Figure 26.17 Os trigonum.

TRIAGE AND SCREENING

Triage and screening is a necessary component of the examination process to complete prior to continuing with the examination. Ruling out serious pathology (refer to chapter 6, Triage and Differential Diagnosis) and pain generation from other related (or close-proximity) structures assists the clinician in more accurately determining the necessity of continuing with the other examination components to identify the actual source of the client's pain. Additionally, clinicians should implement strong screening tests (tests of high SN and low –LR) at this point in the examination to narrow down the competing diagnoses of the respective body region (lower leg, ankle, or foot in this case) when this is applicable.

Ruling Out Serious Pathology: Red Flags

At this point, the clinician must decide whether or not to continue with the examination. The cli-

nician should determine whether to continue examining the client or to potentially refer them to a physician at this stage of the examination procedure. A careful subjective history and observation of the client will help the clinician with the triage process.

Tests for fractures and stress fractures include the following:

- Ottawa Ankle Rules: for screening or diagnosing the ankle fracture
  - Pooled **SN 96.4–99.6** (combined assessment), pooled SP 26.3 (combined assessment); **–LR 0.08**
  - For children, pooled –LR was **0.07**. The pooled **SN 99.6** < 48 hours post injury was **SN 96.4** when combining studies that included both the foot and ankle.
- Bernese Ankle Rules: indirect malleolar stress test
  - **SN 100, SP 91**, using radiographs as the reference standard[34]

Client Position	Supine with the lower extremities relaxed
Clinician Position	Standing at the side of the lower extremity to be assessed, directly the facing client
Movement	The clinician places a stethoscope on the fibular head. The clinician taps and places the tuning fork on the lateral malleolus.
Assessment	A (+) test is a diminished or absent sound.

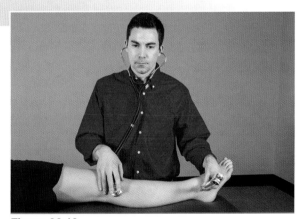

Figure 26.18

Statistics
- Placement over bony landmark: SN 83, SP 80, +LR 4.2, –LR 0.21, QUADAS 6, in a study of 37 clients (19 men, 18 women) with various locations and types of fractures, using a reference standard of radiography[54]
- Placement (stethoscope) over swelling area: SN 83, SP 92, +LR 10.4, –LR 0.2, in the same study[54]
- SN 75, SP 67, +LR 2.3, –LR 0.3, QUADAS 9, in a study of 52 clients with a history and physical examination suggestive of tibial stress fracture, using bone scan as a reference standard[55]

PLANTAR PERCUSSION TEST

Client Position	Sitting or supine with foot in dorsiflexion
Clinician Position	Standing at the side of the lower extremity to be assessed, directly facing the client
Movement	The client extends the toes to full range of motion. The clinician taps the region plantar/volar surface between the 2nd and 3rd metatarsal heads.
Assessment	A (+) test is reproduction of neurological findings, such as tingling.
Statistics	SN 62, QUADAS 7, in a study of 116 feet (76 treated operatively for Morton's neuroma and 40 feet with different pathologies; mean age 51 ± 12 years; 60 women; mean duration of symptoms not reported [NR]), using MRI as a reference standard[56]

FOOT SQUEEZE TEST (MORTON'S TEST)

Client Position	Sitting or supine
Clinician Position	Standing at the side of the lower extremity to be assessed, directly facing the client
Movement	The clinician applies a squeeze to the metatarsal heads from lateral to medial toward the midline.
Assessment	A test is (+) if the client's symptoms are reproduced.
Statistics	SN 88, QUADAS 7, in a study of 116 feet (76 treated operatively for Morton's neuroma and 40 feet with different pathologies; mean age 51 ± 12 years; 60 women; mean duration of symptoms NR), using MRI as a reference standard[56]

WEB SPACE TENDERNESS

Client Position	Sitting or supine
Clinician Position	Standing at the side of the lower extremity to be assessed, directly facing the client
Movement	The clinician applies a force between the 2nd and 3rd metatarsals using the tip or side of their thumb.
Assessment	A test is (+) if the client's symptoms are reproduced.
Statistics	SN 95, QUADAS 7, in a study of 116 feet (76 treated operatively for Morton's neuroma and 40 feet with different pathologies; mean age 51 ± 12 years; 60 women; mean duration of symptoms NR), using MRI as a reference standard[56]

Ruling Out Pain Generation From Other Related Structures

Once red flags are ruled out, an efficient way to begin to differentiate the many potential pain referral sources is through the lower quarter screening examination. The traditional lower quarter screen consists of testing dermatomes, myotomes, deep tendon reflexes, and possible upper motor involvement. The clinician should differentially diagnose the potential contribution of the sacroiliac joint and pelvic girdle, lumbar spine, hip and knee (whichever are relevant) as the primary pain generator for the client's pain in the lower leg, ankle, or foot. Screening tests for these areas are employed to limit the extent of the differential diagnosis for pathology contributing to the client's pain. A systematic approach to ruling out these other areas is suggested. The key points of this approach are listed here. Refer to chapters 19 (Lumbar Spine) and 20 (Sacroiliac Joint and Pelvic Girdle) for greater detail regarding these examination procedures.

Rule Out the Lumbar Spine

The following section lists suggested special tests for ruling out the lumbar spine as a potential pain generator for the client with presentation of pain in the lower leg, ankle, or foot. The details of each of these tests can be found in chapter 19.

Radiculopathy or Discogenic-Related Pathology

This is ruled out with a combination of range of motion (ROM) and special tests assessments.

Repeated Motions (ROM)

- Centralization and peripheralization: 5-20 reps
  - **SN 92 (NR)**, SP 64 (NR), +LR 2.6, **−LR 0.12,** QUADAS 12[57]
  - SN 40 (28-54), **SP 94 (73-99), +LR 6.7,** −LR 0.64, QUADAS 13[58]

Special Tests

- Straight leg raise test
  - **SN 97 (NR)**, SP 57 (NR), +LR 2.3, **−LR 0.05,** QUADAS 10[59]
  - Pooled analysis: **SN 92 (87-95)**, SP 28 (18-40), +LR 2.9, **−LR 0.29**[60]
- Slump test
  - **SN 83 (NR)**, SP 55 (NR), +LR 1.8, **−LR 0.32,** QUADAS 11[61]

Facet Joint Dysfunction

This is ruled out with the seated extension–rotation test. As noted in the lumbar spine chapter, facet joint dysfunction is ruled in with posterior-to-anterior spinal joint-play assessments eliciting stiffness and concordant pain.

- Seated extension–rotation: **SN 100 (NR)**, SP 22 (NR), +LR 1.3, **−LR 0.0,** QUADAS 11[62]

Rule Out SI Joint Dysfunction

The following section lists suggested special tests to utilize for the purpose of ruling out the sacroiliac joint (SIJ) as a potential pain generator for the client with presentation of lower leg, ankle, and foot pain. The details of each of these tests can be found in chapter 20.

- Pain provocation cluster testing:[63] **SN 91 (62-98), SP 83 (68-96), +LR 6.97, −LR 0.11,** QUADAS 13
- Thigh thrust test: **SN 88 (64-97)**, SP 69 (47-82), +LR 2.80, **−LR 0.18,** QUADAS 12[64]

Rule Out Hip Joint Dysfunction

Hip ROM limitations should be ruled out in all planes (see chapter 24). Intra-articular hip joint involvement is ruled out with the flexion-adduction-internal rotation (FADDIR) test:

- **Pooled SN 94 (88-97)**, SP 8 (2-20), +LR 1.02, **−LR 0.48,** across four studies with 128 clients (MRA reference standard)[65]
- **Pooled SN 99 (95-100)**, SP 7 (0-34), +LR 1.06, **−LR 0.15,** across two studies with 157 clients (arthroscopy reference standard)[65]

Additionally, as with any joint, clearing AROM with or without overpressure is necessary. AROM of all motions as per the lower quarter screen described in chapter 7 should be implemented. In order to fully clear the lumbar spine, SI joint, or hip joint, full AROM (with overpressure if pain-free) must be present.

Sensitive Tests: Knee

The following section lists suggested special tests for ruling out the knee joint as a potential pain generator for the client with presentation of lower leg, ankle, and foot pain. The details of each of these tests can be found in chapter 25.

- Ottawa Knee Rules for screening or diagnosing knee fracture
  - Pooled analysis: **SN 99 (93-100)**, SP 49 (43-51), +LR 1.9, **−LR 0.02,** across six studies with 4,249 adult clients (radiography reference standard)[66]
  - **SN 100 (96-100)**, SP 52 (49-55), +LR 2.1, **−LR 0.01** for identifying fractures of the knee and allowing clinicians to reduce the use of radiography in clients with acute knee injuries[67]

Deep Venous Thrombosis

See chapter 6 (Triage and Differential Diagnosis) for details on deep venous thrombosis.

Additionally, as with any joint, clearing AROM with or without overpressure is necessary. In order to fully clear the lower leg, ankle, and foot, full AROM (with overpressure if pain-free) must be present. Details in this regard are described in the following section.

MOTION TESTS

Motion assessment is a very important aspect of the examination for the orthopedic client. Motion dysfunction can be used to differentiate contractile versus non-contractile tissue (see chapter 9). Assessment of end-feel, potential capsular patterns, and ROM norm values can give the clinician an appreciation of the potential impairments for the orthopedic client they are assessing. Active ROM, PROM, and joint-play assessments are necessary to determine not only the presence or absence of joint dysfunction but also the precise aspects of the motion that are dysfunctional. Table 26.2 identifies the close-packed and resting capsular positions, as well as ROM and end-feel for the lower leg, ankle, and foot.

TABLE 26.2   Lower Leg, Ankle, and Foot Arthrology

Joint	Close-packed position	Resting position	Capsular pattern	ROM norms	End-feel
HINDFOOT					
Tibiofibular	Full dorsiflexion	Plantarflexion	Pain on stress		
Talocrural	Full dorsiflexion	10° of plantar flexion midway between inversion and eversion	Plantarflexion > dorsiflexion	Plantarflexion: 30–50° Dorsiflexion: 20°	Dorsiflexion is firm; plantarflexion is firm or hard
Subtalar	Supination	Pronation	Supination > pronation, inversion > eversion (varus > valgus)	Supination (hindfoot inversion): 20° Pronation (hindfoot eversion): 10°	Inversion is firm; eversion is either firm due to soft tissue or hard due to abutment of the calcaneus and sinus tarsi
MIDFOOT					
Midtarsal	Supination	Mid-range	Dorsiflexion > plantarflexion		Same as subtalar
FOREFOOT					
Tarsometatarsal	Supination	Midway between end ranges of flexion and extension	None		Firm
Metatarsophalangeal	Full extension	10° extension	Big toe: extension > flexion Toes 2-5: none	Big toe flexion: 45° Toe flexion: 40° Big toe extension:70° Toe extension: 40°	Firm for all motions
Interphalangeal	Full flexion	Slight flexion	Flexion > extension	Big toe flexion: 90° Toe flexion: PIP 35°, DIP 60° Big toe extension: 0° Toe extension: PIP 0°, DIP 30°	Firm for all motions

Passive and Active ROMs

Passive accessory motion assessment is essential in determining the potential for joint-play dysfunction in the joints being examined. The following section details individual component assessments of passive joint mobility for the lower leg, foot, and ankle joints.

Ample evidence supports the intrarater reliability of dorsiflexion range of motion measurements (reported intraclass correlation coefficient [ICC] for active assessment varies from 0.64 to 0.92; ICC for passive assessment varies from 0.74 to 0.98). Some evidence supports interrater reliability with reported ICC varying from 0.29 to 0.81.[68]

Critical Clinical Pearls

When performing PROM of the midtarsal joints (talonavicular, calcaneocuboid joints), keep the following in mind:

- The longitudinal axis is 15° from the transverse plane in the sagittal plane and 9° from the sagittal plane in the transverse plane.
- Motion along the longitudinal axis is rotational inversion and eversion.
- The oblique axis is 52° from the transverse plane in the sagittal plane and 57° from the sagittal plane in the transverse plane.
- Motion along the oblique axis is forefoot dorsiflexion and abduction, forefoot plantarflexion and adduction.

TALOCRURAL DORSIFLEXION

Client Position	Sitting with the distal leg off the edge of the table, foot in neutral inversion or eversion
Clinician Position	Standing directly to the side of the client
Goniometer Alignment	The clinician positions the fulcrum over the lateral aspect of the lateral malleolus and aligns the proximal arm with the lateral midline of the fibula and the distal arm parallel to the lateral aspect of the fifth metatarsal.
Movement	The clinician stabilizes the client's distal tibia with their proximal hand and grasps the client's foot with their distal hand. The clinician then passively moves the client's foot into dorsiflexion to end range (end-feel is firm due to tension in the posterior capsule and Achilles tendon). This motion can be performed similarly actively by the client (without assistance from the clinician). Active range of motion should be performed prior to PROM to determine the client's willingness to move and so on.
Assessment	Clinician assesses for amount of ROM, end-feel, quality of the movement, client response, potential difference between AROM and PROM, and so on.

TALOCRURAL PLANTARFLEXION

Client Position	Sitting with the distal leg off the edge of the table, foot in neutral inversion or eversion
Clinician Position	Standing directly to the side of the client
Goniometer Alignment	The clinician positions the fulcrum over the lateral aspect of the lateral malleolus and aligns the proximal arm with the lateral midline of the fibula and the distal arm parallel to the lateral aspect of the fifth metatarsal.
Movement	The clinician stabilizes the client's distal tibia with their proximal hand and grasps the client's foot with their distal hand. The clinician then passively moves the client's foot into plantarflexion to end range (end-feel is firm due to tension of anterior capsule and anterior musculature and ligaments). This motion can be performed similarly actively by the client (without assistance from the clinician). Active range of motion should be performed prior to PROM to determine the client's willingness to move and so on.
Assessment	Clinician assesses for amount of ROM, end-feel, quality of the movement, client response, potential difference between AROM and PROM, and so on.

TARSAL JOINT INVERSION

Client Position	Sitting with the distal leg off the edge of the table, foot in neutral inversion or eversion
Clinician Position	Standing directly to the side of the client
Goniometer Alignment	The clinician positions the fulcrum over the anterior aspect of the client's ankle midway between the medial and lateral malleoli and aligns the proximal arm with the midline of the anterior leg and tibial tuberosity and the distal arm with the second metatarsal of the foot.
Movement	The clinician stabilizes the client's distal leg with one hand to prevent lower leg internal and external rotation. With the other hand, the clinician passively moves the client's foot into plantarflexion and adduction, and turns the sole of the foot into supination, producing eversion to end range (end-feel is firm due to tension in the joint capsule and ligamentous structures). This motion can be performed similarly actively by the client (without assistance from the clinician). Active range of motion should be performed prior to PROM to determine the client's willingness to move and so on.
Assessment	Clinician assesses for amount of ROM, end-feel, quality of the movement, client response, potential difference between AROM and PROM, and so on.

TARSAL JOINT EVERSION

Client Position	Sitting with the distal leg off the edge of the table, foot in neutral inversion or eversion
Clinician Position	Standing directly to the side of the client
Goniometer Alignment	The clinician positions the fulcrum over the anterior aspect of the client's ankle midway between the medial and lateral malleoli and aligns the proximal arm with the midline of the anterior leg and tibial tuberosity and the distal arm with the second metatarsal of the foot.
Movement	The clinician stabilizes the client's distal leg with one hand to prevent lower-leg internal and external rotation. With the other hand, the clinician passively moves the foot into dorsiflexion and abduction, and turns the lateral side of the foot into pronation, producing eversion to end range (end-feel may be hard due to contact of calcaneus and sinus tarsi or it may be firm due to tension in the joint capsule and deltoid ligament). This motion can be performed similarly actively by the client (without assistance from the clinician). Active range of motion should be performed prior to PROM to determine the client's willingness to move and so on.
Assessment	Clinician assesses for amount of ROM, end-feel, quality of the movement, client response, potential difference between AROM and PROM, and so on.

SUBTALAR JOINT (REARFOOT) INVERSION

Client Position	Prone on table, hip and knee in neutral and foot off the edge of the table
Clinician Position	Standing directly to the side of the client
Goniometer Alignment	The clinician positions the fulcrum over the posterior aspect of the client's ankle midway between the medial and lateral malleoli and aligns the proximal arm with the midline of posterior lower leg and the distal arm with the midline of the posterior calcaneus.
Movement	The clinician stabilizes the distal tibia and fibula with one hand. With the other hand, the clinician moves the client's calcaneus into adduction and rotates it into supination, producing inversion to end range (end-feel is firm due to the tension of the lateral joint capsule and ligaments). This motion can be performed similarly actively by the client (without assistance from the clinician). Active range of motion should be performed prior to PROM to determine the client's willingness to move and so on.
Assessment	Clinician assesses for amount of ROM, end-feel, quality of the movement, client response, potential difference between AROM and PROM, and so on.

SUBTALAR JOINT (REARFOOT) EVERSION

Client Position	Prone on table, with the hip and knee in neutral and the foot off the edge of the table
Clinician Position	Standing directly to the side of the client
Goniometer Alignment	The clinician positions the fulcrum over the posterior aspect of the client's ankle midway between medial and lateral malleoli and aligns the proximal arm with the midline of the posterior lower leg and the distal arm with the midline of the posterior calcaneus.
Movement	The clinician stabilizes the client's distal tibia and fibula with one hand. With the other hand, the clinician moves the client's calcaneus into abduction and rotates it into pronation, producing inversion to end range (end-feel is hard due to contact between calcaneus and sinus tarsi, or may be firm due to the tension of the deltoid ligament). This motion can be performed similarly actively by the client (without assistance from the clinician). Active range of motion should be performed prior to PROM to determine the client's willingness to move and so on.
Assessment	Clinician assesses for amount of ROM, end-feel, quality of the movement, client response, potential difference between AROM and PROM, and so on.

METATARSOPHALANGEAL JOINT FLEXION

Client Position	Supine or sitting, with the foot in neutral dorsiflexion or plantarflexion and inversion or eversion
Clinician Position	Standing directly to the side of the client
Goniometer Alignment	The clinician positions the fulcrum over the dorsal/anterior aspect of the MTP joint and aligns the proximal arm with the medial midline of the first metatarsal and the distal arm with the medial midline of the proximal phalanx of the first toe. If a toe goniometer is not available, the clinician can use a small goniometer with the medial side of the MTP joint as the fulcrum.
Movement	The clinician stabilizes the first metatarsal with one hand, while the other hand passively moves the big toe into flexion (or downward, avoiding interphalangeal flexion) to end range (end-feel is firm due to tension in the dorsal/anterior joint capsule and ligaments). This motion can be performed similarly actively by the client (without assistance from the clinician). Active range of motion should be performed prior to PROM to determine the client's willingness to move and so on.
Assessment	Clinician assesses for amount of ROM, end-feel, quality of the movement, client response, potential difference between AROM and PROM, and so on.

METATARSOPHALANGEAL JOINT EXTENSION

Client Position	Supine or sitting, with the foot in neutral dorsiflexion or plantarflexion and inversion or eversion
Clinician Position	Standing directly to the side of the client
Goniometer Alignment	The clinician positions the fulcrum over the dorsal/anterior aspect of MTP joint and aligns the proximal arm with the medial midline of the first metatarsal and the distal arm with the medial midline of the proximal phalanx of the first toe. If a toe goniometer is not available, the clinician can use a small goniometer with the medial side of the MTP joint as the fulcrum.
Movement	The clinician stabilizes the first metatarsal with one hand, while the other hand passively moves the big toe into extension (or upward, avoiding interphalangeal extension) to end range (end-feel is firm due to tension in the plantar/posterior joint capsule and muscles). This motion can be performed similarly actively by the client (without assistance from the clinician). Active range of motion should be performed prior to PROM to determine the client's willingness to move and so on.
Assessment	Clinician assesses for amount of ROM, end-feel, quality of the movement, client response, potential difference between AROM and PROM, and so on.

METATARSOPHALANGEAL JOINT ABDUCTION

Client Position	Supine or sitting, with the foot in neutral dorsiflexion or plantarflexion and inversion or eversion
Clinician Position	Standing directly to the side of the client
Goniometer Alignment	The clinician positions the fulcrum over the dorsal/anterior aspect of the MTP joint and aligns the proximal arm with the dorsal/ anterior midline of the metatarsal and the distal arm with the dorsal/ anterior midline of the proximal phalanx.
Movement	The clinician stabilizes the first metatarsal with one hand and uses the other hand to passively move the client's phalanx laterally away from midline (into abduction) to end range (end-feel is firm due to tension of the joint capsule and collateral ligaments). This motion can be performed similarly actively by the client (without assistance from the clinician). Active range of motion should be performed prior to PROM to determine the client's willingness to move and so on.
Assessment	Clinician assesses for amount of ROM, end-feel, quality of the movement, client response, potential difference between AROM and PROM, and so on.

INTERPHALANGEAL JOINT MOTIONS

A finger or toe goniometer is required for these measurements.

Client Position	Supine or sitting, with the foot in neutral dorsiflexion or plantarflexion and inversion or eversion
Clinician Position	Standing directly to the side of the client
Goniometer Alignment	The clinician positions the fulcrum over the dorsal/anterior aspect of the joint to be assessed and aligns the proximal arm over the dorsal/anterior aspect of the bone proximal to joint and the distal arm over the dorsal/anterior aspect of the bone distal to the joint.
Movement	The clinician's proximal hand stabilizes the client's foot proximally to the joint while the other hand moves the bone distal to the joint into flexion to end range (end-feel is firm due to tension in the capsule and soft tissues). This motion can be performed similarly actively by the client (without assistance from the clinician). Active range of motion should be performed prior to PROM to determine the client's willingness to move and so on.
Assessment	Clinician assesses for amount of ROM, end-feel, quality of the movement, client response, potential difference between AROM and PROM, and so on.

Passive Accessories

Passive accessory motion assessment is essential for determining the potential for joint-play dysfunction in the joints being examined. The following section details distinct component assessments of passive joint mobility for the lower leg, ankle, and foot.

PROXIMAL TIBIOFIBULAR JOINT POSTERIOR GLIDE

Client Position	Supine on table with the knee slightly flexed for comfort
Clinician Position	Standing facing the client at the client's side to be assessed
Stabilization	The rest of the client's body on the table serves as a stabilizing force. The clinician's stabilizing hand (right as shown) purchases the medial proximal tibia (anteriorly).
Movement and Direction of Force	The heel of the clinician's assessing hand (left as shown) purchases the anterior surface of the fibular head. With their assessing hand, the clinician glides the fibula in a posterior direction along the plane of the joint.
Assessment	Assessment is done for joint play/passive accessory motion, client response, and end-feel. Reproduction of concordant pain suggests dysfunction. Impaired joint mobility or end-feel may also suggest dysfunction if concordant pain is also reproduced.

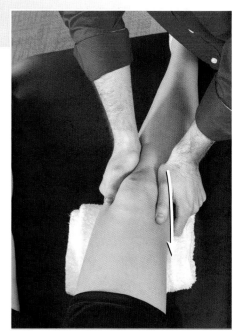

Figure 26.19

PROXIMAL TIBIOFIBULAR JOINT ANTERIOR GLIDE

Client Position	Prone on the table with the knee slightly flexed for comfort
Clinician Position	Standing at the client's side to be assessed
Stabilization	The rest of the client's body on the table serves as a stabilizing force. The clinician's stabilizing hand (left as shown) purchases the medial proximal tibia (posteriorly).
Movement and Direction of Force	The heel of the clinician's assessing hand (right as shown) purchases the posterior surface of the fibular head. The clinician uses their assessing hand to glide the fibula in an anterior direction along the plane of the joint.
Assessment	Assessment is done for joint play/passive accessory motion, client response, and end-feel. Reproduction of concordant pain suggests dysfunction. Impaired joint mobility or end-feel may also suggest dysfunction if concordant pain is also reproduced.

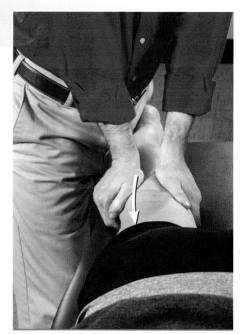

Figure 26.20

DISTAL TIBIOFIBULAR JOINT POSTERIOR GLIDE

Client Position	Supine on the table, with the knee to be assessed slightly flexed for comfort (if desired) and the opposite knee bent to assist the clinician's position
Clinician Position	Standing at the client's ankle to be assessed
Stabilization	The rest of the client's body on the table serves as a stabilizing force. The clinician's stabilizing hand (right as shown) purchases the medial distal portion of tibia (anteriorly).
Movement and Direction of Force	The heel of the clinician's assessing hand (right as shown) purchases the anterior surface of the distal fibula. Using their assessing hand, the clinician glides the fibula in a posterior direction along the plane of the joint.
Assessment	Assessment is done for joint play/passive accessory motion, client response, and end-feel. Reproduction of concordant pain suggests dysfunction. Impaired joint mobility or end-feel may also suggest dysfunction if concordant pain is also reproduced.

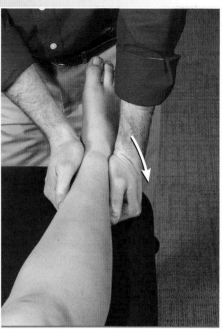

Figure 26.21

DISTAL TIBIOFIBULAR ANTERIOR GLIDE

Client Position	Prone on table
Clinician Position	Standing at the client's ankle to be assessed
Stabilization	The rest of the client's body on the table serves as a stabilizing force. The clinician's stabilizing hand (left as shown) purchases the medial distal portion of tibia (posteriorly).
Movement and Direction of Force	The heel of the clinician's assessing hand (right as shown) purchases the posterior surface of the distal fibula. Using their assessing hand, the clinician glides the fibula in an anterior direction along the plane of the joint.

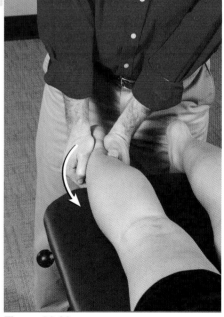

Figure 26.22

DISTAL TIBIOFIBULAR SUPERIOR GLIDE

Client Position	Supine on table, with the opposite knee bent if desired
Clinician Position	Sitting at the distal end of the client's ankle to be assessed, directly facing client
Stabilization	The rest of the client's body on the table serves as a stabilizing force. The clinician's stabilizing hand (right as shown) purchases the distal portion of the tibia (inferiorly).
Movement and Direction of Force	The heel of the clinician's assessing hand (left as shown) purchases the inferior surface of the distal fibula. Using their assessing hand, the clinician glides the fibula in a superior direction along the plane of the joint.
Assessment	Assessment is done for joint play/passive accessory motion, client response, and end-feel. Reproduction of concordant pain suggests dysfunction. Impaired joint mobility or end-feel may also suggest dysfunction if concordant pain is also reproduced.

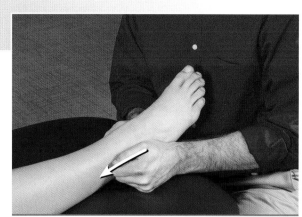

Figure 26.23

TALOCRURAL JOINT DISTRACTION

Client Position	Supine on the table
Clinician Position	Standing at the client's ankle to be assessed
Stabilization	The rest of the client's body on the table serves as a stabilizing force. With one hand (right as shown), the clinician purchases the joint anteriorly over the talus and with the other hand (left as shown), the clinician purchases it posteriorly (directly proximal to posterior calcaneus).
Movement and Direction of Force	Keeping their arms in line with the long axis of lower leg, the clinician leans away from the joint, distracting the talus distally. The clinician performs direct distraction of the talus (inferior direction) from the distal tibia and fibula.
Assessment	Assessment is done for joint play/passive accessory motion, client response, and end-feel. Reproduction of concordant pain suggests dysfunction. Impaired joint mobility or end-feel may also suggest dysfunction if concordant pain is also reproduced.

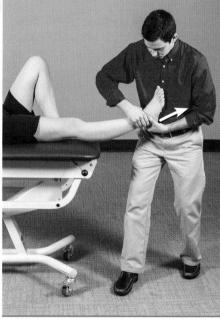

Figure 26.24

TALOCRURAL JOINT POSTERIOR GLIDE

 Video 26.25 **in the web resource shows a demonstration of this test.**

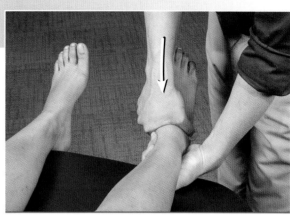

Figure 26.25

Client Position	Supine on the table
Clinician Position	Standing at the client's ankle to be assessed
Stabilization	The rest of the client's body on the table serves as a stabilizing force. The clinician's stabilizing hand (left as shown) purchases the posterior portion of the distal tibia and fibula.
Movement and Direction of Force	The clinician's assessing hand (right as shown) purchases the proximal talus anteriorly in the web space between the thumb and index finger. Using their assessing hand, the clinician glides the talus in a posterior direction along the plane of the joint.
Assessment	Assessment is done for joint play/passive accessory motion, client response, and end-feel. Reproduction of concordant pain suggests dysfunction. Impaired joint mobility or end-feel may also suggest dysfunction if concordant pain is also reproduced.

TALOCRURAL JOINT ANTERIOR GLIDE

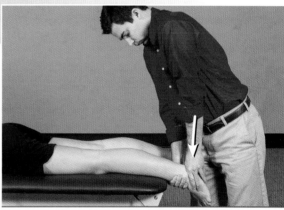

Figure 26.26

Client Position	Prone on the table, with the distal tibia and fibula off the table to assist the clinician's position
Clinician Position	Standing at the client's ankle to be assessed
Stabilization	The rest of the client's body on the table serves as a stabilizing force. The clinician's stabilizing hand (right as shown) purchases the anterior portion of the distal tibia and fibula.
Movement and Direction of Force	The clinician's assessing hand (left as shown) purchases the proximal talus posteriorly in the web space between the thumb and index finger. Using their assessing hand, the clinician glides the talus in an anterior direction along the plane of the joint.
Assessment	Assessment is done for joint play/passive accessory motion, client response, and end-feel. Reproduction of concordant pain suggests dysfunction. Impaired joint mobility or end-feel may also suggest dysfunction if concordant pain is also reproduced.

SUBTALAR JOINT DISTRACTION

Client Position	Prone on the table, with the distal tibia and fibula off the table to assist the clinician's position
Clinician Position	Sitting at the distal end of the client's ankle to be assessed
Stabilization	The rest of the client's body on the table serves as a stabilizing force. The clinician's stabilizing hand (left as shown) purchases the talus anteriorly with the web space of the hand.
Movement and Direction of Force	The clinician's assessing hand (right as shown) purchases the calcaneus on the posterior surface with the ulnar border of the hand. The clinician uses their stabilizing hand to maintain the position of the talus while using their assessing hand to glide the calcaneus distally (inferior direction).
Assessment	Assessment is done for joint play/passive accessory motion, client response, and end-feel. Reproduction of concordant pain suggests dysfunction. Impaired joint mobility or end-feel may also suggest dysfunction if concordant pain is also reproduced.

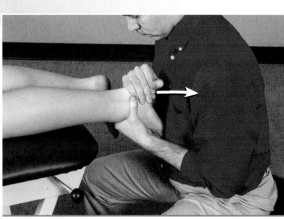

Figure 26.27

SUBTALAR JOINT LATERAL GLIDE (CALCANEUS VARUS TILT)

Client Position	Side lying on the table, with the medial surface of the leg facing the ceiling and the opposite knee bent to assist with the clinician's position
Clinician Position	Standing at the client's ankle to be assessed
Stabilization	The rest of the client's body on the table serves as a stabilizing force. The clinician's stabilizing hand (right as shown) purchases the talus with the web space of the hand and a combination of the thumb and index finger.
Movement and Direction of Force	The clinician's assessing hand (left as shown) purchases the calcaneus on the superior-medial surface with the heel of the hand. The clinician uses their stabilizing hand to maintain the position of the talus and their assessing hand to simultaneously glide the superior portion of the calcaneus laterally and the inferior portion of the calcaneus medially, gliding the calcaneus in a varus direction.
Assessment	Assessment is done for joint play/passive accessory motion, client response, and end-feel. Reproduction of concordant pain suggests dysfunction. Impaired joint mobility or end-feel may also suggest dysfunction if concordant pain is also reproduced.

Figure 26.28

SUBTALAR JOINT MEDIAL GLIDE (CALCANEUS VALGUS TILT)

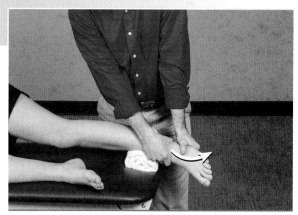

Client Position	Side lying on table, with the lateral surface of the leg facing the ceiling and the opposite knee bent to assist with clinician's position. A towel can be used as shown.
Clinician Position	Standing at the client's ankle to be assessed
Stabilization	The rest of the client's body on the table serves as a stabilizing force. The clinician's stabilizing hand (right as shown) purchases the talus with the web space of the hand and a combination of the thumb and index finger.

Figure 26.29

Movement and Direction of Force	The clinician's assessing hand (left as shown) purchases the calcaneus on the superior-lateral surface with the heel of the hand. The clinician uses their stabilizing hand to maintain position of talus and their assessing hand to simultaneously glide the superior portion of the calcaneus medially and the inferior portion of the calcaneus laterally, gliding the calcaneus in a valgus direction.
Assessment	Assessment is done for joint play/passive accessory motion, client response, and end-feel. Reproduction of concordant pain suggests dysfunction. Impaired joint mobility or end-feel may also suggest dysfunction if concordant pain is also reproduced.

TALONAVICULAR JOINT ANTERIOR (NAVICULAR DORSAL) GLIDE

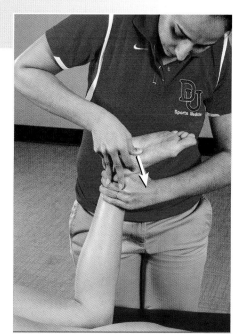

Client Position	Prone on the table with the knee flexed to 90°
Clinician Position	Standing at the client's ankle to be assessed
Stabilization	The rest of the client's body on the table serves as a stabilizing force. The clinician's stabilizing hand (left as shown) purchases the neck of the talus on the anterior surface with their web space.
Movement and Direction of Force	The clinician's assessing hand (right as shown) purchases the posterior (plantar) surface of the navicular bone with their thumb and index finger on the anterior (dorsal) surface. The clinician uses their stabilizing hand to maintain the position of the talus and their assessing hand to glide the navicular bone in an anterior (dorsal) direction.
Assessment	Assessment is done for joint play/passive accessory motion, client response, and end-feel. Reproduction of concordant pain suggests dysfunction. Impaired joint mobility or end-feel may also suggest dysfunction if concordant pain is also reproduced.

Figure 26.30

TALONAVICULAR JOINT POSTERIOR (NAVICULAR PLANTAR) GLIDE

Client Position	Supine on the table
Clinician Position	Sitting at the client's ankle to be assessed
Stabilization	The rest of the client's body on the table serves as a stabilizing force. Additional stabilization of client's leg is achieved by placing their leg against the clinician's trunk. The clinician's stabilizing hand (right as shown) purchases the neck of the talus with their web space.
Movement and Direction of Force	The clinician's assessing hand (left as shown) purchases the anterior (dorsal) surface of the navicular bone with their thumb and index finger on the posterior (plantar) surface. The clinician uses their stabilizing hand to maintain the position of the talus and their assessing hand to glide the navicular bone in a posterior (plantar) direction.
Assessment	Assessment is done for joint play/passive accessory motion, client response, and end-feel. Reproduction of concordant pain suggests dysfunction. Impaired joint mobility or end-feel may also suggest dysfunction if concordant pain is also reproduced.

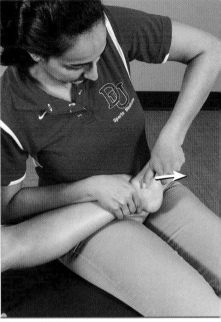

Figure 26.31

CALCANEOCUBOID JOINT ANTERIOR (CUBOID DORSAL) GLIDE

Client Position	Prone on table with knee flexed to 90°
Clinician Position	Standing at the client's ankle to be assessed
Stabilization	The rest of the client's body on the table serves as a stabilizing force. Additional stabilization of the client's leg is achieved by placing their leg against the clinician's trunk. The clinician's stabilizing hand (right) purchases the calcaneus with their web space.
Movement and Direction of Force	The clinician's assessing hand (left as shown) purchases the posterior (plantar) surface of the cuboid bone with their thumb and index finger on the anterior (dorsal) surface. The clinician uses their stabilizing hand to maintain the position of the calcaneus and their assessing hand to glide the cuboid in an anterior (dorsal) direction.
Assessment	Assessment is done for joint play/passive accessory motion, client response, and end-feel. Reproduction of concordant pain suggests dysfunction. Impaired joint mobility or end-feel may also suggest dysfunction if concordant pain is also reproduced.

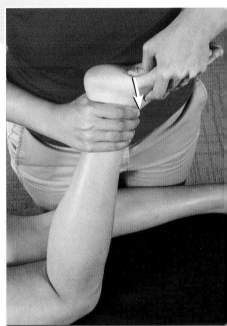

Figure 26.32

CALCANEOCUBOID JOINT POSTERIOR (CUBOID PLANTAR) GLIDE

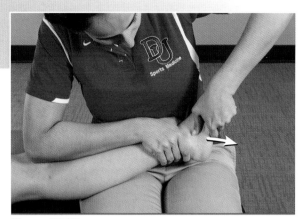

Figure 26.33

Client Position	Supine on the table
Clinician Position	Sitting at the client's ankle to be assessed
Stabilization	The rest of the client's body on the table serves as a stabilizing force. Additional stabilization of the client's leg is achieved by placing their leg against the clinician's trunk. The clinician's stabilizing hand (right as shown) purchases the calcaneus.
Movement and Direction of Force	The clinician's thumb of the assessing hand purchases the anterior (dorsal) aspect of the cuboid, and the index finger purchases the posterior (plantar) surface of the cuboid. The clinician uses their stabilizing hand to maintain the position of the calcaneus and their assessing hand to glide the cuboid in a posterior (plantar) direction.
Assessment	Assessment is done for joint play/passive accessory motion, client response, and end-feel. Reproduction of concordant pain suggests dysfunction. Impaired joint mobility or end-feel may also suggest dysfunction if concordant pain is also reproduced.

TARSOMETATARSAL JOINT ANTERIOR (DORSAL) GLIDE

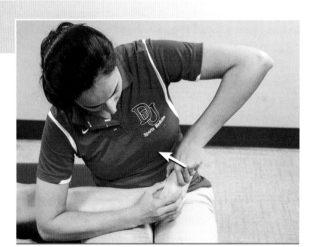

Figure 26.34

Client Position	Supine on the table with the ankle to be assessed in the clinician's lap
Clinician Position	Sitting with the client's ankle in their lap
Stabilization	The rest of the client's body on the table serves as a stabilizing force. Additional stabilization of the client's leg is achieved by placing their leg against the clinician's trunk or lap. The clinician's stabilizing hand (right as shown) purchases the respective tarsal bone, with their thumb on the dorsum and their index finger on the posterior (plantar) aspect.
Movement and Direction of Force	The clinician's assessing hand (left as shown) purchases the metatarsal with their thumb on the anterior (dorsal) aspect and their index finger on the posterior (plantar) aspect of the metatarsal. The clinician uses their stabilizing hand to maintain the tarsal bone in position and their assessing hand to glide the first metatarsal in an anterior (dorsal) direction on the first cuneiform, the second metatarsal anterior (dorsal) on the second cuneiform, the third metatarsal in an anterior (dorsal) direction on the cuboid, and the fourth and fifth metatarsals in an anterior (dorsal) direction on the cuboid.
Assessment	Assessment is done for joint play/passive accessory motion, client response, and end-feel. Reproduction of concordant pain suggests dysfunction. Impaired joint mobility or end-feel may also suggest dysfunction if concordant pain is also reproduced.

TARSOMETATARSAL JOINT POSTERIOR (PLANTAR) GLIDE

Client Position	Supine on the table, with the ankle to be assessed in the clinician's lap
Clinician Position	Sitting with the client's ankle to be assessed in their lap
Stabilization	The rest of the client's body on the table serves as a stabilizing force. Additional stabilization of the client's leg is achieved by placing their leg against clinician's trunk and lap. The clinician's stabilizing hand (right as shown) purchases the respective tarsal bone with their thumb on the dorsum and their index finger on the posterior (plantar) aspect.

Figure 26.35

Movement and Direction of Force	The clinician's assessing hand (left as shown) purchases the metatarsal with their thumb on the anterior (dorsal) aspect and their index finger on the posterior (plantar) aspect of the metatarsal. The clinician uses their stabilizing hand to maintain the tarsal bone in position and their assessing hand to glide the first metatarsal in a posterior (plantar) direction on the first cuneiform, the second metatarsal posterior (plantar) on the second cuneiform, the third metatarsal in a posterior (plantar) direction on the cuboid, and the fourth and fifth metatarsals in a posterior (plantar) direction on the cuboid.
Assessment	Assessment is done for joint play/passive accessory motion, client response, and end-feel. Reproduction of concordant pain suggests dysfunction. Impaired joint mobility or end-feel may also suggest dysfunction if concordant pain is also reproduced.

METATARSOPHALANGEAL JOINT ANTERIOR (DORSAL) GLIDE

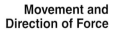

Client Position	Supine on the table with the ankle to be assessed in the clinician's lap
Clinician Position	Sitting on the table with the client's ankle in their lap
Stabilization	The rest of the client's body on the table serves as a stabilizing force. Additional stabilization of the client's leg is achieved by placing it against the clinician's trunk and lap. The clinician's stabilizing hand (right as shown) purchases the respective metatarsal with their thumb on the dorsum and their index finger on the posterior (plantar) aspect.

Figure 26.36

Movement and Direction of Force	The clinician's assessing hand (left as shown) purchases the proximal phalanx with their thumb on the anterior (dorsal) aspect and their index finger on the posterior (plantar) aspect of the metatarsal. The clinician uses their stabilizing hand to maintain the metatarsal bone in position and their assessing hand to glide the phalanx in an anterior (dorsal) direction on the respective metatarsal.
Assessment	Assessment is done for joint play/passive accessory motion, client response, and end-feel. Reproduction of concordant pain suggests dysfunction. Impaired joint mobility or end-feel may also suggest dysfunction if concordant pain is also reproduced.

METATARSOPHALANGEAL JOINT POSTERIOR (PLANTAR) GLIDE

Client Position	Supine on the table with their ankle to be assessed in the clinician's lap
Clinician Position	Sitting on the table with the client's ankle in their lap
Stabilization	The rest of the client's body on the table serves as a stabilizing force. Additional stabilization of the client's leg is achieved by placing it against the clinician's trunk and lap. The clinician's stabilizing hand (right as shown) purchases the respective metatarsal with their thumb on the dorsum and their index finger on the posterior (plantar) aspect.

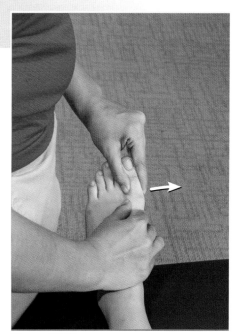

Figure 26.37

Movement and Direction of Force	The clinician's assessing hand (left as shown) purchases the proximal phalanx with their thumb on the anterior (dorsal) aspect and their index finger on the posterior (plantar) aspect of the metatarsal. The clinician uses their stabilizing hand to maintain the metatarsal bone in position and their assessing hand to glide the phalanx in a posterior (plantar) direction on the respective metatarsal.
Assessment	Assessment is done for joint play/passive accessory motion, client response, and end-feel. Reproduction of concordant pain suggests dysfunction. Impaired joint mobility or end-feel may also suggest dysfunction if concordant pain is also reproduced.

METATARSOPHALANGEAL JOINT MEDIAL GLIDE

Client Position	Supine on the table
Clinician Position	Standing at the side of the client's ankle to be assessed
Stabilization	The rest of the client's body on the table serves as a stabilizing force. The clinician's stabilizing hand (right as shown) purchases the respective metatarsal with their thumb on the lateral and their index finger on the medial aspect.
Movement and Direction of Force	The clinician's assessing hand (left as shown) purchases the proximal phalanx with their thumb on the lateral aspect and their index finger on the medial aspect of the metatarsal. The clinician uses their stabilizing hand to maintain the metatarsal bone in position and their assessing hand (thumb) to glide the phalanx in a medial direction on the respective metatarsal.
Assessment	Assessment is done for joint play/passive accessory motion, client response, and end-feel. Reproduction of concordant pain suggests dysfunction. Impaired joint mobility or end-feel may also suggest dysfunction if concordant pain is also reproduced.

Figure 26.38

METATARSOPHALANGEAL JOINT LATERAL GLIDE

Client Position	Supine on the table
Clinician Position	Standing in front of the foot to be assessed
Stabilization	The rest of the client's body on the table serves as a stabilizing force. The clinician's stabilizing hand (left as shown) purchases the respective metatarsal with their thumb on the medial and their index finger on the lateral aspect.
Movement and Direction of Force	The clinician's assessing hand (right as shown) purchases the proximal phalanx with their thumb on the medial aspect and their index finger on the lateral aspect of the metatarsal. The clinician uses their stabilizing hand to maintains the metatarsal bone in position and their assessing hand (thumb) to glide the phalanx in a lateral direction on the respective metatarsal.
Assessment	Assessment is done for joint play/passive accessory motion, client response, and end-feel. Reproduction of concordant pain suggests dysfunction. Impaired joint mobility or end-feel may also suggest dysfunction if concordant pain is also reproduced.

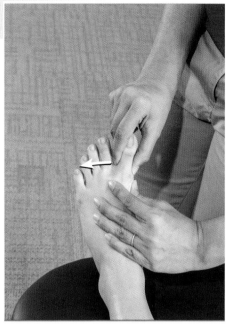

Figure 26.39

INTERPHALANGEAL JOINT GLIDES

All glides, including distraction, are performed as per metatarsal-phalangeal joint assessments, with the exception of those performed at each interphalangeal joint.

Flexibility

As detailed in chapter 8, flexibility is the motion that a particular joint is capable of. Assessment of flexibility can assist the clinician in determining the potential presence of soft-tissue dysfunction.[69] A review of the anatomy can be found in table 26.3.

TABLE 26.3 Gastroc-Soleus Muscle Group

Muscle	Origin	Insertion	Action	Innervation
Gastrocnemius	Posterior surface of femur (medial and lateral condyles), capsule of knee joint	Calcaneus via Achilles tendon (tendo calcaneus), posterior calcaneus	Plantarflexion of foot, flexion of knee	Tibial nerve S1-S2
Soleus	Fibula (head, posterior aspect, and proximal third of shaft), tibia (popliteal line), aponeurosis between tibia and fibula	Calcaneus via Achilles tendon (tendo calcaneus), posterior calcaneus	Plantarflexion of foot	Tibial nerve S1-S2

GASTROCNEMIUS ASSESSMENT

Client Position	Supine with hip and knee extended
Clinician Position	Sitting, facing client
Movement	The clinician maintains the knee in full extension and passively dorsiflexes the client's ankle.
Assessment	The clinician aligns the goniometer's stationary arm in line with the head of the fibula, placing the axis at the lateral malleolus and the moving arm parallel to the fifth metatarsal. Maintaining the joint in subtalar neutral, the clinician passively dorsiflexes the client's ankle to end range and measures the amount of range of motion.
Statistics	There are no known normative data for this flexibility measure. However, Piva and colleagues found an ICC of 0.92 in their study.[70] Wang and colleagues[71] examined lower extremity flexibility in long distance runners and found that intratester reliability of gastrocnemius measurements for 10 subjects, in supine, was 0.98 for both the dominant and nondominant lower extremities.

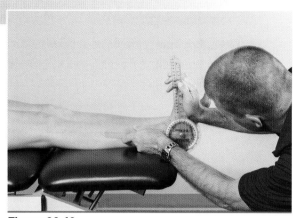

Figure 26.40

MUSCLE PERFORMANCE TESTING

Muscle performance testing helps the clinician identify strength impairments that may be causing or contributing to a client's injury. Strength impairments can be easily addressed to help the client and prevent further injury or reinjury to the lower leg, ankle, and foot. Ankle sprains are a common injury in sports and can often lead to chronic ankle instability. When looking at the isokinetic strength, concentric and eccentric, of ankle everters and invertors, clients with ankle instability were found to have dynamic strength imbalance when compared to the control that may lead to recurrent injury.[72] The calf-raise test assesses the properties of the calf muscle-tendon unit through repetitive concentric–eccentric muscle action of the plantar flexors in unipedal stance. No consistent evaluation purpose, test parameters, outcome measurements, normative values, or reliability and validity values are currently documented for the calf-raise test. Clinicians can rely only on level 5 evidence until universally accepted standardization of the calf-raise test is achieved and used to determine normative values in healthy people and in clients with pathology. [73]

ANKLE PLANTARFLEXION

Client Position	Standing, holding onto a solid surface with no more than two fingers used for balance
Clinician Position	Standing directly to the side of the client
Movement and Assessment[266]	The client performs as many heel raises under control as they can.

- Grade 5: 25 complete heel raises
- Grade 4: 2-24 complete heel raises (at a consistent rate of one rise every 2 seconds, correct form)
- Grade 3: 1 complete heel raise correctly
- Grade 2: Unable to lift the heel from the floor in standing, completes plantarflexion in non-weight bearing against clinician resistance at metatarsal heads
- Grade 1: prone; muscle activity without movement
- Grade 0: prone; no muscle activity

Primary Muscles	Gastrocnemius
	Soleus
Secondary Muscles	Posterior tibialis
	Peroneus longus and brevis
	Plantaris
	Flexor digitorum longus
	Flexor hallucis longus
Primary Nerve	Tibial nerve (S1-2)

FOOT DORSIFLEXION AND INVERSION

Client Position	Sitting with leg off the edge of table, ankle in neutral
Clinician Position	Standing directly to the side of the client
Movement and Assessment	The clinician's proximal hand stabilizes just above the client's malleoli while the other hand gives resistance to the dorsum and medial border of foot as the client attempts to dorsiflex and invert the foot.

- Grade 5: completes full range with maximal resistance
- Grade 4: completes full range with strong resistance
- Grade 3: completes full range without resistance
- Grade 2: completes only partial range
- Grade 1: muscle activity without movement
- Grade 0: no muscle activity

Primary Muscles	Anterior tibialis
Secondary Muscles	Extensor digitorum longus
	Extensor hallucis longus
	Peroneus tertius
Primary Nerve	Deep peroneal nerve (L4-S1)

FOOT INVERSION

Client Position	Sitting with leg off edge of table, ankle in neutral
Clinician Position	Standing directly to the side of the client
Movement and Assessment	The clinician's proximal hand stabilizes just above the malleoli while the other hand gives resistance to the dorsum and medial border of the foot as the client attempts to invert the foot.

- Grade 5: completes full range with maximal resistance
- Grade 4: completes full range with strong resistance
- Grade 3: completes full range without resistance
- Grade 2: completes only partial range
- Grade 1: muscle activity without movement
- Grade 0: no muscle activity

Primary Muscle	Posterior tibialis
Secondary Muscles	Anterior tibialis
	Flexor digitorum longus
	Flexor hallucis longus
	Soleus
	Extensor hallucis longus
Primary Nerve	Tibial nerve (L4-S1)

FOOT EVERSION WITH PLANTARFLEXION

Client Position	Sitting with leg off edge of table, ankle in neutral
Clinician Position	Standing directly to the side of the client
Movement and Assessment	The clinician's proximal hand stabilizes just above the client's malleoli while the other hand gives resistance to the dorsum and lateral border of foot as the client attempts to evert the foot.

- Grade 5: completes full range with maximal resistance
- Grade 4: completes full range with strong resistance
- Grade 3: completes full range without resistance
- Grade 2: completes only partial range
- Grade 1: muscle activity without movement
- Grade 0: no muscle activity

Primary Muscles	Peroneus longus (with plantarflexion)
	Peroneus brevis (with plantarflexion)
	Extensor digitorum longus (with dorsiflexion)
	Peroneus tertius (with dorsiflexion)
Secondary Muscle	Gastrocnemius
Primary Nerve	Superficial peroneal nerve (L5-S1)

HALLUX AND TOE MP, PIP, AND DIP FLEXION

Client Position	Supine with ankle in neutral
Clinician Position	Standing directly to the side of the client on the side to be assessed
Movement and Assessment	The clinician uses one hand to stabilize above the joint to be assessed; the other hand provides proximal resistance.

- Grade 5: completes full range with strong resistance
- Grade 4: completes full range with mild to moderate resistance
- Grade 3: completes full range without resistance
- Grade 2: completes only partial range
- Grade 1: muscle activity without movement
- Grade 0: no muscle activity

Primary Muscles	Lumbricales
	Flexor hallucis longus (IP of hallux)
	Flexor digitorum brevis (PIP of toes)
	Flexor digitorum longus (DIP of toes)
Primary Nerves	Tibial nerve; medial and lateral plantar nerve (L5-S2)

HALLUX AND TOE MP AND IP EXTENSION

Client Position	Supine with ankle in neutral
Clinician Position	Standing directly to the side of client
Movement and Assessment	The clinician uses one hand to stabilize the metatarsals and the thumb of the other hand to give resistance over the dorsal surface of the proximal phalanges of the toes.

- Grades 5 and 4: extends toes against resistance full range with variable resistance
- Grades 3 and 2: complete range without resistance
- Grade 1: muscle activity without movement
- Grade 0: no muscle activity

Primary Muscles	Extensor digitorum longus
	Extensor digitorum brevis
	Extensor hallucis longus
Primary Nerve	Deep peroneal nerve (L5-S1)

SPECIAL TESTS

As mentioned in chapter 10 (Special Tests), in many cases the clinician is overly dependent on the performance and interpretation of special test findings with respect to differential diagnosis of the client's presenting pain. Utilization of special tests for ruling in (or helping to diagnose) a particular pathology should occur at this point in the examination pro-cess. The clinician have a much clearer picture of the client's presentation prior to this point in the examination and will therefore depend minimally on special test findings with respect to diagnosis of the client's pain.

When examining the lower leg, ankle, and foot it is important to rule out the potential contribution of the client's pain originating from related structures such as the lumbar spine, hip, SIJ or pelvic girdle, and knee. The triage and screening section of this chapter provides more information on this. Specific tests to rule in lower leg, ankle, and foot pathologies are listed in this section with descriptions. Remember that the special tests are a very small component of the overall examination and reliance of findings on special testing alone is inadequate clinical practice.

Index of Special Tests

Common Observation Tests and Measures

Edema: Figure 8 Test

Subtalar Joint Neutral (open chain)

Subtalar Joint Neutral (closed chain)

Tibial Torsion

Navicular Drop

Navicular Height

Navicular Position Test (NPT) or Modified Feiss Line

Arch Ratio

Rearfoot Orientation (standing)

Talar Bulge

Forefoot-to-Rearfoot Alignment

Big Toe Extension

Mobility Impairments

First Ray Mobility

Muscle Dysfunction

Posterior Tibial Tendon Dysfunction

Posterior Tibial Edema Sign

Medial Tibial Stress Syndrome (MTSS)

Shin Palpation Test

Shin Edema Test

Achilles Tendinopathy

Palpation for Tenderness Test

Arc Sign

Royal London Hospital Test

Single-Leg Heel Raise Test

Hop Test

Achilles Tendon Rupture

Thompson Test or Calf Squeeze Test

Matles Test

Palpation of Gap in Achilles Tendon

Copeland Test

Tissue Length

Windlass Test

Ligamentous Laxity or Instability

Ankle Lateral Ligament Integrity

Anterior Drawer Test

Talar Tilt (Varus) Stress Test (lateral ligaments)

Medial Subtalar Glide Test

Ankle Medial Ligament Integrity

Talar Tilt (Valgus) Stress Test (medial ligaments)

Medial Tenderness

(continued)

Index of Special Tests *(continued)*

Syndesmotic Integrity

Cotton Test

External Rotation and Dorsiflexion
  External Rotation Test

Fibular Translation Test

Syndesmotic Squeeze Test

Dorsiflexion Lunge with Compression Test

Ankle Impingement

Forced Dorsiflexion Test

Clinical Prediction Rule of Impingement

Nerve Entrapment

Foot Squeeze Test (Morton's Test)

Web Space Tenderness

Plantar Percussion Test

Toe Tip Sensation Deficit

Tuning Fork

Tarsal Tunnel Syndrome

Tinel's Sign

Triple Compression Stress Test
  (side lying and long sitting)

Dorsiflexion-Eversion Test

Case Studies

Go to www.HumanKinetics.com/OrthopedicClinicalExamination and complete these case studies for chapter 26:

- Case study 1 discusses a 34-year-old postpartum female whose ankle gave out while walking down the stairs.
- Case study 2 discusses a 25-year-old female with a diagnosis of right medial ankle pain of 1 month duration.

Abstract Links

Go to www.HumanKinetics.com/OrthopedicClinicalExamination to access abstract links on these issues:

Anterior drawer test

Cotton test

Dorsiflexion-eversion test

Fibular translation test

Forced dorsiflexion test

Palpation for tenderness test

Plantar percussion test

Posterior tibial edema sign

Shin palpation test

Syndesmosis squeeze test

Thompson test

Tinel's sign

Toe tip sensation deficit

Triple compression stress test (long sitting)

Windlass test

COMMON OBSERVATION TESTS AND MEASURES

EDEMA: FIGURE 8 TEST

Client Position	Supine or long sitting
Clinician Position	Standing directly to the side of the leg to be assessed
Assessment	The zero point of the spring tape measure is positioned in the groove at the edge of the lateral malleolus, approximately midway between the prominence of the lateral malleolus and the tibialis anterior tendon. The tape measure is then drawn medially across the instep, pulled laterally toward the base of the fifth metatarsal, drawn toward the medial malleolus and across the Achilles tendon to the lateral malleolus, and finally brought around to meet the original zero point; 3 measures are taken and averaged.[74] (Highest agreement with water volumetry, R = 0.96.)[75]
Statistics	NR
Normative Values	• Difference from side to side is a positive finding (mean 1.77).[76]
	• Figure-of-eight-20 method: minimal detectable change for swollen ankle 9.6 mm without skin marks and 7.3 mm with marks. The differences between affected and unaffected ankle, average of three measures by three testers for edema was: mild 27.4 mm, moderate 29.1 mm, severe 41.7 mm, whole group 33.8 mm.[74]

SUBTALAR JOINT NEUTRAL (OPEN CHAIN)

Client Position	Prone on table
Clinician Position	Standing distal to the leg to be assessed
Assessment	The clinician assesses calcaneal position with respect to the tibia to determine amount of supination or pronation in subtalar neutral.[77]
Statistics	NR
Normative Values	• No normative values: The subtalar joint should line up with the tibia.
	• A study done by Astrom and Arvidson[78] reported that in women, subtalar neutral (ideal foot) had a mean of 2° of valgus (in relation to the calf).[78]

SUBTALAR JOINT NEUTRAL (CLOSED CHAIN)

Client Position	Standing
Clinician Position	Kneeling behind the leg to be assessed
Assessment	The clinician places the client in subtalar neutral (medial and lateral aspects are felt equally). The clinician then measures the position of the calcaneus with the inclinometer (ICC 0.95).[77]
Statistics	NR
Normative Values	NR

TIBIAL TORSION

Client Position	Supine with femur positioned so that a line between the epicondyles is parallel to the horizontal plane
Clinician Position	Standing directly to the side of the leg to be assessed
Assessment	Using a goniometer, the angle formed by a line that bisects the bimalleolar axis relative to the vertical plane is measured.[79]
Statistics	Inter rater reliability 0.84[267]
Normative Values	External tibial torsion averages 0° to 20° at birth; however, it has been suggested that >30° may lead to the client's having clinical symptoms (patella subluxation) and eventually needing surgery (tibial rotational osteotomy and distal tuberosity transfer).[80]

NAVICULAR DROP

Client Position	Standing shifting from non-weight-bearing to weight-bearing leg. It has also been described as moving from seated to standing.
Clinician Position	Kneeling on the medial side of the leg to be assessed
Assessment	The clinician palpates the inferior displacement of the navicular tubercle as the client shifts from non–weight bearing to full weight bearing.[42] Piva and colleagues suggested examining the navicular in subtalar neutral and a relaxed position; a greater difference in mm between positions would signify greater pronation.[70]
Statistics	Intratester reliability 0.61-0.79 and ICC 0.57[268]
Normative Values	• A mean of 5.9 mm (ICC 0.93) is considered normal.[70] • Abnormal > 10–15 mm.[81, 82]

NAVICULAR HEIGHT

Client Position	Standing
Clinician Position	Standing on the medial side of the leg to be assessed
Assessment	The client stands in a relaxed position. The clinician palpates the medial most prominence of the navicular tuberosity and marks the position. Next, the clinician measures the height of the navicular from the ground.[83]
Statistics	NR
Normative Values	Navicular height has been seen to most accurately represent the skeletal alignment of the medial longitudinal arch when compared to radiology gold standard.[83] • 0.316 normal arch • 0.35 high arch • 0.275 low arch • ICC: 0.94 • Inter tester: 0.81[84]

NAVICULAR POSITION TEST (NPT) OR MODIFIED FEISS LINE

Client Position	Standing in an upright position with toes pointing forward and the foot being tested behind the foot not being tested so that the heel of the non-tested foot and the big toe of the tested foot are in the same transverse plane. The knee is aligned with a position between the first and second toes of the foot being tested. The client can hold onto something for support.

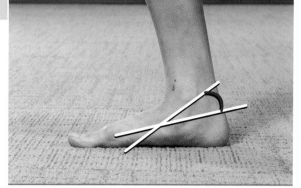

Figure 26.41

Clinician Position	Standing directly to the medial side of the leg to be assessed
Assessment	Markings are made on the medial side of the first metatarsal bone, the navicular tuberosity, and the Achilles. (The clinician marks the Achilles by marking the apex of the medial malleolus, then measuring the height from the floor and projecting posteriorly to a point horizontal to the dorsal/anterior edge of the Achilles tendon.) Measurements are then taken with the center of the goniometer on the navicular tuberosity, with its arms in line with the metatarsal and Achilles markings.[85]
Statistics	ICC of 0.94 and –0.91[85]
Normative Values	Mean NPT was 0.91; 0° represents a neutral foot, negative numbers represent a pes planus foot, and positive numbers represent a pes cavus foot.[85]

ARCH RATIO

Client Position	Standing
Clinician Position	Standing on the medial side of the leg to be assessed
Assessment	The clinician measures the height to the dorsum of the client's foot from the floor (at 50% of the foot length) and divides it by the client's truncated foot length (the length of the foot from the most posterior portion of the calcaneus to the medial joint space of the first metatarsal phalangeal joint).[86]
Statistics	NR
Normative Values	NR

REARFOOT ORIENTATION (STANDING)

Client Position	Standing in non–weight bearing and shifting weight onto single leg to simulate single limb support during stance phase of gait[42]
Clinician Position	Standing behind the leg to be assessed
Assessment	Using a goniometer, the clinician measures the acute angle between the line representing the distal third of the lower leg and the posterior aspect of the rearfoot.[42]
Statistics	NR
Normative Values	NR

TALAR BULGE

Client Position	Standing
Clinician Position	Standing on the side of the leg to be assessed
Assessment	The talar head protrudes excessively on the medial side of midfoot with the client in weight bearing.
Statistics	NR
Normative Values	NR

FOREFOOT-TO-REARFOOT ALIGNMENT

Client Position	Prone with distal leg off table
Clinician Position	Distal to the leg being assessed
Assessment	Neutral alignment: A line representing the plantar/posterior aspect of metatarsal heads is perpendicular to the line bisecting the rearfoot.
Statistics	NR
Normative Values	• Forefoot varus: inversion of the forefoot away from neutral orientation • Forefoot valgus: everted forefoot position[42] • Forefoot varus 7.8°, forefoot valgus 4.7°[42]

BIG TOE EXTENSION

Client Position	Sitting
Clinician Position	Sitting to the side of the leg being assessed
Assessment	The clinician stabilizes the first metatarsal with one hand, while the other hand passively moves the big toe into extension (or upward, avoiding interphalangeal extension) to end range (end-feel is firm due to tension in the plantar/posterior joint capsule and muscles). Goniometer alignment: The clinician places the fulcrum over the dorsal/anterior aspect of the MTP joint, and aligns the proximal arm with the medial midline of the first metatarsal and the distal arm with the medial midline of the proximal phalanx of the first toe.
Statistics	NR
Normative Values	The ruler method, which is also used to perform this test, showed poor reliability and validity when compared to a valid and reliable mechanical device.[87, 88]

MOBILITY IMPAIRMENTS

FIRST RAY MOBILITY

Client Position	Supine or long sitting, with ankle in neutral and bolster under knee
Clinician Position	Standing directly to the side of the leg to be assessed
Movement	The clinician stabilizes the client's second through fifth digits with one hand while using the other hand to stabilize the first ray, distal to the metatarsophalangeal joint. The clinician then applies a dorsal/anterior and plantar/posterior force to the first ray to determine its mobility.

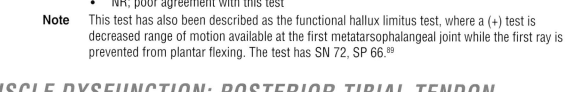

Figure 26.42

Assessment	A (+) test is a reduction of motion into dorsiflexion or plantarflexion. Movement is usually normal or hypomobile.
Statistics	• ICC: 0.05 poor reliability with use of a ruler[88]
	• NR; poor agreement with this test
Note	This test has also been described as the functional hallux limitus test, where a (+) test is decreased range of motion available at the first metatarsophalangeal joint while the first ray is prevented from plantar flexing. The test has SN 72, SP 66.[89]

MUSCLE DYSFUNCTION: POSTERIOR TIBIAL TENDON DYSFUNCTION

POSTERIOR TIBIAL EDEMA SIGN

Client Position	Sitting with lower leg off table
Clinician Position	Standing at medial side of the leg being tested
Movement	The clinician observes pitting edema present along the course of the posterior tibial tendon.
Assessment	A (+) test is if edema is present along the course of the posterior tibial tendon with no associated acute trauma or other areas of edema.
Statistics	SN 86 (74-91), SP 100 (56-100), +LR Inf, –LR 0.14 (0.7–0.3), QUADAS 7, in a study of 49 clients (71% women; mean age 69 years) with posterior tibialis tendon dysfunction, and MRI as a reference standard[90]

MUSCLE DYSFUNCTION: MEDIAL TIBIAL STRESS SYNDROME (MTSS)

SHIN PALPATION TEST

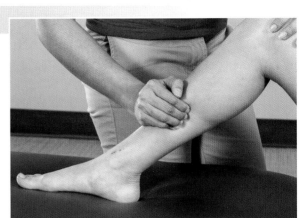

Figure 26.43

Client Position	Supine with involved leg in hook-lying position.
Clinician Position	Standing to the side of leg to be tested.
Movement	The clinician palpates the distal two-thirds of the posteromedial lower leg, including the posteromedial border of the tibia and associated musculature. The clinician uses fingers as shown, with enough pressure to squeeze out a wet sponge.
Assessment	A (+) test is reproduction of concordant pain.
Statistics	To determine the future development of MTSS: SN 34 (24-46), SP 90 (86-93), +LR 3.4, –LR 0.8, QUADAS 9, in a study of 384 (age 17-19 years; 96 women; duration of symptoms NR) asymptomatic officer cadet clients compared to 693 injuries later reported by 326 of the officer cadets, and using diagnosis by a physician or physiotherapist as a reference standard[91]

SHIN EDEMA TEST

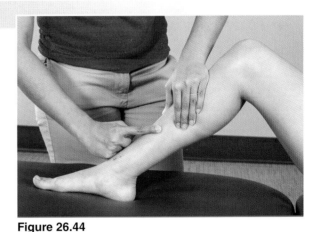

Figure 26.44

Client Position	Supine with involved leg in hook-lying position
Clinician Position	Standing to the side of leg to be tested
Movement	The clinician uses the finger as shown to apply sustained palpation (5-second hold) of the distal two-thirds of the medial tibia.
Assessment	A (+) test was any signs of pitting edema.
Statistics	To determine the future development of MTSS:

- **SN 92 (62-100), SP 87 (84-91), +LR 7.3, –LR 0.09,** QUADAS 9, in a study of 384 asymptomatic officer cadet clients compared to 693 injuries later reported by 326 of the officer cadets, and using diagnosis by a physician or physiotherapist as a reference standard [91]
- Shin palpation and shin edema test together: **SN 87 (84-91), SP 88 (84-91), +LR 7.9, –LR < 0.001**[91]

MUSCLE DYSFUNCTION: ACHILLES TENDINOPATHY

PALPATION FOR TENDERNESS TEST

Client Position	Prone with legs extended and relaxed
Clinician Position	Standing at the client's feet
Movement	The clinician gently palpates the whole length of the Achilles tendon in a proximal to distal direction, gently squeezing the tendon between the thumb and the index finger. The client is asked to state whether palpation tenderness was present or absent.
Assessment	The presence of tenderness during testing is a (+) test.

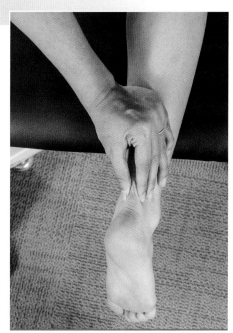

Figure 26.45

Statistics
- Pooled analysis: SN 64 (44-81), SP 81 (65-91), +LR 3.2, –LR 0.48, across two studies with 45 clients[92]

- SN 58 (39-75), SP 85 (75-91), +LR 3.5, –LR 0.50, QUADAS 8, in a study of 10 clients with Achilles tendinopathy (mean age 28.5 ± 6.8 years; all male athletes; duration of symptoms NR) and 14 control clients (mean age 27.1 ± 7.4 years), with US findings and histological findings after surgical exploration as a reference standard[93]

- **SN 84 (68-98)**, SP 73 (53-92), +LR 4.9, **–LR 0.22**, QUADAS 10, in a study of 21 clients with and without Achilles tendinopathy (10 clients with tendinopathy: mean age 48 years; 4 women; duration symptoms NR; Controls: mean age 54 years), and US as a reference standard[94]

ARC SIGN

Client Position	Prone with legs extended and relaxed
Clinician Position	Standing at the client's feet
Movement	The client is asked to dorsiflex and plantar flex the ankle. In tendinopathy of the main body of the tendon, the area of swelling evidenced by palpation moves with dorsiflexion and plantarflexion of the ankle. If no swelling was present, the test is performed selecting an area in the tendon 3 cm proximal to its calcaneal insertion.
Assessment	A (+) test is if the area of swelling moved with dorsiflexion and plantarflexion.

Statistics
- Pooled analysis: SN 42 (23-62), SP 88 (74-96), +LR 3.2, –LR 0.68, across two studies with 45 clients[92]

- SN 53 (35-70), SP 83 (72-91), +LR 2.0, –LR 0.57, QUADAS 8, in a study of 10 clients with Achilles tendinopathy (mean age 28.5 ± 6.8 years; all male athletes; duration of symptoms NR) and 14 control clients (mean age 27.1 ± 7.4 years), with US findings and histological findings after surgical exploration as a reference standard[93]

- SN 25 (9-44), **SP 100 (100-100), +LR Inf**, –LR 0.75, QUADAS 10, in a study of 21 clients with and without Achilles tendinopathy (10 clients with tendinopathy: mean age 48 years, 4 women, and duration symptoms NR; controls: mean age 54 years), and US as a reference standard[94]

ROYAL LONDON HOSPITAL TEST

Client Position	Prone with legs extended and relaxed
Clinician Position	Standing at the client's feet
Movement	Once the clinician has elicited local tenderness by palpating the tendon with the ankle in neutral position or slightly plantar flexed, the client is asked to actively dorsiflex and plantarflex the ankle. With the ankle in maximum dorsiflexion and in maximum plantarflexion, the portion of the tendon originally found to be tender is palpated again.

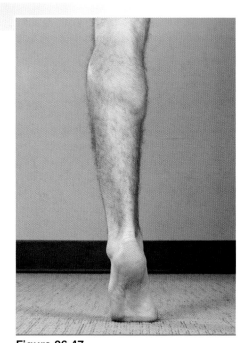

Figure 26.46

Assessment	A (+) test is no tenderness present on palpation during dorsiflexion of the ankle.
Statistics	• Pooled analysis: SN 54 (34-73), SP 86 (72-95), +LR 3.8, –LR 0.54, across two studies with 45 clients[92]
	• SN 54 (35-73), SP 91 (86-95), +LR 6.8, –LR 0.51, QUADAS 8, in a study of 10 clients with Achilles tendinopathy (mean age 28.5 ± 6.8 years; all male athletes; duration of symptoms NR) and 14 control clients (mean age 27.1 ± 7.4 years), with US findings and histological findings after surgical exploration as a reference standard[93]
	• SN 51 (33-70), **SP 93 (83-100)**, **+LR Inf**, –LR 0.51, QUADAS 10, in a study of 21 clients with and without Achilles tendinopathy (10 clients with tendinopathy: mean age 48 years, 4 women, and duration symptoms NR; controls: mean age 54 years), and US as a reference standard[94]
Combined Tests (Palpation, Arc Sign, Royal London Test)	SN 59 (47-74), SP 83 (76-89), +LR 3.5, –LR 0.50[93]

SINGLE-LEG HEEL RAISE TEST

Client Position	Standing on leg to be assessed
Clinician Position	Monitoring from the side or in front of client
Movement	The client is asked to rise up onto tiptoes of leg to be assessed, and then lower themselves back down (heel to floor).
Assessment	A (+) test is complaints of pain either on the up or downward movement.
Statistics	SN 22 (8-36), SP 93 (82-100), +LR 3.1, –LR 0.19, QUADAS 10, in a study of 21 clients with and without Achilles tendinopathy (10 clients with tendinopathy: mean age 48 years, 4 women, and duration symptoms NR; controls: mean age 54 years), and US as a reference standard[94]

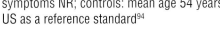

Figure 26.47

HOP TEST

Client Position	Standing on one leg
Clinician Position	Monitoring from the side, or in front of client
Movement	The client is asked to hop forward on one leg over a line marked on the floor.
Assessment	A (+) test is complaint of pain in the mid-Achilles tendon during movement.
Statistics	SN 43 (27-95), SP 87 (74-98), +LR 3.3, –LR 0.66, QUADAS 10, in a study of 21 clients with and without Achilles tendinopathy (10 clients with tendinopathy: mean age 48 years, 4 women, and duration symptoms NR; controls: mean age 54 years), and US as a reference standard[94]

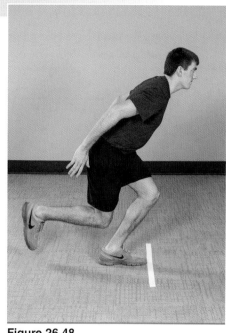

Figure 26.48

MUSCLE DYSFUNCTION: ACHILLES TENDON RUPTURE

THOMPSON TEST OR CALF SQUEEZE TEST

 Video 26.49 **in the web resource shows a demonstration of this test.**

Client Position	Prone with bilateral legs relaxed
Clinician Position	Standing directly next to the side of the leg to be assessed
Movement	The clinician gently squeezes the client's calf muscles with their hands.
Assessment	A (+) test is when the ankle remains still or only minimal plantarflexion occurs.

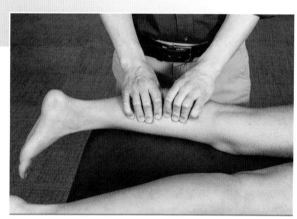

Figure 26.49

Statistics	• SN 96 (93-99), SP 93 (75-99), +LR 13.7, –LR 0.04, QUADAS 7, in a study of 133 clients (mean age 42.5 ± 11.6 years; 25 women; mean duration of symptoms 0-28 days), using surgical repair as a reference standard[95] • SN 40, SP NT, QUADAS 7[96]

MATLES TEST

Client Position	Prone with bilateral legs relaxed
Clinician Position	Standing directly to the side of the leg to be assessed
Movement	The client flexes their knee to 90°. The position of the ankles and feet are observed during flexion of the knee.
Assessment	A (+) test is when the foot on the affected side falls into neutral or dorsiflexion.
Statistics	SN 88 (78-94), SP 85 (66-95), +LR 6.3, –LR 0.14, QUADAS 7, in a study of 133 clients (mean age 42.5 ± 11.6 years; 25 women; duration of symptoms 0-28 days), using surgical repair as a reference standard[95]

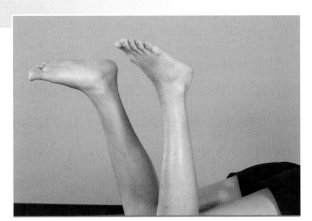

Figure 26.50

PALPATION OF GAP IN ACHILLES TENDON

Client Position	Prone with bilateral legs relaxed
Clinician Position	Standing directly to the side of the leg to be assessed
Movement	The clinician gently palpates the course of the Achilles tendon, feeling for a gap in the continuity of the tendon.
Assessment	A (+) test is the presence of a gap in the tendon.
Statistics	SN 73 (65-81), SP 89 (71-97), +LR 6.6, –LR 0.30, QUADAS 7, in a study of 133 clients (mean age 42.5 ± 11.6 years; 25 women; mean duration of symptoms 0-28 days), using surgical repair as a reference standard[95]

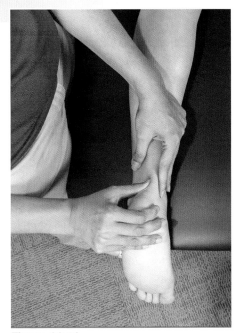

Figure 26.51

COPELAND TEST

Client Position	Prone with legs relaxed and fully extended, feet hanging off table
Clinician Position	Standing directly to the side of the leg to be assessed
Movement	The clinician places a sphygmomanometer cuff around the middle of the calf and inflates it to 100 mmHg. The clinician then dorsiflexes the ankle.
Assessment	A (+) test is little or no pressure rise in the sphygmomanometer.
Statistics	SN 78 (49-94), SP NR, QUADAS 7, in a study of 133 clients (mean age 42.5 ± 11.6 years; 25 women; duration of symptoms 0-28 days), using surgical repair as a reference standard[95]

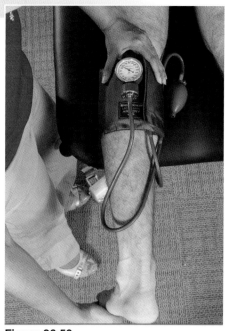

Figure 26.52

TISSUE LENGTH

WINDLASS TEST

Client Position	The test is performed in both non-weight-bearing *(a)* and weight-bearing *(b)* positions. The weight-bearing test is performed with the toes hanging off the edge of a step stool. The non-weight bearing test is performed sitting with toes hanging off the edge of the table.
Clinician Position	Sitting or kneeling directly next to the client's lower extremity to be assessed
Movement	In the non-weight-bearing test, the first toe is maximally dorsiflexed (toe extension) passively at the MTP joint (allowing the IP joint to flex) to end range, with the ankle stabilized *(a)*. The weight-bearing test is performed with the toes hanging off the edge of a step stool. Here, passive dorsiflexion of the first MTP is performed to end range *(b)*.
Assessment	A (+) test is if concordant pain was reproduced during or at the end of the range of MTP extension.

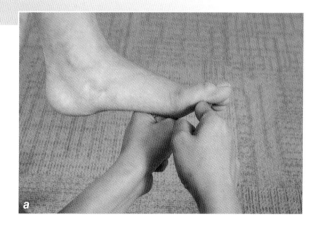

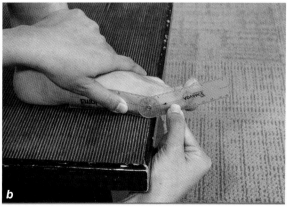

Figure 26.53

(continued)

Windlass Test *(continued)*

Statistics
- Weight-bearing: SN 33 (NR), **SP 99 (NR)**, **+LR 28.7**, –LR 0.68, QUADAS 9, in a study of 22 patients with plantar fasciitis, 23 clients with other types of foot pain, and 30 clients in a control group (mean age 49.1 ± 15.6 years; 12 women with plantar fasciitis, 14 women with other foot pain, and 20 women in the control group; duration of symptoms 88.9 weeks for plantar fasciitis, 232.4 weeks for other foot pain), using diagnosis determined by orthopedic surgeon based on both history and physical exam as a reference standard.[97]
- Non-weight-bearing: SN 18, **SP 99**, **+LR 16.2**, –LR 0.83.[97]
- The strain on the plantar fascia, tibial nerve, lateral plantar nerve, and medial plantar nerve when performing the windlass test with full MTP flexion were significant.[98]

LIGAMENTOUS LAXITY OR INSTABILITY: ANKLE LATERAL LIGAMENT INTEGRITY

ANTERIOR DRAWER TEST

Client Position	Supine or sitting with the ankle prepositioned into slight plantarflexion
Clinician Position	Standing directly in front of leg to be assessed
Movement	The clinician provides anterior glide of the calcaneus and talus on the tibia.
Assessment	A (+) test is excessive translation of one ankle in comparison to the other lower extremity. A dimple or sulcus sign near the anterior talofibular ligament area will likely be seen. A 4-point scale has been described to grade laxity: 0 = no laxity, 1 = mild laxity, 2 = moderate laxity, and 3 = gross laxity.[99]

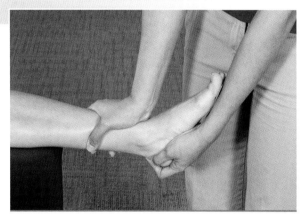

Figure 26.54

Statistics
- SN 58 (29-84), SP 100 (60-100), +LR Inf, –LR 0.42, QUADAS 2, in a study of 20 clients with injury (12 had suffered an average of 2.24 ankle sprains to their injured ankle; average age 21.6; 9 women) and 8 asymptomatic clients (average age 21.25; 5 women), using stress fluoroscopy as the reference standard[99]
- At 2.3 mm [SN 74 (58-86), SP 38 (24-56), +LR 1.2, –LR 0.66] and at 3.7 mm [SN 83 (64-93), SP 40 (27-56), +LR 1.4, –LR 0.41] QUADAS 9, in a study of 66 clients with a history of lateral ankle sprains (average age 22.7 ± 3.6; 31 women in injured group, 12 men and 8 women in control group; duration of symptoms 5.9 ± 4.5 days after the injury)], using diagnostic ultrasound as the reference standard[100]

TALAR TILT (VARUS) STRESS TEST (LATERAL LIGAMENTS)

Client Position	Supine with feet off table or seated at edge of table
Clinician Position	Standing directly in front of leg to be assessed
Movement	Clinician stabilizes the tibia superiorly while gripping the talocrural joint and calcaneus on the plantar aspect. The clinician then applies a quick lateral (varus) tilt to the subtalar joint.
Assessment	A (+) test is gross laxity, diagnostic of joint instability. A scale of 1 to 5 has also been used to denote laxity where 1 is very hypomobile, 2 is hypomobile, 3 is normal, 4 is hypermobile, and 5 is very hypermobile.[100, 101]

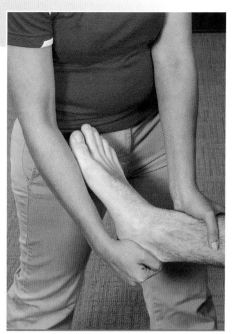

Figure 26.55

Statistics	• SN 50 (29-84), SP 88 (47-99), +LR 4.0, –LR 0.57, QUADAS 2, in a study of 20 clients, 12 (average age 21.6, 9 women) of whom had suffered an average of 2.24 ankle sprains to their injured ankle and 8 (average age 21.25, 5 women) clients who were asymptomatic. Stress fluoroscopy was used as the reference standard.[99, 102]

• The combination of pain with palpation of the anterior talofibular ligament, lateral hematoma, and a positive anterior drawer on examination 5 days after injury: **SN 100**, SP 75, +LR 4.13, **–LR 0.01**, QUADAS 10, to identify lateral ligament rupture in a 160 patients, using arthrography as the reference standard.[103]

• SP 82 (69-90), SN 49 (34-64), +LR 2.65, –LR 0.63, QUADAS 12, in a study of 88 clients (mean age 21; 45 were women), using the self-reported functional questionnaire as the reference standard (Cumberland ankle instability tool).[101]

MEDIAL SUBTALAR GLIDE TEST

Client Position	Supine with ankle being assessed off the table
Clinician Position	Standing directly in front of leg to be assessed
Movement	The clinician stabilizes the talus in subtalar neutral superiorly while gripping the calcaneus at the plantar/posterior aspect of the foot. The clinician then applies a medial glide of the calcaneus on the fixed talus.
Assessment	A (+) test is gross laxity, diagnostic of subtalar joint instability (after lateral ankle sprain).

Figure 26.56

Statistics	SN 58 (29-84), SP 88 (47-99), +LR 4.7, –LR 0.48, QUADAS 2, in a study of 20 clients, 12 (average age 21.6; 9 women) of whom had suffered average of 2.24 lateral ankle sprains to their injured ankle and 8 (average age 21.25; 5 women) clients who were asymptomatic. Stress fluoroscopy was used as the reference standard.[99, 102]

LIGAMENTOUS LAXITY OR INSTABILITY: ANKLE MEDIAL LIGAMENT INTEGRITY

TALAR TILT (VALGUS) STRESS TEST (MEDIAL LIGAMENTS)

Client Position	Sitting or supine
Clinician Position	Standing directly facing the leg to be assessed
Movement	The clinician grasps the ankle of the client at the malleoli, stabilizing the tibia superiorly. The clinician then applies a quick medial (valgus) tilt to the subtalar joint.
Assessment	A (+) test is excessive laxity when compared to the noninjured extremity.
Statistics	NR

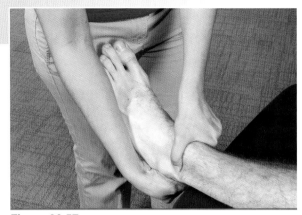

Figure 26.57

MEDIAL TENDERNESS

Client Position	Sitting or supine
Clinician Position	Standing directly to the side of the leg to be assessed
Movement	The clinician places pressure around the deltoid ligament.
Assessment	A (+) test is pain during pressure placement.
Statistics	SN 57 (NR), SP 59 (NR), +LR 1.4, –LR 0.72, QUADAS 8 in a study of 55 clients (26 tender medially and 29 non tender medially; mean age 42; 29 women), using ankle fractures (Weber B lateral malleolar fractures with normal medial clear space over) and stress radiograph as a reference standard[104]

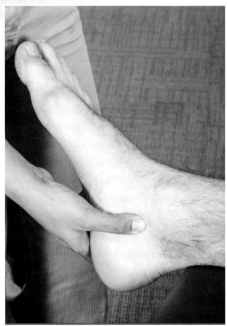

Figure 26.58

LIGAMENTOUS LAXITY OR INSTABILITY: SYNDESMOTIC INTEGRITY

COTTON TEST

Client Position	Supine
Clinician Position	Standing directly in front of leg to be assessed
Movement	The clinician stabilizes the tibia with one hand and applies a lateral force to the ankle with the other hand. Occasionally dorsiflexion is added to increase the sensitivity of the test. Stabilization of the tibia is important to correctly perform the test.
Assessment	A (+) test is lateral translation of the ankle.
Statistics	SN 25, SP NR[102, 105]

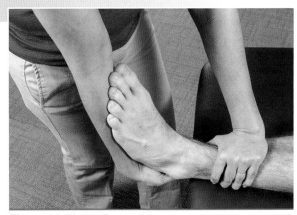

Figure 26.59

EXTERNAL ROTATION AND DORSIFLEXION EXTERNAL ROTATION TEST

Client Position	Supine with the knee flexed to 90°
Clinician Position	Standing directly next to foot to be assessed
Movement	The clinician cradles the ankle in neutral, then externally rotates it. Dorsiflexion is added for the dorsiflexion external rotation test.
Assessment	A (+) test is reproduction of concordant pain.
Statistics	• SN 20, SP 85, +LR 1.3, –LR 0.94, QUADAS 8, in a study of 56 clients (mean age 32 ± 13 years; gender NR; mean duration of symptoms 6.6 ± 2.3 days), using MRI as a reference standard[106]

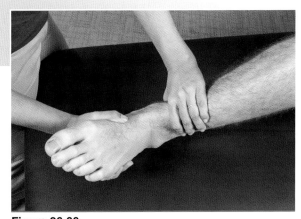

Figure 26.60

• External rotation and dorsiflexion test: SN 71 (55-83), SP 63 (49-75), +LR 1.93, –LR 0.46, QUADAS 9, in a study of 87 clients with acute ankle injury, 37 with ankle syndesmosis injury (75% men; average age 24.6 ± 6.5 years; duration of symptoms 2 weeks), using MRI as a reference standard[107]

FIBULAR TRANSLATION TEST

Client Position	Side lying, leg relaxed, opposite lower extremity knee bent
Clinician Position	Standing directly in front of leg to be assessed
Movement	The clinician applies an anterior to posterior force on the fibula at the level of the syndesmosis.
Assessment	A (+) test is reproduction of concordant pain and increased translation as compared to the contralateral side.
Statistics	**SN 82, SP 88, +LR 6.8, –LR 0.20,** QUADAS 9, in a study of 12 clients (3 suspected of a chronic syndesmotic rupture and 9 healthy volunteers with asymptomatic ankles, demographic data NR), using arthroscopy as a reference standard for the 3 clients[105]

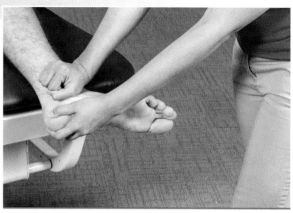

Figure 26.61

SYNDESMOSIS SQUEEZE TEST

Client Position	Supine or side lying with leg relaxed
Clinician Position	Standing directly facing the leg to be tested
Movement	The clinician applies a manual squeeze, compressing the fibula and tibia (applying the force at the midpoint of the calf).
Assessment	A (+) test is reproduction of concordant distal pain at (or near) the syndesmosis.
Statistics	• SN 30, SP 94, +LR 5.0, –LR 0.74, QUADAS 8, in a study of 56 clients with sprained ankle (mean age 32 ± 13 years; gender NR; duration of symptoms 6.6 ± 2.3 days), and MRI as a reference standard[106] • SN 26 (15-42), SP 88 (76-94), +LR 2.15, –LR 0.84, QUADAS 9, in a study of 87 clients with acute ankle injury, 37 with ankle syndesmosis injury (mean age 24.6 ± 6.5 years; 25% women; duration of symptoms 2 weeks), and using MRI as a reference standard[108]

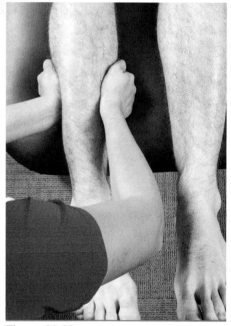

Figure 26.62

DORSIFLEXION LUNGE WITH COMPRESSION TEST

Client Position	Ready to do a lunge
Clinician Position	Kneeling behind lunge leg
Movement	The client performs a lunge forward, moving as far as possible on the injured leg. The lunge is repeated with manual compression provided by the examiner across the ankle syndesmosis.
Assessment	A (+) test is an increase in the ankle range of motion or decreased pain when compression is added.
Statistics	SN 69 (53-82), SP 41 (28-56), +LR 1.18, –LR 0.74, QUADAS 9, in a study of 87 clients with acute ankle injury, 37 with ankle syndesmosis injury (mean age 24.6 ± 6.5 years; 25% women; duration of symptoms 2 weeks), using MRI as a reference standard[108]

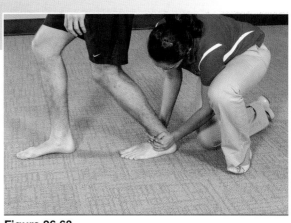

Figure 26.63

LIGAMENTOUS LAXITY OR INSTABILITY: ANKLE IMPINGEMENT

FORCED DORSIFLEXION TEST

 Video 26.64 **in the web resource shows a demonstration of this test.**

Client Position	Sitting or supine
Clinician Position	Seated to the side of the client's lower extremity to be assessed
Movement	Stabilizing the distal aspect of the tibia, the clinician places their thumb on the anterolateral aspect of the talus near the lateral gutter. Next, the clinician applies pressure, followed by a forceful dorsiflexion movement.
Assessment	A (+) test is reproduction of concordant pain at the anterolateral aspect of the foot during forced dorsiflexion.
Statistics	SN 95 (81-99), SP 88 (72-96), +LR 8.06, –LR 0.06, QUADAS 8, in a study of 73 clients with painful giving way without clinical laxity or with persistent pain after a sprain (mean age 39 years; 27 women; duration of symptoms NR), using arthroscopy as a reference standard[109]

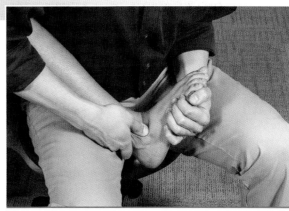

Figure 26.64

CLINICAL PREDICTION RULE OF IMPINGEMENT[110]

- Anterolateral joint tenderness
- Anterolateral ankle joint swelling
- Pain with forced dorsiflexion
- Pain with single leg squat on affected side
- Pain with activities
- Absence of ankle instability

Assessment	A (+) test for anterior ankle impingement is five out of six of the previously mentioned symptoms.
Statistics	SN 94 (73-99), SP 75 (19-99), +LR 3.8, –LR 0.08, QUADAS 7, in a study of 22 clients (average age 28 years; 7 women; duration of symptoms 3-13 months), with arthroscopy as the reference standard[110]

NERVE ENTRAPMENT

FOOT SQUEEZE TEST (MORTON'S TEST)

Client Position	Sitting or supine
Clinician Position	Standing at the side of the lower extremity to be assessed, directly facing client
Movement	The clinician applies a squeeze to the metatarsal heads from lateral to medial toward the midline.
Assessment	A test is (+) if the client's symptoms are reproduced.
Statistics	SN 88, QUADAS 7, in a study of 116 feet (76 treated operatively for Morton's neuroma and 40 feet with different pathologies; mean age 51 ± 12 years; 60 were women; mean duration of symptoms NR), and MRI as a reference standard[56]

WEB SPACE TENDERNESS

Client Position	Sitting or supine
Clinician Position	Standing at the side of the lower extremity to be assessed, directly facing client
Movement	The clinician applies a force between the 2nd and 3rd metatarsals using the tip or side of their thumb.
Assessment	A (+) test is if the client's symptoms are reproduced.
Statistics	SN 95, QUADAS 7, in a study of 116 feet (76 treated operatively for Morton's neuroma and 40 feet with different pathologies; mean age 51 ± 12 years; 60 were women; mean duration of symptoms NR), and MRI as a reference standard[56]

PLANTAR PERCUSSION TEST

Client Position	Sitting or supine with foot in dorsiflexion
Clinician Position	Standing at the side of the lower extremity to be assessed, directly facing client
Movement	The clinician extends the toes to full range. The clinician taps the region between the 2nd and 3rd metatarsal heads.
Assessment	A (+) test is reproduction of neurological findings, such as tingling.
Statistics	SN 62, QUADAS 7, in a study of 116 feet (76 treated operatively for Morton's neuroma and 40 feet with different pathologies; mean age 51 ± 12 years; 60 were women; mean duration of symptoms NR), and MRI as a reference standard[56]

TOE TIP SENSATION DEFICIT

Client Position	Supine or sitting
Clinician Position	Standing directly in front of the leg to be assessed
Movement	The clinician applies light touch sensibility assessment to client's 2nd and 3rd toes.
Assessment	A (+) test is if the client reports paresthesia or anesthesia. Metatarsalgia may cause a false-positive finding in clients.[111]
Statistics	SN 49 (NR), QUADAS 7, in a study of 116 feet (76 treated operatively for Morton's neuroma; 60 women, 10 men; mean age 51; 40 feet with different pathologies), using MRI as a reference standard[56]

TUNING FORK

Refer to the Triage and Screening section of this chapter for a description of this test.

Statistics	• Placement over bony landmark: SN 83, SP 80, +LR 4.2, –LR 0.21, QUADAS 6, in a study of 37 clients (19 men, 18 women), with various locations and types of fractures, using radiography as a reference standard[54]
	• Placement (stethoscope) over swelling area: SN 83, SP 92, +LR 10.4, –LR 0.2, in the same study[54]
	• SN 75, SP 67, +LR 2.3, –LR 0.3, QUADAS 9, in a study of 52 clients with a history and physical examination suggestive of tibial stress fracture, and a reference standard of a bone scan[55]

NERVE ENTRAPMENT: TARSAL TUNNEL SYNDROME

TINEL'S SIGN

Client Position	Side lying with lower extremity relaxed
Clinician Position	Directly next to the client's lower extremity to be assessed
Movement	The clinician applies a tapping force to the posterior-medial aspect of the ankle (just posterior to the medial malleolus).
Assessment	A (+) test is reproduction of numbness or tingling during the test.
Statistics	SN 58, QUADAS 5, in a study of 19 consecutive cases of flexor hallucis longus stenosing tenosynovitis (age, gender, and duration of symptoms NR), with operative tenolysis as a reference standard[102, 112]

TRIPLE COMPRESSION STRESS TEST (SIDE LYING)

Client Position	Side lying with lower extremity relaxed
Clinician Position	Directly next to the client's lower extremity to be assessed
Movement	The clinician applies a tapping force to the posterior-medial aspect of the ankle (just posterior to the medial malleolus).
Assessment	A (+) test is reproduction of numbness or tingling during the test.
Statistics	SN 58 (NR), QUADAS 5, in a study of 19 feet with flexor hallucis longus stenosing tenosynovitis (age, gender, and duration of symptoms NR), with operative tenolysis as a reference standard[102, 112]

TRIPLE COMPRESSION STRESS TEST (LONG SITTING)

Client Position	Long sitting
Clinician Position	Standing beside the client's lower extremity to be assessed
Movement	The clinician places the ankle in full planter flexion and the foot in inversion, applying even, constant digital pressure over the posterior tibial nerve.
Assessment	A (+) test is the provocation of client's concordant symptoms.
Statistics	SN 86 (76-92), SP 100 (93-100), +LR Inf, –LR 0.14, QUADAS 8, in a study of 145 feet (80 asymptomatic and 65 symptomatic feet; mean age 37 years; 23 women; duration of symptoms NR), and basic motor nerve conduction at the tibial nerve as a reference standard[113]

DORSIFLEXION-EVERSION TEST

 Video 26.65 **in the web resource shows a demonstration of this test.**

Client Position	Sitting, lower extremities relaxed
Clinician Position	Kneeling at the side of the client's lower extremity to be assessed
Movement	The clinician maximally dorsiflexes the ankle, everts the foot, and extends the toes, maintaining the position for 5 to 10 seconds, while tapping over the region of the tarsal tunnel to determine if a positive Tinel's sign is present or if the client complains of local nerve tenderness.
Assessment	A (+) test is local tenderness over the nerve or numbness and pain along the nerve distribution.
Statistics	SN 81 (NR), SP 99 (NR), +LR 82.7, –LR 0.19, QUADAS 8, in a study of 50 normal and 37 symptomatic clients (44 feet) with tarsal tunnel syndrome (average age 31 years; 20 women; mean duration of symptoms 4 months), with surgery as a reference standard[114]

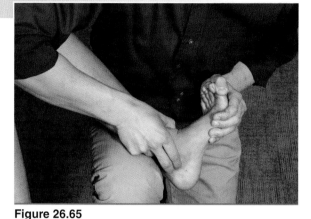

Figure 26.65

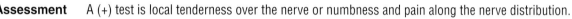

PALPATION

When palpating the lower leg, foot, and ankle complex, the clinician should get some direction from the information collected up to this point in the exam. The clinician should use clinical reasoning to determine if other areas need to be assessed based on referred pain, mechanism of injury, and so on.

Anterior Aspect

Bony Structures

• **Syndesmosis:** The clinician should locate the medial malleolus and palpate laterally. The anterior talofibular can be palpated between the distal tibia and fibula immediately proximal to the talus.

Soft-Tissue Structures

• **Tibialis anterior:** This structure is most prominent and medial. It can be more visible when client dorsiflexes and inverts the foot.

• **Extensor hallucis:** This is located lateral to the tibialis anterior. It is more prominent when the big toe is extended.

• **Extensor digitorum:** This is prominent when the toes are extended. It is located lateral to the extensor hallucis.

• **Dorsalis pedal artery:** This is located between the extensor hallucis and the extensor digitorum tendons.

Lateral Aspect

Bony Structures

• **Fifth metatarsal:** The clinician should start at the MTP of the lateral side. Proximal to its wide base is the styloid process.

• **Cuboid:** The clinician can palpate proximal to the base of the fifth metatarsal when palpating along the fifth metatarsal shaft.

• **Sinus tarsi:** The clinician should palpate the depression just anterior to the lateral malleolus.

Soft-Tissue Structures

• **ATFL:** This is palpable in the sinus tarsi.

• **CFL:** This is palpable from the fibula to the lateral wall of the calcaneus, posterior to peroneal tubercle.

• **PTFL:** The clinician can palpate the posterior edge of the lateral malleolus to the posterior aspect of talus.

• **Peroneus longus and brevis:** The clinician can palpate immediately behind the lateral malleolus. To palpate them more easily, they can have the client evert and plantar flex.

Medial Aspect

Bony Structures

• **First ray and metatarsophalangeal joint:** These are palpable at the ball of the foot. From the joint, the clinician can palpate the medial shaft of the metatarsal bone and first ray.

• **First metatarsocuneiform:** This is located where the first ray meets the first cuneiform.

• **Navicular tubercle:** The clinician can move proximally from the cuneiform: The next large bony prominence is the tubercle.

• **Head of talus:** The medial side of the talar head is immediately proximal to the navicular.

• **Sustentaculum tali:** The clinician can palpate 1 finger's breadth from the distal end of the malleolus toward the bottom of the foot.

Soft-Tissue Structures

• **Deltoid ligament:** This can be palpated from the inferior to medial malleolus.

• **Post tibialis tendon:** This is most palpable when the client inverts and plantar flexes the foot.

• **Flexor hallucis longus:** This is located deep to other muscles. It is hard to palpate, although it runs along the posterior aspect of the tibia and grooves.

• **Flexor digitorum longus:** This is found behind the tibialis posterior. It is most palpable when the client resists toe flexion.

Posterior Aspect

• **Achilles tendon:** The clinician can palpate the lower third of the calf to the calcaneus.

• **Retrocalcaneal bursa:** This is located between the anterior surface of the Achilles tendon and the posterior surface of calcaneus.

Plantar Aspect

• **Sesamoid bones:** The clinician should press on the base of the distal end of the first metatarsal.

PHYSICAL PERFORMANCE MEASURES

Physical performance measures related to the lower leg, ankle, and foot can be found in table 26.4. For detailed information about measures, refer to chapters 24 (Hip), 25 (Knee), and 12 (Physical Performance Measures).

COMMON ORTHOPEDIC CONDITIONS OF THE LOWER LEG, ANKLE, AND FOOT

While it is impossible to distinctly describe various pathological presentations of the lower leg, ankle, and foot, there are evidence-based findings supportive of particular pathologies of this region of the body. Therefore, the intent of this section of the chapter is to present current evidence-supported findings suggestive of lower leg, ankle, and foot pathologies. As previously described in chapter 4 (Evidence-Based Practice and Client Examination), though, not all examination findings are absolutely supported with clinical evidence, and the clinician should also rely on clinical experience and input from the client when performing differential diagnosis of a client's presentation of pain and dysfunction.

Lower leg, ankle, and foot pathologies, much like other joint pathology, can have variable presentations. These pathological presentations can also have similarities in their presentation. Differentiating among their clinical findings is helpful for the clinician to determine not only the appropriate clinical intervention but also the necessity of referral to other potentially more appropriate health care clinicians.

Ankle Sprain

ICD-9: 845.00 (sprain of ankle, unspecified site)

ICD-10: S93.409A (sprain of unspecified ligament of unspecified ankle, initial encounter)

ICD-10: S96.919A (strain of unspecified muscle and tendon at ankle and foot level, unspecified foot, initial encounter)

Twenty percent of all athletic injuries consist of trauma to the ankle and foot, where sprains contribute to 85% of all ankle injuries.[115] Without even accounting for the 70% re-injury rate, 850,000 new sprains are reported in the United States each year.[116, 117] No musculotendinous insertions exist on the talus, and the ankle ligaments provide passive support to the talocrural joint.[118] An acute ankle sprain generally includes clients 72 hours post injury, and they may present with significant swelling, pain, limited weight bearing, and gait

TABLE 26.4   Physical Performance Measure Suggestions for the Lower Leg, Ankle, and Foot

Discrete physical parameter	Potential physical performance measurements for the lower-level client (if appropriate)	Potential physical performance measurements for the higher-level client (if appropriate)
Balance	Single-leg stance test Romberg test Four square step test Functional reach test Sidestep test Tandem walking Tinetti test	Any of the tests appropriate for the lower-level client Star excursion balance test Y-balance test Multiple single-leg hop stabilization test
Fundamental movement	Deep squat test Sit-to-stand test Self-paced walking test Timed up and go test	Any of the tests appropriate for the lower-level client Rotational stability Trunk stability push-up
Strength and power	1RM leg press Lunge test Knee bending in 30 s	Any of the tests appropriate for the lower-level client Jump and hop tests
Lower extremity anaerobic power	Only if appropriate and necessary	Any of the tests appropriate for the lower-level client Wingate anaerobic power test Lower extremity functional test
SAQ	Only if appropriate and necessary	Any of the tests appropriate for the lower-level client Edgren sidestep test Illinois agility test Pro agility test Zigzag run test

SAQ = speed, agility, and quickness

deviations. *Chronic ankle instability* (CAI) is the term used for clients with ankle instability whose impairments are instability, weakness, limited balance, and swelling from time to time.[33]

I. Client Interview

Subjective History

- Incidence of ankle injury and ankle sprain was high in court games and team sports, such as rugby, soccer, volleyball, handball, and basketball.[119]
- Clients will describe pain in the ankle (especially inferior-laterally), stiffness, and some difficulty with walking,

depending on the acuteness of the injury.[120, 121]

- The client may describe giving way of joint.[120-122]
- History of previous sprain.[33]
- The Cumberland ankle instability tool can be used to further diagnose severity of functional ankle instability. ICC 0.96, SN 82.9, SP 74.7 in a study with 236 participants with or without functional ankle instability (no demographic data reported) with the LEFS as the reference standard.[123]

Outcome Measures

- The foot and ankle ability measure, foot and ankle disability measure, and LEFS have been seen to be reliable and to show a minimal detectable change (MDC).[33]
- LEFS: When looking at acute ankle sprains, reliability was 0.87, with an MDC of 9.4 over a 1-week interval.[124] There was a significant difference between changes in scores over a 1-week period when comparing those occurring ≥6 days after the ankle sprain to those within 5 days.

Diagnostic Imaging

- MRI has been reliable in helping in detecting tears to the anterior talofibular ligament and calcaneofibular ligament after acute injury.[125-127]
- MRI and CT can accurately help detect osteochondral lesions of the talus.[127, 128]
- With CAI, the fibula was found to have a more lateral position on CT.[129]

II. Observation

- If a hematoma is present accompanied by local pressure pain at palpation, a positive anterior drawer test is present, or both, it is most likely that a (partial) lateral ankle ligament rupture exists.[130]
- The client has pain or antalgic gait, or difficulty with weight bearing.[120-122]
- The client may have ecchymosis and post-traumatic edema, especially an acutely injured client. [120-122]

III. Triage and Screening

- Foot and ankle fractures can be helped to be **ruled out** with Ottawa Ankle Rules (pooled SN 96.4, −LR 0.08) in clients of all ages;[31] for children aged 5 years or older (pooled SN 98.5, −LR 0.11;[32] pooled SN 99, −LR 0.02[131]).
- Foot and ankle stress fractures: Tuning fork (SN 83, −LR 0.21)[54] and plantar percussion test (SN 62)[56] have less than good ability to rule out these fractures.
- The Ottawa Ankle Rules will dictate if radiographs are warranted.[132]

- The Bernese Ankle Rules have ideal ability to help **rule out** (SN 100, −LR 0) and **rule in** (SP 91, +LR 11.1) fractures.[34]

IV. Motion Tests

- Depending on the severity and acuteness of the injury, clients are likely to have limited ROM, especially for inversion.[120, 121]

V. Muscle Performance Testing

- Depending on severity and acuteness of the injury, clients are likely to have limited muscle performance, especially for inversion or eversion strength.[120, 121]

VI. Special Tests

- Clinicians with limited clinical experience produced more accurate results when physical examination was performed 5 days after the injury, rather than within 48 hours. The SN and SP of delayed physical examination for the presence or absence of a lesion of an ankle ligament were found to be 96 and 84, respectively. The utilization of a delayed physical examination was better at helping **ruling out** (SN 96) versus **ruling in** (SP 84) the presence of a lesion of the ankle ligament.[133]
- Anterior drawer test: A (+) test had poor ability to help rule in (SP 100, +LR Inf) a lateral ankle sprain in one study of high bias.[99]
- Medial subtalar glide: A (+) test had poor ability to help rule in (SP 88, +LR 4.67) a lateral ankle sprain in one study of high bias.[99]
- Talar tilt stress test: A (+) test had poor ability to help rule in (SP 88, +LR 4.0) a lateral ankle sprain in one study of high bias.[99]
- Five days after injury, a (−) anterior drawer test, no lateral hematoma, and no pain with palpation of the ATFL help **rule out** (SN 100, −LR 0.01) a lateral ankle sprain.[103]

VII. Palpation

- Clinicians should look for tenderness to palpation of involved ligaments and potentially the surrounding bone.[120-122]

V. Physical Performance Measures

- Acutely injured clients may have diminished proprioception and altered weight bearing,[120-122] and therefore may be unable to perform any of these measures early in rehabilitation.

- Clinicians may use single-leg hop tests with diagonal and lateral movements as well as direction change; moderate evidence shows that exercises such as side hop, 6 m crossover hop, lateral hopping for distance, figure-eight hop, and hopping course help discriminate clients with continued dysfunction due to ankle sprain.[33]

- Clients may have reduced performance on the star excursion balance test.[134]

Martin and colleagues recommended the grading system for lateral ankle sprains first described by Malliaropoulos and colleagues.[33] This system is shown in table 26.5.

POTENTIAL TREATMENT-BASED CLASSIFICATIONS

Acute

- Pain or immobility: Client may need external support, lace-up brace, or semirigid ankle support.[135] If pain is severe, immobilization or semirigid bracing may be used.[136]

- The clinician can recommend cryotherapy and therapeutic exercises.[33]

- Mobility: should restore pain-free ankle and foot mobility.[33, 137]

Chronic

- Strength and conditioning, with a focus on balance and other proprioception exercises [138-141]

- Dynamic stability through balance training[118]

- Mobility[137, 142]

TABLE 26.5   Grading System for Lateral Ankle Sprains[33]

	Grade I	Grade II	Grade III
Loss of function	None	Some	Near total loss
Ligamentous laxity	None	(+) anterior drawer (−) talar tilt	(+) anterior drawer (+) talar tilt
Hemorrhaging	Little to none	Present	Present
Point tenderness	None	Present	Extreme
Decrease in ankle motion	≤5°	>5° but <10°	>10°
Swelling	≤0.5 cm	>0.5 cm but <2.0 cm	>2.0 cm
Time to full athletic recovery	7.2 ± 1.6 days	15.0 ± 2.1 days	30.7 ± 3.1 (IIIA) days; 55.4 ± 4.9 (IIIB) days

Critical Clinical Pearls

In an inversion ankle sprain, clinicians should also evaluate the following structures:

- Superficial and deep fibular nerves may have been tractioned during injury.
- The cuboid can sublux or dislocate due to the contraction of the fibularis muscles.
- The medial side can incur compression during an inversion sprain.

High Ankle Sprain or Syndesmotic Ankle Injury

ICD-9: 845.00 (sprain of ankle, unspecified site)

ICD-10: S93.409A (sprain of unspecified ligament of unspecified ankle, initial encounter)

ICD -10: S96.919A (strain of unspecified muscle and tendon at ankle and foot level, unspecified foot, initial encounter)

One to eighteen percent of all ankle injuries involve the syndesmosis. The incidence of high ankle sprains has been seen to be 29% in professional American football.[143] These injuries may be differentially diagnosed from lateral ankle sprains due to the external rotation component involved during trauma.[144] These injuries are often hard to diagnose compared to a medial or lateral ankle sprain, and recovery is lengthy and frustrating for the client.[145]

I. Client Interview

Subjective History

- The method of injury (MOI) most commonly includes an external rotation moment at the ankle with the foot in a dorsiflexed and pronated position; however, other positions have been reported to cause a high ankle sprain. The force causes a widening of the mortise and rupture of the ligamentous structures that stabilize the joint.[145]

- Clients who engage in skiing, American football, soccer, and other turf sports (due to greater risk for cutting) may have these injuries.[143, 146]

Outcome Measures

- Any appropriate foot and ankle measure may be used.

Diagnostic Imaging

- The client may need radiographs if triage tests are positive for possible fracture; radiographs showing >1 mm widening may indicate a need for surgical fixation.[145]

- MRI is the gold standard for this type of injury.[147] It has been seen to have similar sensitivity and specificity as arthroscopy.[127, 148-150]

II. Observation

- Less swelling is present in this condition than with lateral ankle sprain.[147] If swelling is notable, the clinician should do figure-eight measurements.

- The client has difficulty with walking and bearing weight.

III. Triage and Screening

- Fibular fractures may be present.[151, 152]

- Foot and ankle fractures can be **ruled out** with the Ottawa Ankle Rules (pooled SN 96.4, −LR 0.08) in clients of all ages;[31] for children aged 5 years or older (pooled SN 98.5, −LR 0.11;[32] pooled SN 99, −LR 0.02[131]).

- Foot and ankle stress fractures: Tuning fork (SN 83, −LR 0.21)[54] and plantar percussion test (SN 62)[56] have less than good ability to rule out these fractures.

- The Ottawa Ankle Rules will dictate if radiographs are warranted.[132]

- The Bernese Ankle Rules have ideal ability to help **rule out** (SN 100, −LR 0) and **rule in** (SP 91, +LR 11.1) fractures.[34]

IV. Motion Tests

- Loss of full plantarflexion[147]

- Pain with active or passive ER of the foot; pain with active or passive forced dorsiflexion[145]

V. Muscle Performance Testing

- Antalgic gait pattern may be present with heel raised instead of heel-toe pattern.[145]

VI. Special Tests

- Syndesmosis squeeze test: A (+) test has less than good ability to help rule in (SP 94, +LR 5.0) a high ankle sprain.[106]

- External rotation test: A (+) external rotation test has less than good ability to help rule in (SP 85, +LR 1.3) a high ankle sprain.[106]

- External rotation test with dorsiflexion: A (+) test has less than good ability to help rule out (SN 71, −LR 0.46) a high ankle sprain.[107]

- Cotton test: A (+) cotton test has very poor ability to help rule out (SN 25) a high ankle sprain.[105]

- Fibular translation test: Both a (−) test (SN 82, −LR 0.20) and a (+) test (SP 88, +LR 6.8) have good ability to **rule out** and **rule in**, respectively, a high ankle sprain.[105]

- Dorsiflexion lunge with compression test: has poor ability to either rule out or rule in a high ankle sprain.[107]

VII. Palpation

- The anterior inferior tibiofibular ligament (AITFL) and proximally along the interosseous membrane will be tender to palpation.[145, 153]

- Isolated syndesmotic ligament injuries are uncommon; therefore, the deltoid ligament may be affected.[151, 152, 154]

- Pain with palpation of the AITFL and PITFL transverse ligament, interosseous ligament, interosseous membrane, and deltoid ligament helps **rule out** (SN 92, −LR 0.28) ankle syndesmosis injury.[108]

VIII. Physical Performance Measures

- A (−) single-leg hop test has good ability to help **rule out** (SN 90, −LR 0.37) syndesmotic pathology.[107]

POTENTIAL TREATMENT-BASED CLASSIFICATIONS

- For sprain with latent diastasis, the clinician should use immobility.

- Phase I: Pain control, edema management, and immobility.[145]

- Phase II: Gait or exercise and conditioning: The clinician should focus on low-level balance training and strength training.[145]

- Phase III: Exercise and conditioning: The clinician should focus on unilateral balance and high-level strength.

- Phase IV: Return to sport.

Achilles Tendon Rupture

ICD-9: 727.67 (nontraumatic rupture of Achilles tendon)

ICD-10: M66.369 (spontaneous rupture of flexor tendons, unspecified lower leg)

The most frequently ruptured tendon in the body is the Achilles tendon.[269] The incidence of rupture has been on the rise since the 1980s with the most rapid increase in males ages 30-50 years,[270] classically the beginner athlete in his fourth decade engaging in an atypical athletic activity.[270] The most common site of rupture is 3 to 6 cm above the calcaneal insertion due to the poor vascularization. Histologically there is significant collagen degeneration observed in clients who have had a tear.[271, 272] Some risk factors include oral ingestion and intratendinous injection of steroids, hypercholesterolemia, gout, rheumatoid arthritis, long term dialysis, and renal transplant.[273]

I. Client Interview

Subjective History

- Clients have acute onset.[155]

- This injury is more common in men aged 30 to 50 years.[156]

- Strenuous physical activity is a common mechanism.[157]

Differential Diagnosis of High Ankle Sprain and Ankle Sprain

- The method of injury in a high ankle sprain will include external rotation moment at the ankle with the foot in a dorsiflexed and pronated position.[145]
- Radiographs will show widening of the mortise in a high ankle sprain.
- Client with high ankle sprain will have loss of full plantarflexion.[147]
- The fibular translation test can both **rule in** (SP 88, +LR 6.8) and **rule out** (SN 82, −LR 0.20) a high ankle sprain.[105]
- A client with a high ankle sprain will have pain with palpation of AITFL and PITFL, the transverse ligament or interosseous membrane, and the deltoid ligament.[107]

- Clients often describe feeling as if they'd been kicked in posterior ankle, feeling or hearing a pop, and experiencing inability to continue activity.[155]

Outcome Measures

- The Achilles Tendon Total Rupture Score (ARTS) has high reliability and validity in clients with a total Achilles tendon rupture.[158]

Diagnostic Imaging

- MRI is helpful for **ruling out** (SN 91) partial tears and complete Achilles tendon tears (SN 94) when not shown on imaging.[24]
- No recommendation exists for or against the routine use of MRI, ultrasound (ultrasonography), and radiograph (roentgenograms, X-rays) to confirm the diagnosis of acute Achilles tendon rupture.[159]

II. Observation

- The client will likely not be able to continue with weight-bearing activity.[155]

III. Triage and Screening

- Foot and ankle fractures can be **ruled out** with the Ottawa Ankle Rules (pooled SN 96.4, −LR 0.08) in clients of all ages;[31] for children aged 5 years or older (pooled SN 98.5, −LR 0.11;[32] pooled SN 99, −LR 0.02[131]).
- Foot and ankle stress fractures: Tuning fork (SN 83, −LR 0.21)[54] and plantar percussion test (SN 62)[56] have less than good ability to rule out these fractures.
- The Ottawa Ankle Rules will dictate if radiographs are warranted.[132]
- The Bernese Ankle Rules have ideal ability to help **rule out** (SN 100, −LR 0) and **rule in** (SP 91, +LR 11.1) fractures.[34]
- Achilles tendon reflex is weak or absent.[155]

IV. Motion Tests

- Increased passive ankle dorsiflexion[159]

V. Muscle Performance Testing

- Clients have loss of true gastrocnemius and soleus strength for plantarflexion.[155, 159]

VI. Special Tests

- Thompson test: A (−) test (SN 96, −LR 0.04) and a (+) test (SP 93, +LR 13.7) have only fair to good ability to rule out and rule in, respectively, Achilles tendon tear in one high-bias study.[95]
- Matles test: A (−) test (SN 88, −LR 0.14) and a (+) test (SP 85, +LR 6.3) have only fair to good ability to rule out and rule in, respectively, Achilles tendon tear.[95]
- Copeland test: A (−) test has less than good ability to help rule out (SN 78) an Achilles tendon tear.[95]
- Palpable of gap in Achilles tendon: A (+) test has fair to good ability to help rule in (SP 89, +LR 6.6) an Achilles tendon tear.[95]

VII. Palpation

- Clinicians may be unable to palpate the Achilles tendon or a palpable defect.[155, 159]
- Clients may have a small bulge at the proximal Achilles tendon.[155]

VIII. Physical Performance Measures

- Only lower-level testing is suggested if this type of testing is appropriate at all in the acute assessment of this pathology.

POTENTIAL TREATMENT-BASED CLASSIFICATIONS

- Pain control
- Stabilization exercises
- Protection of repair if reconstructed
- Mobility or exercise and conditioning when client is ready to return to recreational activities or sport

Achilles Tendinopathy

ICD-9: 727.06 (tenosynovitis of foot and ankle); 726.71 (Achilles bursitis or tendinitis)

ICD-10: M65.879 (other synovitis and tenosynovitis, unspecified ankle and foot); M76.6 (Achilles tendinitis or bursitis)

Achilles tendon dysfunction is a common overuse injury that is often reported by active people participating in activity at a recreational or competitive level.[160] Risk factors that could lead to this dysfunction include abnormal ankle dorsiflexion, decreased plantarflexion strength, increased foot pronation, abnormal tendon structure, obesity, hypertension, hyperlipidemia, and diabetes (moderate evidence). As the client ages, the Achilles tendon goes through morphological and biomechanical changes, making it weaker and stiffer.[161]

I. Client Interview

Subjective History

- Achilles tendinitis can occur in any age, while tendinosis is more likely to occur in those over the age of 35 years.[155]

- Achilles tendinitis is more likely in high-mileage runners and jumpers, ballet dancers, and sedentary and obese people.[119]

- Achilles tendinitis is of acute onset, and it can be prevalent with activity; it elicits pain in the heel and causes stiffness.[119, 155]

- Achilles tendinosis is of chronic nature, and pain along the Achilles tendon can be elicited with loading the tendon. It may or may not have clinical symptoms with activity, and often does not respond to anti-inflammatory modalities or medications.[119, 155, 162-164]

- If the client does *not* report pain located 2 to 6 cm above the insertion of the Achilles tendon, this has fair ability to rule out (SN 78, −LR 0.30) Achilles tendinopathy; if the client reports pain *in this location,* this is fairly helpful for ruling in (SP 77, +LR 3.4) the condition.[94]

- If the client does *not* report that pain is usually worse during the first few steps in the morning, this has good ability to rule out (SN 89, −LR 0.19) Achilles tendinopathy.[94]

Outcome Measures

- The Foot and Ankle Ability Measure or the Victorian Institute of Sport assessment may be used.[161]

Diagnostic Imaging

- Thicker Achilles tendons were associated more often with chronic symptoms (tendinosis).[165]

II. Observation

- Nodules may be noted on the Achilles tendon in resistant cases.[155, 162-164]

III. Triage and Screening

- Foot and ankle fractures can be **ruled out** with the Ottawa Ankle Rules (pooled SN 96.4, −LR 0.08) in clients of all ages;[31] for children aged 5 years or older (pooled SN 98.5, −LR 0.11;[32] pooled SN 99, −LR 0.02[131]).

- Foot and ankle stress fractures: Tuning fork (SN 83, −LR 0.21)[54] and plantar percussion test (SN 62)[56] have less than good ability to rule out these fractures.

- The Ottawa Ankle Rules will dictate if radiographs are warranted.[132]

- The Bernese Ankle Rules have ideal ability to help **rule out** (SN 100, −LR 0) and **rule in** (SP 91, +LR 11.1) fractures.[34]

IV. Motion Tests

- Clients with Achilles tendinitis are more likely to have pain with passive lengthening (or stretching into dorsiflexion) of the involved tendon than those with tendinosis.

V. Muscle Performance Testing

- Clients with Achilles tendinitis will often have pain and weakness with push-off or plantarflexion type of activities, while those with tendinosis may or may not with these activities.[155, 164]

VI. Special Tests

- Palpation for tenderness test: A (+) test had less than good ability to help rule in (SP 81, +LR 3.2) or rule out

(SN 64, −LR 0.48) Achilles tendinopathy in pooled analysis[92] but had good ability to help **rule out** (SN 84, −LR 0.22) Achilles tendinopathy in one high-quality study.[94]

- Royal London Hospital Test: In pooled analysis, this test demonstrated less than good ability to rule out or rule in Achilles tendinopathy[92] but ideal ability to **rule in** (SP 93, +LR Inf) Achilles tendinopathy in one high-quality study.[94]

- Arc sign: A (+) test has fair to good ability to rule in (SP 83, +LR 2.0)[92] Achilles tendinopathy in pooled analysis but had ideal ability to **rule it in** (SP 100, +LR Inf) in one high-quality study.[94]

- Single-leg heel raise test: A (+) test has fair to good ability to help **rule in** (SP 93, +LR 3.1) Achilles tendinopathy.[94]

- Hop test: A (+) test has fair to good ability to help **rule in** (SP 87, +LR 3.3) Achilles tendinopathy.[94]

- Pain with passive dorsiflexion test: A (+) test has fair to good ability to help rule in (SP 87, +LR 0.93) Achilles tendinopathy.[94]

- Combined testing (palpation, arc sign, and Royal London test) have fair to good ability to help rule in (SP 83, +LR 3.5) Achilles tendinopathy.[93]

VII. Palpation

- Tendinitis tends to elicit well-localized tenderness that is similar in quality and location to the pain experienced during activity.[166]

- In clients with tendinosis, clinicians may notice a painless, palpable nodule on the Achilles tendon.[155, 162-164]

- Thickness of the Achilles tendon between 2 and 6 cm above the insertion with gently squeezing the tendon between thumb and index finger helps **rule in** (SP 90, +LR 9.83) Achilles tendinopathy.[94]

- Palpation of crepitus ("wet leather" sign) of the Achilles tendon between 2 and 6 cm above the insertion helps

rule in (SP 100, +LR Inf) Achilles tendinopathy.[94]

- Tenderness to palpation of the tendon has fair to good ability to help rule in (SP 85, +LR 3.5) Achilles tendinopathy,[93] and not having tenderness to palpation of the tendon has good ability to helps **rule out** (SN 84, −LR 0.22)[94] Achilles tendinopathy to a moderate degree.

VIII. Physical Performance Measures

- Stair descent, unilateral heel raise, single-limb hop movements, and recreational activity participation are suggested, based on moderate evidence.[161]

POTENTIAL TREATMENT-BASED CLASSIFICATIONS[161]

- Exercise and conditioning: eccentric loading exercises (strong evidence)

- Pain control: low-level laser, iontophoresis (moderate evidence)

- Stretching, foot orthosis night splint (weak evidence)

- Mobility: possibly manual therapy and taping (expert opinion)[161]

Plantar Fasciitis

ICD-9: 728.71 (plantar fascial fibromatosis)

ICD-10: M72.2 (plantar fascial fibromatosis)

Plantar fasciitis accounts for 15% of all adult complaints related to the foot that require professional help in both athletic and nonathletic populations.[167] Risk factors include decreased ankle dorsiflexion, obesity, and work-related weight bearing.[168] Plantar heel pain may be neural in origin; therefore, ruling out nerve involvement is important.[169] Baxter and Pfeiffer reported that tenderness under the base of the second metatarsal as well as the insertion of the plantar fascia on the calcaneus would be plantar fasciitis; however, pain at the bottom at the heel was more indicative of heel pad atrophy and medial foot pain was more indicative of entrapment of the first branch of the plantar nerve.[170]

I. Client Interview

Subjective History

- People who spend the majority of their workday on their feet and those whose body mass index is >30 kg/m² are at increased risk for the development of plantar fasciitis.[172]

- Pain for this condition appears in the plantar medial heel region. It is most noticeable with initial steps after a period of inactivity but is also worse following prolonged weight bearing and is often precipitated by a recent increase in weight-bearing activity.[168]

- Pain tends to be present with increasing levels of activity (i.e., walking, running), but will tend to worsen toward the end of the day.[168]

- Often the client will have had a change in activity level, such as increased distance with walking or running, or an employment change that requires more time[167] standing or walking.[168]

- Localized pain occurs under the anteromedial aspect of the plantar/posterior surface of the heel, with paresthesias being uncommon.[168]

- In clients with posterior heel pain of neural origin, pain is usually characterized as burning, sharp, shooting, shocklike, electric, localized, or radiating either proximally or distally.[169]

Outcome Measures

- Only the Foot and Ankle Ability Measure has been validated in a physical therapy practice setting for plantar fasciitis.[11]

Diagnostic Imaging

- Imaging studies are typically not necessary for the diagnosis of plantar fasciitis.[168]

II. Observation

- In some cases, the pain is so severe that the client ambulates with an antalgic gait.[168]

- Longitudinal arch angle measure, navicular position test, and big toe extension may provide further information.

III. Triage and Screening

- Foot and ankle fractures can be **ruled out** with Ottawa Ankle Rules (pooled SN 96.4, −LR 0.08) in clients of all ages;[31] for children aged 5 years or older (pooled SN 98.5, −LR 0.11[32] pooled SN 99, −LR 0.02[131]).

- Foot and ankle stress fractures: Tuning fork (SN 83, −LR 0.21)[54] and plantar percussion test (SN 62)[56] have less than good ability to rule out these fractures.

- The Ottawa Ankle Rules will dictate if radiographs are warranted.[132]

- The Bernese Ankle Rules have ideal ability to help **rule out** (SN 100, −LR 0) and **rule in** (SP 91, +LR 11.1) fractures.[34]

- Neurodynamic tests such as the straight leg raise can help rule out neurological plantar heel pain.[169]

IV. Motion Tests

- Clients may have less than 10° dorsiflexion; the risk of plantar fasciitis increases as the range of ankle dorsiflexion decreases.[171] Reduced ankle dorsiflexion appears to be the most important risk factor for developing plantar fasciits.[172]

V. Muscle Performance Testing

- Posterior tibialis weakness may be seen due to excessive pronation.[173]

- The flexor digitorum longus, flexor hallucis longus, peroneus longus, and Achilles tendon assist with the supination needed with the windlass mechanism and should therefore be tested.[173]

- Proximal muscle weakness from the gluteus medius, gluteus minimus, tensor fasciae latae, or quadriceps muscles can contribute to plantar fasciae abnormalities.[174]

VI. Special Tests

- Dorsiflexion-eversion test: A (+) test (SP 99, +LR 82.7) and (−) test (SN 81, −LR 0.19) had less than good ability to rule in and rule out tarsal tunnel syndrome in one study of medium bias.[114]

- Windlass test: A (+) test helps **rule in** (SP 99, +LR 28.7) both weight-bearing and (SP 99, +LR 16.2) non-weight-bearing plantar fasciitis.[97]

- Tinel's sign: has limited ability to help rule out (SN 58) tarsal tunnel syndrome.[112]

- Triple compression stress test in long sitting: A (−) test (SN 86, −LR 0.14) and a (+) test (SP 100, +LR Inf) have less than good ability to rule out or rule in, respectively, tarsal tunnel syndrome.[113]

VII. Palpation

- Clients may have pain with palpation of proximal insertion of the plantar fascia.[175]

- Palpation over the abductor hallucis or on the medial calcaneal tuberosity reproduced symptoms in clients with suspected neurological plantar heel pain.[169]

- The diagnosis of entrapment of the first branch of the lateral plantar nerve should not be made without the presence of maximal tenderness over the nerve, although the entire heel and the proximal plantar fascia may also be tender.[169]

- Diagnosis of entrapment of the anterior branch of the medial calcaneal nerve can be substantiated by the following palpatory findings: maximal tenderness over the medial anterior part of the heel fat pad and abductor hallucis, distally radiating pain with pressure on the nerve, and only minimal tenderness over the plantar fascia origin.[169]

- With medial plantar nerve entrapment, tenderness is typically located over the plantar aspect of the medial arch around the navicular tuberosity.[169]

VIII. Physical Performance Measures

- None is specific to plantar fasciitis.

- Performance measures addressing ankle dorsiflexion ROM (such as bilateral and single-leg squat, star excursion balance test, and lunge testing), balance and proprioception (single-leg balance testing), and progression to jumping and hopping tests are recommended for clients who use these activities in their ADLs or work or sport activity.

POTENTIAL TREATMENT-BASED CLASSIFICATIONS

- Pain, activity modification: Low-dye taping improved first-step pain over the short term (1-week period) when compared to sham intervention; adverse effects in 28% may affect compliance.[176] Clients may have some pain relief from dry needling.[177]

- Mobility
  - Tissue-specific stretching demonstrated superior pain relief compared to calf stretching.[178]
  - Soft-tissue mobilization may provide short-term pain relief in clients with heel pain.[179]

Differential Diagnosis of Plantar Fasciitis and Heel Pain

A client with PF will

- report a recent increase in weight-bearing activity;[168]
- report pain with first few steps out of bed in the morning as well as after a period of inactivity;[168]
- have a positive Windlass test in weight-bearing and non-weight-bearing activities;[97]
- have less than 10° of ankle dorsiflexion;[171] and
- will not have an ankle fracture per Ottawa Ankle Rules.[31]

Medial Tibial Stress Syndrome

ICD-9: 844.9 (sprain of knee and leg NOS)

ICD-10: S83.90XA (sprain of unspecified site of unspecified knee, initial encounter); S86.919A (strain of unspecified muscles and tendons at lower leg level, unspecified leg, initial encounter)

Shin splints can also be defined as MTSS, which is different from stress fractures and compartment syndrome. MTSS is a bony overload injury where the tibial bone bends, and strain is caused during weight-bearing activities.[180, 181, 182] Tibial osteopenia can result from microdamage in the bone as bony formation is outpaced by bone reabsorption.[183, 184] Before diagnosing MTSS, tibial stress fracture (pain more local) and exertional compartment syndrome should be excluded.[183]

Chronic exertional compartment syndrome is commonly diagnosed by the measurement of raised intramuscular pressures in the lower limb. The pathophysiology of the condition is poorly understood, and the criteria used to make the diagnosis are based on small sample sizes of symptomatic clients. Although all intracompartmental pressure (ICP) measurement, magnetic resonance imaging, and near-infrared spectroscopy seem to be useful in confirming the diagnosis of chronic exertional compartment syndrome (CECS), no standard diagnostic procedure is currently universally accepted.[185] In fact, intramuscular pressure values have also been shown to vary in relation to a number of factors other than the presence of CECS.[186]

I. Client Interview

Subjective History

- Clients may do activities that involve a lot of jumping and running; rhythmic gymnasts and military personnel are also at risk.[183, 187, 188]
- Pain is exercise related.[183]
- Pain is localized over the distal two-thirds of the posteromedial tibia.[189]
- Symptoms present on starting activity and subside with continued exercise; however, later on, the pain continues to be present during activity.[183] At worst, the pain can be felt when activity ceases.[190]

Outcome Measures

- Any appropriate outcome measure may be used.

Diagnostic Imaging

- MRI is useful in evaluating shin splints, early osseous stress injuries, and overt stress fracture.[191]
- MRI has SN 79-88, SP 33-100, +LR 1.18, −LR 0.64.[192, 193]
- Bone scintigraphy with MRI is widely used to confirm diagnosis.[194]
- When diagnosis is unclear, bone scan and MRI have approximately the same SN and SP. CT and SN are lower with a higher SP.[183]

II. Observation

- Mild swelling of tibia may be present.[190, 195]
- Female gender and increased BMI were found to be related to MTSS.[189]
- Level I evidence is used for excessive pronation and female gender; level II evidence is used for increased internal and external hip ROM, BMI, previous history of MTSS, and leaner calf girth.[183]

III. Triage and Screening

- Foot and ankle fractures can be **ruled out** with the Ottawa Ankle Rules (pooled SN 96.4, −LR 0.08) in clients of all ages;[31] for children aged 5 years or older (pooled SN 98.5, −LR 0.11;[32] pooled SN 99, −LR 0.02[131]).
- Foot and ankle stress fractures: Tuning fork (SN 83, −LR 0.21)[54] and plantar percussion test (SN 62)[56] have less than good ability to rule out these fractures.
- The Ottawa Ankle Rules will dictate if radiographs are warranted.[132]
- The Bernese Ankle Rules have ideal ability to help **rule out** (SN 100, −LR 0) and **rule in** (SP 91, +LR 11.1) fractures.[34]
- If compartment syndrome is suspected, the clinician should perform compartment testing where pressures are

read before (at rest), during, and after exercise. A delay of pressures returning to normal resting state 6 to 30 minutes after exercise has diagnostic value.[196]

IV. Motion Tests

- Lack of talocrural mobility, decreased ankle dorsiflexion[197]

V. Muscle Performance Testing

- Weak foot intrinsic muscles (pronation, navicular drop), hip weakness

VI. Special Tests

- Shin palpation test: A (+) test has fair to good ability to rule in (SP 90, +LR 3.4) MTSS.[91]

- Shin edema test: A (+) test **rules out** (SN 92, −LR 0.95) MTSS.[91]

- Utilizing both the shin palpation and shin edema test together **rules in** (SP 88, +LR 7.9) MTSS.[91]

VII. Palpation

- Clients may have pain along the posteromedial border of the tibia over a length of 5 or more consecutive cm.[198]

VIII. Physical Performance Measures

- Only lower level testing is suggested if this type of testing is appropriate at all in the acute assessment of this pathology.

POTENTIAL TREATMENT-BASED CLASSIFICATIONS

- Mobility (ankle), shoe insert; exercise and conditioning (hip); and improved running technique[197]

- Modalities: Iontophoresis, phonophoresis, ice massage, ultrasound, periosteal pecking, and extracorporeal shockwave therapy are effective (Level 3 to 4 of evidence—none of the studies were free from some methodological bias).[199]

Tibialis Posterior Tendon Dysfunction

ICD-9: 726.72 (posterior tibial tendonitis)

ICD-10: M76.829 (posterior tibial tendinitis, unspecified leg)

Dysfunction in the tibialis posterior tendon (TPT) has been described as a loss of strength in the tendon that occurs either suddenly or over time.[200] The muscle eccentrically contracts at heel strike to resist internal rotation of the tibia and pronation.[201] At heel rise, the TPT locks the bones of the arch and rearfoot, converting the foot into a rigid lever.[202] The TPT is the main stabilizer of the medial longitudinal arch.[203] TPT dysfunction has been histopathologically seen to be tendinosis[204] from repetitive microtrauma and chronic microdegenration[205] and with degeneration could eventually rupture.[206] It can be broken down into type I, where there is primary tendon inflammation, and type II, tendon dysfunction and elongation, where the client develops flat foot deformity[207] (table 26.6).

I. Client Interview

Subjective History

- Pain occurs in medial ankle on weight bearing, or in the lateral subtalar joint.

- The client is >50 years old, obese, and has a history of diabetes, previous foot ankle surgery or trauma, local steroid injections, or inflammatory diseases (rheumatoid arthritis).

- The client plays basketball, tennis, soccer, or hockey.

- This injury is commonly related to running.[213]

- The client has difficulty walking, with diminished endurance for long periods of time, as well as difficulty with athletic activity. Over time, flattening of the arch and widening of the foot occur, which may affect footwear and gait.[212]

Outcome Measures

- Any appropriate outcome measure may be used.

Diagnostic Imaging

- Radiographs can assess the magnitude of the deformity as well as degenerative changes (anteroposterior and lateral weight-bearing views of the ankle and anteroposterior, lateral, and oblique weight-bearing views of the foot are required).[212]

- In cases where inhomogeneity or partial tears of the posterior tibial tendon

TABLE 26.6   Stages of Posterior Tibial Tendon Dysfunction

	Stage I[208]	Stage II[208]	Stage III[208]	Stage IV[209]
Subjective	Medial focal pain	Pain along course of tendon	Lateral pain (impingement of calcaneus and lateral malleolus)	
Observation	Deformity absent	Heel in valgus; forefoot abducts (too many toes sign)	Marked hindfoot valgus; severe arch collapse	Valgus deformity at the tibiotalar joint due to attenuation of deltoid ligament
Motion	Joints are mobile	Mobility of subtalar joint increases	Hindfoot fixed, loss of subtalar motion; fixed forefoot supination	
Muscle performance	Resisted inversion painful	Weak inversion	Significant weakness	
Physical measures	Can perform single-heel raise (may have discomfort)	Weak heel raise	Unable to perform single heel raise	
Treatment	Cast immobilization for 6 weeks and orthotics[210] Strengthen weak tendon when symptoms resolve[211]		Molded orthotics or solid or articulated ankle foot orthosis, depending on degeneration[212]	Solid foot ankle orthosis[210]

may not be evident clinically, MRI is very SN.[214]

II. Observation

- Flat foot deformity.[215]
- Loss of medial arch height.
- Edema of the medial ankle.
- Runners with stage I PTTD exhibited significant differences in rear foot pronation during walking gait, along with normal inversion ankle muscle strength and foot posture when compared to healthy clients.[216]
- Ipsilateral valgus deformity of the knee.[217]

III. Triage and Screening

- Foot and ankle fractures can be **ruled out** with the Ottawa Ankle Rules (pooled SN 96.4, −LR 0.08) in clients of all ages;[31] for children aged 5 years or older (pooled SN 98.5, −LR 0.11;[32] pooled SN 99, −LR 0.02[131]).

- Foot and ankle stress fractures: Tuning fork (SN 83, −LR 0.21)[54] and plantar percussion test (SN 62)[56] have less than good ability to rule out these fractures.
- The Ottawa Ankle Rules will dictate if radiographs are warranted.[132]
- The Bernese Ankle Rules have ideal ability to help **rule out** (SN 100, −LR 0) and **rule in** (SP 91, +LR 11.1) fractures. [34]

IV. Motion Tests

- See table 26.6 for different stages and effects on motion.
- Clients may have lack of talocrural mobility and decreased ankle dorsiflexion.[187]

V. Muscle Performance Testing

- The peroneus brevis, anterior tibial, and gastrocnemius muscles are weak due to synergistic contraction with the TPT and these muscles.[218]

- Clients have significant concentric and eccentric ankle invertor strength reductions for the involved ankle compared to the uninvolved one.[218]

VI. Special Tests

- Posterior tibial edema sign: A (+) test has good ability to rule in (SP 100, +LR Inf) post-tibial tendon dysfunction.

VII. Palpation

- The medial ankle TPT may be tender to palpation.

VIII. Physical Performance Measures

- Any appropriate physical performance measure may be used.

POTENTIAL TREATMENT-BASED CLASSIFICATIONS

- Pain control and activity modification: conservatively treated despite clinical stage.[210]

- Clinicians should prevent pain and inflammation, promote healing while off loading and rehabbing TPT itself, and prevent progression of foot deformity.[215]

- Clients may need surgery depending on scope of dysfunction and potential disability,[201] although double upright ankle foot orthosis may be an alternative to surgery.[219]

Lisfranc Injury (Midfoot)

ICD-9: 838.03 (closed dislocation of tarsometatarsal joint); 838.13 (open dislocation of tarsometatarsal joint)

ICD-10-CM: S93.326A (dislocation of tarsometatarsal joint of unspecified foot, initial encounter)

Injury to the Lisfranc joint is often missed due to the complexity of the anatomy in the foot and the rarity of the injury.[220] It was originally noticed in soldiers who got thrown off their horses with their feet still stuck in the stirrup. This external rotation with compression at the Lisfranc joint can lead to Lisfranc injury or dislocation. Currently this has been seen in automobile accidents and sports injuries, specifically among football players, gymnasts, and ballet dancers.[221]

I. Client Interview

Subjective History

- The MOI is external rotation force combined with compression due to direct (dropping something on midfoot) or indirect trauma (midfoot twisting after getting caught on something).[220]
- Client has difficulty bearing weight.[222]
- Running on the toes and the push-off phase of running are painful.[223]

Outcome Measures

- Any appropriate outcome measure may be used.

Diagnostic Imaging

- X-rays: lateral, anteroposterior, and 30° internal oblique projections in weight bearing should be taken.[224]
- CT is used for more complex injuries where there are multiple fractures or a dislocation, or when adequate foot position cannot be obtained.[225, 226]

II. Observation

- Minimal swelling over midfoot[222]
- Difficulty with weight bearing[222]
- Pain, edema, tenderness over the tarsometatarsal joint, and ecchymosis at the plantar/posterior aspect of the midfoot[227-230]
- Plantar ecchymosis (disruption to soft tissue)[231]

III. Triage and Screening

- Foot and ankle fractures can be **ruled out** with the Ottawa Ankle Rules (pooled SN 96.4, −LR 0.08) in clients of all ages;[31] for children aged 5 years or older (pooled SN 98.5, −LR 0.11;[32] pooled SN 99, −LR 0.02[131]).
- Foot and ankle stress fractures: Tuning fork (SN 83, −LR 0.21)[54] and plantar percussion test (SN 62)[56] have less than good ability to rule out these fractures.
- The Ottawa Ankle Rules will dictate if radiographs are warranted.[132]
- The Bernese Ankle Rules have ideal ability to help **rule out** (SN 100, −LR 0) and **rule in** (SP 91, +LR 11.1) fractures.[34]

- If the clinician suspects a fracture, they should perform immediate imaging because delayed diagnosis is associated with increased morbidity.[224, 231]

IV. Motion Tests

- Clients have increased pain with passive abduction and pronation of the forefoot.[232, 233]

V. Muscle Performance Testing

- No muscle performance testing is reported particular to this diagnosis.

VI. Special Tests

- No special tests are reported particular to this diagnosis.

VII. Palpation

- The clinician should palpate the first three metatarsal bases articulating with each of the cuneiforms and the lateral two metatarsals articulating with the cuboid.[224]

VIII. Physical Performance Measures

- Only lower-level testing is suggested if this type of testing is appropriate at all in the acute assessment of this pathology.

POTENTIAL TREATMENT-BASED CLASSIFICATIONS

- Immobilization or activity modification: After 6 to 8 weeks of immobilization, the clinician can progress to mobility and strength and conditioning.[222]

- If a fracture is present, the client may need surgery.[234]

Plantar Plate Abnormality

The plantar plate aides with stability and prevents hyperextension of the metatarsophalangeal joints in the forefoot.[235-237] The plantar is made up of fibrocollagen and Type 1 collagen, and it attaches to the base of the phalanx and the metatarsal. It is essential for securing the proximal phalanx of the lesser toes. Injury to the ligament can lead to metatarsalgia, plantar swelling, deformities such as hammer toe, and lesser toe subluxation.[238-240] Significant foot pain can result from degeneration or partial or full tears in the plantar plate, which can significantly affect gait and foot function.[235, 241, 242] These tears are often missed on initial examination. Ninety-five percent of clients with tears presented with onset of forefoot pain (SN 93), edema at the second metatarsal head (SN 95.8), and posterior drawer sign (SN 80.6, SP 99.8; 109 feet from clients who underwent plantar plate repair). Crossover toes (SP 88.9) is a physical sign for **ruling out** this diagnosis.[243] MRI is often used for diagnosis because it has good diagnostic value (SN 95, **SP 100, +LR 100**, −LR 67).[240] Depending on the severity of injury, clients may be able to rest, use ice and anti-inflammatory medications, use orthotics to change pressure distribution, or change their shoes. If conservative treatment fails, surgery is performed.[244]

Turf Toe

This condition is usually seen in American football players who play on turf or artificial surfaces.[245] Typically hyperextension of the MTP joint is due to an axial load when the foot is in fixed equinus position at the ankle and the big toe is in extension at the MTP joint.[246] This hyperextension leads to disruption or attenuation of the capsular ligamentous complex that is supporting the joint. Depending on the vector of force variations from the classic hyperextension, injury can occur such as a traumatic hallux valgus or damage to the medial and plantar medial structures.[247-249] The client will first report MTP joint pain (point tenderness) and swelling. Observation of swelling, ecchymosis, and any malalignment should be performed. Radiographs are usually taken and may include a forced dorsiflexion lateral view. Manual muscle testing (MMT) may reveal a weakness in active flexion, suggesting disruption of the plantar plate of the flexor hallucis brevis. Initial treatment will include immobility and pain and edema control. Limiting hallux motion as the client returns to sport with taping or an orthotic (stiff sole with a turf toe plate insert or custom with a Morton's extension), along with gentle ROM, is recommended.[246] Surgery may be performed in cases where there is a large capsular avulsion making the MTP unstable, as well as with diastasis of the bipartite sesamoid, diastasis of sesamoid fracture, retraction of the sesamoid, traumatic hallux deformity, vertical instability, loose body in MTP joint, chondral injury in MTP joint, or failed conservative treatment.[246, 250]

Hallux Valgus

Stephens[251] describes the development of hallux valgus and states that the weakening of tissues on the medial side of the MTP joint and erosion of the ridge on the metatarsal head between the sesamoids occur early. The proximal phalanx drifts into valgus and the MT head drifts into varus. A groove appears on the medial side of the articular cartilage of the MT head as it atrophies from the lack of normal pressures, which gives rise to the prominence of bony exostosis. A medial bursa can develop as a result of pressure from footwear over the prominence. The extensor hallucis longus and flexor hallucis brevis change direction with the phalanx, and start adducting and making the deformity worse.[252]

The client subjectively will complain of pain, aesthetic concerns, and inability to wear certain shoes. Extrinsic factors include low BMI with high heel use among women aged 20 to 64 years, high BMI, and pes planus.[253] This condition is more prevalent in women and the elderly.[254] Physical examination would include looking at the forefoot and hindfoot because tightness in the gastroc-soleus complex can make the pain under the forefoot worse. The clinician should note range of motion of the MTP joint, and whether there is pronation. They should examine other toes and the metatarsal heads for calluses and deformities. Movement of the MT greater than 9 mm in a plantar lateral to dorsomedial direction indicates hypermobility.[255] Weight-bearing radiographs are used to assess the deformity. Orthoses and accommodative footwear have been seen to help symptoms; however, there is no evidence to show prevention of progression.[256] Hallux valgus has been seen to significantly affect gait, and it can lead to instability and falls in older people when walking on uneven terrain.[7]

Tarsal Tunnel Syndrome

This syndrome involves entrapment of the tibial nerve as it passes through the tunnel between the flexor retinaculum and medial malleolus. Depending on the severity of the entrapment, the terminal branches (medial and lateral plantar nerve) may also be involved.[6] Causes of the entrapment can range from participation in repetitive or strenuous activities, such as jogging or running, or trauma, such as sprains, strains, or fractures.[257, 258] Subjectively the client may report increased symptoms at night or with prolonged activity like standing or walking. On observation, this client may have pes planus. On MMT, there may be some weakness in the abductors and flexors, typically starting with the first metatarsal. The special tests to diagnose this condition include Tinel's sign (SN 58), triple compression test (SP 100, +LR Inf),[113] and the dorsiflexion eversion test (SP 99, +LR 82.7).[114, 257] This condition is very often misdiagnosed as plantar fasciitis due to its presentation; polyneuropathy, radiculopathy, deep flexor compartment syndrome, and Morton's metatarsalgia are often differential diagnoses.[259, 260] This client will benefit from early intervention to decrease pain and inflammation, followed by strengthening and exercise and conditioning.

Fibular or Peroneal Nerve

- **Superficial:** Injury to this nerve is relatively rare. It can be stretched with inversion sprains (lateral) or can become entrapped as it pierces the deep fascia where it becomes subcutaneous above the lateral malleolus. With increased activity, clients will complain of diminished sensation on the posterior aspect of the foot.[6]

- **Deep fibular nerve:** Injury involves compression to the deep fibular nerve as it travels beneath the posterior tibialis and the extensor hallucis brevis tendons and above the first and second cuneiforms, where is it not protected as well as in other places.[261] Weakness (extensor digitorum brevis), pain (deep aching in the medial and posterior aspect of the foot, burning around the nail of the big toe, and pins and needles around the borders of the 1st and 2nd toes that increases with plantarflexion), and sensory changes to the foot and ankle are some symptoms present with this entrapment.[261] Conservative management focuses on removing or reducing the external compression on the nerve,[262] whether through a change in footwear or orthotics, as well as with NSAIDs.[261]

Sural Nerve

The sural nerve runs between the heads of the gastrocnemius muscle and runs deep and distally to the lateral side of the leg, from the peroneal tendon sheath to the lateral tuberosity of the 5th toe. This pathway includes an anatomic fibrous arcade (superficial sural aponeurosis). The nerve runs superficially in the distal third of the leg. With entrapment, the client has acute localized tenderness over the nerve itself. Reproduction of the client's symptoms occurs with gentle pressure on the nerve, and complaints of chronic pain in the posterior aspect of the leg get worse with exertion.[263] Diminished sensation with or without paresthesia in the distribution of the nerve as well as the presence of a tender ganglion usually help to diagnose this condition.[264]

CONCLUSION

The clinician's goals are to address the impairments and to aim to restore a client's function. This chapter provides integration of the best evidence and a systematic examination approach that will help the clinician accomplish these goals. This systematic, evidence-based funnel approach stresses the importance of each part of the examination process. With the lower leg, ankle, and foot, it is important to rule out or screen for competing pathologies early in the examination process and to rule in or diagnose certain pathologies later in the process. Because this area is the distal-most joint, pathology may be the result of compensation.

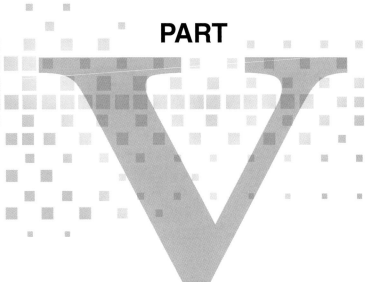

PART

V

Examination of Special Populations

Part V covers special populations as related to the orthopedic client. While clinicians who work with athletic, geriatric, and pediatric clients are all likely to benefit from the detailed, evidence-based examination procedures and sequences provided in the chapters in parts III and IV, these clients are often unique, and their examinations require special focus. Each of these three chapters provides the clinician with the best evidence examinations unique to the clients covered in part V. Special considerations, unique situations, respective pathologies, and the approaches necessary for examining these special populations are described in detail for the athletic client requiring an emergency sport examination (chapter 27), the geriatric client (chapter 28), and the pediatric client (chapter 29).

EMERGENCY SPORT EXAMINATION

John DeWitt, PT, DPT, SCS, ATC
Mitch Salsbery, PT, DPT, SCS, CSCS

The majority of sports-related dysfunction encountered in the sports training room and clinic is of traditional musculoskeletal dysfunction, not of the emergent type. The treating clinician should also be cognizant of the fact that musculoskeletal dysfunction is likely to be fairly prevalent and will be more common in athletes than in nonathletes. In fact, in a prevalence study, athletes reported having the highest pain frequency in the lumbar spine (68%), cervical spine (55%), knee (44%), thoracic spine (33%), ankle (25%), hip (23%), shoulder (21%), wrist (8%), and elbow (7%).[1] Athletes reported a higher percentage of pain in almost all body regions when compared to age-matched nonathletes.[1] Therefore, the majority of the sports-trained clinician's practice will be dealing with traditional musculoskeletal dysfunction. The sports-trained clinician, though, will have training in and experience with emergency sport examination and treatment. This chapter details the specifics of such an examination.

SPORTS-RELATED CONCUSSION

Sports-related mild traumatic brain injury (mTBI) or concussion is a common and challenging injury to diagnose, with a constellation of signs and symptoms that can evolve over hours or days after a concussive episode.[2] Note that players who sustain severe head trauma causing a loss of consciousness (LOC) require prompt, on-the-field assessment of airway, breathing, and circulation, as well as immediate stabilization of the neck with any equipment near the head (e.g., helmet and shoulder pads) left in place. A comprehensive examination of suspected cervical spine injury is beyond the scope of this section. Cervical spine examination is discussed further in this chapter as well as in chapter 17 (Cervical Spine).

Awareness of mTBI in athletic competition has increased drastically over the past two decades due to advances in research, clinical practice guideline development, and legislative changes.[3] Despite increased awareness and improvements in assessment and management of concussion, best practice guidelines still need to be validated as noted in the 4th Consensus Statement on Concussion in Sport, "While agreement exists pertaining to principal messages conveyed within this document, the authors acknowledge that the science of concussion is evolving, and therefore management and return to play decisions remain in the realm of clinical judgment on an individualized basis."[3]

The Centers for Disease Control estimates that more than 170,000 sport- or activity-related concussions occur every year.[4] However, this number only represents people who were admitted to an emergency department and is mostly likely an underrepresentation of true incidence. Of this number, American football contributes the highest rates (55,007; 0.47 per 1,000 athlete exposures) followed by girls' soccer (29,167; 0.36 per 1,000 athlete exposures).[5] Despite an increased awareness in recognition and management, rates of concussion in sport continue to rise.[5] This may be attributed to greater awareness as well as an increase in sport involvement; nonetheless, it is paramount that sideline health care providers utilize high-quality examination techniques to enhance efficacious management of this potentially life-threatening injury.

Health care professionals should be knowledgeable about risk factors for sports-related concussion. Several studies have identified gender, age, fatigue, concussion history, sport, history of migraines, and learning disabilities as potential factors.[4, 5] Genetic factors, including carriers of the apolipoprotein E epsilon 4 allele (APoE-4), may also contribute to greater susceptibility; however, this correlation has yet to be determined in sports-related concussion.[6]

When a TBI is suspected during play, it is paramount to first assess vitals and rule out a cervical spine injury (chapters 6 and 17 detail red flags and screening of the cervical spine). Each year in American football, an estimated 11,000 neck injuries occur that require transport to the emergency room.[7] Proper recognition and early management is critical for preventing catastrophic events. Initiation of the emergency response is required for safely transporting the athletes to the proper medical facility. Those athletes who have persistent LOC or alteration of consciousness should be kept in a stable position and rapidly transported on a back-

board by ambulance to an emergency room. It is important to remember, however, that most athletes will not suffer LOC following a concussion; in this case, they may be evaluated on the sidelines.[2]

Sideline evaluation of a suspected concussion should incorporate a battery of tests to assess cognitive, neuropsychological, and balance abilities. The Sport Concussion Assessment Tool, 3rd edition (SCAT3) is a multimodal tool recommended by the 4th International Conference on Concussion to evaluate these parameters (figure 27.1).[3] The SCAT3 includes the Glasgow Coma Scale, Graded Symptom Checklist, Maddocks' questions, Standardized Assessment of Concussion (SAC), and the Balance Error Scoring System. While the SCAT3 has not been validated, components of the tool have been studied individually. The SCAT3 can be used on athletes 13 years and older, while younger athletes should be tested using the Child SCAT3.

- **Glasgow Coma Scale:** neurologic injury rating scale based on client responses. A score of $\geq 13/15$ indicates a mild traumatic injury consistent with concussion.

- **Graded Symptoms Checklist:** The postconcussive checklist has been validated for both ongoing cerebral hemodynamic abnormality as well as mild cognitive impairment.[8] Due to the multifactorial nature of concussion, however, it is not sufficient to provide return-to-play criteria as a stand-alone test.

- **Maddocks' questions:** Maddocks' questions were first proposed by David Maddocks in 1989.[9] A follow-up study in 1995 demonstrated acceptable sensitivity (SN) compared to age-matched controls.[10, 11]

- **Standardized Assessment of Concussion (SAC):** First described by McCrea in 1998, the SAC has been validated in the sideline diagnosis of concussion.[12] The SAC has demonstrated 94% sensitivity (SN) and 76% specificity (SP) in diagnosing concussion when posttesting is 1 point lower than baseline levels.[13]

- **Balance Error Scoring System (BESS):** The BESS consists of six 20-second balance tests in various positions and surfaces, and has been validated with other measures of stability (figure 27.2).[14, 15] Stances are performed with the eyes closed, and errors are defined as opening eyes, lifting hands off hips, lifting forefoot or heel, abducting hip by more than 30°, failing to return to the test position within 5 seconds, or stepping, stumbling, or falling out of

SCAT3™

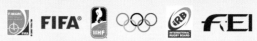

Sport Concussion Assessment Tool – 3rd Edition

For use by medical professionals only

Name

Date/Time of Injury:
Date of Assessment:

Examiner:

What is the SCAT3?[1]

The SCAT3 is a standardized tool for evaluating injured athletes for concussion and can be used in athletes aged from 13 years and older. It supersedes the original SCAT and the SCAT2 published in 2005 and 2009, respectively[2]. For younger persons, ages 12 and under, please use the Child SCAT3. The SCAT3 is designed for use by medical professionals. If you are not qualified, please use the Sport Concussion Recognition Tool[1]. Preseason baseline testing with the SCAT3 can be helpful for interpreting post-injury test scores.

Specific instructions for use of the SCAT3 are provided on page 3. If you are not familiar with the SCAT3, please read through these instructions carefully. This tool may be freely copied in its current form for distribution to individuals, teams, groups and organizations. Any revision or any reproduction in a digital form requires approval by the Concussion in Sport Group.

NOTE: The diagnosis of a concussion is a clinical judgment, ideally made by a medical professional. The SCAT3 should not be used solely to make, or exclude, the diagnosis of concussion in the absence of clinical judgement. An athlete may have a concussion even if their SCAT3 is "normal".

What is a concussion?

A concussion is a disturbance in brain function caused by a direct or indirect force to the head. It results in a variety of non-specific signs and/or symptoms (some examples listed below) and most often does not involve loss of consciousness. Concussion should be suspected in the presence of **any one or more** of the following:

- Symptoms (e.g., headache), or
- Physical signs (e.g., unsteadiness), or
- Impaired brain function (e.g. confusion) or
- Abnormal behaviour (e.g., change in personality).

SIDELINE ASSESSMENT

Indications for Emergency Management

NOTE: A hit to the head can sometimes be associated with a more serious brain injury. Any of the following warrants consideration of activating emergency procedures and urgent transportation to the nearest hospital:

- Glasgow Coma score less than 15
- Deteriorating mental status
- Potential spinal injury
- Progressive, worsening symptoms or new neurologic signs

Potential signs of concussion?

If any of the following signs are observed after a direct or indirect blow to the head, the athlete should stop participation, be evaluated by a medical professional and **should not be permitted to return to sport the same day** if a concussion is suspected.

Any loss of consciousness?	Y	N
"If so, how long?"		
Balance or motor incoordination (stumbles, slow/laboured movements, etc.)?	Y	N
Disorientation or confusion (inability to respond appropriately to questions)?	Y	N
Loss of memory:	Y	N
"If so, how long?"		
"Before or after the injury?"		
Blank or vacant look:	Y	N
Visible facial injury in combination with any of the above:	Y	N

---

1 Glasgow coma scale (GCS)

Best eye response (E)

No eye opening	1
Eye opening in response to pain	2
Eye opening to speech	3
Eyes opening spontaneously	4

Best verbal response (V)

No verbal response	1
Incomprehensible sounds	2
Inappropriate words	3
Confused	4
Oriented	5

Best motor response (M)

No motor response	1
Extension to pain	2
Abnormal flexion to pain	3
Flexion/Withdrawal to pain	4
Localizes to pain	5
Obeys commands	6

Glasgow Coma score (E + V + M)	of 15

GCS should be recorded for all athletes in case of subsequent deterioration.

2 Maddocks Score[3]

"I am going to ask you a few questions, please listen carefully and give your best effort."

Modified Maddocks questions (1 point for each correct answer)

What venue are we at today?	0	1
Which half is it now?	0	1
Who scored last in this match?	0	1
What team did you play last week/game?	0	1
Did your team win the last game?	0	1
Maddocks score		of 5

Maddocks score is validated for sideline diagnosis of concussion only and is not used for serial testing.

Notes: Mechanism of Injury ("tell me what happened"?):

Any athlete with a suspected concussion should be **REMOVED FROM PLAY**, medically assessed, monitored for deterioration (i.e., should not be left alone) and should not drive a motor vehicle until cleared to do so by a medical professional. No athlete diagnosed with concussion should be returned to sports participation on the day of Injury.

Figure 27.1 SCAT3 assessment form.   *(continued)*

McCrory P, Meeuwisse W, Aubry M, Cantu RC, Dvorak J, Echemendia R, Engebretsen L, Johnston K, Kutcher J, Raftery M, Sills A, Benson B, Davis G, Ellenbogen R, Guskeiwicz K, Herring SA, Iverson G, Jordan B, Kissick J, McCrea M, McIntosh A, Maddocks D, Makdissi M, Purcell L, Putukian M, Schneider K, Tator C, Turner M. SCAT3. *Br J Sports Med* 2013; 47(5): 259.

BACKGROUND

Name: _____ Date: _____
Examiner: _____
Sport/team/school: _____ Date/time of injury: _____
Age: _____ Gender: _____ M F
Years of education completed: _____
Dominant hand: _____ right left neither
How many concussions do you think you have had in the past? _____
When was the most recent concussion? _____
How long was your recovery from the most recent concussion? _____

Have you ever been hospitalized or had medical imaging done for a head injury?	Y N
Have you ever been diagnosed with headaches or migraines?	Y N
Do you have a learning disability, dyslexia, ADD/ADHD?	Y N
Have you ever been diagnosed with depression, anxiety or other psychiatric disorder?	Y N
Has anyone in your family ever been diagnosed with any of these problems?	Y N
Are you on any medications? If yes, please list:	Y N

SCAT3 to be done in resting state. Best done 10 or more minutes post excercise.

SYMPTOM EVALUATION

3

How do you feel?

"You should score yourself on the following symptoms, based on how you feel now".

	none	mild		moderate		severe	
Headache	0	1	2	3	4	5	6
"Pressure in head"	0	1	2	3	4	5	6
Neck Pain	0	1	2	3	4	5	6
Nausea or vomiting	0	1	2	3	4	5	6
Dizziness	0	1	2	3	4	5	6
Blurred vision	0	1	2	3	4	5	6
Balance problems	0	1	2	3	4	5	6
Sensitivity to light	0	1	2	3	4	5	6
Sensitivity to noise	0	1	2	3	4	5	6
Feeling slowed down	0	1	2	3	4	5	6
Feeling like "in a fog"	0	1	2	3	4	5	6
"Don't feel right"	0	1	2	3	4	5	6
Difficulty concentrating	0	1	2	3	4	5	6
Difficulty remembering	0	1	2	3	4	5	6
Fatigue or low energy	0	1	2	3	4	5	6
Confusion	0	1	2	3	4	5	6
Drowsiness	0	1	2	3	4	5	6
Trouble falling asleep	0	1	2	3	4	5	6
More emotional	0	1	2	3	4	5	6
Irritability	0	1	2	3	4	5	6
Sadness	0	1	2	3	4	5	6
Nervous or Anxious	0	1	2	3	4	5	6

Total number of symptoms (Maximum possible 22) _____
Symptom severity score (Maximum possible 132) _____

Do the symptoms get worse with physical activity? Y N
Do the symptoms get worse with mental activity? Y N

- self rated   self rated and clinician monitored
- clinician interview   self rated with parent input

Overall rating: If you know the athlete well prior to the injury, how different is the athlete acting compared to his/her usual self?
Please circle one response:

no different   very different   unsure   N/A

Scoring on the SCAT3 should not be used as a stand-alone method to diagnose concussion, measure recovery or make decisions about an athlete's readiness to return to competition after concussion. Since signs and symptoms may evolve over time, it is important to consider repeat evaluation in the acute assessment of concussion.

COGNITIVE & PHYSICAL EVALUATION

4

Cognitive assessment
Standardized Assessment of Concussion (SAC)[4]

Orientation (1 point for each correct answer)

What month is it?	0	1
What is the date today?	0	1
What is the day of the week?	0	1
What year is it?	0	1
What time is it right now? (within 1 hour)	0	1

Orientation score   of 5

Immediate memory

List	Trial 1	Trial 2	Trial 3	Alternative word list		
elbow	0 1	0 1	0 1	candle	baby	finger
apple	0 1	0 1	0 1	paper	monkey	penny
carpet	0 1	0 1	0 1	sugar	perfume	blanket
saddle	0 1	0 1	0 1	sandwich	sunset	lemon
bubble	0 1	0 1	0 1	wagon	iron	insect
Total						

Immediate memory score total   of 15

Concentration: Digits Backward

List	Trial 1	Alternative digit list		
4-9-3	0 1	6-2-9	5-2-6	4-1-5
3-8-1-4	0 1	3-2-7-9	1-7-9-5	4-9-6-8
6-2-9-7-1	0 1	1-5-2-8-6	3-8-5-2-7	6-1-8-4-3
7-1-8-4-6-2	0 1	5-3-9-1-4-8	8-3-1-9-6-4	7-2-4-8-5-6
Total of 4				

Concentration: Month in Reverse Order (1 pt. for entire sequence correct)
Dec-Nov-Oct-Sept-Aug-Jul-Jun-May-Apr-Mar-Feb-Jan   0   1

Concentration score   of 5

5

Neck Examination:

Range of motion   Tenderness   Upper and lower limb sensation & strength
Findings: _____

6

Balance examination

Do one or both of the following tests.
Footwear (shoes, barefoot, braces, tape, etc.)

Modified Balance Error Scoring System (BESS) testing[5]
Which foot was tested (i.e. which is the **non-dominant** foot)   Left   Right
Testing surface (hard floor, field, etc.)
Condition
Double leg stance: Errors
Single leg stance (non-dominant foot):   Errors
Tandem stance (non-dominant foot at back):   Errors
And/Or
Tandem gait[6,7]
Time (best of 4 trials): _____   seconds

7

Coordination examination
Upper limb coordination
Which arm was tested: Left   Right
Coordination score   of 1

8

SAC Delayed Recall[4]
Delayed recall score   of 5

SCAT3 SPORT CONCUSSION ASSESMENT TOOL 3 | PAGE 2   © 2013 Concussion in Sport Group

---

Figure 27.1   *(continued)*

948

INSTRUCTIONS

Words in *Italics* throughout the SCAT3 are the instructions given to the athlete by the tester.

Symptom Scale

"You should score yourself on the following symptoms, based on how you feel now".

To be completed by the athlete. In situations where the symptom scale is being completed after exercise, it should still be done in a resting state, at least 10 minutes post exercise.
For total number of symptoms, maximum possible is 22.
For Symptom severity score, add all scores in table, maximum possible is 22 x 6 = 132.

SAC[4]

Immediate Memory

"I am going to test your memory. I will read you a list of words and when I am done, repeat back as many words as you can remember, in any order."

Trials 2 & 3:

"I am going to repeat the same list again. Repeat back as many words as you can remember in any order, even if you said the word before."

Complete all 3 trials regardless of score on trial 1 & 2. Read the words at a rate of one per second. **Score 1 pt. for each correct response.** Total score equals sum across all 3 trials. Do not inform the athlete that delayed recall will be tested.

Concentration
Digits backward

"I am going to read you a string of numbers and when I am done, you repeat them back to me backwards, in reverse order of how I read them to you. For example, if I say 7-1-9, you would say 9-1-7."

If correct, go to next string length. If incorrect, read trial 2. **One point possible for each string length.** Stop after incorrect on both trials. The digits should be read at the rate of one per second.

Months in reverse order

"Now tell me the months of the year in reverse order. Start with the last month and go backward. So you'll say December, November ... Go ahead"

1 pt. for entire sequence correct

Delayed Recall

The delayed recall should be performed after completion of the Balance and Coordination Examination.

"Do you remember that list of words I read a few times earlier? Tell me as many words from the list as you can remember in any order."

Score 1 pt. for each correct response

Balance Examination

Modified Balance Error Scoring System (BESS) testing[5]

This balance testing is based on a modified version of the Balance Error Scoring System (BESS)[5]. A stopwatch or watch with a second hand is required for this testing.

"I am now going to test your balance. Please take your shoes off, roll up your pant legs above ankle (if applicable), and remove any ankle taping (if applicable). This test will consist of three twenty second tests with different stances."

(a) Double leg stance:

"The first stance is standing with your feet together with your hands on your hips and with your eyes closed. You should try to maintain stability in that position for 20 seconds. I will be counting the number of times you move out of this position. I will start timing when you are set and have closed your eyes."

(b) Single leg stance:

"If you were to kick a ball, which foot would you use? [This will be the dominant foot] Now stand on your non-dominant foot. The dominant leg should be held in approximately 30 degrees of hip flexion and 45 degrees of knee flexion. Again, you should try to maintain stability for 20 seconds with your hands on your hips and your eyes closed. I will be counting the number of times you move out of this position. If you stumble out of this position, open your eyes and return to the start position and continue balancing. I will start timing when you are set and have closed your eyes."

(c) Tandem stance:

"Now stand heel-to-toe with your non-dominant foot in back. Your weight should be evenly distributed across both feet. Again, you should try to maintain stability for 20 seconds with your hands on your hips and your eyes closed. I will be counting the number of times you move out of this position. If you stumble out of this position, open your eyes and return to the start position and continue balancing. I will start timing when you are set and have closed your eyes."

Balance testing – types of errors

1. Hands lifted off iliac crest
2. Opening eyes
3. Step, stumble, or fall
4. Moving hip into > 30 degrees abduction
5. Lifting forefoot or heel
6. Remaining out of test position > 5 sec

Each of the 20-second trials is scored by counting the errors, or deviations from the proper stance, accumulated by the athlete. The examiner will begin counting errors only after the individual has assumed the proper start position. **The modified BESS is calculated by adding one error point for each error during the three 20-second tests. The maximum total number of errors for any single condition is 10.** If an athlete commits multiple errors simultaneously, only one error is recorded but the athlete should quickly return to the testing position, and counting should resume once subject is set. Subjects that are unable to maintain the testing procedure for a minimum of **five seconds** at the start are assigned the highest possible score, ten, for that testing condition.

OPTION: For further assessment, the same 3 stances can be performed on a surface of medium density foam (e.g., approximately 50 cm x 40 cm x 6 cm).

Tandem Gait[6,7]

Participants are instructed to stand with their feet together behind a starting line (the test is best done with footwear removed). Then, they walk in a forward direction as quickly and as accurately as possible along a 38mm wide (sports tape), 3 meter line with an alternate foot heel-to-toe gait ensuring that they approximate their heel and toe on each step. Once they cross the end of the 3m line, they turn 180 degrees and return to the starting point using the same gait. A total of 4 trials are done and the best time is retained. Athletes should complete the test in 14 seconds. Athletes fail the test if they step off the line, have a separation between their heel and toe, or if they touch or grab the examiner or an object. In this case, the time is not recorded and the trial repeated, if appropriate.

Coordination Examination

Upper limb coordination
Finger-to-nose (FTN) task:

"I am going to test your coordination now. Please sit comfortably on the chair with your eyes open and your arm (either right or left) outstretched (shoulder flexed to 90 degrees and elbow and fingers extended), pointing in front of you. When I give a start signal, I would like you to perform five successive finger to nose repetitions using your index finger to touch the tip of the nose, and then return to the starting position, as quickly and as accurately as possible."

Scoring: 5 correct repetitions in < 4 seconds = 1
Note for testers: Athletes fail the test if they do not touch their nose, do not fully extend their elbow or do not perform five repetitions. **Failure should be scored as 0.**

References & Footnotes

1. This tool has been developed by a group of international experts at the 4th International Consensus meeting on Concussion in Sport held in Zurich, Switzerland in November 2012. The full details of the conference outcomes and the authors of the tool are published in The BJSM Injury Prevention and Health Protection, 2013, Volume 47, Issue 5. The outcome paper will also be co-published in other leading biomedical journals with the copyright held by the Concussion in Sport Group, to allow unrestricted distribution, providing no alterations are made.

2. McCrory P et al., Consensus Statement on Concussion in Sport – the 3rd International Conference on Concussion in Sport held in Zurich, November 2008. British Journal of Sports Medicine 2009; 43: i76-89.

3. Maddocks, DL; Dicker, GD; Saling, MM. The assessment of orientation following concussion in athletes. Clinical Journal of Sport Medicine. 1995; 5(1): 32–3.

4. McCrea M. Standardized mental status testing of acute concussion. Clinical Journal of Sport Medicine. 2001; 11: 176–181.

5. Guskiewicz KM. Assessment of postural stability following sport-related concussion. Current Sports Medicine Reports. 2003; 2: 24–30.

6. Schneiders, A.G., Sullivan, S.J., Gray, A., Hammond-Tooke, G. & McCrory, P. Normative values for 16-37 year old subjects for three clinical measures of motor performance used in the assessment of sports concussions. Journal of Science and Medicine in Sport. 2010; 13(2): 196–201.

7. Schneiders, A.G., Sullivan, S.J., Kvarnstrom, J.K., Olsson, M., Yden. T. & Marshall, S.W. The effect of footwear and sports-surface on dynamic neurological screening in sport-related concussion. Journal of Science and Medicine in Sport. 2010; 13(4): 382–386

Figure 27.1 *(continued)*

ATHLETE INFORMATION

Any athlete suspected of having a concussion should be removed from play, and then seek medical evaluation.

Signs to watch for

Problems could arise over the first 24–48 hours. The athlete should not be left alone and must go to a hospital at once if they:

- Have a headache that gets worse
- Are very drowsy or can't be awakened
- Can't recognize people or places
- Have repeated vomiting
- Behave unusually or seem confused; are very irritable
- Have seizures (arms and legs jerk uncontrollably)
- Have weak or numb arms or legs
- Are unsteady on their feet; have slurred speech

Remember, it is better to be safe.
Consult your doctor after a suspected concussion.

Return to play

Athletes should not be returned to play the same day of injury.
When returning athletes to play, they should be **medically cleared and then follow a stepwise supervised program,** with stages of progression.

For example:

Rehabilitation stage	Functional exercise at each stage of rehabilitation	Objective of each stage
No activity	Physical and cognitive rest	Recovery
Light aerobic exercise	Walking, swimming or stationary cycling keeping intensity, 70% maximum predicted heart rate. No resistance training	Increase heart rate
Sport-specific exercise	Skating drills in ice hockey, running drills in soccer. No head impact activities	Add movement
Non-contact training drills	Progression to more complex training drills, eg passing drills in football and ice hockey. May start progressive resistance training	Exercise, coordination, and cognitive load
Full contact practice	Following medical clearance participate in normal training activities	Restore confidence and assess functional skills by coaching staff
Return to play	Normal game play	

There should be at least 24 hours (or longer) for each stage and if symptoms recur the athlete should rest until they resolve once again and then resume the program at the previous asymptomatic stage. Resistance training should only be added in the later stages.

If the athlete is symptomatic for more than 10 days, then consultation by a medical practitioner who is expert in the management of concussion, is recommended.

Medical clearance should be given before return to play.

Scoring Summary:

Test Domain	Score		
	Date:	Date:	Date:
Number of Symptoms of 22			
Symptom Severity Score of 132			
Orientation of 5			
Immediate Memory of 15			
Concentration of 5			
Delayed Recall of 5			
SAC Total			
BESS (total errors)			
Tandem Gait (seconds)			
Coordination of 1			

Notes:

CONCUSSION INJURY ADVICE

(To be given to the **person monitoring** the concussed athlete)

This patient has received an injury to the head. A careful medical examination has been carried out and no sign of any serious complications has been found. Recovery time is variable across individuals and the patient will need monitoring for a further period by a responsible adult. Your treating physician will provide guidance as to this timeframe.

If you notice any change in behaviour, vomiting, dizziness, worsening head-ache, double vision or excessive drowsiness, please contact your doctor or the nearest hospital emergency department immediately.

Other important points:

- Rest (physically and mentally), including training or playing sports until symptoms resolve and you are medically cleared
- No alcohol
- No prescription or non-prescription drugs without medical supervision. Specifically:
  - No sleeping tablets
  - Do not use aspirin, anti-inflammatory medication or sedating pain killers
- Do not drive until medically cleared
- Do not train or play sport until medically cleared

Clinic phone number

Patient's name

Date/time of injury

Date/time of medical review

Treating physician

Contact details or stamp

Figure 27.1 *(continued)*

position. Moderate (0.70) test–retest reliability has been established as well as sufficient interrater (0.57) and intrarater reliability (0.74).[14, 15] The modified BESS is similar to the original test, excluding the foam surface. It is currently used in the SCAT3 and

demonstrates acceptable reliability compared to the original.[16] Enhanced efficiency of the test may be more appropriate for the sideline evaluation; however, delayed postural testing is warranted to limit effects of fatigue with outcomes.

 Video 27.2 **in the web resource shows a demonstration of the BESS balance tests.**

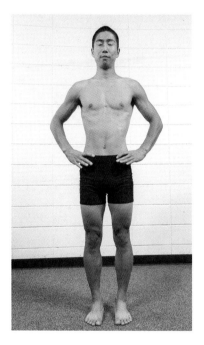
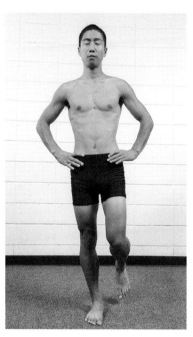
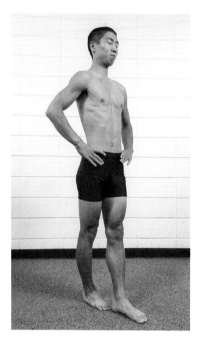

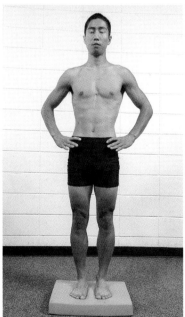
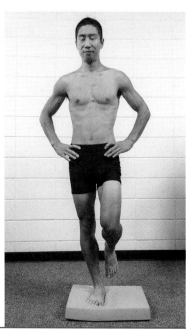
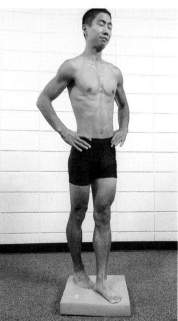

Figure 27.2   BESS balance tests.

Cognitive testing is an important aspect of both baseline and postinjury assessment to diagnose injury. Several testing paradigms exist including ImPACT, which has been shown to be effective in assessing concussion with an SN of 82% and SP of 89.4% in concussed high school athletes.[17] Giza and colleagues also reported high SN regardless of pencil and paper or computerized administration (SN 71–88%).[14] Addition of computerized neurocognitive testing increases the SN of diagnosing concussion from 64% to 83%, and this type of testing is better able to measure neurocognitive deficits in athletes who are asymptomatic or who denied symptoms following injury.[18, 19] ImPACT scores in correlation with symptom clusters have also been shown to predict protracted recovery in postconcussive clients.[20]

CERVICAL SPINE INJURIES

Spinal cord injuries occur approximately 12,000 times per year, 8.2% of which are due to collision sports.[22] High-impact sports, such as American football, rugby, snowboarding, and ice hockey have been identified as high-risk sports for cervical injuries.[23, 24] While rare, disabling and catastrophic events do result from cervical neck injuries. Approximately 1.10 injuries per 100,000 high school athletes and 4.72 injuries per 100,000 college football athletes lead to a catastrophic event, including quadriplegia, central cord syndrome, Brown-Séquard syndrome, and other permanent neurologic conditions.[25] Poor tackling technique and the presence of cervical spinal stenosis may predispose an athlete to spinal cord injury; these should be addressed prior to participation in sport.[23]

Airway, breathing, and circulation (ABCs) should be immediately assessed for any athlete suspected of having a significant cervical spine injury or found unconscious.[24] Immediate immobilization should be utilized for an athlete experiencing bilateral neurologic symptoms or signs of spinal or vascular instability followed by activation of the emergency response system.[23] A secondary neurological examination and fracture assessment may be performed if no life-threatening conditions are present. Diagnostic imaging is the gold standard for cervical spine injuries. To date, no validated sideline assessment exists. Cervical fracture screening is described later in the chapter.

Cervical Cord Neurapraxia

Cervical cord neurapraxia is a less sinister injury, defined as a transient neurological deficit following cervical spinal cord trauma.[27] By definition, clients or athletes with neurapraxia should return to baseline neurologic levels with no residual symptoms. Typical symptoms include acute bilateral burning pain, tingling, loss of sensation, and weakness to complete paralysis. While symptoms vary, resolution typically occurs from several minutes up to 48 hours.[27] A grading system developed by Torg and colleagues[27] is based on the duration of symptoms: grade I (<15 min), grade II (15 min to 24 hrs), and grade III (>24 hrs). The grading system may be helpful for classifying the severity of the injury; however, its application in on-the-field or sideline evaluation is limited.

Critical Clinical Pearls

Consider the following risk factors of concussion:

Predisposed to concussion
- Female gender
- History of concussion

Delayed recovery
- Age (<18 years old)
- Female gender
- History of concussion
- Learning disability
- History of migraines or depression
- Prolonged loss of consciousness (>1 min)
- Amnesia

Brachial Plexus Injury Stingers

Stingers, also known as *burners,* are the most frequent cervical spine injury in athletics, particularly in American football at a rate of 7.7% per year, and have been reported as high as 65% over the course of one's career.[28, 29] Mechanism of injury typically falls into two categories: tensile or compressive. Tensile injuries occur when the neck is rapidly flexed to the contralateral side, which may or may not be accompanied by shoulder depression. Compressive injuries typically occur from rapid extension and lateral flexion on the ipsilateral side, which may involve the nerve root along with the brachial plexus. Poorer outcomes are associated with extension and compression stingers, which involve increased rates of prolonged symptoms and a delayed return to activity.[30]

As with cervical cord neurapraxia, ruling out a spinal cord injury is the first step in an acute evaluation of the brachial plexus. Presence of significant arm pain, altered mental status, bilateral symptoms, or cervical neck pain should be ruled out.[31] Currently no validated on-the-field or sideline assessments exist for a brachial plexus injuries, and current diagnosis is based on mechanism of injury and symptoms presentation.

CARDIAC DISORDERS

By far the most common cause of sudden death in sport is cardiovascular (CV) injury. A study evaluating 1,866 sudden deaths in athletes from 1986 to 2006 reported that over half (56%) were due to CV causes.[32] Due to the high incidence of CV in sudden death, it is essential to recognize signs and symptoms of CV anomalies as well as use appropriate assessment and management strategies.

Hypertrophic cardiomyopathy (HCM) is the number one cause of cardiovascular death in athletes.[33] This condition is caused by asymmetrical ventricular thickening affecting one side of the heart and is typically genetic in nature. Athletes suffering from HCM may report symptoms including dizziness, chest pain, fainting, shortness of breath, and fatigue.[34] Unfortunately, 55% to 80% of athletes are often asymptomatic, contributing to the difficulty of detection until a catastrophic event occurs. Thus, this condition can be challenging to detect in a preparticipation evaluation, and it is usually only when reporting symptoms that athletes are referred

to the appropriate medical professional for further diagnostic testing, such as an echocardiogram.[35]

The second leading cause of sudden cardiovascular death in athletes is attributed to coronary artery abnormalities.[33] Anomalous origin of the left main coronary artery and the right coronary artery are the most common manifestations detected.[36] While coronary circulation differs among people, variability greater than 1% of the normal population is considered abnormal.[36] Coronary artery abnormality is exceedingly rare with an incidence of only 1.2% in the general population, and it is diagnosed more often in children than in adults (4–15% and 1%, respectively).[36] Similar to HCM, many athletes present asymptomatically; however, syncope, angina, and cardiac arrhythmia may be reported, warranting a thorough history during preparticipation examinations (PPE). Unlike HCM, there is no clear genetic or family history link for anomalous coronary arteries.

The importance of screening athletes to mitigate risk of sudden cardiac death is a widely accepted standard of practice; however, controversy exists regarding standardization.[35, 36] The current debate focuses on whether or not to include mandatory 12-lead electrocardiogram (ECG) into the PPE. The International Olympic Committee (IOC) and European Sports Coalition (ESC) advocate the systematic use of a noninvasive diagnostics test (i.e., ECG) in screening procedures. This premise is based on a 25-year Italian study that suggested a significant decrease in CV deaths in athletes when using ECGs during the preparticipation exam.[37] Concerns from an American perspective questioning the low incidence of disease and rate of false positives of an ECG increasing health care costs due to unnecessary follow-up testing have raised concerns on the appropriateness of its systematic use during preparticipation exams.[35] Overall, ECG SN has been reported at 50%; false positive rates of 40% and a 4% to 5% false negative rate limit the validity of this approach.[36] Additionally, with a significantly larger population, the already overburdened United States health care system may come to a standstill if diagnostic testing were mandated for all athletes. Considering epidemiologic, societal, and economic concerns, the American Heart Association (AHA) does not currently endorse the systematic use of ECG diagnostic testing within its screening guidelines.[34, 37, 38] The AHA currently recommends screening guidelines

AHA Recommendations for Preparticipation Cardiovascular Screening of Competitive Athletes[34]

The risk of serious cardiovascular disease should always be a concern for the practicing clinician. The AHA suggests clinicians evaluate several elements during preparticipation screening for competitive athletes. The elements fall into three areas: personal history, family history, and a physical exam.

When taking the athlete's **personal history**, the clinician should ask if the athlete has experienced any of the following during exercise: chest pain or discomfort, fainting or near fainting, becoming very out of breath, or fatigued. The clinician should determine if a medical professional has diagnosed a heart murmur in the past and should check for elevated systemic blood pressure.

After ascertaining the athlete's personal history, the clinician should investigate the athlete's **family history**. Questions such as the following are instructive:

- Has more than one person in your family died suddenly from heart disease before age 50?
- Do any of your close relatives under age 50 have a disability related to heart disease?
- Do you know if any family members have structural or electrical cardiac conditions? Examples could include hypertrophic cardiomyopathy, Marfan syndrome, long-QT syndrome, and so on.

Finally, a qualified health care clinician should do a **physical exam** to check for evidence of a heart murmur or physical attributes of Marfan syndrome. Taking the femoral pulses to make sure there is no aortic coarctation and taking the athlete's blood pressure, preferably in both arms, are also important physical checks. Any one or more positive findings warrants referral for a cardiovascular evaluation.

that do not include advanced diagnostic testing as part of a preparticipation physical in the United States.[37] Instead, a major focus of the guidelines used in the United States includes symptom recognition and family history to identify those athletes at high risk to warrant further diagnostic testing.[35]

COMPARTMENT SYNDROME

Compartment syndrome can occur in any closed fascial compartment; however, the anterior compartment in the lower leg is the most common site of injury.[39] The mechanism may be due to acute trauma or chronic exertion. Acute compartment syndrome due to a direct blow causes a quick onset of pressure, creating an emergent condition that necessitates immediate action. More commonly, compartment syndrome will develop as the result of chronic exertion, creating elevated compartmental pressure in response to repetitive microtrauma. Elevated pressure causing pain in an enclosed compartment may cause neurovascular symptoms

and is often exacerbated with onset of activity. Incidence rates have been reported ranging from 27% to 33% to as high as 40% in active people.[40, 41] Chronic exertional compartment syndrome (CECS) is second only to medial tibial stress syndrome as the underlying cause of lower leg pain.[40] Anatomic risk factors, including muscle hypertrophy, chronic fascial thickening, poor tissue compliance, and limited capillary density, have been suggested.[42] Within the military population, female sex, increasing chronological age, Caucasian race, junior enlisted rank, and Army branch of service were identified as risk factors for onset.[43]

Differential diagnosis of bone or musculotendon involvement, nerve entrapment, vascular occlusion, and infection should be ruled out prior to suspicion for CECS. Pain and tightness with palpation of soft tissue rather than bony structures, as well as sensory changes, can be helpful in diagnosing CECS; however, distal pulses are typically normal.[43, 44] Definitive diagnosis is typically performed through intracompartmental pressure (ICP) testing. While ICP testing before and after exercise is considered a gold standard, protocol variability limits utility for best practice recommendations.[45] To date, no valid sideline examination exists for the diagnosis of CECS. Health care professionals must rely on a thorough history and symptom presentation to appropriately assess and manage the syndrome.

ASTHMA

Asthma is a common pulmonary condition shown to exist in both endurance and power athletes. The incidence of asthma in athletes has been shown to be highest in elite endurance athletes such as swimmers, long-distance runners, and cross-country skiers.[46] Studies have demonstrated prevalence rates between 15% and 55% for endurance athletes.[47-52] Cold weather endurance athletes, including cross-country skiers, have demonstrated the highest rates of asthma.[47, 51] Multiple studies have found speed and power athletes to have asthma rates between approximately 15% and 20%.[52, 54, 55]

Asthma is defined as a chronic inflammatory disease of the airways that causes a cascade of symptoms including wheezing, breathlessness, chest tightness, and coughing due to the inability to inhale and exhale. Airway hyperinflation and airway smooth muscle constriction may occur at the same time. Asthmatic exacerbations can be brought on by several factors including cold, allergens, odors, existing viral infection, emotional upset, changes in barometric pressure, or a combination of multiple factors.[56, 57] Failure to act quickly and appropriately can result in loss of consciousness, severe asthmatic exacerbation, and ultimately death due to respiratory arrest.

While asthma is a chronic condition occurring on and off the field, several pulmonary diagnoses regularly occur only on the field of play. Exercise-induced bronchoconstriction (EIB) is diagnosed when an athlete demonstrates more than a 10% reduction in forced expiratory volume in 1 second (FEV1) occurring after a standardized exercise test. Symptoms are similar to those of asthma but occur exclusively after activity. Exercise-induced bronchoconstriction commonly presents between 6 and 10 minutes after heavy exercise and with significant difficulty exhaling.[58] If the athlete is having difficulty with inspiration, exercise-induced vocal cord dysfunction (VCD) may be a more likely diagnosis.[46] It is important to note that EIB and VCD may occur at the same time. Athletes competing or practicing are more likely to present with EIB versus asthma, since exercise will serve as the trigger for EIB.

It is imperative to review each athlete's medical history in order to identify those at risk for an asthmatic incident. On-field assessment for athletes presenting with difficult breathing should include evaluation of an open airway, breathing quality, and circulation. If the athlete is not able to inhale or exhale, the emergency medical system (EMS) should be activated. Circulation should be assessed by taking the athlete's pulse and looking for changes to blue or gray in the lips and nail beds. The athlete's mental state can be determined while ABCs are being evaluated. A differential diagnosis list including airway obstruction, inhaled foreign body, anaphylaxis, vocal cord dysfunction, anxiety or panic, spontaneous pneumothorax, chronic obstructive pulmonary disease (COPD), and cardiac failure should be considered when evaluating the athlete.

Once the athlete can be moved safely, they should be transferred to a safe, cool, and quiet spot for further examination. The athlete should be placed in a seated position to allow maximal inhalation and should be supported in the event that they become unconscious. Simple questions needing short answers can be used to obtain necessary information. Pertinent questions may include the following:

- Was there contact that led to your shortness of breath?

- Do you have new pain anywhere?

- Has this happened before?

Physical examination of the throat, chest, and lower ribs should be included to rule out pneumothorax and other orthopedic injuries. Once cleared, diagnosis can be made based on a cluster of symptoms. As previously mentioned, common signs of respiratory distress and asthma include coughing, wheezing, shortness of breath, accessory breathing, chest tightness, confusion, and dizziness. Signs of pending respiratory failure include cyanosis, confusion, sweating, and poor air movement. Use of a finger pulse oximeter may be beneficial for monitoring the oxygen perfusion. Values under 95% have been shown to need medical management.[59]

Severity of asthma exacerbation can be generalized as mild, moderate, severe, or respiratory arrest by tracking several factors including pulse, position, ability to talk, alertness, breathlessness, use of accessory muscles, and wheezing volume (table 27.1). Peak expiratory flow rate using a peak flow meter can be used to determine response once treatment has been initiated, but proper use requires knowledge of an athlete's premorbid max effort. It is important to understand that all symptoms may not present. For example, an athlete coming out of a competition will likely have an elevated heart rate and increased respiratory rate. This should be considered when determining severity of exacerbation.[60]

Athletes who have previously been diagnosed with asthma or EIB may carry inhaled medications they can administer themselves. Medical staff who are consistently present with the same team should carry an inhaler in the training kit to be used as needed. This chapter does not go into specific treatments. Once medication is administered, evaluation of symptoms should continue. Athletes should be continuously monitored for all of the categories listed in table 27.1. Pulse, respiratory rate, alertness, and general ABCs require no equipment and are easy to monitor routinely. Signs of respiratory shock should be closely monitored, especially if EMS is not activated.

PNEUMOTHORAX

Pneumothorax occurs when air from the lung is able to escape into the surrounding pleural space. The rupture of the lung tissue can occur spontaneously or traumatically. Predisposing factors of a spontaneous pneumothorax include tall and thin males, smokers, asthmatics, those with history of pneumothorax, and those diagnosed with Marfan syndrome, chronic obstructive pulmonary disorder,

cystic fibrosis, tuberculosis, or whooping cough.[61, 62] A traumatic pneumothorax may occur when the pleural space is punctured by an object such as a fractured rib or torn due to a collision. Oxygen delivery is comprised, which may result in increased respiratory effort and further complications due to poor delivery to vital organs.[63]

Assessment should begin with the ABCs. The athlete will likely be breathing hard from participation, but breathing rate and pulse may not return to normal after cessation of activity. Breathing quality may be slow, shallow, and diminished. The secondary assessment should include palpation of the clavicles, sternum, and ribs to identify any deformity, open wounds, tenderness, or swelling. While symptoms may be similar to asthma, inclusion of chest pain and dyspnea are consistent with pneumothorax. If a pneumothorax is suspected, EMS should be activated and vitals monitored until support arrives.

The two most distinct identifiers of a pneumothorax are distended veins in the anterior cervical region and tracheal deviation. Vein distention occurs secondary to inability of venous blood to return from the head due to the increased pressure in the chest cavity. Tracheal deviation to the opposite side also occurs due to increased chest cavity pressure. This shift can increase pressure on the uninjured lung and heart, which will reduce their function, potentially leading to failure.[64] Additional signs and symptoms include difficulty breathing, paleness or bluish appearance of skin, dizziness, nausea, and pain in the chest, thoracic region, or upper extremities.[65]

TABLE 27.1   Severity of Asthma Exacerbation

Condition	Mild	Moderate	Severe	Respiratory arrest imminent
Breathlessness	Walking	Talking	At rest	
Preferred position	Able to lie supine	Sitting	Hunched/slouched	
Talks in	Sentences	Phrases	Words	
Alertness	May be agitated	Usually agitated	Agitated	Confused/fatigued
Respiratory rate	Increased	Increased	Over 30 breaths/min	
Accessory muscle use	Not typical	Typical	Typical	Paradoxical thoracoabdominal motion
Wheeze	Moderate	Loud	Loud	Usually none
Pulse	<100	100-120	>120	Bradycardia

Based on Lougheed et al. 2012.[60]

HEAT-RELATED ILLNESS

Heat-related illnesses, including heat cramps, heat exhaustion, and heat stroke, are a common concern for the health care professional working with athletes.[66] A majority of these injuries occur primarily in sports exposed to higher environmental temperature, with a majority of heat-related deaths associated with American football, wrestling, and cross country and track.[67] Of these sports, football suffers the highest rate of catastrophic events, with 35 reported heat-related deaths between 1995 and 2010.[67] An epidemiological study on U.S. high school athletes reported that exertional heat illness occurred at a rate of 1.20 per 100,000 athlete exposures, with heat-related illness occurring at 11.4 times greater rate with football compared to all other sports combined.[68] Of concern, approximately 33.6% of the time, medical professionals were not on site, emphasizing the importance for educational and preventive programs.[68]

Recognizing those at risk for heat-related illness is essential for preventing and reducing occurrence. Many intrinsic and extrinsic risk factors exist, and specific populations, including the elderly, children, and those with comorbid conditions, are more prone to heat-related illnesses.[66] Heat cramps associated with muscle cramping commonly occur in the quadriceps, hamstrings, gastrocnemius, and abdominal muscle groups after prolonged activity.[69] Heat exhaustion presents with continuation of muscle cramping, but also includes malaise, nausea, vomiting, and dizziness. The more sinister condition of heat stroke can include any of the previously mentioned symptoms; however, the distinguishable feature is a change in cognition. Heat stroke is defined by core body temperatures of >40 °C (104 °F) and central nervous system (CNS) dysfunction.[66] Oral, axillary, tympanic, and forehead measurements do not accurately assess core temperature in athletes.[70] A recent clinical recommendation suggests the use of rectal temperature as the most reliable way to assess core temperature and asserts that sports medicine staff must be prepared and willing to implement it.[71] By far, the quickest and most effective treatment for heatstroke is immediate removal from the heat, ice-water immersion, and activation of EMS.[69]

Hyponatremia is also considered a heat-related illness; however, the underlying mechanism causing symptoms is different than the dehydrated state of the previously mentioned heat illness. By definition, serum levels of <130 mmol/L constitute hyponatremia.[66] Hyponatremia is caused by excessive ingestion of water over a relatively long period of time, contributing to a sodium imbalance. The condition can have a similar presentation to heat stroke; however, it can be distinguished from that condition by a normal core body temperature.[66]

FRACTURES

The skeletal system's primary responsibility is protection of soft tissue and organs in the body. It is responsible for absorbing forces when the soft-tissue structures cannot handle the magnitude of force imparted on them. Bones can be injured by several forces, including compressive, tensile, shearing, and torsional forces. Each of these can produce a variety of fractures. Fractures are classified as open or closed, with open fractures creating an open wound through the skin and closed remaining below the skin surface. Fractures are also classified as complete or incomplete. A complete fracture will be either displaced or nondisplaced, which refers to the position of the two sides of the fracture. A displaced fracture is often more identifiable due to the malalignment of the fractured ends of the bone.

Critical Clinical Pearls

Immediate removal from the heat and cold immersion is recommended to prevent heat-related illnesses from progressing. Emergency Medical Services should be activated if the athlete has any of the following:[66]

- Altered mental status
- Rectal temperature > 104 °F
- Persistent vomiting

Assessment of airway, breathing, and circulation is the first step in the on-field evaluation when a cervical fracture is suspected. Unconscious athletes should be assumed to have an unstable cervical spine fracture and should be immobilized immediately. Secondary assessment of severe bleeding can help direct the caregiver to the injury site if the athlete is not able to answer questions. More importantly, the presence of severe bleeding should cue the caregiver to prepare for the potential for the athlete to go into shock.

Once the initial assessment is complete and the athlete is cleared of life-threatening emergencies, the secondary assessment can begin. A full assessment of the athlete's body, starting with the head and moving distally toward the feet, should be completed. The acronym DOTS (deformity, open injury, tenderness, swelling) is an easy mnemonic to assist with thorough observation.[72] Any suspected fracture should be compared to the opposite side to assist in diagnosis of injury. Other signs and symptoms of fracture include pain, fear, and loss of movement. The clinician should remain calm during evaluation, especially in the presence of a visual deformity or open fracture. A quality examination and quick treatment will help in protection against and avoidance of further injury.

The physical examination begins with observation for bruising, swelling, and bleeding. Restrictive equipment should be removed if the fracture site can be adequately stabilized to avoid putting the athlete at risk for further injury. In the area of the head and neck, the caregiver should observe and palpate for crepitus, softness, and deformities. Areas that protrude from the skull and neck, including the zygomatic bone, orbits, spinous processes, and mandible, should be carefully examined. Palpable tenderness over the cervical spinous processes should be treated as a potential cervical fracture and immobilized immediately.

In the area of the chest and thoracic spine, the clinician should pay special attention to palpation and observation of each rib, the spinous processes, the clavicles, and the sternum. When two or more ribs on the same side are fractured, there exists the potential for respiratory distress due to flail chest. A fractured rib may protrude inward and pierce the lungs, causing a hemothorax or pneumothorax, both of which can be life-threatening emergencies.

Fractures in the thighs and pelvis are rare but very serious situations. Femur fractures are typically obvious, with the fractured limb presenting as shortened and externally rotated. Other findings suggestive of a femur fracture include significant pain and a palpable strong quadriceps contraction. A femur stress fracture may present with non-specific anterior thigh pain that is made during and after activity. Pelvic fractures are most likely to occur in high-impact sports as well as in skiing and equestrian sports. Due to the ring-shaped nature of the pelvis and force of injury common with this injury, multiple fractures may be present. Additional injuries to the abdomen, genitourinary structures, and neurovascular structures should be screened. Thorough palpation, neurovascular examination of the proximal and distal structures, and monitoring for signs of shock are imperative to averting a potentially life-threatening outcome.

If a fracture is suspected in an extremity, distal pulses should be taken to ensure that local circulation has not been compromised. Sensation in the distal extremity should be grossly assessed with light touch, pressure, vibration, or temperature changes to ensure that the neurologic system is grossly intact. Once the athlete has been treated and immobilized, regular assessments should continue, including taking proximal and distal pulses, monitoring for signs of shock, and assessing neurological function by monitoring sensation.

American College of Radiology (ACR) and clinical practice rules exist to assist in determining if imaging is necessary to confirm a fracture once an athlete has been transferred from the field or play. These rules should not be used to return an athlete to play, but they can be used in determining how to manage the care of an athlete after a suspected fracture on the field. The Ottawa Ankle Rules, Ottawa Knee Rules, and Canadian Cervical Spine Rules aim to reduce the number of radiographs unnecessarily taken and the waiting time spent in emergency departments. These rules are discussed in their respective chapters earlier in this book.

Ottawa Ankle Rules

Ankle injuries make up between 6% and 12% of clients seen in emergency rooms.[73] Of these clients, the majority will undergo advanced imaging to rule in or rule out a fracture. It has been shown that less than 15% of these clients actually have a fracture.[74] Stiell and colleagues[75] developed the Ottawa Ankle Rules in 1992 to assist in screening acute ankle injuries. They have been found to be highly SN (97-100) but modestly SP (30-40).[76, 77] The Ottawa

Ankle Rules is a highly SN test identifying 97% to 100% of ankle fractures but also 60% to 70% of clients who do not have a fracture. While this may seem low, it is an improvement over the 15% of positive radiographs previously reported.[74] Clients must meet one of the following:[75]

- Tenderness on distal 6 cm posterior tibia or malleolus
- Tenderness on distal 6 cm posterior fibula or malleolus
- Tenderness on base of 5th metatarsal
- Tenderness on navicular
- Inability to bear weight for four steps at initial injury and in emergency department exam

Ottawa Knee Rules

The Ottawa Knee Rules were developed by Stiell and colleagues[78] in 1995 to assist in determining the need for radiographs for clients with knee injuries. Their initial prospective study found that 69% of all acute knee injuries were referred for radiographs, but only 6.6% of radiographs were positive for fracture.[78] Due to these data, a list of simple objective criteria was developed.[79] The Ottawa Knee Rules have demonstrated an SN of 99 to 100 and an SP of 49 to 54.[80] These data can be interpreted to state that nearly all clients who are positive for the Ottawa Knee Rules will be identified, but 45% to 50% of those imaged will be negative for a knee fracture. Clients must meet one of the following:[77]

- Age 55 years or older
- Isolated tenderness of patella (no other bone tenderness around knee)

- Tenderness at head of fibula
- Inability to flex 90°
- Inability to bear weight for four steps at initial injury and in emergency department exam

Canadian C-Spine Rules

The Canadian Cervical Spine Rules were developed by Stiell and colleagues[81] as an algorithm to determine necessity of cervical spine radiographs. Studies have shown that only 1% of clients reporting to emergency departments with cervical spine injury and intact neurological status actually have a cervical fracture.[82-84] When radiographs are taken, approximately 98% are negative for fracture.[85-87] The Canadian Cervical Spine Rules have demonstrated an SN of 90 to 100 and an SP of 0.1 to 77.[88] The rules are to be used only when the client is alert (Glasgow Coma Scale = 15) and stable. The Canadian Cervical Spine Rules[81] are described in detail in chapter 17 (Cervical Spine).

ENDOCRINE EMERGENCIES

Diabetes mellitus (DM) is defined as a group of metabolic disorders demonstrating altered glycemic levels. The two types of DM, type 1 and type 2, each involve changes in the body's glycemic levels outside of normal ranges. Health care professionals must be aware of signs and symptoms of both hyper- and hypoglycemia, because misdiagnosis and incorrect treatment of one type could turn a nonemergent, treatable situation into a life-threatening emergency. Regardless of type, the

---

Critical Clinical Pearls

When assessing an athlete for suspected fracture, keep the following in mind:

- Remember the DOTS acronym for initial assessment: deformity, open injury, tenderness, and swelling.
- Always stabilize the cervical spine of an athlete who is unconscious or has suspicion of neck injury. If the suspected fracture is to the cervical spine, ankle, or knee, then the appropriate fracture rules should be employed to help determine if radiographs are appropriate (Canadian C-Spine, Ottawa Ankle, Ottawa Knee).
- If the fracture is in the extremity, always check the distal pulse to ensure that blood flow is not impeded.
- Fractures of the thigh and pelvis should always be treated as life-threatening situations.

staff should know the athlete's history, and should be prepared to administer treatment as needed. A thorough athlete history prior to competition will speed the examination and allow treatment to be administered to the athlete more quickly and accurately. Health care professionals should closely monitor those athletes known to have blood glucose issues and should ensure that they are appropriately taking medications and nutrients to sustain glucose levels.

Signs and symptoms of hypoglycemia and hyperglycemia must be known to the health care staff. The athlete's ABCs should be monitored immediately on examination. Specifically, the athlete's respiratory rate should meet the demands of their effort on the field for the day. Monitoring circulation will determine if the athlete is tachycardic. Observation of sweating, demeanor, mood, and reactions should be assessed for clues of glycemic complication. Questions and simple motor tasks can be included to assess the athlete's physical and mental capabilities compared to their typical abilities. If the athlete is new to the health care staff, a person familiar with the athlete should be included in the examination.

Type 1 Diabetes Mellitus

While only 5% to 10% of diabetics are diagnosed as type 1, the condition may be encountered more often in a healthy, fit, and youthful population. Type 1 diabetes mellitus can be caused by several conditions, the most common as a result an autoimmune dysfunction at the cellular level that destroys the beta cells found in the pancreas. Loss of insulin production inhibits the athlete's ability to regulate the blood glucose levels.[89]

Type 2 Diabetes Mellitus

The most common type of DM in society today is type 2, in which people demonstrate hyperglycemia.[89] This is caused by reduction in the sensitivity of cells to insulin. The body continues to produce insulin, but it does not have the same blood glucose regulatory effects as those without type 2 DM. Type 2 DM is common in the elderly, sedentary, and obese populations. Athletes with the condition should be closely monitored for signs and symptoms because they may have other comorbidities present that put them at a higher risk for emergency situations.[89] Reminding athletes to administer insulin

regularly can help to mitigate or prevent life-threatening emergencies.

Hypoglycemia (blood glucose below 70 mg/dl) is more common than hyperglycemia, and typically occurs in response to poor dosage of insulin during and after participation in sport; this is more common in people with type 1 DM.[90] Initial symptoms reported by a hypoglycemic athlete include tachycardia, hunger, headache, abnormal sweating, heart palpitations, and dizziness.[88] More severe symptoms may present, including visual disturbances, abnormal fatigue, poor motor control, aggressive behavior, seizures, difficulty processing information, and potentially unconsciousness.[89, 90] If symptoms are assessed properly and efficiently, the athlete may be treated on the sidelines. If the athlete is severely hypoglycemic and unconscious, the health care staff should active EMS immediately. The athlete should be kept in a safe location, and ABCs should be monitored regularly.[89]

Hyperglycemia (blood glucose above 180 mg/dl) may occur in athletes with both types of DM; however, it is much more common in those with type 2 DM. Symptoms of hyperglycemia include slowed mental processing, nausea, fatigue, and decreased or slowed performance. If blood sugar levels are allowed to rise further, the body may begin to use fatty-acid metabolism as the preferred energy system. This can be identified by increased fatigue, fruity-scented breath, increased thirst, more frequent urination, and shorter than appropriate breaths known as Kussmaul respirations.[90] Health care staff should look for this cluster of unusual symptoms to identify the state of the athlete's blood glucose. The American Diabetes Association is a good reference for health care staff, athletes, coaches, and families to enhance their overall knowledge of diabetes identification, intervention, safety, and exercise.[89]

Once signs and symptoms have been assessed, the athlete's blood glucose level should be monitored by the athlete or health care staff. This should be done using a blood glucose monitor and testing strips. These should accompany the sports medicine team to every practice and game. When assessing blood glucose, a lancet is used to puncture the tip of the finger and a single drop of blood is placed on the testing strip. This is then inserted into the testing device for analysis. Lancets and all contaminated materials must be placed in a biohazard bag or sharps container.[90]

CONCLUSION

Serious and catastrophic injuries are an inherent risk accepted by each athlete participating in sport and their health care team. A thorough understanding of basic emergency care, risk factors, and each athlete's history can assist the sports medicine staff when faced with a crisis. Efficient decision-making based on current guidelines, position statements, training, and evidence-based tests is paramount for mitigating risk and preventing further, more serious injury. Development and practice of a step-by-step process of examination and management should be part of training for any health care professional providing on-field care.

28

GERIATRIC EXAMINATION

Michael Schmidt, PT, DPT, OCS, FAAOMPT
Charles Sheets, PT, OCS, SCS, Dip MDT
Tasala Rufai, PT, DPT, GCS

In 2012, there were 43.1 million people aged 65 and older in the United States, accounting for 13.7% of the U.S. population, a 21% increase since 2002. The number of people moving into the 65 and older age group in the next two decades increased by 24% from 2002 to 2012.[1] As the U.S. population continues to age, it is expected that the number of musculoskeletal impairments will follow the same trend; an increase in population age is suggestive of an increase in the frequency of musculoskeletal diseases.[2] In the reporting period of 1996 to 1998 until 2004 to 2006, the prevalence of people aged 65 and older who reported a musculoskeletal disease (spine, arthritis and joint pain, osteoporosis, injuries, other) increased from 21.7% to 23.1%.[2] In 2008, the proportion of people who reported a musculoskeletal condition increased with age: 37.9% (42 million) and 56.0% (43.3 million) for those 18 to 44 and 45 to 64 respectively, compared to 65.8% (13 million) of those 65 to 74 and 69.1% (12 million) of those 75 and older.[2]

From 2002 to 2004 in the United States, medical care expenditures for musculoskeletal-related diseases and disorders in those 65 and older were approximately $10,000 per person compared to an average cost of $5,824 for all ages. They also accounted for $195.2 billion, or 38.2% of total aggregate health care costs, for musculoskeletal diseases in that same time span.[2] Musculoskeletal-related diseases occur more frequently with increasing age,[2] while active lifestyle is a contributor to chronic joint pain and arthritis. For example, increasing age is a predictor of chronic joint pain and arthritis.[3] In 2008, 7 in 10 clients aged 65 and older reported one or both of these conditions. In the United States, 1 in every 2 clients aged 65 and older is affected by some form of arthritis.[2] Osteoarthritis and rheumatoid arthritis are the most common diagnoses requiring total joint replacements,[4] and they are increasing in frequency in aging populations,[2] with baby boomers accounting for more than 50% of those procedures.[4] Osteoporosis, which is discussed in detail later in this chapter, is estimated to affect 19% of clients over the age of 65; in 2004, the medical expenditure for osteoporosis-related fractures was estimated at $19.1 billion.[4] In combination, these factors will create a larger patient population with higher health care costs and an increased cost of care associated with musculoskeletal diseases in the future as the population continues to age.[2]

This chapter highlights the important factors to consider when evaluating the geriatric client. It includes valuable information on the influence age has as a diagnostic decision tool and a thorough explanation of the numerous physiological changes that occur throughout every tissue as a result of aging. The influence age plays on the feeling of pain is also highlighted, with special focus on osteoarthritis of the knee and spinal pain. This chapter also focuses on the diagnosis of osteoporosis and the contribution that various diagnosis and medications play on the progression of the disease. Finally, it discusses the examination of balance with use of diverse outcome measures.

INFLUENCE OF AGE ON DIAGNOSIS

In addition to the effect of aging on potential anatomic and physiologic processes, age itself can be a factor in making orthopedic diagnostic decisions. A relatively simple way to identify the influence of age is to observe how often age is a contributing factor in common diagnoses. Table 28.1 provides a review of clinical prediction rules (CPRs) or decision rules that have been developed for musculoskeletal diagnosis and triage. Age is an important predictor across a broad spectrum of diagnoses, including screening for fracture, osteoporosis, and pulmonary embolism, as well as diagnosis of rotator cuff tears,

TABLE 28.1 Influence of Age on Orthopedic Diagnostic Decision Tools

Decision tool (if applicable)	Diagnosis	Age variable
Ottawa Knee Rules[7]	Fracture	>55
Pittsburgh Knee Rules[8]	Fracture	>50
Canadian Cervical Spine Rule[9]	Cervical spine fracture	>65
	Osteoporotic vertebral compression fracture or wedge deformity	>52
	The development of a clinical decision making algorithm for detection of osteoporotic vertebral compression fracture or wedge deformity[10]	
Osteoporosis Risk Assessment Instrument[11]	Osteoporosis	1 of 3 variables assessed: points if >75, 65-74, 55-64
Simple Calculated Osteoporosis Risk Estimation[12]	Osteoporosis	1 of 6 variables assessed (3 points for each decade)
Osteoporosis Self-Assessment Tool[13]	Osteoporosis	Weight (kg): age / 5
Male Osteoporosis Risk Estimation Score[14]	Osteoporosis	1 of 3 variables assessed: points if >75, 55-74
	Cancer in patients with low back pain	≥50
Revised Geneva Score[15]	Pulmonary embolism[5]	>65
	Cervical myelopathy[6]	>45
	Rotator cuff tear[16]	>65
	Carpal tunnel syndrome[17]	>45
	Lumbar spinal stenosis[18]	60-70, 70
	Ankylosing spondylitis[5]	Onset < 40
American College of Rheumatology Criteria for Classification of Osteoarthritis of the Hip[19]	Hip osteoarthritis	>50
American College of Rheumatology Criteria for Classification of Osteoarthritis of the Knee[20]	Knee osteoarthritis	>50

carpal tunnel syndrome, lumbar spinal stenosis, and cervical myelopathy. The youngest value identified in these represented decision rules was 40 years old; onset of symptoms after this time is likely to rule out a diagnosis of ankylosing spondylitis.[5] Younger age is also useful in a decision rule for cervical myelopathy. Age greater than 45 had minimal effect on diagnosis (+LR 1.2), and younger clients had a moderate decrease in the likelihood of cervical myelopathy (−LR 0.48).[6]

The diagnosis of ankylosing spondylitis was unique in that increased age was associated with a decreased likelihood of diagnosis. For the majority of the tools, single-age cutoffs were used, whereby a positive result is an age greater than the cutoff; ages range from 50 to 65. The osteoporosis scales tend to use age in a different manner, identifying the increased risk with age progression. In two osteoporosis scales, age is graded on an ordinal scale, with clients in older age groups scoring higher (greater risk) than those in younger groups.[11, 14] In another scale, additional points are scored for each additional decade,[12] while in a fourth scale, age is a variable in a simple calculation with weight.[13] Inclusion of age in the CPRs was determined for most of the rules through either regression analysis[6] or clinician decision.[17]

When specific pathoanatomic diagnoses cannot be made, clinical prediction rules have also been utilized to classify clients into categories thought to best direct treatment. These are split almost evenly among those that demonstrate better outcomes for younger clients (use of joint mobilization and trigger point therapy for tension-type headache [<44.5 years old],[21] response to mobilization with movement for lateral epicondylalgia [<49 years old],[22] lumbar stabilization for low back pain [<40 years old], and response to physical therapy for clients with soft-tissue shoulder disorders [outcome worsened with each decade])[23] and those with better outcomes for older clients (foot orthoses for patellofemoral pain [>25 years old],[24] cervical traction and exercise for neck pain [≥55 years old],[25] manual therapy for neck pain [>50 years old],[26] lumbar traction for low back pain [>30 years old]).[27] While the development of these rules provides some support for the influence of age on ability to classify clients to provide the best outcome, clinicians implementing these prediction rules should proceed with caution.[28] The majority of these rules have been used only to develop hypotheses; validation testing has frequently yielded disappointing results.[29-31]

The ability of age to accurately classify clients for particular treatments remains in question.

CHANGE IN TISSUE PROPERTIES AS A RESULT OF AGING

The entire human body system is affected in some capacity as we age, but increased age does not necessarily mean a decline in physical function.[32] A large degree of variability exists among the elderly population with respect to physical function compared to any other age group. For this reason, chronological age is a poor indicator of physical and cognitive function. Approximately 50% of decreased function in the older adult has been attributed to pathologic changes rather than normal consequences of aging.[33] It is difficult to fully define the physiological changes that do occur—whether they are from age alone or from a combination of the interactions of aging, disease, and lifestyle. The most common reason for declined functional capabilities in the older client is inactivity or immobility.[32] This section focuses on all the human body systems and the changes that occur as we age.

Cardiovascular System

An estimated 83.6 million American adults have one or more types of cardiovascular disease.[34] In 2009, the total cost for cardiovascular disease was determined to be $115.0 billion for clients over the age of 65, and it totaled 36.5% of overall costs for cardiovascular-related health care.[34] Cardiovascular disease, coronary heart disease, angina, stroke, high blood pressure, and heart failure are the most common diseases that affect the cardiovascular system in the older client. The common cardiovascular system changes that occur as a result of aging are as follows:[42]

Decreased

- Arterial elasticity
- Cardiac output
- Cardiac reserve
- Response to physical stress

Increased

- Blood pressure
- Breakdown of cardiac tissue

The geriatric population is prone to heart arrhythmias and demonstrates high rates of cardiovascular disease. Baseline vital signs including blood pressure and heart rate should be taken prior to, during, and after therapeutic exercise programs. Cardiac medication should be taken into consideration when evaluating cardiac-related vital signs.

Vascular Factors

The most common vascular change that occurs with aging is an increase in overall blood pressure.[34] Blood pressure changes occur due to increased vascular impedance from increased aortic stiffness, increased peripheral vascular resistance, increased viscosity of the blood, and decreased elastic properties of the blood vessels.[35] These four factors lead to an increase in early stages of atherosclerosis with plaque buildup along the arterial walls.

Baroreceptor regulation in the blood stream is also affected with age. Baroreceptors become less sensitive to changes in blood pressure; pathology such as atherosclerosis and hypertension have also been linked to a decrease in the baroreceptor reflex.[36] Decreased sensitivity of the baroreceptors have been implicated in the increased experience of postural hypotension in the older client as well.[36, 37]

Cardiac-Related Factors

Age-associated changes in cardiac tissue include increased thickness of the left ventricle wall with an accompanying increase in myocyte size and decrease in myocyte number.[35, 37, 38] These structural changes prolong the contraction of the heart muscle, decreasing the velocity and power of contraction, which allows for less blood to be distributed throughout the body to working tissues.[35] The decreased number of myocytes and decreased autonomic regulation has been hypothesized to account for the high prevalence of dysrhythmias in the older client.[39]

Resting heart rate does not change significantly during aging, but the maximal heart rate capacity does progressively decrease over time. The maximum heart rate is reduced by almost 33% between 20 and 85 years of age.[35] The heart has a decreased ejection fraction and decreased ability to quickly accelerate the heart during a bout of physical exertion or stress. Stroke volume does not significantly change over time, which allows for no change in cardiac output at rest. However, cardiac output has been shown to decrease by as much as 30% with exercise due to the decreased heart rate

that is observed during submaximal and maximal exercise.[35]

Reduced physical activity has been shown to exaggerate these age-related changes in cardiovascular structures. The function of the cardiac system and all body systems can be affected by a lack of regular physical activity.[32, 35] A lack of physical activity can increase atherosclerotic vascular disease, hypertension, and the likelihood of cardiac disease.[34, 35]

Pulmonary System

Pulmonary diseases are consistently in the top 10 causes for mortality in the elderly population.[40] Changes in the pulmonary system can be classified into changes in mechanical properties, flow, volume, gas exchange, and deficiencies in the lung defense system. The common pulmonary system changes that occur as a result of aging are as follows:[42]

Decreased

- Chest wall compliance
- Diaphragm, intercostal, and accessory breathing muscle strength
- Elastic recoil
- Maximal voluntary ventilation
- Respiratory gas exchange
- Vital capacity

Increased

- Residual volume

Chest wall compliance decreases with calcification of the ribs and a loss of elastic tissue that decreases the expansion of the ribs in the thoracic cavity. A kyphotic posture in the thoracic spine can reduce the compliance and expansion capacity of the lungs. Significant decline also occurs in the diaphragm, intercostal, and accessory musculature strength, which increases the work required for breathing.[41]

Maximum volume of voluntary ventilation and expiratory flow has been shown to decrease with aging, leading to the primary complications of obstructive and restrictive lung diseases.[42] A total decline in the lung capacity, vital capacity, and oxygen exchange occurs as a result of all these physiological changes to the body. Finally, there is decreased cilia activity and diminished effectiveness of mitochondria activity within the lungs, affecting the body's ability to remove inhaled particles.[42]

This leads to the strikingly high mortality rates of pneumonia in the geriatric population.[43]

Consideration of the client's respiratory rate and perceived exertion levels should be considered at baseline and during activity. Clients suspicious of having pneumonia may present with symptoms such as cough, fever, chills, and shortness of breath.[44] These clients should be assessed by a primary care physician as soon as possible due to the high prevalence of mortality in the elderly population.

Musculoskeletal System

Musculoskeletal changes are of primary concern for the orthopedic clinician. A multitude of cellular and physiological changes occur to the muscle tissue, bone, and cartilage as people age. Examination of, and subsequent intervention with, the client must be undertaken with these changes in mind. The common musculoskeletal system changes that occur as a result of aging are as follows:[42]

Muscle
- Decreased muscle mass and strength
- Decreased recruitment of motor units
- Decreased speed of movement

Bone
- Decreased calcium
- Decreased density
- Decreased strength
- Decreased vitamin D

Cartilage
- Increased deterioration
- Decreased elasticity
- Decreased hydration

The geriatric client demonstrates numerous orthopedic-related changes that need to be taken into account during the examination process. Special attention will need to be made to the common tissue changes and their relation to function. The decline of the musculoskeletal system is not entirely irreversible and can be altered with physical activity and education.

Muscle

Sarcopenia has been defined as the age-related reduction of muscle mass and strength.[42, 45] There is a decrease in active functional units within con-tractile muscle tissue and a decrease in the number of fiber types (both Type I slow-twitch and Type II fast-twitch) with age.[46] It is hypothesized that these conditions are due to the lack of vigorous exercise and reduction of physical activity that commonly occur with aging. Moreover, the loss of muscle tissue is hypothetically caused by age-related decrease in growth hormones, insulin-like growth factor, estrogen levels, and testosterone levels.[47, 48] As these hormone levels drop, muscle mass is likely to decrease as well.

Muscle wasting can also occur due to functional nonuse or disuse as a secondary problem from arthritic or pain changes. Inhibition of muscle contraction due to painful or arthritic joints can allow for progressive decline in muscle cross-sectional area, strength,[49] and reduced overall tissue quality due to fatty infiltration into the muscle.[50] These deleterious effects have been shown to be modifiable with appropriate training.[48, 51, 52]

The elastic properties of ligaments, tendons, and muscle tissue have all been shown to decrease over time.[42, 53] The variation in elastic properties results in increased rigidity of the tissue, causing less resistance to lengthening and increased injury risk.

Bone

As we age, there is an imbalance in the regulation of bone production and absorption. Osteoblast activity diminishes and osteoclast activity remains relatively unchanged, which increases bone absorption, leading to frail and brittle bones, [42] resulting in a calcium-related loss of mass and density of the bone structure. A decline in circulating levels of active vitamin D_3, which is used for absorption of calcium from the intestinal tract, increases absorption of calcium from the bone to meet the needs of the body. Postmenopausal women are especially more vulnerable due to a decrease in estrogen levels, which increases bone reabsorption. The rate of bone loss is about 1% per year for women starting at age 30 to 35 years and for men at age 50 to 55 years.[42] This bone-related change can predispose the elderly population to osteoporosis, which is highlighted in a later section.

Changes in the bony structure of the human body can have a profound effect on postural changes that occur with aging. These changes typically include forward head posture and rounded shoulders, commonly termed *upper crossed syndrome*.[54] Thoracic kyphosis, decreased lordosis, and increased hip and knee flexion are also common, resulting in a flexed, stooped posture. These changes in posture are typically common in clients with known decreased bone mineral density and osteoporosis.

Cartilage

Hyaline, elastic, and articular cartilage is found to become dehydrated, display decreased elastic properties, and get thinner in weight-bearing areas as people age.[42] Cartilage does not have a blood supply, so destruction of the cartilage is irreparable. The production of chondroitin sulfate, a compound that is found to give cartilage its compressive properties, has been shown to be reduced as one ages.[55] Reduced chondroitin sulfate results in decreased ability of the cartilage matrix to attract and retain fluids for lubrication to the joint.

A compressive load placed on the cartilage squeezes extra fluid out of the cartilage matrix, causing less fluid and nutrients to enter. For this reason, compressive loads need to be altered in order for proper lubrication to occur.[42] Normal activity allows for alternating compression and noncompressive forces through the cartilage matrix, allowing for optimal cartilage health. With inactivity, cartilage can be converted to fibrocartilage, which increases stiffness and decreases compressive capabilities of the joint.[56] The alternation of compressive and noncompressive forces is highly important in the older client to enhance overall health of the cartilage and preserve the viability of the joints.

The articular surfaces of synovial joints are covered by hyaline cartilage. Compression in these joints release chemicals that aid in joint lubrication. As people age, less of these chemicals are released, affecting the lubrication properties and dispersion of compressive forces.[57] The decrease in lubrication of the joint surface leads to increased degeneration of the cartilage surface. These changes are irreversible, and a program focused on compressive and noncompressive forces is required for maintaining cartilage health in the geriatric population.[56]

The weight-bearing joint surfaces are common areas of cartilage deterioration. Symptoms of cartilage deterioration can go unnoticed for a length of time due to the lack of vascular and neural supply. Erosion of the joint surface can advance before symptoms of stiffness, pain, and crepitus occur. The lack of lubrication and increased fibrous outgrowth within the joint contributes to reduced function and pain leading to osteoarthritis (OA).[49]

Neuromuscular and Neurosensory System

The nervous system is the driving force behind many of the physiological processes that occur in the human body. A decline in this system as we age leads to a deterioration in nearly every body system. As we age, the nervous system is affected through its conduction velocity, sensory acuity, balance, and hemostatic regulation. The common neuromuscular and neurosensory system changes that occur as a result of aging are as follows:[42]

Decreased

- Balance
- Basal metabolic rate
- Blood flow to brain and nerves
- Hearing
- Nerve conduction velocity
- Proprioception
- Quantity of nerve fibers
- Reaction time
- Reflexes
- Smell and taste
- Sweat glands
- Thermoregulation
- Visual acuity

Reflex examination will typically be diminished in the older client, and this is a normal clinical finding. Balance can be affected due to vestibular, proprioceptive, or vision changes. All of these changes must be evaluated for proper understanding of impairments related to balance and falls. Temperature changes should be monitored in the geriatric client due to alterations in thermoregulation properties that occur with aging.

Neuromuscular

Neuronal cells decline in number and efficiency of function with age. The diminished efficiency of the nervous system decreases the impulsive conduction velocity and cerebral transmission of information.[58] Neurotransmitter release has also been shown to decline with age, which impairs the efficiency of the system.[59] Neural cell number and myelin sheath thickness are reduced, leading to a decrease in conduction velocity to skeletal muscle.[42] Deep tendon reflexes are reduced due to these neuronal changes.[60]

Neurosensory

The neurosensory system is also diminished due to the decline and efficiency of neuronal cells. The neurosensory system includes the nervous system and five senses (hearing, taste, smell, vision, and touch). Hearing loss is one of the most common findings in the older client.[61] Speaking in a slow, medium-pitched voice with face-to-face communication is necessary for the older client to better receive verbal information due to transmission impairments of high- and lower-frequency-level sounds from the inner ear to the brain for processing.[42] Touch, pressure vibration, temperature acuity, proprioception, and body awareness,[42] as well as vision-related age changes (visual acuity, macular degeneration, cataracts, diabetic eye disease, glaucoma, dry eye, and low vision),[62] are all variables that must be considered during examination of the geriatric client.

Balance

The entire neurosensory system and the senses are affected with aging, and they play a pivotal role in balance. Within the inner ear, the otolith organs and semicircular canals demonstrate degenerative-related changes that affect the vestibular system.[42] Declining function in the vestibular system, vision, and proprioception contribute to balance-related impairments. Therefore, the geriatric client has an increased risk of falling.[63] Objective testing measures for balance will be touched on at the end of this chapter.

Homeostatic Regulation

Homeostatic regulation within the hypothalamus becomes less sensitive to physiological feedback with aging. The decreased regulatory capabilities of the hypothalamus have been correlated to the age-related increase in heat stroke, hypothermia, and age-related deaths due to a compromised thermoregulation system.[42, 64] This can be a serious problem when considering the older client maintaining regulation of this system during exercise conditions. The decreased thermoregulation is also accompanied by a slower reactivity of the autonomic nervous system to altering skin hydration and circulation.[64]

Other Body Systems

Almost every body system is affected in some capacity as people age. This section highlights some other systems that can be affected with age but may not be the primary concern for examination in the orthopedic physical therapy clinic setting. The common changes that occur in other body systems as a result of aging are as follows:[42]

Decreased

- Gastrointestinal function
  Metabolic absorption
  Motility in esophagus, stomach, and intestines
- Renal
  Structural size and overall function
- Hepatic
  Excretion and reabsorption capabilities
- Urinary
  Ability to fully empty the bladder
- Integumentary
  Healing time of damaged tissue
  Tensile strength

A clear understanding of the geriatric client's medication list is of vital importance. These body systems can be difficult to examine, so a thorough subjective report is necessary for complete understanding of all these systems. Due to the complexity of these body systems, referral to other health care providers may be warranted.

Gastrointestinal

Digestion and absorption of nutrients can become compromised due to a reduction in blood supply, motility, and absorbing cells within the gastrointestinal tract.[42, 65] Reduced gastric emptying, smell, and taste lead to appetite changes within the elderly population.[65] The slow motility of solid material within the colon and a lack of hydration can increase the occurrence of constipation, which leads to fecal impaction and bowel obstruction. A thorough subjective interview is necessary to ensure that proper bowel function and nutritional needs are being met by the geriatric client.

Renal

With age, an overall reduction in kidney size has been identified. This is most prominent during the later decades of life.[66] By the age of 85, the remaining function of the nephrons may be decreased by as much as 40% compared to their function in youth.[42] Treatments to support kidney health such as dialysis may alter baseline physiological function and should be considered during examination.[67]

Hepatic

The liver mass and blood perfusion within the liver declines with age.[42] Two of the more serious effects with the aging liver include alterations of protein binding and prolongation of drug effects within the body. The half-life and elimination of drugs from the liver have been shown to take 50% to 75% longer in people over the age of 65.[68] The prolongation of drug effects and deficiency in eliminating these drugs should be considered during examination of clients who are taking medications that could potentially alter examination findings, such as cardiovascular, diabetic, or pain medication. Communication with the primary care physician and pharmacist is paramount for proper care of a client with multiple medication sources.

Urinary

A loss of urine concentration abilities occurs within the urinary system with aging. More residual urine within the ureters increases the likelihood of bacterial growth.[42] Resulting urinary tract infections, both symptomatic and asymptomatic, are frequent in the older client.[69] The diagnosis of a urinary tract infection can be very difficult to make, and it is commonly overdiagnosed and overtreated.[70] A comprehensive assessment is indicated, and clients with any suspicion of an infection should be referred immediately.

Integumentary

With age, the dermis of the skin becomes very thin, with a loss of elastic properties to the tissue and a diminished vascular supply. The loss of tissue support results in fragile and easily bruised skin and compromises tissue repair.[42] The appearance of age-related spots and increased risk for neoplastic development are common among the geriatric population. A thorough examination of the integumentary system is necessary to screen for potential tissue compromise or neoplastic activity.

INFLUENCE OF AGE ON PAIN

Aging is commonly assumed to have consistent association with pain, degenerative changes, and functional decline. For example, one in three people over age 40 can be expected to develop knee pain over a 12-year period.[71] Age has been identified as a major risk factor for knee OA in nearly all studies, with few exceptions.[72] Despite this association, the relationship between advancing age and pain is far from linear, and a number of clinical factors play an important role in modifying this relationship between advancing age and the symptoms described.

A consistent risk factor for development of painful lower extremity arthritis, particularly in the knees, is obesity.[71] The effect of obesity appears to be pronounced when developed at a young age and sustained into later years.[73] This may limit the effect of weight management as a treatment tool for the obese older client with knee OA, particularly if the obesity has been long standing. However, clinical studies have identified weight loss as effective for pain control throughout the age spectrum,[74] making observation and counseling about weight a potentially key aspect of examination for any client with lower extremity OA.

Excessive weight leading to advanced OA is consistent with one of the two primary hypotheses of the cause of exercise-related OA, namely wear and tear of the articular cartilage versus muscle dysfunction.[75] Obesity appears to be a stronger predictor of bilateral OA,[76] while previous knee injury is a stronger predictor of unilateral OA.[76, 77] Shrier and colleagues, noting the association of major injuries with high rates of OA, speculated that because muscles provide stability during movement, some signs of OA may be an attempt by the body to reduce joint instability due to muscle dysfunction.[75] Given

Critical Clinical Pearls

Here are some reminders about the change in tissue properties that occur as a result of aging:

- Chronological age is a poor indicator of physical and cognitive function.
- The most common reason for declined functional capabilities in the older client is inactivity or immobility.
- Every body system is affected in some capacity with increased age.

Critical Clinical Pearls

Here are some myths of aging and pain:

- Increased age does not demonstrate a linear relationship with pain.
- Pain associated with degenerative processes does not necessarily increase over time.
- Clinical studies have identified weight loss as effective for pain control throughout the age spectrum.
- Spinal-related pain demonstrates increased prevalence from the age of 30-65 and gradually declines in age >65.

the improvements consistently seen with a variety of exercise programs for clients with painful OA,[78] clients (and clinicians) should be mindful that OA may not necessarily become progressively degenerated and painful; improved strength and motor control can have significant effects on a client's function, pain, and quality of life.

Clinicians should feel particularly confident in providing this information to clients with spinal pain. The incidence of low back pain is highest in the third decade, and overall prevalence increases with age until the 60- to 65-year age group and then gradually declines.[79] This result has been found to be similar for all spinal pain, with no increase from approximately 45 years old into the 60s, with most studies identifying a decline in reported pain in the oldest group.[80] The proposed anatomic bases for these changes are described previously in this section. The key message for clients and the general public is that aging need not be seen as a time when pain, particularly pain due to degenerative processes, must necessarily increase over time.

PHYSICAL REQUIREMENTS FOR ACTIVITIES OF DAILY LIVING

The ability to complete activities of daily living (ADLs) has been correlated with quality of life as well as functional status. Oftentimes the physical limitations that affect older clients go unnoticed until there is a decline in their ability to independently ambulate or complete ADLs. There are also many implications specific to admission to skilled nursing facilities or long-term care facilities, eligibility for hospital services or paid home care services, insurance coverage, as well as mortality. The contributing factors that allow for one to complete ADLs include muscle strength, joint range of motion (ROM), and metabolic equivalents (METs).

While it has been documented that strength decreases with increasing age,[32] there is not an absolute standard for the muscle strength requirements for the completion of ADLs. Absolute and relative strength values have been documented using modified sphygmomanometers and dynamometers for muscle actions involved with functional movements, and these may be used as reference values. Measured values that fall outside of the normal range may be deemed as abnormal, which may correlate to a client's inability to complete a functional activity or task. Andrews and colleagues provide reference values for the normal strength of 10 extremity muscle actions.[81] Any value less than two standard deviations below the mean value is considered to be an impairment or a below-normal force measure.[81] Ultimately, the use of functional tools along with the observation of a client completing specified tasks may be the most accurate approach for determining how the presence of strength deficits may limit the client's ability to complete ADLs.

The American Association of Orthopaedic Surgeons and the American Medical Association have established normative ROM values for the joints in the body, but studies have shown that clients with less than normal ROM can preserve the functional ROM necessary to complete ADLs.[82] Aging clients tend to have less joint ROM on average than their younger counterparts,[42] but they are still able to maintain functional ROM,[82] which allows them to continue to function at an independent level.

Complex motions of the joints of the spine and upper and lower extremities are required for completion of instrumental and basic ADLs. Each activity requires that a joint or combination of joints move into a singular plane of motion or that joints move into multiple planes. Variability in joint ROM and required ROM for a specific functional task persists between clients, regardless of age,[82] so normative values should be used only as a general frame of reference. A ROM measurement that falls short of the normative value should only be classified as contributing to a client's functional limitation if it directly alters the ability to complete an ADL or functional task at an independent level; otherwise, it can be deemed a decreased joint ROM without functional implications.

For each ADL, there is an associated metabolic cost or equivalent. The ADLs related to self-care (e.g., bathing, feeding, dressing, toileting, and grooming) are categorized as light physical activity, requiring fewer than three METs for completion in the average healthy client.[83] However, with older clients, METs for functional activities have been found to be different compared to normative criteria. Also, older clients with mobility impairments, a state which may lend itself to poor efficiency with movement patterns or co-activation of antagonistic muscle groups, require more METs for completing ADLs.[84] Thus, it is extremely difficult to estimate the METs requirement on an individualized basis for the older client, but trends suggest that in the presence of mobility impairments, which are more prevalent in older clients, the metabolic cost and demand for completion of ADLs are elevated.[84]

OSTEOPOROSIS

Osteoporosis is a chronic condition of the bone characterized by low bone mass and structural deterioration of bone tissue with resultant increase in the fragility of bone and consequently an increase in the bone's susceptibility to fracture.[85] This condition results when the rate of formation of new bone mass is less than that of the reabsorption of old bone, leaving the bone structurally weak. The World Health Organization diagnostic classification of osteoporosis is a bone mineral density (BMD) at or below 2.5 standard deviations. While bone mineral content peaks in the third or fourth decade of life and gradually declines as part of normal aging thereafter, the extensive bone loss that characterizes

osteoporosis is not the inevitable fate of the aging client. Many factors influence the rate of bone mineral loss across the life cycle, including nutrition-, endocrine-, and exercise-related factors.[42]

In the United States, an estimated 10 million people are living with osteoporosis, and another 34 million have low bone mass and are at risk for developing osteoporosis.[85] While osteoporosis affects Caucasians and women at a higher rate than other groups, the incidences in all racial groups will continue to rise as the population ages. An estimated one in two Americans over the age of 50 will be diagnosed with, or will be at risk of developing, osteoporosis of the hip by 2020.[86] This statistic does not account for cases of undiagnosed osteoporosis.[86]

In completing a comprehensive examination of the aging client, a good history can reveal risk factors that increase one's likelihood of developing osteoporosis. Female gender, menopause, family history of osteoporosis, low body mass with small stature, personal or family history of fractures, and other diseases that may cause bone loss (e.g., diabetes mellitus, rheumatoid arthritis) are the more common nonmodifiable risk factors that can increase the likelihood of developing osteoporosis. Modifiable risk factors include inactive lifestyle, smoking, alcohol abuse, diet (e.g., low calcium and vitamin D intake; excessive protein, sodium, and caffeine intake), and medications such as steroids and some anticonvulsants.[85] The following sidebar contains a comprehensive list of conditions, diseases, and medications that cause or contribute to osteoporosis and osteoporosis-related fractures.

Osteoporosis is one of the leading causes of fractures in the United States, particularly in the elderly population, and it often leads to an increase in both morbidity and mortality. Osteoporosis-related fractures, traumatic or nontraumatic, are the most prevalent musculoskeletal condition that requires hospitalization amongst Medicare enrollees.[86] Often referred to as a silent disease, it is not uncommon for osteoporosis to go undiagnosed until a client experiences a fall with a resultant fracture. Osteoporosis increases the likelihood of a fracture, and it accounted for nearly 2 million fractures in 2005 alone. An estimated one in two Caucasian women and one in five Caucasian men will experience an osteoporosis-related fracture within their lifetime.[85] Hip and vertebral fractures are associated with increased morbidity and mortality.[87] The total incidences of osteoporosis-related fractures by skeletal site include vertebrae (27%),

Conditions, Diseases, and Medications That Cause or Contribute to Osteoporosis and Fractures

Genetic Factors

Cystic fibrosis	Homocystinuria	Osteogenesis imperfect
Ehlers-Danlos syndrome	Hypophosphatasia	Porphyria
Gaucher's disease	Idiopathic hypercalciuria	Riley-Day syndrome
Glycogen storage diseases	Marfan syndrome	
Hemochromatosis	Menkes steely hair syndrome	

Hypogonadal States

Androgen insensitivity	Hyperprolactinemia	Turner's and Klinefelter's syndrome
Anorexia nervosa	Panhypopituitarism	
Athletic amenorrhea	Premature ovarian failure	

Endocrine Disorders

Acromegaly	Cushing's syndrome	Hyperparathyroidism
Adrenal insufficiency	Diabetes mellitus (type 1)	Thyrotoxicosis

Gastrointestinal Diseases

Celiac disease	Inflammatory bowel disease	Primary biliary cirrhosis
Gastrectomy	Malabsorption	

Hematologic Disorders

Hemophilia	Multiple myeloma	Systemic mastocytosis
Leukemia and lymphomas	Sickle-cell disease	Thalassemia

Rheumatic and Autoimmune Diseases

Ankylosing spondylitis	Lupus	Rheumatoid arthritis

Miscellaneous

Alcoholism	Emphysema	Multiple sclerosis
Amyloidosis	End-stage renal disease	Muscular dystrophy
Chronic metabolic acidosis	Epilepsy	Post-transplant bone disease
Congestive heart failure	Idiopathic scoliosis	Sarcoidosis
Depression	Immobilization	

Medications

Anticoagulants (heparin)	Glucocorticoids (and ACTH)	Methotrexate
Anticonvulsants	Gonadotropin-releasing hormone agonists	Parenteral nutrition
Cyclosporine A and Tacrolimus		Thyroxine
Cancer chemotherapeutic drugs	Lithium	

Reprinted from Office of the Surgeon General, 2004, *Bone health and osteoporosis: A report of the Surgeon General* (Rockville, MD: Office of the Surgeon General). Available: www.ncbi.nlm.nih.gov/books/NBK45513/

wrist (19%), hip (14%), pelvis (7%), and other (33%).[85] One's future fracture risk increases 2.5-fold after a fracture, while vertebral fractures are predictive of future fractures at other sites by 2- to 3-fold.[85] In clients aged 65 years and older in the United States, greater than 90% of hip fractures are the direct result of a fall.[85]

A comprehensive examination of the older client should also include measurements and observation of posture, height, thoracic kyphosis, and decreased spinal extensibility due to the correlation between vertebral compression fractures and osteoporosis. The presence and degree of thoracic kyphosis may limit a client's ability to complete functional tasks that require bending and reaching. Height measurements may be taken using a stadiometer, and the presence and degree of kyphosis can be measured using a flexicurve. A crude measure of the presence or absence of height loss due to osteoporosis-related vertebral compression fractures is the rib-to-pelvis distance using fingerbreadths. A distance of less than two fingerbreadths between the inferior margin of the ribs and the superior surface of the pelvis in the midaxillary line has been suggestive of indicating the presence of a vertebral compression fracture in clients with osteoporosis.[88] For additional detail on vertebral compression fractures, refer to chapter 18 (Thoracic Spine).

EXAMINATION OF BALANCE

One of the key assessments in the geriatric population is falls risk. One-third of people 65 and older fall each year, with one in five falls causing a serious injury such as head trauma or fracture.[89] Dozens of scales have been developed to address differing aspects of balance, gait, attention, and cognition in an attempt to assess and predict risk of falling. While these scales can be used to set baseline balance scores and assess for clinically meaningful change over time, a more frequent use of these tests is to determine whether the client's score lies above or below a certain cutoff point (or range) within the scale that has been determined to be predictive of falls risk. The majority of these scales are in use for a variety of populations, including community elderly, nursing home residents, and those recovering from a variety of neurologic injuries.

Several factors must be considered in choosing the correct measure for a particular client or setting.

Correct interpretation of a client's results requires an understanding of the population on which the measure has been tested and validated. Cutoff scores for fall prediction can vary on the same scale depending on the population. For example, using the Dynamic Gait Index, cutoff scores (out of a maximum of 24) for increased falls risk were below 19, 16, and 12 points, for community elderly,[90] multiple sclerosis,[91] and Parkinson's disease,[92] respectively. The majority of the measures listed in tables 28.2 and 28.3 have been tested in populations such as post-CVA or vestibular disorders; the results from those populations should specifically be applied only to those populations and not to community elderly in general. The measures presented are included here because data exist to guide interpretation of scores for falls risk of those most likely to be seen in an outpatient orthopedic setting: community elderly with no specific comorbidities. References are provided to assist with guidance on score interpretation for alternate populations.

Another concern in choosing a measure is understanding the requirements of the test and the goal of the assessment. For example, the Timed Up and Go, 10-Meter Walk, 5 Times Sit to Stand, and Functional Reach Test can all be administered in less than 1 minute, and may be appropriate for a community screening event or as part of a general medical screening examination. If more specific information is required, such as details of gait or cognitive status, tests such as the Functional Gait Assessment or Dual-Task Timed Up and Go, respectively, may be more appropriate.

A related concern is a concept of ceiling effects, in which a test may not have sufficient range to identify those who are still at risk of falls. In this case, a large proportion of community elderly may score at the top of the scale, resulting in an inability to identify improvements in those scoring at or near the top of the scale at baseline, as well as to discriminate fallers in this population. As described previously, cutoff points for falls in community elderly may be higher than in other populations, and in some cases the scale may not be able to identify a potential faller who presents to a standard outpatient clinic. Table 28.4 provides a general understanding of the activities involved in common balance screens; activities at the top of the scale are easier, becoming progressively more difficult as they reach the bottom. In some cases, a stepped assessment may be useful. For example, if the goal is to assess a client's gait, the

TABLE 28.2 Physical Performance Balance Measures

Measure	Purpose	Cutoff for increased falls risk in community elderly	Maximum score	SN/SP	Study prevalence	95% CI of post-test probability with (+) test	Client demographics
Four-Step Square Test	Clinically assesses the person's ability to change directions while stepping	15 s	NR	85/88	0.33 (27/81)	0.58–0.88	Community elderly >65[95]
Berg Balance Scale	Assess static balance and fall risk in adult populations	History of falls: ≤51 No history of falls: ≤42	56	91/82	0.50 (22/44)	0.64–0.93	Community elderly, average age 76.5[96]
Short-Form Berg Balance Scale	Assess static and dynamic balance and fall risk in adult and geriatric population	<23	28	NA[97]			
Dynamic Gait Index	Assesses client's ability to modify balance while walking in the presence of external demands	<19	24	59/64	0.50 (22/44)	0.40–0.79	Community elderly > 65[96]
Functional Gait Assessment	Assesses postural stability during various walking tasks	<22	30	100/76	0.49 (17/35)	0.59–0.92	Community elderly (60-90)[98]
10 m walk test	Assesses walking speed in meters per second over a short duration	>0.8 m/s for community ambulation >1.2 m/s required to cross street	NR[99]				
Timed Up and Go	Assesses mobility, balance, walking ability, and fall risk in older adults	≥13.5 s	NR	80/100	0.50 (15/30)	0.75–1.0	Community elderly (mean age 78)[100]
Clinical Test of Sensory Interaction and Balance	Assesses client's balance under a variety of conditions to infer the source of instability	Composite score <260 s Average score <81 s in compliant surface conditions	NR	44/90 Age-adjusted odds ratio 8.67	0.52 (16/31)	0.44–0.93	Community elderly (mean age 80.5)[101]

(continued)

Table 28.2 *(continued)*

Measure	Purpose	Cutoff for increased falls risk in community elderly	Maximum score	SN/SP	Study prevalence	95% CI of post-test probability with (+) test	Client demographics
Functional Reach Test	Assesses a patient's stability by measuring the maximum distance a client can reach forward while standing in a fixed position	<7 in. (18 cm)	NR	NA			Community elderly (mean age 78)[102]
Community Balance and Mobility Scale	Used to detect high-level balance and mobility deficits based on tasks that are commonly encountered in community environments	Not established Mean 60-69: 65 Mean 70-79: 50	85	NA[103]			
Five Times Sit to Stand Test	A measure of functional lower limb muscle strength	>12 s	NR	66/55	0.22 (80/362)	0.23–0.36	Community elderly (mean age 80.4)[104]
Tinetti Performance-Oriented Mobility Assessment	Measure balance (including fall risk) and gait function in elderly: total, balance, and gait	POMA-T < 19 POMA-B < 10 POMA-G < 9	Total = 32 Balance = 18 Gait = 14	64/66 64/66 64/63	0.31 (25/81)	0.30–0.62 0.30–0.62 0.28–0.59	Community elderly (mean age 84.9)[105]
Dual-Task Timed Up and Go	A dual-task dynamic measure for identifying clients who are at risk for falls. Clients are asked to complete the test while counting backward by threes from a randomly selected number between 20 and 100.	≥15 s	NR	80/93	0.50 (15/30)	0.66–0.98	Community elderly (mean age 78)[100]

Measure	Purpose	Cutoff for increased falls risk in community elderly	Maximum score	SN/SP	Study prevalence	95% CI of post-test probability with (+) test	Client demographics
Fullerton Advanced Balance Scale	Test of both static and dynamic balance under varying sensory conditions; measures balance in higher-functioning active older adults	<25	40	75/53	0.31 (59/192)	0.32–0.50	Community elderly (mean age 77)[106]
Walking While Talking	To predict falls by way of a divided attention task during walking WWT-simple: walking while reciting the alphabet aloud WWT-complex: walking while reciting alternate letters of the alphabet aloud	≥20 s for WWT-simple ≥33 s for WWT-complex	NR	46/89 39/96	0.22 (13/60)	0.26–0.78 0.34–0.91	Community-dwelling elderly without dementia (mean age 80)[107]
Physical Performance Test	Multiple domains of physical function using observed performance of tasks that simulate activities of daily living of various degrees of difficulty in elderly persons	32-36 = not frail 25-32 = mild frailty 17-24 = moderate frailty <17 = unlikely to be able to function in the community	36	NA[108]			

CI = confidence intervals; NA = not applicable; SN = sensitivity; SP = specificity; NR = not reported

TABLE 28.3 Self-Report Balance Measures

Measure	Purpose	Cutoff for increased falls risk in community elderly	Maximum score	SN/SP	Study prevalence	95% CI of post-test probability with (+) test	Client demographics
Tinetti Falls Efficacy Scale	Assesses perception of balance and stability during activities of daily living Assesses fear of falling in the elderly population	>80	100	NR[109]	------	------	Volunteer community sample
Activity-Specific Balance Confidence Scale	Subjective measure of confidence in performing various ambulatory activities without falling	<67	100	84/88	0.36 (45/125)	0.65–0.88	Community elderly[110]

CI = confidence interval; NR = not reported; SN = sensitivity; SP = specificity

clinician may start with a measure such as the Tinetti Performance-Oriented Mobility Assessment, which is a very quick (~3 min) screen that has known ceiling effects. If the client scores at the top of the scale, the clinician can utilize a more challenging tool such as the Dynamic Gait Index, on which the client is less likely to score at the top of the scale, and therefore has more potential to demonstrate responsiveness, recording changes in balance over time.

A final caveat lies in the interpretation of the score itself. An ideal measure would have 100% diagnostic accuracy for predicting fallers with a single cutoff point. In this ideal situation, everyone who falls would score below the determined cutoff point, while all non-fallers would score above the same cutoff point. In reality, there is often a fair amount of overlap in scores between the groups of fallers and non-fallers. To better understand the post-test probability of falling based on a particular score relative to the established cutoff, clinicians are encouraged to become familiar with the concepts of population prevalence, diagnostic accuracy, and positive and negative likelihood ratios as discussed in previous chapters. The precision of the point estimate of the post-test probability of risk of falling is influenced by the sample size of the study assessing the balance measure. Table 28.2 contains information regarding diagnostic accuracy, sample size, and fall prevalence in the referenced study. Each of these influences the confidence interval of the post-test probability, provided in column 7.

While most of the measures used to assess falls risk involve physical performance measures where the client's abilities are directly tested by the clinician (table 28.2), self-report measures have also been developed (table 28.3). These often address similar constructs to the physical performance measures. They have been validated in identifying those at risk of falling, and they may be particularly useful for large population screens.

Given the challenges to diagnostic accuracy with any single falls risk tool, as well as the structural

TABLE 28.4 Components of Common Balance Assessments

	Tinetti	5 × sit-to-stand	TUG	Short physical performance battery	Berg	Physical performance	Dynamic gait	Functional assessment	BEST test	10 m walk	6 min walk
Postural observation									X		
Write a sentence						X					
Simulated eating						X					
Sitting balance	X				X						
Standing/sitting	X	X	X	X	X				X		
Standing balance	X				X				X		
Hip strength									X		
Ankle strength									X		
Lift book and put it on a shelf						X					
Transfer					X						
Put on and remove a jacket						X					
Perturbations	X								X		
Stand with eyes closed	X				X				X		
Stand with feet together				X	X				X		
Reach with outstretched arm					X				X		
Pick up object from floor					X	X					
Turn to look over shoulder					X	X					
Turn 360°	X				X	X					
Turn around while walking			X	X					X		
Place foot on stool					X				X		
Change in gait speed							X	X	X		

(continued)

Table 28.4 *(continued)*

	Tinetti	5 × sit-to-stand	TUG	Short physical performance battery	Berg	Physical performance	Dynamic gait	Functional assessment	BEST test	10 m walk	6 min walk
Stand with one foot in front of the other				X	X						
Stand on one foot					X				X		
Stairs						X	X	X			
Floor-to-stand transfer									X		
Stand on foam									X		
Inclined standing									X		
Gait with horizontal head turns							X	X	X		
Gait with vertical head turns							X	X			
Gait with rapid pivot turn							X	X	X		
Step over obstacle							X	X	X		
Step around obstacle							X				
Gait with narrow base of support								X			
Gait with eyes closed								X			
Timed up and go with counting									X		
Ambulate backwards								X			
Stand on foam, eyes closed									X		
Gait evaluation	X						X	X			
Walking speed			X	X		X	X	X	X	X	X
Endurance		X		X		X			X		X

Critical Clinical Pearls

Things to consider before choosing a balance-related outcome measure:

- Determine if a physical performance or a self-report measure should be utilized.
- Understand what population the outcome measure was validated for.
- Understand requirements of the test and the goal of the assessment to limit ceiling effects.
- Understand the diagnostic properties of the test.

---

challenges of screening large populations, a combination of self-report and physical performance testing may be ideal for most accurately capturing an elderly person's risk of falling. The Center for Disease control has created the STEADI program, which utilizes an algorithm[93] involving a client questionnaire, specific clinical questions, and three physical performance tests to assist with determination of falls risk. Readers are encouraged to visit the STEADI Tool Kit website[94] for more information about this algorithm.

Because measures related to falls are frequently developed, validated, and updated, clinicians are recommended to utilize dedicated websites such as www.rehabmeasures.org, www.strokengine.ca, and www.PTNow.org (APTA subscription required to access specific information about individual measures on www.PTNow.org) to remain abreast of the most current status of the various available tools. These sites utilize slightly different search strategies and present slightly different content related to the key properties of each measure. Information on all of the measures listed in tables 28.2 and 28.3, including diagnostic accuracy for specific populations, can be found there in greater detail.

CONCLUSION

The geriatric client examination can be considered fairly complex with the multitude of comorbidities and age-related changes that can occur throughout life. Proper understanding of these age-related changes is paramount for optimal examination of a geriatric client. Understanding of the physiological responses that the body can have on aging and the effect of medication management on the geriatric client is of most importance. Time should be taken to thoroughly evaluate a geriatric client due to the multifactorial nature of orthopedic diagnosis.

PEDIATRIC EXAMINATION

Dora J. Gosselin, PT, DPT, PCS, C/NDT

Musculoskeletal pain complaints were the reason for 25.7% to 36.1% of primary care visits for children aged 14.[1] As physical therapists expand their roles as practitioners of health and wellness, clinicians who may not consider themselves pediatric therapists will likely gain more experience with evaluating, and possibly treating, children with musculoskeletal pathology.

The goal of this chapter is to provide information about common musculoskeletal disorders in children and to suggest strategies for examination. While children are not small adults, many examination techniques used in the adult population are appropriate, some requiring modifications, in the pediatric population.

CHILD'S MUSCULOSKELETAL SYSTEM

Transitioning to the area of pediatric musculoskeletal assessment brings a few particular challenges. First, children are generally less able to provide specific descriptions of their injury, their pain (type and exact location), and aggravating and alleviating factors. Second, the majority of a child's life occurs in tandem with a maturing and changing musculoskeletal system. Girls are generally skeletally mature around 15 years of age, while boys generally complete their skeletal development 2 or 3 years later.[2, 3] Growth and change provide unique considerations in a pediatric client's examination, prognosis, and intervention. Clinicians who are consistently working with skeletally immature girls and boys must be keenly aware of typical multisystem developmental changes through puberty. Last, but certainly not least, is that reliability of examination can be difficult when a child does not understand specific directions or is scared to interact with a new face. Clinicians have a variety of ways to make examination kid-centric. When examination occurs in the setting of a very upset child or a child who is not interactive, the clinician must closely assess the validity of findings. Children enjoy showing far more than following. For example, if the clinician needs to see if a child is able to bear weight on an extremity, the clinician can ask them to pretend to kick a soccer ball rather than asking them if they can stand on one leg.

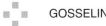

Critical Clinical Pearls

Children are not just small adults.

- Their musculoskeletal system is immature and changing.
- They may have difficulty accurately identifying precipitating and alleviating factors of pain and dysfunction.
- They are susceptible to unique disorders of the musculoskeletal system.

MULTISYSTEM PATHOLOGIES

A subset of pathologies that could primarily present as musculoskeletal may have multisystem etiologies. This section reviews the most common multisystem pathologies affecting the pediatric client. It discusses examination of children with juvenile idiopathic arthritis, muscular dystrophies, and inherited disorders of connective tissue.

Juvenile Idiopathic Arthritis

A variety of rheumatologic diseases may affect the pediatric client. Arthritic conditions are some of the most common chronic diseases of childhood, afflicting between 6.6 and 15 per 100,000 children.[4] The International League of Associations for Rheumatology (ILAR) describes seven classifications of the most common type of arthritis in children, juvenile idiopathic arthritis (JIA).[5] Consistent within the subtypes of JIA is that the symptoms present before 16 years of age, persist for longer than six weeks, and are of unknown origin. The most common subtype of JIA is oligoarthritis, which affects nearly 50% of all children with JIA.[4]

Other subtypes include systemic, rheumatoid factor positive polyarthritis, rheumatoid factor negative polyarthritis, enthesitis-related arthritis, psoriatic arthritis, and undifferentiated arthritis (table 29.1). Other less common arthritic conditions in children include juvenile dermatomyositis, juvenile spondyloarthropathies, childhood lupus, and scleroderma.

JIA should be considered when children under the age of 16 present with greater than six weeks of joint pain. Of significance is that the joint pain often does not have an identifiable cause. Disease presentation is dependent on the type and severity of disease. Primary clinical findings range from musculoskeletal impairments to visual impairments. Secondary impairments are common and include decreased joint range of motion (ROM), osteopenia, and osteoporosis due to chronic steroid use and fatigue. Limitations in activities of daily living and difficulty with participation are common. Within each of the seven types of JIA, there are clinical criteria for diagnosis that include the number of joints involved, which joints are involved, and other systemic manifestations (table 29.2).

Numerous outcome assessments are available to use with this patient population. Many address system-level impairments, for example, ROM and strength. Gait assessment, endurance measures,

TABLE 29.1 Presentations of Juvenile Idiopathic Arthritis

Type of JIA	Age of onset	Gender
Systemic arthritis	Throughout childhood	50% male, 50% female
Oligoarthritis	Early childhood	Mostly female
RF+ polyarthritis	Late childhood or adolescence	Mostly female
RF– polyarthritis	Early peak 2-4 yr; later peak 6-12 yr	Mostly female
Enthesitis-related arthritis	Late childhood or adolescence	Mostly male
Psoriatic arthritis	Early peak 2-4 yr; later peak 9-11 yr	Female slightly more

TABLE 29.2   Diagnostic Criteria for Juvenile Idiopathic Arthritis

Type of JIA	Diagnostic criteria
Systemic arthritis	Pain in one or more joints with a fever for at least 2 weeks duration and one or more of the following: erythematous rash, lymph node enlargement, hepatomegaly, or splenomegaly or serositis.
Oligoarthritis	Pain in 1-4 joints during the first 6 months of the disease.
RF+/RF− polyarthritis	Pain in 5 or more joints during the first 6 months of the disease.
Enthesitis-related arthritis	Arthritis and enthesitis or arthritis or enthesitis with at least two of the following: history of sacroiliac joint or lumbar pain, +HLA-B27 antigen, onset in boy over 6 years of age, acute uveitis, or a positive related history in a first-degree relative.
Psoriatic arthritis	Arthritis and psoriasis or arthritis and at least two of the following: dactylitis, nail pitting, or psoriasis in a first-degree relative.

and pain levels are also important portions of the examination.

Muscular Dystrophy

Neuromuscular diseases include those of the motor neuron, neuromuscular junction, and muscle. The most common neuromuscular diseases in children are muscular dystrophy (MD) and spinal muscular atrophy (SMA). In the pediatric setting, clinicians are likely quite astute at identifying the early signs of MD and SMA; however, in a general outpatient setting, all clinicians must be able to identify the early signs of these progressive and devastating diseases. If there is a concern about potential progressive neuromuscular diseases, the child must be referred back to the physician for further testing.

Duchenne muscular dystrophy (DMD) is the most common form of MD, affecting 1 in 3,500 live male births.[6] DMD is an X-linked genetic disorder, thereby almost exclusively affecting only boys. Boys usually receive a diagnosis of DMD by 5 years of age. The loss of walking usually occurs between 8 and 12 years of age, although this is variable. The life expectancy of boys with DMD is increasing due to improved medical management, and many men are living into their mid- to late 20s.[7, 8] Respiratory disease is almost always the cause of death in DMD. Becker muscular dystrophy (BMD) is the second most common type of MD with an incidence of 1 in 20,000 births. The life expectancy of men with BMD is into the 40s, and death is most commonly due to dilated cardiomyopathy.[9] Both DMD and BMD are the result of a missing or defective protein, dystrophin, which is responsible for protecting muscle fibers from injury as muscles contract and relax.

With the exception of cystic fibrosis, SMA is the most common fatal autosomal recessive disease in childhood.[10] SMA occurs when the cells in the anterior horn of the spinal cord are reduced in number and experience progressive degeneration, resulting in progressive weakness and loss of function. SMA is categorized into four presentations according to time of onset and severity. Generally the more severe and earlier identifiable forms, Types I and II, are diagnosed within the first few months of life. They would rarely be encountered sans diagnosis in an outpatient setting. Type IV is adult-onset. Type III generally presents between 5 and 10 years of age and would be much more likely to be undiagnosed in its earliest stages.

Clumsiness and delayed gross motor skills are common early indications of neuromuscular disease in children. A variety of clinical presentations exist that also may confirm or refute the presence of a neuromuscular disease. Early clinical signs and symptoms of DMD include, but are not limited to, head lag when the child is pulled to sitting position, inability to hop and jump, difficulty running, and a positive Gower's maneuver (pushing on thighs to assume an upright standing position). Gait is characterized by an anterior pelvic tilt, lumbar lordosis, excessive frontal plane motion of the trunk during gait, and an outward foot progression angle. Toe walking may also be present in some children. Pseudohypertrophy of the gastrocnemius muscle is a common clinical finding.

Children and parents often report fatigue that is significant compared to age-matched peers.[11] Later signs and symptoms include significant weakness with compensatory movement patterns, as well as decreasing independence. Respiratory assessment in the clinic may include rib cage expansion and incentive spirometry. Screening for or assessment of scoliosis should be frequent.

Many other, less common types of muscular dystrophy exist, as well as other neuromuscular diseases that present in childhood. As a general rule, when seeing a pediatric client, if a child is not making progress with intervention or if their gross motor skills are falling further behind age-matched peers, neuromuscular disease should be ruled out.

Obesity

In the United States, obesity is a leading chronic pediatric disorder. Musculoskeletal impairments, along with other well-known multisystemic complications, are well documented in adults who are obese. According to data from the Centers for Disease Control and prevention (CDC), in 2011 to 2012, 8.4% of 2- to 5-year-olds were obese compared with 17.7% of 6- to 11-year-olds and 20.5% of 12- to 19-year-olds.[12] With the increasing prevalence of childhood overweightedness and obesity, more focus has been given to the effects of increased weight on immature body systems. Common musculoskeletal impairments in children who are obese are malalignment of the lower extremity,[13] slipped capital femoral epiphysis,[14] Blount's disease,[13] and increased fracture risk.[15] A 2014 review found that chronic pain and a reduction in physical activity likely contribute to the cycle of weight gain and increasing disability that obese children experience.[16]

Calculation of body mass index (BMI) for children and adolescents and adults is the same; however, the interpretation of the BMI is different between the two groups. The BMI of children and adolescents is assessed as a percentile representative of the BMI for age, which is specific for a child's age and sex. Children and adolescents are considered to be underweight if their BMI for age is less than the 5th percentile. Children and adolescents with BMI for age between the 5th and 85th percentiles are considered to be a healthy weight. Children and adolescents with a BMI between the 85th and 95th percentiles are considered overweight, and those with a BMI for age above the 95th percentile are obese. Growth charts and a BMI calculator for children and adolescents are available at the CDC website.

Inherited Connective Tissue Disorders

Common heritable disorders of connective tissue in children include Marfan syndrome (MS), Ehler-Danlos syndrome (EDS), and osteogenesis imperfecta (OI). While it may be rare that a clinician working with a mainly adult population encounters a child with one of these disorders, having knowledge of the clinical features of each is essential. MS is a disorder that involves abnormalities in fibrillin. Fibrillin is vital for the integrity of connective tissue. MS affects about 1 in every 5,000 people.[17] Common musculoskeletal findings in MS are extraordinarily long extremities, pes planus, malalignment of the spine (scoliosis and kyphosis), and deformity of the chest wall.[17, 18] While the outward presentation of the musculoskeletal impairments may be quite evident, other systemic complications may be life threatening, including common cardiac anomalies: mitral valve prolapse and increased risk for aortic aneurysm and aortic dissection.

EDS is a disorder of collagen that is as common as MS, affecting 1 in 5,000 people.[17] A combination of impairments in the integumentary system (increased skin extensibility, tendency to bruise easily, poor wound healing, and hypertrophic scarring) and the musculoskeletal system (mainly joint hypermobility) may lead a clinician to consider EDS in the differential diagnosis.[17] Refer to chapter 8 (Range of Motion Assessment) for detail on the Beighton scale for generalized ligamentous laxity.

OI is a less common collagen disorder that affects between 25,000 and 50,000 people in the United States.[19] The deficiency is in the synthesis or structure of Type I collagen. While many classes of OI are severe and identifiable in utero or at birth, Type I OI, the most common type, is not associated with deformity or severe medical complications. People with Type I OI rarely have identified fractures at birth, and may reach nearly normal height. Clinical findings may include a mild scoliosis due to vertebral fractures as well as blue sclera. Most fractures in people with this most mild form of OI occur during childhood and adolescence and decrease after puberty.

With the increasing emphasis on client-centered goals and functional and participation outcomes, clinicians should consider using a measure of physical function or performance for children with chronic illnesses. See table 29.3 for common pediatric quality-of-life assessments.

PATHOLOGIES OF THE SPINE

Pathology in the immature and developing spine has a variety of causes. Nearly all pathologies fit into one of the following categories: congenital, acquired idiopathic, acquired positional, or progressive changes. Knowledge of the changes that spinal structures undergo from the early embryological period through adolescence is critical for understanding and examining pathologies of the spine in children. During the first weeks of pregnancy, mesodermal tissue proliferates to form 29 pairs of somites. Somites then differentiate further, and eventually sclerotomal cells produce early vertebral structures that will ossify during the fetal period and after birth to create the mature portions of the spine: the cervical spine, thoracic spine, lumbar spine, sacrum, and coccyx. The spine of a child born full-term is flexed. Through typical movement experiences and selective and coordinated recruitment of muscles, the development of cervical and lumbar lordosis occurs. Growth of the spine occurs through adolescence. A significant increase in growth occurs in conjunction with puberty. Girls experience this growth between the ages of 8 and 14, whereas boys generally experience it between 11 and 16 years of age.

Kyphosis

Kyphosis is a posterior convexity of a spinal segment. A normal adult value of thoracic kyphosis is 20° to 40°. Spinal kyphoses can occur in children with a variety of disorders that are not primarily problems of the musculoskeletal system, for example, in children with a myelomeningocele. Congenital kyphosis occurs when the structure of the anterior portion of the thoracic vertebrae is atypical.[20] Scheuermann's disease is the most common kyphosis in adolescents and typically occurs just before or in tandem with puberty.[21]

While kyphosis is often the result of a problem on the anterior portion of the vertebrae, lordosis, an anterior convexity of the spine, can be caused by structural failure or anomaly of the posterior portion of the vertebrae. As mentioned previously, lordosis of the lumbar spine is common in children with neuromuscular problems.

A thorough and systematic postural assessment—anterior and posterior and lateral—must be conducted. Asymmetries should be documented and quantified, when possible.

Spinal cord compression and resultant neurological impairments occur in about 10% of children with kyphosis. Most children with neurological impairment demonstrate an apex at the mid or lower thoracic region.[20] Examination must include a complete and accurate upper motor neuron screening.

A definite diagnosis of Scheuermann's disease is based on radiography. Plain films of the thoracic spine will demonstrate irregular vertebral

TABLE 29.3 Pediatric Quality-of-Life Assessments

Measure	Ages (yr)	Description
Pediatric Quality of Life Inventory (PedsQL)	2-18 (4 age groups)	Physical, emotional, school functioning
KINDL	4-16 (2 age groups)	Physical and psychological well-being, self-esteem, family and social functioning
KIDSCREEN-52	8-18	Physical and psychological well-being, moods and emotion, self-perception, autonomy, parent relationship and home life, social support and peers, social acceptance and bullying, school environment, financial resources
Child Health and Illness Profile (CHIP)	6-17 (2 age groups)	Satisfaction, comfort, resilience, risk avoidance, achievement

Data from K. Kenzik, S. Tuli, D. Revicki, et al. Comparison of four pediatric health-related quality-of-life instruments: A study on a Medicaid population. *Medical Decision Making.* 2014; DOI: 10.1177/0272989X14529846.

end plates, narrowing of the disc space between the vertebrae, anterior wedging of 5° for three or more consecutive vertebrae, and a kyphosis of greater than 40° that is uncorrected with active hyperextension. In the clinic, clinicians can determine whether or not there is any correction in the kyphotic curve by asking the client to actively extend their spine while in prone.

Flexibility and strength assessments in most children with kyphosis will demonstrate tight anterior chest musculature with overlengthened and weak dorsal musculature. Refer to chapters 18 (Thoracic Spine) and 19 (Lumbar Spine) for greater detail on examination of Scheuermann's disease, scoliosis, kyphosis, and lordosis.

Scoliosis

Scoliosis is a multiplanar deformity of the spine and is defined by a curvature of greater than 10°. Scoliosis can be broadly classified into two groups: idiopathic and nonidiopathic. The incidence of idiopathic scoliosis is 0.47% to 5.2%.[22] Girls are more likely than boys to have idiopathic scoliosis, and the severity of curves in girls is more than those in boys.[22] Nonidiopathic scoliosis includes congenital scoliosis, neuromuscular scoliosis, and mesenchymal scoliosis. Congenital scoliosis can result from atypical formation or growth of vertebrae. Neuromuscular scoliosis is a secondary impairment resulting from some type of neuromuscular disease. The highest rates of neuromuscular scoliosis occur in muscular dystrophies, myelomeningocele, and cerebral palsy. Mesenchymal scoliosis is the result of insufficiency of the passive tissue stabilizers of the spine, and occurs as a secondary impairment of connective tissue disorders like osteogenesis imperfecta and Marfan syndrome.[22]

Regardless of the etiology of the child's scoliosis, examination should begin with a big-picture observation of asymmetries of the trunk, shoulder, and pelvis. Children with asymmetry should be referred for a baseline orthopedic evaluation. The gold standard for quantifying scoliosis is the Cobb method, by which an anterior–posterior or posterior–anterior coronal plane spinal radiograph is used to quantify the amount of scoliotic curvature.[23] A systematic standing postural examination should be followed by the Adam's forward bend test (AFBT). When performing the AFBT, the clinician should instruct the client to place their feet shoulder-width apart, extend their arms with the hands placed together, and bend forward slowly. The AFBT is positive if the clinician observes a rib hump.[24] The rib hump forms on the side of the convexity as a result of the rib's articulation with the vertebrae. A scoliometer can be used to measure the amount of asymmetry. The reliability of scoliometric data for outcomes measures is in question, however. For examination and quantification of baseline asymmetry, a scoliometer may be a helpful tool.

In addition to the previously mentioned assessments, other more conventional examinations of posture should be completed in children with scoliosis or with suspected scoliosis. These measurements should include quantification of asymmetries, including leg-length measurement.[25, 26] As with any pathology of the spine, assessments for changes in bowel and bladder function as well as sensory and strength testing should be thorough.

Congenital Muscular Torticollis

Congenital muscular torticollis (CMT) is a common postural deformity of the head and neck that is identifiable at birth or shortly after birth. The incidence of CMT has been reported between 0.3% and 1.9%;[27] however, recent data have shown it to be as high as 16%[28] in some newborns. Some hypothesize that the increase in CMT is due to the recommendation by the National Institute of Child Health and Human Development's 1994 Back to Sleep Campaign that all children sleep in supine as a way to try to decrease the incidence of sudden infant death syndrome.[29] Many theories exist about the etiology of CMT, including intrauterine positioning, birth trauma, and ischemia. CMT is generally classified as postural CMT, muscular CMT, or CMT related to fibrotic thickening of the sternocleidomastoid (SCM).[27, 29, 30, 31] The SCM has two major portions: the sternal head, which arises from the manubrium, and the clavicular head, which arises from the medial one-third of the clavicle. Both portions of the SCM attach to the mastoid process and, via a think aponeurosis, to the superior nuchal line of the occipital bone. Conditions associated with CMT include plagiocephaly, changes in the craniofacial structure, brachial plexus injury, and hip dysplasia.[27, 29-31]

Recently the American Physical Therapy Association's Section on Pediatrics published clinical practice guidelines for the physical therapy management of CMT.[31] The guidelines were developed after an extensive review of literature and survey of current clinical practices. With regard to examination, specific recommendations are made that include assessment of the infant's posture and tolerance in a variety of positions: passive and active cervical rotation and lateral flexion, passive and active range of motion of the upper and lower extremities, as well as an assessment of pain or discomfort at rest and during passive and active movement. There is an increased incidence of hip dysplasia in children with CMT. (For examination of hip dysplasia in infants, refer to the section Lower Extremity Pathology.) Furthermore the guidelines recommend that clinicians should observe skin integrity and skin folds, as well the sternocleidomastoid's mass, size, and shape.

Plagiocephaly coexists with CMT in up to 90% of children.[27] An examination of the child's craniofacial features must also be completed. The most common craniofacial anomalies in children with CMT include posterior position of the ipsilateral ear, posterior regression of the ipsilateral cheek and forehead, mandibular deviation toward the involved side, and an ipsilateral eye position that is lower compared to the contralateral side.

The Muscle Function Scale (MFS)[32] for torticollis is an ordinal visual scale that interprets an infant's righting responses. The MFS is easy and quick to administer. In front of a mirror, the infant is brought to the horizontal position. The head position is observed and given a score of 0 to 5 depending on the righting response. The MFS can also be used with objective measurements of degrees of head righting, and it is a valid tool to measure muscle function of the lateral neck flexors in infants (figure 29.1).

Critical to the outcome of torticollis are early identification and early intervention. The most significant gross motor delays occur in children with CMT under the age of 10 months.[33] Additionally, the ability for improvement or resolution of anomalies of craniofacial structures in children with CMT is correlated to early intervention.

Neural Tube Defects

Genetic, environmental, and nutritional factors, in some combination, are likely the cause of neural tube defects, which occur as the structures of the spine and cranium develop during the first month of pregnancy. While it would be impossible for an open NTD to go unnoticed, some NTDs are more subtle, hidden, or closed. These are less easily identifiable, and may be identified only if and when a person demonstrates difficulty or changes in their movement. A combination of changes in function

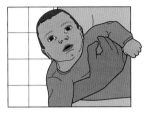

5. Head very high above the horizontal line, almost vertical position

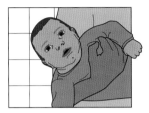

4. Head high above the horizontal line and more than 45°

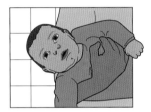

3. Head high above the horizontal line but below 45°

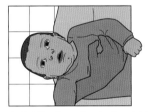

2. Head slightly above the horizontal line

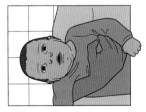

1. Head on the horizontal line

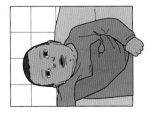

0. Head below the horizontal line

Figure 29.1 Muscle Function Scale.

and cutaneous findings may lead a clinician to consider an NTD as a differential diagnosis. A tethering of the spinal cord due to the skeletal abnormality may result in upper motor neuron signs, while peripheral nerve anomalies will result in atypical findings in a lower motor neuron assessment. Cutaneous findings that are associated with this type of NTD are a subcutaneous lipoma, a hairy patch, skin discoloration, and a hemangioma. If a clinician suspects an NTD as a cause for changing or loss of function in a child, they should immediately refer the child to a physician.

UPPER EXTREMITY PATHOLOGY

Neonates begin to use their upper extremities in a purposeful way almost immediately postnatally when they soothe themselves by sucking on their hands and fingers. Less than halfway through the first year of life, babies are purposefully reaching to interact with their environments. When children of any age experience a pathology involving their upper extremity, the functional consequences can be great. In this section discussion focuses on examination of three common pathologies: brachial plexus injuries, Little League elbow, and nursemaid's elbow.

Brachial Plexus Injury

Brachial plexus injuries (BPI) in children are common during birth. Birth weight greater than 7.7 lbs (3.5 kg), difficult delivery of the shoulder, breech delivery, prolonged labor, and maternal diabetes are all risk factors for an obstetric brachial plexus injury (OBPI). Other injuries of the neck and shoulder may result in BPI; however, examination would be similar between groups. Therefore, discussion in this section focuses on OBPI. The literature reports a range of incidences of OBPI between 1 and 4 per 1,000 births.[34] BPI are classified into three types, dependent on the root levels that are involved. The most common injury is to the C5 and C6 roots. Injury to the upper roots is termed Erb's palsy, and is characterized by impaired shoulder function with preservation of hand and wrist flexor function. Klumpke's palsy involves the lower roots of the brachial plexus, specifically C7-T1, and is characterized by intact shoulder and elbow function with loss of function more distal. Injury of the upper and lower roots is called Erb-Klumpke palsy. Dermatomal

sensory loss is also present in some capacity in most BPIs. Importantly, if a child suffers an avulsion of the T1 root, Horner's syndrome may occur. While Horner's syndrome occurs in less than 10%[35] of cases of OBPI, a variety of visual impairments may occur and must be managed. Most children with OBPI demonstrate some amount of spontaneous recovery within the first few months of life; however, those with persisting symptoms may have impairment and possible functional limitation throughout the life span.

As with any physical therapy examination, assessment should commence with a big-picture assessment to look grossly for symmetry of movements. Assessment of strength is a critical component of examination of a child with a BPI. In children with BPI, clinicians should use a variety of assessments, from observation of functional skills to manual muscle testing and dynamometry, to observe the strength in the involved upper extremity. Likewise, a combination of functional observation, estimation, and goniometric measurement can be used to examine the range of motion of the neck, shoulder, elbow, hand, and wrist of children with BPI. In addition to focusing on the affected upper extremity, clinicians must also assess the influence that the weakness or paralysis of that upper extremity has on the child's overall posture, gross motor skill acquisition, and symmetry of gross motor skill acquisition.

The Hospital for Sick Children proposed an Active Movement Scale (AMS)[36] for children with OBPI. The scale was created to identify small but meaningful changes in active upper extremity motion (table 29.4). The AMS has been found to have

TABLE 29.4 Hospital for Sick Children Active Movement Scale

Observation	Muscle grade
GRAVITY ELIMINATED	
No contraction	0
Contraction, no motion	1
Motion ≤ 50% range	2
Motion ≥ 50% range	3
Full motion	4
AGAINST GRAVITY	
Motion ≤ 50% range	5
Motion ≥ 50% range	6
Full motion	7

Based on H.M. Clarke and G.C. Curtis. An approach to obstetrical brachial plexus injuries. *Hand Clinics.* 1995;11(4):567.

nearly perfect intrarater reliability and excellent interrater reliability.[37] The Mallet classification of upper extremity function uses a 5-point scale (0, no movement to 5, full movement) to score five upper extremity movements: abduction, external rotation, hand to the nape of the neck, hand to back, and hand to mouth (figure 29.2). Both the intrarater and interobserver reliability of the Mallet classification are excellent.[37]

The strategy for sensory assessment of the involved extremity will be different depending on the age of the child being examined. For a younger child, the clinician will use various forms of touch

in different dermatomal areas to see if the child responds. Older children will be able to more accurately respond validly to typical dermatomal assessment of light touch sensation.

Little League Elbow

As mentioned in the introduction of this chapter, the possibility for physeal injuries in the immature musculoskeletal system presents unique considerations exclusive to children and adolescents. Little League elbow describes the separation of the medial epicondyle from the humerus due to the valgus

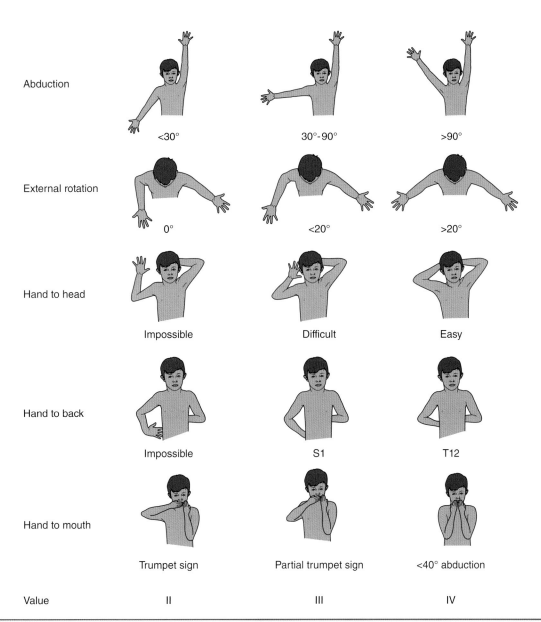

Abduction	<30°	30°-90°	>90°
External rotation	0°	<20°	>20°
Hand to head	Impossible	Difficult	Easy
Hand to back	Impossible	S1	T12
Hand to mouth	Trumpet sign	Partial trumpet sign	<40° abduction
Value	II	III	IV

Figure 29.2 Mallet classification.

stress that is placed on the epicondyles during the throwing motion. If throwing is not ceased, Little League elbow can develop into osteochondritis of the capitellum and possible avascular necrosis of the radial head. Little League elbow likely results from a combination of skeletal maturity, number of throws, and throwing mechanics.

The most commonly reported symptom of Little League elbow is pain in the inner elbow. This pain will be reported as coming on abruptly or increasing over time. In the clinic, pain can be recreated with the throwing motion.[38]

Nursemaid's Elbow

Nursemaid's elbow (NE) occurs when there is a subluxation of the radial head. The cause of NE is usually traction of the distal extremity, often when holding a child's hand and pulling them along while walking or lifting them up into the air by one or both hands. The annular ligament, which helps support the radial head in its articulation with the capitulum, is not fully developed and strong until the age of 5, so NE generally occurs in children under the age of 5. The movement of the radial head occurs as the ligament stretches, but generally does not tear.

A child with NE will likely be under the age of 5. Children will present with a slightly flexed elbow, held in some pronation. The child will likely want to support their involved extremity with the contralateral arm. Older children will report pain at the distal wrist. Reduction of the dislocation is generally completed quite easily and with a dramatic alleviation of symptoms; however, if the reduction is complete and the pain persists for more than 30 minutes, children should be seen by a physician for radiography to rule out a fracture or tear of the annular ligament.[39]

Fractures in the Upper Extremity

A British study found that about one-third of children experience fracture before the age of 17.[40] The most common upper extremity fractures in children occur at the distal radius and usually result from a fall on an outstretched arm. Other common upper extremity fractures in children include the distal humerus and proximal ulna and radius as well as the clavicle. Additionally, the presence of a proximal humeral fracture needs to be considered in any child with chronic or acute onset of shoulder pain without a mechanism of injury. As with any fracture, examination should include an assessment of pain and neurovascular status as well as an assessment of and management of swelling. Immobilization should be carried out with immediate referral to a physician.

LOWER EXTREMITY PATHOLOGY

The musculoskeletal system evolves and changes in utero but also changes dramatically during childhood and then more slowly toward adolescence. Fetal alignment of the lower extremity differs from that of an adult in a number of ways. Diverse and frequent movement experiences with typical muscle recruitment patterns and introduction of forces to bones must occur for fetal alignment to become typical, mature lower-extremity alignment (see table 29.5 for a brief overview of skeletal changes in the lower extremity).

Bipedal gait is important for function and participation in one's world. Moreover, it is a symbol of system maturation, more specifically, multisystem

Critical Clinical Pearls

When examining a child with a complaint of dorsal wrist pain, clinicians should do the following:

- Examine all of the articulations at the elbow and wrist thoroughly.
- Consider a fracture of the distal radius, which is the most common fracture in children.
- Rule out nursemaid's elbow (a subluxation of the radial head).

TABLE 29.5 Changes in Skeletal Alignment With Maturation

	Neonate	Childhood trend	Adulthood/mature
Hip	Anteversion: 60°	Decreasing anteversion	
	Antetorsion: 30°	Decreasing antetorsion	12° anteversion/torsion
	Coxa valga	Less valgum	Coxa vara
Knee	Varus	1-2 yr: straight	Female: slight valgus
		2-4 yr: valgum	Male: slight varus
Leg	Tibial internal torsion	Decreasing IR	20° external torsion
	Tibial varum (bowing)	Decreasing varum (bowing)	Aligned

Data from M. Tachdjian, 1972, *Pediatric orthopedics,* Volume 2. (Philadelphia: Saunders); S. Campbell, R. Palisano, and N. Orlin, 2012, *Physical therapy for children,* 4th ed. (St. Louis: Elsevier).

integration. Babies are more often referred to as children once they walk, and parents scramble to document the first steps that their little one takes. This chapter does not discuss the development of gait through pregait movement and experiences because it is almost exclusively within the domain of pediatric physical therapy. However, changes in gait that define immature and mature gait are important for all clinicians to know.

The mean age for the onset of independent walking (defined as taking a minimum of five unaided steps) is 13 months.[41] Gait in the new walker is characterized by a wide base of support, excessive trunk movement, and arms held in high guard— all strategies for inventing stability in an unstable system.[42, 43] New walkers also demonstrate high cadence and do not demonstrate heel strike. In general, the kinematic and kinetic variables of gait are adultlike by 7 years of age.[42] Gait assessment in children can be challenging. Children's gait is more variable than adult gait. Clinicians may develop the most accurate gait assessment by using one of the many readily available devices that has video capabilities.

Hip Dysplasia

Developmental dysplasia of the hip (DDH) describes any anomaly of the femoral head, acetabulum, or articulation between the femoral head and acetabulum. A distinction must be made between a hip that is dislocated, dislocatable, subluxed, or subluxable. Clinicians must also be aware that DDH is present at birth and is different from the atypical hip development that may occur in some diseases, for example, cerebral palsy. DDH occurs in approximately 1 per 100 live births. In comparison, dislocated hips are present in 1 in 1,000 births. Significant risk factors for DDH include being female, a breech uterine position, and genetic factors.[44]

Development of a mature hip joint begins in utero and relies on normal differentiation of the mesenchymal tissue during the first trimester. The architecture of the joint is dependent on the relationship of the femoral head and acetabulum of the pelvis in utero, in infancy, and during upright weight-bearing activities. Early detection of DDH is critical so that structural alignment between the femoral head and acetabulum can be provided as early as possible.

Clinical signs and symptoms of DDH are a crucial component of newborn examination. The Galeazzi sign is assessed with the infant in supine. The clinician flexes the hips and knees to 90°. The Galeazzi sign is considered to be positive if the knee on the dislocated side appears to be lower than the one on the intact side. The Galeazzi sign is not valid on children with bilateral DDH, and other confirmatory clinical examinations should accompany it.[44]

The clinician should assess the symmetry of the gluteal and thigh folds. Although a finding of asymmetric folds may be a false positive, in the setting of other positive tests, it may add to body of evidence to support or refute the diagnosis.

Normal hip abduction range in a neonate is between 60° and 80°. There has been some thought that all infants, despite their age, with less than 60° of hip abduction may have DDH; however, a recent article has suggested that this measurement is less accurate prior to 8 weeks of age, but after 8 weeks of age a finding of limited hip abduction should warrant further imaging.[45]

The Ortolani and Barlow maneuvers are dynamic assessments of hip stability. The Ortolani test is to detect dislocated hips that can be relocated. It is performed with an infant in supine and with their contralateral hip stabilized. The clinician flexes the infant's hips to 90° and then abducts the thigh while maintaining a finger over the great trochanter. A clunking sound is a sign of a positive test. The clunk is the result of the femoral head moving over the posterior rim of the acetabulum and the hip relocating as the femoral head is brought into approximation with the acetabulum.

The Barlow test differs from the Ortolani because it identifies an unstable hip that would likely demonstrate a negative Ortolani test. The infant is also in supine for the Barlow test. During this test the clinician moves the infant's hip from a position of 90° of flexion and hip abduction toward hip adduction with a simultaneous posterior direction of pressure. A positive test occurs if the clinician feels the unstable hip sliding over the posterior rim of the acetabulum as they provide a compressive force posteriorly.

The aforementioned assessments are appropriate for children under the age of 4 months. While the previously discussed findings should be collaborated by imaging, older infants and children may have negative tests but abnormal movement. Screening for DDH in older children should include radiography, not ultrasounds, as well as a gait assessment in ambulatory children. Gait in children with DDH can be characterized by a number of atypical findings, including toe walking on the involved side and increased frontal plane movement of the pelvis and hip.

Other Common Conditions of the Hip

Other common conditions of the hip joint in children are Legg-Calvé-Perthes disease (LCP), transient synovitis (TS), and slipped capital femoral epiphysis (SCFE). See table 29.6 for a comparison of these conditions.

LCP is the result of necrosis of the center of the ossification site of the femoral head, and it usually occurs in children, usually boys, between the ages of 4 and 8. Signs and symptoms of LCP include limping and intermittent pain in the groin, hip, or knee. Range of motion will be limited in abduction and internal rotation. Early identification of LCP is critical for a successful outcome.[46]

TS must be immediately differentiated from septic arthritis (SA; discussed in the next section). TS is most common in children under the age of 10 and afflicts boys more often than girls. Clinical findings include a limp or pain with weight bearing, limited motion, and joint effusion. Laboratory findings may also be abnormal and will be the deciding factor in differentiating TS and SA. Because of the common presentation of TS and SA, if clinicians suspect TS, they must refer the child to a physician to rule out SA.[47]

TABLE 29.6 Disorders of the Pediatric Hip Joint

Hip condition	Common demographic	Presentation
Legg-Calvé-Perthes disease	Boys > girls Ages 4-8 yr	• Limping and intermittent pain in the groin, hip, or knee • Decreased abduction and internal rotation ROM
Transient synovitis	Boys > girls Usually younger than 10 yr	• Less acute pain and less ROM restriction compared to SA • Afebrile
Slipped capital femoral epiphysis	Boys > girls Pubertal period Associated with obesity	• Groin pain and anteromedial pain of the thigh and knee • Strong preference for maintaining the hip in external rotation
Septic arthritis	Usually under the age of 3 yrs	• Pain with movement of joint in any direction • Atypical blood work • Inability to bear weight • Febrile

SCFE is a common condition of the hip that occurs when the growth plate of the proximal femoral physis weakens and becomes displaced. SCFE can be acute, acute on chronic, or chronic. The cause of SCFE is unclear, but it is likely due to both mechanical and endocrine factors.[48] Two-thirds of adolescents with SCFE are obese.[14] SCFE can be unilateral or bilateral. It occurs in boys more than girls and is most likely to present during the pubertal growth phase. Clinical signs of SCFE include reports groin pain and anteromedial pain of the thigh and knee, an antalgic gait, and a strong preference for maintaining the hip in external rotation.

Septic Arthritis

Septic arthritis (SA) is the inflammation of a joint due to a bacterial organism. If SA is suspected, a child must be immediately referred to a physician because joint destruction can occur within 48 hours. Most cases of SA occur in children under the age of 3. SA can occur in the upper extremity, but the vast majority of cases occur in the knee and hip.

While hip aspiration is the gold standard for diagnosing septic arthritis, a variety of laboratory tests may also lead to a diagnosis of septic arthritis. Clinical examinations may show symptoms similar to transient synovitis (TS), decreased range of motion, and difficulty with weight bearing; however, a clinical prediction rule exists to differentiate between TS and SA. The clinical prediction rule proposes four predictors for SA: a history of fever, refusal to bear weight, and two abnormal blood work results (elevated erythrocyte sedimentation rate and white blood count).[49]

Blount's Disease

Blount's disease (BD) is a progressive varus deformity of the tibia. The infantile and adolescent forms of BD are most common. The infantile form occurs in children between the ages of 2 and 5 years. The adolescent form occurs in older children and is much more related to obesity. The exact cause of the structural changes is debatable; however, in both forms, there is clear and persistent degeneration of the medial tibial physis.[13]

Clinicians must assess the stability of the knee joint as well as the leg length. Because there may be some possibility of nonsurgical management of the infantile form, early identification and referral to orthopedics are critical. The later-onset adolescent form requires extensive surgical intervention to restore alignment.

Osgood-Schlatter Disease

Osgood-Schlatter disease (OS) is a common condition in girls between the ages of 8 and 12 and in boys between the ages of 12 and 15. While the condition is more common in boys, both groups report pain at the tibial tuberosity.[50] The pain is often the result of repetitive pull of the quadriceps tendon on the skeletally immature tibial tuberosity. The repetitive trauma may result in apophysitis and avulsion of the tibial tuberosity. The majority of cases of OS occur in children and adolescents involved in sports.

Children and adolescents, either prepubescent and or in early pubescence, will report a slow onset of local pain at the tendon's insertion on the tibial tuberosity. Pain will be reported as more significant during and after activity. The pain can be reproduced with resisted knee extension and sometimes with palpation of the tibial tuberosity, which may appear more prominent.

Idiopathic Clubfoot

Idiopathic clubfoot (IC), also known as talipes equinovarus, affects 1 in 1,000 babies, and is twice as common in boys. About half of the cases of IC are

---

Critical Clinical Pearls

Hip pain in children can be complicated:

- Legg-Calvé-Perthes syndrome, transient synovitis, and slipped capital femoral epiphysis are more common in boys.
- Children with transient synovitis are afebrile.
- Children with suspected slipped capital femoral epiphysis need to be seen immediately by an orthopedic surgeon.

bilateral.[51] Clubfoot is associated with many neuromuscular and genetic syndromes; however, this information is related to idiopathic clubfoot in an otherwise typical baby. The cause of IC is unknown, but current prevailing theories include some combination of environmental and genetic factors.[51] Several studies have shown that there are many abnormal tissues in the clubfoot.[52]

Clubfoot is a multiplanar deformity of the foot and ankle that includes the cavus, adductus, varus, and equinus components, sometimes referred to with the acronym CAVE. Most cases of clubfoot are diagnosed in utero via ultrasound; however, when in-utero diagnosis is not made, early identification and intervention are critical. Clubfoot must be differentiated from metatarsus adductus, another common deformity of the newborn foot.

Clubfoot examination should begin with an overall assessment of lower extremity alignment. Palpation of the foot, particularly of the position of the talus, is critical. Because of the high incidence of clubfoot with other disorders, thorough examination of the neuromuscular system and all other joints must occur. Gross assessment will reveal small feet, positioned in equinus and varus. A crease on the medial side of the foot is often present. The calf muscle is often small.

A variety of classification systems exist for the clubfoot. The most common classification systems (Ponseti and Smoley, Harold and Walker, Catterall and Diméglio) all consider the position or the amount of correction of various components of the clubfoot. The Diméglio classification has been found to be the most reliable method for classifying clubfoot.[53] The Diméglio method uses a scale of 0 to 20 to assess the reducibility of sagittal plane equinus, frontal plane varus, adduction of the forefoot in the horizontal plane, and derotation around the talus of the calcaneo-forefoot unit. Each motion is scored on a 4-point scale, with 4 being the most reducible and 0 being the least reducible. A cumulative score of all four positions provides a category of severity between grade I (benign) and grade IV (very severe).[54]

As mentioned previously, distinguishing clubfoot from metatarsus adductus is important. Notably, metatarsus adductus does not involve the hindfoot. As such, the equinus position is not present in metatarsus adductus.

Other Conditions of the Foot and Ankle

Other common conditions of the foot and ankle in children include flat foot, congenital vertical talus, Kohler syndrome, and Sever's disease.

Occurrence of flat feet (FF) in children is common, reportedly between 7% and 22%, and is frequently a reason for referral to physical therapy and orthopedics. The Pediatric Orthopedic Society of America reports that most cases of FF resolve with age. The development of the medial arch occurs as children have developmental experiences, specifically, a lateral weight shift through the foot between ages 2 and 6.[55] Prior to age 6, the presence of FF may be considered typical.[56] Examination should include an assessment of the flexibility of the calcaneal tendon, medial arch constitution with heel rise, proximal kinetic chain alignment, and wear patterns on shoes. Because FF may be the result of a child with weakness attempting to increase their base of support, a strength assessment is also warranted.

Congenital vertical talus (CVT) occurs in 1 in 10,000 births. Of babies with CVT, 50% of those cases are considered idiopathic.[57] CVT will present as a rigid, convex flat foot due to a variety of anatomical anomalies in the foot. Some of these anomalies include a vertical talus and dorsal translation of the forefoot that is thought to be due to the failure of the foot's intrinsic muscles and resultant overpull of the dorsiflexors.

Kohler syndrome is osteochondrosis of the navicular, which may be caused by avascular necrosis or mechanical compression. It generally occurs in children between the ages of 2 and 8. Children often describe pain that is localized at the navicular. There may be swelling and redness on the dorsum of the foot. Due to the presentation, infection may be a differential diagnosis with this presentation. Pain may or may not influence gait mechanics.

Sever's disease is essentially due to overuse that results in calcaneal apophysitis. It occurs in children between 7 and 14 years of age. Children will present with tenderness on the posterior aspect of the calcaneus. Pain may be reproduced at this site with resisted plantar flexion.

Fractures in the Lower Extremity

As described earlier in the chapter, fractures in children are rather common; in fact, nearly half of boys will experience a fracture during their childhood.[40]

The most common fracture in the pediatric lower extremity is of the tibia; however, presence of a fracture in the fibula should be ruled out. Another newer presentation of fractures in the lower extremity in older children is stress fractures. With the earlier and more intense sporting activities that many children are participating in, stress fractures are becoming more common.

While this is rare, anytime a child has a fracture without a clear and reliable mechanism, child abuse must be ruled out. Most large medical centers have programs in place to systematically rule out abuse. In a more distant setting, clinicians should defer to a cautionary reaction and contact their local Department of Social Services immediately when there is even a remote possibility of child abuse.

CONCLUSION

Musculoskeletal injuries in children and adolescents are more common than one might think. Children are susceptible to musculoskeletal pathologies that are also common in adults, but the immature mus-

culoskeletal system is vulnerable to a specific set of pathologies that are exclusive to the immature system. When examining a child with a complaint or confirmed diagnosis of the musculoskeletal system, therapists can rely on many examination techniques that they are familiar with in the adult population. Therapists must appreciate where the child's musculoskeletal system is along its journey for maturation and how immaturity has influenced the child's presentation. Therapists must also have some familiarity with diagnoses that are exclusive to the pediatric population.

The goal of this chapter is to provide clinicians who are not primarily pediatric therapists with information about the immature musculoskeletal system, to identify common musculoskeletal pathologies in children, and to describe physical therapy examination of children who present with musculoskeletal complaints. When clinicians encounter a child with a musculoskeletal impairment, they must appreciate how the impairment affects the child's function and participation as they would when working with the adult population.

References

Chapter 1

1. Palmer KT, Cooper C. Work-related disorders of the upper limb. *Arthritis Research Campaign: Topical Reviews.* 2006;10:1-7.

2. Raisz LG. Physiology and pathophysiology of bone remodeling. *Clin Chem.* 1999;45(8)(part 2):1353-1358.

3. Clarke B. Normal bone anatomy and physiology. *Clin J Am Soc Nephrol.* 2008;3(suppl 3):S131-S139.

4. Väänänen HK, Zhao H, Mulari M, Halleen JM. The cell biology of osteoclast function. *J Cell Sci.* 2000;113(part 3):377-381.

5. Rho JY, Kuhn-Spearing L, Zioupos P. Mechanical properties and the hierarchical structure of bone. *Med Eng Phys.* 1998;20(2):92-102.

6. Augat P, Schorlemmer S. The role of cortical bone and its microstructure in bone strength. *Age Ageing.* 2006;35(suppl 2):ii27-ii31.

7. Jee WS. Principles in bone physiology. *J Musculoskelet Neuronal Interact.* 2000;1(1):11-13.

8. Comarr AE, Hutchinson RH, Bors E. Extremity fractures of patients with spinal cord injuries. *Am J Surg.* 1962;103:732-739.

9. Chappard D, Baslé MF, Legrand E, Audran M. Trabecular bone microarchitecture: A review. *Morphologie.* 2008;92(299):162-170.

10. Frost HM. A 2003 update of bone physiology and Wolff's Law for clinicians. *Angle Orthod.* 2004;74(1):3-15.

11. Hasegawa K, Turner CH, Burr DB. Contribution of collagen and mineral to the elastic anisotropy of bone. *Calcif Tissue Int.* 1994;55(5):381-386.

12. Yamashita J, Li X, Furman BR, Rawls HR, Wang X, Agrawal CM. Collagen and bone viscoelasticity: A dynamic mechanical analysis. *J Biomed Mater Res.* 2002;63(1):31-36.

13. Burr DB, Turner CH, Naick P, et al. Does microdamage accumulation affect the mechanical properties of bone? *J Biomech.* 1998;31(4):337-345.

14. Ralphs JR, Benjamin M. The joint capsule: Structure, composition, ageing and disease. *J Anat.* 1994;184(part 3):503-509.

15. Piette E. Anatomy of the human temporomandibular joint. An updated comprehensive review. *Acta Stomatol Belg.* 1993;90(2):103-127.

16. Unsworth A, Dowson D, Wright V. 'Cracking joints'. A bioengineering study of cavitation in the metacarpophalangeal joint. *Ann Rheum Dis.* 1971;30(4):348-358.

17. Malghem J, Omoumi P, Lecouvet FE, Vande Berg BC. Presumed intraarticular gas microbubbles resulting from a vacuum phenomenon: Visualization with ultrasonography as hyperechoic microfoci. *Skeletal Radiol.* 2011;40(10):1287-1293.

18. Kawchuk GN, Fryer J, Jaremko JL, Zeng H, Rowe L, Thompson R. Real-time visualization of joint cavitation. *PLoS One.* 2015;10(4):e0119470.

19. James CB, Uhl TL. A review of articular cartilage pathology and the use of glucosamine sulfate. *J Athl Train.* 2001;36(4):413-419.

20. Jackson DW, Scheer MJ, Simon TM. Cartilage substitutes: Overview of basic science and treatment opti ons. *J Am Acad Orthop Surg.* 2001;9(1):37-52.

21. Mankin H, Brandt K. *Textbook of Rheumatology.* 3rd ed. Philadelphia, PA: Saunders; 1989.

22. Buckwalter JA, Mankin HJ. Articular cartilage: Tissue design and chondrocyte-matrix interactions. *Instr Course Lect.* 1998;47:477-486.

23. Jurvelin JS, Buschmann MD, Hunziker EB. Mechanical anisotropy of the human knee articular cartilage in compression. *Proc Inst Mech Eng H.* 2003;217(3):215-219.

24. Mow VC, Holmes MH, Lai WM. Fluid transport and mechanical properties of articular cartilage: A review. *J Biomech.* 1984;17(5):377-394.

25. Nordin M, Frankel V. *Basic Biomechanics of the Musculoskeletal System.* 2nd ed. Philadelphia, PA: Lea & Febiger; 1989.

26. Suh JK, Li Z, Woo SL. Dynamic behavior of a biphasic cartilage model under cyclic compressive loading. *J Biomech.* 1995;28(4):357-364.

27. Mansour J. *Kinesiology: The Mechanics and Pathomechanics of Human Movement.* 2nd ed. Philadelphia, PA: Lippincott, Williams and Wilkins; 2008.

28. Frank CB, Hart DA, Shrive NG. Molecular biology and biomechanics of normal and healing ligaments—a review. *Osteoarthr Cartilage.* 1999;7(1):130-140.

29. Netti P, D'Amore A, Ronca D, Ambrosio L, Nicolais L. Structure-mechanical properties relationship of natural tendons and ligaments. *J Mater Sci—Mater M.* 1996;7(9):525-530.

30. Quapp KM, Weiss JA. Material characterization of human medial collateral ligament. *J Biomech Eng.* 1998;120(6):757-763.

31. Crowninshield RD, Pope MH. The strength and failure characteristics of rat medial collateral ligaments. *J Trauma.* 1976;16(2):99-105.

32. Hsu AT, Chang JH, Chang CH. Determining the resting position of the glenohumeral joint: A cadaver study. *J Orthop Sports Phys Ther.* 2002;32(12):605-612.

33. Barak T, Rosen E, Sofa R. Mobility: Passive orthopedic manual therapy. In: Gould J, Davies G, eds. *Orthopedic and Sports Physical Therapy.* St. Louis, MO: CV Mosby Co.; 1990:195-206.

34. Grieve G. *Common vertebral joint problems.* 2nd ed. Edinburgh: Churchill Livingstone; 1988.

35. Kaltenborn F. *Manual Mobilization of the Extremity Joints.* 4th ed. Minneapolis, MN: OPTP; 1989.

36. Baeyens J-P, Van Roy P, Clarys JP. Intra-articular kinematics of the normal glenohumeral joint in the late preparatory phase of throwing: Kaltenborn's rule revisited. *Ergonomics.* 2000;43(10):1726-1737.

37. Baeyens JP, Van Roy P, De Schepper A, Declercq G, Clarijs JP. Glenohumeral joint kinematics related to minor anterior instability of the shoulder at the end of the late preparatory phase of throwing. *Clin Biomech (Bristol, Avon).* 2001;16(9):752-757.

38. Cattrysse E, Baeyens JP, Van Roy P, Van de Wiele O, Roosens T, Clarys JP. Intra-articular kinematics of the upper limb joints: A six degrees of freedom study of coupled motions. *Ergonomics.* 2005;48(11-14):1657-1671.

39. Johnson AJ, Godges JJ, Zimmerman GJ, Ounanian LL. The effect of anterior versus posterior glide joint mobilization on external rotation range of motion in patients with shoulder adhesive capsulitis. *J Orthop Sports Phys Ther.* 2007;37(3):88-99.

40. Schomacher J. The convex-concave rule and the lever law. *Man Ther.* 2009;14(5):579-582.

41. Hopkins P. Skeletal muscle physiology. *Continuing Education in Anaesthesia, Critical Care & Pain.* 2006;6(1):1-6.

42. Lorenz T, Campello M. Biomechanics of skeletal muscle. In: Nordin M, Frankel V, eds. *Basic Biomechanics of the Musculoskeletal System.* 3rd ed. Philadelphia, PA: Lippincott, Williams and Wilkins; 2000.

43. Williams PL, Warwick R, Dyson M. *Gray's Anatomy.* Vol. 37. London, England: Churchill Livingstone; 1995.

44. Noonan TJ, Garrett WE. Injuries at the myotendinous junction. *Clin Sports Med.* 1992;11(4):783-806.

45. Gamble JG. *Musculoskeletal System: Physiological Basics.* New York. NY: Raven Press; 1988.

46. The motor unit. In: Purves D, Augustine G, Fitzpatrick D, et al., eds. *Neuroscience.* 2nd ed. Sunderland, MA: Sinauer Associates; 2001.

47. Huxley H, Hanson J. Changes in the cross-striations of muscle during contraction and stretch and their structural interpretation. *Nature.* 1954;173(4412):973-976.

48. Lieber RL. *Skeletal Muscle Structure and Function: Implications for Rehabilitation and Sports Medicine.* Baltimore, MD: Williams & Wilkins; 1992.

49. Lieber RL, Fridén J. Functional and clinical significance of skeletal muscle architecture. *Muscle Nerve.* 2000;23(11):1647-1666.

50. Billeter R, Oetliker H, Hoppeler H. Structural basis of muscle performance. *Adv Vet Sci Comp Med.* 1994;38A:57-124.

51. Ikai M, Fukunaga T. Calculation of muscle strength per unit cross-sectional area of human muscle by means of ultrasonic measurement. *Int Z Angew Physiol.* 1968;26(1):26-32.

52. Tabary JC, Tardieu C, Tabary C, Lombard M, Gagnard L, Tardieu G. [Neural regulation and adaptation of the number of sarcomeres of the muscle fiber to the length imposed upon it]. *J Physiol (Paris).* 1972;65(suppl 1):168A.

53. Deusinger RH. Biomechanics in clinical practice. *Phys Ther.* 1984;64(12):1860-1868.

54. Cavagna GA, Dusman B, Margaria R. Positive work done by a previously stretched muscle. *J Appl Physiol.* 1968;24(1):21-32.

55. Van Ingen Schenau G. An alternative view of the concept of utilisation of elastic energy in human movement. *Human Movement Science.* 1984;3:301-336.

56. Enoka RM. Eccentric contractions require unique activation strategies by the nervous system. *J Appl Physiol (1985).* 1996;81(6):2339-2346.

57. Häkkinen K, Häkkinen A. Neuromuscular adaptations during intensive strength training in middle-aged and elderly males and females. *Electromyogr Clin Neurophysiol.* 1995;35(3):137-147.

58. Fitzgerald GK. Open versus closed kinetic chain exercise: Issues in rehabilitation after anterior cruciate ligament reconstructive surgery. *Phys Ther.* 1997;77(12):1747-1754.

59. Birch HL. Tendon matrix composition and turnover in relation to functional requirements. *Int J Exp Pathol.* 2007;88(4):241-248.

60. Vogel KG, Koob TJ. Structural specialization in tendons under compression. *Int Rev Cytol.* 1989;115:267-293.

61. Kannus P. Structure of the tendon connective tissue. *Scand J Med Sci Sports.* 2000;10(6):312-320.

62. Wang JH. Mechanobiology of tendon. *J Biomech.* 2006;39(9):1563-1582.

63. Jung HJ, Fisher MB, Woo SL. Role of biomechanics in the understanding of normal, injured, and healing ligaments and tendons. *Sports Med Arthrosc Rehabil Ther Technol.* 2009;1(1):9.

Chapter 2

1. Waxman S. *Correlative Neuroanatomy.* 24th ed. New York, NY: McGraw-Hill; 1996.

2. Lee MW, McPhee RW, Stringer MD. An evidence-based approach to human dermatomes. *Clin Anat.* 2008;21(5):363-373.

3. Thomas P, Olsson Y. Microscopic anatomy and function of the connective tissue components of peripheral nerve. In: Dyck P, Thomas P, Lambert E, eds. *Peripheral Neuropathy.* Philadelphia, PA: Saunders; 1984.

4. Henneman E, Somjen G, Carpenter DO. Functional significance of cell size in spinal motoneurons. *J Neurophysiol.* 1965;28:560-580.

5. Linnamo V, Moritani T, Nicol C, Komi PV. Motor unit activation patterns during isometric, concentric and eccentric actions at different force levels. *J Electromyogr Kinesiol.* 2003;13(1):93-101.

6. Howell JN, Fuglevand AJ, Walsh ML, Bigland-Ritchie B. Motor unit activity during isometric and concentric-eccentric contractions of the human first dorsal interosseus muscle. *J Neurophysiol.* 1995;74(2):901-904.

7. Van Vliet PM, Heneghan NR. Motor control and the management of musculoskeletal dysfunction. *Man Ther.* 2006;11(3):208-213.

8. Borsa P, Lephart S, Kocher M. Functional assessment and rehabilitation of shoulder proprioception for glenohumeral instability. *J Sport Rehabil.* 1994;3:84-104.

9. McCloskey DI. Kinesthetic sensibility. *Physiol Rev.* 1978;58(4):763-820.

10. Wyke B. Articular neurology—a review. *Physiotherapy.* 1972;58(3):94-99.

11. Milne RJ, Foreman RD, Giesler GJ, Willis WD. Convergence of cutaneous and pelvic visceral nociceptive inputs onto primate spinothalamic neurons. *Pain.* 1981;11(2):163-183.

12. Vierck CJ, Greenspan JD, Ritz LA. Long-term changes in purposive and reflexive responses to nociceptive stimulation following anterolateral chordotomy. *J Neurosci.* 1990;10(7):2077-2095.

13. Gardner E. Reflex muscular response to stimulation of articular nerves in the cat. *Am J Physiol.* 1950;161(1):133-141.

14. Carpenter M. *Human Neuroanatomy.* 7th ed. Philadelphia, PA: Williams & Wilkins; 1977.

15. Prochazka A, Gorassini M. Ensemble firing of muscle afferents recorded during normal locomotion in cats. *J Physiol.* 1998;507(part 1):293-304.

16. Prosperini L, Petsas N, Raz E, et al. Balance deficit with opened or closed eyes reveals involvement of different structures of the central nervous system in multiple sclerosis. *Mult Scler.* 2014;20(1):81-90.

17. Kloos A. Mechanics and control of posture and balance. In: Hughes C, ed. *Movement Disorders and Neuromuscular Interventions for the Trunk and Extremities—Independent Study Course.* La Crosse, WI: Orthopaedic Section, APTA, Inc.; 2008:1-26.

18. Horak FB, Nashner LM. Central programming of postural movements: Adaptation to altered support-surface configurations. *J Neurophysiol.* 1986;55(6):1369-1381.

19. Halle J. Neuromusculoskeletal scan examination with selected related topics. In: Flynn T, ed. *The Thoracic Spine and Rib Cage Musculoskeletal Evaluation and Treatment.* Boston, MA: Butterworth-Heinemann; 1996:121-146.

20. Virani SN, Ferrari R, Russell AS. Physician resistance to the late whiplash syndrome. *J Rheumatol.* 2001;28(9):2096-2099.

21. Moseley G. Reconceptualising pain according to modern pain science. *Phys Ther Rev.* 2007;12:169-178.

22. Sloan TJ, Walsh DA. Explanatory and diagnostic labels and perceived prognosis in chronic low back pain. *Spine (Phila Pa 1976).* 2010;35(21):E1120-E1125.

23. Wall P, Melzack R. *Textbook of Pain.* London, England: Elsevier; 2005.

24. Louw A. *Why Do I Hurt? A Neuroscience Approach to Pain.* Minneapolis, MN: OPTP; 2013.

25. Puentedura EJ, Louw A. A neuroscience approach to managing athletes with low back pain. *Phys Ther Sport.* 2012;13(3):123-133.

26. Louw A, Puentedura E. *Therapeutic Neuroscience Education.* Minneapolis, MN: OPTP; 2013.

27. Moseley GL. A pain neuromatrix approach to patients with chronic pain. *Man Ther.* 2003;8(3):130-140.

28. Kovacs FM, Seco J, Royuela A, Peña A, Muriel A, Network SBPR. The correlation between pain, catastrophizing, and disability in subacute and chronic low back pain: A study in the routine clinical practice of the Spanish National Health Service. *Spine (Phila Pa 1976).* 2011;36(4):339-345.

29. Waddell G, Newton M, Henderson I, Somerville D, Main CJ. A Fear-Avoidance Beliefs Questionnaire (FABQ) and the role of fear-avoidance beliefs in chronic low back pain and disability. *Pain.* 1993;52(2):157-168.

30. Cleland JA, Fritz JM, Childs JD. Psychometric properties of the Fear-Avoidance Beliefs Questionnaire and Tampa Scale of Kinesiophobia in patients with neck pain. *Am J Phys Med Rehabil.* 2008;87(2):109-117.

31. Mintken PE, Cleland JA, Whitman JM, George SZ. Psychometric properties of the Fear-Avoidance Beliefs Questionnaire and Tampa Scale of Kinesiophobia in patients with shoulder pain. *Arch Phys Med Rehabil.* 2010;91(7):1128-1136.

32. George SZ, Valencia C, Zeppieri G, Robinson ME. Development of a self-report measure of fearful activities for patients with low back pain: The Fear of Daily Activities Questionnaire. *Phys Ther.* 2009;89(9):969-979.

33. García-Campayo J, Serrano-Blanco A, Rodero B, et al. Effectiveness of the psychological and pharmacological treatment of catastrophization in patients with fibromyalgia: A randomized controlled trial. *Trials.* 2009;10:24.

34. Melzack R, Wall PD. Pain mechanisms: A new theory. *Science.* 1965;150(3699):971-979.

35. Carter R. *The Human Brain Book.* New York, NY: Kindersley Limited; 2009.

36. Delcomyn F. *Foundations of Neurobiology.* New York, NY: W.H. Freeman; 1998.

37. Melzack R. Pain—An overview. *Acta Anaesthesiol Scand.* 1999;43(9):880-884.

38. Melzack R. Pain and the neuromatrix in the brain. *J Dent Educ.* 2001;65(12):1378-1382.

39. Melzack R. From the gate to the neuromatrix. *Pain.* 1999;6:S121-S126.

40. Melzack R. Gate control theory: On the evolution of pain. *Pain Forum.* 1996;5:128-138.

41. Latremoliere A, Woolf CJ. Central sensitization: A generator of pain hypersensitivity by central neural plasticity. *J Pain.* 2009;10(9):895-926.

42. Meeus M, Vervisch S, De Clerck LS, Moorkens G, Hans G, Nijs J. Central sensitization in patients with rheumatoid arthritis: A systematic literature review. *Semin Arthritis Rheu.* 2012;41(4):556-567.

43. Woolf CJ, Salter MW. Plasticity and pain: The role of the dorsal horn. In: McMahon S, Koltzenburg M, eds. *Wall and Melzack's Textbook of Pain.* 5th ed. Edinburgh, Scotland: Elsevier; 2005.

44. Woolf CJ, Mannion RJ. Neuropathic pain: Aetiology, symptoms, mechanisms, and management. *Lancet.* 1999;353(9168):1959-1964.

45. Villaneuva L, Fields HL. Endogenous central mechanisms of pain modulation. In: Villaneuva L, Dickenson A, Ollat H, eds. *The Pain System in Normal and Pathological States*. Seattle, WA: IASP Press; 2004.

46. Woolf CJ. Central sensitization: Uncovering the relation between pain and plasticity. *Anesthesiology.* 2007;106(4):864-867.

47. Woolf CJ, Doubell TP. The pathophysiology of chronic pain: Increased sensitivity to low threshold A beta fibre inputs. *Curr Opin Neurobiol.* 1994;4:525-534.

48. Doubell TP, Mannion R, Woolf CJ. The dorsal horn: State dependent sensory processing, plasticity and the generation of pain. In: Wall PD, Melzack R, eds. *Textbook of Pain*. 4th ed. Edinburgh, Scotland: Churchill Livingstone; 1999.

49. Fukuoka T, Tokunaga A, Kondo E, Miki K, Tachibana T, Noguchi K. Change in mRNAs for neuropeptides and the GABA(A) receptor in dorsal root ganglion neurons in a rat experimental neuropathic pain model. *Pain.* 1998;78(1):13-26.

50. Woolf CJ. Pain. *Neurobiol Dis.* 2000;7(5):504-510.

51. Bear M, Connors B, Paradiso M. *Neuroscience: Exploring the Brain*. Baltimore, MD: Williams & Wilkins; 1996.

52. Juan S. *The Odd Brain: Mysteries of Our Weird and Wonderful Brains Explained*. New York, NY: MJF Books; 2006.

53. Flor H. The functional organization of the brain in chronic pain. *Prog Brain Res.* 2000;129:313-322.

54. Flor H. Remapping somatosensory cortex after injury. *Adv Neurol.* 2003;93:195-204.

55. Sapolsky RM. *Why Zebras Don't Get Ulcers: An Updated Guide to Stress, Stress-Related Diseases, and Coping*. New York, NY: W.H. Freeman and Co; 1998.

56. Riva R, Mork PJ, Westgaard RH, Okkenhaug Johansen T, Lundberg U. Catecholamines and heart rate in female fibromyalgia patients. *J Psychosom Res.* 2012;72(1):51-57.

57. Larsson SE, Cai H, Zhang Q, Larsson R, Oberg PA. Microcirculation in the upper trapezius muscle during sustained shoulder load in healthy women—An endurance study using percutaneous laser-Doppler flowmetry and surface electromyography. *Eur J Appl Physiol Occup Physiol.* 1995;70(5):451-456.

58. Hodges PW, Richardson CA. Delayed postural contraction of transversus abdominis in low back pain associated with movement of the lower limb. *J Spinal Disord.* 1998;11(1):46-56.

59. Moseley GL. Evidence for a direct relationship between cognitive and physical change during an education intervention in people with chronic low back pain. *Eur J Pain.* 2004;8(1):39-45.

60. Stephens R, Atkins J, Kingston A. Swearing as a response to pain. *Neuroreport.* 2009;20(12):1056-1060.

61. Riva R, Mork PJ, Westgaard RH, Lundberg U. Comparison of the cortisol awakening response in women with shoulder and neck pain and women with fibromyalgia. *Psychoneuroendocrino.* 2012;37(2):299-306.

62. Segal TY, Hindmarsh PC, Viner RM. Disturbed adrenal function in adolescents with chronic fatigue syndrome. *J Pediatr Endocrinol Metab.* 2005;18(3):295-301.

63. Van Houdenhove B, Van Den Eede F, Luyten P. Does hypothalamic-pituitary-adrenal axis hypofunction in chronic fatigue syndrome reflect a 'crash' in the stress system? *Med Hypotheses.* 2009;72(6):701-705.

64. Geiss A, Rohleder N, Kirschbaum C, Steinbach K, Bauer HW, Anton F. Predicting the failure of disc surgery by a hypofunctional HPA axis: Evidence from a prospective study on patients undergoing disc surgery. *Pain.* 2005;114(1-2):104-117.

65. Mohs R, Mease P, Arnold LM, et al. The effect of duloxetine treatment on cognition in patients with fibromyalgia. *Psychosom Med.* 2012;74(6):628-634.

66. Dinarello CA. Overview of cytokines and their role in pain. In: Watkins LR, Maier SF, eds. *Cytokines and Pain*. Basel, Switzerland: Birkhauser; 1999.

67. Nippoldt T. Mayo Clinic office visit. Adrenal fatigue. An interview with Todd Nippoldt, M.D. *Mayo Clin Womens Healthsource.* 2010;14(3):6.

68. Devor M. Response of nerves to injury in relation to neuropathic pain. In: McMahon S, Koltzenburg M, eds. *Melzack and Wall's Textbook of Pain*. Edinburgh, Scotland: Elsevier; 2005.

69. Schweinhardt P, Sauro KM, Bushnell MC. Fibromyalgia: A disorder of the brain? *Neuroscientist.* 2008;14(5):415-421.

70. Bradley LA. Pathophysiologic mechanisms of fibromyalgia and its related disorders. *J Clin Psychiatry.* 2008;69(suppl 2):6-13.

71. Sarzi-Puttini P, Atzeni F, Diana A, Doria A, Furlan R. Increased neural sympathetic activation in fibromyalgia syndrome. *Ann NY Acad Sci.* 2006;1069:109-117.

72. Bennett RM, Goldenberg DL. Fibromyalgia, myofascial pain, tender points and trigger points: Splitting or lumping? *Arthritis Res Ther.* 2011;13(3):117.

73. Edmondston SJ, Chan HY, Ngai GC, et al. Postural neck pain: An investigation of habitual sitting posture, perception of 'good' posture and cervicothoracic kinaesthesia. *Man Ther.* 2007;12(4):363-371.

74. Moseley GL, Hodges PW. Are the changes in postural control associated with low back pain caused by pain interference? *Clin J Pain.* 2005;21(4):323-329.

75. Moseley GL, Nicholas MK, Hodges PW. Does anticipation of back pain predispose to back trouble? *Brain.* 2004;127(part 10):2339-2347.

76. Moseley GL, Hodges PW. Reduced variability of postural strategy prevents normalization of motor changes induced by back pain: A risk factor for chronic trouble? *Behav Neurosci.* 2006;120(2):474-476.

77. Sapolsky RM. *Why Zebras Don't Get Ulcers*. New York, NY: Freeman; 1994.

78. Meeus M, Nijs J. Central sensitization: A biopsychosocial explanation for chronic widespread pain in patients with fibromyalgia and chronic fatigue syndrome. *Clin Rheumatol.* 2007;26(4):465-473.

79. Togo F, Natelson BH, Adler GK, et al. Plasma cytokine fluctuations over time in healthy controls and patients with fibromyalgia. *Exp Biol Med (Maywood)*. 2009;234(2):232-240.

80. Miller GE, Cohen S, Ritchey AK. Chronic psychological stress and the regulation of pro-inflammatory cytokines: A glucocorticoid-resistance model. *Health Psychol*. 2002;21(6):531-541.

81. Thacker MA, Clark AK, Marchand F, McMahon SB. Pathophysiology of peripheral neuropathic pain: Immune cells and molecules. *Anesth Analg*. 2007;105(3):838-847.

82. Weissbecker I, Floyd A, Dedert E, Salmon P, Sephton S. Childhood trauma and diurnal cortisol disruption in fibromyalgia syndrome. *Psychoneuroendocrino*. 2006;31(3):312-324.

Chapter 3

1. Prentice WE. Understanding and managing the healing process. In: Prentice WE, Voight ML, eds. *Techniques in Musculoskeletal Rehabilitation*. New York, NY: McGraw-Hill; 2001:x, 780.

2. Wong ME, Hollinger JO, Pinero GJ. Integrated processes responsible for soft tissue healing. *Oral Surg Oral Med O*. 1996;82(5):475-492.

3. Garrett WE, Jr. Muscle strain injuries: Clinical and basic aspects. *Med Sci Sports Exerc*. 1990;22(4):436-443.

4. Jarvinen TA, Jarvinen TL, Kaariainen M, et al. Muscle injuries: Optimising recovery. *Best Pract Res Clin Rheumatol*. 2007;21(2):317-331.

5. Jarvinen TA, Jarvinen TL, Kaariainen M, Kalimo H, Jarvinen M. Muscle injuries: Biology and treatment. *Am J Sports Med*. 2005;33(5):745-764.

6. Noonan TJ, Garrett WE, Jr. Injuries at the myotendinous junction. *Clin Sports Med*. 1992;11(4):783-806.

7. Tidball JG. Myotendinous junction injury in relation to junction structure and molecular composition. *Exerc Sport Sci Rev*. 1991;19:419-445.

8. Pollock N, James SL, Lee JC, Chakraverty R. British athletics muscle injury classification: A new grading system. *Brit J Sport Med*. 2014;48(18):1347-1351.

9. Trojian TH. Muscle contusion (thigh). *Clin Sports Med*. 2013;32(2):317-324.

10. Bentley S. Exercise-induced muscle cramp. Proposed mechanisms and management. *Sports Med*. 1996;21(6):409-420.

11. Khan KM, Cook JL, Bonar F, Harcourt P, Astrom M. Histopathology of common tendinopathies. Update and implications for clinical management. *Sports Med*. 1999;27(6):393-408.

12. Wang JH, Guo Q, Li B. Tendon biomechanics and mechanobiology—A minireview of basic concepts and recent advancements. *J Hand Ther*. 2012;25:133-141.

13. Maffulli N, Khan KM, Puddu G. Overuse tendon conditions: Time to change a confusing terminology. *Arthroscopy*. 1998;14(8):840-843.

14. Kvist MH, Lehto MU, Jozsa L, Jarvinen M, Kvist HT. Chronic Achilles paratenonitis. An immunohistologic study of fibronectin and fibrinogen. *Am J Sports Med*. 1988;16(6):616-623.

15. Hope M, Saxby TS. Tendon healing. *Foot Ankle Clin*. 2007;12(4):553-567, v.

16. Lin TW, Cardenas L, Soslowsky LJ. Biomechanics of tendon injury and repair. *J Biomech*. 2004;37(6):865-877.

17. Sharma P, Maffulli N. Basic biology of tendon injury and healing. *Surgeon*. 2005;3(5):309-316.

18. Sharma P, Maffulli N. Biology of tendon injury: Healing, modeling and remodeling. *J Musculoskelet Neuronal Interact*. 2006;6(2):181-190.

19. Hildebrand KA, Frank CB. Scar formation and ligament healing. *Can J Surg*. 1998;41(6):425-429.

20. Woo SL, Abramowitch SD, Kilger R, Liang R. Biomechanics of knee ligaments: Injury, healing, and repair. *J Biomech*. 2006;39(1):1-20.

21. Woo SL, Chan SS, Yamaji T. Biomechanics of knee ligament healing, repair and reconstruction. *J Biomech*. 1997;30(5):431-439.

22. Beynnon BD, Johnson RJ, Abate JA, Fleming BC, Nichols CE. Treatment of anterior cruciate ligament injuries, part I. *Am J Sports Med*. 2005;33(10):1579-1602.

23. Johnson DL, Bealle DP, Brand JC, Jr., Nyland J, Caborn DN. The effect of a geographic lateral bone bruise on knee inflammation after acute anterior cruciate ligament rupture. *Am J Sports Med*. 2000;28(2):152-155.

24. Cruess RL, Dumont J. Fracture healing. *Can J Surg*. 1975;18(5):403-413.

25. Dimitriou R, Tsiridis E, Giannoudis PV. Current concepts of molecular aspects of bone healing. *Injury*. 2005;36(12):1392-1404.

26. Issa SN, Sharma L. Epidemiology of osteoarthritis: An update. *Curr Rheumatol Rep*. 2006;8(1):7-15.

27. Brittberg M, Winalski CS. Evaluation of cartilage injuries and repair. *J Bone Joint Surg*. 2003;85-A(suppl 2):58-69.

28. Athanasiou KA, Shah AR, Hernandez RJ, LeBaron RG. Basic science of articular cartilage repair. *Clin Sports Med*. 2001;20(2):223-247.

29. O'Driscoll SW. The healing and regeneration of articular cartilage. *J Bone Joint Surg*. 1998;80(12):1795-1812.

Chapter 4

1. Sackett DL, Rosenberg WM, Gray JA, Haynes RB, Richardson WS. Evidence based medicine: What it is and what it isn't. *BMJ*. 1996;312(7023):71-72.

2. Armijo-Olivo S, Warren S, Fuentes J, Magee DJ. Clinical relevance vs. statistical significance: Using neck outcomes in patients with temporomandibular disorders as an example. *Man Ther*. 2011;16(6):563-572.

3. Jaeschke R, Guyatt GH, Sackett DL. Users' guides to the medical literature. III. How to use an article about a diagnostic test. B. What are the results and will they help me in caring for my patients? The Evidence-Based Medicine Working Group. *JAMA*. 1994;271(9):703-707.

4. Deville WL, van der Windt DA, Dzaferagic A, Bezemer PD, Bouter LM. The test of Lasègue: Systematic review of the accuracy in diagnosing herniated discs. *Spine (Phila Pa 1976)*. 2000;25(9):1140-1147.

5. Sackett DL. Evidence-based medicine. *Spine (Phila Pa 1976)*. 1998;23(10):1085-1086.

6. Domholdt E. *Physical Therapy Research*. 2nd ed. Philadelphia, PA: WB Saunders; 2000.

7. Rothstein JM, Echternach JL. *Primer on Measurement: An Introductory Guide to Measurement Issues*. Alexandria, VA.: American Physical Therapy Association; 1999.

8. Sackett DL, Haynes RB. The architecture of diagnostic research. *BMJ*. 2002;324(7336):539-541.

9. Obuchowski NA, Graham RJ, Baker ME, Powell KA. Ten criteria for effective screening: Their application to multislice CT screening for pulmonary and colorectal cancers. *AJR Am J Roentgenol*. 2001;176(6):1357-1362.

10. Stiell IG, Wells GA, Vandemheen KL, et al. The Canadian C-spine rule for radiography in alert and stable trauma patients. *JAMA*. 2001;286(15):1841-1848.

11. Cook C. *Differential Diagnosis*. San Antonio, TX: American Academy of Orthopaedic and Manual Physical Therapists; 2010.

12. Phillips B, Ball C, Sackett D, et al. *Levels of Evidence*. Oxford, UK: University of Oxford; 2009.

13. Whiting P, Rutjes AW, Reitsma JB, Bossuyt PM, Kleijnen J. The development of QUADAS: A tool for the quality assessment of studies of diagnostic accuracy included in systematic reviews. *BMC Med Res Methodol*. 2003;3:25.

14. Jaeschke R, Guyatt G, Sackett DL. Users' guides to the medical literature. III. How to use an article about a diagnostic test. A. Are the results of the study valid? Evidence-Based Medicine Working Group. *JAMA*. 1994;271(5):389-391.

15. Bossuyt PM. The quality of reporting in diagnostic test research: Getting better, still not optimal. *Clin Chem*. 2004;50(3):465-466.

16. Lijmer JG, Mol BW, Heisterkamp S, et al. Empirical evidence of design-related bias in studies of diagnostic tests. *JAMA*. 1999;282(11):1061-1066.

17. Smidt N, Rutjes AW, van der Windt DA, et al. The quality of diagnostic accuracy studies since the STARD statement: Has it improved? *Neurology*. 2006;67(5):792-797.

18. Whiting PF, Weswood ME, Rutjes AW, Reitsma JB, Bossuyt PN, Kleijnen J. Evaluation of QUADAS, a tool for the quality assessment of diagnostic accuracy studies. *BMC Med Res Methodol*. 2006;6:9.

19. Hegedus EJ, Goode A, Campbell S, et al. Physical examination tests of the shoulder: A systematic review with meta-analysis of individual tests. *Brit J Sports Med*. 2008;42(2):80-92; discussion 92.

20. Reiman MP, Goode AP, Hegedus EJ, Cook CE, Wright AA. Diagnostic accuracy of clinical tests of the hip: A systematic review with meta-analysis. *Brit J Sport Med*. 2013;47(14):893-902.

21. Reiman MP, Loudon JK, Goode AP. Diagnostic accuracy of clinical tests for assessment of hamstring injury: A systematic review. *J Orthop Sports Phys Ther*. 2013;43(4):223-231.

22. Cook C, Mabry L, Reiman MP, Hegedus EJ. Best tests/clinical findings for screening and diagnosis of patellofemoral pain syndrome: A systematic review. *Physiotherapy*. 2012;98(2):93-100.

23. Hegedus EJ, Stern B, Reiman MP, Tarara D, Wright AA. A suggested model for physical examination and conservative treatment of athletic pubalgia. *Phys Ther Sport*. 2013;14(1):3-16.

24. Jaeschke R, Guyatt G, Lijmer JG. *User's Guide to the Medical Literature: Essentials of Evidence-Based Practice*. Chicago, IL: AMA Press; 2002.

25. Levine R, Shore K, Lubalin J, Garfinkel S, Hurtado M, Carman K. Comparing physician and patient perceptions of quality in ambulatory care. *Int J Qual Health Care*. 2012;24(4):348-356.

26. Duffy FD, Gordon GH, Whelan G, et al. Assessing competence in communication and interpersonal skills: The Kalamazoo II report. *Acad Med*. 2004;79(6):495-507.

27. Benbassat J, Baumal R, Heyman SN, Brezis M. Viewpoint: Suggestions for a shift in teaching clinical skills to medical students: The reflective clinical examination. *Acad Med*. 2005;80(12):1121-1126.

28. Moosapour H, Raza M, Rambod M, Soltani A. Conceptualization of category-oriented likelihood ratio: A useful tool for clinical diagnostic reasoning. *BMC Med Educ*. 2011;11:94.

29. Croskerry P. A universal model of diagnostic reasoning. *Acad Med*. 2009;84(8):1022-1028.

30. Hampton JR, Harrison MJ, Mitchell JR, Prichard JS, Seymour C. Relative contributions of history-taking, physical examination, and laboratory investigation to diagnosis and management of medical outpatients. *Brit Med J*. 1975;2(5969):486-489.

31. Peterson MC, Holbrook JH, Von Hales D, Smith NL, Staker LV. Contributions of the history, physical examination, and laboratory investigation in making medical diagnoses. *West J Med*. 1992;156(2):163-165.

32. Portal JM, Romano PE. Major review: Ocular sighting dominance: A review and a study of athletic proficiency and eye-hand dominance in a collegiate baseball team. *Binocul Vis Strabismus Q*. 1998;13(2):125-132.

33. Carey DP. Vision research: Losing sight of eye dominance. *Curr Biol*. 2001;11(20):R828-830.

34. Hong W, Earnest A, Sultana P, Koh Z, Shahidah N, Ong ME. How accurate are vital signs in predicting clinical outcomes in critically ill emergency department patients. *Eur J Emerg Med*. 2013;20(1):27-32.

35. Barfod C, Lauritzen MM, Danker JK, et al. Abnormal vital signs are strong predictors for Intensive Care Unit admission and in-hospital mortality in adults triaged in the Emergency Department—A prospective cohort study. *Scand J Trauma Resusc Emerg Med*. 2012;20(1):28.

36. Ley EJ, Singer MB, Clond MA, et al. Elevated admission systolic blood pressure after blunt trauma predicts delayed pneumonia and mortality. *J Trauma.* 2011;71(6):1689-1693.

37. Kerry R, Taylor AJ. Cervical arterial dysfunction assessment and manual therapy. *Man Ther.* 2006;11(4):243-253.

38. Kerry R, Taylor AJ. Cervical arterial dysfunction: Knowledge and reasoning for manual physical therapists. *J Orthop Sports Phys Ther.* 2009;39(5):378-387.

39. Woolf AD. How to assess musculoskeletal conditions. History and physical examination. *Best Pract Res Clin Rheumatol.* 2003;17(3):381-402.

40. Cyriax J. *Textbook of Orthopaedic Medicine, Diagnosis of Soft Tissue Lesions.* 8th ed. London, England: Bailliere Tindall; 1982.

Chapter 5

1. Rubinstein SM, van Tulder M. A best-evidence review of diagnostic procedures for neck and low-back pain. *Best Pract Res Clin Rheumatol.* 2008;22(3):471-482.

2. Maitland G. *Maitland's Vertebral Manipulation.* 6th ed. London, England: Butterworth-Heinemann; 2001.

3. Hampton JR, Harrison MJ, Mitchell JR, Prichard JS, Seymour C. Relative contributions of history-taking, physical examination, and laboratory investigation to diagnosis and management of medical outpatients. *Brit Med J.* 1975;2(5969):486-489.

4. Peterson MC, Holbrook JH, Von Hales D, Smith NL, Staker LV. Contributions of the history, physical examination, and laboratory investigation in making medical diagnoses. *West J Med.* 1992;156(2):163-165.

5. Schmitt BP, Kushner MS, Wiener SL. The diagnostic usefulness of the history of the patient with dyspnea. *J Gen Intern Med.* 1986;1(6):386-393.

6. Sandler G. Costs of unnecessary tests. *Brit Med J.* 1979;2(6181):21-24.

7. Feddock CA, Bailey PD, Griffith CH, Lineberry MJ, Wilson JF. Is time spent with the physician associated with parent dissatisfaction due to long waiting times? *Eval Health Prof.* 2010;33(2):216-225.

8. Kong MC, Camacho FT, Feldman SR, Anderson RT, Balkrishnan R. Correlates of patient satisfaction with physician visit: Differences between elderly and non-elderly survey respondents. *Health Qual Life Outcomes.* 2007;5:62.

9. Fuertes JN, Mislowack A, Bennett J, et al. The physician-patient working alliance. *Patient Educ Couns.* 2007;66(1):29-36.

10. Dalia S, Schiffman FJ. Who's my doctor? First-year residents and patient care: Hospitalized patients' perception of their "main physician". *J Grad Med Educ.* 2010;2(2):201-205.

11. Mourad M, Auerbach AD, Maselli J, Sliwka D. Patient satisfaction with a hospitalist procedure service: Is bedside procedure teaching reassuring to patients? *J Hosp Med.* 2011;6(4):219-224.

12. Beckman HB, Frankel RM. The effect of physician behavior on the collection of data. *Ann Intern Med.* 1984;101(5):692-696.

13. Marvel MK, Epstein RM, Flowers K, Beckman HB. Soliciting the patient's agenda: Have we improved? *JAMA.* 1999;281(3):283-287.

14. Duffy FD, Gordon GH, Whelan G, et al. Assessing competence in communication and interpersonal skills: The Kalamazoo II report. *Acad Med.* 2004;79(6):495-507.

15. Kurtz SM. Doctor-patient communication: Principles and practices. *Can J Neurol Sci.* 2002;29(suppl 2):S23-S29.

16. Teutsch C. Patient-doctor communication. *Med Clin North Am.* 2003;87(5):1115-1145.

17. Frohna JG, Kalet A, Kachur E, et al. Assessing residents' competency in care management: Report of a consensus conference. *Teach Learn Med.* 2004;16(1):77-84.

18. Oh J, Segal R, Gordon J, Boal J, Jotkowitz A. Retention and use of patient-centered interviewing skills after intensive training. *Acad Med.* 2001;76(6):647-650.

19. Fallowfield L, Jenkins V, Farewell V, Solis-Trapala I. Enduring impact of communication skills training: Results of a 12-month follow-up. *Brit J Cancer.* 2003;89(8):1445-1449.

20. Boissonnault WG. *Primary Care for the Physical Therapist: Examination and Triage.* 2nd ed. St. Louis, MO: Saunders; 2011.

21. Levinson W, Roter DL, Mullooly JP, Dull VT, Frankel RM. Physician-patient communication. The relationship with malpractice claims among primary care physicians and surgeons. *JAMA.* 1997;277(7):553-559.

22. Adamson TE, Tschann JM, Gullion DS, Oppenberg AA. Physician communication skills and malpractice claims. A complex relationship. *West J Med.* 1989;150(3):356-360.

23. Sandler G. The importance of the history in the medical clinic and the cost of unnecessary tests. *Am Heart J.* 1980;100(6)(part 1):928-931.

24. Richards T. Chasms in communication. *BMJ.* 1990;301(6766):1407-1408.

25. Levine R, Shore K, Lubalin J, Garfinkel S, Hurtado M, Carman K. Comparing physician and patient perceptions of quality in ambulatory care. *Int J Qual Health Care.* 2012;24(4):348-356.

26. Hasnain M, Bordage G, Connell KJ, Sinacore JM. History-taking behaviors associated with diagnostic competence of clerks: An exploratory study. *Acad Med.* 2001;76(suppl 10):S14-S17.

27. Hall AM, Ferreira PH, Maher CG, Latimer J, Ferreira ML. The influence of the therapist-patient relationship on treatment outcome in physical rehabilitation: A systematic review. *Phys Ther.* 2010;90(8):1099-1110.

28. Bruera E, Sweeney C, Calder K, Palmer L, Benisch-Tolley S. Patient preferences versus physician perceptions of treatment decisions in cancer care. *J Clin Oncol.* 2001;19(11):2883-2885.

29. Dierckx K, Deveugele M, Roosen P, Devisch I. Implementation of shared decision making in physical therapy: Observed level of involvement and patient preference. *Phys Ther.* 2013;93(10):1321-1330.

30. Ferreira PH, Ferreira ML, Maher CG, Refshauge KM, Latimer J, Adams RD. The therapeutic alliance between clinicians and patients predicts outcome in chronic low back pain. *Phys Ther.* 2013;93(4):470-478.

31. Roberts LC, Whittle CT, Cleland J, Wald M. Measuring verbal communication in initial physical therapy encounters. *Phys Ther.* 2013;93(4):479-491.

32. Thornquist E. Body communication is a continuous process. The first encounter between patient and physiotherapist. *Scand J Prim Health Care.* 1991;9(3):191-196.

33. Caris-Verhallen WM, Kerkstra A, Bensing JM. Non-verbal behaviour in nurse-elderly patient communication. *J Adv Nurs.* 1999;29(4):808-818.

34. Lurie JD. What diagnostic tests are useful for low back pain? *Best Pract Res Clin Rheumatol.* 2005;19(4):557-575.

35. Jensen GM, Shepard KF, Gwyer J, Hack LM. Attribute dimensions that distinguish master and novice physical therapy clinicians in orthopedic settings. *Phys Ther.* 1992;72(10):711-722.

36. Roter DL, Frankel RM, Hall JA, Sluyter D. The expression of emotion through nonverbal behavior in medical visits. Mechanisms and outcomes. *J Gen Intern Med.* 2006;21(suppl 1):S28-S34.

37. Bartlett EE, Grayson M, Barker R, Levine DM, Golden A, Libber S. The effects of physician communications skills on patient satisfaction, recall, and adherence. *J Chronic Dis.* 1984;37(9-10):755-764.

38. Beck RS, Daughtridge R, Sloane PD. Physician-patient communication in the primary care office: A systematic review. *J Am Board Fam Pract.* 2002;15(1):25-38.

39. Baker LH, O'Connell D, Platt FW. "What else?" Setting the agenda for the clinical interview. *Ann Intern Med.* 2005;143(10):766-770.

40. White J, Levinson W, Roter D. "Oh, by the way ...": The closing moments of the medical visit. *J Gen Intern Med.* 1994;9(1):24-28.

41. Rodondi PY, Maillefer J, Suardi F, Rodondi N, Cornuz J, Vannotti M. Physician response to "by-the-way" syndrome in primary care. *J Gen Intern Med.* 2009;24(6):739-741.

42. Schillinger D, Piette J, Grumbach K, et al. Closing the loop: Physician communication with diabetic patients who have low health literacy. *Arch Intern Med.* 2003;163(1):83-90.

43. Gross DA, Zyzanski SJ, Borawski EA, Cebul RD, Stange KC. Patient satisfaction with time spent with their physician. *J Fam Pract.* 1998;47(2):133-137.

44. Stewart MA, McWhinney IR, Buck CW. The doctor/patient relationship and its effect upon outcome. *J R Coll Gen Pract.* 1979;29(199):77-81.

45. Levinson W, Gorawara-Bhat R, Lamb J. A study of patient clues and physician responses in primary care and surgical settings. *JAMA.* 2000;284(8):1021-1027.

46. Manzoni GC, Torelli P. The patient-physician relationship in the approach to therapeutic management. *Neurol Sci.* 2007;28(suppl 2):S130-S133.

47. Maguire P, Pitceathly C. Key communication skills and how to acquire them. *BMJ.* 2002;325(7366):697-700.

48. Redelmeier DA, Schull MJ, Hux JE, Tu JV, Ferris LE. Problems for clinical judgement: 1. Eliciting an insightful history of present illness. *CMAJ.* 2001;164(5):647-651.

49. Engel GL. Editorial: Are medical schools neglecting clinical skills? *JAMA.* 1976;236(7):861-863.

50. Fletcher C. Listening and talking to patients. II: The clinical interview. *Brit Med J.* 1980;281(6245):931-933.

51. Leibold MR, Huijbregts PA, Jensen R. Concurrent criterion-related validity of physical examination tests for hip labral lesions: A systematic review. *J Man Manip Ther.* 2008;16(2):E24-E41.

52. Laslett M, Young SB, Aprill CN, McDonald B. Diagnosing painful sacroiliac joints: A validity study of a McKenzie evaluation and sacroiliac provocation tests. *Aust J Physiother.* 2003;49(2):89-97.

53. Altman R, Alarcon G, Appelrouth D, et al. The American College of Rheumatology criteria for the classification and reporting of osteoarthritis of the hip. *Arthritis and Rheumatism.* 1991;34(5):505-514.

54. Katz JN, Dalgas M, Stucki G, et al. Degenerative lumbar spinal stenosis. Diagnostic value of the history and physical examination. *Arthritis Rheum.* 1995;38(9):1236-1241.

55. Revel M, Poiraudeau S, Auleley GR, et al. Capacity of the clinical picture to characterize low back pain relieved by facet joint anesthesia. Proposed criteria to identify patients with painful facet joints. *Spine (Phila Pa 1976).* 1998;23(18):1972-1976; discussion 1977.

56. Revel ME, Listrat VM, Chevalier XJ, et al. Facet joint block for low back pain: Identifying predictors of a good response. *Arch Phys Med Rehab.* 1992;73(9):824-828.

57. Fortin JD, Falco FJ. The Fortin finger test: An indicator of sacroiliac pain. *Am J Orthop (Belle Mead NJ).* 1997;26(7):477-480.

58. Sizer PS, Jr., Brismee JM, Cook C. Medical screening for red flags in the diagnosis and management of musculoskeletal spine pain. *Pain Practice.* 2007;7(1):53-71.

59. Coronado RA, Alappattu MJ, Hart DL, George SZ. Total number and severity of comorbidities do not differ based on anatomical region of musculoskeletal pain. *J Orthop Sports Phys Ther.* 2011;41(7):477-485.

60. Grieve G. *Common Vertebral Joint Problems.* 2nd ed. Edinburgh, Scotland: Churchill Livingstone; 1988.

61. Melzack R. Pain—An overview. *Acta Anaesthesiol Scand.* 1999;43(9):880-884.

62. Moseley GL. A pain neuromatrix approach to patients with chronic pain. *Man Ther.* 2003;8(3):130-140.

63. Jensen MC, Brant-Zawadzki MN, Obuchowski N, Modic MT, Malkasian D, Ross JS. Magnetic resonance imaging of the lumbar spine in people without back pain. *N Engl J Med.* 1994;331(2):69-73.

64. Jarvik JG, Deyo RA. Diagnostic evaluation of low back pain with emphasis on imaging. *Ann Intern Med.* 2002;137(7):586-597.

65. Deyo RA, Rainville J, Kent DL. What can the history and physical examination tell us about low back pain? *JAMA.* 1992;268(6):760-765.

66. Turk DC. The role of psychological factors in chronic pain. *Acta Anaesthesiol Scand.* 1999;43(9):885-888.

67. Baker K. Recent advances in the neurophysiology of chronic pain. *Emerg Med Australas.* 2005;17(1):65-72.

68. Cimmino MA, Ferrone C, Cutolo M. Epidemiology of chronic musculoskeletal pain. *Best Pract Res Clin Rheumatol.* 2011;25(2):173-183.

69. Woolf AD, Vos T, March L. How to measure the impact of musculoskeletal conditions. *Best Pract Res Clin Rheumatol.* 2010;24(6):723-732.

70. Woolf AD, Akesson K. Understanding the burden of musculoskeletal conditions. The burden is huge and not reflected in national health priorities. *BMJ.* 2001;322(7294):1079-1080.

71. Woolf AD, Pfleger B. Burden of major musculoskeletal conditions. *B World Health Organ.* 2003;81(9):646-656.

72. Brooks PM. The burden of musculoskeletal disease—A global perspective. *Clin Rheumatol.* 2006;25(6):778-781.

73. Turk DC. Customizing treatment for chronic pain patients: Who, what, and why. *Clin J Pain.* 1990;6(4):255-270.

74. Garratt A, Schmidt L, Mackintosh A, Fitzpatrick R. Quality of life measurement: Bibliographic study of patient assessed health outcome measures. *BMJ.* 2002;324(7351):1417.

75. Maly MR, Costigan PA, Olney SJ. Determinants of self-report outcome measures in people with knee osteoarthritis. *Arch Phys Med Rehabil.* 2006;87(1):96-104.

76. Lee CE, Simmonds MJ, Novy DM, Jones S. Self-reports and clinician-measured physical function among patients with low back pain: A comparison. *Arch Phys Med Rehabil.* 2001;82(2):227-231.

77. Reneman MF, Jorritsma W, Schellekens JM, Goeken LN. Concurrent validity of questionnaire and performance-based disability measurements in patients with chronic nonspecific low back pain. *J Occup Rehabil.* 2002;12(3):119-129.

78. Bellamy N, Kirwan J, Boers M, et al. Recommendations for a core set of outcome measures for future phase III clinical trials in knee, hip, and hand osteoarthritis. Consensus development at OMERACT III. *J Rheumatol.* 1997;24(4):799-802.

79. Terwee CB, van der Slikke RM, van Lummel RC, Benink RJ, Meijers WG, de Vet HC. Self-reported physical functioning was more influenced by pain than performance-based physical functioning in knee-osteoarthritis patients. *J Clin Epidemiol.* 2006;59(7):724-731.

80. Stratford PW, Kennedy DM, Maly MR, Macintyre NJ. Quantifying self-report measures' overestimation of mobility scores postarthroplasty. *Phys Ther.* 2010;90(9):1288-1296.

81. Stratford PW, Kennedy DM, Woodhouse LJ. Performance measures provide assessments of pain and function in people with advanced osteoarthritis of the hip or knee. *Phys Ther.* 2006;86(11):1489-1496.

82. Parent E, Moffet H. Comparative responsiveness of locomotor tests and questionnaires used to follow early recovery after total knee arthroplasty. *Arch Phys Med Rehabil.* 2002;83(1):70-80.

83. Filho IT, Simmonds MJ, Protas EJ, Jones S. Back pain, physical function, and estimates of aerobic capacity: What are the relationships among methods and measures? *Am J Phys Med Rehabil.* 2002;81(12):913-920.

84. Simmonds MJ. Measuring and managing pain and performance. *Man Ther.* 2006;11(3):175-179.

85. Westaway MD, Stratford PW, Binkley JM. The patient-specific functional scale: Validation of its use in persons with neck dysfunction. *J Orthop Sports Phys Ther.* 1998;27(5):331-338.

86. Stratford P, Gill C, Westaway M, Binkley J. Assessing disability and change on individual patients: A report of a patient-specific measure. *Physiother Can.* 1995;47:258.

87. Kamper SJ, Maher CG, Mackay G. Global rating of change scales: A review of strengths and weaknesses and considerations for design. *J Man Manip Ther.* 2009;17(3):163-170.

88. Mattingly C, Flemming M. *Clinical Reasoning: Forms of Inquiry in a Therapeutic Practice.* Philadelphia, PA: FA Davis Company; 1994.

89. Higgs J, Jones M. *Clinical Reasoning in the Health Professions.* 2nd ed. Oxford, England: Butterworth-Heinemann; 2000.

90. Cook C. *Orthopedic Manual Therapy: An Evidenced-Based Approach.* 2nd ed. Boston, MA: Pearson; 2012.

91. Borrell-Carrió F, Suchman AL, Epstein RM. The biopsychosocial model 25 years later: Principles, practice, and scientific inquiry. *Ann Fam Med.* 2004;2(6):576-582.

92. Charon R. The patient-physician relationship. Narrative medicine: A model for empathy, reflection, profession, and trust. *JAMA.* 2001;286(15):1897-1902.

93. Epstein RM. Mindful practice. *JAMA.* 1999;282(9):833-839.

94. Jones MA. Clinical reasoning in manual therapy. *Physical Therapy.* 1992;72(12):875-884.

95. Haynes RB, Devereaux PJ, Guyatt GH. Physicians' and patients' choices in evidence based practice. *BMJ.* 2002;324(7350):1350.

96. Mamede S, Splinter TA, van Gog T, Rikers RM, Schmidt HG. Exploring the role of salient distracting clinical features in the emergence of diagnostic errors and the mechanisms through which reflection counteracts mistakes. *BMJ Qual Saf.* 2012;21(4):295-300.

97. Elstein AS, Schwartz A, Schwarz A. Clinical problem solving and diagnostic decision making: Selective review of the cognitive literature. *BMJ.* 2002;324(7339):729-732.

98. Norman G. Research in clinical reasoning: Past history and current trends. *Med Educ.* 2005;39(4):418-427.

99. Engel GL. The need for a new medical model: A challenge for biomedicine. *Science.* 1977;196(4286):129-136.

100. Engel GL. The clinical application of the biopsychosocial model. *Am J Psychiatry.* 1980;137(5):535-544.

101. Eva KW. What every teacher needs to know about clinical reasoning. *Med Educ.* 2005;39(1):98-106.

102. Kassirer JP. Teaching clinical reasoning: Case-based and coached. *Acad Med.* 2010;85(7):1118-1124.

103. Epstein RM, Hundert EM. Defining and assessing professional competence. *JAMA.* 2002;287(2):226-235.

104. Resnik L, Jensen GM. Using clinical outcomes to explore the theory of expert practice in physical therapy. *Phys Ther.* 2003;83(12):1090-1106.

105. Ericsson KA. Deliberate practice and acquisition of expert performance: A general overview. *Acad Emerg Med.* 2008;15(11):988-994.

106. Ericsson KA. Deliberate practice and the acquisition and maintenance of expert performance in medicine and related domains. *Acad Med.* 2004;79(suppl 10):S70-S81.

107. Ericsson K, Prietula M, Cokely E. The making of an expert. *Harvard Bus Rev.* 2007:115-121.

108. Krampe RT, Ericsson KA. Maintaining excellence: Deliberate practice and elite performance in young and older pianists. *J Exp Psychol Gen.* 1996;125(4):331-359.

109. Simon H, Chase W. Skill in chess. *Am Sci.* 1973;61:394-403.

110. Jones M, Jensen G, Edwards I. Clinical reasoning in physiotherapy. In: Higgs J, Jones, M, eds. *Clinical Reasoning in the Health Professions.* 2nd ed. Oxford, England: Butterworth Heinemann; 2000.

111. Wainwright SF, Shepard KF, Harman LB, Stephens J. Novice and experienced physical therapist clinicians: A comparison of how reflection is used to inform the clinical decision-making process. *Phys Ther.* 2010;90(1):75-88.

112. Klein JG. Five pitfalls in decisions about diagnosis and prescribing. *BMJ.* 2005;330(7494):781-783.

Chapter 6

1. Chipman M, Hackley BE, Spencer TS. Triage of mass casualties: Concepts for coping with mixed battlefield injuries. *Mil Med.* 1980;145(2):99-100.

2. American Physical Therapy Association. *Guide to Physical Therapist Practice.* 2nd ed. Alexandria, VA: Author; 2003.

3. Goodman CC, Snyder TE. *Differential Diagnosis for Physical Therapists: Screening for Referral.* 4th ed. St. Louis, MO: Saunders Elsevier; 2007.

4. Boissonnault WG, Ross MD. Physical therapists referring patients to physicians: A review of case reports and series. *J Orthop Sports Phys Ther.* 2012;42(5):446-454.

5. Sizer PS, Jr., Brismee JM, Cook C. Medical screening for red flags in the diagnosis and management of musculoskeletal spine pain. *Pain Pract.* 2007;7(1):53-71.

6. Pineda CJ, Guerra J, Jr., Weisman MH, Resnick D, Martinez-Lavin M. The skeletal manifestations of clubbing: A study in patients with cyanotic congenital heart disease and hypertrophic osteoarthropathy. *Semin Arthritis Rheum.* 1985;14(4):263-273.

7. Zyluk A, Ostrowski P. An analysis of factors influencing accuracy of the diagnosis of acute appendicitis. *Pol Przegl Chir.* 2011;83(3):135-143.

8. Henschke N, Maher CG, Refshauge KM, et al. Prevalence of and screening for serious spinal pathology in patients presenting to primary care settings with acute low back pain. *Arthritis Rheum.* 2009;60(10):3072-3080.

9. Bishop PB, Wing PC. Knowledge transfer in family physicians managing patients with acute low back pain: A prospective randomized control trial. *Spine J.* 2006;6(3):282-288.

10. Jette DU, Ardleigh K, Chandler K, McShea L. Decision-making ability of physical therapists: Physical therapy intervention or medical referral. *Phys Ther.* 2006;86(12):1619-1629.

11. Barr JB. Integration of imaging into physical therapy practice. In: McKinnis LN, ed. *Fundamentals of Musculoskeletal Imaging.* Philadelphia, PA: FA Davis; 2005.

12. Beltrame V, Stramare R, Rebellato N, Angelini F, Frigo AC, Rubaltelli L. Sonographic evaluation of bone fractures: A reliable alternative in clinical practice? *Clin Imaging.* 2012;36(3):203-208.

13. Menashe L, Hirko K, Losina E, et al. The diagnostic performance of MRI in osteoarthritis: A systematic review and meta-analysis. *Osteoarthr Cartilage.* 2012;20(1):13-21.

14. Suter LG, Fraenkel L, Braithwaite RS. Role of magnetic resonance imaging in the diagnosis and prognosis of rheumatoid arthritis. *Arthrit Care Res (Hoboken).* 2011;63(5):675-688.

15. Butalia S, Palda VA, Sargeant RJ, Detsky AS, Mourad O. Does this patient with diabetes have osteomyelitis of the lower extremity? *JAMA.* 2008;299(7):806-813.

16. Termaat MF, Raijmakers PG, Scholten HJ, Bakker FC, Patka P, Haarman HJ. The accuracy of diagnostic imaging for the assessment of chronic osteomyelitis: A systematic review and meta-analysis. *J Bone Joint Surg Am.* 2005;87(11):2464-2471.

17. Cappello ZJ, Kasdan ML, Louis DS. Meta-analysis of imaging techniques for the diagnosis of complex regional pain syndrome type I. *J Hand Surg Am.* 2012;37(2):288-296.

18. Samad Z, Hakeem A, Mahmood SS, et al. A meta-analysis and systematic review of computed tomography angiography as a diagnostic triage tool for patients with chest pain presenting to the emergency department. *J Nucl Cardiol.* 2012;19(2):364-376.

19. Jaarsma C, Leiner T, Bekkers SC, et al. Diagnostic performance of noninvasive myocardial perfusion imaging using single-photon emission computed tomography, cardiac magnetic resonance, and positron emission tomography imaging for the detection of obstructive coronary artery disease: A meta-analysis. *J Am Coll Cardiol.* 2012;59(19):1719-1728.

20. Romero J, Xue X, Gonzalez W, Garcia MJ. CMR imaging assessing viability in patients with chronic ventricular dysfunction due to coronary artery disease: A meta-analysis of prospective trials. *JACC Cardiovasc Imaging.* 2012;5(5):494-508.

21. Collins R, Cranny G, Burch J, et al. A systematic review of duplex ultrasound, magnetic resonance angiography and computed tomography angiography for the diagnosis and assessment of symptomatic, lower limb peripheral arterial disease. *Health Technol Assess.* 2007;11(20):iii-iv, xi-xiii, 1-184.

22. Thomas SM, Goodacre SW, Sampson FC, van Beek EJ. Diagnostic value of CT for deep vein thrombosis: Results of a systematic review and meta-analysis. *Clin Radiol.* 2008;63(3):299-304.

23. Sampson FC, Goodacre SW, Thomas SM, van Beek EJ. The accuracy of MRI in diagnosis of suspected deep vein thrombosis: Systematic review and meta-analysis. *Eur Radiol.* 2007;17(1):175-181.

24. Goodacre S, Sampson F, Thomas S, van Beek E, Sutton A. Systematic review and meta-analysis of the diagnostic accuracy of ultrasonography for deep vein thrombosis. *BMC Med Imaging.* 2005;5:6.

25. Segal JB, Eng J, Tamariz LJ, Bass EB. Review of the evidence on diagnosis of deep venous thrombosis and pulmonary embolism. *Ann Fam Med.* 2007;5(1):63-73.

26. Mustafa BO, Rathbun SW, Whitsett TL, Raskob GE. Sensitivity and specificity of ultrasonography in the diagnosis of upper extremity deep vein thrombosis: A systematic review. *Arch Intern Med.* 2002;162(4):401-404.

27. Kory PD, Pellecchia CM, Shiloh AL, Mayo PH, DiBello C, Koenig S. Accuracy of ultrasonography performed by critical care physicians for the diagnosis of DVT. *Chest.* 2011;139(3):538-542.

28. Locker T, Goodacre S, Sampson F, Webster A, Sutton AJ. Meta-analysis of plethysmography and rheography in the diagnosis of deep vein thrombosis. *Emerg Med J.* 2006;23(8):630-635.

29. Rubano E, Mehta N, Caputo W, Paladino L, Sinert R. Systematic review: Emergency department bedside ultrasonography for diagnosing suspected abdominal aortic aneurysm. *Acad Emerg Med.* 2013;20(2):128-138.

30. Biancari F, Paone R, Venermo M, D'Andrea V, Perälä J. Diagnostic accuracy of computed tomography in patients with suspected abdominal aortic aneurysm rupture. *Eur J Vasc Endovasc Surg.* 2013;45(3):227-230.

31. Rathbun SW, Raskob GE, Whitsett TL. Sensitivity and specificity of helical computed tomography in the diagnosis of pulmonary embolism: A systematic review. *Ann Intern Med.* 2000;132(3):227-232.

32. Stengel D, Ottersbach C, Matthes G, et al. Accuracy of single-pass whole-body computed tomography for detection of injuries in patients with major blunt trauma. *CMAJ.* 2012;184(8):869-876.

33. Nishijima DK, Simel DL, Wisner DH, Holmes JF. Does this adult patient have a blunt intra-abdominal injury? *JAMA.* 2012;307(14):1517-1527.

34. Holmes JF, Harris D, Battistella FD. Performance of abdominal ultrasonography in blunt trauma patients with out-of-hospital or emergency department hypotension. *Ann Emerg Med.* 2004;43(3):354-361.

35. Stephen AE, Segev DL, Ryan DP, et al. The diagnosis of acute appendicitis in a pediatric population: To CT or not to CT. *J Pediatr Surg.* 2003;38(3):367-371; discsussion 367-371.

36. Bachar I, Perry Z, Dukhno L, Mizrahi S, Kirshtein B. Diagnostic value of laparoscopy, abdominal computed tomography, and ultrasonography in acute appendicitis. *J Laparoendosc Adv S.* 2013;23(12):982-989.

37. Navarro Fernandez JA, Tarraga Lopez PJ, Rodriguez Montes JA, Lopez Cara MA. Validity of tests performed to diagnose acute abdominal pain in patients admitted at an emergency department. *Rev Esp Enferm Dig.* 2009;101(9):610-618.

38. Linguraru MG, Sandberg JK, Jones EC, Petrick N, Summers RM. Assessing hepatomegaly: Automated volumetric analysis of the liver. *Acad Radiol.* 2012;19(5):588-598.

39. Wong KW, Leong JC, Chan MK, Luk KD, Lu WW. The flexion-extension profile of lumbar spine in 100 healthy volunteers. *Spine (Phila Pa 1976).* 2004;29(15):1636-1641.

40. Kellgren JH, Lawrence JS. Radiological assessment of osteo-arthrosis. *Ann Rheum Dis.* 1957;16(4):494-502.

41. Modic MT, Masaryk TJ, Mulopulos GP, Bundschuh C, Han JS, Bohlman H. Cervical radiculopathy: Prospective evaluation with surface coil MR imaging, CT with metrizamide, and metrizamide myelography. *Radiology.* 1986;161(3):753-759.

42. Laker SR, Concannon LG. Radiologic evaluation of the neck: A review of radiography, ultrasonography, computed tomography, magnetic resonance imaging, and other imaging modalities for neck pain. *Phys Med Rehabil Clin N Am.* 2011;22(3):411-428, vii-viii.

43. Hong W, Earnest A, Sultana P, Koh Z, Shahidah N, Ong ME. How accurate are vital signs in predicting clinical outcomes in critically ill emergency department patients. *Eur J Emerg Med.* 2013;20(1)-27-32.

44. Barfod C, Lauritzen MM, Danker JK, et al. Abnormal vital signs are strong predictors for Intensive Care Unit admission and in-hospital mortality in adults triaged in the Emergency Department—A prospective cohort study. *Scand J Trauma Resusc Emerg Med.* 2012;20(1):28.

45. Ley EJ, Singer MB, Clond MA, et al. Elevated admission systolic blood pressure after blunt trauma predicts delayed pneumonia and mortality. *J Trauma.* 2011;71(6):1689-1693.

46. Khan KM, Thompson AM, Blair SN, et al. Sport and exercise as contributors to the health of nations. *Lancet.* 2012;380(9836):59-64.

47. Simel D. Approach to the patient: History and physical examination. In: Goldman L, Schafer A, eds. *Goldman's Cecil Medicine.* Philadelphia, PA: Saunders Elsevier; 2011.

48. Fraser S, Roberts L, Murphy E. Cauda equina syndrome: A literature review of its definition and clinical presentation. *Arch Phys Med Rehabil.* 2009;90(11):1964-1968.

49. Balasubramanian K, Kalsi P, Greenough CG, Kuskoor Seetharam MP. Reliability of clinical assessment in diagnosing cauda equina syndrome. *Brit J Neurosurg.* 2010;24(4):383-386.

50. Haj-Hassan TA, Thompson MJ, Mayon-White RT, et al. Which early 'red flag' symptoms identify children with meningococcal disease in primary care? *Brit J Gen Pract.* 2011;61(584):e97-e104.

51. Hong YH, Lee YS, Park SH. Headache as a predictive factor of severe systolic hypertension in acute ischemic stroke. *Can J Neurol Sci.* 2003;30(3):210-214.

52. Bruce MG, Rosenstein NE, Capparella JM, Shutt KA, Perkins BA, Collins M. Risk factors for meningococcal disease in college students. *JAMA.* 2001;286(6):688-693.

53. Sobri M, Lamont AC, Alias NA, Win MN. Red flags in patients presenting with headache: clinical indications for neuroimaging. *Brit J Radiol.* 2003;76(908):532-535.

54. Borg J, Holm L, Cassidy JD, et al. Diagnostic procedures in mild traumatic brain injury: Results of the WHO Collaborating Centre Task Force on Mild Traumatic Brain Injury. *J Rehabil Med.* 2004;(suppl 43):61-75.

55. Harmon KG, Drezner JA, Gammons M, et al. American Medical Society for Sports Medicine position statement: Concussion in sport. *Brit J Sport Med.* 2013;47(1):15-26.

56. Forsyth PA, Posner JB. Headaches in patients with brain tumors: A study of 111 patients. *Neurology.* 1993;43(9):1678-1683.

57. Zaki A, Natarajan N, Mettlin CJ. Patterns of presentation in brain tumors in the United States. *J Surg Oncol.* 1993;53(2):110-112.

58. Snyder H, Robinson K, Shah D, Brennan R, Handrigan M. Signs and symptoms of patients with brain tumors presenting to the emergency department. *J Emerg Med.* 1993;11(3):253-258.

59. Rao G, Fisch L, Srinivasan S, et al. Does this patient have Parkinson disease? *JAMA.* 2003;289(3):347-353.

60. Friedman JH, Abrantes AM. The Glabellar reflex is a poor measure of Parkinson motor severity. *Int J Neurosci.* 2013;123(6):417-419.

61. Knol W, Keijsers CJ, Jansen PA, et al. Validity and reliability of the Simpson-Angus Scale (SAS) in drug induced Parkinsonism in the elderly. *Int J Geriatr Psychiatry.* 2009;24(2):183-189.

62. Scherer K, Bedlack RS, Simel DL. Does this patient have myasthenia gravis? *JAMA.* 2005;293(15):1906-1914.

63. Benatar M. A systematic review of diagnostic studies in myasthenia gravis. *Neuromuscul Disord.* 2006;16(7):459-467.

64. Cook CE, Hegedus E, Pietrobon R, Goode A. A pragmatic neurological screen for patients with suspected cord compressive myelopathy. *Phys Ther.* 2007;87(9):1233-1242.

65. Steurer J, Held U, Schmid D, Ruckstuhl J, Bachmann LM. Clinical value of diagnostic instruments for ruling out acute coronary syndrome in patients with chest pain: A systematic review. *Emerg Med J.* 2010;27(12):896-902.

66. Whiting P, Rutjes AW, Reitsma JB, Bossuyt PM, Kleijnen J. The development of QUADAS: A tool for the quality assessment of studies of diagnostic accuracy included in systematic reviews. *BMC Med Res Methodol.* 2003;3:25.

67. Selker HP, Griffith JL, D'Agostino RB. A tool for judging coronary care unit admission appropriateness, valid for both real-time and retrospective use. A time-insensitive predictive instrument (TIPI) for acute cardiac ischemia: A multicenter study. *Med Care.* 1991;29(7):610-627.

68. Selker HP, Griffith JL, D'Agostino RB. A time-insensitive predictive instrument for acute myocardial infarction mortality: A multicenter study. *Med Care.* 1991;29(12):1196-1211.

69. Seyal JM, Clark EN, Macfarlane PW. Diagnosis of acute myocardial ischaemia using probabilistic methods. *J Cardiovasc Risk.* 2002;9(2):115-121.

70. Miller CD, Lindsell CJ, Anantharaman V, et al. Performance of a population-based cardiac risk stratification tool in Asian patients with chest pain. *Acad Emerg Med.* 2005;12(5):423-430.

71. Mitchell AM, Garvey JL, Chandra A, Diercks D, Pollack CV, Kline JA. Prospective multicenter study of quantitative pretest probability assessment to exclude acute coronary syndrome for patients evaluated in emergency department chest pain units. *Ann Emerg Med.* 2006;47(5):447.

72. Kellett J. Early diagnosis of acute myocardial infarction by either electrocardiogram or a logistic regression model: Portability of a predictive instrument of acute cardiac ischemia to a small rural coronary care unit. *Can J Cardiol.* 1997;13(11):1033-1038.

73. Sanchis J, Bodí V, Núñez J, et al. New risk score for patients with acute chest pain, non-ST-segment deviation, and normal troponin concentrations: A comparison with the TIMI risk score. *J Am Coll Cardiol.* 2005;46(3):443-449.

74. Haasenritter J, Bösner S, Vaucher P, et al. Ruling out coronary heart disease in primary care: External validation of a clinical prediction rule. *Brit J Gen Pract.* 2012;62(599):e415-e421.

75. Bruyninckx R, Aertgeerts B, Bruyninckx P, Buntinx F. Signs and symptoms in diagnosing acute myocardial infarction and acute coronary syndrome: A diagnostic meta-analysis. *Brit J Gen Pract.* 2008;58(547):105-111.

76. Goodacre S, Locker T, Morris F, Campbell S. How useful are clinical features in the diagnosis of acute, undifferentiated chest pain? *Acad Emerg Med.* 2002;9(3):203-208.

77. Goodacre SW, Angelini K, Arnold J, Revill S, Morris F. Clinical predictors of acute coronary syndromes in patients with undifferentiated chest pain. *QJM.* 2003;96(12):893-898.

78. Wang CS, FitzGerald JM, Schulzer M, Mak E, Ayas NT. Does this dyspneic patient in the emergency department have congestive heart failure? *JAMA.* 2005;294(15):1944-1956.

79. Wells PS, Anderson DR, Bormanis J, et al. Value of assessment of pretest probability of deep-vein thrombosis in clinical management. *Lancet.* 1997;350(9094):1795-1798.

80. Goodacre S, Sutton AJ, Sampson FC. Meta-analysis: The value of clinical assessment in the diagnosis of deep venous thrombosis. *Ann Intern Med.* 2005;143(2):129-139.

81. Khan NA, Rahim SA, Anand SS, Simel DL, Panju A. Does the clinical examination predict lower extremity peripheral arterial disease? *JAMA.* 2006;295(5):536-546.

82. Lederle FA, Simel DL. The rational clinical examination. Does this patient have abdominal aortic aneurysm? *JAMA.* 1999;281(1):77-82.

83. Cosford PA, Leng GC. Screening for abdominal aortic aneurysm. *Cochrane Db Syst Rev.* 2007(2):CD002945.

84. Lynch RM. Accuracy of abdominal examination in the diagnosis of non-ruptured abdominal aortic aneurysm. *Accid Emerg Nurs.* 2004;12(2):99-107.

85. Smetana GW, Shmerling RH. Does this patient have temporal arteritis? *JAMA.* 2002;287(1):92-101.

86. West J, Goodacre S, Sampson F. The value of clinical features in the diagnosis of acute pulmonary embolism: Systematic review and meta-analysis. *QJM.* 2007;100(12):763-769.

87. Le Gal G, Righini M, Roy PM, et al. Prediction of pulmonary embolism in the emergency department: The revised Geneva score. *Ann Intern Med.* 2006;144(3):165-171.

88. Klok FA, Kruisman E, Spaan J, et al. Comparison of the revised Geneva score with the Wells rule for assessing clinical probability of pulmonary embolism. *J Thromb Haemost.* 2008;6(1):40-44.

89. Calisir C, Yavas US, Ozkan IR, et al. Performance of the Wells and Revised Geneva scores for predicting pulmonary embolism. *Eur J Emerg Med.* 2009;16(1):49-52.

90. Lucassen W, Geersing GJ, Erkens PM, et al. Clinical decision rules for excluding pulmonary embolism: A meta-analysis. *Ann Intern Med.* 2011;155(7):448-460.

91. Stein PD, Woodard PK, Weg JG, et al. Diagnostic pathways in acute pulmonary embolism: Recommendations of the PIOPED II Investigators. *Radiology.* 2007;242(1):15-21.

92. Holmes JF, Wisner DH, McGahan JP, Mower WR, Kuppermann N. Clinical prediction rules for identifying adults at very low risk for intra-abdominal injuries after blunt trauma. *Ann Emerg Med.* 2009;54(4):575-584.

93. Wagner JM, McKinney WP, Carpenter JL. Does this patient have appendicitis? *JAMA.* 1996;276(19):1589-1594.

94. Yeh B. Evidence-based emergency medicine/rational clinical examination abstract. Does this adult patient have appendicitis? *Ann Emerg Med.* 2008;52(3):301-303.

95. Bundy DG, Byerley JS, Liles EA, Perrin EM, Katznelson J, Rice HE. Does this child have appendicitis? *JAMA.* 2007;298(4):438-451.

96. Alvarado A. A practical score for the early diagnosis of acute appendicitis. *Ann Emerg Med.* 1986;15(5):557-564.

97. Tzanakis NE, Efstathiou SP, Danulidis K, et al. A new approach to accurate diagnosis of acute appendicitis. *World J Surg.* 2005;29(9):1151-1156, discussion 1157.

98. Trowbridge RL, Rutkowski NK, Shojania KG. Does this patient have acute cholecystitis? *JAMA.* 2003;289(1):80-86.

99. Naylor CD. The rational clinical examination. Physical examination of the liver. *JAMA.* 1994;271(23):1859-1865.

100. Joshi R, Singh A, Jajoo N, Pai M, Kalantri SP. Accuracy and reliability of palpation and percussion for detecting hepatomegaly: A rural hospital-based study. *Indian J Gastroenterol.* 2004;23(5):171-174.

101. Ralphs DN, Venn G, Khan O, Palmer JG, Cameron DE, Hobsley M. Is the undeniably palpable liver ever 'normal'? *Ann R Coll Surg Engl.* 1983;65(3):159-160.

102. Larson SM, Tuell SH, Moores KD, Nelp WB. Dimensions of the normal adult spleen scan and prediction of spleen weight. *J Nucl Med.* 1971;12(3):123-126.

103. Berris B. The incidence of palpable liver and spleen in the postpartum period. *Can Med Assoc J.* 1966;95(25):1318-1319.

104. Barkun AN, Grover SA, Muir A. *Make the Diagnosis: Splenomegaly.* New York, NY: McGraw-Hill; 2009.

105. Barkun AN, Camus M, Green L, et al. The bedside assessment of splenic enlargement. *Am J Med.* 1991;91(5):512-518.

106. Bent S, Nallamothu BK, Simel DL, Fihn SD, Saint S. Does this woman have an acute uncomplicated urinary tract infection? *JAMA.* 2002;287(20):2701-2710.

107. Simel DL. *Make the Diagnosis: Upper Gastrointestinal Bleed.* New York, NY: McGraw-Hill; 2013.

108. Agréus L, Talley NJ, Svärdsudd K, Tibblin G, Jones MP. Identifying dyspepsia and irritable bowel syndrome: The value of pain or discomfort, and bowel habit descriptors. *Scand J Gastroenterol.* 2000;35(2):142-151.

109. Manning AP, Thompson WG, Heaton KW, Morris AF. Towards positive diagnosis of the irritable bowel. *Br Med J.* 1978;2(6138):653-654.

110. Kruis W, Thieme C, Weinzierl M, Schüssler P, Holl J, Paulus W. A diagnostic score for the irritable bowel syndrome. Its value in the exclusion of organic disease. *Gastroenterology.* 1984;87(1):1-7.

111. Tibble JA, Sigthorsson G, Foster R, Forgacs I, Bjarnason I. Use of surrogate markers of inflammation and Rome criteria to distinguish organic from nonorganic intestinal disease. *Gastroenterology.* 2002;123(2):450-460.

112. Simel DL. *Make the Diagnosis: Irritable Bowel Syndrome.* New York, NY: McGraw-Hill; 2009.

113. Margaretten ME, Kohlwes J, Moore D, Bent S. Does this adult patient have septic arthritis? *JAMA.* 2007;297(13):1478-1488.

114. Ludewig PM, Lawrence RL, Braman JP. What's in a name? Using movement system diagnoses versus pathoanatomic diagnoses. *J Orthop Sports Phys Ther.* 2013;43(5):280-283.

115. Green S, Buchbinder R, Glazier R, Forbes A. Systematic review of randomised controlled trials of interventions for painful shoulder: Selection criteria, outcome assessment, and efficacy. *BMJ.* 1998;316(7128):354-360.

116. Schellingerhout JM, Verhagen AP, Thomas S, Koes BW. Lack of uniformity in diagnostic labeling of shoulder pain: Time for a different approach. *Man Ther.* 2008;13(6):478-483.

117. Van Tulder MW, Koes BW, Bouter LM. Conservative treatment of acute and chronic nonspecific low back pain. A systematic review of randomized controlled trials of the most common interventions. *Spine (Phila Pa 1976).* 1997;22(18):2128-2156.

118. Delitto A, Erhard RE, Bowling RW. A treatment-based classification approach to low back syndrome: Identifying and staging patients for conservative treatment. *Phys Ther.* 1995;75(6):470-485; discussion 485-479.

119. Spratt KF, Weinstein JN, Lehmann TR, Woody J, Sayre H. Efficacy of flexion and extension treatments incorporating braces for low-back pain patients with retrodisplacement, spondylolisthesis, or normal sagittal translation. *Spine (Phila Pa 1976).* 1993;18(13):1839-1849.

120. Fritz JM, Brennan GP, Clifford SN, Hunter SJ, Thackeray A. An examination of the reliability of a classification algorithm for subgrouping patients with low back pain. *Spine (Phila Pa 1976).* 2006;31(1):77-82.

121. BenDebba M, Torgerson WS, Long DM. A validated, practical classification procedure for many persistent low back pain patients. *Pain.* 2000;87(1):89-97.

122. Binkley J, Finch E, Hall J, Black T, Gowland C. Diagnostic classification of patients with low back pain: Report on a survey of physical therapy experts. *Phys Ther.* 1993;73(3):138-150; discussion 150-155.

123. Heiss DG, Fitch DS, Fritz JM, Sanchez WJ, Roberts KE, Buford JA. The interrater reliability among physical therapists newly trained in a classification system for acute low back pain. *J Orthop Sports Phys Ther.* 2004;34(8):430-439.

124. Fritz JM, Cleland JA, Childs JD. Subgrouping patients with low back pain: Evolution of a classification approach to physical therapy. *J Orthop Sports Phys Ther.* 2007;37(6):290-302.

125. Fritz JM, Delitto A, Erhard RE. Comparison of classification-based physical therapy with therapy based on clinical practice guidelines for patients with acute low back pain: A randomized clinical trial. *Spine (Phila Pa 1976).* 2003;28(13):1363-1371; discussion 1372.

126. Fritz JM, George S. The use of a classification approach to identify subgroups of patients with acute low back pain. Interrater reliability and short-term treatment outcomes. *Spine (Phila Pa 1976).* 2000;25(1):106-114.

127. Brennan GP, Fritz JM, Hunter SJ, Thackeray A, Delitto A, Erhard RE. Identifying subgroups of patients with acute/subacute "nonspecific" low back pain: Results of a randomized clinical trial. *Spine (Phila Pa 1976).* 2006;31(6):623-631.

128. Stanton TR, Fritz JM, Hancock MJ, et al. Evaluation of a treatment-based classification algorithm for low back pain: A cross-sectional study. *Phys Ther.* 2011;91(4):496-509.

Chapter 7

1. Lee MW, McPhee RW, Stringer MD. An evidence-based approach to human dermatomes. *Clin Anat.* 2008;21(5):363-373.

2. Wolff AP, Groen GJ, Crul BJ. Diagnostic lumbosacral segmental nerve blocks with local anesthetics: A prospective double-blind study on the variability and interpretation of segmental effects. *Reg Anesth Pain Med.* 2001;26(2):147-155.

3. Slipman CW, Plastaras CT, Palmitier RA, Huston CW, Sterenfeld EB. Symptom provocation of fluoroscopically guided cervical nerve root stimulation. Are dynatomal maps identical to dermatomal maps? *Spine (Phila Pa 1976).* 1998;23(20):2235-2242.

4. Sizer PS, Jr., Brismee JM, Cook C. Medical screening for red flags in the diagnosis and management of musculoskeletal spine pain. *Pain Practice.* 2007;7(1):53-71.

5. Gemici C. Lhermitte's sign: Review with special emphasis in oncology practice. *Crit Rev Oncol Hematol.* 2010;74(2):79-86.

6. Suri P, Hunter DJ, Katz JN, Li L, Rainville J. Bias in the physical examination of patients with lumbar radiculopathy. *BMC Musculoskelet Disord.* 2010;11:275.

7. Louw A, Mintken P. Neurophysiologic effects of neural mobilization maneuvers. In: Fernandez-de-Las-Penas C, Arendt-Nielson L, Gerwin R, eds. *Tension-Type and Cervicogenic Headache.* Boston, MA: Jones and Bartlett; 2009:231-245.

8. Reiman MP, Manske RC. *Functional Testing in Human Performance.* Champaign, IL: Human Kinetics; 2009.

9. Butler DA. *Mobilisation of the Nervous System.* Melbourne, Australia: Churchille Livingstone; 1991.

10. Butler D. *The Sensitive Nervous System.* Prussia, PA: NOI Group; 2000.

11. Olaleye D, Perkins BA, Bril V. Evaluation of three screening tests and a risk assessment model for diagnosing peripheral neuropathy in the diabetes clinic. *Diabetes Res Clin Pract.* 2001;54(2):115-128.

12. Perkins BA, Olaleye D, Zinman B, Bril V. Simple screening tests for peripheral neuropathy in the diabetes clinic. *Diabetes Care.* 2001;24(2):250-256.

13. Wainner RS, Fritz JM, Irrgang JJ, Boninger ML, Delitto A, Allison S. Reliability and diagnostic accuracy of the clinical examination and patient self-report measures for cervical radiculopathy. *Spine (Phila Pa 1976).* 2003;28(1):52-62.

14. Lauder TD, Dillingham TR, Andary M, et al. Predicting electrodiagnostic outcome in patients with upper limb symptoms: Are the history and physical examination helpful? *Arch Phys Med Rehabil.* 2000;81(4):436-441.

15. Matsumoto M, Fujimura Y, Toyama Y. Usefulness and reliability of neurological signs for level diagnosis in cervical myelopathy caused by soft disc herniation. *J Spinal Disord.* 1996;9(4):317-321.

16. Matsumoto M, Ishikawa M, Ishii K, et al. Usefulness of neurological examination for diagnosis of the affected level in patients with cervical compressive myelopathy: Prospective comparative study with radiological evaluation. *J Neurosurg Spine.* 2005;2(5):535-539.

17. Berger JR, Fannin M. The "bedsheet" Babinski. *South Med J.* 2002;95(10):1178-1179.

18. Kerr RS, Cadoux-Hudson TA, Adams CB. The value of accurate clinical assessment in the surgical management of the lumbar disc protrusion. *J Neurol Neurosur Ps.* 1988;51(2):169-173.

19. Stankovic R, Johnell O, Maly P, Willner S. Use of lumbar extension, slump test, physical and neurological examination in the evaluation of patients with suspected herniated nucleus pulposus. A prospective clinical study. *Man Ther.* 1999;4(1):25-32.

20. Peeters GG, Aufdemkampe G, Oostendorp RA. Sensibility testing in patients with a lumbosacral radicular syndrome. *J Manip Physiol Ther.* 1998;21(2):81-88.

21. Mayo Clinic. *Clinical Examinations in Neurology.* 6th ed. St. Louis, MO: Mosby; 1991.

22. Impallomeni M, Kenny RA, Flynn MD, Kraenzlin M, Pallis CA. The elderly and their ankle jerks. *Lancet.* 1984;1(8378):670-672.

23. Marin R, Dillingham TR, Chang A, Belandres PV. Extensor digitorum brevis reflex in normals and patients with radiculopathies. *Muscle Nerve.* 1995;18(1):52-59.

24. Rico RE, Jonkman EJ. Measurement of the Achilles tendon reflex for the diagnosis of lumbosacral root compression syndromes. *J Neurol Neurosurg Psychiatry.* 1982;45(9):791-795.

25. Cook C, Roman M, Stewart KM, Leithe LG, Isaacs R. Reliability and diagnostic accuracy of clinical special tests for myelopathy in patients seen for cervical dysfunction. *J Orthop Sports Phys Ther.* 2009;39(3):172-178.

26. Miller TM, Johnston SC. Should the Babinski sign be part of the routine neurologic examination? *Neurology.* 2005;65(8):1165-1168.

27. Cook C, Brown C, Isaacs R, Roman M, Davis S, Richardson W. Clustered clinical findings for diagnosis of cervical spine myelopathy. *J Man Manip Ther.* 2010;18(4):175-180.

28. Rhee JM, Heflin JA, Hamasaki T, Freedman B. Prevalence of physical signs in cervical myelopathy: A prospective, controlled study. *Spine (Phila Pa 1976).* 2009;34(9):890-895.

29. Glaser JA, Curé JK, Bailey KL, Morrow DL. Cervical spinal cord compression and the Hoffmann sign. *Iowa Orthop J.* 2001;21:49-52.

30. Shacklock M. *Clinical Neurodynamics.* Edinburgh, Scotland: Elsevier; 2005.

31. Coppieters MW, Butler DS. Do 'sliders' slide and 'tensioners' tension? An analysis of neurodynamic techniques and considerations regarding their application. *Man Ther.* 2008;13(3):213-221.

32. Dilley A, Lynn B, Greening J, DeLeon N. Quantitative in vivo studies of median nerve sliding in response to wrist, elbow, shoulder and neck movements. *Clin Biomech (Bristol, Avon).* 2003;18(10):899-907.

33. Greening J, Smart S, Leary R, Hall-Craggs M, O'Higgins P, Lynn B. Reduced movement of median nerve in carpal tunnel during wrist flexion in patients with non-specific arm pain. *Lancet.* 1999;354(9174):217-218.

34. Yuan Q, Dougherty L, Margulies SS. In vivo human cervical spinal cord deformation and displacement in flexion. *Spine (Phila Pa 1976).* 1998;23(15):1677-1683.

35. Breig A. *Biomechanics of the Central Nervous System.* Stockholm, Sweden: Almqvist and Wiksell; 1960.

36. Troup JD. Biomechanics of the lumbar spinal canal. *Clin Biomech (Bristol, Avon).* 1986;1(1):31-43.

37. Millesi H, Zöch G, Reihsner R. Mechanical properties of peripheral nerves. *Clin Orthop Relat Res.* 1995(314):76-83.

38. McCracken LM, Gross RT, Sorg PJ, Edmands TA. Prediction of pain in patients with chronic low back pain: Effects of inaccurate prediction and pain-related anxiety. *Behav Res Ther.* 1993;31(7):647-652.

39. Beneciuk JM, Bishop MD, George SZ. Pain catastrophizing predicts pain intensity during a neurodynamic test for the median nerve in healthy participants. *Man Ther.* 2010;15(4):370-375.

40. Coppieters M, Ryan L. Do patients beliefs based on widespread medical information hinder accurate diagnosis? Sydney: 11th Annual World Congress on Pain; 2005.

41. Shacklock M. Neurodynamics. *Physiotherapy.* 1995;81:9-16.

42. Walsh J, Flatley M, Johnston N, Bennett K. Slump test: Sensory responses in asymptomatic subjects. *J Man Manip Ther.* 2007;15(4):231-238.

43. Walsh J, Hall T. Agreement and correlation between the straight leg raise and slump tests in subjects with leg pain. *J Manip Physiol Ther.* 2009;32(3):184-192.

44. Wainner RS, Fritz JM, Irrgang JJ, Delitto A, Allison S, Boninger ML. Development of a clinical prediction rule for the diagnosis of carpal tunnel syndrome. *Arch Phys Med Rehabil.* 2005;86(4):609-618.

45. Majlesi J, Togay H, Unalan H, Toprak S. The sensitivity and specificity of the Slump and the Straight Leg Raising tests in patients with lumbar disc herniation. *J Clin Rheumatol.* 2008;14(2):87-91.

46. Van der Windt DA, Simons E, Riphagen, II, et al. Physical examination for lumbar radiculopathy due to disc herniation in patients with low-back pain. *Cochrane Db Syst Rev.* 2010(2):CD007431.

47. Deville WL, van der Windt DA, Dzaferagic A, Bezemer PD, Bouter LM. The test of Lasègue: Systematic review of the accuracy in diagnosing herniated discs. *Spine (Phila Pa 1976).* 2000;25(9):1140-1147.

48. Vroomen PC, de Krom MC, Wilmink JT, Kester AD, Knottnerus JA. Diagnostic value of history and physical examination in patients suspected of lumbosacral nerve root compression. *J Neurol Neurosurg Psychiatry.* 2002;72(5):630-634.

49. Kosteljanetz M, Bang F, Schmidt-Olsen S. The clinical significance of straight-leg raising (Lasègue's sign) in the diagnosis of prolapsed lumbar disc. Interobserver variation and correlation with surgical finding. *Spine (Phila Pa 1976).* 1988;13(4):393-395.

50. Nadler SF, Malanga GA, Ciccone DS. Positive straight-leg raising in lumbar radiculopathy: Is documentation affected by insurance coverage? *Arch Phys Med Rehabil.* 2004;85(8):1336-1338.

51. Scham SM, Taylor TK. Tension signs in lumbar disc prolapse. *Clin Orthop Relat Res.* 1971;75:195-204.

52. Cram RH. A sign of sciatic nerve foot pressure. *J Bone Joint Surg Br.* 1953;35-B(2):192-195.

53. Summers B, Mishra V, Jones JM. The flip test: A reappraisal. *Spine.* 2009;34(15):1585-1589.

54. Rabin A, Gerszten PC, Karausky P, Bunker CH, Potter DM, Welch WC. The sensitivity of the seated straight-leg raise test compared with the supine straight-leg raise test in patients presenting with magnetic resonance imaging evidence of lumbar nerve root compression. *Arch Phys Med Rehabil.* 2007;88(7):840-843.

55. MacDermid JC, Wessel J. Clinical diagnosis of carpal tunnel syndrome: A systematic review. *J Hand Ther.* 2004;17(2):309-319.

56. Fernández-de-Las-Peñas C, Coppieters MW, Cuadrado ML, Pareja JA. Patients with chronic tension-type headache demonstrate increased mechano-sensitivity of the supra-orbital nerve. *Headache.* 2008;48(4):570-577.

57. Fernández-de-las-Peñas C, Arendt-Nielsen L, Cuadrado ML, Pareja JA. Generalized mechanical pain sensitivity over nerve tissues in patients with strictly unilateral migraine. *Clin J Pain.* 2009;25(5):401-406.

58. Khambati FA, Shetty VP, Ghate SD, Capadia GD. Sensitivity and specificity of nerve palpation, monofilament testing and voluntary muscle testing in detecting peripheral nerve abnormality, using nerve conduction studies as gold standard; a study in 357 patients. *Lepr Rev.* 2009;80(1):34-50.

59. Letchuman R, Gay RE, Shelerud RA, VanOstrand LA. Are tender points associated with cervical radiculopathy? *Arch Phys Med Rehabil.* 2005;86(7):1333-1337.

60. Schmid AB, Brunner F, Luomajoki H, et al. Reliability of clinical tests to evaluate nerve function and mechanosensitivity of the upper limb peripheral nervous system. *BMC Musculoskelet Disord.* 2009;10:11.

Chapter 8

1. Loudon JK, Manske RC, Reiman MP. *Clinical Mechanics and Kinesiology.* Champaign, IL: Human Kinetics; 2013.

2. Kaltenborn F. *Manual Mobilization of the Extremity Joints.* 4th ed. Minneapolis, MN: OPTP; 1989.

3. Kaltenborn F. *Manual Mobilization of the Joints. The Kaltenborn Method of Joint Mobilization and Treatment.* Oslo, Norway: Olaf Norlis Bokhandel; 1999.

4. Mennell J. *Back Pain: Diagnosis and Treatment Using Manipulative Techniques.* Boston. MD: Little, Brown; 1960.

5. Abbott JH, McCane B, Herbison P, Moginie G, Chapple C, Hogarty T. Lumbar segmental instability: A criterion-related validity study of manual therapy assessment. *BMC Musculoskel Dis.* 2005;6:56.

6. Zito G, Jull G, Story I. Clinical tests of musculoskeletal dysfunction in the diagnosis of cervicogenic headache. *Man Ther.* 2006;11(2):118-129.

7. Jull G, Bogduk N, Marsland A. The accuracy of manual diagnosis for cervical zygapophysial joint pain syndromes. *Med J Aust.* 1988;148(5):233-236.

8. Macconaill MA. Joint movement. *Physiotherapy.* 1964;50:359-367.

9. McClure PW, Flowers KR. Treatment of limited shoulder motion: A case study based on biomechanical considerations. *Phys Ther.* 1992;72(12):929-936.

10. Cyriax J. *Textbook of Orthopaedic Medicine, Diagnosis of Soft Tissue Lesions.* 8th ed. London, England: Bailliere Tindall; 1982.

11. Cyriax J, Cyriax P. *Cyriax's Illustrated Manual of Orthopaedic Medicine.* Boston, MA: Butterworth-Heinemann; 1993.

12. Norkin C, White D. *Measurement of Joint Motion: A Guide to Goniometry.* Philadelphia, PA: F.A. Davis Company; 2003.

13. Magee DJ. *Orthopedic Physical Assessment.* Philadelphia, PA: Saunders; 2002.

14. Klassbo M, Harms-Ringdahl K, Larsson G. Examination of passive ROM and capsular patterns in the hip. *Physiother Res Int.* 2003;8(1):1-12.

15. Bijl D, Dekker J, van Baar ME, et al. Validity of Cyriax's concept capsular pattern for the diagnosis of osteoarthritis of hip and/or knee. *Scand J Rheumatol.* 1998;27(5):347-351.

16. Fritz JM, Delitto A, Erhard RE, Roman M. An examination of the selective tissue tension scheme, with evidence for the concept of a capsular pattern of the knee. *Phys Ther.* 1998;78(10):1046-1056; discussion 1057-1061.

17. Schollmeier G, Sarkar K, Fukuhara K, Uhthoff HK. Structural and functional changes in the canine shoulder after cessation of immobilization. *Clin Orthop Relat Res.* 1996(323):310-315.

18. Freeman M, Wyke B. An experimental study of articular neurology. *J Bone Joint Surg.* 1967;49B:185.

19. Maitland G. *Maitland's Vertebral Manipulation.* 6th ed. London, England: Butterworth-Heinemann; 2001.

20. Laslett M, Young SB, Aprill CN, McDonald B. Diagnosing painful sacroiliac joints: A validity study of a McKenzie evaluation and sacroiliac provocation tests. *Aust J Physiother.* 2003;49(2):89-97.

21. Grahame R. Hypermobility and hypermobility syndrome. In: Keer R, Grahame R, eds. *Hypermobility Syndrome—Recognition and Management for Physiotherapists.* London, England: Butterworth-Heinemann; 2003.

22. Birrell FN, Adebajo AO, Hazleman BL, Silman AJ. High prevalence of joint laxity in West Africans. *Brit J Rheumatol.* 1994;33(1):56-59.

23. Jessee EF, Owen DS, Jr., Sagar KB. The benign hypermobile joint syndrome. *Arthritis Rheum.* 1980;23(9):1053-1056.

24. Murray KJ. Hypermobility disorders in children and adolescents. *Best Pract Res Clin Rheumatol.* 2006;20(2):329-351.

25. Qvindesland A, Jonsson H. Articular hypermobility in Icelandic 12-year-olds. *Rheumatology (Oxford).* 1999;38(10):1014-1016.

26. Remvig L, Jensen DV, Ward RC. Epidemiology of general joint hypermobility and basis for the proposed criteria for benign joint hypermobility syndrome: Review of the literature. *J Rheumatol.* 2007;34(4):804-809.

27. Russek LN. Hypermobility syndrome. *Phys Ther.* 1999;79(6):591-599.

28. Tofts LJ, Elliott EJ, Munns C, Pacey V, Sillence DO. The differential diagnosis of children with joint hypermobility: A review of the literature. *Pediatr Rheumatol Online J.* 2009;7:1.

29. Juul-Kristensen B, Rogind H, Jensen DV, Remvig L. Inter-examiner reproducibility of tests and criteria for generalized joint hypermobility and benign joint hypermobility syndrome. *Rheumatology (Oxford).* 2007;46(12):1835-1841.

30. Remvig L, Jensen DV, Ward RC. Are diagnostic criteria for general joint hypermobility and benign joint hypermobility syndrome based on reproducible and valid tests? A review of the literature. *J Rheumatol.* 2007;34(4):798-803.

31. Baumhauer JF, Alosa DM, Renstrom AF, Trevino S, Beynnon B. A prospective study of ankle injury risk factors. *Am J Sports Med.* 1995;23(5):564-570.

32. Beynnon BD, Renstrom PA, Alosa DM, Baumhauer JF, Vacek PM. Ankle ligament injury risk factors: A prospective study of college athletes. *J Orthop Res.* 2001;19(2):213-220.

33. Hiller CE, Refshauge KM, Herbert RD, Kilbreath SL. Intrinsic predictors of lateral ankle sprain in adolescent dancers: A prospective cohort study. *Clin J Sport Med.* 2008;18(1):44-48.

34. Hopper DM, Hopper JL, Elliott BC. Do selected kinanthropometric and performance variables predict injuries in female netball players? *J Sports Sci.* 1995;13(3):213-222.

35. Decoster LC, Bernier JN, Lindsay RH, Vailas JC. Generalized joint hypermobility and its relationship to injury patterns among NCAA lacrosse players. *J Athl Train.* 1999;34(2):99-105.

36. Acasuso Diaz M, Collantes Estevez E, Sanchez Guijo P. Joint hyperlaxity and musculoligamentous lesions: Study of a population of homogeneous age, sex and physical exertion. *Brit J Rheumatol.* 1993;32(2):120-122.

37. Soderman K, Alfredson H, Pietila T, Werner S. Risk factors for leg injuries in female soccer players: A prospective investigation during one outdoor season. *Knee Surg Sports Traumatol Arthrosc.* 2001;9(5):313-321.

38. Uhorchak JM, Scoville CR, Williams GN, Arciero RA, St Pierre P, Taylor DC. Risk factors associated with noncontact injury of the anterior cruciate ligament: A prospective four-year evaluation of 859 West Point cadets. *Am J Sports Med.* 2003;31(6):831-842.

39. Hakim AJ, Grahame R. A simple questionnaire to detect hypermobility: An adjunct to the assessment of patients with diffuse musculoskeletal pain. *Int J Clin Pract.* 2003;57(3):163-166.

40. Adib N, Davies K, Grahame R, Woo P, Murray KJ. Joint hypermobility syndrome in childhood. A not so benign multisystem disorder? *Rheumatology (Oxford).* 2005;44(6):744-750.

41. Klemp P, Stevens JE, Isaacs S. A hypermobility study in ballet dancers. *J Rheumatol.* 1984;11(5):692-696.

42. Kalenak A, Morehouse CA. Knee stability and knee ligament injuries. *JAMA.* 1975;234(11):1143-1145.

43. Huston LJ, Greenfield ML, Wojtys EM. Anterior cruciate ligament injuries in the female athlete. Potential risk factors. *Clin Orthop Relat Res.* 2000(372):50-63.

44. Murphy DF, Connolly DA, Beynnon BD. Risk factors for lower extremity injury: A review of the literature. *Brit J Sport Med.* 2003;37(1):13-29.

45. Donaldson PR. Does generalized joint hypermobility predict joint injury in sport? A review. *Clin J Sport Med.* 2012;22(1):77-78.

46. Pacey V, Nicholson LL, Adams RD, Munn J, Munns CF. Generalized joint hypermobility and risk of lower limb joint injury during sport: A systematic review with meta-analysis. *Am J Sports Med.* 2010;38(7):1487-1497.

47. Heyward V. *Advanced Fitness and Exercise Prescription.* 5th ed. Champaign, IL: Human Kinetics; 2006.

48. Williams PE, Goldspink G. Connective-tissue changes in immobilized muscle. *Journal of Anatomy.* 1984;138(MAR):343-350.

49. Goldspink DF, Cox VM, Smith SK, et al. Muscle growth in response to mechanical stimuli. *Am J Physiol.* 1995;268(2)(part 1):E288-E297.

50. Leivseth G, Torstensson J, Reikerås O. Effect of passive muscle stretching in osteoarthritis of the hip. *Clin Sci (Lond).* 1989;76(1):113-117.

51. Wessling KC, DeVane DA, Hylton CR. Effects of static stretch versus static stretch and ultrasound combined on triceps surae muscle extensibility in healthy women. *Phys Ther.* 1987;67(5):674-679.

52. Weldon SM, Hill RH. The efficacy of stretching for prevention of exercise-related injury: A systematic review of the literature. *Man Ther.* 2003;8(3):141-150.

53. Janda V. *Muscle Function Testing.* London, England: Butterworth; 1983.

54. Kendall FP, McCreary EK, Provance PG, Rodgers MM, Romani WA. *Muscles: Testing and Function with Posture and Pain.* 5th ed. Baltimore, MD: Lippincott Williams & Wilkins; 2005.

55. Sahrmann S. *Diagnosis and Treatment of Movement Impairment Syndromes.* St. Louis, MO: Mosby; 2002.

56. Bell RD, Hoshizaki TB. Relationships of age and sex with range of motion of seventeen joint actions in humans. *Can J Appl Sport Sci.* 1981;6(4):202-206.

57. Walker JM, Sue D, Miles-Elkousy N, Ford G, Trevelyan H. Active mobility of the extremities in older subjects. *Phys Ther.* 1984;64(6):919-923.

58. Beighton P, Solomon L, Soskolne CL. Articular mobility in an African population. *Ann Rheum Dis.* 1973;32(5):413-418.

Chapter 9

1. Hall C, Thein-Brody L. Functional approach to therapeutic exercise for physiologic impairments. In: Hall C, Thein-Brody L, eds. *Therapeutic Exercise: Moving Toward Function.* Philadelphia, PA: Lippincott Williams & Wilkins; 1999.

2. Kraemer WJ, Adams K, Cafarelli E, et al. American College of Sports Medicine position stand. Progression models in resistance training for healthy adults. *Med Sci Sport Exer.* 2002;34(2):364-380.

3. Fleck SJ, Kraemer WJ. *Designing Resistance Training Programs.* 3rd ed. Champaign, IL: Human Kinetics; 2004.

4. Wilson GJ, Newton RU, Murphy AJ, Humphries BJ. The optimal training load for the development of dynamic athletic performance. *Med Sci Sport Exer.* 1993;25(11):1279-1286.

5. Kawamori N, Haff GG. The optimal load for the development of muscular power. *J Strength Cond Res.* 2004;18(3):675-684.

6. Powers SK, Howley ET. *Exercise Physiology: Theory and Application.* Boston, MA: McGraw-Hill; 2001.

7. Lieber RL, Fridén J. Clinical significance of skeletal muscle architecture. *Clin Orthop Relat Res.* 2001(383):140-151.

8. Lieber RL. *Skeletal Muscle Structure and Function: Implications for Rehabilitation and Sports Medicine.* Baltimore, MD: Williams & Wilkins; 1992.

9. Baratta RV, Solomonow M, Best R, D'Ambrosia R. Isotonic length/force models of nine different skeletal muscles. *Med Biol Eng Comput.* 1993;31(5):449-458.

10. Ikai M, Fukunaga T. Calculation of muscle strength per unit cross-sectional area of human muscle by means of ultrasonic measurement. *Int Z Angew Physiol.* 1968;26(1):26-32.

11. LaStayo PC, Woolf JM, Lewek MD, Snyder-Mackler L, Reich T, Lindstedt SL. Eccentric muscle contractions: Their contribution to injury, prevention, rehabilitation, and sport. *J Orthop Sports Phys Ther.* 2003;33(10):557-571.

12. Granacher U, Gollhofer A, Hortobágyi T, Kressig RW, Muehlbauer T. The importance of trunk muscle strength for balance, functional performance, and fall prevention in seniors: A systematic review. *Sports Med.* 2013;43(7):627-641.

13. Den Ouden ME, Schuurmans MJ, Arts IE, van der Schouw YT. Physical performance characteristics related to disability in older persons: A systematic review. *Maturitas.* 2011;69(3):208-219.

14. Daly RM, Rosengren BE, Alwis G, Ahlborg HG, Sernbo I, Karlsson MK. Gender specific age-related changes in bone density, muscle strength and functional performance in the elderly: A 10-year prospective population-based study. *BMC Geriatr.* 2013;13(1):71.

15. Glenmark B, Hedberg G, Kaijser L, Jansson E. Muscle strength from adolescence to adulthood—Relationship to muscle fibre types. *Eur J Appl Physiol Occup Physiol.* 1994;68(1):9-19.

16. Laubach LL. Comparative muscular strength of men and women: A review of the literature. *Aviat Space Environ Med.* 1976;47(5):534-542.

17. Glenmark B. Skeletal muscle fibre types, physical performance, physical activity and attitude to physical activity in women and men. A follow-up from age 16 to 27. *Acta Physiol Scand Suppl.* 1994;623:1-47.

18. Cooper H, Doods WN, Adams ID. Use and misuse of the tape measure as a means of assessing muscle strength and power. *Rheumatological Rehabilitation.* 1981;20(4):211-218.

19. Hortobagyi T, Katch FI, Katch VL. Relationships of body size, segmental dimensions, and ponderal equivalents to muscular strength in high-strength and low-strength subjects. *IntJ Sports Med.* 1990;11(5):349-356.

20. Kendall FP, McCreary EK, Provance PG, Rodgers MM, Romani WA. *Muscles: Testing and Function with Posture and Pain.* 5th ed. Baltimore, MD: Lippincott Williams & Wilkins; 2005.

21. White D. Musculoskeletal examination. In: O'Sullivan S, Schmitz T, eds. *Physical Rehabilitation.* 5th ed. Philadelphia, PA: FA Davis; 2007:159-192.

22. Wessel J, Kaup C, Fan J, et al. Isometric strength measurements in children with arthritis: Reliability and relation to function. *Arthritis Care Res.* 1999;12(4):238-246.

23. Bohannon RW. Test-retest reliability of hand-held dynamometry during a single session of strength assessment. *Phys Ther.* 1986;66(2):206-209.

24. Bohannon RW, Andrews AW. Interrater reliability of hand-held dynamometry. *Phys Ther.* 1987;67(6):931-933.

25. Bohannon RW, Larkin PA, Smith MB, Horton MG. Relationship between static muscle strength deficits and spasticity in stroke patients with hemiparesis. *Phys Ther.* 1987;67(7):1068-1071.

26. Wadsworth C, Nielsen DH, Corcoran DS, Phillips CE, Sannes TL. Interrater reliability of hand-held dynamometry: Effects of rater gender, body weight, and grip strength. *J Orthop Sports Phys Ther.* 1992;16(2):74-81.

27. DeLorme T, Wilkins A. *Progressive Resistance Exercises.* New York, NY: Appleton-Century-Crofts; 1951.

28. Sale DG. Testing strength and power. In: MacDougall JD, Wenger HA, Green HJ, eds. *Physiological Testing of the High Performance Athlete.* 2nd ed. Champaign, IL: Human Kinetics; 1991.

29. Escamilla R, Wickham R. Exercise-based conditioning and rehabilitation. In: Kolt GS, Snyder-Mackler L, eds. *Physical Therapies in Sports and Exercise.* London, England: Churchill Livingstone; 2003.

30. Davies G. *Compendium of Isokinetics in Clinical Usage and Rehabilitation Techniques.* Onalaska, WI: S&S Publishers; 1992.

31. Davies G, Wilk K, Ellenbecker TS. Assessment of strength. In: Malone TR, McPhoil T, Nitz AJ, eds. *Orthopedic and Sports Physical Therapy.* 3rd ed. St. Louis, MO: Mosby; 1997.

32. Wilk KE, Andrews JR. Current concepts in the treatment of anterior cruciate ligament disruption. *J Orthop Sports Phys Ther.* 1992;15(6):279-293.

33. Cyriax J. *Textbook of Orthopaedic Medicine, Diagnosis of Soft Tissue Lesions.* 8th ed. London, England: Bailliere Tindall; 1982.

34. Franklin ME, Conner-Kerr T, Chamness M, Chenier TC, Kelly RR, Hodge T. Assessment of exercise-induced minor muscle lesions: The accuracy of Cyriax's diagnosis by selective tension paradigm. *J Orthop Sports Phys Ther.* 1996;24(3):122-129.

35. Garrett WE, Seaber AV, Boswick J, Urbaniak JR, Goldner JL. Recovery of skeletal muscle after laceration and repair. *J Hand Surg Am.* 1984;9(5):683-692.

36. Garrett WE. Muscle strain injuries. *Am J Sports Med.* 1996;24(suppl 6):S2-S8.

Chapter 10

1. Cook C, Hegedus E. Diagnostic utility of clinical tests for spinal dysfunction. *Man Ther.* 2011;16(1):21-25.

2. Cook C, Hegedus E, Hawkins R, Scovell F, Wyland D. Diagnostic accuracy and association to disability of clinical test findings associated with patellofemoral pain syndrome. *PhysiotherCan.* 2010;62(1):17-24.

3. Cook C, Massa L, Harm-Ernandes I, et al. Interrater reliability and diagnostic accuracy of pelvic girdle pain classification. *J Manip Physiol Ther.* 2007;30(4):252-258.

4. Cook CE, Wilhelm M, Cook AE, Petrosino C, Isaacs R. Clinical tests for screening and diagnosis of cervical spine myelopathy: A systematic review. *J Manip Physiol Ther.* 2011;34(8):539-546.

5. Cook JL, Khan KM, Kiss ZS, Purdam CR, Griffiths L. Reproducibility and clinical utility of tendon palpation to detect patellar tendinopathy in young basketball players. Victorian Institute of Sport tendon study group. *Brit J Sport Med.* 2001;35(1):65-69.

6. Goode A, Hegedus EJ, Sizer P, Brismee JM, Linberg A, Cook CE. Three-dimensional movements of the sacroiliac joint: A systematic review of the literature and assessment of clinical utility. *J Man Manip Ther.* 2008;16(1):25-38.

7. Hegedus EJ, Cook C, Hasselblad V, Goode A, McCrory DC. Physical examination tests for assessing a torn meniscus in the knee: A systematic review with meta-analysis. *J Orthop Sports Phys Ther.* 2007;37(9):541-550.

8. Hegedus EJ, Goode AP, Cook CE, et al. Which physical examination tests provide clinicians with the most value when examining the shoulder? Update of a systematic review with meta-analysis of individual tests. *Brit J Sport Med.* 2012;46(14):964-978.

9. Reneker J, Paz J, Petrosino C, Cook C. Diagnostic accuracy of clinical tests and signs of temporomandibular joint disorders: A systematic review of the literature. *J Orthop Sports Phys Ther.* 2011;41(6):408-416.

10. Reiman MP, Goode AP, Hegedus EJ, Cook CE, Wright AA. Diagnostic accuracy of clinical tests of the hip: A systematic review with meta-analysis [Published online ahead of print July 7 2012]. *Brit J Sport Med.* 2012.

11. Reiman MP, Loudon JK, Goode AP. Diagnostic accuracy of clinical tests for assessment of hamstring injury: A systematic review. *J Orthop Sports Phys Ther.* 2013;43(4):223-231.

12. Reiman MP, Goode AP, Hegedus EJ, Cook CE, Wright AA. Diagnostic accuracy of clinical tests of the hip: A systematic review with meta-analysis. *Brit J Sport Med.* 2013;47(14):893-902.

13. Deville WL, van der Windt DA, Dzaferagic A, Bezemer PD, Bouter LM. The test of Lasègue: Systematic review of the accuracy in diagnosing herniated discs. *Spine (Phila Pa 1976).* 2000;25(9):1140-1147.

14. Klein JG. Five pitfalls in decisions about diagnosis and prescribing. *BMJ.* 2005;330(7494):781-783.

15. Sackett DL, Rosenberg WM, Gray JA, Haynes RB, Richardson WS. Evidence based medicine: What it is and what it isn't. *BMJ.* 1996;312(7023):71-72.

16. McGinn TG, Guyatt GH, Wyer PC, Naylor CD, Stiell IG, Richardson WS. Users' guides to the medical literature: XXII: How to use articles about clinical decision rules. Evidence-Based Medicine Working Group. *JAMA.* 2000;284(1):79-84.

17. Stiell IG, Wells GA, Vandemheen KL, et al. The Canadian C-spine rule for radiography in alert and stable trauma patients. *JAMA.* 2001;286(15):1841-1848.

Chapter 11

1. Cyriax J. *Textbook of Orthopaedic Medicine, Diagnosis of Soft Tissue Lesions.* 8th ed. London, England: Bailliere Tindall; 1982.

2. Toprak U, Ustuner E, Ozer D, et al. Palpation tests versus impingement tests in Neer stage I and II subacromial impingement syndrome. *Knee Surg Sports Traumatol Arthrosc.* 2013;21(2):424-429.

3. Mancini F, Sambo CF, Ramirez JD, Bennett DL, Haggard P, Iannetti GD. A fovea for pain at the fingertips. *Curr Biol.* 2013;23(6):496-500.

4. Kassirer JP. Teaching clinical reasoning: Case-based and coached. *Acad Med.* 2010;85(7):1118-1124.

5. Gomes MB, Guimaraes JP, Guimaraes FC, Neves AC. Palpation and pressure pain threshold: Reliability and validity in patients with temporomandibular disorders. *Cranio.* 2008;26(3):202-210.

6. Fu R, Iqbal CW, Jaroszewski DE, St Peter SD. Costal cartilage excision for the treatment of pediatric slipping rib syndrome. *J Pediatr Surg.* 2012;47(10):1825-1827.

7. Stochkendahl MJ, Christensen HW. Chest pain in focal musculoskeletal disorders. *Med Clin N Am.* 2010;94(2):259-273.

8. Boissonnault WG, Thein-Nissenbaum JM. Differential diagnosis of a sacral stress fracture. *J Orthop Sports Phys Ther.* 2002;32(12):613-621.

9. Heyworth BE, Williams RJ, III Internal impingement of the shoulder. *Am J Sports Med.* 2009;37(5):1024-1037.

10. Hegedus EJ, Goode A, Campbell S, et al. Physical examination tests of the shoulder: A systematic review with meta-analysis of individual tests. *Brit J Sport Med.* 2008;42(2):80-92; discussion 92.

11. Hsu SH, Moen TC, Levine WN, Ahmad CS. Physical examination of the athlete's elbow. *Am J Sports Med.* 2012;40(3):699-708.

12. Gurney B, Boissonnault WG, Andrews R. Differential diagnosis of a femoral neck/head stress fracture. *J Orthop Sport Phys.* 2006;36(2):80-88.

13. Jansen JA, Mens JM, Backx FJ, Stam HJ. Diagnostics in athletes with long-standing groin pain. *Scand J Med Sci Sports.* 2008;18(6):679-690.

14. Tibor LM, Sekiya JK. Differential diagnosis of pain around the hip joint. *Arthroscopy.* 2008;24(12):1407-1421.

15. Kerkhoffs GM, van Es N, Wieldraaijer T, Sierevelt IN, Ekstrand J, van Dijk CN. Diagnosis and prognosis of acute hamstring injuries in athletes. *Knee Surg Sports Traumatol Arthrosc.* 2013;21(2):500-509.

16. Konan S, Rayan F, Haddad FS. Do physical diagnostic tests accurately detect meniscal tears? *Knee Surg Sports Traumatol Arthrosc.* 2009;17(7):806-811.

17. Logerstedt DS, Snyder-Mackler L, Ritter RC, Axe MJ. Knee pain and mobility impairments: Meniscal and articular cartilage lesions. *J Orthop Sport Phys.* 2010;40(6):A1-A35.

18. Carcia CR, Martin RL, Houck J, Wukich DK. Achilles pain, stiffness, and muscle power deficits: Achilles tendinitis. *J Orthop Sports Phys Ther.* 2010;40(9):A1-A26.

19. Hopper DM, Strauss GR, Boyle JJ, Bell J. Functional recovery after anterior cruciate ligament reconstruction: A longitudinal perspective. *Arch Phys Med Rehabil.* 2008;89(8):1535-1541.

20. Hutchison AM, Evans R, Bodger O, et al. What is the best clinical test for Achilles tendinopathy? *Foot Ankle Surg.* 2013;19(2):112-117.

21. McPoil TG, Martin RL, Cornwall MW, Wukich DK, Irrgang JJ, Godges JJ. Heel pain—plantar fasciitis: Clinical practice guidelines linked to the international classification of function, disability, and health from the orthopaedic section of the American Physical Therapy Association. *J Orthop Sport Phys.* 2008;38(4):A1-A18.

22. Sman AD, Hiller CE, Refshauge KM. Diagnostic accuracy of clinical tests for diagnosis of ankle syndesmosis injury: A systematic review. *Brit J Sport Med.* 2013;47(10):620-628.

23. Thomas JL, Christensen JC, Kravitz SR, et al. The diagnosis and treatment of heel pain: A clinical practice guideline-revision 2010. *J Foot Ankle Surg.* 2010;49(suppl 3):S1-19.

24. Wuerz TH, Gurd DP. Pediatric physeal ankle fracture. *J Am Acad Orthop Surg.* 2013;21(4):234-244.

25. Montazem A. Secondary tinnitus as a symptom of instability of the upper cervical spine: Operative management. *International Tinnitus Journal.* 2000;6(2):130-133.

26. Joensen J, Couppe C, Bjordal JM. Increased palpation tenderness and muscle strength deficit in the prediction of tendon hypertrophy in symptomatic unilateral shoulder tendinopathy: An ultrasonographic study. *Physiotherapy.* 2009;95(2):83-93.

27. Mattingly GE, Mackarey PJ. Optimal methods for shoulder tendon palpation: A cadaver study. *Phys Ther.* 1996;76(2):166-173.

28. Alvarez DJ, Rockwell PG. Trigger points: Diagnosis and management. *Am Fam Physician.* 2002;65(4):653-660.

29. Lucas N, Macaskill P, Irwig L, Moran R, Bogduk N. Reliability of physical examination for diagnosis of myofascial trigger points: A systematic review of the literature. *Clin J Pain.* 2009;25(1):80-89.

30. Bron C, Dommerholt JD. Etiology of myofascial trigger points. *Curr Pain Headache Rep.* 2012;16(5):439-444.

31. Lavelle ED, Lavelle W, Smith HS. Myofascial trigger points. *Med Clin North Am.* 2007;91(2):229-239.

32. Myburgh C, Larsen AH, Hartvigsen J. A systematic, critical review of manual palpation for identifying myofascial trigger points: Evidence and clinical significance. *Arch Phys Med Rehabil.* 2008;89(6):1169-1176.

33. Petho G, Reeh PW. Sensory and signaling mechanisms of bradykinin, eicosanoids, platelet-activating factor, and nitric oxide in peripheral nociceptors. *Physiol Rev.* 2012;92(4):1699-1775.

34. Wang H, Ehnert C, Brenner GJ, Woolf CJ. Bradykinin and peripheral sensitization. *Biol Chem.* 2006;387(1):11-14.

35. Haage P, Krings T, Schmitz-Rode T. Nontraumatic vascular emergencies: Imaging and intervention in acute venous occlusion. *Eur Radiol.* 2002;12(11):2627-2643.

36. Mant J, Doust J, Roalfe A, et al. Systematic review and individual patient data meta-analysis of diagnosis of heart failure, with modelling of implications of different diagnostic strategies in primary care. *Health Technol Assess.* 2009;13(32):1-207, iii.

37. Trayes KP, Studdiford JS, Pickle S, Tully AS. Edema: Diagnosis and management. *Am Fam Physician.* 2013;88(2):102-110.

38. Standring S, Gray H. *Gray's Anatomy: The Anatomical Basis of Clinical Practice.* 40th ed. Edinburgh, Scotland: Churchill Livingstone/Elsevier; 2008.

39. Cools AM, Struyf F, De Mey K, Maenhout A, Castelein B, Cagnie B. Rehabilitation of scapular dyskinesis: From the office worker to the elite overhead athlete. *Brit J Sport Med.* 2014;48(8):692-697.

40. Freeman S, Mascia A, McGill S. Arthrogenic neuromusculature inhibition: A foundational investigation of existence in the hip joint. *Clin Biomech (Bristol, Avon).* 2013;28(2):171-177.

41. Rice DA, McNair PJ. Quadriceps arthrogenic muscle inhibition: Neural mechanisms and treatment perspectives. *Semin Arthritis Rheum.* 2010;40(3):250-266.

42. Delitto A, George SZ, Van Dillen LR, et al. Low back pain. *J Orthop Sports Phys Ther.* 2012;42(4):A1-A57.

43. Sedaghat N, Latimer J, Maher C, Wisbey-Roth T. The reproducibility of a clinical grading system of motor control in patients with low back pain. *J Manipulative Physiol Ther.* 2007;30(7):501-508.

44. Hides J, Stanton W, Mendis MD, Sexton M. The relationship of transversus abdominis and lumbar multifidus clinical muscle tests in patients with chronic low back pain. *Man Ther.* 2011;16(6):573-577.

45. Macedo LG, Latimer J, Maher CG, et al. Effect of motor control exercises versus graded activity in patients with chronic nonspecific low back pain: A randomized controlled trial. *Phys Ther.* 2012;92(3):363-377.

46. Venes D, Taber CW. *Taber's Cyclopedic Medical Dictionary.* 21st ed. Philadelphia, PA: Davis; 2009.

47. Altman R, Asch E, Bloch D, et al. Development of criteria for the classification and reporting of osteoarthritis. Classification of osteoarthritis of the knee. Diagnostic and Therapeutic Criteria Committee of the American Rheumatism Association. *Arthritis Rheum.* 1986;29(8):1039-1049.

48. Hayes KW, Petersen C, Falconer J. An examination of Cyriax's passive motion tests with patients having osteoarthritis of the knee. *Phys Ther.* 1994;74(8):697-707; discussion 707-709.

49. Woolf AD, Pfleger B. Burden of major musculoskeletal conditions. *B World Health Organ.* 2003;81(9):646-656.

50. Kibler WB, Putukian M. Selected issues for the master athlete and the team physician: A consensus statement. *Med Sci Sports Exerc.* 2010;42(4):820-833.

51. Gluck GS, Heckman DS, Parekh SG. Tendon disorders of the foot and ankle, part 3: The posterior tibial tendon. *Am J Sports Med.* 2010;38(10):2133-2144.

52. Rudzki JR, Paletta GA, Jr. Juvenile and adolescent elbow injuries in sports. *Clin Sports Med.* 2004;23(4):581-608, ix.

53. Williams GR, Jr. Painful shoulder after surgery for rotator cuff disease. *J Am Acad Orthop Surg.* 1997;5(2):97-108.

54. Batteson R, Hammond A, Burke F, Sinha S. The de Quervain's screening tool: Validity and reliability of a measure to support clinical diagnosis and management. *Musculoskeletal Care.* 2008;6(3):168-180.

55. Wilk KE, Obma P, Simpson CD, Cain EL, Dugas JR, Andrews JR. Shoulder injuries in the overhead athlete. *J Orthop Sports Phys Ther.* 2009;39(2):38-54.

56. Loudon JK, Wiesner D, Goist-Foley HL, Asjes C, Loudon KL. Intrarater reliability of functional performance tests for subjects with patellofemoral pain syndrome. *J Athl Train.* 2002;37(3):256-261.

57. Reneker J, Paz J, Petrosino C, Cook C. Diagnostic accuracy of clinical tests and signs of temporomandibular joint disorders: A systematic review of the literature. *J Orthop Sports Phys.* 2011;41(6):408-416.

58. Kaale BR, Krakenes J, Albrektsen G, Wester K. Clinical assessment techniques for detecting ligament and membrane injuries in the upper cervical spine region—A comparison with MRI results. *Man Ther.* 2008;13(5):397-403.

59. Osmotherly PG, Rivett DA, Rowe LJ. Construct validity of clinical tests for alar ligament integrity: An evaluation using magnetic resonance imaging. *Phys Ther.* 2012;92(5):718-725.

60. Magee DJ. *Orthopedic Physical Assessment.* Philadelphia, PA: Saunders; 2002.

61. Malanga GA, Andrus S, Nadler SF, McLean J. Physical examination of the knee: A review of the original test description and scientific validity of common orthopedic tests. *Arch Phys Med Rehabil.* 2003;84(4):592-603.

62. Wolf EM, Agrawal V. Transdeltoid palpation (the rent test) in the diagnosis of rotator cuff tears. *J Shoulder Elbow Surg.* 2001;10(5):470-473.

63. Devereaux MW, ElMaraghy AW. Improving the rapid and reliable diagnosis of complete distal biceps tendon rupture: A nuanced approach to the clinical examination. *Am J Sports Med.* 2013;41(9):1998-2004.

64. Karachalios T, Hantes M, Zibis AH, Zachos V, Karantanas AH, Malizos KN. Diagnostic accuracy of a new clinical test (the Thessaly test) for early detection of meniscal tears. *J Bone Joint Surg.* 2005;87(5):955-962.

65. LaStayo P, Howell J. Clinical provocative tests used in evaluating wrist pain: A descriptive study. *J Hand Ther.* 1995;8(1):10-17.

66. American Board of Physical Therapy Specialties. *Description of Specialty Practice: Orthopaedic Physical Therapy.* Alexandria, VA: Author; 2002.

67. LeBlond RF, DeGowin RL, Brown DD. *DeGowin's Diagnostic Examination.* 9th ed. New York, NY: McGraw-Hill Medical; 2009.

68. Nuzzaci G, Giuliano G, Righi D, Baroncelli T, Lotti A, Marinoni M. A study of the semeiological reliability of dorsalis pedis artery and posterior tibial artery in the diagnosis of lower limb arterial occlusive disease. *Angiology.* 1984;35(12):767-772.

69. Greenman PE. *Principles of Manual Medicine.* 2nd ed. Baltimore, MD: Williams & Wilkins; 1996.

70. Fukui S, Ohseto K, Shiotani M, Ohno K, Karasawa H, Naganuma Y. Distribution of referred pain from the lumbar zygapophyseal joints and dorsal rami. *Clin J Pain.* 1997;13(4):303-307.

71. Kravetz RE. To touch or not to touch: That is the question. *Am J Gastroenterol.* 2009;104(9):2143-2144.

Chapter 12

1. Reiman MP, Manske RC. *Functional Testing in Human Performance.* Champaign, IL: Human Kinetics; 2009.

2. Cook G, Burton L, Kiesel K, Rose G, Bryant M. *Movement: Functional Movement Systems.* Santa Cruz, CA; On Target Publications: 2010.

3. Minick KI, Kiesel K, Burton L, Taylor A, Plisky P, Butler RJ. Inter-rater reliability of the functional movement screen. *J Strength Cond Res.* 2010;4:479-486.

4. Onate JA, Dewey T, Kollock RO, et al. Real-time intersession and interrater reliability of the functional movement screen. *J Strength Cond Res.* 2012;26:408-415.

5. Teyhen DS, Shaffer SW, Lorenson CL, et al. The Functional Movement Screen: A reliability study. *J Ortho Sports Phys Ther.* 2012;42:530-540.

6. O'Connor FG, Deuster PA, Davis J, Pappas CG, Knapik JJ. Functional movement screening: Predicting injuries in officer candidates. *Med Sci Sports Exerc.* 2011;43:2224-2230.

7. Butler RJ, Contreras M, Burton LC, Plisky PJ, Kiesel KB. Modifiable risk factors predict injuries in firefighters during training academies. *Work.* 2013; 46:11-17.

8. Kiesel KB, Plisky PJ, Butler RJ. Fundamental movement limitations and asymmetries relate to injury risk in professional football players. *J Sports Rehabil.* 2014:23:88-94.

9. Glaws KR, Juneau CM, Becker LC, Di Stasi SL, Hewett TE. Intra- and inter-rater reliability of the Selective Functional Movement Assessment (SFMA). *Int J Sports Phys Ther.* 2014;9:195-208.

10. Piva SR, Fitzgerald GK, Irrgang JJ, et al. Reliability of measures of impairments associated with patellofemoral pain syndrome. *BMC Musculoskelet Disord.* 2006;7:33.

11. Piva SR, Fitzgerald GK, Irrgang JI, et al. Associates of physical function and pain in patients with patellofemoral pain syndrome. *Arch Phys Med Rehabil.* 2009;90:285-295.

12. McMullen KL, Cosby NL, Hertel J, Ingersoll CD, Hart JM. Lower extremity neuromuscular control immediately after fatiguing hip-abduction exercise. *J Athl Train.* 2011;46(6):607-614.

13. Bohannon RW. One-legged balance test times. *Percept Motor Skills.* 1994;78:101-102.

14. Gribble PA, Hertel J, Plisky P. Using the Star Excursion Balance Test to assess dynamic postural-control deficits and outcomes in lower extremity injury: A literature and systematic review. *J Athl Train.* 2012;47:339-357.

15. Hertel J, Braham RA, Hale SA, Olmsted-Kramer LC. Simplifying the star excursion balance test: Analyses of subjects with and without chronic ankle instability. *J Ortho Sports Phys Ther.* 2006;36:131-137.

16. Plisky PJ, Gorman PP, Butler RJ, Kiesel KB, Underwood FB, Elkins B. The reliability of an instrumented device for measuring components of the Star Excursion Balance Test. *N Am J Sport Phys Ther.* 2009;4:92-99.

17. Plisky PJ, Rauh MJ, Kaminski TW, Underwood FB. Star Excursion Balance Test as a predictor of lower extremity injury in high school basketball players. *J Ortho Sports Phys Ther.* 2006; 36:911-919.

18. de Noronha M, França LC, Haupenthal A, Nunes GS. Intrinsic predictive factors for ankle sprain in active university students: A prospective study. *Scand J Med Sci Sports.* 2013;23:541-547.

19. Butler RJ, Lehr ME, Fink ML, Kiesel KB, Plisky PJ. Dynamic balance performance and noncontact lower extremity injury in college football players: An initial study. *Sports Health.* 2013;5:417-422.

20. Seminick DVM. Testing protocols and procedures. In: Baechle TR, ed. *Esssentials of Strength Training and Conditioning.* 1st ed. Champaign, IL: Human Kinetics; 1994.

21. Myer GD, Schmitt LC, Brent JL, et al. Utilization of modified NFL combine testing to identify functional deficits in athletes following ACL reconstruction. *J Ortho Sports Phys Ther.* 2011;41:377-387.

22. Teyhen DS, Riebel MA, McArthur DR, et al. Normative data and the influence of age and gender on power, balance, flexibility, and functional movement in healthy service members. *Mil Med.* 2014;179:413-420.

23. Considine WJ, Sullivan WJ. Relationship of selected tests of leg strength and leg power on college men. *Res Q.* 1973;44:404-416.

24. Markovic G, Dizdar D, Jukic I, Cardinale M. Reliability and factorial validity of squat and countermovement jump tests. *J Strength Cond Res.* 2004;18:551-555.

25. Witvrouw E, Lysens R, Bellemans J, Cambier D, Vanderstraeten G. Intrinsic risk factors for the development of anterior knee pain in an athletic population. A two-year prospective study. *Am J Sports Med.* 2000;28:480-489.

26. Reid A, Birmingham TB, Stratford PW, Alcock GK, Giffin JR. Hop testing provides a reliable and valid outcome measure during rehabilitation after anterior cruciate ligament reconstruction. *Phys Ther.* 2007;87:337-349.

27. Petschnig R, Baron R, Albrecht M. The relationship between isokinetic quadriceps strength test and hop tests for distance and one-legged vertical jump test following anterior cruciate ligament reconstruction. *J Ortho Sports Phys Ther*. 1998;28:23-31.

28. Juris PM, Phillips EM, Dalpe C, Edwards C, Gotlin RS, Kane DJ. A dynamic test of lower extremity function following anterior cruciate ligament reconstruction and rehabilitation. *J Ortho Sports Phys Ther*. 1997;26:184-191.

29. Myer GD, Ford KR, Khoury J, Succop P, Hewett TE. Development and validation of a clinic-based prediction tool to identify female athletes at high risk for anterior cruciate ligament injury. *Am J Sports Med*. 2010;38:2025-2033.

30. Hewett TE, Myer GD, Ford KR, et al. Biomechanical measures of neuromuscular control and valgus loading of the knee predict anterior cruciate ligament injury risk in female athletes: A prospective study. *Am J Sports Med*. 2005;33:492-501.

31. Pfile KR, Hart JM, Herman DC, Hertel J, Kerrigan DC, Ingersoll CD. Different exercise training interventions and drop-landing biomechanics in high school female athletes. *J Athl Train*. 2013;48:450-462.

32. Brosky JA Jr, Nitz AJ, Malone TR, Caborn DN, Rayens MK. Intrarater reliability of selected clinical outcome measures following anterior cruciate ligament reconstruction. *J Orthop Sports Phys Ther*. 1999;29:39-48.

33. Harman E, Garhammer J, Pandorf C. Administration, scoring and interpretation of selected tests. In: Baechle TR, Earle RW, eds. *Essentials of Strength Training and Conditioning*. 2nd ed. Champaign, IL: Human Kinetics; 2000.

34. Wilk KE, Romaniello WT, Soscia SM, Arrigo CA, Andrews JR. The relationship between subjective knee scores, isokinetic testing, and functional testing in the ACL-reconstructed knee. *J Ortho Sports Phys Ther*. 1994;20:60-73.

35. Hoffman J. *Norms for Fitness, Performance, and Health*. Champaign, IL: Human Kinetics; 2006.

36. Gillam GM. 300 yard shuttle. *NSCA J*. 1983;5:46.

37. Sporis G, Ruzic L, Leko G. The anaerobic endurance of elite soccer players improved after a high-intensity training intervention in the 8-week conditioning program. *J Strength Cond Res*. 2008;22:559-566.

38. Brumitt J, Heiderscheit BC, Manske RC, Niemuth PE, Rauh MJ. Lower extremity functional tests and risk of injury in Division III collegiate athletes. *Int J Sports Phys Ther*. 2013;8:216-227.

39. Davies GJ, Heiderscheit BC, Clark M. The scientific and clinical rationale for the use of open and closed kinetic chain rehabilitation. In: Ellenbecker TS, ed. *Knee Ligament Rehabilitation*. Philadelphia, PA: Churchill Livingstone; 2000: 291-300.

40. Tabor MA, Davies GJ, Kernozek TW, Negrete RJ, Hudson V. A multicenter study of the test-retest reliability of the lower extremity functional test. *J Sports Rehab*. 2002;11:190-201.

41. Ramsbottom R, Brewer J, Williams C. A progressive shuttle run test to estimate maximal oxygen uptake. *Brit J Sport Med*. 1988;22:141-144.

42. Léger L, Gadoury C. Validity of the 20 m shuttle run test with 1 min stages to predict $\dot{V}O_2$max in adults. *Can J Sport Sci*. 1989;14:21-26.

43. Shvartz E, Reibold RC. Aerobic fitness norms for males and females aged 6 to 75 years: A review. *Aviat Space Environ Med*. 1990;61:3-11.

44. Vernillo G, Silvestri A, Torre AL. The yo-yo intermittent recovery test in junior basketball players according to performance level and age group. *J Strength Cond Res*. 2012;26:2490-2494.

45. Roush JR, Kitamura J, Waits MC. Reference values for the Closed Kinetic Chain Upper Extremity Stability Test (CKCUEST) for collegiate baseball players. *N Am J Sports Phys Ther*. 2007;2:159-163.

46. Westrick RB, Miller JM, Carow SD, Gerber JP. Exploration of the Y-balance test for assessment of upper quarter closed kinetic chain performance. *Int J Sports Phys Ther*. 2012;7:139-147.

47. Tucci HT, Martins J, de Carvallo Sposito G, Camarini PM, de Oliveira AS. Closed Kinetic Chain Upper Extremity Stability test (CKCUES test): A reliability study in persons with and without shoulder impingement syndrome. *BMC Musculoskelet Disord*. 2014;15:1.

48. Gorman PP, Butler RJ, Plisky PJ, Kiesel KB. Upper Quarter Y Balance Test: Reliability and performance comparison between genders in active adults. *J Strength Cond Res*. 2012; 26:3043-3048.

49. Falsone SA, Gross MT, Guskiewicz KM, Schneider RA. One-arm hop test: Reliability and effects of arm dominance. *J Orthop Sports Phys Ther*. 2002;32(3):98-103.

50. Mayhew JL, Ware JS, Johns RA, Bemben MG. Changes in upper body power following heavy-resistance strength training in college men. *Int J Sports Med*. 1997;18(7):516-520.

51. Mayhew JL, Bemben MG, Rohrs DM, Ware J, Bemben DA. Seated shot put as a measure of upper body power in college males. *J Hum Mvmt Stud*. 1991;21:137-148.

52. Schellenberg KL, Lang JM, Chan KM, Burnham RS. A clinical tool for office assessment of lumbar spine stabilization endurance: Prone and supine bridge maneuvers. *Am J Phys Med Rehabil*. 2007;86:380-386.

53. McGill SM. Low back exercises: Prescription for the healthy back when recovering from injury. In: American College of Sports Medicine, ed. *ACSM's Resources Manual for Guidelines for Exercise Testing and Prescription*. 3rd ed. Baltimore. MD: Williams & Wilkins; 1998.

54. Reiman MP, Manske RC. The assessment of function, part 1—How is it measured? A clinical perspective. *J Man Manip Ther*. 2011;19(3):91-99.

Chapter 13

1. Murray MP. Gait as a total pattern of movement. *Am J Phys Med*. 1967;46(1):290-333.

2. Judge JO, Ounpuu S, Davis RB, III. Effects of age on the biomechanics and physiology of gait. *Clin Geriatr Med*. 1996;12(4):659-678.

3. Perry J. *Gait Analysis: Normal and Pathological Function*. New York, NY: Slack; 1992.

4. Kadaba MP, Ramakrishnan HK, Wootten ME, Gainey J, Gorton G, Cochran GV. Repeatability of kinematic, kinetic, and electromyographic data in normal adult gait. *J Orthop Res*. 1989;7(6):849-860.

5. Rodgers MM. 1995. Dynamic foot mechanics. *J Orthop Sports Phys Ther*. 1995; 21(6):306-316.

6. LaFortune MA, Cavanagh PR, Sommer HJ, Kalenak A. 1992. Three-dimensional kinematics of the human knee during walking. *J Biomech*. 1992;25(4):347-357.

7. Sekiya N. Nagasaki H, Ito H, Furuna T. Optimal walking in terms of variability in step length. *J Orthop Sports Phys Ther*. 1997;26(5):266-272.

8. Oatis CA. *Kinesiology: The Mechanics and Pathomechanics of Human Movement*. Baltimore, MD: Williams & Wilkins; 2004.

9. Craik RL, Dutterer L. Spatial and temporal characteristics of foot fall patterns. In: Craik RL, Oatis CA, eds. *Gait Analysis: Theory and Application*. St. Louis: Mosby-Year Book, 1995.

10. Finley FR, Cody KA. Locomotion characteristics of urban pedestrians. *Arch Phys Med Rehabil*. 1970;51(7):423-426.

11. Ostrosky KM, Van Swearingen JM, Burdett RG, Gee Z. A comparison of gait characteristics in young and old subjects. *Phys Ther*. 1994;74(7):637-646.

12. Hasegawa H, Yamauchi T, Kraemer WJ. Foot strike patterns of runners at the 15-km point during an elite-level half marathon. *J Strength Cond Res*. 2007;21(3):888-893.

13. Goss DL, Gross MT. Relationship among self-reported shoe type, footstrike pattern, and injury incidence. *US Army Med Dep J*. 2012;Oct-Dec:25-30.

14. Arendse RE, Noakes TD, Azvedo LB, Romanov N, Schwellnus MP, Fletcher G. Reduced eccentric loading of the knee with the pose running method. *Med Sci Sports Exerc*. 2004;36(2):272-277.

15. Kulmala JP, Avela J, Pasanen K, Parkkari J. Forefoot strikers exhibit lower running-induced knee loading than rearfoot strikers. *Med Sci Sports Exerc*. 2013;45(12):2306-2313.

16. Novacheck T. The biomechanics of running. *Gait Posture*. 1998;7(1):77-95.

17. Cavanagh PR. *Biomechanics of Distance Running*. Champaign, IL: Human Kinetics; 1990.

18. Schache AG, Bennell KL, Blanch PD, Wrigley TV. The coordinated movement of the lumbo-pelvic-hip complex during running: A literature review. *Gait Posture*. 1999;10(1):30-47.

19. Elliott BC, Banksby BA. The synchronization of muscle activity and body segment movements during a running cycle. *Med Sci Sports Exerc*. 1979;11(4):322-327.

20. Ferber R, Noehren B, Hamill J, Davis I. Competitive female runners with a history of iliotibial band syndrome demonstrate atypical hip and knee kinematics. *J Orthop Sports Phys Ther*. 2010;40(2):52-58.

21. Hinrichs RN. Upper extremity function in distance running. In: Cavanagh PR. ed. *Biomechanics of Distance Running*. Champaign, IL: Human Kinetics; 1990.

22. Gerringer SR. The biomechanics of running. *J Back Musculoskeletal Rehabil*. 1995;5(4):273-279.

23. Winter D. Moments of force and mechanical power in jogging. *J Biomech*. 1983;16(1):91-97.

24. James SL, Brubaker CE. Biomechanics of running. *Orthop Clin North Am*. 1973;4(3):605-615.

25. Sinning WE, Forsyth HL. Lower-limb actions while running at different velocities. *Med Sci Sports*.1970;2(1):28-34.

26. Mann RA, Moran GT, Dougherty SE. Comparative electromyography of the lower extremity in jogging, running and sprinting. *Am J Sports Med*. 1986;14(6):501-510.

27. Dierks TA, Manal KT, Hamill J, Davis IS. Proximal and distal influences on hip and knee kinematics in runners with patellofemoral pain during a prolonged run. *J Orthop Sports Phys Ther*. 2008;38(8):448-456.

28. Lieberman DE, Raichlen DA, Pontzer H, Bramble DM, Cutright-Smith E. The human gluteus maximus and its role in running. *J Exp Biol*. 2006;209(11):2143-2155.

29. VanGent RN, Siem D, van Middelkoop M, van Os AG, Bierma-Zeinstra SM, Koes BW. Incidence and determinants of lower extremity running injuries in long distance runners: A systematic review. *Brit J Sport Med*. 2007;41(8):469-480.

30. Nigg BM. Biomechanics, load analysis and sports injuries in the lower extremity. *Sports Med*. 1985;2(5):367-379.

31. Cook SD, Kester MA, Brunet ME, Haddad RJ, Jr. Biomechanics of running shoe performance. *Clin Sports Med*. 1985;4(4):619-626.

32. Williams DS, III, McClay IS, Hamill J. 2001. Arch structure and injury patterns in runners. *Clin Biomech*. 2001;16(4):341-347.

33. Tong JWK, Kong PW. Association between foot type and lower extremity injuries. Systematic literature review with meta-analysis. *J Orthop Sports Phys Ther*. 2013;43(10):700-715.

34. Thijs Y. DeClercq D, Roosen P, Witvrouw E. Gait-related intrinsic factors for patellofemoral pain in novice recreational runners. *Brit J Sport Med*. 2008;42(6):466-471.

35. Dierks TA, Davis I. Discrete and continuous joint coupling relationships in uninjured recreational runners. *Clin Biomech*. 2007; 22:581-591.

36. Stergiou N, Bates BT, James SL. Asynchrony between subtalar and knee joint function during running. *Med Sci Sports Exerc*. 1999;31:1645-1655.

37. Tiberio D. The effect of excessive subtalar joint pronation and patellofemoral mechanics: A theoretical model. *J Orthop Sports Phys Ther*. 1987;9(4):160-165.

38. Willson JD, Davis IS. Lower extremity mechanics of females with and without patellofemoral pain across activities with progressively greater task demands. *Clin Biomech.* 2008;23(2):203-211.

39. Milner CE, Hamill J, Davis IS. Distinct hip and rearfoot kinematics in female runners with a history of tibial stress fracture. *J Orthop Sports Phys Ther.* 2010;40(2):59-66.

40. Macera CA, Pate RR, Powell KE, Jackson KL, Kendrick JS, Craven TE. Predicting lower-extremity injuries among habitual runners. *Arch Intern Med.* 1989;149(11):2565-2568.

41. Milner CE, Ferber R, Pollard CD, Hamill J, Davis IS. Biomechanical factors associated with tibial stress fracture in female runners. *Med Sci Sports Exerc.* 2006;38(2):323-328.

Chapter 14

1. Kendall FP, McCreary EK, Provance PG, Rodgers MM, Romani WA. *Muscles: Testing and Function with Posture and Pain.* 5th ed. Baltimore, MD: Lippincott Williams & Wilkins; 2005.

2. Sahrmann S. *Movement System Impairment Syndromes.* St. Louis, MO: Mosby; 2002.

3. Adams MA, Hutton WC. The effect of posture on the lumbar spine. *J Bone Joint Surg Br.* 1985;67(4):625-629.

4. Claus A, Hides J, Moseley GL, Hodges P. Sitting versus standing: Does the intradiscal pressure cause disc degeneration or low back pain? *J Electromyogr Kinesiol.* 2008;18(4):550-558.

5. Wilke HJ, Neef P, Caimi M, Hoogland T, Claes LE. New in vivo measurements of pressures in the intervertebral disc in daily life. *Spine (Phila Pa 1976).* 1999;24(8):755-762.

6. Nachemson AL. Disc pressure measurements. *Spine (Phila Pa 1976).* 1981;6(1):93-97.

7. Janda V. Muscles and motor control in low back pain: Assessment and management. In: Twomey LT, ed. *Physical Therapy of the Low Back.* New York, NY: Churchill Livingstone; 1987.

8. Magee DJ. *Orthopedic Physical Assessment.* Philadelphia, PA: Saunders; 2002.

9. Norkin C. Posture. In: Levangie P, Norkin C, eds. *Joint Structure and Function: A Comprehensive Analysis.* 5th ed. Philadelphia, PA: F.A. Davis; 2011:483-523.

10. Kim H, Kim HS, Moon ES, et al. Scoliosis imaging: What radiologists should know. *Radiographics.* 2010;30(7):1823-1842.

11. Keynan O, Fisher CG, Vaccaro A, et al. Radiographic measurement parameters in thoracolumbar fractures: A systematic review and consensus statement of the spine trauma study group. *Spine (Phila Pa 1976).* 2006;31(5):E156-E165.

12. Christensen ST, Hartvigsen J. Spinal curves and health: A systematic critical review of the epidemiological literature dealing with associations between sagittal spinal curves and health. *J Manip Physiol Ther.* 2008;31(9):690-714.

13. Ferber R, Noehren B, Hamill J, Davis IS. Competitive female runners with a history of iliotibial band syndrome demonstrate atypical hip and knee kinematics. *J Orthop Sports Phys Ther.* 2010;40(2):52-58.

14. Noehren B, Davis I, Hamill J. ASB clinical biomechanics award winner 2006 prospective study of the biomechanical factors associated with iliotibial band syndrome. *Clin Biomech (Bristol, Avon).* 2007;22(9):951-956.

15. Souza RB, Powers CM. Differences in hip kinematics, muscle strength, and muscle activation between subjects with and without patellofemoral pain. *J Orthop Sports Phys Ther.* 2009;39(1):12-19.

16. Souza RB, Powers CM. Predictors of hip internal rotation during running: An evaluation of hip strength and femoral structure in women with and without patellofemoral pain. *Am J Sports Med.* 2009;37(3):579-587.

17. Powers CM. The influence of abnormal hip mechanics on knee injury: A biomechanical perspective. *J Orthop Sports Phys Ther.* 2010;40(2):42-51.

Chapter 15

1. Practice parameter: The management of concussion in sports (summary statement). Report of the Quality Standards Subcommittee. *Neurology.* 1997;48(3):581-585.

2. Nonfatal traumatic brain injuries related to sports and recreation activities among persons aged ≤19 years—United States, 2001-2009. *MMWR. Morb Mortal Wkly Rep.* 2011;60(39):1337-1342.

3. Sports-related recurrent brain injuries—United States. *MMWR. Morb Mortal Wkly Rep.* 1997;46(10):224-227.

4. Guskiewicz KM. Balance assessment in the management of sport-related concussion. *Clin Sports Med.* 2011;30(1):89-102, ix.

5. Guskiewicz KM. Assessment of postural stability following sport-related concussion. *Curr Sports Med Rep.* 2003;2(1):24-30.

6. Guskiewicz KM, Marshall SW, Bailes J, et al. Association between recurrent concussion and late-life cognitive impairment in retired professional football players. *Neurosurgery.* 2005;57(4):719-726; discussion 719-726.

7. Guskiewicz KM, McCrea M, Marshall SW, et al. Cumulative effects associated with recurrent concussion in collegiate football players: The NCAA Concussion Study. *JAMA.* 2003;290(19):2549-2555.

8. Register-Mihalik J, Guskiewicz KM, Mann JD, Shields EW. The effects of headache on clinical measures of neurocognitive function. *Clin J Sport Med.* 2007;17(4):282-288.

9. Iinuma T, Hirota Y, Ishio K. Orbital wall fractures. Conventional views and CT. *Rhinology.* 1994;32(2):81-83.

10. Rowe LD, Miller E, Brandt-Zawadzki M. Computed tomography in maxillofacial trauma. *Laryngoscope.* 1981;91(5):745-757.

11. Salvolini U. Traumatic injuries: Imaging of facial injuries. *Eur Radiol.* 2002;12(6):1253-1261.

12. Jager L, Reiser M. CT and MR imaging of the normal and pathologic conditions of the facial nerve. *Eur J Radiol.* 2001;40(2):133-146.

13. Jank S, Emshoff R, Etzelsdorfer M, Strobl H, Nicasi A, Norer B. The diagnostic value of ultrasonography in the detection of orbital floor fractures with a curved array transducer. *Int J Oral Maxillofac Surg.* 2004;33(1):13-18.

14. Adeyemo WL, Akadiri OA. A systematic review of the diagnostic role of ultrasonography in maxillofacial fractures. *Int J Oral Maxillofac Surg.* 2011;40(7):655-661.

15. Stengel D, Ottersbach C, Matthes G, et al. Accuracy of single-pass whole-body computed tomography for detection of injuries in patients with major blunt trauma. *CMAJ.* 2012;184(8):869-876.

16. Ogunmuyiwa SA, Fatusi OA, Ugboko VI, Ayoola OO, Maaji SM. The validity of ultrasonography in the diagnosis of zygomaticomaxillary complex fractures. *Int J Oral Maxillofac Surg.* 2012;41(4):500-505.

17. Javadrashid R, Khatoonabad M, Shams N, Esmaeili F, Jabbari Khamnei H. Comparison of ultrasonography with computed tomography in the diagnosis of nasal bone fractures. *Dentomaxillofac Radiol.* 2011;40(8):486-491.

18. Atighechi S, Baradaranfar MH, Karimi G, et al. Diagnostic value of ultrasonography in the diagnosis of nasal fractures. *J Craniofac Surg.* 2014;25(1):e51-e53.

19. Marshman LA, Polkey CE, Penney CC. Unilateral fixed dilation of the pupil as a false-localizing sign with intracranial hemorrhage: Case report and literature review. *Neurosurgery.* 2001;49(5):1251-1255; discussion 1255-1256.

20. Pretto Flores L, De Almeida CS, Casulari LA. Positive predictive values of selected clinical signs associated with skull base fractures. *J Neurosurg Sci.* 2000;44(2):77-82; discussion 82-73.

21. McPheeters RA, White S, Winter A. Raccoon eyes. *West J Emerg Med.* 2010;11(1):97.

22. Herbella FA, Mudo M, Delmonti C, Braga FM, Del Grande JC. 'Raccoon eyes' (periorbital haematoma) as a sign of skull base fracture. *Injury.* 2001;32(10):745-747.

23. Perez R, Oeltjen JC, Thaller SR. A review of mandibular angle fractures. *Craniomaxillofac Trauma Reconstr.* 2011;4(2):69-72.

24. Perez-Guisado J, Maclennan P. Clinical evaluation of the nose: A cheap and effective tool for the nasal fracture diagnosis. *Eplasty.* 2012;12:e3.

25. Perry JJ, Stiell IG, Sivilotti ML, et al. Clinical decision rules to rule out subarachnoid hemorrhage for acute headache. *JAMA.* 2013;310(12):1248-1255.

26. Pandor A, Goodacre S, Harnan S, et al. Diagnostic management strategies for adults and children with minor head injury: A systematic review and an economic evaluation. *Health Technol Assess.* 2011;15(27):1-202.

27. Harnan SE, Pickering A, Pandor A, Goodacre SW. Clinical decision rules for adults with minor head injury: A systematic review. *J Trauma.* 2011;71(1):245-251.

28. Lyttle MD, Cheek JA, Blackburn C, et al. Applicability of the CATCH, CHALICE and PECARN paediatric head injury clinical decision rules: Pilot data from a single Australian centre. *Emerg Med J.* 2013;30(10):790-794.

29. Lyttle MD, Crowe L, Oakley E, Dunning J, Babl FE. Comparing CATCH, CHALICE and PECARN clinical decision rules for paediatric head injuries. *Emerg Med J.* 2012;29(10):785-794.

30. Shah KC, Rajshekhar V. Reliability of diagnosis of soft cervical disc prolapse using Spurling's test. *Brit J Neurosurg.* 2004;18(5):480-483.

31. Wainner RS, Fritz JM, Irrgang JJ, Boninger ML, Delitto A, Allison S. Reliability and diagnostic accuracy of the clinical examination and patient self-report measures for cervical radiculopathy. *Spine (Phila Pa 1976).* 2003;28(1):52-62.

32. Gumina S, Carbone S, Albino P, Gurzi M, Postacchini F. Arm Squeeze Test: A new clinical test to distinguish neck from shoulder pain. *Eur Spine J.* 2013;22(7):1558-1563.

33. Halker RB, Barrs DM, Wellik KE, Wingerchuk DM, Demaerschalk BM. Establishing a diagnosis of benign paroxysmal positional vertigo through the Dix-Hallpike and side-lying maneuvers: A critically appraised topic. *Neurologist.* 2008;14(3):201-204.

34. Teitelbaum JS, Eliasziw M, Garner M. Tests of motor function in patients suspected of having mild unilateral cerebral lesions. *Can J Neurol Sci.* 2002;29(4):337-344.

35. Anderson NE, Mason DF, Fink JN, Bergin PS, Charleston AJ, Gamble GD. Detection of focal cerebral hemisphere lesions using the neurological examination. *J Neurol Neurosurg Psychiatry.* 2005;76(4):545-549.

36. Bagai A, Thavendiranathan P, Detsky AS. Does this patient have hearing impairment? *JAMA.* 2006;295(4):416-428.

37. Browning GG, Swan IR. Sensitivity and specificity of Rinne tuning fork test. *BMJ.* 1988;297(6660):1381-1382.

38. Rubinstein SM, van Tulder M. A best-evidence review of diagnostic procedures for neck and low-back pain. *Best Pract Res Clin Rheumatol.* 2008;22(3):471-482.

39. Anderson PA, Muchow RD, Munoz A, Tontz WL, Resnick DK. Clearance of the asymptomatic cervical spine: A meta-analysis. *J Orthop Trauma.* 2010;24(2):100-106.

40. Michaleff ZA, Maher CG, Verhagen AP, Rebbeck T, Lin CW. Accuracy of the Canadian C-spine rule and NEXUS to screen for clinically important cervical spine injury in patients following blunt trauma: A systematic review. *CMAJ.* 2012;184(16):E867-E876.

41. Bandiera G, Stiell IG, Wells GA, et al. The Canadian C-spine rule performs better than unstructured physician judgment. *Ann Emerg Med.* 2003;42(3):395-402.

42. Kaale BR, Krakenes J, Albrektsen G, Wester K. Clinical assessment techniques for detecting ligament and membrane injuries in the upper cervical spine region—A comparison with MRI results. *Man Ther.* 2008;13(5):397-403.

43. Uitvlugt G, Indenbaum S. Clinical assessment of atlantoaxial instability using the Sharp-Purser test. *Arthritis Rheum.* 1988;31(7):918-922.

44. Petersen B, von Maravic M, Zeller JA, Walker ML, Kompf D, Kessler C. Basilar artery blood flow during head rotation in vertebrobasilar ischemia. *Acta Neurol Scand.* 1996;94(4):294-301.

45. Sakaguchi M, Kitagawa K, Hougaku H, et al. Mechanical compression of the extracranial vertebral artery during neck rotation. *Neurology.* 2003;61(6):845-847.

46. Society IH. The International Classification of Headache Disorders, 2nd edition. *Cephalalgia.* 2004;24(suppl 1):S9-S160.

47. The International Classification of Headache Disorders, 3rd edition (beta version). *Cephalalgia.* 2013;33(9):629-808.

48. Society TIH. IHS Classification ICHD-II. Available at: http://ihs-classification.org/en/. Accessed September 1, 2013.

49. Esposito CJ, Crim GA, Binkley TK. Headaches: A differential diagnosis. *Cranio.* 1986;4(4):317-322.

50. Spierings EL. Acute, subacute, and chronic headache. *Otolaryngol Clin North Am.* 2003;36(6):1095-1107, vi.

51. Simel DL. *Make the Diagnosis: Does This Patient With Headaches Have a Migraine or Need Neuroimaging?* New York, NY: McGraw-Hill; 2010.

52. Láinez MJ, Domínguez M, Rejas J, et al. Development and validation of the Migraine Screen Questionnaire (MS-Q). *Headache.* 2005;45(10):1328-1338.

53. Láinez MJ, Castillo J, Domínguez M, Palacios G, Díaz S, Rejas J. New uses of the Migraine Screen Questionnaire (MS-Q): Validation in the Primary Care setting and ability to detect hidden migraine. MS-Q in Primary Care. *BMC Neurol.* 2010;10:39.

54. Dreyfuss P, Rogers J, Dreyer S, Fletcher D. Atlanto-occipital joint pain. A report of three cases and description of an intraarticular joint block technique. *Reg Anesth.* 1994;19(5):344-351.

55. Trevor-Jones R. Osteo-arthritis of the paravertebral joints of the second and third cervical vertebrae as a cause of occipital headaches. *S Afr Med J.* 1964;38:392-394.

56. Bogduk N, Marsland A. On the concept of third occipital headache. *J Neurol Neurosurg Psychiatry.* 1986;49(7):775-780.

57. Bovim G. Cervicogenic headache, migraine, and tension-type headache. Pressure-pain threshold measurements. *Pain.* 1992;51(2):169-173.

58. Hall T, Robinson K. The flexion-rotation test and active cervical mobility—A comparative measurement study in cervicogenic headache. *Man Ther.* 2004;9(4):197-202.

59. Zito G, Jull G, Story I. Clinical tests of musculoskeletal dysfunction in the diagnosis of cervicogenic headache. *Man Ther.* 2006;11(2):118-129.

60. Treleaven J, Jull G, Sterling M. Dizziness and unsteadiness following whiplash injury: Characteristic features and relationship with cervical joint position error. *J Rehabil Med.* 2003;35(1):36-43.

61. Carvalho TB, Cancian LR, Marques CG, Piatto VB, Maniglia JV, Molina FD. Six years of facial trauma care: An epidemiological analysis of 355 cases. *Braz J Otorhinolaryngol.* 2010;76(5):565-574.

62. Reilly MJ, Davison SP. Open vs. closed approach to the nasal pyramid for fracture reduction. *Arch Facial Plast Surg.* 2007;9(2):82-86.

63. Batista AM, Ferreira Fde O, Marques LS, Ramos-Jorge ML, Ferreira MC. Risk factors associated with facial fractures. *Braz Oral Res.* 2012;26(2):119-125.

64. Tuli T, Hachl O, Hohlrieder M, Grubwieser G, Gassner R. Dentofacial trauma in sport accidents. *Gen Dent.* 2002;50(3):274-279.

65. Sun GH, Shoman NM, Samy RN, Pensak ML. Analysis of carotid artery injury in patients with basilar skull fractures. *Otol Neurotol.* 2011;32(5):882-886.

66. Huh YE, Kim JS. Bedside evaluation of dizzy patients. *J Clin Neurol.* 2013;9(4):203-213.

Chapter 16

1. Shaffer SM, Brismee JM, Sizer P, Courtney CA. Temporomandibular disorders. Part 1: Anatomy and examination/diagnosis. *J Man Manip Ther.* 2014;22(2):2-12.

2. Jerjes W, Upile T, Abbas S, et al. Muscle disorders and dentition-related aspects in temporomandibular disorders: Controversies in the most commonly used treatment modalities. *Int Arch Med.* 2008;1(1):23.

3. Lobbezoo F, Drangsholt M, Peck C, Sato H, Kopp S, Svensson P. Topical review: New insights into the pathology and diagnosis of disorders of the temporomandibular joint. *J Orofac Pain.* 2004;18(3):181-191.

4. Kafas P, Chiotaki N, Stavrianos C, Stavrianou I. Temporomandibular joint pain: Diagnostic characteristics of chronicity. *J Med Sci.* 2007;7:1088-1092.

5. Neumann DA. *Kinesiology of the Musculoskeletal System: Foundations for Rehabilitation.* 2nd ed. St Louis, MO: Mosby Elsevier; 2010.

6. Ugboko VI, Oginni FO, Ajike SO, Olasoji HO, Adebayo ET. A survey of temporomandibular joint dislocation: Aetiology, demographics, risk factors and management in 96 Nigerian cases. *Int J Oral Maxillofac Surg.* 2005;34(5):499-502.

7. Koh KJ, List T, Petersson A, Rohlin M. Relationship between clinical and magnetic resonance imaging diagnoses and findings in degenerative and inflammatory temporomandibular joint diseases: A systematic literature review. *J Orofac Pain.* 2009;23(2):123-139.

8. Pullinger AG, Seligman DA. Trauma history in diagnostic groups of temporomandibular disorders. *Oral Surg Oral Med Oral Pathol.* 1991;71(5):529-534.

9. How CK. Orthodontic treatment has little to do with temporomandibular disorders. *Evid Based Dent.* 2004;5(3):75.

10. Dahlstrom L, Kahnberg KE, Lindahl L. 15 years follow-up on condylar fractures. *Int J Oral Maxillofac Surg.* 1989;18(1):18-23.

11. Kasch H, Hjorth T, Svensson P, Nyhuus L, Jensen TS. Temporomandibular disorders after whiplash injury: A controlled, prospective study. *J Orofac Pain.* 2002;16(2):118-128.

12. Fernandez CE, Amiri A, Jaime J, Delaney P. The relationship of whiplash injury and temporomandibular disorders: A narrative literature review. *J Chiropr Med.* 2009;8(4):171-186.

13. Trott JP. *Examination of the Temporomandibular Joint.* Edinburgh, Scotland: Churchill Livingstone; 1986.

14. Manfredini D, Basso D, Salmaso L, Guarda-Nardini L. Temporomandibular joint click sound and magnetic resonance-depicted disk position: Which relationship? *J Dent.* 2008;36(4):256-260.

15. Manfredini D, Tognini F, Zampa V, Bosco M. Predictive value of clinical findings for temporomandibular joint effusion. *Oral Surg Oral Med Oral Pathol Oral Radiol Endod.* 2003;96(5):521-526.

16. Stegenga B, de Bont LG, van der Kuijl B, Boering G. Classification of temporomandibular joint osteoarthrosis and internal derangement. 1. Diagnostic significance of clinical and radiographic symptoms and signs. *Cranio.* 1992;10(2):96-106; discussion 116-107.

17. Uşümez S, Oz F, Güray E. Comparison of clinical and magnetic resonance imaging diagnoses in patients with TMD history. *J Oral Rehabil.* 2004;31(1):52-56.

18. Lavigne GJ, Khoury S, Abe S, Yamaguchi T, Raphael K. Bruxism physiology and pathology: An overview for clinicians. *J Oral Rehabil.* 2008;35(7):476-494.

19. Pergamalian A, Rudy TE, Zaki HS, Greco CM. The association between wear facets, bruxism, and severity of facial pain in patients with temporomandibular disorders. *J Prosthet Dent.* 2003;90(2):194-200.

20. Fearon CG, Serwatka WJ. Stress: A common denominator for nonorganic TMJ pain-dysfunction. *J Prosthet Dent.* 1983;49(6):805-808.

21. Speculand B, Goss AN, Hughes A, Spence ND, Pilowsky I. Temporo-mandibular joint dysfunction: Pain and illness behaviour. *Pain.* 1983;17(2):139-150.

22. Aghabeigi B, Feinmann C, Harris M. Prevalence of post-traumatic stress disorder in patients with chronic idiopathic facial pain. *Brit J Oral Max Surg.* 1992;30(6):360-364.

23. Kinney RK, Gatchel RJ, Ellis E, Holt C. Major psychological disorders in chronic TMD patients: Implications for successful management. *J Am Dent Assoc.* 1992;123(10):49-54.

24. List T, Wahlund K, Wenneberg B, Dworkin SF. TMD in children and adolescents: Prevalence of pain, gender differences, and perceived treatment need. *J Orofac Pain.* 1999;13(1):9-20.

25. Macfarlane TV, Blinkhorn AS, Davies RM, Kincey J, Worthington HV. Predictors of outcome for orofacial pain in the general population: A four-year follow-up study. *J Dent Res.* 2004;83(9):712-717.

26. Dworkin SF, LeResche L. Research diagnostic criteria for temporomandibular disorders: Review, criteria, examinations and specifications, critique. *J Craniomandib Disord.* 1992;6(4):301-355.

27. Ohrbach R, Turner JA, Sherman JJ, et al. The Research Diagnostic Criteria For Temporomandibular Disorders. IV: Evaluation of psychometric properties of the Axis II measures. *J Orofac Pain.* 2010;24(1):48-62.

28. Truelove E, Pan W, Look JO, et al. The Research Diagnostic Criteria for Temporomandibular Disorders. III: Validity of Axis I diagnoses. *J Orofac Pain.* 2010;24(1):35-47.

29. Manfredini D. Ultrasonography has an acceptable diagnostic efficacy for temporomandibular disc displacement. *Evid Based Dent.* 2012;13(3):84-85.

30. Li C, Su N, Yang X, Shi Z, Li L. Ultrasonography for detection of disc displacement of temporomandibular joint: A systematic review and meta-analysis. *J Oral Maxillofac Surg.* 2012;70(6):1300-1309.

31. Tasaki MM, Westesson PL. Temporomandibular joint: Diagnostic accuracy with sagittal and coronal MR imaging. *Radiology.* 1993;186(3):723-729.

32. Melis M, Secci S, Ceneviz C. Use of ultrasonography for the diagnosis of temporomandibular joint disorders: A review. *Am J Dent.* 2007;20(2):73-78.

33. Liedberg J, Panmekiate S, Petersson A, Rohlin M. Evidence-based evaluation of three imaging methods for the temporomandibular disc. *Dentomaxillofac Rad.* 1996;25(5):234-241.

34. Santler G, Karcher H, Simbrunner J. MR imaging of the TMJ. MR diagnosis and intraoperative findings. *J Craniomaxillofac. Surg.* 1993;21(7):284-288.

35. Zain-Alabdeen EH, Alsadhan RI. A comparative study of accuracy of detection of surface osseous changes in the temporomandibular joint using multidetector CT and cone beam CT. *Dentomaxillofac Rad.* 2012;41(3):185-191.

36. Manfredini D, Lobbezoo F. Relationship between bruxism and temporomandibular disorders: A systematic review of literature from 1998 to 2008. *Oral Surg Oral Med Oral Pathol Oral Radiol Endod.* 2010;109(6):e26-e50.

37. Buckingham RB, Braun T, Harinstein DA, et al. Temporomandibular joint dysfunction syndrome: A close association with systemic joint laxity (the hypermobile joint syndrome). *Oral Surg Oral Med Oral Pathol.* 1991;72(5):514-519.

38. Adair SM, Hecht C. Association of generalized joint hypermobility with history, signs, and symptoms of temporomandibular joint dysfunction in children. *Pediatr Dent.* 1993;15(5):323-326.

39. Dijkstra PU, Kropmans TJ, Stegenga B. The association between generalized joint hypermobility and temporomandibular joint disorders: A systematic review. *J Dent Res.* 2002;81(3):158-163.

40. Shah KC, Rajshekhar V. Reliability of diagnosis of soft cervical disc prolapse using Spurling's test. *Brit J Neurosurg.* 2004;18(5):480-483.

41. Wainner RS, Fritz JM, Irrgang JJ, Boninger ML, Delitto A, Allison S. Reliability and diagnostic accuracy of the clinical examination and patient self-report measures for cervical radiculopathy. *Spine (Phila Pa 1976).* 2003;28(1):52-62.

42. Reneker J, Paz J, Petrosino C, Cook C. Diagnostic accuracy of clinical tests and signs of temporomandibular joint disorders: A systematic review of the literature. *J Orthop Sports Phys Ther.* 2011;41(6):408-416.

43. Chaput E, Gross A, Stewart R, Nadeau G, Goldsmith CH. The diagnostic validity of clinical tests in temporomandibular internal derangement: A systematic review and meta-analysis. *Physiother Can.* 2012;64(2):116-134.

44. Yatani H, Suzuki K, Kuboki T, Matsuka Y, Maekawa K, Yamashita A. The validity of clinical examination for diagnosing anterior disk displacement without reduction. *Oral Surg Oral Med Oral Pathol Oral Radiol Endod.* 1998;85(6):654-660.

45. Holmlund AB, Axelsson S. Temporomandibular arthropathy: Correlation between clinical signs and symptoms and arthroscopic findings. *Int J Oral Maxillofac Surg.* 1996;25(3):178-181.

46. Orsini MG, Kuboki T, Terada S, Matsuka Y, Yatani H, Yamashita A. Clinical predictability of temporomandibular joint disc displacement. *J Dent Res.* 1999;78(2):650-660.

47. Seligman DA, Pullinger AG, Solberg WK. Temporomandibular disorders. Part III: Occlusal and articular factors associated with muscle tenderness. *J Prosthet Dent.* 1988;59(4):483-489.

48. De Leeuw PW. *Orofacial Pain: Guidelines for Assessment, Diagnosis and Management.* 4th ed. Oxford, UK: Quintessence; 2008.

49. Liu F, Steinkeler A. Epidemiology, diagnosis, and treatment of temporomandibular disorders. *Dent Clin North Am.* 2013;57(3):465-479.

50. Wiese M, Svensson P, Bakke M, et al. Association between temporomandibular joint symptoms, signs, and clinical diagnosis using the RDC/TMD and radiographic findings in temporomandibular joint tomograms. *J Orofac Pain.* 2008;22(3):239-251.

51. Turp JC, Minagi S. Palpation of the lateral pterygoid region in TMD—Where is the evidence? *J Dent.* 2001;29(7):475-483.

52. Stratmann U, Mokrys K, Meyer U, et al. Clinical anatomy and palpability of the inferior lateral pterygoid muscle. *J Prosthet Dent.* 2000;83(5):548-554.

53. Conti PC, Dos Santos Silva R, Rossetti LM, De Oliveira Ferreira Da Silva R, Do Valle AL, Gelmini M. Palpation of the lateral pterygoid area in the myofascial pain diagnosis. *Oral Surg Oral Med Oral Pathol Oral Radiol Endod.* 2008;105(3):e61-e66.

54. Solberg WK, Woo MW, Houston JB. Prevalence of mandibular dysfunction in young adults. *J Am Dent Assoc.* 1979;98(1):25-34.

55. Seligman DA, Pullinger AG, Solberg WK. The prevalence of dental attrition and its association with factors of age, gender, occlusion, and TMJ symptomatology. *J Dent Res.* 1988;67(10):1323-1333.

56. Pimenta e Silva Machado L, de Macedo Nery MB, de Gois Nery C, Leles CR. Profiling the clinical presentation of diagnostic characteristics of a sample of symptomatic TMD patients. *BMC Oral Health.* 2012;12:26.

Chapter 17

1. Jette AM, Smith K, Haley SM, Davis KD. Physical therapy episodes of care for patients with low back pain. *Phys Ther.* 1994;74(2):101-110, discussion 110-105.

2. Picavet HS, Schouten JS. Musculoskeletal pain in the Netherlands: Prevalences, consequences and risk groups, the DMC(3)-study. *Pain.* 2003;102(1-2):167-178.

3. Wright A, Mayer TG, Gatchel RJ. Outcomes of disabling cervical spine disorders in compensation injuries. A prospective comparison to tertiary rehabilitation response for chronic lumbar spinal disorders. *Spine (Phila Pa 1976).* 1999;24(2):178-183.

4. van der Donk J, Schouten JS, Passchier J, van Romunde LK, Valkenburg HA. The associations of neck pain with radiological abnormalities of the cervical spine and personality traits in a general population. *J Rheumatol.* 1991;18(12):1884-1889.

5. Holmstrom EB, Lindell J, Moritz U. Low back and neck/shoulder pain in construction workers: Occupational workload and psychosocial risk factors. Part 2: Relationship to neck and shoulder pain. *Spine (Phila Pa 1976).* 1992;17(6):672-677.

6. Cote P, Cassidy JD, Carroll LJ, Kristman V. The annual incidence and course of neck pain in the general population: A population-based cohort study. *Pain.* 2004;112(3):267-273.

7. Bovim G, Schrader H, Sand T. Neck pain in the general population. *Spine (Phila Pa 1976).* 1994;19(12):1307-1309.

8. Cote P, Cassidy JD, Carroll L. The factors associated with neck pain and its related disability in the Saskatchewan population. *Spine (Phila Pa 1976).* 2000;25(9):1109-1117.

9. Croft PR, Lewis M, Papageorgiou AC, et al. Risk factors for neck pain: A longitudinal study in the general population. *Pain.* 2001;93(3):317-325.

10. Andersson HI. The epidemiology of chronic pain in a Swedish rural area. *Qual Life Res.* 1994;3(suppl 1):S19-S26.

11. Childs JD, Cleland JA, Elliott JM, et al. Neck pain: Clinical practice guidelines linked to the International Classification of Functioning, Disability, and Health from the Orthopedic Section of the American Physical Therapy Association. *J Orthop Sport Phys.* 2008;38(9):A1-A34.

12. Mercer S, Bogduk N. Intra-articular inclusions of the cervical synovial joints. *Brit J Rheumatol.* 1993;32(8):705-710.

13. Bland JH, Boushey DR. Anatomy and physiology of the cervical spine. *Semin Arthritis Rheu.* 1990;20(1):1-20.

14. White AA III, Johnson RM, Panjabi MM, Southwick WO. Biomechanical analysis of clinical stability in the cervical spine. *Clin Orthop Relat R.* 1975;109:85-96.

15. Cloward RB. Cervical diskography. A contribution to the etiology and mechanism of neck, shoulder and arm pain. *Ann Surg.* 1959;150:1052-1064.

16. Grubb SA, Kelly CK. Cervical discography: Clinical implications from 12 years of experience. *Spine (Phila Pa 1976).* 2000;25(11):1382-1389.

17. Ohnmeiss DD, Vanharanta H, Ekholm J. Relation between pain location and disc pathology: A study of pain drawings and CT/discography. *Clin J Pain.* 1999;15(3):210-217.

18. Wainner RS, Fritz JM, Irrgang JJ, Boninger ML, Delitto A, Allison S. Reliability and diagnostic accuracy of the clinical examination and patient self-report measures for cervical radiculopathy. *Spine (Phila Pa 1976).* 2003;28(1):52-62.

19. Fukui S, Ohseto K, Shiotani M, et al. Referred pain distribution of the cervical zygapophyseal joints and cervical dorsal rami. *Pain.* 1996;68(1):79-83.

20. Dreyfuss P, Rogers J, Dreyer S, Fletcher D. Atlan-to-occipital joint pain. A report of three cases and description of an intraarticular joint block technique. *Reg Anesth.* 1994;19(5):344-351.

21. Trevor-Jones R. Osteo-arthritis of the paravertebral joints of the second and third cervical vertebrae as a cause of occipital headaches. *S Afr Med J.* 1964;38:392-394.

22. Bogduk N, Marsland A. On the concept of third occipital headache. *J Neurol Neurosur Ps.* 1986;49(7):775-780.

23. Bovim G. Cervicogenic headache, migraine, and tension-type headache. Pressure-pain threshold measurements. *Pain.* 1992;51(2):169-173.

24. Hall T, Robinson K. The flexion-rotation test and active cervical mobility—A comparative measurement study in cervicogenic headache. *Man Ther.* 2004;9(4):197-202.

25. Grieve GP. *Common Vertebral Joint Problems.* 2nd ed. Philadelphia, PA: Elsevier Health Sciences; 1989.

26. Stiell IG, Wells GA, Vandemheen KL, et al. The Canadian C-spine rule for radiography in alert and stable trauma patients. *JAMA.* 2001;286(15):1841-1848.

27. Hoffman JR, Wolfson AB, Todd K, Mower WR. Selective cervical spine radiography in blunt trauma: Methodology of the National Emergency X-Radiography Utilization Study (NEXUS). *Ann Emerg Med.* 1998;32(4):461-469.

28. Kaale BR, Krakenes J, Albrektsen G, Wester K. Head position and impact direction in whiplash injuries: Associations with MRI-verified lesions of ligaments and membranes in the upper cervical spine. *J Neurotraum.* 2005;22(11):1294-1302.

29. Ivancic PC, Ito S, Tominaga Y, Carlson EJ, Rubin W, Panjabi MM. Effect of rotated head posture on dynamic vertebral artery elongation during simulated rear impact. *Clin Biomech (Bristol, Avon).* 2006;21(3):213-220.

30. Fritz JM, Brennan GP. Preliminary examination of a proposed treatment-based classification system for patients receiving physical therapy interventions for neck pain. *Phys Ther.* 2007;87(5):513-524.

31. Jull G, Bogduk N, Marsland A. The accuracy of manual diagnosis for cervical zygapophysial joint pain syndromes. *Med J Aust.* 1988;148(5):233-236.

32. Nystrom A, Ginsburg GM, Stuberg W, Dejong S. Pre- and post-operative gait analysis for evaluation of neck pain in chronic whiplash. *J Brachial Plex Peripher Nerve Inj.* 2009;4:10.

33. Cook C, Brown C, Isaacs R, Roman M, Davis S, Richardson W. Clustered clinical findings for diagnosis of cervical spine myelopathy. *J Man Manip Ther.* 2010;18(4):175-180.

34. Society IH. The international classification of headache disorders, 2nd edition. *Cephalalgia.* 2004;24(suppl 1):S9-S160.

35. Nordin M, Carragee EJ, Hogg-Johnson S, et al. Assessment of neck pain and its associated disorders: Results of the Bone and Joint Decade 2000-2010 Task Force on Neck Pain and Its Associated Disorders. *Spine (Phila Pa 1976).* 2008;33(4)(suppl):S101-S122.

36. Vernon H, Mior S. The Neck Disability Index: A study of reliability and validity. *J Manip Physiol Ther.* 1991;14(7):409-415.

37. MacDermid JC, Walton DM, Avery S, et al. Measurement properties of the neck disability index: A systematic review. *J Orthop Sports Phys.* 2009;39(5):400-417.

38. Jette DU, Jette AM. Physical therapy and health outcomes in patients with spinal impairments. *Phys Ther.* 1996;76(9):930-941, discussion 942-935.

39. Riddle DL, Stratford PW. Use of generic versus region-specific functional status measures on patients with cervical spine disorders. *Phys Ther.* 1998;78(9):951-963.

40. Cleland JA, Childs JD, Whitman JM. Psychometric properties of the Neck Disability Index and Numeric Pain Rating Scale in patients with mechanical neck pain. *Arch Phys Med Rehab.* 2008;89(1):69-74.

41. Young IA, Michener LA, Cleland JA, Aguilera AJ, Snyder AR. Manual therapy, exercise, and traction for patients with cervical radiculopathy: A randomized clinical trial. *Phys Ther.* 2009;89(7):632-642.

42. Cleland JA, Fritz JM, Whitman JM, Palmer JA. The reliability and construct validity of the Neck Disability Index and patient specific functional scale in patients with cervical radiculopathy. *Spine (Phila Pa 1976).* 2006;31(5):598-602.

43. Kamper SJ, Maher CG, Mackay G. Global rating of change scales: A review of strengths and weaknesses and considerations for design. *J Man Manip Ther.* 2009;17(3):163-170.

44. Guzman J, Haldeman S, Carroll LJ, et al. Clinical practice implications of the Bone and Joint Decade 2000-2010 Task Force on Neck Pain and Its Associated Disorders: From concepts and findings to recommendations. *Spine (Phila Pa 1976).* 2008;33(4)(suppl):S199-S213.

45. Mutze S, Rademacher G, Matthes G, Hosten N, Stengel D. Blunt cerebrovascular injury in patients with blunt multiple trauma: Diagnostic accuracy of duplex Doppler US and early CT angiography. *Radiology.* 2005;237(3):884-892.

46. Stengel D, Rademacher G, Hanson B, Ekkernkamp A, Mutze S. Screening for blunt cerebrovascular injuries: The essential role of computed tomography angiography. *Semin Ultrasound CT.* 2007;28(2):101-108.

47. Cher LM, Chambers BR, Smidt V. Comparison of transcranial Doppler with DSA in vertebrobasilar ischaemia. *Clin Exp Neurol.* 1992;29:143-148.

48. Panczykowski DM, Tomycz ND, Okonkwo DO. Comparative effectiveness of using computed tomography alone to exclude cervical spine injuries in obtunded or intubated patients: Meta-analysis of 14,327 patients with blunt trauma. *J Neurosurg.* 2011;115(3):541-549.

49. Holmes JF, Akkinepalli R. Computed tomography versus plain radiography to screen for cervical spine injury: A meta-analysis. *J Trauma.* 2005;58(5):902-905.

50. Offerman SR, Holmes JF, Katzberg RX, Richards JR. Utility of supine oblique radiographs in detecting cervical spine injury. *J Emerg Med.* 2006;30(2):189-195.

51. Harnan SE, Pickering A, Pandor A, Goodacre SW. Clinical decision rules for adults with minor head injury: A systematic review. *J Trauma.* 2011;71(1):245-251.

52. Anderson SE, Boesch C, Zimmermann H, et al. Are there cervical spine findings at MR imaging that are specific to acute symptomatic whiplash injury? A prospective controlled study with four experienced blinded readers. *Radiology.* 2012;262(2):567-575.

53. Rubinstein SM, van Tulder M. A best-evidence review of diagnostic procedures for neck and low-back pain. *Best Pract Res Clin Rheumatol.* 2008;22(3):471-482.

54. van Tulder M, Becker A, Bekkering T, et al. Chapter 3. European guidelines for the management of acute nonspecific low back pain in primary care. *Eur Spine J.* 2006;15(suppl 2):S169-S191.

55. Laker SR, Concannon LG. Radiologic evaluation of the neck: A review of radiography, ultrasonography, computed tomography, magnetic resonance imaging, and other imaging modalities for neck pain. *Phys Med Rehabil Cli.* 2011;22(3):411-428, vii-viii.

56. Henschke N, Maher CG, Refshauge KM, et al. Prevalence of and screening for serious spinal pathology in patients presenting to primary care settings with acute low back pain. *Arthritis Rheum.* 2009;60(10):3072-3080.

57. Daffner RH, Dalinka MK, Alazraki N, et al. Chronic neck pain. American College of Radiology. ACR Appropriateness Criteria. *Radiology.* 2000;215(suppl):345-356.

58. Michaleff ZA, Maher CG, Verhagen AP, Rebbeck T, Lin CW. Accuracy of the Canadian C-spine rule and NEXUS to screen for clinically important cervical spine injury in patients following blunt trauma: A systematic review. *CMAJ.* 2012;184(16):E867-E876.

59. Bandiera G, Stiell IG, Wells GA, et al. The Canadian C-spine rule performs better than unstructured physician judgment. *Ann Emerg Med.* 2003;42(3):395-402.

60. Anderson PA, Muchow RD, Munoz A, Tontz WL, Resnick DK. Clearance of the asymptomatic cervical spine: A meta-analysis. *J Orthop Trauma.* 2010;24(2):100-106.

61. Swischuk LE, John SD, Hendrick EP. Is the open-mouth odontoid view necessary in children under 5 years? *Pediatr Radiol.* 2000;30(3):186-189.

62. Buhs C, Cullen M, Klein M, Farmer D. The pediatric trauma C-spine: Is the 'odontoid' view necessary? *J Pediatr Surg.* 2000;35(6):994-997.

63. Duane TM, Cross J, Scarcella N, et al. Flexion-extension cervical spine plain films compared with MRI in the diagnosis of ligamentous injury. *Am Surg.* 2010;76(6):595-598.

64. Taniguchi D, Tokunaga D, Hase H, et al. Evaluation of lateral instability of the atlanto-axial joint in rheumatoid arthritis using dynamic open-mouth view radiographs. *Clin Rheumatol.* 2008;27(7):851-857.

65. Gale SC, Gracias VH, Reilly PM, Schwab CW. The inefficiency of plain radiography to evaluate the cervical spine after blunt trauma. *J Trauma.* 2005;59(5):1121-1125.

66. Bailitz J, Starr F, Beecroft M, et al. CT should replace three-view radiographs as the initial screening test in patients at high, moderate, and low risk for blunt cervical spine injury: A prospective comparison. *J Trauma.* 2009;66(6):1605-1609.

67. Kuijper B, Beelen A, van der Kallen BF, et al. Interobserver agreement on MRI evaluation of patients with cervical radiculopathy. *Clin Radiol.* 2011;66(1):25-29.

68. Bono CM, Ghiselli G, Gilbert TJ, et al. An evidence-based clinical guideline for the diagnosis and treatment of cervical radiculopathy from degenerative disorders. *Spine J.* 2011;11(1):64-72.

69. Vaillancourt C, Stiell IG, Beaudoin T, et al. The out-of-hospital validation of the Canadian C-Spine Rule by paramedics. *Ann Emerg Med.* 2009;54(5):663-671, e661.

70. Dickinson G, Stiell IG, Schull M, et al. Retrospective application of the NEXUS low-risk criteria for cervical spine radiography in Canadian emergency departments. *Ann Emerg Med.* 2004;43(4):507-514.

71. Chin KR, Eiszner JR, Huang JL, Huang JI, Roh JS, Bohlman HH. Myelographic evaluation of cervical spondylosis: Patient tolerance and complications. *J Spinal Disord Tech.* 2008;21(5):334-337.

72. Fassett DR, Dailey AT, Vaccaro AR. Vertebral artery injuries associated with cervical spine injuries: A review of the literature. *J Spinal Disord Tech.* 2008;21(4):252-258.

73. Brewin J, Hill M, Ellis H. The prevalence of cervical ribs in a London population. *Clin Anat.* 2009;22(3):331-336.

74. Wang P, Lou L, Song L. Design and efficacy of surgery for horizontal idiopathic nystagmus with abnormal head posture and strabismus. *J Huazhong U Sci-Med.* 2011;31(5):678-681.

75. Dumitrescu AV, Moga DC, Longmuir SQ, Olson RJ, Drack AV. Prevalence and characteristics of abnormal head posture in children with Down syndrome: A 20-year retrospective, descriptive review. *Ophthalmology.* 2011;118(9):1859-1864.

76. Lewis RF, Priesol AJ, Nicoucar K, Lim K, Merfeld DM. Dynamic tilt thresholds are reduced in vestibular migraine. *J Vestib Res.* 2011;21(6):323-330.

77. Staab JP. Clinical clues to a dizzying headache. *J Vestib Res.* 2011;21(6):331-340.

78. Ventura LM, Golubev I, Lee W, et al. Head-down posture induces PERG alterations in early glaucoma [published online ahead of print December 1 2011]. *J Glaucoma.* 2011.

79. Okuro RT, Morcillo AM, Sakano E, Schivinski CI, Ribeiro MA, Ribeiro JD. Exercise capacity, respiratory mechanics and posture in mouth breathers. *Braz J Otorhinolaryngol.* 2011;77(5):656-662.

80. Sizer PS, Jr., Brismee JM, Cook C. Medical screening for red flags in the diagnosis and management of musculoskeletal spine pain. *Pain Pract.* 2007;7(1):53-71.

81. Cook CE, Wilhelm M, Cook AE, Petrosino C, Isaacs R. Clinical tests for screening and diagnosis of cervical spine myelopathy: A systematic review. *J Manip Physiol Ther.* 2011;34(8):539-546.

82. Hong YH, Lee YS, Park SH. Headache as a predictive factor of severe systolic hypertension in acute ischemic stroke. *Can J Neurol Sci.* 2003;30(3):210-214.

83. Ohkuma H, Tabata H, Suzuki S, Islam MS. Risk factors for aneurysmal subarachnoid hemorrhage in Aomori, Japan. *Stroke.* 2003;34(1):96-100.

84. Hurwitz EL, Aker PD, Adams AH, Meeker WC, Shekelle PG. Manipulation and mobilization of the cervical spine. A systematic review of the literature. *Spine (Phila Pa 1976).* 1996;21(15):1746-1759, discussion 1759-1760.

85. Bruce MG, Rosenstein NE, Capparella JM, Shutt KA, Perkins BA, Collins M. Risk factors for meningococcal disease in college students. *JAMA.* 2001;286(6):688-693.

86. Haj-Hassan TA, Thompson MJ, Mayon-White RT, et al. Which early 'red flag' symptoms identify children with meningococcal disease in primary care? *Brit J Gen Pract.* 2011;61(584):e97-e104.

87. Sobri M, Lamont AC, Alias NA, Win MN. Red flags in patients presenting with headache: Clinical indications for neuroimaging. *Brit J Radiol.* 2003;76(908):532-535.

88. Borg J, Holm L, Cassidy JD, et al. Diagnostic procedures in mild traumatic brain injury: Results of the WHO Collaborating Centre Task Force on Mild Traumatic Brain Injury. *J Rehabil Med.* 2004(43)(suppl):61-75.

89. Snyder H, Robinson K, Shah D, Brennan R, Handrigan M. Signs and symptoms of patients with brain tumors presenting to the emergency department. *J Emerg Med.* 1993;11(3):253-258.

90. Zaki A, Natarajan N, Mettlin CJ. Patterns of presentation in brain tumors in the United States. *J Surg Oncol.* 1993;53(2):110-112.

91. Forsyth PA, Posner JB. Headaches in patients with brain tumors: A study of 111 patients. *Neurology.* 1993;43(9):1678-1683.

92. Slipman CW, Patel RK, Botwin K, et al. Epidemiology of spine tumors presenting to musculoskeletal physiatrists. *Arch Phys Med Rehab.* 2003;84(4):492-495.

93. Rushton A, Rivett D, Carlesso L, Flynn T, Hing W, Kerry R. International framework for examination of the cervical region for potential of cervical arterial dysfunction prior to orthopaedic manual therapy intervention. New Zealand: International Federation of Orthopaedic Manipulative Physical Therapists; 2012.

94. Carlson EJ, Tominaga Y, Ivancic PC, Panjabi MM. Dynamic vertebral artery elongation during frontal and side impacts. *Spine J.* 2007;7(2):222-228.

95. Cook C, Brismee JM, Fleming R, Sizer PS Jr. Identifiers suggestive of clinical cervical spine instability: A Delphi study of physical therapists. *Phys Ther.* 2005;85(9):895-906.

96. Arnold M, Bousser MG. Carotid and vertebral dissection. *Pract Neurol.* 2005;5:100-109.

97. Kerry R, Taylor AJ, Mitchell J, McCarthy C. Cervical arterial dysfunction and manual therapy: A critical literature review to inform professional practice. *Man Ther.* 2008;13(4):278-288.

98. Rubinstein SM, Peerdeman SM, van Tulder MW, Riphagen I, Haldeman S. A systematic review of the risk factors for cervical artery dissection. *Stroke.* 2005;36(7):1575-1580.

99. Thomas LC, Rivett DA, Attia JR, Parsons M, Levi C. Risk factors and clinical features of craniocervical arterial dissection. *Man Ther.* 2011;16(4):351-356.

100. Kerry R, Taylor AJ. Cervical arterial dysfunction assessment and manual therapy. *Man Ther.* 2006;11(4):243-253.

101. Kerry R, Taylor AJ. Cervical arterial dysfunction: Knowledge and reasoning for manual physical therapists. *J Orthop Sport Phys.* 2009;39(5):378-387.

102. Cook CE, Hegedus EJ. *Orthopedic Physical Examination Tests: An Evidence-Based Approach.* Upper Saddle River, NJ: Pearson Prentice Hall; 2008.

103. Rushton A, Rivett D, Carlesso L, Flynn T, Hing W, Kerry R. International framework for examination of the cervical region for potential of Cervical Arterial Dysfunction prior to Orthopaedic Manual Therapy intervention [published online ahead of print November 23 2013]. *Man Ther.* 2013.

104. Sorimachi Y, Iizuka H, Ara T, et al. Atlanto-axial joint of atlanto-axial subluxation patients due to rheumatoid arthritis before and after surgery: Morphological evaluation using CT reconstruction. *Eur Spine J.* 2011;20(5):798-803.

105. Brockmeyer D. Down syndrome and craniovertebral instability. Topic review and treatment recommendations. *Pediatr Neurosurg.* 1999;31(2):71-77.

106. Hankinson TC, Anderson RC. Craniovertebral junction abnormalities in Down syndrome. *Neurosurgery.* 2010;66(3)(suppl):32-38.

107. Kaale BR, Krakenes J, Albrektsen G, Wester K. Clinical assessment techniques for detecting ligament and membrane injuries in the upper cervical spine region—A comparison with MRI results. *Man Ther.* 2008;13(5):397-403.

108. Uitvlugt G, Indenbaum S. Clinical assessment of atlantoaxial instability using the Sharp-Purser test. *Arthritis Rheum.* 1988;31(7):918-922.

109. Cattrysse E, Swinkels RA, Oostendorp RA, Duquet W. Upper cervical instability: Are clinical tests reliable? *Man Ther.* 1997;2(2):91-97.

110. Asavasopon S, Jankoski J, Godges JJ. Clinical diagnosis of vertebrobasilar insufficiency: Resident's case problem. *J Orthop Sport Phys.* 2005;35(10):645-650.

111. Sweeney A, Doody C. The clinical reasoning of musculoskeletal physiotherapists in relation to the assessment of vertebrobasilar insufficiency: A qualitative study. *Man Ther.* 2010;15(4):394-399.

112. Hutting N, Verhagen AP, Vijverman V, Keesenberg MD, Dixon G, Scholten-Peeters GG. Diagnostic accuracy of premanipulative vertebrobasilar insufficiency tests: A systematic review [published online ahead of print November 3 2012]. *Man Ther.* 2012.

113. Mitchell J. Vertebral artery blood flow velocity changes associated with cervical spine rotation: A meta-analysis of the evidence with implications for professional practice. *J Man Manip Ther.* 2009;17(1):46-57.

114. Thomas LC, Rivett DA, Bateman G, Stanwell P, Levi CR. Effect of selected manual therapy interventions for mechanical neck pain on vertebral and internal carotid arterial blood flow and cerebral inflow [published online ahead of print June 27 2013]. *Phys Ther.* 2013.

115. Petersen B, von Maravic M, Zeller JA, Walker ML, Kompf D, Kessler C. Basilar artery blood flow during head rotation in vertebrobasilar ischemia. *Acta Neurol Scand.* 1996;94(4):294-301.

116. Li YK, Zhang YK, Lu CM, Zhong SZ. Changes and implications of blood flow velocity of the vertebral artery during rotation and extension of the head. *J Manip Physiol Ther.* 1999;22(2):91-95.

117. Sakaguchi M, Kitagawa K, Hougaku H, et al. Mechanical compression of the extracranial vertebral artery during neck rotation. *Neurology.* 2003;61(6):845-847.

118. Bhattacharyya N, Baugh RF, Orvidas L, et al. Clinical practice guideline: Benign paroxysmal positional vertigo. *Otolaryng. Head Neck.* 2008;139(5)(suppl 4):S47-S81.

119. Halker RB, Barrs DM, Wellik KE, Wingerchuk DM, Demaerschalk BM. Establishing a diagnosis of benign paroxysmal positional vertigo through the Dix-Hallpike and side-lying maneuvers: A critically appraised topic. *Neurologist.* 2008;14(3):201-204.

120. Sobel JB, Sollenberger P, Robinson R, Polatin PB, Gatchel RJ. Cervical nonorganic signs: A new clinical tool to assess abnormal illness behavior in neck pain patients: A pilot study. *Arch Phys Med Rehab.* 2000;81(2):170-175.

121. Langdon J, Way A, Heaton S, Bernard J, Molloy S. Vertebral compression fractures—New clinical signs to aid diagnosis. *Ann R Coll Surg Engl.* 2010;92(2):163-166.

122. Shah KC, Rajshekhar V. Reliability of diagnosis of soft cervical disc prolapse using Spurling's test. *Brit J Neurosurg.* 2004;18(5):480-483.

123. Gumina S, Carbone S, Albino P, Gurzi M, Postacchini F. Arm Squeeze Test: A new clinical test to distinguish neck from shoulder pain. *Eur Spine J.* 2013;22(7):1558-1563.

124. Hoving JL, Pool JJ, van Mameren H, et al. Reproducibility of cervical range of motion in patients with neck pain. *BMC Musculoskel Dis.* 2005;6:59.

125. Antonaci F, Ghirmai S, Bono G, Nappi G. Current methods for cervical spine movement evaluation: A review. *Clin Exp Rheumatol.* 2000;18(2)(suppl 19):S45-S52.

126. Fletcher JP, Bandy WD. Intrarater reliability of CROM measurement of cervical spine active range of motion in persons with and without neck pain. *J Orthop Sport Phys.* 2008;38(10):640-645.

127. Shahidi B, Johnson CL, Curran-Everett D, Maluf KS. Reliability and group differences in quantitative cervicothoracic measures among individuals with and without chronic neck pain. *BMC Musculoskel Disord.* 2012;13:215.

128. Kaale BR, Krakenes J, Albrektsen G, Wester K. Active range of motion as an indicator for ligament and membrane lesions in the upper cervical spine after a whiplash trauma. *J Neurotraum.* 2007;24(4):713-721.

129. Hall TM, Briffa K, Hopper D, Robinson KW. The relationship between cervicogenic headache and impairment determined by the flexion-rotation test. *J Manip Phys Ther.* 2010;33(9):666-671.

130. Kuhlman KA. Cervical range of motion in the elderly. *Arch Phys Med Rehab.* 1993;74(10):1071-1079.

131. Salo PK, Hakkinen AH, Kautiainen H, Ylinen JJ. Quantifying the effect of age on passive range of motion of the cervical spine in healthy working-age women. *J Orthop Sport Phys.* 2009;39(6):478-483.

132. Ogince M, Hall T, Robinson K, Blackmore AM. The diagnostic validity of the cervical flexion-rotation test in C1/2-related cervicogenic headache. *Man Ther.* 2007;12(3):256-262.

133. Zito G, Jull G, Story I. Clinical tests of musculoskeletal dysfunction in the diagnosis of cervicogenic headache. *Man Ther.* 2006;11(2):118-129.

134. King W, Lau P, Lees R, Bogduk N. The validity of manual examination in assessing patients with neck pain. *Spine J.* 2007;7(1):22-26.

135. Sandmark H, Nisell R. Validity of five common manual neck pain provoking tests. *Scand J Rehabil Med.* 1995;27(3):131-136.

136. Jull G, Treleaven J, Verace G. Manual examination: Is pain provocation a major cue for spinal dysfunction? *Aust J Physiother.* 1994;40:159-165.

137. Cleland JA, Childs JD, Fritz JM, Whitman JM. Interrater reliability of the history and physical examination in patients with mechanical neck pain. *Arch Phys Med Rehab.* 2006;87(10):1388-1395.

138. Humphreys BK, Delahaye M, Peterson CK. An investigation into the validity of cervical spine motion palpation using subjects with congenital block vertebrae as a 'gold standard'. *BMC Musculoskel Dis.* 2004;5:19.

139. Greenman PE. *Principles of Manual Medicine.* 2nd ed. Baltimore, MD: Williams & Wilkins; 1996.

140. Viikari-Juntura E, Porras M, Laasonen EM. Validity of clinical tests in the diagnosis of root compression in cervical disc disease. *Spine (Phila Pa 1976).* 1989;14(3):253-257.

141. Ruggieri PM. Cervical radiculopathy. *Neuroimag Clin N Am.* 1995;5(3):349-366.

142. Malanga GA, Landes P, Nadler SF. Provocative tests in cervical spine examination: Historical basis and scientific analyses. *Pain Physician.* 2003;6(2):199-205.

143. Uchihara T, Furukawa T, Tsukagoshi H. Compression of brachial plexus as a diagnostic test of cervical cord lesion. *Spine (Phila Pa 1976).* 1994;19(19):2170-2173.

144. Anekstein Y, Blecher R, Smorgick Y, Mirovsky Y. What is the best way to apply the Spurling test for cervical radiculopathy? [published online ahead of print July 18 2012]. *Clin Orthop Relat Res.* 2012.

145. Sizer PS Jr, Phelps V, Dedrick G, Matthijs O. Differential diagnosis and management of spinal nerve root-related pain. *Pain Pract.* 2002;2(2):98-121.

146. Farshad M, Min K. Abduction extension cervical nerve root stress test: Anatomical basis and clinical relevance. *Eur Spine J.* 2013;22(7):1522-1525.

147. Jull GA, O'Leary SP, Falla DL. Clinical assessment of the deep cervical flexor muscles: The craniocervical flexion test. *J Manip Physiol Ther.* 2008;31(7):525-533.

148. Grimmer K. Measuring the endurance capacity of the cervical short flexor muscle group. *Aust J Physiother.* 1994;40:251-254.

149. Harris KD, Heer DM, Roy TC, Santos DM, Whitman JM, Wainner RS. Reliability of a measurement of neck flexor muscle endurance. *Phys Ther.* 2005;85(12):1349-1355.

150. de Koning CH, van den Heuvel SP, Staal JB, Smits-Engelsman BC, Hendriks EJ. Clinimetric evaluation of methods to measure muscle functioning in patients with non-specific neck pain: A systematic review. *BMC Musculoskel Dis.* 2008;9:142.

151. Borghouts JA, Koes BW, Bouter LM. The clinical course and prognostic factors of non-specific neck pain: A systematic review. *Pain.* 1998;77(1):1-13.

152. Quek J, Pua YH, Clark RA, Bryant AL. Effects of thoracic kyphosis and forward head posture on cervical range of motion in older adults [published online ahead of print September 5 2012]. *Man Ther.* 2012.

153. Honet JC, Puri K. Cervical radiculitis: Treatment and results in 82 patients. *Arch Phys Med Rehab.* 1976;57(1):12-16.

154. Kellgren JH, Lawrence JS. Radiological assessment of osteo-arthrosis. *Ann Rheum Dis.* 1957;16(4):494-502.

155. Fukui S, Ohseto K, Shiotani M, Ohno K, Karasawa H, Naganuma Y. Distribution of referred pain from the lumbar zygapophyseal joints and dorsal rami. *Clin J Pain.* 1997;13(4):303-307.

156. Brown S, Guthmann R, Hitchcock K, Davis JD. Clinical inquiries. Which treatments are effective for cervical radiculopathy? *J Fam Pract.* 2009;58(2):97-99.

157. Harrop JS, Hanna A, Silva MT, Sharan A. Neurological manifestations of cervical spondylosis: An overview of signs, symptoms, and pathophysiology. *Neurosurgery.* 2007;60(1)(suppl 1):S14-S20.

158. Matsuda Y, Miyazaki K, Tada K, et al. Increased MR signal intensity due to cervical myelopathy. Analysis of 29 surgical cases. *J Neurosurg.* 1991;74(6):887-892.

159. Bednarik J, Kadanka Z, Dusek L, et al. Presymptomatic spondylotic cervical cord compression. *Spine (Phila Pa 1976).* 2004;29(20):2260-2269.

160. Chiles BW III, Leonard MA, Choudhri HF, Cooper PR. Cervical spondylotic myelopathy: Patterns of neurological deficit and recovery after anterior cervical decompression. *Neurosurgery.* 1999;44(4):762-769, discussion 769-770.

161. Lev N, Maimon S, Rappaport ZH, Melamed E. Spinal dural arteriovenous fistulae—A diagnostic challenge. *Isr Med Assoc J.* 2001;3(7):492-496.

162. Good DC, Couch JR, Wacaser L. "Numb, clumsy hands" and high cervical spondylosis. *Surg Neurol.* 1984;22(3):285-291.

163. Dalitz K, Vitzthum HE. Evaluation of five scoring systems for cervical spondylogenic myelopathy [published online ahead of print September 5 2008]. *Spine J.* 2008.

164. Vitzthum HE, Dalitz K. Analysis of five specific scores for cervical spondylogenic myelopathy. *Eur Spine J.* 2007;16(12):2096-2103.

165. Polston DW. Cervical radiculopathy. *Neurol Clin.* 2007;25(2):373-385.

166. Rhee JM, Heflin JA, Hamasaki T, Freedman B. Prevalence of physical signs in cervical myelopathy: A prospective, controlled study. *Spine (Phila Pa 1976).* 2009;34(9):890-895.

167. Sung RD, Wang JC. Correlation between a positive Hoffmann's reflex and cervical pathology in asymptomatic individuals. *Spine (Phila Pa 1976).* 2001;26(1):67-70.

168. Cook C, Roman M, Stewart KM, Leithe LG, Isaacs R. Reliability and diagnostic accuracy of clinical special tests for myelopathy in patients seen for cervical dysfunction. *J Orthop Sport Phys.* 2009;39(3):172-178.

169. Kimura A, Seichi A, Endo T, et al. Tally counter test as a simple and objective assessment of cervical myelopathy. *Eur Spine J.* 2013;22(1):183-188.

170. Numasawa T, Ono A, Wada K, et al. Simple foot tapping test as a quantitative objective assessment of cervical myelopathy. *Spine (Phila Pa 1976).* 2012;37(2):108-113.

171. Wolff MW, Levine LA. Cervical radiculopathies: Conservative approaches to management. *Phys Med Rehabi Cli.* 2002;13(3):589-608, vii.

172. Davidson RI, Dunn EJ, Metzmaker JN. The shoulder abduction test in the diagnosis of radicular pain in cervical extradural compressive monoradiculopathies. *Spine (Phila Pa 1976).* 1981;6(5):441-446.

173. Yoss RE, Corbin KB, Maccarty CS, Love JG. Significance of symptoms and signs in localization of involved root in cervical disk protrusion. *Neurology.* 1957;7(10):673-683.

174. Marshall GL, Little JW. Deep tendon reflexes: A study of quantitative methods. *J Spinal Cord Med.* 2002;25(2):94-99.

175. Rubinstein SM, Pool JJ, van Tulder MW, Riphagen II, de Vet HC. A systematic review of the diagnostic accuracy of provocative tests of the neck for diagnosing cervical radiculopathy. *Eur Spine J.* 2007;16(3):307-319.

176. Lauder TD, Dillingham TR, Andary M, et al. Predicting electrodiagnostic outcome in patients with upper limb symptoms: Are the history and physical examination helpful? *Arch Phys Med Rehab.* 2000;81(4):436-441.

177. Osmotherly PG, Rivett DA, Rowe LJ. Construct validity of clinical tests for alar ligament integrity: An evaluation using magnetic resonance imaging. *Phys Ther.* 2012;92(5):718-725.

178. Osmotherly PG, Rivett DA, Rowe LJ. The anterior shear and distraction tests for craniocervical instability. An evaluation using magnetic resonance imaging. *Man Ther.* 2012;17(5):416-421.

179. Scott D, Jull G, Sterling M. Widespread sensory hypersensitivity is a feature of chronic whiplash-associated disorder but not chronic idiopathic neck pain. *Clin J Pain.* 2005;21(2):175-181.

180. Treleaven J, Jull G, Lowchoy N. Standing balance in persistent whiplash: A comparison between subjects with and without dizziness. *J Rehabil Med.* 2005;37(4):224-229.

181. Treleaven J, Jull G, LowChoy N. Smooth pursuit neck torsion test in whiplash-associated disorders: Relationship to self-reports of neck pain and disability, dizziness and anxiety. *J Rehabil Med.* 2005;37(4):219-223.

182. Dall'Alba PT, Sterling MM, Treleaven JM, Edwards SL, Jull GA. Cervical range of motion discriminates between asymptomatic persons and those with whiplash. *Spine (Phila Pa 1976).* 2001;26(19):2090-2094.

183. Woodhouse A, Vasseljen O. Altered motor control patterns in whiplash and chronic neck pain. *BMC Musculoskel Dis.* 2008;9:90.

184. Woodhouse A, Liljeback P, Vasseljen O. Reduced head steadiness in whiplash compared with non-traumatic neck pain. *J Rehabil Med.* 2010;42(1):35-41.

185. Sterling M, Kenardy J. Physical and psychological aspects of whiplash: Important considerations for primary care assessment. *Man Ther.* 2008;13(2):93-102.

186. Nederhand MJ, Hermens HJ, IJzerman MJ, Turk DC, Zilvold G. Cervical muscle dysfunction in chronic whiplash-associated disorder grade 2: The relevance of the trauma. *Spine (Phila Pa 1976).* 2002;27(10):1056-1061.

187. Wenzel HG, Haug TT, Mykletun A, Dahl AA. A population study of anxiety and depression among persons who report whiplash traumas. *J Psychosom Res.* 2002;53(3):831-835.

188. Wenzel HG, Vasseljen O, Mykletun A, Nilsen TI. Pre-injury health-related factors in relation to self-reported whiplash: Longitudinal data from the HUNT study, Norway. *Eur Spine J.* 2012;21(8):1528-1535.

189. Kongsted A, Bendix T, Qerama E, et al. Acute stress response and recovery after whiplash injuries. A one-year prospective study. *Eur J Pain.* 2008;12(4):455-463.

190. Sterling M, Jull G, Vicenzino B, Kenardy J, Darnell R. Development of motor system dysfunction following whiplash injury. *Pain.* 2003;103(1-2):65-73.

191. Sterling M, Kenardy J, Jull G, Vicenzino B. The development of psychological changes following whiplash injury. *Pain.* 2003;106(3):481-489.

192. Kamper SJ, Rebbeck TJ, Maher CG, McAuley JH, Sterling M. Course and prognostic factors of whiplash: A systematic review and meta-analysis. *Pain.* 2008;138(3):617-629.

193. Antepohl W, Kiviloog L, Andersson J, Gerdle B. Cognitive impairment in patients with chronic whiplash-associated disorder—A matched control study. *Neurorehabilitation.* 2003;18(4):307-315.

194. Treleaven J, Jull G, Sterling M. Dizziness and unsteadiness following whiplash injury: Characteristic features and relationship with cervical joint position error. *J Rehabil Med.* 2003;35(1):36-43.

195. Sterling M. Whiplash-associated disorder: Musculoskeletal pain and related clinical findings. *J Man Manip Ther.* 2011;19(4):194-200.

196. Elliott J, Jull G, Noteboom JT, Darnell R, Galloway G, Gibbon WW. Fatty infiltration in the cervical extensor muscles in persistent whiplash-associated disorders: A magnetic resonance imaging analysis. *Spine (Phila Pa 1976).* 2006;31(22):E847-E855.

197. Kasch H, Qerama E, Bach FW, Jensen TS. Reduced cold pressor pain tolerance in non-recovered whiplash patients: A 1-year prospective study. *Eur J Pain.* 2005;9(5):561-569.

198. Kristjansson E, Leivseth G, Brinckmann P, Frobin W. Increased sagittal plane segmental motion in the lower cervical spine in women with chronic whiplash-associated disorders, grades I-II: A case-control study using a new measurement protocol. *Spine (Phila Pa 1976)*. 2003;28(19):2215-2221.

199. Henry P, Dartigues JF, Puymirat C, Peytour P, Lucas J. The association cervicalgia-headaches: An epidemiologic study. *Cephalalgia*. 1987;7 (suppl 6):189-190.

200. Sjaastad O, Fredriksen TA, Pfaffenrath V. Cervicogenic headache: Diagnostic criteria. The Cervicogenic Headache International Study Group. *Headache*. 1998;38(6):442-445.

201. Niere K, Robinson P. Determination of manipulative physiotherapy treatment outcome in headache patients. *Man Ther*. 1997;2(4):199-205.

202. Treleaven J, Jull G, Atkinson L. Cervical musculoskeletal dysfunction in post-concussional headache. *Cephalalgia*. 1994;14(4):273-279, discussion 257.

203. Zwart JA. Neck mobility in different headache disorders. *Headache*. 1997;37(1):6-11.

204. Jull G, Amiri M, Bullock-Saxton J, Darnell R, Lander C. Cervical musculoskeletal impairment in frequent intermittent headache. Part 1: Subjects with single headaches. *Cephalalgia*. 2007;27(7):793-802.

205. Hall TM, Briffa K, Hopper D, Robinson K. Comparative analysis and diagnostic accuracy of the cervical flexion-rotation test. *J Headache Pain*. 2010;11(5):391-397.

206. Cleland JA, Childs JD, McRae M, Palmer JA, Stowell T. Immediate effects of thoracic manipulation in patients with neck pain: A randomized clinical trial. *Man Ther*. 2005;10(2):127-135.

207. Kanlayanaphotporn R, Chiradejnant A, Vachalathiti R. The immediate effects of mobilization technique on pain and range of motion in patients presenting with unilateral neck pain: A randomized controlled trial. *Arch Phys Med Rehabil*. 2009;90(2):187-192.

208. Sehgal N, Dunbar EE, Shah RV, Colson J. Systematic review of diagnostic utility of facet (zygapophysial) joint injections in chronic spinal pain: An update. *Pain Physician*. 2007;10(1):213-228.

209. Fejer R, Kyvik KO, Hartvigsen J. The prevalence of neck pain in the world population: A systematic critical review of the literature. *Eur Spine J*. 2006;15(6):834-848.

210. Cote P, van der Velde G, Cassidy JD, et al. The burden and determinants of neck pain in workers: Results of the Bone and Joint Decade 2000-2010 Task Force on Neck Pain and Its Associated Disorders. *J Manip Physiol Ther*. 2009;32(2)(suppl):S70-S86.

211. Carroll LJ, Holm LW, Hogg-Johnson S, et al. Course and prognostic factors for neck pain in whiplash-associated disorders (WAD): Results of the Bone and Joint Decade 2000-2010 Task Force on Neck Pain and Its Associated Disorders. *J Manip Physiol Ther*. 2009;32(2)(suppl):S97-S107.

212. Hogg-Johnson S, van der Velde G, Carroll LJ, et al. The burden and determinants of neck pain in the general population: Results of the Bone and Joint Decade 2000-2010 Task Force on Neck Pain and Its Associated Disorders. *J Manip Physiol Ther*. 2009;32(2)(suppl):S46-S60.

213. Carroll LJ, Hogg-Johnson S, Cote P, et al. Course and prognostic factors for neck pain in workers: Results of the Bone and Joint Decade 2000-2010 Task Force on Neck Pain and Its Associated Disorders. *J Manip Physiol Ther*. 2009;32(2)(suppl):S108S116.

214. Siegenthaler A, Eichenberger U, Schmidlin K, Arendt-Nielsen L, Curatolo M. What does local tenderness say about the origin of pain? An investigation of cervical zygapophysial joint pain. *Anesth Analg*. 2010;110(3):923-927.

215. Cyriax J. *Textbook of Orthopaedic Medicine, Diagnosis of Soft Tissue Lesions*. 8th ed. London, England: Bailliere Tindall; 1982.

216. Wrisley DM, Sparto PJ, Whitney SL, Furman JM. Cervicogenic dizziness: A review of diagnosis and treatment. *J Orthop Sport Phys*. 2000;30(12):755-766.

217. Al Saif A, Al Nakhli H, Alsenany S. Physical therapy exmaination for patients with cervicogenic dizziness. *Journal of Novel Physiotherapies*. 2013;3(3):149-152.

Chapter 18

1. Briggs AM, Smith AJ, Straker LM, Bragge P. Thoracic spine pain in the general population: Prevalence, incidence and associated factors in children, adolescents and adults. A systematic review. *BMC Musculoskel Dis*. 2009;10:77.

2. Briggs AM, Bragge P, Smith AJ, Govil D, Straker LM. Prevalence and associated factors for thoracic spine pain in the adult working population: A literature review. *J Occup Health*. 2009;51(3):177-192.

3. Singh V, Manchikanti L, Shah RV, Dunbar EE, Glaser SE. Systematic review of thoracic discography as a diagnostic test for chronic spinal pain. *Pain Physician*. 2008;11(5):631-642.

4. Gregory PL, Biswas AC, Batt ME. Musculoskeletal problems of the chest wall in athletes. *Sports Med*. 2002;32(4):235-250.

5. Disla E, Rhim HR, Reddy A, Karten I, Taranta A. Costochondritis. A prospective analysis in an emergency department setting. *Arch Intern Med*. 1994;154(21):2466-2469.

6. Lips P. Epidemiology and predictors of fractures associated with osteoporosis. *Am J Med*. 1997;103(2A):3S-8S, discussion 8S-11S.

7. Naves M, Diaz-Lopez JB, Gomez C, Rodriguez-Rebollar A, Cannata-Andia JB. Determinants of incidence of osteoporotic fractures in the female Spanish population older than 50. *Osteoporosis Int*. 2005;16(12):2013-2017.

8. Roux C, Priol G, Fechtenbaum J, Cortet B, Liu-Leage S, Audran M. A clinical tool to determine the necessity of spine radiography in postmenopausal women with osteoporosis presenting with back pain. *Ann Rheum Dis*. 2007;66(1):81-85.

9. Grados F, Fechtenbaum J, Flipon E, Kolta S, Roux C, Fardellone P. Radiographic methods for evaluating osteoporotic vertebral fractures. *Joint Bone Spine.* 2009;76(3):241-247.

10. Miller NH. Cause and natural history of adolescent idiopathic scoliosis. *Orthop Clin N Am.* 1999;30(3):343-352, vii.

11. Roach JW. Adolescent idiopathic scoliosis. *Orthop Clin N Am.* 1999;30(3):353-365, vii-viii.

12. Freeston J, Karim Z, Lindsay K, Gough A. Can early diagnosis and management of costochondritis reduce acute chest pain admissions? *J Rheumatol.* 2004;31(11):2269-2271.

13. Grindstaff TL, Beazell JR, Saliba EN, Ingersoll CD. Treatment of a female collegiate rower with costochondritis: A case report. *J Man Manip Ther.* 2010;18(2):64-68.

14. Bahm J. Critical review of pathophysiologic mechanisms in thoracic outlet syndrome (TOS). *Acta Neurochir Suppl.* 2007;100:137-139.

15. Lindgren KA, Leino E, Manninen H. Cervical rotation lateral flexion test in brachialgia. *Arch Phys Med. Rehab.* 1992;73(8):735-737.

16. Lindgren KA. Thoracic outlet syndrome with special reference to the first rib. *Ann Chir Gynaecol.* 1993;82(4):218-230.

17. Sanders RJ, Hammond SL, Rao NM. Diagnosis of thoracic outlet syndrome. *J Vasc Surg.* 2007;46(3):601-604.

18. Sanders RJ, Hammond SL, Rao NM. Thoracic outlet syndrome: A review. *Neurologist.* 2008;14(6):365-373.

19. Huang JH, Zager EL. Thoracic outlet syndrome. *Neurosurgery.* 2004;55(4):897-902, discussion 902-903.

20. Cooke RA. Thoracic outlet syndrome—Aspects of diagnosis in the differential diagnosis of hand-arm vibration syndrome. *Occup Med (Lond).* 2003;53(5):331-336.

21. Tones MJ, Moss ND. The impact of patient self assessment of deformity on HRQL in adults with scoliosis. *Scoliosis.* 2007;2:14.

22. Asher MA, Lai SM, Glattes RC, Burton DC, Alanay A, Bago J. Refinement of the SRS-22 Health-Related Quality of Life questionnaire function domain. *Spine (Phila Pa 1976).* 2006;31(5):593-597.

23. Haher TR, Gorup JM, Shin TM, et al. Results of the Scoliosis Research Society instrument for evaluation of surgical outcome in adolescent idiopathic scoliosis. A multicenter study of 244 patients. *Spine (Phila Pa 1976).* 1999;24(14):1435-1440.

24. Bridwell KH, Cats-Baril W, Harrast J, et al. The validity of the SRS-22 instrument in an adult spinal deformity population compared with the Oswestry and SF-12: A study of response distribution, concurrent validity, internal consistency, and reliability. *Spine (Phila Pa 1976).* 2005;30(4):455-461.

25. Sanders JO, Polly DW Jr, Cats-Baril W, et al. Analysis of patient and parent assessment of deformity in idiopathic scoliosis using the Walter Reed Visual Assessment Scale. *Spine (Phila Pa 1976).* 2003;28(18):2158-2163.

26. Pineda S, Bago J, Gilperez C, Climent JM. Validity of the Walter Reed Visual Assessment Scale to measure subjective perception of spine deformity in patients with idiopathic scoliosis. *Scoliosis.* 2006;1:18.

27. Bago J, Climent JM, Pineda S, Gilperez C. Further evaluation of the Walter Reed Visual Assessment Scale: Correlation with curve pattern and radiological deformity. *Scoliosis.* 2007;2:12.

28. Bago J, Climent JM, Perez-Grueso FJ, Pellise F. Outcome instruments to assess scoliosis surgery. *Eur Spine J.* 2013;22(suppl 2):195-202.

29. Kim YM, Demissie S, Genant HK, et al. Identification of prevalent vertebral fractures using CT lateral scout views: A comparison of semi-automated quantitative vertebral morphometry and radiologist semi-quantitative grading. *Osteoporosis Int.* 2012;23(3):1007-1016.

30. Bazzocchi A, Spinnato P, Fuzzi F, et al. Vertebral fracture assessment by new dual-energy X-ray absorptiometry. *Bone.* 2012;50(4):836-841.

31. Diacinti D, Guglielmi G, Pisani D, et al. Vertebral morphometry by dual-energy X-ray absorptiometry (DXA) for osteoporotic vertebral fractures assessment (VFA). *Radiol Med.* 2012;117(8):1374-1385.

32. Oh CH, Kim CG, Lee MS, Yoon SH, Park HC, Park CO. Usefulness of chest radiographs for scoliosis screening: A comparison with thoraco-lumbar standing radiographs. *Yonsei Med J.* 2012;53(6):1183-1189.

33. O'Connor E, Walsham J. Review article: Indications for thoracolumbar imaging in blunt trauma patients: A review of current literature. *Emerg Med Australas.* 2009;21(2):94-101.

34. Keynan O, Fisher CG, Vaccaro A, et al. Radiographic measurement parameters in thoracolumbar fractures: A systematic review and consensus statement of the spine trauma study group. *Spine (Phila Pa 1976).* 2006;31(5):E156-E165.

35. Kim H, Kim HS, Moon ES, et al. Scoliosis imaging: What radiologists should know. *Radiographics.* 2010;30(7):1823-1842.

36. Venkatesan M, Fong A, Sell PJ. CT scanning reduces the risk of missing a fracture of the thoracolumbar spine. *J Bone Joint Surg Br.* 2012;94(8):1097-1100.

37. Inaba K, Munera F, McKenney M, et al. Visceral torso computed tomography for clearance of the thoracolumbar spine in trauma: A review of the literature. *J Traum.* 2006;60(4):915-920.

38. Quek J, Pua YH, Clark RA, Bryant AL. Effects of thoracic kyphosis and forward head posture on cervical range of motion in older adults [published online ahead of print September 5 2012]. *Man Ther.* 2012.

39. Boyles RE, Ritland BM, Miracle BM, et al. The short-term effects of thoracic spine thrust manipulation on patients with shoulder impingement syndrome. *Man Ther.* 2009;14(4):375-380.

40. Handrakis JP, Friel K, Hoeffner F, et al. Key characteristics of low back pain and disability in college-aged adults: A pilot study. *Arch Phys Med Rehab.* 2012;93(7):1217-1224.

41. Henschke N, Maher CG, Refshauge KM, et al. Prevalence of and screening for serious spinal pathology in patients presenting to primary care settings with acute low back pain. *Arthritis Rheum.* 2009;60(10):3072-3080.

42. Roman M, Brown C, Richardson W, Isaacs R, Howes C, Cook C. The development of a clinical decision making algorithm for detection of osteoporotic vertebral compression fracture or wedge deformity. *J Man Manip Ther.* 2010;18(1):44-49.

43. Langdon J, Way A, Heaton S, Bernard J, Molloy S. Vertebral compression fractures—New clinical signs to aid diagnosis. *Ann R Coll Surg Engl.* 2010;92(2):163-166.

44. Siminoski K, Warshawski RS, Jen H, Lee KC. The accuracy of clinical kyphosis examination for detection of thoracic vertebral fractures: Comparison of direct and indirect kyphosis measures. *J Musculoskelet Neuronal Interact.* 2011;11(3):249-256.

45. Shah KC, Rajshekhar V. Reliability of diagnosis of soft cervical disc prolapse using Spurling's test. *Brit J Neurosurg.* 2004;18(5):480-483.

46. Wainner RS, Fritz JM, Irrgang JJ, Boninger ML, Delitto A, Allison S. Reliability and diagnostic accuracy of the clinical examination and patient self-report measures for cervical radiculopathy. *Spine (Phila Pa 1976).* 2003;28(1):52-62.

47. Donelson R, Aprill C, Medcalf R, Grant W. A prospective study of centralization of lumbar and referred pain. A predictor of symptomatic discs and anular competence. *Spine (Phila Pa 1976).* 1997;22(10):1115-1122.

48. Laslett M, Oberg B, Aprill CN, McDonald B. Centralization as a predictor of provocation discography results in chronic low back pain, and the influence of disability and distress on diagnostic power. *Spine J.* 2005;5(4):370-380.

49. Vroomen PC, de Krom MC, Wilmink JT, Kester AD, Knottnerus JA. Diagnostic value of history and physical examination in patients suspected of lumbosacral nerve root compression. *J Neurol Neurosurg Psychiatry.* 2002;72(5):630-634.

50. van der Windt DA, Simons E, Riphagen II, et al. Physical examination for lumbar radiculopathy due to disc herniation in patients with low-back pain. *Cochrane Db Syst Rev.* 2010;2:CD007431.

51. Deville WL, van der Windt DA, Dzaferagic A, Bezemer PD, Bouter LM. The test of Lasegue: Systematic review of the accuracy in diagnosing herniated discs. *Spine (Phila Pa 1976).* 2000;25(9):1140-1147.

52. Stankovic R, Johnell O, Maly P, Willner S. Use of lumbar extension, slump test, physical and neurological examination in the evaluation of patients with suspected herniated nucleus pulposus. A prospective clinical study. *Man Ther.* 1999;4(1):25-32.

53. Majlesi J, Togay H, Unalan H, Toprak S. The sensitivity and specificity of the Slump and the Straight Leg Raising tests in patients with lumbar disc herniation. *J Clin Rheumatol.* 2008;14(2):87-91.

54. Laslett M, Aprill CN, McDonald B, Oberg B. Clinical predictors of lumbar provocation discography: A study of clinical predictors of lumbar provocation discography. *Eur Spine J.* 2006;15(10):1473-1484.

55. Schwarzer AC, Derby R, Aprill CN, Fortin J, Kine G, Bogduk N. Pain from the lumbar zygapophysial joints: A test of two models. *J Spinal Disord.* 1994;7(4):331-336.

56. Cote P, Kreitz BG, Cassidy JD, Dzus AK, Martel J. A study of the diagnostic accuracy and reliability of the Scoliometer and Adam's forward bend test. *Spine (Phila Pa 1976).* 1998;23(7):796-802, discussion 803.

57. Gravina AR, Ferraro C, Frizziero A, Ferraro M, Masiero S. Goniometer evaluation of thoracic kyphosis and lumbar lordosis in subjects during growth age: A validity study. *Stud Health Technol Inform.* 2012;176:247-251.

58. Smedmark V, Wallin M, Arvidsson I. Inter-examiner reliability in assessing passive intervertebral motion of the cervical spine. *Man Ther.* 2000;5(2):97-101.

59. Kelly TR. Thoracic outlet syndrome: Current concepts of treatment. *Ann Surg.* 1979;190(5):657-662.

60. Sobey AV, Grewal RP, Hutchison KJ, Urschel JD. Investigation of nonspecific neurogenic thoracic outlet syndrome. *J Cardiovasc Surg (Torino).* 1993;34(4):343-345.

61. Urschel HC Jr, Paulson DL, McNamara JJ. Thoracic outlet syndrome. *Ann Thorac Surg.* 1968;6(1):1-10.

62. Fechter JD, Kuschner SH. The thoracic outlet syndrome. *Orthopedics.* 1993;16(11):1243-1251.

63. Karachalios T, Sofianos J, Roidis N, Sapkas G, Korres D, Nikolopoulos K. Ten-year follow-up evaluation of a school screening program for scoliosis. Is the forward-bending test an accurate diagnostic criterion for the screening of scoliosis? *Spine (Phila Pa 1976).* 1999;24(22):2318-2324.

64. Plewa MC, Delinger M. The false-positive rate of thoracic outlet syndrome shoulder maneuvers in healthy subjects. *Acad Emerg Med.* 1998;5(4):337-342.

65. Lee AD, Agarwal S, Sadhu D. Doppler Adson's test: Predictor of outcome of surgery in non-specific thoracic outlet syndrome. *World J Surg.* 2006;30(3):291-292.

66. Gillard J, Perez-Cousin M, Hachulla E, et al. Diagnosing thoracic outlet syndrome: Contribution of provocative tests, ultrasonography, electrophysiology, and helical computed tomography in 48 patients. *Joint Bone Spine.* 2001;68(5):416-424.

67. Howard M, Lee C, Dellon AL. Documentation of brachial plexus compression (in the thoracic inlet) utilizing provocative neurosensory and muscular testing. *J Reconstr Microsurg.* 2003;19(5):303-312.

68. Frost M, Wraae K, Abrahamsen B, et al. Osteoporosis and vertebral fractures in men aged 60-74 years. *Age Ageing.* 2012;41(2):171-177.

69. Diaz JJ Jr, Cullinane DC, Altman DT, et al. Practice management guidelines for the screening of thoracolumbar spine fracture. *J Traum.* 2007;63(3):709-718.

70. Inaba K, DuBose JJ, Barmparas G, et al. Clinical examination is insufficient to rule out thoracolumbar spine injuries. *J Traum.* 2011;70(1):174-179.

71. Seo MR, Park SY, Park JS, Jin W, Ryu KN. Spinous process fractures in osteoporotic thoracolumbar vertebral fractures. *Brit J Radiol.* 2011;84(1007):1046-1049.

72. Siminoski K, Lee KC, Jen H, et al. Anatomical distribution of vertebral fractures: Comparison of pediatric and adult spines. *Osteoporosis Int.* 2012;23(7):1999-2008.

73. Westrick RB, Zylstra E, Issa T, Miller JM, Gerber JP. Evaluation and treatment of musculoskeletal chest wall pain in a military athlete. *Int J Sports Phys Ther.* 2012;7(3):323-332.

74. Yelland MJ. Back, chest and abdominal pain. How good are spinal signs at identifying musculoskeletal causes of back, chest or abdominal pain? *Aust Fam Physician.* 2001;30(9):908-912.

75. Stochkendahl MJ, Christensen HW. Chest pain in focal musculoskeletal disorders. *Med Clin N Am.* 2010;94(2):259-273.

76. Mendelson G, Mendelson H, Horowitz SF, Goldfarb CR, Zumoff B. Can (99m) technetium methylene diphosphonate bone scans objectively document costochondritis? *Chest.* 1997;111(6):1600-1602.

77. Kane WJ. Scoliosis prevalence: A call for a statement of terms. *Clin Orthop Relat Res.* 1977(126):43-46.

78. Lonstein JE, Carlson JM. The prediction of curve progression in untreated idiopathic scoliosis during growth. *J Bone Joint Surg Am.* 1984;66(7):1061-1071.

79. Lonstein JE. Natural history and school screening for scoliosis. *Orthop Clin N Am.* 1988;19(2):227-237.

80. Fong DY, Lee CF, Cheung KM, et al. A meta-analysis of the clinical effectiveness of school scoliosis screening. *Spine (Phila Pa 1976).* 2010;35(10):1061-1071.

81. Luk KD, Lee CF, Cheung KM, et al. Clinical effectiveness of school screening for adolescent idiopathic scoliosis: A large population-based retrospective cohort study. *Spine (Phila Pa 1976).* 2010;35(17):1607-1614.

82. Kellgren JH, Lawrence JS. Radiological assessment of osteo-arthrosis. *Ann Rheum Dis.* 1957;16(4):494-502.

83. Roux C, Fechtenbaum J, Briot K, Cropet C, Liu-Leage S, Marcelli C. Inverse relationship between vertebral fractures and spine osteoarthritis in postmenopausal women with osteoporosis. *Ann Rheum Dis.* 2008;67(2):224-228.

84. Rochlin DH, Gilson MM, Likes KC, et al. Quality-of-life scores in neurogenic thoracic outlet syndrome patients undergoing first rib resection and scalenectomy. *J Vasc Surg.* 2013;57(2):436-443.

85. Brewin J, Hill M, Ellis H. The prevalence of cervical ribs in a London population. *Clin Anat.* 2009;22(3):331-336.

86. Sanders RJ. Recurrent neurogenic thoracic outlet syndrome stressing the importance of pectoralis minor syndrome. *Vasc Endovasc Surg.* 2011;45(1):33-38.

87. Kai Y, Oyama M, Kurose S, Inadome T, Oketani Y, Masuda Y. Neurogenic thoracic outlet syndrome in whiplash injury. *J Spinal Disord.* 2001;14(6):487-493.

Chapter 19

1. Woolf AD, Pfleger B. Burden of major musculoskeletal conditions. *B World Health Organ.* 2003;81(9):646-656.

2. Jonasson P, Halldin K, Karlsson J, et al. Prevalence of joint-related pain in the extremities and spine in five groups of top athletes. *Knee Surg Sport Tra A.* 2011;19(9):1540-1546.

3. Picavet HS, Schouten JS. Musculoskeletal pain in the Netherlands: Prevalences, consequences and risk groups, the DMC(3)-study. *Pain.* 2003;102(1-2):167-178.

4. Deyo RA, Weinstein JN. Low back pain. *N Engl J Med.* 1 2001;344(5):363-370.

5. Deyo RA, Rainville J, Kent DL. What can the history and physical examination tell us about low back pain? *JAMA.* 1992;268(6):760-765.

6. Bogduk N. The causes of low back pain. *Med J Aust.* 1992;156(3):151-153.

7. Sembrano JN, Polly DW Jr. How often is low back pain not coming from the back? *Spine (Phila Pa 1976).* 2009;34(1):E27-E32.

8. Depalma MJ, Ketchum JM, Trussell BS, Saullo TR, Slipman CW. Does the location of low back pain predict its source? *Pm R.* 2011;3(1):33-39.

9. Schwarzer AC, April CN, Bogduk N. The sacroiliac joint in chronic low back pain. *Spine (Phila Pa 1976).* 1995;20(1):31-37.

10. Laslett M, Young SB, April CN, McDonald B. Diagnosing painful sacroiliac joints: A validity study of a McKenzie evaluation and sacroiliac provocation tests. *Aust J Physiother.* 2003;49(2):89-97.

11. Bogduk N. The anatomical basis for spinal pain syndromes. *J Manip Physiol Ther.* 1995;18(9):603-605.

12. Hoy D, Brooks P, Blyth F, Buchbinder R. The epidemiology of low back pain. *Best Pract Res Clin Rheumatol.* 2010;24(6):769-781.

13. Hestbaek L, Leboeuf-Yde C, Manniche C. Low back pain: What is the long-term course? A review of studies of general patient populations. *Eur Spine J.* 2003;12(2):149-165.

14. Pengel LH, Herbert RD, Maher CG, Refshauge KM. Acute low back pain: Systematic review of its prognosis. *BMJ.* 2003;327(7410):323.

15. da CMCL, Maher CG, Hancock MJ, McAuley JH, Herbert RD, Costa LO. The prognosis of acute and persistent low-back pain: A meta-analysis. *CMAJ.* 2012;184(11):E613-E624.

16. Wai EK, Howse K, Pollock JW, Dornan H, Vexler L, Dagenais S. The reliability of determining "leg dominant pain". *Spine J.* 2009;9(6):447-453.

17. Chou R, Qaseem A, Snow V, et al. Diagnosis and treatment of low back pain: A joint clinical practice guideline from the American College of Physicians and the American Pain Society. *Ann Intern Med.* 2007;147(7):478-491.

18. Fukui S, Ohseto K, Shiotani M, Ohno K, Karasawa H, Naganuma Y. Distribution of referred pain from the lumbar zygapophyseal joints and dorsal rami. *Clin J Pain.* 1997;13(4):303-307.

19. Dworkin GE. Advanced concepts in interventional spine care. *J Am Osteopath Assoc.* 2002;102(9)(suppl 3):S8-S11.

20. Schwarzer AC, Derby R, Aprill CN, Fortin J, Kine G, Bogduk N. Pain from the lumbar zygapophysial joints: A test of two models. *J Spinal Disord.* 1994;7(4):331-336.

21. Vroomen PC, de Krom MC, Wilmink JT, Kester AD, Knottnerus JA. Diagnostic value of history and physical examination in patients suspected of lumbosacral nerve root compression. *J Neurol Neurosur Ps.* 2002;72(5):630-634.

22. Vroomen PC, de Krom MC, Knottnerus JA. Diagnostic value of history and physical examination in patients suspected of sciatica due to disc herniation: A systematic review. *J Neurol.* 1999;246(10):899-906.

23. Slipman CW, Jackson HB, Lipetz JS, Chan KT, Lenrow D, Vresilovic EJ. Sacroiliac joint pain referral zones. *Arch Phys Med Rehab.* 2000;81(3):334-338.

24. Katz JN, Dalgas M, Stucki G, et al. Degenerative lumbar spinal stenosis. Diagnostic value of the history and physical examination. *Arthritis Rheum.* 1995;38(9):1236-1241.

25. Lyle MA, Manes S, McGuinness M, Ziaei S, Iversen MD. Relationship of physical examination findings and self-reported symptom severity and physical function in patients with degenerative lumbar conditions. *Phys Ther.* 2005;85(2):120-133.

26. Tomkins CC, Battie MC, Hu R. Construct validity of the physical function scale of the Swiss Spinal Stenosis Questionnaire for the measurement of walking capacity. *Spine (Phila Pa 1976).* 2007;32(17):1896-1901.

27. Rubinstein SM, van Tulder M. A best-evidence review of diagnostic procedures for neck and low-back pain. *Best Pract Res Clin Rheumatol.* 2008;22(3):471-482.

28. O'Sullivan PB, Mitchell T, Bulich P, Waller R, Holte J. The relationship beween posture and back muscle endurance in industrial workers with flexion-related low back pain. *Man Ther.* 2006;11(4):264-271.

29. DePalma MJ, Ketchum JM, Saullo T. What is the source of chronic low back pain and does age play a role? *Pain Med.* 2011;12(2):224-233.

30. Jarvik JG, Deyo RA. Diagnostic evaluation of low back pain with emphasis on imaging. *Ann Intern Med.* 2002;137(7):586-597.

31. Fritz JM, Erhard RE, Delitto A, Welch WC, Nowakowski PE. Preliminary results of the use of a two-stage treadmill test as a clinical diagnostic tool in the differential diagnosis of lumbar spinal stenosis. *J Spinal Disord.* 1997;10(5):410-416.

32. Suri P, Rainville J, Kalichman L, Katz JN. Does this older adult with lower extremity pain have the clinical syndrome of lumbar spinal stenosis? *JAMA.* 2010;304(23):2628-2636.

33. Dionne CE, Von Korff M, Koepsell TD, Deyo RA, Barlow WE, Checkoway H. Formal education and back pain: A review. *J Epidemiol Commun H.* 2001;55(7):455-468.

34. Lawrence RC, Helmick CG, Arnett FC, et al. Estimates of the prevalence of arthritis and selected musculoskeletal disorders in the United States. *Arthritis Rheum.* 1998;41(5):778-799.

35. Matsui H, Maeda A, Tsuji H, Naruse Y. Risk indicators of low back pain among workers in Japan. Association of familial and physical factors with low back pain. *Spine (Phila Pa 1976).* 1997;22(11):1242-1247, discussion 1248.

36. Bener A, Alwash R, Gaber T, Lovasz G. Obesity and low back pain. *Coll Antropol.* 2003;27(1):95-104.

37. Chou YC, Shih CC, Lin JG, Chen TL, Liao CC. Low back pain associated with sociodemographic factors, lifestyle and osteoporosis: A population-based study [published online ahead of print October 11 2012]. *J Rehabil Med.* 2012.

38. Osman A, Barrios FX, Gutierrez PM, Kopper BA, Merrifield T, Grittmann L. The Pain Catastrophizing Scale: Further psychometric evaluation with adult samples. *J Behav Med.* 2000;23(4):351-365.

39. Latza U, Kohlmann T, Deck R, Raspe H. Influence of occupational factors on the relation between socioeconomic status and self-reported back pain in a population-based sample of German adults with back pain. *Spine (Phila Pa 1976).* 2000;25(11):1390-1397.

40. Cook C, Brismee JM, Sizer PS Jr. Subjective and objective descriptors of clinical lumbar spine instability: A Delphi study. *Man Ther.* 2006;11(1):11-21.

41. Hicks GE, Fritz JM, Delitto A, Mishock J. Interrater reliability of clinical examination measures for identification of lumbar segmental instability. *Arch Phys Med Rehab.* 2003;84(12):1858-1864.

42. Hicks GE, Fritz JM, Delitto A, McGill SM. Preliminary development of a clinical prediction rule for determining which patients with low back pain will respond to a stabilization exercise program. *Arch Phys Med Rehab.* 2005;86(9):1753-1762.

43. Fritz JM, Piva SR, Childs JD. Accuracy of the clinical examination to predict radiographic instability of the lumbar spine. *Eur Spine J.* 2005;14(8):743-750.

44. Fritz JM, Whitman JM, Childs JD. Lumbar spine segmental mobility assessment: An examination of validity for determining intervention strategies in patients with low back pain. *Arch Phys Med Rehab.* 2005;86(9):1745-1752.

45. Abbott JH, McCane B, Herbison P, Moginie G, Chapple C, Hogarty T. Lumbar segmental instability: A criterion-related validity study of manual therapy assessment. *BMC Musculoskel Dis.* 2005;6:56.

46. Kasai Y, Morishita K, Kawakita E, Kondo T, Uchida A. A new evaluation method for lumbar spinal instability: Passive lumbar extension test. *Phys Ther.* 2006;86(12):1661-1667.

47. Maigne JY, Lapeyre E, Morvan G, Chatellier G. Pain immediately upon sitting down and relieved by standing up is often associated with radiologic lumbar instability or marked anterior loss of disc space. *Spine (Phila Pa 1976).* 2003;28(12):1327-1334.

48. Cook C, Brown C, Michael K, et al. The clinical value of a cluster of patient history and observational findings as a diagnostic support tool for lumbar spine stenosis [published online ahead of print November 11 2010]. *Physiother Res Int.* 2010.

49. Young S, Aprill C, Laslett M. Correlation of clinical examination characteristics with three sources of chronic low back pain. *Spine J.* 2003;3(6):460-465.

50. Delitto A, George SZ, Van Dillen LR, et al. Low back pain. *J Orthop Sport Phys.* 2012;42(4):A1-A57.

51. Fairbank JC, Couper J, Davies JB, O'Brien JP. The Oswestry low back pain disability questionnaire. *Physiotherapy.* 1980;66(8):271-273.

52. Fritz JM, Irrgang JJ. A comparison of a modified Oswestry Low Back Pain Disability Questionnaire and the Quebec Back Pain Disability Scale. *Phys Ther.* 2001;81(2):776-788.

53. Frost H, Lamb SE, Stewart-Brown S. Responsiveness of a patient specific outcome measure compared with the Oswestry Disability Index v2.1 and Roland and Morris Disability Questionnaire for patients with subacute and chronic low back pain. *Spine (Phila Pa 1976).* 2008;33(22):2450-2457, discussion 2458.

54. Ostelo RW, Deyo RA, Stratford P, et al. Interpreting change scores for pain and functional status in low back pain: Towards international consensus regarding minimal important change. *Spine (Phila Pa 1976).* 2008;33(1):90-94.

55. Roland M, Morris R. A study of the natural history of back pain. Part I: Development of a reliable and sensitive measure of disability in low-back pain. *Spine (Phila Pa 1976).* 1983;8(2):141-144.

56. Chou R, Shekelle P. Will this patient develop persistent disabling low back pain? *JAMA.* 2010;303(13):1295-1302.

57. Heitz CA, Hilfiker R, Bachmann LM, et al. Comparison of risk factors predicting return to work between patients with subacute and chronic non-specific low back pain: Systematic review. *Eur Spine J.* 2009;18(12):1829-1835.

58. Di Iorio D, Henley E, Doughty A. A survey of primary care physician practice patterns and adherence to acute low back problem guidelines. *Arch Fam Med.* 2000;9(10):1015-1021.

59. Webster BS, Courtney TK, Huang YH, Matz S, Christiani DC. Physicians' initial management of acute low back pain versus evidence-based guidelines. Influence of sciatica. *J Gen Intern Med.* 2005;20(12):1132-1135.

60. Webster BS, Courtney TK, Huang YH, Matz S, Christiani DC. Survey of acute low back pain management by specialty group and practice experience. *J Occup Environ Med.* 2006;48(7):723-732.

61. Finestone AS, Raveh A, Mirovsky Y, Lahad A, Milgrom C. Orthopaedists' and family practitioners' knowledge of simple low back pain management. *Spine (Phila Pa 1976).* 2009;34(15):1600-1603.

62. Lurie JD. What diagnostic tests are useful for low back pain? *Best Pract Res Clin Rheumatol.* 2005;19(4):557-575.

63. Weber U, Maksymowych WP. Sensitivity and specificity of magnetic resonance imaging for axial spondyloarthritis. *Am J Med Sci.* 2011;341(4):272-277.

64. Carragee EJ, Paragioudakis SJ, Khurana S. 2000 Volvo Award winner in clinical studies: Lumbar high-intensity zone and discography in subjects without low back problems. *Spine (Phila Pa 1976).* 2000;25(23):2987-2992.

65. Carragee E, Alamin T, Cheng I, Franklin T, van den Haak E, Hurwitz E. Are first-time episodes of serious LBP associated with new MRI findings? *Spine J.* 2006;6(6):624-635.

66. Jensen MC, Brant-Zawadzki MN, Obuchowski N, Modic MT, Malkasian D, Ross JS. Magnetic resonance imaging of the lumbar spine in people without back pain. *N Engl J Med.* 1994;331(2):69-73.

67. Borenstein DG, O'Mara JW Jr, Boden SD, et al. The value of magnetic resonance imaging of the lumbar spine to predict low-back pain in asymptomatic subjects: A seven-year follow-up study. *J Bone Joint Surg Am.* 2001;83-A(9):1306-1311.

68. Maus T. Imaging the back pain patient. *Phys Med Rehabil Clin N Am.* 2010;21(4):725-766.

69. Modic MT, Obuchowski NA, Ross JS, et al. Acute low back pain and radiculopathy: MR imaging findings and their prognostic role and effect on outcome. *Radiology.* 2005;237(2):597-604.

70. Zeifang F, Schiltenwolf M, Abel R, Moradi B. Gait analysis does not correlate with clinical and MR imaging parameters in patients with symptomatic lumbar spinal stenosis. *BMC Musculoskel Dis.* 2008;9:89.

71. Steurer J, Roner S, Gnannt R, Hodler J. Quantitative radiologic criteria for the diagnosis of lumbar spinal stenosis: A systematic literature review. *BMC Musculoskel Dis.* 2011;12:175.

72. de Graaf I, Prak A, Bierma-Zeinstra S, Thomas S, Peul W, Koes B. Diagnosis of lumbar spinal stenosis: A systematic review of the accuracy of diagnostic tests. *Spine (Phila Pa 1976).* 2006;31(10):1168-1176.

73. Carragee EJ, Don AS, Hurwitz EL, Cuellar JM, Carrino JA, Herzog R. 2009 ISSLS Prize Winner: Does discography cause accelerated progression of degeneration changes in the lumbar disc: A ten-year matched cohort study. *Spine (Phila Pa 1976).* 2009;34(21):2338-2345.

74. Wassenaar M, van Rijn RM, van Tulder MW, et al. Magnetic resonance imaging for diagnosing lumbar spinal pathology in adult patients with low back pain or sciatica: A diagnostic systematic review. *Eur Spine J.* 2012;21(2):220-227.

75. van Rijn RM, Wassenaar M, Verhagen AP, et al. Computed tomography for the diagnosis of lumbar spinal pathology in adult patients with low back pain or sciatica: A diagnostic systematic review. *Eur Spine J.* 2012;21(2):228-239.

76. Aota Y, Niwa T, Yoshikawa K, Fujiwara A, Asada T, Saito T. Magnetic resonance imaging and magnetic resonance myelography in the presurgical diagnosis of lumbar foraminal stenosis. *Spine (Phila Pa 1976).* 2007;32(8):896-903.

77. Tervonen O, Lahde S, Vanharanta H. Ultrasound diagnosis of lumbar disc degeneration. Comparison with computed tomography/discography. *Spine (Phila Pa 1976).* 1991;16(8):951-954.

78. Cho WI, Chang UK. Comparison of MR imaging and FDG-PET/CT in the differential diagnosis of benign and malignant vertebral compression fractures. *J Neurosurg Spine.* 2011;14(2):177-183.

79. Thariat J, Toubeau M, Ornetti P, et al. Sensitivity and specificity of thallium-201 scintigraphy for the diagnosis of malignant vertebral fractures. *Eur J Radiol.* 2004;51(3):274-278.

80. Bazzocchi A, Spinnato P, Fuzzi F, et al. Vertebral fracture assessment by new dual-energy X-ray absorptiometry. *Bone.* 2012;50(4):836-841.

81. Savelli G, Maffioli L, Maccauro M, De Deckere E, Bombardieri E. Bone scintigraphy and the added value of SPECT (single photon emission tomography) in detecting skeletal lesions. *Q J Nucl Med.* 2001;45(1):27-37.

82. Han LJ, Au-Yong TK, Tong WC, Chu KS, Szeto LT, Wong CP. Comparison of bone single-photon emission tomography and planar imaging in the detection of vertebral metastases in patients with back pain. *Eur J Nucl Med.* 1998;25(6):635-638.

83. Ganiyusufoglu AK, Onat L, Karatoprak O, Enercan M, Hamzaoglu A. Diagnostic accuracy of magnetic resonance imaging versus computed tomography in stress fractures of the lumbar spine. *Clin Radiol.* 2010;65(11):902-907.

84. Kepler CK, Pavlov H, Herzog RJ, Rawlins BA, Endo Y, Green DW. Comparison of a fluoroscopic 3-dimensional imaging system and conventional CT in detection of pars fractures in the cadaveric lumbar spine [published online ahead of print March 15 2012]. *J Spinal Disord Tech.* 2012.

85. D'Agostino MA, Aegerter P, Bechara K, et al. How to diagnose spondyloarthritis early? Accuracy of peripheral enthesitis detection by power Doppler ultrasonography. *Ann Rheum Dis.* 2011;70(8):1433-1440.

86. Weber U, Lambert RG, Ostergaard M, Hodler J, Pedersen SJ, Maksymowych WP. The diagnostic utility of magnetic resonance imaging in spondylarthritis: An international multicenter evaluation of one hundred eighty-seven subjects. *Arthritis Rheum.* 2010;62(10):3048-3058.

87. Li AL, Yen D. Effect of increased MRI and CT scan utilization on clinical decision-making in patients referred to a surgical clinic for back pain. *Can J Surg.* 2011;54(2):128-132.

88. Ash LM, Modic MT, Obuchowski NA, Ross JS, Brant-Zawadzki MN, Grooff PN. Effects of diagnostic information, per se, on patient outcomes in acute radiculopathy and low back pain. *AJNR Am J Neuroradiol.* 2008;29(6):1098-1103.

89. Chou D, Samartzis D, Bellabarba C, et al. Degenerative magnetic resonance imaging changes in patients with chronic low back pain: A systematic review. *Spine (Phila Pa 1976).* 2011;36(21 suppl):S43-S53.

90. Carragee EJ, Alamin TF, Miller JL, Carragee JM. Discographic, MRI and psychosocial determinants of low back pain disability and remission: A prospective study in subjects with benign persistent back pain. *Spine J.* 2005;5(1):24-35.

91. Takatalo J, Karppinen J, Niinimaki J, et al. Prevalence of degenerative imaging findings in lumbar magnetic resonance imaging among young adults. *Spine (Phila Pa 1976).* 2009;34(16):1716-1721.

92. Kjaer P, Leboeuf-Yde C, Korsholm L, Sorensen JS, Bendix T. Magnetic resonance imaging and low back pain in adults: A diagnostic imaging study of 40-year-old men and women. *Spine (Phila Pa 1976).* 2005;30(10):1173-1180.

93. Jarvik JG, Hollingworth W, Heagerty PJ, Haynor DR, Boyko EJ, Deyo RA. Three-year incidence of low back pain in an initially asymptomatic cohort: Clinical and imaging risk factors. *Spine (Phila Pa 1976).* 2005;30(13):1541-1548, discussion 1549.

94. Leone A, Cianfoni A, Cerase A, Magarelli N, Bonomo L. Lumbar spondylolysis: A review. *Skeletal Radiol.* 2011;40(6):683-700.

95. Standaert CJ, Herring SA. Spondylolysis: A critical review. *Brit J Sport Med.* 2000;34(6):415-422.

96. Rainville J, Smeets RJ, Bendix T, Tveito TH, Poiraudeau S, Indahl AJ. Fear-avoidance beliefs and pain avoidance in low back pain—Translating research into clinical practice. *Spine J.* 2011;11(9):895-903.

97. Hartvigsen J, Leboeuf-Yde C, Lings S, Corder EH. Is sitting-while-at-work associated with low back pain? A systematic, critical literature review. *Scand J Public Health.* 2000;28(3):230-239.

98. Wai EK, Roffey DM, Bishop P, Kwon BK, Dagenais S. Causal assessment of occupational lifting and low back pain: Results of a systematic review. *Spine J.* 2010;10(6):554-566.

99. Inufusa A, An HS, Lim TH, Hasegawa T, Haughton VM, Nowicki BH. Anatomic changes of the spinal canal and intervertebral foramen associated with flexion-extension movement. *Spine (Phila Pa 1976).* 1996;21(21):2412-2420.

100. Fujiwara A, An HS, Lim TH, Haughton VM. Morphologic changes in the lumbar intervertebral foramen due to flexion-extension, lateral bending, and axial rotation: An in vitro anatomic and biomechanical study. *Spine (Phila Pa 1976).* 2001;26(8):876-882.

101. Delitto A, Erhard RE, Bowling RW. A treatment-based classification approach to low back syndrome: Identifying and staging patients for conservative treatment. *Phys Ther.* 1995;75(6):470-485, discussion 485-479.

102. Clare HA, Adams R, Maher CG. Reliability of detection of lumbar lateral shift. *J Manip Physiol Ther.* 2003;26(8):476-480.

103. Panjabi MM. The stabilizing system of the spine. Part I. Function, dysfunction, adaptation, and enhancement. *J Spinal Disord.* 1992;5(4):383-389, discussion 397.

104. Panjabi MM. The stabilizing system of the spine. Part II. Neutral zone and instability hypothesis. *J Spinal Disord.* 1992;5(4):390-396, discussion 397.

105. Pope MH, Panjabi M. Biomechanical definitions of spinal instability. *Spine (Phila Pa 1976).* 1985;10(3):255-256.

106. Henschke N, Maher CG, Refshauge KM, et al. Prevalence of and screening for serious spinal pathology in patients presenting to primary care settings with acute low back pain. *Arthritis Rheum.* 2009;60(10):3072-3080.

107. Henschke N, Maher CG, Refshauge KM. Screening for malignancy in low back pain patients: A systematic review. *Eur Spine J.* 2007;16(10):1673-1679.

108. Henschke N, Maher CG, Refshauge KM. A systematic review identifies five "red flags" to screen for vertebral fracture in patients with low back pain. *J Clin Epidemiol.* 2008;61(2):110-118.

109. Underwood M. Diagnosing acute nonspecific low back pain: Time to lower the red flags? *Arthritis Rheum.* 2009;60(10):2855-2857.

110. Ross MD, Boissonnault WG. Red flags: To screen or not to screen? *J Orthop Sport Phys.* 2010;40(11):682-684.

111. Waldvogel FA, Papageorgiou PS. Osteomyelitis: The past decade. *N Engl J Med.* 1980;303(7):360-370.

112. Crowell MS, Gill NW. Medical screening and evacuation: Cauda equina syndrome in a combat zone. *J Orthop Sport Phys.* 2009;39(7):541-549.

113. Gran JT. An epidemiological survey of the signs and symptoms of ankylosing spondylitis. *Clin Rheumatol.* 1985;4(2):161-169.

114. Fink HA, Lederle FA, Roth CS, Bowles CA, Nelson DB, Haas MA. The accuracy of physical examination to detect abdominal aortic aneurysm. *Arch Intern Med.* 2000;160(6):833-836.

115. Deyo RA, Mirza SK, Turner JA, Martin BI. Overtreating chronic back pain: Time to back off? *J Am Board Fam Med.* 2009;22(1):62-68.

116. Deyo RA, Diehl AK. Cancer as a cause of back pain: Frequency, clinical presentation, and diagnostic strategies. *J Gen Intern Med.* 1988;3(3):230-238.

117. Downie A, Williams CM, Henschke N, et al. Red flags to screen for malignancy and fracture in patients with low back pain: Systematic review. *BMJ.* 2013;347:f7095.

118. Fraser S, Roberts L, Murphy E. Cauda equina syndrome: A literature review of its definition and clinical presentation. *Arch Phys Med Rehab.* 2009;90(11):1964-1968.

119. Balasubramanian K, Kalsi P, Greenough CG, Kuskoor Seetharam MP. Reliability of clinical assessment in diagnosing cauda equina syndrome. *Brit J Neurosurg.* 2010;24(4):383-386.

120. Small SA, Perron AD, Brady WJ. Orthopedic pitfalls: Cauda equina syndrome. *Am J Emerg Med.* 2005;23(2):159-163.

121. Shapiro S. Medical realities of cauda equina syndrome secondary to lumbar disc herniation. *Spine (Phila Pa 1976).* 2000;25(3):348-351, discussion 352.

122. Jalloh I, Minhas P. Delays in the treatment of cauda equina syndrome due to its variable clinical features in patients presenting to the emergency department. *Emerg Med J.* 2007;24(1):33-34.

123. Roman M, Brown C, Richardson W, Isaacs R, Howes C, Cook C. The development of a clinical decision making algorithm for detection of osteoporotic vertebral compression fracture or wedge deformity. *J Man Manip Ther.* 2010;18(1):44-49.

124. Langdon J, Way A, Heaton S, Bernard J, Molloy S. Vertebral compression fractures—New clinical signs to aid diagnosis. *Ann R Coll Surg Engl.* 2010;92(2):163-166.

125. Waddell G, McCulloch JA, Kummel E, Venner RM. Nonorganic physical signs in low-back pain. *Spine (Phila Pa 1976).* 1980;5(2):117-125.

126. Main CJ, Waddell G. Behavioral responses to examination. A reappraisal of the interpretation of "nonorganic signs". *Spine (Phila Pa 1976).* 1998;23(21):2367-2371.

127. Fritz JM, Wainner RS, Hicks GE. The use of nonorganic signs and symptoms as a screening tool for return-to-work in patients with acute low back pain. *Spine (Phila Pa 1976).* 2000;25(15):1925-1931.

128. Kobori S, Takizawa S, Sekiyama S, Takagi S. Ten centimeter elevation of the contralateral leg is enough to evaluate Hoover sign. *Intern Med.* 2007;46(1):55-56.

129. Laslett M, Aprill CN, McDonald B, Young SB. Diagnosis of sacroiliac joint pain: Validity of individual provocation tests and composites of tests. *Man Ther.* 2005;10(3):207-218.

130. Reiman MP, Goode AP, Hegedus EJ, Cook CE, Wright AA. Diagnostic accuracy of clinical tests of the hip: A systematic review with meta-analysis. *Brit J Sport Med.* 2013;47(14):893-902.

131. Altman R, Alarcon G, Appelrouth D, et al. The American College of Rheumatology criteria for the classification and reporting of osteoarthritis of the hip. *Arthritis Rheum.* 1991;34(5):505-514.

132. Pateder DB, Hungerford MW. Use of fluoroscopically guided intra-articular hip injection in differentiating the pain source in concomitant hip and lumbar spine arthritis. *Am J Orthop (Belle Mead NJ).* 2007;36(11):591-593.

133. Donelson R, Aprill C, Medcalf R, Grant W. A prospective study of centralization of lumbar and referred pain. A predictor of symptomatic discs and anular competence. *Spine (Phila Pa 1976).* 1997;22(10):1115-1122.

134. Laslett M, Oberg B, Aprill CN, McDonald B. Centralization as a predictor of provocation discography results in chronic low back pain, and the influence of disability and distress on diagnostic power. *Spine J.* 2005;5(4):370-380.

135. van der Windt DA, Simons E, Riphagen II, et al. Physical examination for lumbar radiculopathy due to disc herniation in patients with low-back pain. *Cochrane Db Syst Rev.* 2010;2:CD007431.

136. Deville WL, van der Windt DA, Dzaferagic A, Bezemer PD, Bouter LM. The test of Lasegue: Systematic review of the accuracy in diagnosing herniated discs. *Spine (Phila Pa 1976).* 2000;25(9):1140-1147.

137. Stankovic R, Johnell O, Maly P, Willner S. Use of lumbar extension, slump test, physical and neurological examination in the evaluation of patients with suspected herniated nucleus pulposus. A prospective clinical study. *Man Ther.* 1999;4(1):25-32.

138. Majlesi J, Togay H, Unalan H, Toprak S. The sensitivity and specificity of the Slump and the Straight Leg Raising tests in patients with lumbar disc herniation. *J Clin Rheumatol.* 2008;14(2):87-91.

139. Laslett M, Aprill CN, McDonald B, Oberg B. Clinical predictors of lumbar provocation discography: A study of clinical predictors of lumbar provocation discography. *Eur Spine J.* 2006;15(10):1473-1484.

140. Cyriax J. *Textbook of Orthopaedic Medicine, Diagnosis of Soft Tissue Lesions.* 8th ed. London, England: Bailliere Tindall; 1982.

141. *American Medical Association: Guides to the Evaluation of Permanent Impairment.* 3rd ed. Chicago, IL: American Medical Association; 1988.

142. Surkitt LD, Ford JJ, Hahne AJ, Pizzari T, McMeeken JM. Efficacy of directional preference management for low back pain: A systematic review. *Phys Ther.* 2012;92(5):652-665.

143. Saur PM, Ensink FB, Frese K, Seeger D, Hildebrandt J. Lumbar range of motion: Reliability and validity of the inclinometer technique in the clinical measurement of trunk flexibility. *Spine (Phila Pa 1976).* 1996;21(11):1332-1338.

144. Janda V. *Muscle Function Testing.* London, England: Butterworth; 1983.

145. Greenman PE. *Principles of Manual Medicine.* 2nd ed. Baltimore, MD: Williams & Wilkins; 1996.

146. Lee D. *The Pelvic Girdle: An Approach to the Examination and Treatment of the Lumbopelvic-Hip Region.* 3rd ed. London, England: Churchill Livingstone; 2004.

147. Barz T, Melloh M, Staub L, et al. The diagnostic value of a treadmill test in predicting lumbar spinal stenosis. *Eur Spine J.* 2008;17(5):686-690.

148. Masci L, Pike J, Malara F, Phillips B, Bennell K, Brukner P. Use of the one-legged hyperextension test and magnetic resonance imaging in the diagnosis of active spondylolysis. *Brit J Sport Med.* 2006;40(11):940-946, discussion 946.

149. Kobayashi A, Kobayashi T, Kato K, Higuchi H, Takagishi K. Diagnosis of radiographically occult lumbar spondylolysis in young athletes by magnetic resonance imaging. *Am J Sport Med.* 2013;41(1):169-176.

150. Collaer JW, McKeough DM, Boissonnault WG. Lumbar isthmic spondylolisthesis detection with palpation: Interrater reliability and concurrent criterion-related validity. *J Man Manip Ther.* 2006;14(1):22-29.

151. Nelson-Wong E, Flynn T, Callaghan JP. Development of active hip abduction as a screening test for identifying occupational low back pain. *J Orthop Sport Phys.* 2009;39(9):649-657.

152. Lee CE, Simmonds MJ, Novy DM, Jones S. Self-reports and clinician-measured physical function among patients with low back pain: A comparison. *Arch Phys Med Rehab.* 2001;82(2):227-231.

153. Handrakis JP, Friel K, Hoeffner F, et al. Key characteristics of low back pain and disability in college-aged adults: A pilot study. *Arch Phys Med Rehab.* 2012;93(7):1217-1224.

154. Flanagan SP, Kulig K. Assessing musculoskeletal performance of the back extensors following a single-level microdiscectomy. *J Orthop Sport Phys.* 2007;37(7):356-363.

155. Weinstein JN, Lurie JD, Olson PR, Bronner KK, Fisher ES. United States' trends and regional variations in lumbar spine surgery: 1992-2003. *Spine (Phila Pa 1976).* 2006;31(23):2707-2714.

156. Iversen MD, Katz JN. Examination findings and self-reported walking capacity in patients with lumbar spinal stenosis. *Phys Ther.* 2001;81(7):1296-1306.

157. Ljunggren AE. A schedule for registration of pain in lumbago sciatica. A diagnostic aid [in Norwegian]. *Tidsskr Nor Laegeforen.* 1991;111(29):3516-3518.

158. Konno S, Hayashino Y, Fukuhara S, et al. Development of a clinical diagnosis support tool to identify patients with lumbar spinal stenosis. *Eur Spine J.* 2007;16(11):1951-1957.

159. Kellgren JH, Lawrence JS. Radiological assessment of osteo-arthrosis. *Ann Rheum Dis.* 1957;16(4):494-502.

160. Lurie JD, Tosteson AN, Tosteson TD, et al. Reliability of readings of magnetic resonance imaging features of lumbar spinal stenosis. *Spine (Phila Pa 1976).* 2008;33(14):1605-1610.

161. Sirvanci M, Bhatia M, Ganiyusufoglu KA, et al. Degenerative lumbar spinal stenosis: Correlation with Oswestry Disability Index and MR imaging. *Eur Spine J.* 2008;17(5):679-685.

162. Sigmundsson FG, Kang XP, Jonsson B, Stromqvist B. Correlation between disability and MRI findings in lumbar spinal stenosis: A prospective study of 109 patients operated on by decompression. *Acta Orthop.* 2011;82(2):204-210.

163. Jonsson B, Annertz M, Sjoberg C, Stromqvist B. A prospective and consecutive study of surgically treated lumbar spinal stenosis. Part I: Clinical features related to radiographic findings. *Spine (Phila Pa 1976).* 1997;22(24):2932-2937.

164. Pratt RK, Fairbank JC, Virr A. The reliability of the Shuttle Walking Test, the Swiss Spinal Stenosis Questionnaire, the Oxford Spinal Stenosis Score, and the Oswestry Disability Index in the assessment of patients with lumbar spinal stenosis. *Spine (Phila Pa 1976).* 2002;27(1):84-91.

165. Heliovaara M, Makela M, Knekt P, Impivaara O, Aromaa A. Determinants of sciatica and low-back pain. *Spine.* 1991;16(6):608-614.

[]

166. Dammers R, Koehler PJ. Lumbar disc herniation: Level increases with age. *Surg Neurol.* 2002;58(3-4):209-212, discussion 212-203.

167. Manchikanti L, Glaser SE, Wolfer L, Derby R, Cohen SP. Systematic review of lumbar discography as a diagnostic test for chronic low back pain. *Pain Physician.* 2009;12(3):541-559.

168. Rainville J, Jouve C, Finno M, Limke J. Comparison of four tests of quadriceps strength in L3 or L4 radiculopathies. *Spine (Phila Pa 1976).* 2003;28(21):2466-2471.

169. Cyron BM, Hutton WC, Troup JD. Spondylolytic fractures. *J Bone Joint Surg Br.* 1976;58-B(4):462-466.

170. McGregor AH, Anderton L, Gedroyc WM, Johnson J, Hughes SP. The use of interventional open MRI to assess the kinematics of the lumbar spine in patients with spondylolisthesis. *Spine (Phila Pa 1976).* 2002;27(14):1582-1586.

171. Watters WC III, Bono CM, Gilbert TJ, et al. An evidence-based clinical guideline for the diagnosis and treatment of degenerative lumbar spondylolisthesis. *Spine J.* 2009;9(7):609-614.

172. Herman MJ, Pizzutillo PD. Spondylolysis and spondylolisthesis in the child and adolescent: A new classification. *Clin Orthop Relat Res.* 2005;434:46-54.

173. Wiltse LL, Newman PH, Macnab I. Classification of spondylolisis and spondylolisthesis. *Clin Orthop Relat Res.* 1976;117:23-29.

174. Wiltse LL, Winter RB. Terminology and measurement of spondylolisthesis. *J Bone Joint Surg Am.* 1983;65(6):768-772.

175. Meyerding HW. Spondylolisthesis. *Surgery, Gynecology and Obstetrics.* 1932;54:371-377.

176. Kalichman L, Kim DH, Li L, Guermazi A, Berkin V, Hunter DJ. Spondylolysis and spondylolisthesis: Prevalence and association with low back pain in the adult community-based population. *Spine (Phila Pa 1976).* 2009;34(2):199-205.

177. McCleary MD, Congeni JA. Current concepts in the diagnosis and treatment of spondylolysis in young athletes. *Curr Sports Med Rep.* 2007;6(1):62-66.

178. Standaert CJ, Herring SA. Expert opinion and controversies in sports and musculoskeletal medicine: The diagnosis and treatment of spondylolysis in adolescent athletes. *Arch Phys Med Rehabil.* 2007;88(4):537-540.

179. Patel DR, Nelson TL. Sports injuries in adolescents. *Med Clin North Am.* 2000;84(4):983-1007, viii.

180. Hatz D, Esposito PW, Schroeder B, Burke B, Lutz R, Hasley BP. The incidence of spondylolysis and spondylolisthesis in children with osteogenesis imperfecta. *J Pediatr Orthop.* 2011;31(6):655-660.

181. Ogon M, Bender BR, Hooper DM, et al. A dynamic approach to spinal instability. Part II: Hesitation and giving-way during interspinal motion. *Spine (Phila Pa 1976).* 1997;22(24):2859-2866.

182. Wood KB, Fritzell P, Dettori JR, Hashimoto R, Lund T, Shaffrey C. Effectiveness of spinal fusion versus structured rehabilitation in chronic low back pain patients with and without isthmic spondylolisthesis: A systematic review. *Spine (Phila Pa 1976).* 2011;36(21)(suppl):S110-S119.

183. Kobayashi A, Kobayashi T, Kato K, Higuchi H, Takagishi K. Diagnosis of radiographically occult lumbar spondylolysis in young athletes by magnetic resonance imaging [published online ahead of print November 7 2012]. *Am J Sports Med.* 2012.

184. Kalpakcioglu B, Altinbilek T, Senel K. Determination of spondylolisthesis in low back pain by clinical evaluation. *J Back Musculoskelet Rehabil.* 2009;22(1):27-32.

185. O'Sullivan PB, Phyty GD, Twomey LT, Allison GT. Evaluation of specific stabilizing exercise in the treatment of chronic low back pain with radiologic diagnosis of spondylolysis or spondylolisthesis. *Spine (Phila Pa 1976).* 1997;22(24):2959-2967.

186. Manchikanti L, Boswell MV, Singh V, Pampati V, Damron KS, Beyer CD. Prevalence of facet joint pain in chronic spinal pain of cervical, thoracic, and lumbar regions. *BMC Musculoskel Dis.* 2004;5:15.

187. Revel ME, Listrat VM, Chevalier XJ, et al. Facet joint block for low back pain: Identifying predictors of a good response. *Arch Phys Med Rehab.* 1992;73(9):824-828.

188. Revel M, Poiraudeau S, Auleley GR, et al. Capacity of the clinical picture to characterize low back pain relieved by facet joint anesthesia. Proposed criteria to identify patients with painful facet joints. *Spine (Phila Pa 1976).* 1998;23(18):1972-1976, discussion 1977.

189. Manchikanti L, Cash KA, Pampati V, Fellows B. Influence of psychological variables on the diagnosis of facet joint involvement in chronic spinal pain. *Pain Physician.* 2008;11(2):145-160.

190. Wilde VE, Ford JJ, McMeeken JM. Indicators of lumbar zygapophyseal joint pain: Survey of an expert panel with the Delphi technique. *Phys Ther.* 2007;87(10):1348-1361.

191. Jackson RP, Jacobs RR, Montesano PX. 1988 Volvo award in clinical sciences. Facet joint injection in low-back pain. A prospective statistical study. *Spine (Phila Pa 1976).* 1988;13(9):966-971.

192. Eubanks JD, Lee MJ, Cassinelli E, Ahn NU. Prevalence of lumbar facet arthrosis and its relationship to age, sex, and race: An anatomic study of cadaveric specimens. *Spine (Phila Pa 1976).* 2007;32(19):2058-2062.

193. Laslett M, McDonald B, Aprill CN, Tropp H, Oberg B. Clinical predictors of screening lumbar zygapophyseal joint blocks: Development of clinical prediction rules. *Spine J.* 2006;6(4):370-379.

194. Keene JS, Albert MJ, Springer SL, Drummond DS, Clancy WG Jr. Back injuries in college athletes. *J Spinal Disord.* 1989;2(3):190-195.

195. Leinonen V, Kankaanpaa M, Airaksinen O, Hanninen O. Back and hip extensor activities during trunk flexion/extension: Effects of low back pain and rehabilitation. *Arch Phys Med Rehab.* 2000;81(1):32-37.

196. Nourbakhsh MR, Arab AM. Relationship between mechanical factors and incidence of low back pain. *J Orthop Sport Phys.* 2002;32(9):447-460.

Chapter 20

1. Vleeming A, Albert HB, Ostgaard HC, Sturesson B, Stuge B. European guidelines for the diagnosis and treatment of pelvic girdle pain. *Eur Spine J.* 2008;17(6):794-819.

2. Laslett M, Aprill CN, McDonald B, Young SB. Diagnosis of sacroiliac joint pain: Validity of individual provocation tests and composites of tests. *Man Ther.* 2005;10(3):207-218.

3. Slipman CW, Jackson HB, Lipetz JS, Chan KT, Lenrow D, Vresilovic EJ. Sacroiliac joint pain referral zones. *Arch Phys Med Rehab.* 2000;81(3):334-338.

4. Fortin JD, Aprill CN, Ponthieux B, Pier J. Sacroiliac joint: Pain referral maps upon applying a new injection/arthrography technique. Part II: Clinical evaluation. *Spine (Phila Pa 1976).* 1994;19(13):1483-1489.

5. Dreyfuss P, Michaelsen M, Pauza K, McLarty J, Bogduk N. The value of medical history and physical examination in diagnosing sacroiliac joint pain. *Spine (Phila Pa 1976).* 1996;21(22):2594-2602.

6. Bogduk N. The anatomical basis for spinal pain syndromes. *J Manip Physiol Ther.* 1995;18(9):603-605.

7. Laslett M, Young SB, Aprill CN, McDonald B. Diagnosing painful sacroiliac joints: A validity study of a McKenzie evaluation and sacroiliac provocation tests. *Aust J Physiother.* 2003;49(2):89-97.

8. Slipman CW, Whyte WS II, Chow DW, Chou L, Lenrow D, Ellen M. Sacroiliac joint syndrome. *Pain Physician.* 2001;4(2):143-152.

9. Cohen SP, Chen Y, Neufeld NJ. Sacroiliac joint pain: A comprehensive review of epidemiology, diagnosis and treatment. *Expert Rev Neurother.* 2013;13(1):99-116.

10. Fortin JD, Dwyer AP, West S, Pier J. Sacroiliac joint: Pain referral maps upon applying a new injection/arthrography technique. Part I: Asymptomatic volunteers. *Spine (Phila Pa 1976).* 1994;19(13):1475-1482.

11. Murakami E, Aizawa T, Noguchi K, Kanno H, Okuno H, Uozumi H. Diagram specific to sacroiliac joint pain site indicated by one-finger test. *J Orthop Sci.* 2008;13(6):492-497.

12. Young S, Aprill C, Laslett M. Correlation of clinical examination characteristics with three sources of chronic low back pain. *Spine J.* 2003;3(6):460-465.

13. Ostgaard HC, Andersson GB, Karlsson K. Prevalence of back pain in pregnancy. *Spine (Phila Pa 1976).* 1991;16(5):549-552.

14. Gutke A, Ostgaard HC, Oberg B. Pelvic girdle pain and lumbar pain in pregnancy: A cohort study of the consequences in terms of health and functioning. *Spine (Phila Pa 1976).* 2006;31(5):E149-E155.

15. Wu WH, Meijer OG, Uegaki K, et al. Pregnancy-related pelvic girdle pain (PPP), I: Terminology, clinical presentation, and prevalence. *Eur Spine J.* 2004;13(7):575-589.

16. Kanakaris NK, Roberts CS, Giannoudis PV. Pregnancy-related pelvic girdle pain: An update. *BMC Med.* 2011;9:15.

17. Laplante BL, Ketchum JM, Saullo TR, DePalma MJ. Multivariable analysis of the relationship between pain referral patterns and the source of chronic low back pain. *Pain Physician.* 2012;15(2):171-178.

18. Gran JT. An epidemiological survey of the signs and symptoms of ankylosing spondylitis. *Clin Rheumatol.* 1985;4(2):161-169.

19. Friberg O. Clinical symptoms and biomechanics of lumbar spine and hip joint in leg length inequality. *Spine (Phila Pa 1976).* 1983;8(6):643-651.

20. Ivanov AA, Kiapour A, Ebraheim NA, Goel V. Lumbar fusion leads to increases in angular motion and stress across sacroiliac joint: A finite element study. *Spine (Phila Pa 1976).* 2009;34(5):E162-E169.

21. Ha KY, Lee JS, Kim KW. Degeneration of sacroiliac joint after instrumented lumbar or lumbosacral fusion: A prospective cohort study over five-year follow-up. *Spine (Phila Pa 1976).* 2008;33(11):1192-1198.

22. Ebraheim NA, Elgafy H, Semaan HB. Computed tomographic findings in patients with persistent sacroiliac pain after posterior iliac graft harvesting. *Spine (Phila Pa 1976).* 2000;25(16):2047-2051.

23. Maigne JY, Planchon CA. Sacroiliac joint pain after lumbar fusion. A study with anesthetic blocks. *Eur Spine J.* 2005;14(7):654-658.

24. Katz V, Schofferman J, Reynolds J. The sacroiliac joint: A potential cause of pain after lumbar fusion to the sacrum. *J Spinal Disord Tech.* 2003;16(1):96-99.

25. Sengupta R, Stone MA. The assessment of ankylosing spondylitis in clinical practice. *Nat Clin Pract Rheumatol.* 2007;3(9):496-503.

26. Weber U, Maksymowych WP. Sensitivity and specificity of magnetic resonance imaging for axial spondyloarthritis. *Am J Med Sci.* 2011;341(4):272-277.

27. Song IH, Brandt H, Rudwaleit M, Sieper J. Limited diagnostic value of unilateral sacroiliitis in scintigraphy in assessing axial spondyloarthritis. *J Rheumatol.* 2010;37(6):1200-1202.

28. Slipman CW, Sterenfeld EB, Chou LH, Herzog R, Vresilovic E. The value of radionuclide imaging in the diagnosis of sacroiliac joint syndrome. *Spine (Phila Pa 1976).* 1996;21(19):2251-2254.

29. Maigne JY, Boulahdour H, Chatellier G. Value of quantitative radionuclide bone scanning in the diagnosis of sacroiliac joint syndrome in 32 patients with low back pain. *Eur Spine J.* 1998;7(4):328-331.

30. Elgafy H, Semaan HB, Ebraheim NA, Coombs RJ. Computed tomography findings in patients with sacroiliac pain. *Clin Orthop Relat Res.* 2001(382):112-118.

31. Arnbak B, Leboeuf-Yde C, Jensen TS. A systematic critical review on MRI in spondyloarthritis. *Arthritis Res Ther.* 2012;14(2):R55.

32. Weber U, Pedersen SJ, Ostergaard M, Rufibach K, Lambert RG, Maksymowych WP. Can erosions on MRI of the sacroiliac joints be reliably detected in patients with ankylosing spondylitis? A cross-sectional study. *Arthritis Res Ther.* 2012;14(3):R124.

33. Weber U, Lambert RG, Ostergaard M, Hodler J, Pedersen SJ, Maksymowych WP. The diagnostic utility of magnetic resonance imaging in spondylarthritis: An international multicenter evaluation of one hundred eighty-seven subjects. *Arthritis Rheum.* 2010;62(10):3048-3058.

34. Song IH, Carrasco-Fernandez J, Rudwaleit M, Sieper J. The diagnostic value of scintigraphy in assessing sacroiliitis in ankylosing spondylitis: A systematic literature research. *Ann Rheum Dis.* 2008;67(11):1535-1540.

35. Sauerland S, Bouillon B, Rixen D, Raum MR, Koy T, Neugebauer EA. The reliability of clinical examination in detecting pelvic fractures in blunt trauma patients: A meta-analysis. *Arch Orthop Trauma Surg.* 2004;124(2):123-128.

36. van Tubergen A, Weber U. Diagnosis and classification in spondyloarthritis: Identifying a chameleon. *Nat Rev Rheumatol.* 2012;8(5):253-261.

37. Pedersen SJ, Weber U, Ostergaard M. The diagnostic utility of MRI in spondyloarthritis. *Best Pract Res Clin Rheumatol.* 2012;26(6):751-766.

38. Lee D. *The Pelvic Girdle: An Approach to the Examination and Treatment of the Lumbopelvic-Hip Region.* 3rd ed. London: Churchill Livingstone; 2004.

39. Sidiropoulos PI, Hatemi G, Song IH, et al. Evidence-based recommendations for the management of ankylosing spondylitis: Systematic literature search of the 3E Initiative in Rheumatology involving a broad panel of experts and practising rheumatologists. *Rheumatology (Oxford).* 2008;47(3):355-361.

40. Machado P, Castrejon I, Katchamart W, et al. Multinational evidence-based recommendations on how to investigate and follow-up undifferentiated peripheral inflammatory arthritis: Integrating systematic literature research and expert opinion of a broad international panel of rheumatologists in the 3E Initiative. *Ann Rheum Dis.* 2011;70(1):15-24.

41. Ince G, Sarpel T, Durgun B, Erdogan S. Effects of a multimodal exercise program for people with ankylosing spondylitis. *Phys Ther.* 2006;86(7):924-935.

42. Sieper J, Braun J, Rudwaleit M, Boonen A, Zink A. Ankylosing spondylitis: An overview. *Ann Rheum Dis.* 2002;61(suppl 3):iii8-18.

43. VanWye WR. Patient screening by a physical therapist for nonmusculoskeletal hip pain. *Phys Ther.* 2009;89(3):248-256.

44. Greenwood MJ, Erhard RE, Jones DL. Differential diagnosis of the hip vs. lumbar spine: Five case reports. *J Orthop Sport Phys.* 1998;27(4):308-315.

45. McCormick JP, Morgan SJ, Smith WR. Clinical effectiveness of the physical examination in diagnosis of posterior pelvic ring injuries. *J Orthop Trauma.* 2003;17(4):257-261.

46. Ham SJ, van Walsum AD, Vierhout PA. Predictive value of the hip flexion test for fractures of the pelvis. *Injury.* 1996;27(8):543-544.

47. Roman M, Brown C, Richardson W, Isaacs R, Howes C, Cook C. The development of a clinical decision making algorithm for detection of osteoporotic vertebral compression fracture or wedge deformity. *J Man Manip Ther.* 2010;18(1):44-49.

48. Langdon J, Way A, Heaton S, Bernard J, Molloy S. Vertebral compression fractures—New clinical signs to aid diagnosis. *Ann R Coll Surg Engl.* 2010;92(2):163-166.

49. Spiegel BM, Farid M, Esrailian E, Talley J, Chang L. Is irritable bowel syndrome a diagnosis of exclusion? A survey of primary care providers, gastroenterologists, and IBS experts. *Am J Gastroenterol.* 2010;105(4):848-858.

50. Donelson R, Aprill C, Medcalf R, Grant W. A prospective study of centralization of lumbar and referred pain. A predictor of symptomatic discs and anular competence. *Spine (Phila Pa 1976).* 1997;22(10):1115-1122.

51. Laslett M, Oberg B, Aprill CN, McDonald B. Centralization as a predictor of provocation discography results in chronic low back pain, and the influence of disability and distress on diagnostic power. *Spine J.* 2005;5(4):370-380.

52. Vroomen PC, de Krom MC, Wilmink JT, Kester AD, Knottnerus JA. Diagnostic value of history and physical examination in patients suspected of lumbosacral nerve root compression. *J Neurol Neurosur Ps.* 2002;72(5):630-634.

53. van der Windt DA, Simons E, Riphagen II, et al. Physical examination for lumbar radiculopathy due to disc herniation in patients with low-back pain. *Cochrane Db Syst Rev.* 2010; 2:CD007431.

54. Deville WL, van der Windt DA, Dzaferagic A, Bezemer PD, Bouter LM. The test of Lasegue: Systematic review of the accuracy in diagnosing herniated discs. *Spine (Phila Pa 1976).* 2000;25(9):1140-1147.

55. Stankovic R, Johnell O, Maly P, Willner S. Use of lumbar extension, slump test, physical and neurological examination in the evaluation of patients with suspected herniated nucleus pulposus. A prospective clinical study. *Man Ther.* 1999;4(1):25-32.

56. Majlesi J, Togay H, Unalan H, Toprak S. The sensitivity and specificity of the Slump and the Straight Leg Raising tests in patients with lumbar disc herniation. *J Clin Rheumatol.* 2008;14(2):87-91.

57. Laslett M, Aprill CN, McDonald B, Oberg B. Clinical predictors of lumbar provocation discography: A study of clinical predictors of lumbar provocation discography. *Eur Spine J.* 2006;15(10):1473-1484.

58. Schwarzer AC, Derby R, Aprill CN, Fortin J, Kine G, Bogduk N. Pain from the lumbar zygapophysial joints: A test of two models. *J Spinal Disord.* 1994;7(4):331-336.

59. Reiman MP, Goode AP, Hegedus EJ, Cook CE, Wright AA. Diagnostic accuracy of clinical tests of the hip: A systematic review with meta-analysis. *Brit J Sport Med.* 2013;47(14):893-902.

60. Altman R, Alarcon G, Appelrouth D, et al. The American College of Rheumatology criteria for the classification and reporting of osteoarthritis of the hip. *Arthritis Rheum.* 1991;34(5):505-514.

61. Hansen HC, McKenzie-Brown AM, Cohen SP, Swicegood JR, Colson JD, Manchikanti L. Sacroiliac joint interventions: A systematic review. *Pain Physician.* 2007;10(1):165-184.

62. Mens JM, Pool-Goudzwaard A, Stam HJ. Mobility of the pelvic joints in pregnancy-related lumbopelvic pain: A systematic review. *Obstet Gynecol Surv.* 2009;64(3):200-208.

63. Mens JM, Vleeming A, Snijders CJ, Koes BW, Stam HJ. Reliability and validity of the active straight leg raise test in posterior pelvic pain since pregnancy. *Spine (Phila Pa 1976).* 2001;26(10):1167-1171.

64. Fishman LM, Zybert PA. Electrophysiologic evidence of piriformis syndrome. *Arch Phys Med Rehab.* 1992;73(4):359-364.

65. Fishman LM, Dombi GW, Michaelsen C, et al. Piriformis syndrome: Diagnosis, treatment, and outcome—a 10-year study. *Arch Phys Med Rehab.* 2002;83(3):295-301.

66. Goode A, Hegedus EJ, Sizer P, Brismee JM, Linberg A, Cook CE. Three-dimensional movements of the sacroiliac joint: A systematic review of the literature and assessment of clinical utility. *J Man Manip Ther.* 2008;16(1):25-38.

67. Walheim GG, Selvik G. Mobility of the pubic symphysis. In vivo measurements with an electromechanic method and a roentgen stereophotogrammetric method. *Clin Orthop Relat Res.* 1984(191):129-135.

68. Meissner A, Fell M, Wilk R, Boenick U, Rahmanzadeh R. [Biomechanics of the pubic symphysis. Which forces lead to mobility of the symphysis in physiological conditions?]. *Unfallchirurg.* 1996;99(6):415-421.

69. Kean Chen C, Nizar AJ. Prevalence of piriformis syndrome in chronic low back pain patients. A clinical diagnosis with modified FAIR test [published online ahead of print August 2 2012]. *Pain Pract.* 2012.

70. Mens JM, Vleeming A, Snijders CJ, Ronchetti I, Stam HJ. Reliability and validity of hip adduction strength to measure disease severity in posterior pelvic pain since pregnancy. *Spine (Phila Pa 1976).* 2002;27(15):1674-1679.

71. Levangie PK. Four clinical tests of sacroiliac joint dysfunction: The association of test results with innominate torsion among patients with and without low back pain. *Phys Ther.* 1999;79(11):1043-1057.

72. Jaeschke R, Guyatt GH, Sackett DL. Users' guides to the medical literature. III. How to use an article about a diagnostic test. B. What are the results and will they help me in caring for my patients? The Evidence-Based Medicine Working Group. *JAMA.* 1994;271(9):703-707.

73. Cyriax J. *Textbook of Orthopaedic Medicine, Diagnosis of Soft Tissue Lesions.* 8th ed. London: Bailliere Tindall; 1982.

74. Fritz JM, Cleland JA, Childs JD. Subgrouping patients with low back pain: Evolution of a classification approach to physical therapy. *J Orthop Sport Phys.* 2007;37(6):290-302.

75. Ozgocmen S, Bozgeyik Z, Kalcik M, Yildirim A. The value of sacroiliac pain provocation tests in early active sacroiliitis. *Clin Rheumatol.* 2008;27(10):1275-1282.

76. Albert H, Godskesen M, Westergaard J. Evaluation of clinical tests used in classification procedures in pregnancy-related pelvic joint pain. *Eur Spine J.* 2000;9(2):161-166.

77. Damen L, Buyruk HM, Guler-Uysal F, Lotgering FK, Snijders CJ, Stam HJ. The prognostic value of asymmetric laxity of the sacroiliac joints in pregnancy-related pelvic pain. *Spine (Phila Pa 1976).* 2002;27(24):2820-2824.

78. Broadhurst NA, Bond MJ. Pain provocation tests for the assessment of sacroiliac joint dysfunction. *J Spinal Disord.* 1998;11(4):341-345.

79. Gutke A, Hansson ER, Zetherstrom G, Ostgaard HC. Posterior pelvic pain provocation test is negative in patients with lumbar herniated discs. *Eur Spine J.* 2009;18(7):1008-1012.

80. Ostgaard HC, Zetherstrom G, Roos-Hansson E, Svanberg B. Reduction of back and posterior pelvic pain in pregnancy. *Spine (Phila Pa 1976).* 1994;19(8):894-900.

81. Vleeming A, de Vries HJ, Mens JM, van Wingerden JP. Possible role of the long dorsal sacroiliac ligament in women with peripartum pelvic pain. *Acta Obstet Gynecol Scand.* 2002;81(5):430-436.

82. Fagevik Olsen M, Gutke A, Elden H, et al. Self-administered tests as a screening procedure for pregnancy-related pelvic girdle pain. *Eur Spine J.* 2009;18(8):1121-1129.

83. Berthelot JM, Labat JJ, Le Goff B, Gouin F, Maugars Y. Provocative sacroiliac joint maneuvers and sacroiliac joint block are unreliable for diagnosing sacroiliac joint pain. *Joint Bone Spine.* 2006;73(1):17-23.

84. Simopoulos TT, Manchikanti L, Singh V, et al. A systematic evaluation of prevalence and diagnostic accuracy of sacroiliac joint interventions. *Pain Physician.* 2012;15(3):E305-E344.

85. DePalma MJ, Ketchum JM, Saullo T. What is the source of chronic low back pain and does age play a role? *Pain Med.* 2011;12(2):224-233.

86. Schwarzer AC, Aprill CN, Bogduk N. The sacroiliac joint in chronic low back pain. *Spine (Phila Pa 1976).* 1995;20(1):31-37.

87. Leadbetter RE, Mawer D, Lindow SW. The development of a scoring system for symphysis pubis dysfunction. *J Obstet Gynaecol.* 2006;26(1):20-23.

88. Stomp-van den Berg SG, Hendriksen IJ, Bruinvels DJ, Twisk JW, van Mechelen W, van Poppel MN. Predictors for postpartum pelvic girdle pain in working women: The Mom@Work cohort study. *Pain.* 2012;153(12):2370-2379.

89. van der Weijden MA, Claushuis TA, Nazari T, Lems WF, Dijkmans BA, van der Horst-Bruinsma IE. High prevalence of low bone mineral density in patients within 10 years of onset of ankylosing spondylitis: A systematic review [published online ahead of print June 16 2012]. *Clin Rheumatol.* 2012.

90. van der Horst-Bruinsma IE, Nurmohamed MT, Landewe RB. Comorbidities in patients with spondyloarthritis. *Rheum Dis Clin N Am.* 2012;38(3):523-538.

91. Kellgren JH, Lawrence JS. Radiological assessment of osteo-arthrosis. *Ann Rheum Dis.* 1957;16(4):494-502.

92. Fukui S, Ohseto K, Shiotani M, Ohno K, Karasawa H, Naganuma Y. Distribution of referred pain from the lumbar zygapophyseal joints and dorsal rami. *Clin J Pain.* 1997;13(4):303-307.

93. Ozgocmen S, Akgul O, Altay Z, et al. Expert opinion and key recommendations for the physical therapy and rehabilitation of patients with ankylosing spondylitis. *Int J Rheum Dis.* 2012;15(3):229-238.

94. Calin A, Porta J, Fries JF, Schurman DJ. Clinical history as a screening test for ankylosing spondylitis. *JAMA.* 1977;237(24):2613-2614.

95. Averns HL, Oxtoby J, Taylor HG, Jones PW, Dziedzic K, Dawes PT. Radiological outcome in ankylosing spondylitis: Use of the Stoke Ankylosing Spondylitis Spine Score (SASSS). *Brit J Rheumatol.* 1996;35(4):373-376.

96. Lee W, Reveille JD, Davis JC Jr, Learch TJ, Ward MM, Weisman MH. Are there gender differences in severity of ankylosing spondylitis? Results from the PSOAS cohort. *Ann Rheum Dis.* 2007;66(5):633-638.

97. Pace JB, Nagle D. Piriform syndrome. *West J Med.* 1976;124(6):435-439.

98. Papadopoulos EC, Khan SN. Piriformis syndrome and low back pain: A new classification and review of the literature. *Orthop Clin N Am.* 2004;35(1):65-71.

Chapter 21

1. Wofford JL, Mansfield RJ, Watkins RS. Patient characteristics and clinical management of patients with shoulder pain in U.S. primary care settings: Secondary data analysis of the National Ambulatory Medical Care Survey. *BMC Musculoskel Dis.* 2005;6:4.

2. Luime JJ, Koes BW, Hendriksen IJ, et al. Prevalence and incidence of shoulder pain in the general population: A systematic review. *Scand J Rheumatol.* 2004;33(2):73-81.

3. Picavet HS, Schouten JS. Musculoskeletal pain in the Netherlands: Prevalences, consequences and risk groups, the DMC(3)-study. *Pain.* 2003;102(1-2):167-178.

4. Michener LA, Walsworth MK, Doukas WC, Murphy KP. Reliability and diagnostic accuracy of 5 physical examination tests and combination of tests for subacromial impingement. *Arch Phys Med Rehab.* 2009;90(11):1898-1903.

5. Massimini DF, Boyer PJ, Papannagari R, Gill TJ, Warner JP, Li G. In-vivo glenohumeral translation and ligament elongation during abduction and abduction with internal and external rotation. *J Orthop Surg Res.* 2012;7:29.

6. Cooper DE, Arnoczky SP, O'Brien SJ, Warren RF, DiCarlo E, Allen AA. Anatomy, histology, and vascularity of the glenoid labrum. An anatomical study. *J Bone Joint Surg. Am.* 1992;74(1):46-52.

7. Ludewig PM, Reynolds JF. The association of scapular kinematics and glenohumeral joint pathologies. *J Orthop Sports Phys Ther.* 2009;39(2):90-104.

8. Balke M, Schmidt C, Dedy N, Banerjee M, Bouillon B, Liem D. Correlation of acromial morphology with impingement syndrome and rotator cuff tears. *Acta Orthop.* 2013;84(2):178-183.

9. Kuijpers T, van der Windt DA, Boeke AJ, et al. Clinical prediction rules for the prognosis of shoulder pain in general practice. *Pain.* 2006;120(3):276-285.

10. Litaker D, Pioro M, El Bilbeisi H, Brems J. Returning to the bedside: Using the history and physical examination to identify rotator cuff tears. *J Am Geriatr Soc.* 2000;48(12):1633-1637.

11. Michener LA, Doukas WC, Murphy KP, Walsworth MK. Diagnostic accuracy of history and physical examination of superior labrum anterior-posterior lesions. *J Athl Train.* 2011;46(4):343-348.

12. Mall NA, Lee AS, Chahal J, et al. Transosseous-equivalent rotator cuff repair: A systematic review on the biomechanical importance of tying the medial row. *Arthroscopy.* 2013;29(2):377-386.

13. Schaeffeler C, Waldt S, Holzapfel K, et al. Lesions of the biceps pulley: Diagnostic accuracy of MR arthrography of the shoulder and evaluation of previously described and new diagnostic signs. *Radiology.* 2012;264(2):504-513.

14. Lewis JS. Rotator cuff tendinopathy. *Brit J Sport Med.* 2009;43(4):236-241.

15. Chang D, Mohana-Borges A, Borso M, Chung CB. SLAP lesions: Anatomy, clinical presentation, MR imaging diagnosis and characterization. *Eur J Radiol.* 2008;68(1):72-87.

16. Wilk KE, Reinold MM, Dugas JR, Arrigo CA, Moser MW, Andrews JR. Current concepts in the recognition and treatment of superior labral (SLAP) lesions. *J Orthop Sports Phys Ther.* 2005;35(5):273-291.

17. Kelley MJ, Shaffer MA, Kuhn JE, et al. Shoulder pain and mobility deficits: Adhesive capsulitis. *J Orthop Sports Phys Ther.* 2013;43(5):A1-A31.

18. Chronopoulos E, Kim TK, Park HB, Ashenbrenner D, McFarland EG. Diagnostic value of physical tests for isolated chronic acromioclavicular lesions. *Am J Sport Med.* 2004;32(3):655-661.

19. Wright AA, Wassinger CA, Frank M, Michener LA, Hegedus EJ. Diagnostic accuracy of scapular physical examination tests for shoulder disorders: A systematic review. *Brit J Sport Med.* 2013;47(14):886-892.

20. van Kampen DA, van den Berg T, van der Woude HJ, Castelein RM, Terwee CB, Willems WJ. Diagnostic value of patient characteristics, history, and six clinical tests for traumatic anterior shoulder instability. *J Shoulder Elb Surg.* 2013;22(10):1310-1319.

21. Roy JS, MacDermid JC, Woodhouse LJ. Measuring shoulder function: A systematic review of four questionnaires. *Arthritis Rheum.* 2009;61(5):623-632.

22. Desai AS, Dramis A, Hearnden AJ. Critical appraisal of subjective outcome measures used in the assessment of shoulder disability. *Ann R Coll Surg Engl.* 2010;92(1):9-13.

23. Rouleau DM, Faber K, MacDermid JC. Systematic review of patient-administered shoulder functional scores on instability. *J Shoulder Elb Surg.* 2010;19(8):1121-1128.

24. Rasmussen JV, Jakobsen J, Olsen BS, Brorson S. Translation and validation of the Western Ontario Osteoarthritis of the Shoulder (WOOS) index—the Danish version. *Patient Relat Outcome Meas.* 2013;4:49-54.

25. Ottenheijm RP, Jansen MJ, Staal JB, et al. Accuracy of diagnostic ultrasound in patients with suspected subacromial disorders: A systematic review and meta-analysis. *Arch Phys Med Rehab.* 2010;91(10):1616-1625.

26. Dinnes J, Loveman E, McIntyre L, Waugh N. The effectiveness of diagnostic tests for the assessment of shoulder pain due to soft tissue disorders: A systematic review. *Health Technol Assess.* 2003;7(29):iii, 1-166.

27. Smith TO, Back T, Toms AP, Hing CB. Diagnostic accuracy of ultrasound for rotator cuff tears in adults: A systematic review and meta-analysis. *Clin Radiol.* 2011;66(11):1036-1048.

28. de Jesus JO, Parker L, Frangos AJ, Nazarian LN. Accuracy of MRI, MR arthrography, and ultrasound in the diagnosis of rotator cuff tears: A meta-analysis. *Am J Roentgenol.* 2009;192(6):1701-1707.

29. Smith TO, Daniell H, Geere JA, Toms AP, Hing CB. The diagnostic accuracy of MRI for the detection of partial- and full-thickness rotator cuff tears in adults. *Magn Reson Imaging.* 2012;30(3):336-346.

30. Oh JH, Kim JY, Choi JA, Kim WS. Effectiveness of multidetector computed tomography arthrography for the diagnosis of shoulder pathology: Comparison with magnetic resonance imaging with arthroscopic correlation. *J Shoulder Elb Surg.* 2010;19(1):14-20.

31. Adams CR, Brady PC, Koo SS, et al. A systematic approach for diagnosing subscapularis tendon tears with preoperative magnetic resonance imaging scans. *Arthroscopy.* 2012;28(11):1592-1600.

32. Walton J, Mahajan S, Paxinos A, et al. Diagnostic values of tests for acromioclavicular joint pain. *J Bone Joint Surg Am.* 2004;86-A(4):807-812.

33. Smith TO, Drew BT, Toms AP. A meta-analysis of the diagnostic test accuracy of MRA and MRI for the detection of glenoid labral injury. *Arch Orthop Trauma Surg.* 2012;132(7):905-919.

34. Phillips JC, Cook C, Beaty S, Kissenberth MJ, Siffri P, Hawkins RJ. Validity of noncontrast magnetic resonance imaging in diagnosing superior labrum anterior-posterior tears. *J Shoulder Elb Surg.* 2013;22(1):3-8.

35. Waldt S, Burkart A, Imhoff AB, Bruegel M, Rummeny EJ, Woertler K. Anterior shoulder instability: Accuracy of MR arthrography in the classification of anteroinferior labroligamentous injuries. *Radiology.* 2005;237(2):578-583.

36. Middernacht B, Winnock de Grave P, Van Maele G, Favard L, Mole D, De Wilde L. What do standard radiography and clinical examination tell about the shoulder with cuff tear arthropathy? *J Orthop Surg Res.* 2011;6:1.

37. Malone T, Hazle C. Diagnostic imaging of the throwing athlete's shoulder. *Int J Sports Phys Ther.* 2013;8(5):641-651.

38. Shahabpour M, Kichouh M, Laridon E, Gielen JL, De Mey J. The effectiveness of diagnostic imaging methods for the assessment of soft tissue and articular disorders of the shoulder and elbow. *Eur J Radiol.* 2008;65(2):194-200.

39. Strobel K, Pfirrmann CW, Zanetti M, Nagy L, Hodler J. MRI features of the acromioclavicular joint that predict pain relief from intraarticular injection. *Am J Roentgenol.* 2003;181(3):755-760.

40. Lenza M, Buchbinder R, Takwoingi Y, Johnston RV, Hanchard NC, Faloppa F. Magnetic resonance imaging, magnetic resonance arthrography and ultrasonography for assessing rotator cuff tears in people with shoulder pain for whom surgery is being considered. *Cochrane Db Syst Rev.* 2013;9:CD009020.

41. Thigpen CA, Padua DA, Michener LA, et al. Head and shoulder posture affect scapular mechanics and muscle activity in overhead tasks. *J Electromyogr Kines.* 2010;20(4):701-709.

42. Lewis JS, Green A, Wright C. Subacromial impingement syndrome: The role of posture and muscle imbalance. *J Shoulder Elb Surg.* 2005;14(4):385-392.

43. Priest JD, Nagel DA. Tennis shoulder. *Am J Sport Med.* 1976;4(1):28-42.

44. Steurer J, Held U, Schmid D, Ruckstuhl J, Bachmann LM. Clinical value of diagnostic instruments for ruling out acute coronary syndrome in patients with chest pain: A systematic review. *Emerg Med J.* 2010;27(12):896-902.

45. Selker HP, Griffith JL, D'Agostino RB. A tool for judging coronary care unit admission appropriateness, valid for both real-time and retrospective use. A time-insensitive predictive instrument (TIPI) for acute cardiac ischemia: A multicenter study. *Med Care.* 1991;29(7):610-627.

46. Adams SL, Yarnold PR, Mathews JJ IV. Clinical use of the olecranon-manubrium percussion sign in shoulder trauma. *Ann Emerg Med.* 1988;17(5):484-487.

47. Moore MB. The use of a tuning fork and stethoscope to identify fractures. *J Athl Train.* 2009;44(3):272-274.

48. Bushnell BD, Creighton RA, Herring MM. The bony apprehension test for instability of the shoulder: A prospective pilot analysis. *Arthroscopy.* 2008;24(9):974-982.

49. Shah KC, Rajshekhar V. Reliability of diagnosis of soft cervical disc prolapse using Spurling's test. *Brit J Neurosurg.* 2004;18(5):480-483.

50. Wainner RS, Fritz JM, Irrgang JJ, Boninger ML, Delitto A, Allison S. Reliability and diagnostic accuracy of the clinical examination and patient self-report measures for cervical radiculopathy. *Spine (Phila Pa 1976).* 2003;28(1):52-62.

51. Gumina S, Carbone S, Albino P, Gurzi M, Postacchini F. Arm Squeeze Test: A new clinical test to distinguish neck from shoulder pain. *Eur Spine J.* 2013;22(7):1558-1563.

52. Docherty MA, Schwab RA, Ma OJ. Can elbow extension be used as a test of clinically significant injury? *South Med J.* 2002;95(5):539-541.

53. Darracq MA, Vinson DR, Panacek EA. Preservation of active range of motion after acute elbow trauma predicts absence of elbow fracture. *Am J Emerg Med.* 2008;26(7):779-782. doi: 710.1016/j.ajem.2007.1011.1005.

54. Alqunaee M, Galvin R, Fahey T. Diagnostic accuracy of clinical tests for subacromial impingement syndrome: A systematic review and meta-analysis. *Arch Phys Med Rehab.* 2012;93(2):229-236.

55. Hegedus EJ, Goode AP, Cook CE, et al. Which physical examination tests provide clinicians with the most value when examining the shoulder? Update of a systematic review with meta-analysis of individual tests. *Brit J Sport Med.* 2012;46(14):964-978.

56. Brandt C, Sole G, Krause MW, Nel M. An evidence-based review on the validity of the Kaltenborn rule as applied to the glenohumeral joint. *Manual Ther.* 2007;12(1):3-11.

57. Schomacher J. The convex-concave rule and the lever law. *Manual Ther.* 2009;14(5):579-582.

58. Rundquist PJ, Anderson DD, Guanche CA, Ludewig PM. Shoulder kinematics in subjects with frozen shoulder. *Arch Phys Med Rehab.* 2003;84(10):1473-1479.

59. Rundquist PJ, Ludewig PM. Patterns of motion loss in subjects with idiopathic loss of shoulder range of motion. *Clin Biomech.* 2004;19(8):810-818.

60. Conway AM. Movements at the sternoclavicular and acromioclavicular joints. *Phys Ther Rev.* 1961;41:421-432.

61. Riddle DL, Rothstein JM, Lamb RL. Goniometric reliability in a clinical setting. Shoulder measurements. *Phys Ther.* 1987;67(5):668-673.

62. Johnson AJ, Godges JJ, Zimmerman GJ, Ounanian LL. The effect of anterior versus posterior glide joint mobilization on external rotation range of motion in patients with shoulder adhesive capsulitis. *J Orthop Sports Phys Ther.* 2007;37(3):88-99.

63. Tyler TF, Nicholas SJ, Lee SJ, Mullaney M, McHugh MP. Correction of posterior shoulder tightness is associated with symptom resolution in patients with internal impingement. *Am J Sports Med.* 2010;38(1):114-119.

64. Reese NB, Bandy WD. *Joint Range of Motion and Muscle Length Testing.* Philadelphia, PA: Saunders; 2002.

65. Wilk KE, Macrina LC, Fleisig GS, et al. Deficits in glenohumeral passive range of motion increase risk of elbow injury in professional baseball pitchers: A prospective study. *Am J Sports Med.* 2014;42(9):2075-2081.

66. Chester R, Smith TO, Hooper L, Dixon J. The impact of subacromial impingement syndrome on muscle activity patterns of the shoulder complex: A systematic review of electromyographic studies. *BMC Musculoskel Dis.* 2010;11:45.

67. Michener LA, Boardman ND, Pidcoe PE, Frith AM. Scapular muscle tests in subjects with shoulder pain and functional loss: Reliability and construct validity. *Phys Ther.* 2005;85(11):1128-1138.

68. Brookham RL, McLean L, Dickerson CR. Construct validity of muscle force tests of the rotator cuff muscles: An electromyographic investigation. *Phys Ther.* 2010;90(4):572-580.

69. Kelly BT, Kadrmas WR, Speer KP. The manual muscle examination for rotator cuff strength. An electromyographic investigation. *Am J Sport Med.* 1996;24(5):581-588.

70. Kelly SM, Brittle N, Allen GM. The value of physical tests for subacromial impingement syndrome: A study of diagnostic accuracy. *Clin Rehabil.* 2010;24(2):149-158.

71. Hegedus EJ, Goode A, Campbell S, et al. Physical examination tests of the shoulder: A systematic review with meta-analysis of individual tests. *Brit J Sport Med.* 2008;42(2):80-92, discussion 92.

72. Hughes PC, Taylor NF, Green RA. Most clinical tests cannot accurately diagnose rotator cuff pathology: A systematic review. *Austr J Physiother.* 2008;54(3):159-170.

73. Munro W, Healy R. The validity and accuracy of clinical tests used to detect labral pathology of the shoulder—A systematic review. *Manual Ther.* 2009;14(2):119-130.

74. Johansson K, Ivarson S. Intra- and interexaminer reliability of four manual shoulder maneuvers used to identify subacromial pain. *Manual Ther.* 2009;14(2):231-239.

75. Nomden JG, Slagers AJ, Bergman GJ, Winters JC, Kropmans TJ, Dijkstra PU. Interobserver reliability of physical examination of shoulder girdle. *Manual Ther.* 2009;14(2):152-159.

76. Beaudreuil J, Nizard R, Thomas T, et al. Contribution of clinical tests to the diagnosis of rotator cuff disease: A systematic literature review. *Joint, Bone, Spine: Revue du Rhumatisme.* 2009;76(1):15-19.

77. Park HB, Yokota A, Gill HS, El Rassi G, McFarland EG. Diagnostic accuracy of clinical tests for the different degrees of subacromial impingement syndrome. *J Bone Joint Surg.* 2005;87(7):1446-1455.

78. Bak K, Sorensen AK, Jorgensen U, et al. The value of clinical tests in acute full-thickness tears of the supraspinatus tendon: Does a subacromial lidocaine injection help in the clinical diagnosis? A prospective study. *Arthroscopy.* 2010;26(6):734-742.

79. Miller CA, Forrester GA, Lewis JS. The validity of the lag signs in diagnosing full-thickness tears of the rotator cuff: A preliminary investigation. *Arch Phys Med Rehab.* 2008;89(6):1162-1168.

80. Castoldi F, Blonna D, Hertel R. External rotation lag sign revisited: Accuracy for diagnosis of full thickness supraspinatus tear. *J. Shoulder Elb Surg.* 2009;18(4):529-534.

81. Calis M, Akgun K, Birtane M, Karacan I, Calis H, Tuzun F. Diagnostic values of clinical diagnostic tests in subacromial impingement syndrome. *Ann Rheum Dis.* 2000;59(1):44-47.

82. MacDonald PB, Clark P, Sutherland K. An analysis of the diagnostic accuracy of the Hawkins and Neer subacromial impingement signs. *J Shoulder Elb Surg.* 2000;9(4):299-301.

83. Zaslav KR. Internal rotation resistance strength test: A new diagnostic test to differentiate intra-articular pathology from outlet (Neer) impingement syndrome in the shoulder. *J Shoulder Elb Surg.* 2001;10(1):23-27.

84. Wolf EM, Agrawal V. Transdeltoid palpation (the rent test) in the diagnosis of rotator cuff tears. *J Shoulder Elb Surg.* 2001;10(5):470-473.

85. Gillooly JJ, Chidambaram R, Mok D. The lateral Jobe test: A more reliable method of diagnosing rotator cuff tears. *Int J Shoulder Surg.* 2010;4(2):41-43.

86. Murrell GA, Walton JR. Diagnosis of rotator cuff tears. *Lancet.* 2001;357(9258):769-770.

87. Itoi E, Kido T, Sano A, Urayama M, Sato K. Which is more useful, the "full can test" or the "empty can test," in detecting the torn supraspinatus tendon? *Am J Sport Med.* 1999;27(1):65-68.

88. Itoi E, Minagawa H, Yamamoto N, Seki N, Abe H. Are pain location and physical examinations useful in locating a tear site of the rotator cuff? *Am J Sport Med.* 2006;34(2):256-264.

89. Walch G, Boulahia A, Calderone S, Robinson AH. The 'dropping' and 'hornblower's' signs in evaluation of rotator-cuff tears. *J Bone Joint Surg Br.* 1998;80(4):624-628.

90. Barth JR, Burkhart SS, De Beer JF. The bear-hug test: A new and sensitive test for diagnosing a subscapularis tear. *Arthroscopy.* 2006;22(10):1076-1084.

91. Meister K, Buckley B, Batts J. The posterior impingement sign: Diagnosis of rotator cuff and posterior labral tears secondary to internal impingement in overhand athletes. *Am J Orthop (Belle Mead, NJ).* 2004;33(8):412-415.

92. Kim SH, Ha KI, Han KY. Biceps load test: A clinical test for superior labrum anterior and posterior lesions in shoulders with recurrent anterior dislocations. *Am J Sport Med.* 1999;27(3):300-303.

93. Guanche CA, Jones DC. Clinical testing for tears of the glenoid labrum. *Arthroscopy.* 2003;19(5):517-523.

94. Nakagawa S, Yoneda M, Hayashida K, Obata M, Fukushima S, Miyazaki Y. Forced shoulder abduction and elbow flexion test: A new simple clinical test to detect superior labral injury in the throwing shoulder. *Arthroscopy.* 2005;21(11):1290-1295.

95. Stetson WB, Templin K. The crank test, the O'Brien test, and routine magnetic resonance imaging scans in the diagnosis of labral tears. *Am J Sport Med.* 2002;30(6):806-809.

96. Liu SH, Henry MH, Nuccion SL. A prospective evaluation of a new physical examination in predicting glenoid labral tears. *Am J Sport Med.* 1996;24(6):721-725.

97. Oh JH, Kim JY, Kim WS, Gong HS, Lee JH. The evaluation of various physical examinations for the diagnosis of type II superior labrum anterior and posterior lesion. *Am J Sport Med.* 2008;36(2):353-359.

98. Kim SH, Ha KI, Ahn JH, Choi HJ. Biceps load test II: A clinical test for SLAP lesions of the shoulder. *Arthroscopy.* 2001;17(2):160-164.

99. Parentis MA, Glousman RE, Mohr KS, Yocum LA. An evaluation of the provocative tests for superior labral anterior posterior lesions. *Am J Sport Med.* 2006;34(2):265-268.

100. McFarland EG, Kim TK, Savino RM. Clinical assessment of three common tests for superior labral anterior-posterior lesions. *American J Sport Med.* 2002;30(6):810-815.

101. Morgan CD, Burkhart SS, Palmeri M, Gillespie M. Type II SLAP lesions: Three subtypes and their relationships to superior instability and rotator cuff tears. *Arthroscopy* 1998;14(6):553-565.

102. Bennett WF. Specificity of the Speed's test: Arthroscopic technique for evaluating the biceps tendon at the level of the bicipital groove. *Arthroscopy.* 1998;14(8):789-796.

103. Kibler WB. Specificity and sensitivity of the anterior slide test in throwing athletes with superior glenoid labral tears. *Arthroscopy.* 1995;11(3):296-300.

104. Holtby R, Razmjou H. Accuracy of the Speed's and Yergason's tests in detecting biceps pathology and SLAP lesions: Comparison with arthroscopic findings. *Arthroscopy* 2004;20(3):231-236.

105. Kim YS, Kim JM, Ha KY, Choy S, Joo MW, Chung YG. The passive compression test: A new clinical test for superior labral tears of the shoulder. *Am J Sport Med.* 2007;35(9):1489-1494.

106. Schlechter JA, Summa S, Rubin BD. The passive distraction test: A new diagnostic aid for clinically significant superior labral pathology. *Arthroscopy.* 2009;25(12):1374-1379.

107. Kim SH, Park JS, Jeong WK, Shin SK. The Kim test: A novel test for posteroinferior labral lesion of the shoulder—a comparison to the jerk test. *Am J Sport Med.* 2005;33(8):1188-1192.

108. Lo IK, Nonweiler B, Woolfrey M, Litchfield R, Kirkley A. An evaluation of the apprehension, relocation, and surprise tests for anterior shoulder instability. *Am J Sport Med.* 2004;32(2):301-307.

109. Farber AJ, Castillo R, Clough M, Bahk M, McFarland EG. Clinical assessment of three common tests for traumatic anterior shoulder instability. *J Bone Joint Surg Am.* 2006;88(7):1467-1474.

110. Gill HS, El Rassi G, Bahk MS, Castillo RC, McFarland EG. Physical examination for partial tears of the biceps tendon. *Am J Sport Med.* 2007;35(8):1334-1340.

111. Ben Kibler W, Sciascia AD, Hester P, Dome D, Jacobs C. Clinical utility of traditional and new tests in the diagnosis of biceps tendon injuries and superior labrum anterior and posterior lesions in the shoulder. *Am J Sport Med.* 2009;37(9):1840-1847.

112. Ardic F, Kahraman Y, Kacar M, Kahraman MC, Findikoglu G, Yorgancioglu ZR. Shoulder impingement syndrome: Relationships between clinical, functional, and radiologic findings. *Am J Phys Med Rehab.* 2006;85(1):53-60.

113. Cadogan A, McNair P, Laslett M, Hing W. Shoulder pain in primary care: Diagnostic accuracy of clinical examination tests for non-traumatic acromioclavicular joint pain. *BMC Musculoskel Dis.* 2013;14:156.

114. Jia X, Ji JH, Petersen SA, Keefer J, McFarland EG. Clinical evaluation of the shoulder shrug sign. *Clin Orthop Relat R.* 2008;466(11):2813-2819.

115. Carbone S, Gumina S, Vestri AR, Postacchini R. Coracoid pain test: A new clinical sign of shoulder adhesive capsulitis. *Int Orthop.* 2010;34(3):385-388.

116. Rabin A, Irrgang JJ, Fitzgerald GK, Eubanks A. The intertester reliability of the Scapular Assistance Test. *J Orthop Sport Phys.* 2006;36(9):653-660.

117. Tate AR, McClure P, Kareha S, Irwin D, Barbe MF. A clinical method for identifying scapular dyskinesis, part 2: Validity. *J Athl Training.* 2009;44(2):165-173.

118. Odom CJ, Taylor AB, Hurd CE, Denegar CR. Measurement of scapular asymetry and assessment of shoulder dysfunction using the Lateral Scapular Slide Test: A reliability and validity study. *Physical Ther.* 2001;81(2):799-809.

119. Shadmehr A, Bagheri H, Ansari NN, Sarafraz H. The reliability measurements of lateral scapular slide test at three different degrees of shoulder joint abduction. *Brit J Sport Med.* 2010;44(4):289-293.

120. Kibler WB, Sciascia A, Dome D. Evaluation of apparent and absolute supraspinatus strength in patients with shoulder injury using the scapular retraction test. *Am J Sport Med.* 2006;34(10):1643-1647.

121. Gumina S, Carbone S, Postacchini F. Scapular dyskinesis and SICK scapula syndrome in patients with chronic type III acromioclavicular dislocation. *Arthroscopy.* 2009;25(1):40-45.

122. Levy O, Relwani JG, Mullett H, Haddo O, Even T. The active elevation lag sign and the triangle sign: New clinical signs of trapezius palsy. *J Shoulder Elb Surg.* 2009;18(4):573-576.

123. Hertel R, Lambert SM, Ballmer FT. The deltoid extension lag sign for diagnosis and grading of axillary nerve palsy. *J Shoulder Elb Surg.* 1998;7(2):97-99.

124. Westrick RB, Miller JM, Carow SD, Gerber JP. Exploration of the y-balance test for assessment of upper quarter closed kinetic chain performance. *Int J Sports Phys Ther.* 2012;7(2):139-147.

125. Roush JR, Kitamura J, Waits MC. Reference values for the Closed Kinetic Chain Upper Extremity Stability Test (CKCUEST) for collegiate baseball players. *N Am J Sports Phys Ther.* 2007;2(3):159-163.

126. Kumta P, MacDermid JC, Mehta SP, Stratford PW. The FIT-HaNSA demonstrates reliability and convergent validity of functional performance in patients with shoulder disorders. *J Orthop Sport Phys.* 2012;42(5):455-464.

127. Reiman MP, Manske RC. *Functional Testing in Human Performance.* Champaign, IL: Human Kinetics; 2009.

128. Wassinger CA, Myers JB, Gatti JM, Conley KM, Lephart SM. Proprioception and throwing accuracy in the dominant shoulder after cryotherapy. *J Athl Training.* 2007;42(1):84-89.

129. Edmondston SJ, Wallumrod ME, Macleid F, Kvamme LS, Joebges S, Brabham GC. Reliability of isometric muscle endurance tests in subjects with postural neck pain. *J Manip Physiol Ther.* 2008;31(5):348-354.

130. Schellingerhout JM, Verhagen AP, Thomas S, Koes BW. Lack of uniformity in diagnostic labeling of shoulder pain: Time for a different approach. *Manual Ther.* 2008;13(6):478-483.

131. van der Windt DA, Koes BW, de Jong BA, Bouter LM. Shoulder disorders in general practice: Incidence, patient characteristics, and management. *Ann Rheum Dis.* 1995;54(12):959-964.

132. Hermans J, Luime JJ, Meuffels DE, Reijman M, Simel DL, Bierma-Zeinstra SM. Does this patient with shoulder pain have rotator cuff disease? The Rational Clinical Examination systematic review. *JAMA.* 2013;310(8):837-847.

133. Hawkins RJ, Abrams JS. Impingement syndrome in the absence of rotator cuff tear (stages 1 and 2). *Orthop Clin N Am.* 1987;18(3):373-382.

134. Jobe FW. Impingement problems in the athlete. *Instr Course Lect.* 1989;38:205-209.

135. Joensen J, Couppe C, Bjordal JM. Increased palpation tenderness and muscle strength deficit in the prediction of tendon hypertrophy in symptomatic unilateral shoulder tendinopathy: An ultrasonographic study. *Physiotherapy.* 2009;95(2):83-93.

136. Wilson JJ, Best TM. Common overuse tendon problems: A review and recommendations for treatment. *Am Fam Physician.* 2005;72(5):811-818.

137. Toprak U, Ustuner E, Ozer D, et al. Palpation tests versus impingement tests in Neer stage I and II subacromial impingement syndrome. *Knee Surg Sport Tr A.* 2013;21(2):424-429.

138. Michener LA, Snyder Valier AR, McClure PW. Defining substantial clinical benefit for patient-rated outcome tools for shoulder impingement syndrome. *Arch Phys Med Rehab.* 2013;94(4):725-730.

139. Warner JJ, Micheli LJ, Arslanian LE, Kennedy J, Kennedy R. Patterns of flexibility, laxity, and strength in normal shoulders and shoulders with instability and impingement. *Am J Sport Med.* 1990;18(4):366-375.

140. Leroux JL, Codine P, Thomas E, Pocholle M, Mailhe D, Blotman F. Isokinetic evaluation of rotational strength in normal shoulders and shoulders with impingement syndrome. *Clin Orthop Relat Res.* 1994;304:108-115.

141. Garofalo R, Karlsson J, Nordenson U, Cesari E, Conti M, Castagna A. Anterior-superior internal impingement of the shoulder: An evidence-based review. *Knee Surg Sport Tr A.* 2010;18(12):1688-1693.

142. Cools AM, Declercq G, Cagnie B, Cambier D, Witvrouw E. Internal impingement in the tennis player: Rehabilitation guidelines. *Brit J Sport Med.* 2008;42(3):165-171.

143. Beach ML, Whitney SL, Dickoff-Hoffman S. Relationship of shoulder flexibility, strength, and endurance to shoulder pain in competitive swimmers. *J Orthop Sport Phys.* 1992;16(6):262-268.

144. Castagna A, Garofalo R, Cesari E, Markopoulos N, Borroni M, Conti M. Posterior superior internal impingement: An evidence-based review [corrected]. *Brit J Sport Med.* 2010;44(5):382-388.

145. Chan YS, Lien LC, Hsu HL, et al. Evaluating hip labral tears using magnetic resonance arthrography: A prospective study comparing hip arthroscopy and magnetic resonance arthrography diagnosis. *Arthroscopy.* 2005;21(10):1250.

146. Edouard P, Degache F, Beguin L, et al. Rotator cuff strength in recurrent anterior shoulder instability. *J Bone Joint Surg Am.* 2011;93(8):759-765.

147. Bak K, Wiesler ER, Poehling GG, Committee IUE. Consensus statement on shoulder instability. *Arthroscopy.* 2010;26(2):249-255.

148. McFarland EG, Kim TK, Park HB, Neira CA, Gutierrez MI. The effect of variation in definition on the diagnosis of multidirectional instability of the shoulder. *J Bone Joint Surg Am.* 2003;85-A(11):2138-2144.

149. Struyf F, Nijs J, Baeyens JP, Mottram S, Meeusen R. Scapular positioning and movement in unimpaired shoulders, shoulder impingement syndrome, and glenohumeral instability. *Scand J Med Sci Spor.* 2011;21(3):352-358.

150. Singh JA, Sperling J, Buchbinder R, McMaken K. Surgery for shoulder osteoarthritis: A Cochrane systematic review. *J Rheumatol.* 2011;38(4):598-605.

151. Izquierdo R, Voloshin I, Edwards S, et al. Treatment of glenohumeral osteoarthritis. *J Am Acad Orthop Sur.* 2010;18(6):375-382.

152. Kellgren JH, Lawrence JS. Radiological assessment of osteo-arthrosis. *Ann Rheum Dis.* 1957;16(4):494-502.

153. Kasten P, Maier M, Wendy P, et al. Can shoulder arthroplasty restore the range of motion in activities of daily living? A prospective 3D video motion analysis study. *J Shoulder Elb Surg.* 2010;19(2)(suppl):59-65.

154. Anakwenze OA, Hsu JE, Kim JS, Abboud JA. Acromioclavicular joint pain in patients with adhesive capsulitis: A prospective outcome study. *Orthopedics.* 2011;34(9):e556-e560.

155. Pennington RG, Bottomley NJ, Neen D, Brownlow HC. Radiological features of osteoarthritis of the acromiclavicular joint and its association with clinical symptoms. *J Orthop Surg (Hong Kong).* 2008;16(3):300-302.

156. Heers G, Hedtmann A. Correlation of ultrasonographic findings to Tossy's and Rockwood's classification of acromioclavicular joint injuries. *Ultrasound Med Biol.* 2005;31(6):725-732.

157. Kibler WB, McMullen J. Scapular dyskinesis and its relation to shoulder pain. *J Am Acad Orthop Surg.* 2003;11(2):142-151.

158. Struyf F, Nijs J, Mottram S, Roussel NA, Cools AM, Meeusen R. Clinical assessment of the scapula: A review of the literature. *Brit J Sport Med.* 2014;48(11):883-890.

159. Chen HS, Lin SH, Hsu YH, Chen SC, Kang JH. A comparison of physical examinations with musculoskeletal ultrasound in the diagnosis of biceps long head tendinitis. *Ultrasound Med Biol.* 2011;37(9):1392-1398.

Chapter 22

1. Webster BS, Snook SH. The cost of compensable upper extremity cumulative trauma disorders. *J Occup Med.* 1994;36(7):713-717.

2. Huisstede BM, Bierma-Zeinstra SM, Koes BW, Verhaar JA. Incidence and prevalence of upper-extremity musculoskeletal disorders. A systematic appraisal of the literature. *BMC Musculoskel Dis.* 2006;7:7.

3. Kryger AI, Lassen CF, Andersen JH. The role of physical examinations in studies of musculoskeletal disorders of the elbow. *Occup Environ Med.* 2007;64(11):776-781.

4. Van Roy P, Baeyens JP, Fauvart D, Lanssiers R, Clarijs JP. Arthro-kinematics of the elbow: Study of the carrying angle. *Ergonomics.* 2005;48(11-14):1645-1656.

5. Paraskevas G, Papadopoulos A, Papaziogas B, Spanidou S, Argiriadou H, Gigis J. Study of the carrying angle of the human elbow joint in full extension: A morphometric analysis. *Surg Radiol Anat.* 2004;26(1):19-23.

6. Martin S, Sanchez E. Anatomy and biomechanics of the elbow joint. *Semin Musculoskel R.* 2013;17(5):429-436.

7. Hariri S, Safran MR. Ulnar collateral ligament injury in the overhead athlete. *Clin Sports Med.* 2010;29(4):619-644. doi: 610.1016/j.csm.2010.1006.1007.

8. Cain EL Jr, Dugas JR, Wolf RS, Andrews JR. Elbow injuries in throwing athletes: A current concepts review. *Am J Sport Med.* 2003;31(4):621-635.

9. Galik K, Baratz ME, Butler AL, Dougherty J, Cohen MS, Miller MC. The effect of the annular ligament on kinematics of the radial head. *J Hand Surg Am.* 2007;32(8):1218-1224.

10. Giang GM. Epidemiology of work-related upper extremity disorders: Understanding prevalence and outcomes to impact provider performances using a practice management reporting tool. *Clin Occup Environ Med.* 2006;5(2):267-283, vi.

11. English CJ, Maclaren WM, Court-Brown C, et al. Relations between upper limb soft tissue disorders and repetitive movements at work. *Am J Ind Med.* 1995;27(1):75-90.

12. Feuerstein M, Miller VL, Burrell LM, Berger R. Occupational upper extremity disorders in the federal workforce. Prevalence, health care expenditures, and patterns of work disability. *J Occup Environ Med.* 1998;40(6):546-555.

13. Bongers PM, Kremer AM, ter Laak J. Are psychosocial factors, risk factors for symptoms and signs of the shoulder, elbow, or hand/wrist? A review of the epidemiological literature. *Am J Ind Med.* 2002;41(5):315-342.

14. Bergqvist U, Wolgast E, Nilsson B, Voss M. Musculoskeletal disorders among visual display terminal workers: Individual, ergonomic, and work organizational factors. *Ergonomics.* 1995;38(4):763-776.

15. Bernard B, Sauter S, Fine L, Petersen M, Hales T. Job task and psychosocial risk factors for work-related musculoskeletal disorders among newspaper employees. *Scand J Work Environ Health.* 1994;20(6):417-426.

16. Engstrom T, Hanse JJ, Kadefors R. Musculoskeletal symptoms due to technical preconditions in long cycle time work in an automobile assembly plant: A study of prevalence and relation to psychosocial factors and physical exposure. *Appl Ergon.* 1999;30(5):443-453.

17. Lagerstrom M, Wenemark M, Hagberg M, Hjelm EW. Occupational and individual factors related to musculoskeletal symptoms in five body regions among Swedish nursing personnel. *Int Arch Occup Environ Health.* 1995;68(1):27-35.

18. Novak CB, Lee GW, Mackinnon SE, Lay L. Provocative testing for cubital tunnel syndrome. *J Hand Surg Am.* 1994;19(5):817-820.

19. MacDermid JC, Michlovitz SL. Examination of the elbow: Linking diagnosis, prognosis, and outcomes as a framework for maximizing therapy interventions. *J Hand Ther.* 2006;19(2):82-97.

20. Crowther M. Elbow pain in pediatrics. *Curr Rev Musculoskelet Med.* 2009;2(2):83-87.

21. Rethnam U, Yesupalan RS, Bastawrous SS. Isolated radial head dislocation, a rare and easily missed injury in the presence of major distracting injuries: A case report. *J Med Case Rep.* 2007;1:38.

22. Tanaka S, Petersen M, Cameron L. Prevalence and risk factors of tendinitis and related disorders of the distal upper extremity among U.S. workers: Comparison to carpal tunnel syndrome. *Am J Ind Med.* 2001;39(3):328-335.

23. Bylak J, Hutchinson MR. Common sports injuries in young tennis players. *Sports Med.* 1998;26(2):119-132.

24. Field LD, Savoie FH. Common elbow injuries in sport. *Sports Med.* 1998;26(3):193-205.

25. Field LD, Altchek DW. Elbow injuries. *Clin Sports Med.* 1995;14(1):59-78.

26. Doornberg JN, Ring D. Coronoid fracture patterns. *J Hand Surg Am.* 2006;31(1):45-52.

27. Beaton DE, Katz JN, Fossel AH, Wright JG, Tarasuk V, Bombardier C. Measuring the whole or the parts? Validity, reliability, and responsiveness of the Disabilities of the Arm, Shoulder and Hand outcome measure in different regions of the upper extremity. *J Hand Ther.* 2001;14(2):128-146.

28. Hudak PL, Amadio PC, Bombardier C. Development of an upper extremity outcome measure: The DASH (disabilities of the arm, shoulder and hand) [corrected]. The Upper Extremity Collaborative Group (UECG). *Am J Ind Med.* 1996;29(6):602-608.

29. SooHoo NF, McDonald AP, Seiler JG III, McGillivary GR. Evaluation of the construct validity of the DASH questionnaire by correlation to the SF-36. *J Hand Surg Am.* 2002;27(3):537-541.

30. Jester A, Harth A, Germann G. Measuring levels of upper-extremity disability in employed adults using the DASH Questionnaire. *J Hand Surg Am.* 2005;30(5):1074.e1-1074.e10.

31. Gummesson C, Atroshi I, Ekdahl C. The disabilities of the arm, shoulder and hand (DASH) outcome questionnaire: Longitudinal construct validity and measuring self-rated health change after surgery. *BMC Musculoskel Dis.* 2003;4:11.

32. Beaton DE, Wright JG, Katz JN, Group UEC. Development of the QuickDASH: Comparison of three item-reduction approaches. *J Bone Joint Surg Am.* 2005;87(5):1038-1046.

33. Polson K, Reid D, McNair PJ, Larmer P. Responsiveness, minimal importance difference and minimal detectable change scores of the shortened disability arm shoulder hand (QuickDASH) questionnaire. *Manual Ther.* 2010;15(4):404-407.

34. Mintken PE, Glynn P, Cleland JA. Psychometric properties of the shortened disabilities of the Arm, Shoulder, and Hand Questionnaire (QuickDASH) and Numeric Pain Rating Scale in patients with shoulder pain. *J Shoulder Elb Surg.* 2009;18(6):920-926.

35. King GJ, Richards RR, Zuckerman JD, et al. A standardized method for assessment of elbow function. Research Committee, American Shoulder and Elbow Surgeons. *J Shoulder Elb Surg.* 1999;8(4):351-354.

36. Cook C, Hegedus E, Goode A, Mina C, Pietrobon R, Higgins LD. Relative validity of the modified American Shoulder and Elbow Surgeons (M-ASES) questionnaire using item response theory. *Rheumatol Int.* 2008;28(3):217-223.

37. Dawson J, Doll H, Boller I, et al. The development and validation of a patient-reported questionnaire to assess outcomes of elbow surgery. *J Bone Joint Surg Br.* 2008;90(4):466-473.

38. The B, Reininga IH, El Moumni M, Eygendaal D. Elbow-specific clinical rating systems: Extent of established validity, reliability, and responsiveness. *J Shoulder Elb Surg.* 2013;22(10):1380-1394.

39. de Haan J, Goei H, Schep NW, Tuinebreijer WE, Patka P, den Hartog D. The reliability, validity and responsiveness of the Dutch version of the Oxford elbow score. *J Orthop Surg Res.* 2011;6:39.

40. MacDermid JC. Outcome evaluation in patients with elbow pathology: Issues in instrument development and evaluation. *J Hand Ther.* 2001;14(2):105-114.

41. Macdermid J. Update: The Patient-Rated Forearm Evaluation Questionnaire is now the Patient-Rated Tennis Elbow Evaluation. *J Hand Ther.* 2005;18(4):407-410.

42. Shahabpour M, Kichouh M, Laridon E, Gielen JL, De Mey J. The effectiveness of diagnostic imaging methods for the assessment of soft tissue and articular disorders of the shoulder and elbow. *Eur J Radiol.* 2008;65(2):194-200.

43. Sasaki K, Tamakawa M, Onda K, et al. The detection of the capsular tear at the undersurface of the extensor carpi radialis brevis tendon in chronic tennis elbow: The value of magnetic resonance imaging and computed tomography arthrography. *J Shoulder Elb Surg.* 2011;20(3):420-425.

44. Brouwer KM, Lindenhovius AL, Dyer GS, Zurakowski D, Mudgal CS, Ring D. Diagnostic accuracy of 2- and 3-dimensional imaging and modeling of distal humerus fractures. *J Shoulder Elb Surg.* 2012;21(6):772-776.

45. Guitton TG, Kinaci A, Ring D. Diagnostic accuracy of 2- and 3-dimensional computed tomography and solid modeling of coronoid fractures. *J Shoulder Elb Surg.* 2013;22(6):782-786.

46. Doornberg JN, Guitton TG, Ring D. Diagnosis of elbow fracture patterns on radiographs: Interobserver reliability and diagnostic accuracy. *Clin Orthop Relat Res.* 2013;471(4):1373-1378.

47. Rabiner JE, Khine H, Avner JR, Friedman LM, Tsung JW. Accuracy of point-of-care ultrasonography for diagnosis of elbow fractures in children. *Ann Emerg Med.* 2013;61(1):9-17.

48. Timmerman LA, Schwartz ML, Andrews JR. Preoperative evaluation of the ulnar collateral ligament by magnetic resonance imaging and computed tomography arthrography. Evaluation in 25 baseball players with surgical confirmation. *Am J Sport Med.* 1994;22(1):26-31, discussion 32.

49. Thompson WH, Jobe FW, Yocum LA, Pink MM. Ulnar collateral ligament reconstruction in athletes: Muscle-splitting approach without transposition of the ulnar nerve. *J Shoulder Elb Surg.* 2001;10(2):152-157.

50. Iwasaki N, Kamishima T, Kato H, Funakoshi T, Minami A. A retrospective evaluation of magnetic resonance imaging effectiveness on capitellar osteochondritis dissecans among overhead athletes. *Am J Sport Med.* 2012;40(3):624-630.

51. Obradov M, Anderson PG. Ultra sonographic findings for chronic lateral epicondylitis. *JBR-BTR.* 2012;95(2):66-70.

52. Lee MH, Cha JG, Jin W, et al. Utility of sonographic measurement of the common tensor tendon in patients with lateral epicondylitis. *Am J Roentgenol.* 2011;196(6):1363-1367.

53. Park GY, Lee SM, Lee MY. Diagnostic value of ultrasonography for clinical medial epicondylitis. *Arch Phys Med Rehab.* 2008;89(4):738-742.

54. Festa A, Mulieri PJ, Newman JS, Spitz DJ, Leslie BM. Effectiveness of magnetic resonance imaging in detecting partial and complete distal biceps tendon rupture. *J Hand Surg Am.* 2010;35(1):77-83.

55. Lobo Lda G, Fessell DP, Miller BS, et al. The role of sonography in differentiating full versus partial distal biceps tendon tears: Correlation with surgical findings. *Am J Roentgenol.* 2013;200(1):158-162.

56. O'Driscoll SW, Goncalves LB, Dietz P. The hook test for distal biceps tendon avulsion. *Am J Sport Med.* 2007;35(11):1865-1869.

57. Bayrak AO, Bayrak IK, Turker H, Elmali M, Nural MS. Ultrasonography in patients with ulnar neuropathy at the elbow: Comparison of cross-sectional area and swelling ratio with electrophysiological severity. *Muscle Nerve.* 2010;41(5):661-666.

58. Pompe SM, Beekman R. Which ultrasonographic measure has the upper hand in ulnar neuropathy at the elbow? *Clin Neurophysiol.* 2013;124(1):190-196.

59. Baumer P, Dombert T, Staub F, et al. Ulnar neuropathy at the elbow: MR neurography—nerve T2 signal increase and caliber. *Radiology.* 2011;260(1):199-206.

60. Ramponi DR, Kaufmann JA. Elbow injuries and fractures. *Adv Emerg Nurs J.* 2012;34(2):99-109, quiz 110-101.

61. Rettig LA, Hastings H II, Feinberg JR. Primary osteoarthritis of the elbow: Lack of radiographic evidence for morphologic predisposition, results of operative debridement at intermediate follow-up, and basis for a new radiographic classification system. *J Shoulder Elb Surg.* 2008;17(1):97-105.

62. Draghi F, Danesino GM, de Gautard R, Bianchi S. Ultrasound of the elbow: Examination techniques and US appearance of the normal and pathologic joint. *J Ultrasound.* 2007;10(2):76-84.

63. Bodor M, Fullerton B. Ultrasonography of the hand, wrist, and elbow. *Phys Med Rehabil Cli.* 2010;21(3):509-531.

64. Radunovic G, Vlad V, Micu MC, et al. Ultrasound assessment of the elbow. *Med Ultrason.* 2012;14(2):141-146.

65. Miller TT, Shapiro MA, Schultz E, Kalish PE. Comparison of sonography and MRI for diagnosing epicondylitis. *J Clin Ultrasound.* 2002;30(4):193-202.

66. Thoirs K, Williams MA, Phillips M. Ultrasonographic measurements of the ulnar nerve at the elbow: Role of confounders. *J Ultrasound Med.* 2008;27(5):737-743.

67. Volpe A, Rossato G, Bottanelli M, et al. Ultrasound evaluation of ulnar neuropathy at the elbow: Correlation with electrophysiological studies. *Rheumatology (Oxford).* 2009;48(9):1098-1101.

68. Wiesler ER, Chloros GD, Cartwright MS, Shin HW, Walker FO. Ultrasound in the diagnosis of ulnar neuropathy at the cubital tunnel. *J Hand Surg Am.* 2006;31(7):1088-1093.

69. Papatheodorou LK, Baratz ME, Sotereanos DG. Elbow arthritis: Current concepts. *J Hand Surg Am.* 2013;38(3):605-613.

70. Harvey C. Compartment syndrome: When it is least expected. *Orthop Nurs.* 2001;20(3):15-23, quiz 24-26.

71. Jawed S, Jawad AS, Padhiar N, Perry JD. Chronic exertional compartment syndrome of the forearms secondary to weight training. *Rheumatology (Oxford).* 2001;40(3):344-345.

72. Major NM, Crawford ST. Elbow effusions in trauma in adults and children: Is there an occult fracture? *Am J Roentgenol.* 2002;178(2):413-418.

73. Moore MB. The use of a tuning fork and stethoscope to identify fractures. *J Athl Train.* 2009;44(3):272-274.

74. Adams SL, Yarnold PR. Clinical use of the patellar-pubic percussion sign in hip trauma. *Am J Emerg Med.* 1997;15(2):173-175.

75. Adams SL, Yarnold PR, Mathews JJ IV. Clinical use of the olecranon-manubrium percussion sign in shoulder trauma. *Ann Emerg Med.* 1988;17(5):484-487.

76. Appelboam A, Reuben AD, Benger JR, et al. Elbow extension test to rule out elbow fracture: Multicentre, prospective validation and observational study of diagnostic accuracy in adults and children. *BMJ.* 2008;337:a2428.(doi):10.1136/bmj.a2428.

77. Bushnell BD, Creighton RA, Herring MM. The bony apprehension test for instability of the shoulder: A prospective pilot analysis. *Arthroscopy.* 2008;24(9):974-982.

78. Docherty MA, Schwab RA, Ma OJ. Can elbow extension be used as a test of clinically significant injury? *South Med J.* 2002;95(5):539-541.

79. Darracq MA, Vinson DR, Panacek EA. Preservation of active range of motion after acute elbow trauma predicts absence of elbow fracture. *Am J Emerg Med.* 2008;26(7):779-782. doi: 710.1016/j.ajem.2007.1011.1005.

80. Yung E, Asavasopon S, Godges JJ. Screening for head, neck, and shoulder pathology in patients with upper extremity signs and symptoms. *J Hand Ther.* 2010;23(2):173-185, quiz 186.

81. Shah KC, Rajshekhar V. Reliability of diagnosis of soft cervical disc prolapse using Spurling's test. *Brit J Neurosurg.* 2004;18(5):480-483.

82. Wainner RS, Fritz JM, Irrgang JJ, Boninger ML, Delitto A, Allison S. Reliability and diagnostic accuracy of the clinical examination and patient self-report measures for cervical radiculopathy. *Spine (Phila Pa 1976).* 2003;28(1):52-62.

83. Gumina S, Carbone S, Albino P, Gurzi M, Postacchini F. Arm Squeeze Test: A new clinical test to distinguish neck from shoulder pain. *Eur Spine J.* 2013;22(7):1558-1563.

84. Alqunaee M, Galvin R, Fahey T. Diagnostic accuracy of clinical tests for subacromial impingement syndrome: A systematic review and meta-analysis. *Arch Phys Med Rehab.* 2012;93(2):229-236.

85. Hegedus EJ, Goode AP, Cook CE, et al. Which physical examination tests provide clinicians with the most value when examining the shoulder? Update of a systematic review with meta-analysis of individual tests. *Brit J Sport Med.* 2012;46(14):964-978.

86. Boone DC, Azen SP. Normal range of motion of joints in male subjects. *J Bone Joint Surg Am.* 1979;61(5):756-759.

87. Soucie JM, Wang C, Forsyth A, et al. Range of motion measurements: Reference values and a database for comparison studies. *Haemophilia.* 2011;17(3):500-507.

88. Blonna D, Zarkadas PC, Fitzsimmons JS, O'Driscoll SW. Accuracy and inter-observer reliability of visual estimation compared to clinical goniometry of the elbow. *Knee Surg Sport Tr A.* 2012;20(7):1378-1385.

89. Yilmaz E, Karakurt L, Belhan O, Bulut M, Serin E, Avci M. Variation of carrying angle with age, sex, and special reference to side. *Orthopedics.* 2005;28(11):1360-1363.

90. Chapleau J, Canet F, Petit Y, Laflamme GY, Rouleau DM. Validity of goniometric elbow measurements: Comparative study with a radiographic method. *Clin Orthop Relat Res.* 2011;469(11):3134-3140.

91. Cozen L. The painful elbow. *Ind Med Surg.* 1962;31:369-371.

92. Fairbank SM, Corlett RJ. The role of the extensor digitorum communis muscle in lateral epicondylitis. *J Hand Surg Br.* 2002;27(5):405-409.

93. Ruland RT, Dunbar RP, Bowen JD. The biceps squeeze test for diagnosis of distal biceps tendon ruptures. *Clin Orthop Relat R.* 2005; 437:128-131.

94. ElMaraghy A, Devereaux M. The "bicipital aponeurosis flex test": Eevaluating the integrity of the bicipital aponeurosis and its implications for treatment of distal biceps tendon ruptures. *J Shoulder Elb Surg.* 2013;22(7):908-914.

95. Devereaux MW, ElMaraghy AW. Improving the rapid and reliable diagnosis of complete distal biceps tendon rupture: A nuanced approach to the clinical examination. *Am J Sports Med.* 2013;41(9):1998-2004.

96. ElMaraghy A, Devereaux M, Tsoi K. The biceps crease interval for diagnosing complete distal biceps tendon ruptures. *Clin Orthop Relat R.* 2008;466(9):2255-2262.

97. O'Driscoll SW, Lawton RL, Smith AM. The "moving valgus stress test" for medial collateral ligament tears of the elbow. *Am J Sport Med.* 2005;33(2):231-239.

98. Regan W, Lapner PC. Prospective evaluation of two diagnostic apprehension signs for posterolateral instability of the elbow. *J Shoulder Elb Surg.* 2006;15(3):344-346.

99. O'Driscoll SW, Bell DF, Morrey BF. Posterolateral rotatory instability of the elbow. *J Bone Joint Surg Am.* 1991;73(3):440-446.

100. O'Driscoll SW, Jupiter JB, King GJ, Hotchkiss RN, Morrey BF. The unstable elbow. *Instr Course Lect.* 2001;50:89-102.

101. Anakwenze OA, Kancherla VK, Iyengar J, Ahmad CS, Levine WN. Posterolateral rotatory instability of the elbow. *Am J Sport Med.* 2014;42(2):485-491.

102. Arvind CH, Hargreaves DG. Table top relocation test—New clinical test for posterolateral rotatory instability of the elbow. *J Shoulder Elb Surg.* 2006;15(4):500-501.

103. Azam MQ, Iraqi AA, Syed A, Abbas M. Posterolateral rotatory instability of elbow: An uncommon entity. *Indian J Orthop.* 2008;42(3):355-356.

104. Cheng CJ, Mackinnon-Patterson B, Beck JL, Mackinnon SE. Scratch collapse test for evaluation of carpal and cubital tunnel syndrome. *J Hand Surg Am.* 2008;33(9):1518-1524.

105. Beekman R, Schreuder AH, Rozeman CA, Koehler PJ, Uitdehaag BM. The diagnostic value of provocative clinical tests in ulnar neuropathy at the elbow is marginal. *J Neurol Neurosur Ps.* 2009;80(12):1369-1374.

106. Buehler MJ, Thayer DT. The elbow flexion test. A clinical test for the cubital tunnel syndrome. *Clin Orthop Relat R.* 1988;233:213-216.

107. Rayan GM, Jensen C, Duke J. Elbow flexion test in the normal population. *J Hand Surg Am.* 1992;17(1):86-89.

108. Paoloni JA, Appleyard RC, Murrell GA. The Orthopaedic Research Institute-Tennis Elbow Testing System: A modified chair pick-up test-interrater and intrarater reliability testing and validity for monitoring lateral epicondylosis. *J Shoulder Elb Surg.* 2004;13(1):72-77.

109. Herd CR, Meserve BB. A systematic review of the effectiveness of manipulative therapy in treating lateral epicondylalgia. *J Man Manip Ther.* 2008;16(4):225-237.

110. Shiri R, Viikari-Juntura E. Lateral and medial epicondylitis: Role of occupational factors. *Best Pract Res Clin Rheumatol.* 2011;25(1):43-57.

111. Wilson JJ, Best TM. Common overuse tendon problems: A review and recommendations for treatment. *Am Fam Physician.* 2005;72(5):811-818.

112. Shukla DR, Morrey BF, Thoreson AR, An KN, O'Driscoll SW. Distal biceps tendon rupture: An in vitro study. *Clin Biomech (Bristol, Avon).* 2012;27(3):263-267.

113. Seiler JG III, Parker LM, Chamberland PD, Sherbourne GM, Carpenter WA. The distal biceps tendon. Two potential mechanisms involved in its rupture: Arterial supply and mechanical impingement. *J Shoulder Elb Surg.* 1995;4(3):149-156.

114. Konin GP, Nazarian LN, Walz DM. US of the elbow: Indications, technique, normal anatomy, and pathologic conditions. *Radiographics.* 2013;33(4):E125-E147.

115. Bernstein AD, Breslow MJ, Jazrawi LM. Distal biceps tendon ruptures: A historical perspective and current concepts. *Am J Orthop (Belle Mead, NJ).* 2001;30(3):193-200.

116. Quach T, Jazayeri R, Sherman OH, Rosen JE. Distal biceps tendon injuries—Current treatment options. *Bull NYU Hosp Jt Dis.* 2010;68(2):103-111.

117. Nesterenko S, Domire ZJ, Morrey BF, Sanchez-Sotelo J. Elbow strength and endurance in patients with a ruptured distal biceps tendon. *J Shoulder Elb Surg.* 2010;19(2):184-189.

118. Kuhn MA, Ross G. Acute elbow dislocations. *Orthop Clin N Am.* 2008;39(2):155-161, v.

119. Chang CW, Wang YC, Chu CH. Increased carrying angle is a risk factor for nontraumatic ulnar neuropathy at the elbow. *Clin Orthop Relat R.* 2008;466(9):2190-2195.

120. Bozentka DJ. Cubital tunnel syndrome pathophysiology. *Clin Orthop Relat R.* 1998(351):90-94.

121. Gruber H, Glodny B, Peer S. The validity of ultrasonographic assessment in cubital tunnel syndrome: The value of a cubital-to-humeral nerve area ratio (CHR) combined with morphologic features. *Ultrasound Med Biol.* 2010;36(3):376-382.

122. Wong AS, Baratz ME. Elbow fractures: Distal humerus. *J Hand Surg Am.* 2009;34(1):176-190.

123. Lamprakis A, Vlasis K, Siampou E, Grammatikopoulos I, Lionis C. Can elbow-extension test be used as an alternative to radiographs in primary care? *Eur J Gen Pract.* 2007;13(4):221-224.

124. Nauth A, McKee MD, Ristevski B, Hall J, Schemitsch EH. Distal humeral fractures in adults. *J Bone Joint Surg Am.* 2011;93(7):686-700.

125. Brouwer KM, Bolmers A, Ring D. Quantitative 3-dimensional computed tomography measurement of distal humerus fractures. *J Shoulder Elb Surg.* 2012;21(7):977-982.

126. Tashjian RZ, Katarincic JA. Complex elbow instability. *J Am Acad Orthop Surg.* 2006;14(5):278-286.

127. Dodds SD, Yeh PC, Slade JF III. Essex-Lopresti injuries. *Hand Clin.* 2008;24(1):125-137.

128. Zeiders GJ, Patel MK. Management of unstable elbows following complex fracture-dislocations—the "terrible triad" injury. *J Bone Joint Surg Am.* 2008;90(suppl 4):75-84.

129. Fern SE, Owen JR, Ordyna NJ, Wayne JS, Boardman ND III. Complex varus elbow instability: A terrible triad model. *J Shoulder Elb Surg.* 2009;18(2):269-274.

130. Lee AT, Daluiski A. Osteoarthritis of the elbow. *J Hand Surg Am.* 2012;37(1):148-150.

131. Kokkalis ZT, Schmidt CC, Sotereanos DG. Elbow arthritis: Current concepts. *J Hand Surg Am.* 2009;34(4):761-768.

132. Kellgren JH, Lawrence JS. Radiological assessment of osteo-arthrosis. *Ann Rheum Dis.* 1957;16(4):494-502.

133. Mosshammer D, Hlobil H, Joos S, Reichert W. A patient with Lyme arthritis presenting in general practice. *Practitioner.* 2013;257(1758):25-27.

Chapter 23

1. Rettig AC. Epidemiology of hand and wrist injuries in sports. *Clin Sports Med.* 1998;17(3):401-406.

2. Barr AE, Barbe MF, Clark BD. Work-related musculoskeletal disorders of the hand and wrist: Epidemiology, pathophysiology, and sensorimotor changes. *J Orthop Sport Phys.* 2004;34(10):610-627.

3. Kiuru MJ, Haapamaki VV, Koivikko MP, Koskinen SK. Wrist injuries: Diagnosis with multidetector CT. *Emerg Radiol.* 2004;10(4):182-185.

4. Owen RA, Melton LJ, Johnson KA, Ilstrup DM, Riggs BL. Incidence of Colles' fracture in a North American community. *Am J Public Health.* 1982;72(6):605-607.

5. Phillips TG, Reibach AM, Slomiany WP. Diagnosis and management of scaphoid fractures. *Am Fam Physician.* 2004;70(5):879-884.

6. Ranney D, Wells R, Moore A. Upper limb musculoskeletal disorders in highly repetitive industries: Precise anatomical physical findings. *Ergonomics.* 1995;38(7):1408-1423.

7. Latko WA, Armstrong TJ, Franzblau A, Ulin SS, Werner RA, Albers JW. Cross-sectional study of the relationship between repetitive work and the prevalence of upper limb musculoskeletal disorders. *Am J Ind Med.* 1999;36(2):248-259.

8. Heijne A, Werner S. Early versus late start of open kinetic chain quadriceps exercises after ACL reconstruction with patellar tendon or hamstring grafts: A prospective randomized outcome study. *Knee Surg Sport Tr A.* 2007;15(4):402-414.

9. Werner RA, Hamann C, Franzblau A, Rodgers PA. Prevalence of carpal tunnel syndrome and upper extremity tendinitis among dental hygienists. *J Dent Hyg.* 2002;76(2):126-132.

10. Katz JN, Larson MG, Sabra A, et al. The carpal tunnel syndrome: Diagnostic utility of the history and physical examination findings. *Ann Intern Med.* 1990;112(5):321-327.

11. Gunnarsson LG, Amilon A, Hellstrand P, Leissner P, Philipson L. The diagnosis of carpal tunnel syndrome. Sensitivity and specificity of some clinical and electrophysiological tests. *J Hand Surg Br.* 1997;22(1):34-37.

12. Hudak PL, Amadio PC, Bombardier C. Development of an upper extremity outcome measure: The DASH (disabilities of the arm, shoulder and hand) [corrected]. The Upper Extremity Collaborative Group (UECG). *Am J Ind Med.* 1996;29(6):602-608.

13. Beaton DE, Wright JG, Katz JN, Group UEC. Development of the QuickDASH: Comparison of three item-reduction approaches. *J Bone Joint Surg Am.* 2005;87(5):1038-1046.

14. Changulani M, Okonkwo U, Keswani T, Kalairajah Y. Outcome evaluation measures for wrist and hand: Which one to choose? *Int Orthop.* 2008;32(1):1-6.

15. Beaton DE, Katz JN, Fossel AH, Wright JG, Tarasuk V, Bombardier C. Measuring the whole or the parts? Validity, reliability, and responsiveness of the Disabilities of the Arm, Shoulder and Hand outcome measure in different regions of the upper extremity. *J Hand Ther.* 2001;14(2):128-146.

16. Roy JS, MacDermid JC, Woodhouse LJ. Measuring shoulder function: A systematic review of four questionnaires. *Arthritis Rheum.* 2009;61(5):623-632.

17. Gummesson C, Ward MM, Atroshi I. The shortened disabilities of the arm, shoulder and hand questionnaire (QuickDASH): Validity and reliability based on responses within the full-length DASH. *BMC Musculoskel Dis.* 2006;7:44.

18. MacDermid JC, Richards RS, Donner A, Bellamy N, Roth JH. Responsiveness of the short form-36, disability of the arm, shoulder, and hand questionnaire, patient-rated wrist evaluation, and physical impairment measurements in evaluating recovery after a distal radius fracture. *J Hand Surg Am.* 2000;25(2):330-340.

19. MacDermid JC, Tottenham V. Responsiveness of the disability of the arm, shoulder, and hand (DASH) and patient-rated wrist/hand evaluation (PRWHE) in evaluating change after hand therapy. *J Hand Ther.* 2004;17(1):18-23.

20. Schmitt JS, Di Fabio RP. Reliable change and minimum important difference (MID) proportions facilitated group responsiveness comparisons using individual threshold criteria. *J Clin Epidemiol.* 2004;57(10):1008-1018.

21. Sartorio F, Bravini E, Vercelli S, et al. The Functional Dexterity Test: Test-retest reliability analysis and up-to date reference norms. *J Hand Ther.* 2013;26(1):62-67, quiz 68.

22. Sorensen AA, Howard D, Tan WH, Ketchersid J, Calfee RP. Minimal clinically important differences of 3 patient-rated outcomes instruments. *J Hand Surg Am.* 2013;38(4):641-649.

23. Polson K, Reid D, McNair PJ, Larmer P. Responsiveness, minimal importance difference and minimal detectable change scores of the shortened disability arm shoulder hand (QuickDASH) questionnaire. *Manual Ther.* 2010;15(4):404-407.

24. Franchignoni F, Vercelli S, Giordano A, Sartorio F, Bravini E, Ferriero G. Minimal clinically important difference of the disabilities of the Arm, Shoulder and Hand outcome measure (DASH) and its shortened version (QuickDASH). *J Orthop Sport Phys.* 2014;44(1):30-39.

25. Mintken PE, Glynn P, Cleland JA. Psychometric properties of the shortened disabilities of the Arm, Shoulder, and Hand Questionnaire (QuickDASH) and Numeric Pain Rating Scale in patients with shoulder pain. *J Shoulder Elb Surg.* 2009;18(6):920-926.

26. Stratford P, Gill C, Westaway M, Binkley J. Assessing disability and change on individual patients: A report on a patient specific measure. *Physiother Can.* 1995;47(5):258-263.

27. Hefford C, Abbott JH, Arnold R, Baxter GD. The patient-specific functional scale: Validity, reliability, and responsiveness in patients with upper extremity musculoskeletal problems. *J Orthop Sport Phys.* 2012;42(2):56-65.

28. Levine DW, Simmons BP, Koris MJ, et al. A self-administered questionnaire for the assessment of severity of symptoms and functional status in carpal tunnel syndrome. *J Bone Joint Surg Am.* 1993;75(11):1585-1592.

29. Katz JN, Gelberman RH, Wright EA, Lew RA, Liang MH. Responsiveness of self-reported and objective measures of disease severity in carpal tunnel syndrome. *Med Care.* 1994;32(11):1127-1133.

30. Ozyürekoğlu T, McCabe SJ, Goldsmith LJ, LaJoie AS. The minimal clinically important difference of the Carpal Tunnel Syndrome Symptom Severity Scale. *J Hand Surg Am.* 2006;31(5):733-738, discussion 739-740.

31. Kim JK, Jeon SH. Minimal clinically important differences in the Carpal Tunnel Questionnaire after carpal tunnel release. *J Hand Surg Eur Vol.* 2013;38(1):75-79.

32. MacDermid JC, Turgeon T, Richards RS, Beadle M, Roth JH. Patient rating of wrist pain and disability: A reliable and valid measurement tool. *J Orthop Trauma.* 1998;12(8):577-586.

33. MacDermid JC, Wessel J, Humphrey R, Ross D, Roth JH. Validity of self-report measures of pain and disability for persons who have undergone arthroplasty for osteoarthritis of the carpometacarpal joint of the hand. *Osteoarthr Cartilage.* 2007;15(5):524-530.

34. Gartland GJ Jr, Werley CW. Evaluation of a healed Colles' fracture. *J Bone Joint Surg.* 1951;33:895-907.

35. Menashe L, Hirko K, Losina E, et al. The diagnostic performance of MRI in osteoarthritis: A systematic review and meta-analysis. *Osteoarthr Cartilage.* 2012;20(1):13-21.

36. Deniz FE, Oksuz E, Sarikaya B, et al. Comparison of the diagnostic utility of electromyography, ultrasonography, computed tomography, and magnetic resonance imaging in idiopathic carpal tunnel syndrome determined by clinical findings. *Neurosurgery.* 2012;70(3):610-616.

37. Tai TW, Wu CY, Su FC, Chern TC, Jou IM. Ultrasonography for diagnosing carpal tunnel syndrome: A meta-analysis of diagnostic test accuracy. *Ultrasound Med Biol.* 2012;38(7):1121-1128.

38. Fowler JR, Gaughan JP, Ilyas AM. The sensitivity and specificity of ultrasound for the diagnosis of carpal tunnel syndrome: A meta-analysis. *Clin Orthop Relat R.* 2011;469(4):1089-1094.

39. Descatha A, Huard L, Aubert F, Barbato B, Gorand O, Chastang JF. Meta-analysis on the performance of sonography for the diagnosis of carpal tunnel syndrome. *Semin Arthritis Rheu.* 2012;41(6):914-922.

40. Abe A, Ishikawa H, Murasawa A, Nakazono K. Extensor tendon rupture and three-dimensional computed tomography imaging of the rheumatoid wrist. *Skeletal Radiol.* 2010;39(4):325-331.

41. Heo YM, Roh JY, Kim SB, et al. Evaluation of the sigmoid notch involvement in the intra-articular distal radius fractures: The efficacy of computed tomography compared with plain X-ray. *Clin Orthop Surg.* 2012;4(1):83-90.

42. Smith TO, Drew B, Toms AP, Jerosch-Herold C, Chojnowski AJ. Diagnostic accuracy of magnetic resonance imaging and magnetic resonance arthrography for triangular fibrocartilaginous complex injury: A systematic review and meta-analysis. *J Bone Joint Surg.* 2012;94(9):824-832.

43. Hobby JL, Tom BD, Bearcroft PW, Dixon AK. Magnetic resonance imaging of the wrist: Diagnostic performance statistics. *Clin Radiol.* 2001;56(1):50-57.

44. Potter HG, Asnis-Ernberg L, Weiland AJ, Hotchkiss RN, Peterson MG, McCormack RR. The utility of high-resolution magnetic resonance imaging in the evaluation of the triangular fibrocartilage complex of the wrist. *J Bone Joint Surg Am.* 1997;79(11):1675-1684.

45. Smith TO, Drew BT, Toms AP, Chojnowski AJ. The diagnostic accuracy of X-ray arthrography for triangular fibrocartilaginous complex injury: A systematic review and meta-analysis. *J Hand Surg Eur Vol.* 2012;37(9):879-887.

46. Yin ZG, Zhang JB, Kan SL, Wang XG. Diagnosing suspected scaphoid fractures: A systematic review and meta-analysis. *Clin Orthop Relat R.* 2010;468(3):723-734.

47. Vrettos BC, Adams BK, Knottenbelt JD, Lee A. Is there a place for radionuclide bone scintigraphy in the management of radiograph-negative scaphoid trauma? *S Afr Med J.* 1996;86(5):540-542.

48. Smith M, Bain GI, Turner PC, Watts AC. Review of imaging of scaphoid fractures. *ANZ J Surg.* 2010;80(1-2):82-90.

49. Gaebler C, Kukla C, Breitenseher M, Trattnig S, Mittlboeck M, Vécsei V. Magnetic resonance imaging of occult scaphoid fractures. *J Trauma.* 1996;41(1):73-76.

50. Buijze GA, Jørgsholm P, Thomsen NO, Bjorkman A, Besjakov J, Ring D. Diagnostic performance of radiographs and computed tomography for displacement and instability of acute scaphoid waist fractures. *J Bone Joint Surg Am.* 2012;94(21):1967-1974.

51. Adey L, Souer JS, Lozano-Calderon S, Palmer W, Lee SG, Ring D. Computed tomography of suspected scaphoid fractures. *J Hand Surg Am.* 2007;32(1):61-66.

52. Cruickshank J, Meakin A, Breadmore R, et al. Early computerized tomography accurately determines the presence or absence of scaphoid and other fractures. *Emerg Med Australas.* 2007;19(3):223-228.

53. Metz VM, Gilula LA. Imaging techniques for distal radius fractures and related injuries. *Orthop Clin N Am.* 1993;24(2):217-228.

54. Jarvik JG, Yuen E, Kliot M. Diagnosis of carpal tunnel syndrome: Electrodiagnostic and MR imaging evaluation. *Neuroimag Clin N Am.* 2004;14(1):93-102, viii.

55. Zaidman CM, Seelig MJ, Baker JC, Mackinnon SE, Pestronk A. Detection of peripheral nerve pathology: Comparison of ultrasound and MRI. *Neurology.* 2013;80(18):1634-1640.

56. Yazdchi M, Tarzemani MK, Mikaeili H, Ayromlu H, Ebadi H. Sensitivity and specificity of median nerve ultrasonography in diagnosis of carpal tunnel syndrome. *Int J Gen Med.* 2012;5:99-103.

57. Bodor M, Fullerton B. Ultrasonography of the hand, wrist, and elbow. *Phys Med Rehabil Cli.* 2010;21(3):509-531.

58. Daniels JM, Zook EG, Lynch JM. Hand and wrist injuries: Part I. Nonemergent evaluation. *Am Fam Physician.* 2004;69(8):1941-1948.

59. Jiang SD, Jiang LS, Dai LY. Cervical spondylotic amyotrophy. *Eur Spine J.* 2011;20(3):351-357.

60. Leard JS, Breglio L, Fraga L, et al. Reliability and concurrent validity of the figure-of-eight method of measuring hand size in patients with hand pathology. *J Orthop Sport Phys.* 2004;34(6):335-340.

61. Moore MB. The use of a tuning fork and stethoscope to identify fractures. *J Athl Train.* 2009;44(3):272-274.

62. Cevik AA, Gunal I, Manisali M, et al. Evaluation of physical findings in acute wrist trauma in the emergency department. *Ulus Travma Acil Cerrahi Derg.* 2003;9(4):257-261.

63. Pershad J, Monroe K, King W, Bartle S, Hardin E, Zinkan L. Can clinical parameters predict fractures in acute pediatric wrist injuries? *Acad Emerg Med.* 2000;7(10):1152-1155.

64. Yung E, Asavasopon S, Godges JJ. Screening for head, neck, and shoulder pathology in patients with upper extremity signs and symptoms. *J Hand Ther.* 2010;23(2):173-185, quiz 186.

65. Shah KC, Rajshekhar V. Reliability of diagnosis of soft cervical disc prolapse using Spurling's test. *Brit J Neurosurg.* 2004;18(5):480-483.

66. Wainner RS, Fritz JM, Irrgang JJ, Boninger ML, Delitto A, Allison S. Reliability and diagnostic accuracy of the clinical examination and patient self-report measures for cervical radiculopathy. *Spine (Phila Pa 1976).* 2003;28(1):52-62.

67. Gumina S, Carbone S, Albino P, Gurzi M, Postacchini F. Arm Squeeze Test: A new clinical test to distinguish neck from shoulder pain. *Eur Spine J.* 2013;22(7):1558-1563.

68. Alqunaee M, Galvin R, Fahey T. Diagnostic accuracy of clinical tests for subacromial impingement syndrome: A systematic review and meta-analysis. *Arch Phys Med Rehab.* 2012;93(2):229-236.

69. Hegedus EJ, Goode AP, Cook CE, et al. Which physical examination tests provide clinicians with the most value when examining the shoulder? Update of a systematic review with meta-analysis of individual tests. *Brit J Sport Med.* 2012;46(14):964-978.

70. Docherty MA, Schwab RA, Ma OJ. Can elbow extension be used as a test of clinically significant injury? *South Med J.* 2002;95(5):539-541.

71. Darracq MA, Vinson DR, Panacek EA. Preservation of active range of motion after acute elbow trauma predicts absence of elbow fracture. *Am J Emerg Med.* 2008;26(7):779-782. doi: 710.1016/j.ajem.2007.1011.1005.

72. van de Pol RJ, van Trijffel E, Lucas C. Inter-rater reliability for measurement of passive physiological range of motion of upper extremity joints is better if instruments are used: A systematic review. *J Physiother.* 2010;56(1):7-17.

73. Carter TI, Pansy B, Wolff AL, et al. Accuracy and reliability of three different techniques for manual goniometry for wrist motion: A cadaveric study. *J Hand Surg Am.* 2009;34(8):1422-1428.

74. Ellis B, Bruton A. A study to compare the reliability of composite finger flexion with goniometry for measurement of range of motion in the hand. *Clin Rehabil.* 2002;16(5):562-570.

75. Groth GN, VanDeven KM, Phillips EC, Ehretsman RL. Goniometry of the proximal and distal interphalangeal joints, part II: Placement prefereces, interrater reliability, and concurrent validity. *J Hand Ther.* 2001;14(1):23-29.

76. LaStayo PC, Wheeler DL. Reliability of passive wrist flexion and extension goniometric measurements: A multicenter study. *Phys Ther.* 1994;74(2):162-174, discussion 174-166.

77. Horger MM. The reliability of goniometric measurements of active and passive wrist motions. *Am J Occup Ther.* 1990;44(4):342-348.

78. Brown A, Cramer LD, Eckhaus D, Schmidt J, Ware L, MacKenzie E. Validity and reliability of the Dexter hand evaluation and therapy system in hand-injured patients. *J Hand Ther.* 2000;13(1):37-45.

79. Adams BD, Grosland NM, Murphy DM, McCullough M. Impact of impaired wrist motion on hand and upper-extremity performance (1). *J Hand Surg Am.* 2003;28(6):898-903.

80. Staes FF, Banks KJ, De Smet L, Daniels KJ, Carels P. Reliability of accessory motion testing at the carpal joints. *Manual Ther.* 2009;14(3):292-298.

81. Wadsworth C, Nielsen DH, Corcoran DS, Phillips CE, Sannes TL. Interrater reliability of hand-held dynamometry: Effects of rater gender, body weight, and grip strength. *J Orthop Sport Phys.* 1992;16(2):74-81.

82. Wadsworth CT, Krishnan R, Sear M, Harrold J, Nielsen DH. Intrarater reliability of manual muscle testing and hand-held dynametric muscle testing. *Phys Ther.* 1987;67(9):1342-1347.

83. Cuthbert SC, Goodheart GJ. On the reliability and validity of manual muscle testing: A literature review. *Chiropr Osteopat.* 2007;15:4.

84. Bohannon RW, Andrews AW. Interrater reliability of hand-held dynamometry. *Phys Ther.* 1987;67(6):931-933.

85. van den Beld WA, van der Sanden GA, Sengers RC, Verbeek AL, Gabreëls FJ. Validity and reproducibility of hand-held dynamometry in children aged 4-11 years. *J Rehabil Med.* 2006;38(1):57-64.

86. Wainner RS, Fritz JM, Irrgang JJ, Delitto A, Allison S, Boninger ML. Development of a clinical prediction rule for the diagnosis of carpal tunnel syndrome. *Arch Phys Med Rehab.* 2005;86(4):609-618.

87. MacDermid JC, Wessel J. Clinical diagnosis of carpal tunnel syndrome: A systematic review. *J Hand Ther.* 2004;17(2):309-319.

88. Szabo RM, Slater RR Jr, Farver TB, Stanton DB, Sharman WK. The value of diagnostic testing in carpal tunnel syndrome. *J Hand Surg Am.* 1999;24(4):704-714.

89. Hansen PA, Micklesen P, Robinson LR. Clinical utility of the flick maneuver in diagnosing carpal tunnel syndrome. *Am J Phys Med Rehab.* 2004;83(5):363-367.

90. Koris M, Gelberman RH, Duncan K, Boublick M, Smith B. Carpal tunnel syndrome. Evaluation of a quantitative provocational diagnostic test. *Clin Orthop Relat R.* 1990; 251:157-161.

91. Bilkis S, Loveman DM, Eldridge JA, Ali SA, Kadir A, McConathy W. Modified Phalen's test as an aid in diagnosing carpal tunnel syndrome. *Arthrit Care Res.* 2012;64(2):287-289.

92. Ma H, Kim I. The diagnostic assessment of hand elevation test in carpal tunnel syndrome. *J Korean Neurosurg S.* 2012;52(5):472-475.

93. de Krom MC, Knipschild PG, Kester AD, Spaans F. Efficacy of provocative tests for diagnosis of carpal tunnel syndrome. *Lancet.* 1990;335(8686):393-395.

94. Practice parameter for carpal tunnel syndrome (summary statement). Report of the Quality Standards Subcommittee of the American Academy of Neurology. *Neurology.* 1993;43(11):2406-2409.

95. El Miedany Y, Ashour S, Youssef S, Mehanna A, Meky FA. Clinical diagnosis of carpal tunnel syndrome: Old tests-new concepts. *Joint Bone Spine.* 2008;75(4):451-457.

96. Mondelli M, Passero S, Giannini F. Provocative tests in different stages of carpal tunnel syndrome. *Clin Neurol Neurosurg.* 2001;103(3):178-183.

97. Meek MF, Dellon AL. Modification of Phalen's wrist-flexion test. *J Neurosci Methods.* 2008;170(1):156-157.

98. Ahn DS. Hand elevation: A new test for carpal tunnel syndrome. *Ann Plast Surg.* 2001;46(2):120-124.

99. Amirfeyz R, Clark D, Parsons B, et al. Clinical tests for carpal tunnel syndrome in contemporary practice. *Arch Orthop Trauma Surg.* 2011;131(4):471-474.

100. Amirfeyz R, Gozzard C, Leslie IJ. Hand elevation test for assessment of carpal tunnel syndrome. *J Hand Surg Br.* 2005;30(4):361-364.

101. Kaul MP, Pagel KJ, Dryden JD. Lack of predictive power of the "tethered" median stress test in suspected carpal tunnel syndrome. *Arch Phys Med Rehab.* 2000;81(3):348-350.

102. MacDermid JC, Doherty T. Clinical and electrodiagnostic testing of carpal tunnel syndrome: A narrative review. *J Orthop Sport Phys.* 2004;34(10):565-588.

103. Karl AI, Carney ML, Kaul MP. The lumbrical provocation test in subjects with median inclusive paresthesia. *Arch Phys Med Rehab.* 2001;82(7):935-937.

104. Kuhlman KA, Hennessey WJ. Sensitivity and specificity of carpal tunnel syndrome signs. *Am J Phys Med Rehab.* 1997;76(6):451-457.

105. Katz JN, Stirrat CR. A self-administered hand diagram for the diagnosis of carpal tunnel syndrome. *J Hand Surg Am.* 1990;15(2):360-363.

106. Calfee RP, Dale AM, Ryan D, Descatha A, Franzblau A, Evanoff B. Performance of simplified scoring systems for hand diagrams in carpal tunnel syndrome screening. *J Hand Surg Am.* 2012;37(1):10-17.

107. Makanji HS, Becker SJ, Mudgal CS, Jupiter JB, Ring D. Evaluation of the scratch collapse test for the diagnosis of carpal tunnel syndrome. *J Hand Surg Eur Vol.* 2014;39(2):181-186.

108. Tetro AM, Evanoff BA, Hollstien SB, Gelberman RH. A new provocative test for carpal tunnel syndrome. Assessment of wrist flexion and nerve compression. *J Bone Joint Surg Br.* 1998;80(3):493-498.

109. Boland RA, Kiernan MC. Assessing the accuracy of a combination of clinical tests for identifying carpal tunnel syndrome. *J Clin Neurosci.* 2009;16(7):929-933.

110. Thüngen T, Sadowski M, El Kazzi W, Schuind F. Value of Gilliatt's pneumatic tourniquet test for diagnosis of carpal tunnel syndrome. *Chir Main.* 2012;31(3):152-156.

111. Hems TE, Miller R, Massraf A, Green J. Assessment of a diagnostic questionnaire and protocol for management of carpal tunnel syndrome. *J Hand Surg Eur Vol.* 2009;34(5):665-670.

112. Heyman P, Gelberman RH, Duncan K, Hipp JA. Injuries of the ulnar collateral ligament of the thumb metacarpophalangeal joint. Biomechanical and prospective clinical studies on the usefulness of valgus stress testing. *Clin Orthop Relat R.* 1993;292:165-171.

113. Alexander RD, Catalano LW, Barron OA, Glickel SZ. The extensor pollicis brevis entrapment test in the treatment of de Quervain's disease. *J Hand Surg Am.* 2002;27(5):813-816.

114. Ruland RT, Hogan CJ. The ECU synergy test: An aid to diagnose ECU tendonitis. *J Hand Surg Am.* 2008;33(10):1777-1782.

115. Esberger DA. What value the scaphoid compression test? *J Hand Surg Br.* 1994;19(6):748-749.

116. Parvizi J, Wayman J, Kelly P, Moran CG. Combining the clinical signs improves diagnosis of scaphoid fractures. A prospective study with follow-up. *J Hand Surg Br.* 1998;23(3):324-327.

117. Freeland P. Scaphoid tubercle tenderness: A better indicator of scaphoid fractures? *Arch Emerg Med.* 1989;6(1):46-50.

118. Powell JM, Lloyd GJ, Rintoul RF. New clinical test for fracture of the scaphoid. *Can J Surg.* 1988;31(4):237-238.

119. Unay K, Gokcen B, Ozkan K, Poyanli O, Eceviz E. Examination tests predictive of bone injury in patients with clinically suspected occult scaphoid fracture. *Injury.* 2009;40(12):1265-1268.

120. van Andel CJ, Roescher WB, Tromp MF, Ritt MJ, Strackee SD, Veeger DH. Quantification of wrist joint laxity. *J Hand Surg Am.* 2008;33(5):667-674.

121. LaStayo P, Howell J. Clinical provocative tests used in evaluating wrist pain: A descriptive study. *J Hand Ther.* 1995;8(1):10-17.

122. Truong NP, Mann FA, Gilula LA, Kang SW. Wrist instability series: Increased yield with clinical-radiologic screening criteria. *Radiology.* 1994;192(2):481-484.

123. Kim JP, Park MJ. Assessment of distal radioulnar joint instability after distal radius fracture: Comparison of computed tomography and clinical examination results. *J Hand Surg Am.* 2008;33(9):1486-1492.

124. Moriya T, Aoki M, Iba K, Ozasa Y, Wada T, Yamashita T. Effect of triangular ligament tears on distal radioulnar joint instability and evaluation of three clinical tests: A biomechanical study. *J Hand Surg Eur Vol.* 2009;34(2):219-223.

125. Lester B, Halbrecht J, Levy IM, Gaudinez R. "Press test" for office diagnosis of triangular fibrocartilage complex tears of the wrist. *Ann Plast Surg.* 1995;35(1):41-45.

126. Nitschke JE, McMeeken JM, Burry HC, Matyas TA. When is a change a genuine change? A clinically meaningful interpretation of grip strength measurements in healthy and disabled women. *J Hand Ther.* 1999;12(1):25-30.

127. Mathiowetz V, Weber K, Volland G, Kashman N. Reliability and validity of grip and pinch strength evaluations. *J Hand Surg Am.* 1984;9(2):222-226.

128. Gerodimos V. Reliability of handgrip strength test in basketball players. *J Hum Kinet.* 2012;31:25-36.

129. Bohannon RW. Hand-grip dynamometry provides a valid indication of upper extremity strength impairment in home care patients. *J Hand Ther.* 1998;11(4):258-260.

130. Bohannon RW. Adequacy of simple measures for characterizing impairment in upper limb strength following stroke. *Percept Mot Skills.* 2004;99(3)(Pt 1):813-817.

131. Metter EJ, Talbot LA, Schrager M, Conwit R. Skeletal muscle strength as a predictor of all-cause mortality in healthy men. *J Gerontol A-Biol.* 2002;57(10):B359-B365.

132. Norman K, Stobäus N, Gonzalez MC, Schulzke JD, Pirlich M. Hand grip strength: Outcome predictor and marker of nutritional status. *Clin Nutr.* 2011;30(2):135-142.

133. Schmidt RT, Toews JV. Grip strength as measured by the Jamar dynamometer. *Arch Phys Med Rehab.* 1970;51(6):321-327.

134. Hamilton A, Balnave R, Adams R. Grip strength testing reliability. *J Hand Ther.* 1994;7(3):163-170.

135. Coldham F, Lewis J, Lee H. The reliability of one vs. three grip trials in symptomatic and asymptomatic subjects. *J Hand Ther.* 2006;19(3):318-326, quiz 327.

136. Peolsson A, Hedlund R, Oberg B. Intra- and inter-tester reliability and reference values for hand strength. *J Rehabil Med.* 2001;33(1):36-41.

137. Bellace JV, Healy D, Besser MP, Byron T, Hohman L. Validity of the Dexter Evaluation System's Jamar dynamometer attachment for assessment of hand grip strength in a normal population. *J Hand Ther.* 2000;13(1):46-51.

138. Kennedy D, Jerosch-Herold C, Hickson M. The reliability of one vs. three trials of pain-free grip strength in subjects with rheumatoid arthritis. *J Hand Ther.* 2010;23(4):384-390, quiz 391.

139. España-Romero V, Artero EG, Santaliestra-Pasias AM, Gutierrez A, Castillo MJ, Ruiz JR. Hand span influences optimal grip span in boys and girls aged 6 to 12 years. *J Hand Surg Am.* 2008;33(3):378-384.

140. Clerke AM, Clerke JP, Adams RD. Effects of hand shape on maximal isometric grip strength and its reliability in teenagers. *J Hand Ther.* 2005;18(1):19-29.

141. España-Romero V, Ortega FB, Vicente-Rodríguez G, Artero EG, Rey JP, Ruiz JR. Elbow position affects handgrip strength in adolescents: Validity and reliability of Jamar, DynEx, and TKK dynamometers. *J Strength Cond Res.* 2010;24(1):272-277.

142. Bohannon R, Peolsson A, Massy-Westropp N, Desrosiers J, Bear-Lehman J. Reference values for adult grip strength measured with a Jamar dynamometer: A descriptive meta-analysis. *Physiotherapy.* 2006;92:11-15.

143. Günther CM, Bürger A, Rickert M, Crispin A, Schulz CU. Grip strength in healthy caucasian adults: Reference values. *J Hand Surg Am.* 2008;33(4):558-565.

144. Hanten WP, Chen WY, Austin AA, et al. Maximum grip strength in normal subjects from 20 to 64 years of age. *J Hand Ther.* 1999;12(3):193-200.

145. Beckman C, Cork S, Gibson G, Parsons J. Assessment of hand function: The relationship between pegboard dexterity and applied dexterity. 1992;59(4):208-213.

146. Yancosek KE, Howell D. A narrative review of dexterity assessments. *J Hand Ther.* 2009;22(3):258-269, quiz 270.

147. Aaron DH, Jansen CW. Development of the Functional Dexterity Test (FDT): Construction, validity, reliability, and normative data. *J Hand Ther.* 2003;16(1):12-21.

148. Tiffin J, Asher EJ. The Purdue pegboard; norms and studies of reliability and validity. *J Appl Psychol.* 1948;32(3):234-247.

149. Gallus J, Mathiowetz V. Test-retest reliability of the Purdue Pegboard for persons with multiple sclerosis. *Am J Occup Ther.* 2003;57(1):108-111.

150. Buddenberg LA, Davis C. Test-retest reliability of the Purdue Pegboard test. *Am J Occup Ther.* 2000;54(5):555-558.

151. Kellor M, Frost J, Silberberg N, Iversen I, Cummings R. Hand strength and dexterity. *Am J Occup Ther.* 1971;25(2):77-83.

152. Svensson E, Häger-Ross C. Hand function in Charcot Marie Tooth: Test-retest reliability of some measurements. *Clin Rehabil.* 2006;20(10):896-908.

153. Oxford Grice K, Vogel KA, Le V, Mitchell A, Muniz S, Vollmer MA. Adult norms for a commercially available Nine Hole Peg Test for finger dexterity. *Am J Occup Ther.* 2003;57(5):570-573.

154. Mathiowetz V, Weber K, Kashman N, Volland G. Adult norms for Nine Hole Peg Test of finger dexterity. *Occup Ther J Res.* 1985;5(1):24-38.

155. Jebsen RH, Taylor N, Trieschmann RB, Trotter MJ, Howard LA. An objective and standardized test of hand function. *Arch Phys Med Rehab.* 1969;50(6):311-319.

156. Mathiowetz V, Volland G, Kashman N, Weber K. Adult norms for the Box and Block Test of manual dexterity. *Am J Occup Ther.* 1985;39(6):386-391.

157. Platz T, Pinkowski C, van Wijck F, Kim IH, di Bella P, Johnson G. Reliability and validity of arm function assessment with standardized guidelines for the Fugl-Meyer Test, Action Research Arm Test and Box and Block Test: A multicentre study. *Clin Rehabil.* 2005;19(4):404-411.

158. Desrosiers J, Bravo G, Hébert R, Dutil E, Mercier L. Validation of the Box and Block Test as a measure of dexterity of elderly people: Reliability, validity, and norms studies. *Arch Phys Med Rehab.* 1994;75(7):751-755.

159. Bickel KD. Carpal tunnel syndrome. *J Hand Surg Am.* 2010;35(1):147-152.

160. Gupta SK, Benstead TJ. Symptoms experienced by patients with carpal tunnel syndrome. *Can J Neurol Sci.* 1997;24(4):338-342.

161. Uemura T, Hidaka N, Nakamura H. Clinical outcome of carpal tunnel release with and without opposition transfer. *J Hand Surg Eur Vol.* 2010;35(8):632-636.

162. Burke DT, Burke MA, Bell R, Stewart GW, Mehdi RS, Kim HJ. Subjective swelling: A new sign for carpal tunnel syndrome. *Am J Phys Med Rehab.* 1999;78(6):504-508.

163. Spahn G, Wollny J, Hartmann B, Schiele R, Hofmann GO. [Metaanalysis for the evaluation of risk factors for carpal tunnel syndrome (CTS) Part I. General factors]. *Z Orthop Unfall.* 2012;150(5):503-515.

164. Spahn G, Wollny J, Hartmann B, Schiele R, Hofmann GO. [Metaanalysis for the evaluation of risk factors for carpal tunnel syndrome (CTS) Part II. Occupational risk factors]. *Z Orthop Unfall.* 2012;150(5):516-524.

165. Atroshi I, Gummesson C, Johnsson R, Ornstein E. Diagnostic properties of nerve conduction tests in population-based carpal tunnel syndrome. *BMC Musculoskel Dis.* 2003;4:9.

166. Bessette L, Keller RB, Lew RA, et al. Prognostic value of a hand symptom diagram in surgery for carpal tunnel syndrome. *J Rheumatol.* 1997;24(4):726-734.

167. Roll SC, Case-Smith J, Evans KD. Diagnostic accuracy of ultrasonography vs. electromyography in carpal tunnel syndrome: A systematic review of literature. *Ultrasound Med Biol.* 2011;37(10):1539-1553.

168. Gerr F, Letz R, Harris-Abbott D, Hopkins LC. Sensitivity and specificity of vibrometry for detection of carpal tunnel syndrome. *J Occup Environ Med.* 1995;37(9):1108-1115.

169. Cherniack MG, Moalli D, Viscolli C. A comparison of traditional electrodiagnostic studies, electroneurometry, and vibrometry in the diagnosis of carpal tunnel syndrome. *J Hand Surg Am.* 1996;21(1):122-131.

170. Graham B, Regehr G, Naglie G, Wright JG. Development and validation of diagnostic criteria for carpal tunnel syndrome. *J Hand Surg Am.* 2006;31(6):919-924.

171. Vanti C, Bonfiglioli R, Calabrese M, et al. Upper Limb Neurodynamic Test 1 and symptoms reproduction in carpal tunnel syndrome. A validity study. *Manual Ther.* 2011;16(3):258-263.

172. Dale AM, Descatha A, Coomes J, Franzblau A, Evanoff B. Physical examination has a low yield in screening for carpal tunnel syndrome. *Am J Ind Med.* 2011;54(1):1-9.

173. Descatha A, Dale AM, Franzblau A, Coomes J, Evanoff B. Diagnostic strategies using physical examination are minimally useful in defining carpal tunnel syndrome in population-based research studies. *Occup Environ Med.* 2010;67(2):133-135.

174. Sachar K. Ulnar-sided wrist pain: Evaluation and treatment of triangular fibrocartilage complex tears, ulnocarpal impaction syndrome, and lunotriquetral ligament tears. *J Hand Surg Am.* 2012;37(7):1489-1500.

175. Palmer AK. Triangular fibrocartilage complex lesions: A classification. *J Hand Surg Am.* 1989;14(4):594-606.

176. Henry MH. Management of acute triangular fibrocartilage complex injury of the wrist. *J Am Acad Orthop Surg.* 2008;16(6):320-329.

177. Zlatkin MB, Rosner J. MR imaging of ligaments and triangular fibrocartilage complex of the wrist. *Radiol Clin N Am.* 2006;44(4):595-623, ix.

178. Palmer AK. The distal radioulnar joint. Anatomy, biomechanics, and triangular fibrocartilage complex abnormalities. *Hand Clin.* 1987;3(1):31-40.

179. Woolf AD, Pfleger B. Burden of major musculoskeletal conditions. *B World Health Organ.* 2003;81(9):646-656.

180. Tay SC, Tomita K, Berger, RA. The "unlar fovea sign" for defining ulnar wrist pain: an analysis of sensitivity and specificity. *J Hand Surg Am.* 2007;32:438-44.

181. Melone CP, Nathan R. Traumatic disruption of the triangular fibrocartilage complex. Pathoanatomy. *Clin Orthop Relat R.* 1992;275:65-73.

182. Wolf JM, Sturdivant RX, Owens BD. Incidence of de Quervain's tenosynovitis in a young, active population. *J Hand Surg Am.* 2009;34(1):112-115.

183. Moore JS. De Quervain's tenosynovitis. Stenosing tenosynovitis of the first dorsal compartment. *J Occup Environ Med.* 1997;39(10):990-1002.

184. Walker MJ. Manual physical therapy examination and intervention of a patient with radial wrist pain: A case report. *J Orthop Sport Phys.* 2004;34(12):761-769.

185. Avci S, Yilmaz C, Sayli U. Comparison of nonsurgical treatment measures for de Quervain's disease of pregnancy and lactation. *J Hand Surg Am.* 2002;27(2):322-324.

186. Schned ES. De Quervain tenosynovitis in pregnant and postpartum women. *Obstet Gynecol.* 1986;68(3):411-414.

187. Schumacher HR, Dorwart BB, Korzeniowski OM. Occurrence of de Quervain's tendinitis during pregnancy. *Arch Intern Med.* 1985;145(11):2083-2084.

188. Read HS, Hooper G, Davie R. Histological appearances in post-partum de Quervain's disease. *J Hand Surg Br.* 2000;25(1):70-72.

189. Marini M, Boni S, Pingi A, De Dominicis C, Cartolari R. De Quervain's disease: Diagnostic imaging. *Chir Organi Mov.* 1994;79(2):219-223.

190. Nagaoka M, Matsuzaki H, Suzuki T. Ultrasonographic examination of de Quervain's disease. *J Orthop Sci.* 2000;5(2):96-99.

191. Glajchen N, Schweitzer M. MRI features in de Quervain's tenosynovitis of the wrist. *Skeletal Radiol.* 1996;25(1):63-65.

192. Wilson JJ, Best TM. Common overuse tendon problems: A review and recommendations for treatment. *Am Fam Physician.* 2005;72(5):811-818.

193. Anderson M, Tichenor CJ. A patient with de Quervain's tenosynovitis: A case report using an Australian approach to manual therapy. *Phys Ther.* 1994;74(4):314-326.

194. Felson DT, Lawrence RC, Dieppe PA, et al. Osteoarthritis: New insights. Part 1: The disease and its risk factors. *Ann Intern Med.* 2000;133(8):635-646.

195. Peyron JG. Epidemiologic and etiologic approach of osteoarthritis. *Semin Arthritis Rheu.* 1979;8(4):288-306.

196. Zhang W, Doherty M, Leeb BF, et al. EULAR evidence-based recommendations for the diagnosis of hand osteoarthritis: Report of a task force of ESCISIT. *Ann Rheum Dis.* 2009;68(1):8-17.

197. Watson HK, Ryu J. Evolution of arthritis of the wrist. *Clin Orthop Relat R.* 1986;202:57-67.

198. Oliveria SA, Felson DT, Reed JI, Cirillo PA, Walker AM. Incidence of symptomatic hand, hip, and knee osteoarthritis among patients in a health maintenance organization. *Arthritis Rheum.* 1995;38(8):1134-1141.

199. Zhang Y, Jordan JM. Epidemiology of osteoarthritis. *Clin Geriatr Med.* 2010;26(3):355-369.

200. Ziebland S, Fitzpatrick R, Jenkinson C, Mowat A. Comparison of two approaches to measuring change in health status in rheumatoid arthritis: The Health Assessment Questionnaire (HAQ) and modified HAQ. *Ann Rheum Dis.* 1992;51(11):1202-1205.

201. Backman C, Mackie H. Arthritis hand function test: Inter-rater reliability among self-trained raters. *Arthrit Care Res.* 1995;8(1):10-15.

202. Meenan RF, Mason JH, Anderson JJ, Guccione AA, Kazis LE. AIMS2. The content and properties of a revised and expanded Arthritis Impact Measurement Scales Health Status Questionnaire. *Arthritis Rheum.* 1992;35(1):1-10.

203. Leeb BF, Sautner J, Andel I, Rintelen B. SACRAH: A score for assessment and quantification of chronic rheumatic affections of the hands. *Rheumatology.* 2003;42(10):1173-1178.

204. Sautner J, Andel I, Rintelen B, Leeb BF. Development of the M-SACRAH, a modified, shortened version of SACRAH (Score for the Assessment and quantification of Chronic Rheumatoid Affections of the Hands). *Rheumatology.* 2004;43(11):1409-1413.

205. Dreiser RL, Maheu E, Guillou GB, Caspard H, Grouin JM. Validation of an algofunctional index for osteoarthritis of the hand. *Rev Rhum Engl Ed.* 1995;62(6)(suppl 1):43S-53S.

206. Dreiser RL, Maheu E, Guillou GB. Sensitivity to change of the functional index for hand osteoarthritis. *Osteoarthr Cartilage.* 2000;8(suppl A):S25-S28.

207. Duruöz MT, Poiraudeau S, Fermanian J, et al. Development and validation of a rheumatoid hand functional disability scale that assesses functional handicap. *J Rheumatol.* 1996;23(7):1167-1172.

208. Poiraudeau S, Chevalier X, Conrozier T, et al. Reliability, validity, and sensitivity to change of the Cochin hand functional disability scale in hand osteoarthritis. *Osteoarthr Cartilage.* 2001;9(6):570-577.

209. Bellamy N, Campbell J, Haraoui B, et al. Clinimetric properties of the AUSCAN Osteoarthritis Hand Index: An evaluation of reliability, validity and responsiveness. *Osteoarthr Cartilage.* 2002;10(11):863-869.

210. Dziedzic KS, Thomas E, Hay EM. A systematic search and critical review of measures of disability for use in a population survey of hand osteoarthritis (OA). *Osteoarthr Cartilage.* 2005;13(1):1-12.

211. Maheu E, Cadet C, Gueneugues S, Ravaud P, Dougados M. Reproducibility and sensitivity to change of four scoring methods for the radiological assessment of osteoarthritis of the hand. *Ann Rheum Dis.* 2007;66(4):464-469.

212. Bijsterbosch J, Haugen IK, Malines C, et al. Reliability, sensitivity to change and feasibility of three radiographic scoring methods for hand osteoarthritis. *Ann Rheum Dis.* 2011;70(8):1465-1467.

213. Kellgren JH, Lawrence JS. Radiological assessment of osteo-arthrosis. *Ann Rheum Dis.* 1957;16(4):494-502.

214. Kloppenburg M, Kwok WY. Hand osteoarthritis—a heterogeneous disorder. *Nat Rev Rheumatol.* 2012;8(1):22-31.

215. Myers HL, Thomas E, Hay EM, Dziedzic KS. Hand assessment in older adults with musculoskeletal hand problems: A reliability study. *BMC Musculoskel Dis.* 2011;12:3.

216. Alexander CJ. Heberden's and Bouchard's nodes. *Ann Rheum Dis.* 1999;58(11):675-678.

217. Jackson DS, Kellgren JH. Hyaluronic acid in Heberden's nodes. *Ann Rheum Dis.* 1957;16(2):238-240.

218. Altman R, Alarcón G, Appelrouth D, et al. The American College of Rheumatology criteria for the classification and reporting of osteoarthritis of the hand. *Arthritis Rheum.* 1990;33(11):1601-1610.

219. Alamanos Y, Drosos AA. Epidemiology of adult rheumatoid arthritis. *Autoimmun Rev.* 2005;4(3):130-136.

220. Costenbader KH, Kountz DS. Treatment and management of early RA: A primary care primer. *J Fam Pract.* 2007;56(7)(suppl):S1-S7, quiz S8.

221. Birch JT, Bhattacharya S. Emerging trends in diagnosis and treatment of rheumatoid arthritis. *Prim Care.* 2010;37(4):779-792, vii.

222. Rindfleisch JA, Muller D. Diagnosis and management of rheumatoid arthritis. *Am Fam Physician.* 2005;72(6):1037-1047.

223. Rheumatoid Arthritis. Available at: http://www.cdc.gov/arthritis/basics/rheumatoid.htm. Accessed November 2, 2014.

224. Anderson J, Caplan L, Yazdany J, et al. Rheumatoid arthritis disease activity measures: American College of Rheumatology recommendations for use in clinical practice. *Arthrit Care Res.* 2012;64(5):640-647.

225. Østergaard M, Pedersen SJ, Døhn UM. Imaging in rheumatoid arthritis—status and recent advances for magnetic resonance imaging, ultrasonography, computed tomography and conventional radiography. *Best Pract Res Clin Rheumatol.* 2008;22(6):1019-1044.

226. Suter LG, Fraenkel L, Braithwaite RS. Role of magnetic resonance imaging in the diagnosis and prognosis of rheumatoid arthritis. *Arthrit Care Res.* 2011;63(5):675-688.

227. Aletaha D, Neogi T, Silman AJ, et al. 2010 rheumatoid arthritis classification criteria: An American College of Rheumatology/European League Against Rheumatism collaborative initiative. *Ann Rheum Dis.* 2010;69(9):1580-1588.

228. Chung KC, Spilson SV. The frequency and epidemiology of hand and forearm fractures in the United States. *J Hand Surg Am.* 2001;26(5):908-915.

229. O'Neill TW, Cooper C, Finn JD, et al. Incidence of distal forearm fracture in British men and women. *Osteoporos Int.* 2001;12(7):555-558.

230. Jessee EF, Owen DS Jr, Sagar KB. The benign hypermobile joint syndrome. *Arthritis Rheum.* 1980;23(9):1053-1056.

231. MacDermid JC, Roth JH, Richards RS. Pain and disability reported in the year following a distal radius fracture: A cohort study. *BMC Musculoskel Dis.* 2003;4:24.

232. Spence LD, Savenor A, Nwachuku I, Tilsley J, Eustace S. MRI of fractures of the distal radius: Comparison with conventional radiographs. *Skeletal Radiol.* 1998;27(5):244-249.

233. Pruitt DL, Gilula LA, Manske PR, Vannier MW. Computed tomography scanning with image reconstruction in evaluation of distal radius fractures. *J Hand Surg Am.* 1994;19(5):720-727.

234. van Onselen EB, Karim RB, Hage JJ, Ritt MJ. Prevalence and distribution of hand fractures. *J Hand Surg Br.* 2003;28(5):491-495.

235. Leslie IJ, Dickson RA. The fractured carpal scaphoid. Natural history and factors influencing outcome. *J Bone Joint Surg Br.* 1981;63-B(2):225-230.

236. van der Molen AB, Groothoff JW, Visser GJ, Robinson PH, Eisma WH. Time off work due to scaphoid fractures and other carpal injuries in the Netherlands in the period 1990 to 1993. *J Hand Surg Br.* 1999;24(2):193-198.

237. Duckworth AD, Jenkins PJ, Aitken SA, Clement ND, Court-Brown CM, McQueen MM. Scaphoid fracture epidemiology. *J Trauma Acute Care Surg.* 2012;72(2):E41-E45.

238. Brooks S, Wluka AE, Stuckey S, Cicuttini F. The management of scaphoid fractures. *J Sci Med Sport.* 2005;8(2):181-189.

239. Van Tassel DC, Owens BD, Wolf JM. Incidence estimates and demographics of scaphoid fracture in the U.S. population. *J Hand Surg Am.* 2010;35(8):1242-1245.

240. Bethel J. Scaphoid fracture: Diagnosis and management. *Emerg Nurse.* 2009;17(4):24-29, quiz 31.

241. Tiel-van Buul MM, van Beek EJ, Borm JJ, Gubler FM, Broekhuizen AH, van Royen EA. The value of radiographs and bone scintigraphy in suspected scaphoid fracture. A statistical analysis. *J Hand Surg Br.* 1993;18(3):403-406.

242. Jørgsholm P, Thomsen NO, Besjakov J, Abrahamsson SO, Björkman A. The benefit of magnetic resonance imaging for patients with posttraumatic radial wrist tenderness. *J Hand Surg Am.* 2013;38(1):29-33.

243. Tiel-van Buul MM, van Beek EJ, Broekhuizen AH, Nooitgedacht EA, Davids PH, Bakker AJ. Diagnosing scaphoid fractures: Radiographs cannot be used as a gold standard! *Injury.* 1992;23(2):77-79.

244. Waizenegger M, Barton NJ, Davis TR, Wastie ML. Clinical signs in scaphoid fractures. *J Hand Surg Br.* 1994;19(6):743-747.

245. Herzberg G, Comtet JJ, Linscheid RL, Amadio PC, Cooney WP, Stalder J. Perilunate dislocations and fracture-dislocations: A multicenter study. *J Hand Surg Am.* 1993;18(5):768-779.

246. Murray PM. Dislocation of the wrist: Carpal instability complex. *J Hand Surg Am.* 2003;3(2):88-99.

247. Bonzar M, Firrell JC, Hainer M, Mah ET, McCabe SJ. Kienböck disease and negative ulnar variance. *J Bone Joint Surg Am.* 1998;80(8):1154-1157.

248. Schuind F, Eslami S, Ledoux P. Kienbock's disease. *J Bone Joint Surg Br.* 2008;90(2):133-139.

249. Allan CH, Joshi A, Lichtman DM. Kienbock's disease: Diagnosis and treatment. *J Am Acad Orthop Surg.* 2001;9(2):128-136.

250. Beredjiklian PK. Kienböck's disease. *J Hand Surg Am.* 2009;34(1):167-175.

251. Garcia-Elias M, Vidal A. Keinbock's disease. *Current Orthopedics.* 1997;11:28-35.

252. Keith PP, Nuttall D, Trail I. Long-term outcome of nonsurgically managed Kienböck's disease. *J Hand Surg Am.* 2004;29(1):63-67.

253. Schmitt R, Heinze A, Fellner F, Obletter N, Strühn R, Bautz W. Imaging and staging of avascular osteonecroses at the wrist and hand. *Eur J Radiol.* 1997;25(2):92-103.

254. Gerber C, Senn E, Matter P. Skier's thumb. Surgical treatment of recent injuries to the ulnar collateral ligament of the thumb's metacarpophalangeal joint. *Am J Sports Med.* 1981;9(3):171-177.

255. Campbell CS. Gamekeeper's thumb. *J Bone Joint Surg Br.* 1955;37-B(1):148-149.

256. Louis DS, Huebner JJ, Hankin FM. Rupture and displacement of the ulnar collateral ligament of the metacarpophalangeal joint of the thumb. Preoperative diagnosis. *J Bone Joint Surg Am.* 1986;68(9):1320-1326.

257. Tsiouri C, Hayton MJ, Baratz M. Injury to the ulnar collateral ligament of the thumb. *Hand (NY).* 2009;4(1):12-18.

258. Newland CC. Gamekeeper's thumb. *Orthop Clin N Am.* 1992;23(1):41-48.

259. Patel S, Potty A, Taylor EJ, Sorene ED. Collateral ligament injuries of the metacarpophalangeal joint of the thumb: A treatment algorithm. *Strategies Trauma Limb Reconstr.* 2010;5(1):1-10.

260. Ritting AW, Baldwin PC, Rodner CM. Ulnar collateral ligament injury of the thumb metacarpophalangeal joint. *Clin J Sport Med.* 2010;20(2):106-112.

261. Peterson JJ, Bancroft LW. Injuries of the fingers and thumb in the athlete. *Clin Sports Med.* 2006;25(3):527-542, vii-viii.

262. Shinohara T, Horii E, Majima M, et al. Sonographic diagnosis of acute injuries of the ulnar collateral ligament of the metacarpophalangeal joint of the thumb. *J Clin Ultrasound.* 2007;35(2):73-77.

263. Malik AK, Morris T, Chou D, Sorene E, Taylor E. Clinical testing of ulnar collateral ligament injuries of the thumb. *J Hand Surg Eur Vol.* 2009;34(3):363-366.

264. Anderson D. Skier's thumb. *Aust Fam Physician.* 2010;39(8):575-577.

265. Jeanmonod RK, Jeanmonod D, Damewood S, Perry C, Powers M, Lazansky V. Punch injuries: Insights into intentional closed fist injuries. *West J Emerg Med.* 2011;12(1):6-10.

266. Gudmundsen TE, Borgen L. Fractures of the fifth metacarpal. *Acta Radiol.* 2009;50(3):296-300.

267. Kjaer-Petersen K, Jurik AG, Petersen LK. Intra-articular fractures at the base of the fifth metacarpal. A clinical and radiographical study of 64 cases. *J Hand Surg Br.* 1992;17(2):144-147.

268. Altizer L. Boxer's fracture. *Orthop Nurs.* 2006;25(4):271-273, quiz 274-275.

269. Aksay E, Yesilaras M, Kilic TY, Tur FC, Sever M, Kaya A. Sensitivity and specificity of bedside ultrasonography in the diagnosis of fractures of the fifth metacarpal [published online ahead of print October 23 2013]. *Emerg Med J.* 2013.

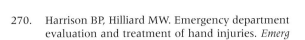

270. Harrison BP, Hilliard MW. Emergency department evaluation and treatment of hand injuries. *Emerg Med Clin North Am.* 1999;17(4):793-822, v.

271. Bragg S. The boxers' fracture. *J Emerg Nurs.* 2005;31(5):473.

272. Souter WA. The problem of boutonniere deformity. *Clin Orthop Relat R.* 1974(104):116-133.

273. Dreyfus JN, Schnitzer TJ. Pathogenesis and differential diagnosis of the swan-neck deformity. *Semin Arthritis Rheu.* 1983;13(2):200-211.

274. Bendre AA, Hartigan BJ, Kalainov DM. Mallet finger. *J Am Acad Orthop Surg.* 2005;13(5):336-344.

275. Foucher G, Binhamer P, Cange S, Lenoble E. Long-term results of splintage for mallet finger. *Int Orthop.* 1996;20(3):129-131.

276. Okafor B, Mbubaegbu C, Munshi I, Williams DJ. Mallet deformity of the finger. Five-year follow-up of conservative treatment. *J Bone Joint Surg Br.* 1997;79(4):544-547.

277. Grundberg AB, Reagan DS. Central slip tenotomy for chronic mallet finger deformity. *J Hand Surg Am.* 1987;12(4):545-547.

278. Akhtar S, Bradley MJ, Quinton DN, Burke FD. Management and referral for trigger finger/thumb. *BMJ.* 2005;331(7507):30-33.

279. Ametewee K. Trigger thumb in adults after hyperextension injury. *Hand.* 1983;15(1):103-105.

280. Best TJ. Post-traumatic stenosing flexor tenosynovitis. *Can J Plast Surg.* 2003;11(3):143-144.

281. Bonnici AV, Spencer JD. A survey of 'trigger finger' in adults. *J Hand Surg Br.* 1988;13(2):202-203.

282. Gorsche R, Wiley JP, Renger R, Brant R, Gemer TY, Sasyniuk TM. Prevalence and incidence of stenosing flexor tenosynovitis (trigger finger) in a meat-packing plant. *J Occup Environ Med.* 1998;40(6):556-560.

283. Trezies AJ, Lyons AR, Fielding K, Davis TR. Is occupation an aetiological factor in the development of trigger finger? *J Hand Surg Br.* 1998;23(4):539-540.

284. Anderson B, Kaye S. Treatment of flexor tenosynovitis of the hand ('trigger finger') with corticosteroids. A prospective study of the response to local injection. *Arch Intern Med.* 1991;151(1):153-156.

285. Weilby A. Trigger finger. Incidence in children and adults and the possibility of a predisposition in certain age groups. *Acta Orthop Scand.* 1970;41(4):419-427.

286. Strom L. Trigger finger in diabetes. *J Med Soc N J.* 1977;74(11):951-954.

287. Stahl S, Kanter Y, Karnielli E. Outcome of trigger finger treatment in diabetes. *J Diabetes Complicat.* 1997;11(5):287-290.

288. Uotani K, Kawata A, Nagao M, Mizutani T, Hayashi H. Trigger finger as an initial manifestation of familial amyloid polyneuropathy in a patient with Ile107Val TTR. *Intern Med.* 2007;46(8):501-504.

289. Makkouk AH, Oetgen ME, Swigart CR, Dodds SD. Trigger finger: Etiology, evaluation, and treatment. *Curr Rev Musculoskelet Med.* 2008;1(2):92-96.

290. Chammas M, Bousquet P, Renard E, Poirier JL, Jaffiol C, Allieu Y. Dupuytren's disease, carpal tunnel syndrome, trigger finger, and diabetes mellitus. *J Hand Surg Am.* 1995;20(1):109-114.

291. Griggs SM, Weiss AP, Lane LB, Schwenker C, Akelman E, Sachar K. Treatment of trigger finger in patients with diabetes mellitus. *J Hand Surg Am.* 1995;20(5):787-789.

292. Moore JS. Flexor tendon entrapment of the digits (trigger finger and trigger thumb). *J Occup Environ Med.* 2000;42(5):526-545.

293. Gottlieb NL. Digital flexor tenosynovitis: Diagnosis and clinical significance. *J Rheumatol.* 1991;18(7):954-955.

294. Ryzewicz M, Wolf JM. Trigger digits: Principles, management, and complications. *J Hand Surg Am.* 2006;31(1):135-146.

295. Rodgers JA, McCarthy JA, Tiedeman JJ. Functional distal interphalangeal joint splinting for trigger finger in laborers: A review and cadaver investigation. *Orthopedics.* 1998;21(3):305-309, discussion 309-310.

296. Patel MR, Bassini L. Trigger fingers and thumb: When to splint, inject, or operate. *J Hand Surg Am.* 1992;17(1):110-113.

297. Freiberg A, Mulholland RS, Levine R. Nonoperative treatment of trigger fingers and thumbs. *J Hand Surg Am.* 1989;14(3):553-558.

298. Newport ML, Lane LB, Stuchin SA. Treatment of trigger finger by steroid injection. *J Hand Surg Am.* 1990;15(5):748-750.

299. Thorpe AP. Results of surgery for trigger finger. *J Hand Surg Br.* 1988;13(2):199-201.

300. Hove LM. Fractures of the hand. Distribution and relative incidence. *Scand J Plast Recons.* 1993;27(4):317-319.

301. Ellis H. Edward Hallarran Bennett: Bennett's fracture of the base of the thumb. *J Perioper Pract.* 2013;23(3):59-60.

302. Cannon SR, Dowd GS, Williams DH, Scott JM. A long-term study following Bennett's fracture. *J Hand Surg Br.* 1986;11(3):426-431.

303. Brownlie C, Anderson D. Bennett fracture dislocation—review and management. *Aust Fam Physician.* 2011;40(6):394-396.

304. Kjaer-Petersen K, Langhoff O, Andersen K. Bennett's fracture. *J Hand Surg Br.* 1990;15(1):58-61.

305. Livesley PJ. The conservative management of Bennett's fracture-dislocation: A 26-year follow-up. *J Hand Surg Br.* 1990;15(3):291-294.

306. Leclère FM, Jenzer A, Hüsler R, et al. 7-year follow-up after open reduction and internal screw fixation in Bennett fractures. *Arch Orthop Trauma Surg.* 2012;132(7):1045-1051.

307. Foster RJ, Hastings H. Treatment of Bennett, Rolando, and vertical intraarticular trapezial fractures. *Clin Orthop Relat R.* 1987;214:121-129.

308. Thurston AJ, Dempsey SM. Bennett's fracture: A medium to long-term review. *Aust N Z J Surg.* 1993;63(2):120-123.

309. Timmenga EJ, Blokhuis TJ, Maas M, Raaijmakers EL. Long-term evaluation of Bennett's fracture. A comparison between open and closed reduction. *J Hand Surg Br.* 1994;19(3):373-377.

310. Gudmundsson KG, Arngrímsson R, Sigfússon N, Björnsson A, Jónsson T. Epidemiology of Dupuytren's disease: Clinical, serological, and social assessment. The Reykjavik Study. *J Clin Epidemiol.* 2000;53(3):291-296.

311. Anthony SG, Lozano-Calderon SA, Simmons BP, Jupiter JB. Gender ratio of Dupuytren's disease in the modern U.S. population. *Hand (NY).* 2008;3(2):87-90.

312. Bayat A, McGrouther DA. Management of Dupuytren's disease—clear advice for an elusive condition. *Ann R Coll Surg Engl.* 2006;88(1):3-8.

313. Burge P, Hoy G, Regan P, Milne R. Smoking, alcohol and the risk of Dupuytren's contracture. *J Bone Joint Surg Br.* 1997;79(2):206-210.

314. Burke FD, Proud G, Lawson IJ, McGeoch KL, Miles JN. An assessment of the effects of exposure to vibration, smoking, alcohol and diabetes on the prevalence of Dupuytren's disease in 97,537 miners. *J Hand Surg Eur Vol.* 2007;32(4):400-406.

315. Noble J, Erat K. In defence of the meniscus. A prospective study of 200 meniscectomy patients. *J Bone Joint Surg Br.* 1980;62-B(1):7-11.

316. Smith SP, Devaraj VS, Bunker TD. The association between frozen shoulder and Dupuytren's disease. *J Shoulder Elb Surg.* 2001;10(2):149-151.

317. Arafa M, Noble J, Royle SG, Trail IA, Allen J. Dupuytren's and epilepsy revisited. *J Hand Surg Br.* 1992;17(2):221-224.

318. Arkkila PE, Kantola IM, Viikari JS. Dupuytren's disease: Association with chronic diabetic complications. *J Rheumatol.* 1997;24(1):153-159.

319. Kelly SA, Burke FD, Elliot D. Injury to the distal radius as a trigger to the onset of Dupuytren's disease. *J Hand Surg Br.* 1992;17(2):225-229.

320. Hart MG, Hooper G. Clinical associations of Dupuytren's disease. *Postgrad Med J.* 2005;81(957):425-428.

Chapter 24

1. Byrd JW, Jones KS. Diagnostic accuracy of clinical assessment, magnetic resonance imaging, magnetic resonance arthrography, and intra-articular injection in hip arthroscopy patients. *Am J Sport Med.* 2004;32(7):1668-1674.

2. McCarthy JC, Busconi BD, Owens BD. Assessment of the painful hip. In: McCarthy JC, ed. *Early Hip Disorders.* New York, NY: Springer; 2003.

3. Tibor LM, Sekiya JK. Differential diagnosis of pain around the hip joint. *Arthroscopy.* 2008;24(12):1407-1421.

4. Martin RL, Irrgang JJ, Sekiya JK. The diagnostic accuracy of a clinical examination in determining intra-articular hip pain for potential hip arthroscopy candidates. *Arthroscopy.* 2008;24(9):1013-1018.

5. Burnett RS, Della Rocca GJ, Prather H, Curry M, Maloney WJ, Clohisy JC. Clinical presentation of patients with tears of the acetabular labrum. *J Bone Joint Surg Am.* 2006;88(7):1448-1457.

6. Martin HD, Kelly BT, Leunig M, et al. The pattern and technique in the clinical evaluation of the adult hip: The common physical examination tests of hip specialists. *Arthroscopy.* 2010;26(2):161-172.

7. Reiman MP, Weisbach PC, Glynn PE. The hips influence on low back pain: A distal link to a proximal problem. *J Sport Rehabil.* 2009;18(1):24-32.

8. Ben-Galim P, Ben-Galim T, Rand N, et al. Hip-spine syndrome: The effect of total hip replacement surgery on low back pain in severe osteoarthritis of the hip. *Spine (Phila Pa 1976).* 2007;32(19):2099-2102.

9. Offierski CM, MacNab I. Hip-spine syndrome. *Spine (Phila Pa 1976).* 1983;8(3):316-321.

10. Yoshimoto H, Sato S, Masuda T, et al. Spinopelvic alignment in patients with osteoarthrosis of the hip: A radiographic comparison to patients with low back pain. *Spine (Phila Pa 1976).* 2005;30(14):1650-1657.

11. Prather H, Hunt D, Fournie A, Clohisy JC. Early intra-articular hip disease presenting with posterior pelvic and groin pain. *Pm R.* 2009;1(9):809-815.

12. Zierenberg A, Sahrmann S, Prather H. End-stage disorders of the hip presenting with posterior pelvic girdle and lateral thigh pain: Two case reports. *PM&R.* 2010;2(4):298-302.

13. McCarthy JC, Noble PC, Schuck MR, Wright J, Lee J. The Otto E. Aufranc Award: The role of labral lesions to development of early degenerative hip disease. *Clin Orthop Relat R.* 2001(393):25-37.

14. McCarthy JC, Busconi B. The role of hip arthroscopy in the diagnosis and treatment of hip disease. *Orthopedics.* 1995;18(8):753-756.

15. Lewis CL, Sahrmann SA, Moran DW. Anterior hip joint force increases with hip extension, decreased gluteal force, or decreased iliopsoas force. *J Biomech.* 2007;40(16):3725-3731.

16. Narvani AA, Tsiridis E, Kendall S, Chaudhuri R, Thomas P. A preliminary report on prevalence of acetabular labrum tears in sports patients with groin pain. *Knee Surg Sport Tr A.* 2003;11(6):403-408.

17. Petersen W, Petersen F, Tillmann B. Structure and vascularization of the acetabular labrum with regard to the pathogenesis and healing of labral lesions. *Arch Orthop Traum Su.* 2003;123(6):283-288.

18. Safran MR, Giordano G, Lindsey DP, et al. Strains across the acetabular labrum during hip motion: A cadaveric model. *Am J Sport Med.* 2011;39(suppl):92S-102S.

19. McCarthy J, Noble P, Aluisio FV, Schuck M, Wright J, Lee JA. Anatomy, pathologic features, and treatment of acetabular labral tears. *Clin Orthop Relat R.* 2003(406):38-47.

20. Myers CA, Register BC, Lertwanich P, et al. Role of the acetabular labrum and the iliofemoral ligament in hip stability: An in vitro biplane fluoroscopy study. *Am J Sport Med.* 2011;39(suppl):85S-91S.

21. Philippon MJ, Schenker ML. Athletic hip injuries and capsular laxity. *Operative Tech Orthop.* 2005;15:261-266.

22. Lewis CL, Sahrmann SA. Acetabular labral tears. *Phys Ther.* 2006;86(1):110-121.

23. Brown MD, Gomez-Marin O, Brookfield KF, Li PS. Differential diagnosis of hip disease versus spine disease. *Clin Orthop Relat R.* 2004;419:280-284.

24. Kelly BT, Buly RL. Hip arthroscopy update. *HSS J.* 2005;1(1):40-48.

25. Askling CM, Tengvar M, Saartok T, Thorstensson A. Acute first-time hamstring strains during high-speed running: A longitudinal study including clinical and magnetic resonance imaging findings. *Am J Sport Med.* 2007;35(2):197-206.

26. Askling CM, Tengvar M, Saartok T, Thorstensson A. Proximal hamstring strains of stretching type in different sports: Injury situations, clinical and magnetic resonance imaging characteristics, and return to sport. *Am J Sport Med.* 2008;36(9):1799-1804.

27. Verrall GM, Slavotinek JP, Barnes PG, Fon GT. Description of pain provocation tests used for the diagnosis of sports-related chronic groin pain: Relationship of tests to defined clinical (pain and tenderness) and MRI (pubic bone marrow oedema) criteria. *Scand J Med Sci Spor.* 2005;15(1):36-42.

28. Verrall GM, Slavotinek JP, Barnes PG, Fon GT. Diagnostic and prognostic value of clinical findings in 83 athletes with posterior thigh injury: Comparison of clinical findings with magnetic resonance imaging documentation of hamstring muscle strain. *Am J Sport Med.* 2003;31(6):969-973.

29. Lesher JM, Dreyfuss P, Hager N, Kaplan M, Furman M. Hip joint pain referral patterns: A descriptive study. *Pain Med.* 2008;9(1):22-25.

30. Arnold DR, Keene JS, Blankenbaker DG, Desmet AA. Hip pain referral patterns in patients with labral tears: Analysis based on intra-articular anesthetic injections, hip arthroscopy, and a new pain "circle" diagram. *Phys Sportsmed.* 2011;39(1):29-35.

31. Byrd JW. Snapping hip. *Oper Techn Sport Med.* 2005;13:303-308.

32. Fitzgerald RH Jr. Acetabular labrum tears. Diagnosis and treatment. *Clin Orthop Relat R.* 1995;311:60-68.

33. Allen WC, Cope R. Coxa saltans: The snapping hip revisited. *J Am Acad Orthop Sur.* 1995;3(5):303-308.

34. Winston P, Awan R, Cassidy JD, Bleakney RK. Clinical examination and ultrasound of self-reported snapping hip syndrome in elite ballet dancers. *Am J Sport Med.* 2007;35(1):118-126.

35. Tijssen M, van Cingel R, van Melick N, de Visser E. Patient-Reported Outcome questionnaires for hip arthroscopy: A systematic review of the psychometric evidence. *BMC Musculoskel Dis.* 2011;12:117.

36. Peter WF, Jansen MJ, Hurkmans EJ, et al. Physiotherapy in hip and knee osteoarthritis: Development of a practice guideline concerning initial assessment, treatment and evaluation. *Acta Reumatol Port.* 2011;36(3):268-281.

37. Wright AA, Hegedus EJ, Baxter GD, Abbott JH. Measurement of function in hip osteoarthritis: Developing a standardized approach for physical performance measures. *Physiother Theory Pract.* 2011;27(4):253-262.

38. Thorborg K, Roos EM, Bartels EM, Petersen J, Holmich P. Validity, reliability and responsiveness of patient-reported outcome questionnaires when assessing hip and groin disability: A systematic review. *Brit J Sport Med.* 2010;44(16):1186-1196.

39. Mohtadi NG, Griffin DR, Pedersen ME, et al. The development and validation of a self-administered quality-of-life outcome measure for young, active patients with symptomatic hip disease: The International Hip Outcome Tool (iHOT-33). *Arthroscopy.* 2012;28(5):595-605, quiz 606-510, e591.

40. Griffin DR, Parsons N, Mohtadi NG, Safran MR. A short version of the International Hip Outcome Tool (iHOT-12) for use in routine clinical practice. *Arthroscopy.* 2012;28(5):611-616, quiz 616-618.

41. Thorborg K, Holmich P, Christensen R, Petersen J, Roos EM. The Copenhagen Hip and Groin Outcome Score (HAGOS): Development and validation according to the COSMIN checklist. *Brit J Sport Med.* 2011;45(6):478-491.

42. Hedbeck CJ, Tidermark J, Ponzer S, Blomfeldt R, Bergstrom G. Responsiveness of the Short Musculoskeletal Function Assessment (SMFA) in patients with femoral neck fractures. *Qual Life Res.* 2011;20(4):513-521.

43. Aguilar CM, Neumayr LD, Eggleston BE, et al. Clinical evaluation of avascular necrosis in patients with sickle cell disease: Children's Hospital Oakland Hip Evaluation Scale—a modification of the Harris Hip Score. *Arch Phys Med Rehab.* 2005;86(7):1369-1375.

44. Silvis ML, Mosher TJ, Smetana BS, et al. High prevalence of pelvic and hip magnetic resonance imaging findings in asymptomatic collegiate and professional hockey players. *Am J Sport Med.* 2011;39(4):715-721.

45. Jung KA, Restrepo C, Hellman M, AbdelSalam H, Morrison W, Parvizi J. The prevalence of cam-type femoroacetabular deformity in asymptomatic adults. *J Bone Joint Surg Br.* 2011;93(10):1303-1307.

46. Gerhardt MB, Romero AA, Silvers HJ, Harris DJ, Watanabe D, Mandelbaum BR. The prevalence of radiographic hip abnormalities in elite soccer players. *Am J Sport Med.* 2012;40(3):584-588.

47. Hartofilakidis G, Bardakos NV, Babis GC, Georgiades G. An examination of the association between different morphotypes of femoroacetabular impingement in asymptomatic subjects and the development of osteoarthritis of the hip. *J Bone Joint Surg Br.* 2011;93(5):580-586.

48. Clohisy JC, Carlisle JC, Trousdale R, et al. Radiographic evaluation of the hip has limited reliability. *Clin Orthop Relat R.* 2009;467(3):666-675.

49. Mamisch TC, Zilkens C, Siebenrock KA, Bittersohl B, Kim YJ, Werlen S. Hip MRI and its implications for surgery in osteoarthritis patients. *Rheum Dis Clin N Am.* 2009;35(3):591-604.

50. Omar IM, Zoga AC, Kavanagh EC, et al. Athletic pubalgia and "sports hernia": Optimal MR imaging technique and findings. *Radiographics.* 2008;28(5):1415-1438.

51. Ansede G, English B, Healy JC. Groin pain: Clinical assessment and the role of MR imaging. *Semin Musculoskel R.* 2011;15(1):3-13.

52. Zajick DC, Zoga AC, Omar IM, Meyers WC. Spectrum of MRI findings in clinical athletic pubalgia. *Semin Musculoskel R.* 2008;12(1):3-12.

53. Bizzini M. The groin area: The Bermuda triangle of sports medicine? *Brit J Sport Med.* 2011;45(1):1.

54. Menashe L, Hirko K, Losina E, et al. The diagnostic performance of MRI in osteoarthritis: A systematic review and meta-analysis. *Osteoarthr Cartilage.* 2012;20(1):13-21.

55. Nishii T, Tanaka H, Sugano N, Miki H, Takao M, Yoshikawa H. Disorders of acetabular labrum and articular cartilage in hip dysplasia: Evaluation using isotropic high-resolutional CT arthrography with sequential radial reformation. *Osteoarthr Cartilage.* 2007;15(3):251-257.

56. Yamamoto Y, Tonotsuka H, Ueda T, Hamada Y. Usefulness of radial contrast-enhanced computed tomography for the diagnosis of acetabular labrum injury. *Arthroscopy.* 2007;23(12):1290-1294.

57. Smith TO, Hilton G, Toms AP, Donell ST, Hing CB. The diagnostic accuracy of acetabular labral tears using magnetic resonance imaging and magnetic resonance arthrography: A meta-analysis. *Eur Radiol.* 2011;21(4):863-874.

58. Jin W, Kim KI, Rhyu KH, et al. Sonographic evaluation of anterosuperior hip labral tears with magnetic resonance arthrographic and surgical correlation. *J. Ultras Med.* 2012;31(3):439-447.

59. Knuesel PR, Pfirrmann CW, Noetzli HP, et al. MR arthrography of the hip: Diagnostic performance of a dedicated water-excitation 3D double-echo steady-state sequence to detect cartilage lesions. *AJR.* 2004;183(6):1729-1735.

60. Schmid MR, Notzli HP, Zanetti M, Wyss TF, Hodler J. Cartilage lesions in the hip: Diagnostic effectiveness of MR arthrography. *Radiology.* 2003;226(2):382-386.

61. Nishii T, Tanaka H, Nakanishi K, Sugano N, Miki H, Yoshikawa H. Fat-suppressed 3D spoiled gradient-echo MRI and MDCT arthrography of articular cartilage in patients with hip dysplasia. *AJR.* 2005;185(2):379-385.

62. Smith TO, Simpson M, Ejindu V, Hing CB. The diagnostic test accuracy of magnetic resonance imaging, magnetic resonance arthrography and computer tomography in the detection of chondral lesions of the hip. *Eur J Orthop Surg Tr.* 2013;23(3):335-344.

63. Matar WY, May O, Raymond F, Beaule PE. Bone scintigraphy in femoroacetabular impingement: A preliminary report. *Clin Orthop Relat R.* 2009;467(3):676-681.

64. Rosenberg ZS, La Rocca Vieira R, Chan SS, et al. Bisphosphonate-related complete atypical subtrochanteric femoral fractures: Diagnostic utility of radiography. *AJR.* 2011;197(4):954-960.

65. Rubin SJ, Marquardt JD, Gottlieb RH, Meyers SP, Totterman SM, O'Mara RE. Magnetic resonance imaging: A cost-effective alternative to bone scintigraphy in the evaluation of patients with suspected hip fractures. *Skeletal Radiol.* 1998;27(4):199-204.

66. Lieberman JR, Berry DJ, Mont MA, et al. Osteonecrosis of the hip: Management in the 21st century. *Instr Cours Lec.* 2003;52:337-355.

67. Markisz JA, Knowles RJ, Altchek DW, Schneider R, Whalen JP, Cahill PT. Segmental patterns of avascular necrosis of the femoral heads: Early detection with MR imaging. *Radiology.* 1987;162(3):717-720.

68. Westacott DJ, Minns JI, Foguet P. The diagnostic accuracy of magnetic resonance imaging and ultrasonography in gluteal tendon tears—a systematic review. *Hip Int.* 2011;21(6):637-645.

69. Cvitanic O, Henzie G, Skezas N, Lyons J, Minter J. MRI diagnosis of tears of the hip abductor tendons (gluteus medius and gluteus minimus). *AJR.* 2004;182(1):137-143.

70. Fearon AM, Scarvell JM, Cook JL, Smith PN. Does ultrasound correlate with surgical or histologic findings in greater trochanteric pain syndrome? A pilot study. *Clin Orthop Relat R.* 2010;468(7):1838-1844.

71. Brukner P. Is there a role for magentic resonance imaging in chronic groin pain? *Aust J Sci Med Sport.* 2004;7:74.

72. Kassarjian A. Hip MR arthrography and femoroacetabular impingement. *Semin Musculoskel R.* 2006;10(3):208-219.

73. Ganz R, Parvizi J, Beck M, Leunig M, Notzli H, Siebenrock KA. Femoroacetabular impingement: A cause for osteoarthritis of the hip. *Clin Orthop Relat R.* 2003;417:112-120.

74. Kumar R, Aggarwal A. Femoroacetabular impingement and risk factors: A study of 50 cases. *Orthop Surg.* 2011;3(4):236-241.

75. Gholve PA, Cameron DB, Millis MB. Slipped capital femoral epiphysis update. *Curr Opin Pediatr.* 2009;21(1):39-45.

76. Croft P, Cooper C, Wickham C, Coggon D. Defining osteoarthritis of the hip for epidemiologic studies. *Am J Epidemiol.* 1990;132(3):514-522.

77. Verrall GM, Slavotinek JP, Fon GT. Incidence of pubic bone marrow oedema in Australian rules football players: Relation to groin pain. *Brit J Sport Med.* 2001;35(1):28-33.

78. Paajanen H, Hermunen H, Karonen J. Pubic magnetic resonance imaging findings in surgically and conservatively treated athletes with osteitis pubis compared to asymptomatic athletes during heavy training. *Am J Sport Med.* 2008;36(1):117-121.

79. Malanga GA, Dentico R, Halperin JS. Ultrasonography of the hip and lower extremity. *Phys Med Rehabil Cli.* 2010;21(3):533-547.

80. Shipman SA, Helfand M, Moyer VA, Yawn BP. Screening for developmental dysplasia of the hip: A systematic literature review for the US Preventive Services Task Force. *Pediatrics.* 2006;117(3):e557-e576.

81. Shorter D, Hong T, Osborn DA. Screening programmes for developmental dysplasia of the hip in newborn infants. *Cochrane Db Syst Rev.* 2011;9:CD004595.

82. Grimaldi A, Richardson C, Durbridge G, Donnelly W, Darnell R, Hides J. The association between degenerative hip joint pathology and size of the gluteus maximus and tensor fascia lata muscles. *Man Ther.* 2009;14(6):611-617.

83. Grimaldi A, Richardson C, Stanton W, Durbridge G, Donnelly W, Hides J. The association between degenerative hip joint pathology and size of the gluteus medius, gluteus minimus and piriformis muscles. *Man Ther.* 2009;14(6):605-610.

84. Pfirrmann CW, Chung CB, Theumann NH, Trudell DJ, Resnick D. Greater trochanter of the hip: Attachment of the abductor mechanism and a complex of three bursae—MR imaging and MR bursography in cadavers and MR imaging in asymptomatic volunteers. *Radiology.* 2001;221(2):469-477.

85. Gottschalk F, Kourosh S, Leveau B. The functional anatomy of tensor fasciae latae and gluteus medius and minimus. *J Anat.* 1989;166:179-189.

86. Lyons K, Perry J, Gronley JK, Barnes L, Antonelli D. Timing and relative intensity of hip extensor and abductor muscle action during level and stair ambulation. An EMG study. *Phys Ther.* 1983;63(10):1597-1605.

87. Hurwitz DE, Foucher KC, Andriacchi TP. A new parametric approach for modeling hip forces during gait. *J Biomech.* 2003;36(1):113-119.

88. Youdas JW, Madson TJ, Hollman JH. Usefulness of the Trendelenburg test for identification of patients with hip joint osteoarthritis. *Physiother.* 2010;26(3):184-194.

89. Song KM, Halliday S, Reilly C, Keezel W. Gait abnormalities following slipped capital femoral epiphysis. *J Pediatr Orthop.* 2004;24(2):148-155.

90. Cahalan TD, Johnson ME, Liu S, Chao EY. Quantitative measurements of hip strength in different age groups. *Clin Orthop Relat R.* 1989;246:136-145.

91. Arnold AS, Salinas S, Asakawa DJ, Delp SL. Accuracy of muscle moment arms estimated from MRI-based musculoskeletal models of the lower extremity. *Comput Aided Surg.* 2000;5(2):108-119.

92. Byrd JW. Physical examination. In: Byrd JW, ed. *Operative Hip Arthroscopy.* 2nd ed. New York, NY: Springer; 2005.

93. Livingston LA, Stevenson JM, Olney SJ. Stairclimbing kinematics on stairs of differing dimensions. *Arch Phys Med Rehab.* 1991;72(6):398-402.

94. McFadyen BJ, Winter DA. An integrated biomechanical analysis of normal stair ascent and descent. *J Biomech.* 1988;21(9):733-744.

95. Magee DJ, ed. *Orthopedic Physical Assessment.* 4th ed. Philadelphia, PA: WB Saunders; 2002.

96. Lamontagne M, Kennedy MJ, Beaule PE. The effect of cam FAI on hip and pelvic motion during maximum squat. *Clin Orthop.* 2009;467(3):645-650.

97. Henschke N, Maher CG, Refshauge KM. Screening for malignancy in low back pain patients: A systematic review. *Eur Spine J.* 2007;16(10):1673-1679.

98. Meyers WC, Foley DP, Garrett WE, Lohnes JH, Mandlebaum BR. Management of severe lower abdominal or inguinal pain in high-performance athletes. PAIN (Performing Athletes with Abdominal or Inguinal Neuromuscular Pain Study Group). *Am J Sport Med.* 2000;28(1):2-8.

99. Gabbe BJ, Bailey M, Cook JL, et al. The association between hip and groin injuries in the elite junior football years and injuries sustained during elite senior competition. *Brit J Sport Med.* 2010;44(11):799-802.

100. Leerar PJ, Boissonnault W, Domholdt E, Roddey T. Documentation of red flags by physical therapists for patients with low back pain. *J Man Manip Ther.* 2007;15(1):42-49.

101. Van den Bruel A, Haj-Hassan T, Thompson M, Buntinx F, Mant D. Diagnostic value of clinical features at presentation to identify serious infection in children in developed countries: A systematic review. *Lancet.* 2010;375(9717):834-845.

102. Wagner JM, McKinney WP, Carpenter JL. Does this patient have appendicitis? *JAMA.* 1996;276(19):1589-1594.

103. Maslowski E, Sullivan W, Forster Harwood J, et al. The diagnostic validity of hip provocation maneuvers to detect intra-articular hip pathology. *PM&R.* 2010;2(3):174-181.

104. Clohisy JC, Knaus ER, Hunt DM, Lesher JM, Harris-Hayes M, Prather H. Clinical presentation of patients with symptomatic anterior hip impingement. *Clin Orthop.* 2009;467(3):638-644.

105. Domb BG, Brooks AG, Byrd JW. Clinical examination of the hip joint in athletes. *J Sport Rehabil.* 2009;18(1):3-23.

106. Woolf AD, Pfleger B. Burden of major musculoskeletal conditions. *B World Health Organ.* 2003;81(9):646-656.

107. Johnson AW, Weiss CB Jr, Wheeler DL. Stress fractures of the femoral shaft in athletes—more common than expected. A new clinical test. *Am J Sport Med.* 1994;22(2):248-256.

108. Kang L, Belcher D, Hulstyn MJ. Stress fractures of the femoral shaft in women's college lacrosse: A report of seven cases and a review of the literature. *Brit J Sport Med.* 2005;39(12):902-906.

109. Reiman MP, Goode AP, Hegedus EJ, Cook CE, Wright AA. Diagnostic accuracy of clinical tests of the hip: A systematic review with meta-analysis. *Brit J Sport Med.* 2013;47(14):893-902.

110. Adams SL, Yarnold PR. Clinical use of the patellar-pubic percussion sign in hip trauma. *Am J Emerg Med.* 1997;15(2):173-175.

111. Bache JB, Cross AB. The Barford test. A useful diagnostic sign in fractures of the femoral neck. *Practitioner.* 1984;228(1389):305-308.

112. Tiru M, Goh SH, Low BY. Use of percussion as a screening tool in the diagnosis of occult hip fractures. *Singapore Med J.* 2002;43(9):467-469.

113. Donelson R, Aprill C, Medcalf R, Grant W. A prospective study of centralization of lumbar and referred pain. A predictor of symptomatic discs and anular competence. *Spine (Phila Pa 1976).* 1997;22(10):1115-1122.

114. Laslett M, Oberg B, Aprill CN, McDonald B. Centralization as a predictor of provocation discography results in chronic low back pain, and the influence of disability and distress on diagnostic power. *Spine J.* 2005;5(4):370-380.

115. Vroomen PC, de Krom MC, Wilmink JT, Kester AD, Knottnerus JA. Diagnostic value of history and physical examination in patients suspected of lumbosacral nerve root compression. *J Neurol Neurosur Ps.* 2002;72(5):630-634.

116. van der Windt DA, Simons E, Riphagen II, et al. Physical examination for lumbar radiculopathy due to disc herniation in patients with low-back pain. *Cochrane Db Syst Rev.* 2010;2:CD007431.

117. Deville WL, van der Windt DA, Dzaferagic A, Bezemer PD, Bouter LM. The test of Lasegue: Systematic review of the accuracy in diagnosing herniated discs. *Spine (Phila Pa 1976).* 2000;25(9):1140-1147.

118. Stankovic R, Johnell O, Maly P, Willner S. Use of lumbar extension, slump test, physical and neurological examination in the evaluation of patients with suspected herniated nucleus pulposus. A prospective clinical study. *Man Ther.* 1999;4(1):25-32.

119. Majlesi J, Togay H, Unalan H, Toprak S. The sensitivity and specificity of the Slump and the Straight Leg Raising tests in patients with lumbar disc herniation. *J Clin Rheumatol.* 2008;14(2):87-91.

120. Laslett M, Aprill CN, McDonald B, Oberg B. Clinical predictors of lumbar provocation discography: A study of clinical predictors of lumbar provocation discography. *Eur Spine J.* 2006;15(10):1473-1484.

121. Schwarzer AC, Derby R, Aprill CN, Fortin J, Kine G, Bogduk N. Pain from the lumbar zygapophysial joints: A test of two models. *J Spinal Disord.* 1994;7(4):331-336.

122. Laslett M, Young SB, Aprill CN, McDonald B. Diagnosing painful sacroiliac joints: A validity study of a McKenzie evaluation and sacroiliac provocation tests. *Aust J Physiother.* 2003;49(2):89-97.

123. Laslett M, Aprill CN, McDonald B, Young SB. Diagnosis of sacroiliac joint pain: Validity of individual provocation tests and composites of tests. *Man Ther.* 2005;10(3):207-218.

124. Altman R, Alarcon G, Appelrouth D, et al. The American College of Rheumatology criteria for the classification and reporting of osteoarthritis of the hip. *Arthritis Rheum.* 1991;34(5):505-514.

125. Pateder DB, Hungerford MW. Use of fluoroscopically guided intra-articular hip injection in differentiating the pain source in concomitant hip and lumbar spine arthritis. *Am J Orthop (Belle Mead NJ).* 2007;36(11):591-593.

126. Holm I, Bolstad B, Lutken T, Ervik A, Rokkum M, Steen H. Reliability of goniometric measurements and visual estimates of hip ROM in patients with osteoarthrosis. *Physiother Res Int.* 2000;5(4):241-248.

127. Lin YC, Davey RC, Cochrane T. Tests for physical function of the elderly with knee and hip osteoarthritis. *Scand J Med Sci Spor.* 2001;11(5):280-286.

128. Pua YH, Wrigley TV, Cowan SM, Bennell KL. Intrarater test-retest reliability of hip range of motion and hip muscle strength measurements in persons with hip osteoarthritis. *Arch Phys Med Rehab.* 2008;89(6):1146-1154.

129. Prather H, Harris-Hayes M, Hunt DM, Steger-May K, Mathew V, Clohisy JC. Reliability and agreement of hip range of motion and provocative physical examination tests in asymptomatic volunteers. *PM&R.* 2010;2(10):888-895.

130. Philippon MJ, Maxwell RB, Johnston TL, Schenker M, Briggs KK. Clinical presentation of femoroacetabular impingement. *Knee Surg Sport Tr A.* 2007;15(8):1041-1047.

131. Birrell F, Croft P, Cooper C, Hosie G, Macfarlane G, Silman A. Predicting radiographic hip osteoarthritis from range of movement. *Rheumatology (Oxford).* 2001;40(5):506-512.

132. Holla JF, van der Leeden M, Roorda LD, et al. Diagnostic accuracy of range of motion measurements in early symptomatic hip and/or knee osteoarthritis. *Arthritis Care Res.* 2012;64(1):59-65.

133. Greenman PE. *Principles of Manual Medicine.* 2nd ed. Baltimore, MD: Williams & Wilkins; 1996.

134. Harvey D. Assessment of the flexibility of elite athletes using the modified Thomas test. *Brit J Sport Med.* 1998;32(1):68-70.

135. Kendall FP, McCreary EK, Provance PG, Rodgers MM, Romani WA. *Muscles: Testing and Function with Posture and Pain.* 5th ed. Baltimore, MD: Lippincott Williams & Wilkins; 2005.

136. Reese NB, Bandy WD. *Joint Range of Motion and Muscle Length Testing.* Philadelphia, PA: Saunders; 2002.

137. Youdas JW, Krause DA, Hollman JH, Harmsen WS, Laskowski E. The influence of gender and age on hamstring muscle length in healthy adults. *J Orthop Sport Phys.* 2005;35(4):246-252.

138. Leibold MR, Huijbregts PA, Jensen R. Concurrent criterion-related validity of physical examination tests for hip labral lesions: A systematic review. *J Man Manip Ther.* 2008;16(2):E24-E41.

139. Burgess RM, Rushton A, Wright C, Daborn C. The validity and accuracy of clinical diagnostic tests used to detect labral pathology of the hip: A systematic review. *Man Ther.* 2011;16(4):318-326.

140. Woodfield HC, Gerstman BB, Olaisen RH, Johnson DF. Interexaminer reliability of supine leg checks for discriminating leg-length inequality. *J Manip Physiol Ther.* 2011;34(4):239-246.

141. Jamaluddin S, Sulaiman AR, Imran MK, Juhara H, Ezane MA, Nordin S. Reliability and accuracy of the tape measurement method with a nearest reading of 5 mm in the assessment of leg length discrepancy. *Singapore Med J.* 2011;52(9):681-684.

142. Neely K, Wallmann HW, Backus CJ. Validity of measuring leg length with a tape measure compared to a computed tomography scan. *Physiother Theory Pract.* 2013;29(6):487-492.

143. Knutson GA. Anatomic and functional leg-length inequality: A review and recommendation for clinical decision-making. Part I, anatomic leg-length inequality: Prevalence, magnitude, effects and clinical significance. *Chiropr Osteopat.* 2005;13:11.

144. Segal NA, Harvey W, Felson DT, et al. Leg-length inequality is not associated with greater trochanteric pain syndrome. *Arthritis Res Ther.* 2008;10(3):R62.

145. Golightly YM, Allen KD, Helmick CG, Renner JB, Jordan JM. Symptoms of the knee and hip in individuals with and without limb length inequality. *Osteoarthr Cartilage.* 2009;17(5):596-600.

146. Hoikka V, Ylikoski M, Tallroth K. Leg-length inequality has poor correlation with lumbar scoliosis. A radiological study of 100 patients with chronic low-back pain. *Arch Orthop Traum Su.* 1989;108(3):173-175.

147. Piva SR, Fitzgerald K, Irrgang JJ, et al. Reliability of measures of impairments associated with patellofemoral pain syndrome. *BMC Musculoskel Dis.* 2006;7:33.

148. Souza RB, Powers CM. Concurrent criterion-related validity and reliability of a clinical test to measure femoral anteversion. *J Orthop Sport Phys.* 2009;39(8):586-592.

149. Bird PA, Oakley SP, Shnier R, Kirkham BW. Prospective evaluation of magnetic resonance imaging and physical examination findings in patients with greater trochanteric pain syndrome. *Arthritis Rheum.* 2001;44(9):2138-2145.

150. Woodley SJ, Nicholson HD, Livingstone V, et al. Lateral hip pain: Findings from magnetic resonance imaging and clinical examination. *J Orthop Sport Phys.* 2008;38(6):313-328.

151. Lequesne M, Mathieu P, Vuillemin-Bodaghi V, Bard H, Djian P. Gluteal tendinopathy in refractory greater trochanter pain syndrome: Diagnostic value of two clinical tests. *Arthritis Rheum.* 2008;59(2):241-246.

152. Fishman LM, Dombi GW, Michaelsen C, et al. Piriformis syndrome: Diagnosis, treatment, and outcome—a 10-year study. *Arch Phys Med Rehab.* 2002;83(3):295-301.

153. Fishman LM, Zybert PA. Electrophysiologic evidence of piriformis syndrome. *Arch Phys Med Rehab.* 1992;73(4):359-364.

154. Cacchio A, Borra F, Severini G, et al. Reliability and validity of three pain provocation tests used for the diagnosis of chronic proximal hamstring tendinopathy [published online ahead of print January 4 2012]. *Brit J Sport Med.* 2012.

155. Zeren B, Oztekin HH. A new self-diagnostic test for biceps femoris muscle strains. *Clin J Sport Med.* 2006;16(2):166-169.

156. Staheli LT. The prone hip extension test: A method of measuring hip flexion deformity. *Clin Orthop Relat R.* 1977;123:12-15.

157. Fearon AM, Scarvell JM, Neeman T, Cook JL, Cormick W, Smith PN. Greater trochanteric pain syndrome: Defining the clinical syndrome. *Brit J Sport Med.* 2013;47(10):649-653.

158. Gajdosik RL, Sandler MM, Marr HL. Influence of knee positions and gender on the Ober test for length of the iliotibial band. *Clin Biomech (Bristol, Avon).* 2003;18(1):77-79.

159. Melchione WE, Sullivan MS. Reliability of measurements obtained by use of an instrument designed to indirectly measure iliotibial band length. *J Orthop Sport Phys.* 1993;18(3):511-515.

160. Reese NB, Bandy WD. Use of an inclinometer to measure flexibility of the iliotibial band using the Ober test and the modified Ober test: Differences in magnitude and reliability of measurements. *J Orthop Sport Phys.* 2003;33(6):326-330.

161. Martin RL, Enseki KR, Draovitch P, Trapuzzano T, Philippon MJ. Acetabular labral tears of the hip: Examination and diagnostic challenges. *J Orthop Sport Phys.* 2006;36(7):503-515.

162. Martin RL, Sekiya JK. The interrater reliability of 4 clinical tests used to assess individuals with musculoskeletal hip pain. *J Orthop Sport Phys.* 2008;38(2):71-77.

163. Cliborne AV, Wainner RS, Rhon DI, et al. Clinical hip tests and a functional squat test in patients with knee osteoarthritis: Reliability, prevalence of positive test findings, and short-term response to hip mobilization. *J Orthop Sport Phys.* 2004;34(11):676-685.

164. Troelsen A, Mechlenburg I, Gelineck J, Bolvig L, Jacobsen S, Soballe K. What is the role of clinical tests and ultrasound in acetabular labral tear diagnostics? *Acta Orthop.* 2009;80(3):314-318.

165. Ross MD, Nordeen MH, Barido M. Test-retest reliability of Patrick's hip range of motion test in healthy college-aged men. *J Strength Cond Res.* 2003;17(1):156-161.

166. Sutlive TG, Lopez HP, Schnitker DE, et al. Development of a clinical prediction rule for diagnosing hip osteoarthritis in individuals with unilateral hip pain. *J Orthop Sport Phys.* 2008;38(9):542-550.

167. Theiler R, Stucki G, Schutz R, et al. Parametric and non-parametric measures in the assessment of knee and hip osteoarthritis: Interobserver reliability and correlation with radiology. *Osteoarthr Cartilage.* 1996;4(1):35-42.

168. Cibulka MT, Threlkeld J. The early clinical diagnosis of osteoarthritis of the hip. *J Orthop Sport Phys.* 2004;34(8):461-467.

169. O'Donnell J, Economopoulos K, Singh P, Bates D, Pritchard M. The ligamentum teres test: A novel and effective test in diagnosing tears of the ligamentum teres [published online ahead of print November 26 2013]. *Am J Sport Med.* 2013.

170. Leunig M, Beck M, Kalhor M, Kim YJ, Werlen S, Ganz R. Fibrocystic changes at anterosuperior femoral neck: Prevalence in hips with femoroacetabular impingement. *Radiology.* 2005;236(1):237-246.

171. Beaule PE, Zaragoza E, Motamedi K, Copelan N, Dorey FJ. Three-dimensional computed tomography of the hip in the assessment of femoroacetabular impingement. *J Orthop Res.* 2005;23(6):1286-1292.

172. Keeney JA, Peelle MW, Jackson J, Rubin D, Maloney WJ, Clohisy JC. Magnetic resonance arthrography versus arthroscopy in the evaluation of articular hip pathology. *Clin Orthop Relat R.* 2004;429:163-169.

173. Leunig M, Werlen S, Ungersbock A, Ito K, Ganz R. Evaluation of the acetabular labrum by MR arthrography. *J Bone Joint Surg Br.* 1997;79(2):230-234.

174. Sink EL, Gralla J, Ryba A, Dayton M. Clinical presentation of femoroacetabular impingement in adolescents. *J Pediatr Orthop.* 2008;28(8):806-811.

175. Chan YS, Lien LC, Hsu HL, et al. Evaluating hip labral tears using magnetic resonance arthrography: A prospective study comparing hip arthroscopy and magnetic resonance arthrography diagnosis. *Arthroscopy.* 2005;21(10):1250.

176. Hase T, Ueo T. Acetabular labral tear: Arthroscopic diagnosis and treatment. *Arthroscopy.* 1999;15(2):138-141.

177. Petersilge CA, Haque MA, Petersilge WJ, Lewin JS, Lieberman JM, Buly R. Acetabular labral tears: Evaluation with MR arthrography. *Radiology.* 1996;200(1):231-235.

178. Jari S, Paton RW, Srinivasan MS. Unilateral limitation of abduction of the hip. A valuable clinical sign for DDH? *J Bone Joint Surg Br.* 2002;84(1):104-107.

179. Kivlan BR, Martin RL. Functional performance testing of the hip in athletes. A systematic review for reliability and validity. *Int J Sports Phys Ther.* 2012;7(4):402-412.

180. Plisky PJ, Rauh MJ, Kaminski TW, Underwood FB. Star Excursion Balance Test as a predictor of lower extremity injury in high school basketball players. *J Orthop Sport Phys.* 2006;36(12):911-919.

181. Robinson R, Gribble P. Kinematic predictors of performance on the Star Excursion Balance Test. *J Sport Rehabil.* 2008;17(4):347-357.

182. Hubbard TJ, Kramer LC, Denegar CR, Hertel J. Correlations among multiple measures of functional and mechanical instability in subjects with chronic ankle instability. *J Athl Train.* 2007;42(3):361-366.

183. Norris B, Trudelle-Jackson E. Hip- and thigh-muscle activation during the star excursion balance test. *J Sport Rehabil.* 2011;20(4):428-441.

184. Crossley KM, Zhang WJ, Schache AG, Bryant A, Cowan SM. Performance on the single-leg squat task indicates hip abductor muscle function. *Am J Sport Med.* 2011;39(4):866-873.

185. Reiman MP, Manske RC. *Functional Testing in Human Performance.* Champaign, IL: Human Kinetics; 2009.

186. Wahoff M, Ryan M. Rehabilitation after hip femoroacetabular impingement arthroscopy. *Clin Sport Med.* 2011;30(2):463-482.

187. Altman RD, Fries JF, Bloch DA, et al. Radiographic assessment of progression in osteoarthritis. *Arthritis Rheum.* 1987;30(11):1214-1225.

188. Cooper C, Inskip H, Croft P, et al. Individual risk factors for hip osteoarthritis: Obesity, hip injury, and physical activity. *Am J Epidemiol.* 1998;147(6):516-522.

189. Yoshimura N, Sasaki S, Iwasaki K, et al. Occupational lifting is associated with hip osteoarthritis: A Japanese case-control study. *J Rheumatol.* 2000;27(2):434-440.

190. Yoshimura N, Nishioka S, Kinoshita H, et al. Risk factors for knee osteoarthritis in Japanese women: Heavy weight, previous joint injuries, and occupational activities. *J Rheumatol.* 2004;31(1):157-162.

191. Stratford PW, Kennedy DM. Performance measures were necessary to obtain a complete picture of osteoarthritic patients. *J Clin Epidemiol.* 2006;59(2):160-167.

192. Stratford PW, Kennedy DM, Woodhouse LJ. Performance measures provide assessments of pain and function in people with advanced osteoarthritis of the hip or knee. *Phys Ther.* 2006;86(11):1489-1496.

193. Terwee CB, van der Slikke RM, van Lummel RC, Benink RJ, Meijers WG, de Vet HC. Self-reported physical functioning was more influenced by pain than performance-based physical functioning in knee-osteoarthritis patients. *J Clin Epidemiol.* 2006;59(7):724-731.

194. van Dijk GM, Veenhof C, Schellevis F, et al. Comorbidity, limitations in activities and pain in patients with osteoarthritis of the hip or knee. *BMC Musculoskel Dis.* 2008;9:95.

195. Kellgren JH, Lawrence JS. Radiological assessment of osteo-arthrosis. *Ann Rheum Dis.* 1957;16(4):494-502.

196. Kennedy MJ, Lamontagne M, Beaule PE. Femoroacetabular impingement alters hip and pelvic biomechanics during gait: Walking biomechanics of FAI. *Gait Posture.* 2009;30(1):41-44.

197. Dekker J, van Dijk GM, Veenhof C. Risk factors for functional decline in osteoarthritis of the hip or knee. *Curr Opin Rheumatol.* 2009;21(5):520-524.

198. van Dijk GM, Dekker J, Veenhof C, van den Ende CH. Course of functional status and pain in osteoarthritis of the hip or knee: A systematic review of the literature. *Arthritis Rheum.* 2006;55(5):779-785.

199. Klassbo M, Harms-Ringdahl K, Larsson G. Examination of passive ROM and capsular patterns in the hip. *Physiother Res Int.* 2003;8(1):1-12.

200. Loureiro A, Mills PM, Barrett RS. Muscle weakness in hip osteoarthritis: A systematic review [published online ahead of print July 25 2012]. *Arthritis Care Res.* 2012.

201. Cibulka MT, White DM, Woehrle J, et al. Hip pain and mobility deficits—hip osteoarthritis: Clinical practice guidelines linked to the international classification of functioning, disability, and health from the orthopaedic section of the American Physical Therapy Association. *J Orthop Sport Phys.* 2009;39(4):A1-A25.

202. Terwee CB, Mokkink LB, Steultjens MP, Dekker J. Performance-based methods for measuring the physical function of patients with osteoarthritis of the hip or knee: A systematic review of measurement properties. *Rheumatology (Oxford).* 2006;45(7):890-902.

203. Groh MM, Herrera J. A comprehensive review of hip labral tears. *Curr Rev Musculoskelet Med.* 2009;2(2):105-117.

204. Hack K, Di Primio G, Rakhra K, Beaule PE. Prevalence of cam-type femoroacetabular impingement morphology in asymptomatic volunteers. *J Bone Joint Surg Am.* 2010;92(14):2436-2444.

205. Dolan MM, Heyworth BE, Bedi A, Duke G, Kelly BT. CT reveals a high incidence of osseous abnormalities in hips with labral tears. *Clin Orthop Relat R.* 2011;469(3):831-838.

206. Kapron AL, Anderson AE, Aoki SK, et al. Radiographic prevalence of femoroacetabular impingement in collegiate football players: AAOS exhibit selection. *J Bone Joint Surg Am.* 2011;93(19):e111(1-10).

207. Lamontagne M, Brisson N, Kennedy MJ, Beaule PE. Preoperative and postoperative lower-extremity joint and pelvic kinematics during maximal squatting of patients with cam femoro-acetabular impingement. *J Bone Joint Surg Am.* 2011;93(suppl 2):40-45.

208. Lodhia P, Slobogean GP, Noonan VK, Gilbart MK. Patient-reported outcome instruments for femoroacetabular impingement and hip labral pathology: A systematic review of the clinimetric evidence. *Arthroscopy.* 2011;27(2):279-286.

209. Lohan DG, Seeger LL, Motamedi K, Hame S, Sayre J. Cam-type femoral-acetabular impingement: Is the alpha angle the best MR arthrography has to offer? *Skeletal Radiol.* 2009;38(9):855-862.

210. Kalberer F, Sierra RJ, Madan SS, Ganz R, Leunig M. Ischial spine projection into the pelvis: A new sign for acetabular retroversion. *Clin Orthop Relat R.* 2008;466(3):677-683.

211. Akhtar M, Campton L. Generalized ligament laxity and hip arthroscopy in an athletic population. *Brit J Sport Med.* 2013;47(17):e4.

212. Kubiak-Langer M, Tannast M, Murphy SB, Siebenrock KA, Langlotz F. Range of motion in anterior femoroacetabular impingement. *Clin Orthop Relat R.* 2007;458:117-124.

213. Audenaert EA, Peeters I, Vigneron L, Baelde N, Pattyn C. Hip morphological characteristics and range of internal rotation in femoroacetabular impingement. *Am J Sport Med.* 2012;40(6):1329-1336.

214. Kelly BT, Bedi A, Robertson CM, Dela Torre K, Giveans MR, Larson CM. Alterations in internal rotation and alpha angles are associated with arthroscopic cam decompression in the hip. *Am J Sport Med.* 2012;40(5):1107-1112.

215. Bedi A, Zaltz I, De La Torre K, Kelly BT. Radiographic comparison of surgical hip dislocation and hip arthroscopy for treatment of cam deformity in femoroacetabular impingement. *Am J Sport Med.* 2011;39(suppl):20S-28S.

216. Lequesne M, Bellaiche L. Anterior femoroacetabular impingement: An update. *Joint Bone Spine.* 2012;79(3):249-255.

217. Casartelli NC, Maffiuletti NA, Item-Glatthorn JF, et al. Hip muscle weakness in patients with symptomatic femoroacetabular impingement. *Osteoarthr Cartilage.* 2011;19(7):816-821.

218. Casartelli NC, Leunig M, Item-Glatthorn JF, Lepers R, Maffiuletti NA. Hip flexor muscle fatigue in patients with symptomatic femoroacetabular impingement. *Int Orthop.* 2012;36(5):967-973.

219. Signorelli C, Lopomo N, Bonanzinga T, et al. Relationship between femoroacetabular contact areas and hip position in the normal joint: An in vitro evaluation. *Knee Surg Sport Tr A.* 2013;21(2):408-414.

220. Vendittoli PA, Young DA, Stitson DJ, Wolfe R, Del Buono A, Maffulli N. Acetabular rim lesions: Arthroscopic assessment and clinical relevance [published online ahead of print June 23 2012]. *Int Orthop.* 2012.

221. Domb BG, Shindle MK, McArthur B, Voos JE, Magennis EM, Kelly BT. Iliopsoas impingement: A newly identified cause of labral pathology in the hip. *HSS J.* 2011;7(2):145-150.

222. Tey M, Alvarez S, Rios JL. Hip labral cyst caused by psoas impingement. *Arthroscopy.* 2012;28(8):1184-1186.

223. Egol KA, Koval KJ, Kummer F, Frankel VH. Stress fractures of the femoral neck. *Clin Orthop Relat R.* 1998;348:72-78.

224. Fredericson M, Jennings F, Beaulieu C, Matheson GO. Stress fractures in athletes. *Top Magn Reson Imag.* 2006;17(5):309-325.

225. Gurney B, Boissonnault WG, Andrews R. Differential diagnosis of a femoral neck/head stress fracture. *J Orthop Sport Phys.* 2006;36(2):80-88.

226. Weishaar MD, McMillian DM, Moore JH. Identification and management of 2 femoral shaft stress injuries. *J Orthop Sport Phys.* 2005;35(10):665-673.

227. Adkins SB III, Figler RA. Hip pain in athletes. *Am Fam Physician.* 2000;61(7):2109-2118.

228. Weistroffer JK, Muldoon MP, Duncan DD, Fletcher EH, Padgett DE. Femoral neck stress fractures: Outcome analysis at minimum five-year follow-up. *J Orthop Trauma.* 2003;17(5):334-337.

229. Lawrence RC, Helmick CG, Arnett FC, et al. Estimates of the prevalence of arthritis and selected musculoskeletal disorders in the United States. *Arthritis Rheum.* 1998;41(5):778-799.

230. Watson RM, Roach NA, Dalinka MK. Avascular necrosis and bone marrow edema syndrome. *Radiol Clin N Am.* 2004;42(1):207-219.

231. Joe GO, Kovacs JA, Miller KD, et al. Diagnosis of avascular necrosis of the hip in asymptomatic HIV-infected patients: Clinical correlation of physical examination with magnetic resonance imaging. *J Back Musculoskelet.* 2002;16:135-139.

232. Brignall CG, Stainsby GD. The snapping hip. Treatment by Z-plasty. *J Bone Joint Surg Br.* 1991;73(2):253-254.

233. Faraj AA, Moulton A, Sirivastava VM. Snapping iliotibial band. Report of ten cases and review of the literature. *Acta Orthop. Belg.* 2001;67(1):19-23.

234. Ilizaliturri VM Jr, Camacho-Galindo J. Endoscopic treatment of snapping hips, iliotibial band, and iliopsoas tendon. *Sports Med Arthrosc.* 2010;18(2):120-127.

235. Jacobs M, Young R. Snapping hip phenomenon among dancers. *Am Correct Ther J.* 1978;32(3):92-98.

236. Deleget A. Overview of thigh injuries in dance. *J Dance Med Sci.* 2010;14(3):97-102.

237. Reid DC. Prevention of hip and knee injuries in ballet dancers. *Sports Med.* 1988;6(5):295-307.

238. Kocher MS, Tucker R. Pediatric athlete hip disorders. *Clin Sport Med.* 2006;25(2):241-253, viii.

239. Kovacevic D, Mariscalco M, Goodwin RC. Injuries about the hip in the adolescent athlete. *Sports Med Arthrosc.* 2011;19(1):64-74.

240. Loder RT, Starnes T, Dikos G. Atypical and typical (idiopathic) slipped capital femoral epiphysis. Reconfirmation of the age-weight test and description of the age-weight and age-height tests. *J Bone Joint Surg Am.* 2006;88(7):1574-1581.

241. Loder RT, Starnes T, Dikos G, Aronsson DD. Demographic predictors of severity of stable slipped capital femoral epiphyses. *J Bone Joint Surg Am.* 2006;88(1):97-105.

242. Lehmann CL, Arons RR, Loder RT, Vitale MG. The epidemiology of slipped capital femoral epiphysis: An update. *J Pediatr Orthop.* 2006;26(3):286-290.

243. Pellecchia GL, Lugo-Larcheveque N, Deluca PA. Differential diagnosis in physical therapy evaluation of thigh pain in an adolescent boy. *J Orthop Sport Phys.* 1996;23(1):51-55.

244. Loder RT, Dietz FR. What is the best evidence for the treatment of slipped capital femoral epiphysis? *J Pediatr Orthop.* 2012;32(suppl 2):S158-S165.

245. McKenzie M, Carlson B, Carlson WO. Evaluating hip pain in children. *S D Med.* 2012;65(8):303-305, 307-308.

246. Kaniklides C, Lonnerholm T, Moberg A, Sahlstedt B. Legg-Calve-Perthes disease. Comparison of conventional radiography, MR imaging, bone scintigraphy and arthrography. *Acta Radiol.* 1995;36(4):434-439.

247. Dillman JR, Hernandez RJ. MRI of Legg-Calve-Perthes disease. *AJR.* 2009;193(5):1394-1407.

248. Bradshaw CJ, Bundy M, Falvey E. The diagnosis of longstanding groin pain: A prospective clinical cohort study. *Brit J Sport Med.* 2008;42(10):851-854.

249. Thorborg K, Serner A, Petersen J, Madsen TM, Magnusson P, Holmich P. Hip adduction and abduction strength profiles in elite soccer players: Implications for clinical evaluation of hip adductor muscle recovery after injury. *Am J Sport Med.* 2011;39(1):121-126.

250. Hrysomallis C. Hip adductors' strength, flexibility, and injury risk. *J Strength Cond Res.* 2009;23(5):1514-1517.

251. Tyler TF, Nicholas SJ, Campbell RJ, McHugh MP. The association of hip strength and flexibility with the incidence of adductor muscle strains in professional ice hockey players. *Am J Sport Med.* 2001;29(2):124-128.

52. Verrall GM, Slavotinek JP, Barnes PG, Esterman A, Oakeshott RD, Spriggins AJ. Hip joint range of motion restriction precedes athletic chronic groin injury. *J Sci Med Sport.* 2007;10(6):463-466.

253. Weir A, de Vos RJ, Moen M, Holmich P, Tol JL. Prevalence of radiological signs of femoroacetabular impingement in patients presenting with long-standing adductor-related groin pain. *Brit J Sport Med.* 2011;45(1):6-9.

254. Holmich P, Thorborg K, Nyvold P, Klit J, Nielsen MB, Troelsen A. Does bony hip morphology affect the outcome of treatment for patients with adductor-related groin pain? Outcome 10 years after baseline assessment [published online ahead of print July 11 2013]. *Brit J Sport Med.* 2013.

55. Verrall GM, Hamilton IA, Slavotinek JP, et al. Hip joint range of motion reduction in sports-related chronic groin injury diagnosed as pubic bone stress injury. *J Sci Med Sport.* 2005;8(1):77-84.

256. Hegedus EJ, Stern B, Reiman MP, Tarara D, Wright AA. A suggested model for physical examination and conservative treatment of athletic pubalgia. *Phys Ther Sport.* 2013;14(1):3-16.

257. Verrall GM, Slavotinek JP, Fon GT, Barnes PG. Outcome of conservative management of athletic chronic groin injury diagnosed as pubic bone stress injury. *Am J Sport Med.* 2007;35(3):467-474.

258. Holmich P, Uhrskou P, Ulnits L, et al. Effectiveness of active physical training as treatment for long-standing adductor-related groin pain in athletes: Randomised trial. *Lancet.* 1999;353(9151):439-443.

259. Woods C, Hawkins RD, Maltby S, Hulse M, Thomas A, Hodson A. The Football Association Medical Research Programme: An audit of injuries in professional football—analysis of hamstring injuries. *Brit J Sport Med.* 2004;38(1):36-41.

260. Gabbett TJ. Incidence of injury in junior and senior rugby league players. *Sports Med.* 2004;34(12):849-859.

261. Verrall GM, Slavotinek JP, Barnes PG, Fon GT, Spriggins AJ. Clinical risk factors for hamstring muscle strain injury: A prospective study with correlation of injury by magnetic resonance imaging. *Brit J Sport Med.* 2001;35(6):435-439, discussion 440.

262. Askling CM, Tengvar M, Saartok T, Thorstensson A. Acute first-time hamstring strains during slow-speed stretching: Clinical, magnetic resonance imaging, and recovery characteristics. *Am J Sport Med.* 2007;35(10):1716-1724.

263. Brooks JH, Fuller CW, Kemp SP, Reddin DB. Incidence, risk, and prevention of hamstring muscle injuries in professional rugby union. *Am J Sport Med.* 2006;34(8):1297-1306.

264. Brooks JH, Fuller CW, Kemp SP, Reddin DB. Epidemiology of injuries in English professional rugby union: part 1 match injuries. *Brit J Sport Med.* 2005;39(10):757-766.

265. Brooks JH, Fuller CW, Kemp SP, Reddin DB. Epidemiology of injuries in English professional rugby union: Part 2 training injuries. *Brit J Sport Med.* 2005;39(10):767-775.

266. Meeuwisse WH, Sellmer R, Hagel BE. Rates and risks of injury during intercollegiate basketball. *Am J Sport Med.* 2003;31(3):379-385.

267. Orchard J, Seward H. Epidemiology of injuries in the Australian Football League, seasons 1997-2000. *Brit J Sport Med.* 2002;36(1):39-44.

268. Schache AG, Dorn TW, Blanch PD, Brown NA, Pandy MG. Mechanics of the human hamstring muscles during sprinting. *Med Sci Sport Exerc.* 2012;44(4):647-658.

269. Petersen J, Holmich P. Evidence based prevention of hamstring injuries in sport. *Brit J Sport Med.* 2005;39(6):319-323.

270. Connell DA, Schneider-Kolsky ME, Hoving JL, et al. Longitudinal study comparing sonographic and MRI assessments of acute and healing hamstring injuries. *AJR.* 2004;183(4):975-984.

271. Slavotinek JP. Muscle injury: The role of imaging in prognostic assignment and monitoring of muscle repair. *Semin Musculoskel R.* 2010;14(2):194-200.

272. Blankenbaker DG, Tuite MJ. Temporal changes of muscle injury. *Semin Musculoskel R.* 2010;14(2):176-193.

273. Silder A, Sherry MA, Sanfilippo J, Tuite MJ, Hetzel SJ, Heiderscheit BC. Clinical and morphological changes following 2 rehabilitation programs for acute hamstring strain injuries: A randomized clinical trial. *J Orthop Sport Phys.* 2013;43(5):284-299.

274. Reurink G, Goudswaard GJ, Tol JL, et al. MRI observations at return to play of clinically recovered hamstring injuries [published online ahead of print November 19 2013]. *Brit J Sport Med.* 2013.

275. Petersen J, Thorborg K, Nielsen MB, et al. The diagnostic and prognostic value of ultrasonography in soccer players with acute hamstring injuries [published online ahead of print December 11 2013]. *Am J Sport Med.* 2013.

276. Askling C, Saartok T, Thorstensson A. Type of acute hamstring strain affects flexibility, strength, and time to return to pre-injury level. *Brit J Sport Med.* 2006;40(1):40-44.

277. Orchard JW, Farhart P, Leopold C. Lumbar spine region pathology and hamstring and calf injuries in athletes: Is there a connection? *Brit J Sport Med.* 2004;38(4):502-504, discussion 502-504.

278. Fousekis K, Tsepis E, Poulmedis P, Athanasopoulos S, Vagenas G. Intrinsic risk factors of non-contact quadriceps and hamstring strains in soccer: A prospective study of 100 professional players. *Brit J Sport Med.* 2011;45(9):709-714.

279. Turl SE, George KP. Adverse neural tension: A factor in repetitive hamstring strain? *J Orthop Sport Phys.* 1998;27(1):16-21.

280. Askling CM, Nilsson J, Thorstensson A. A new hamstring test to complement the common clinical examination before return to sport after injury. *Knee Surg Sport Tr A.* 2010;18(12):1798-1803.

281. Kong A, Van der Vliet A, Zadow S. MRI and US of gluteal tendinopathy in greater trochanteric pain syndrome. *Eur Radiol.* 2007;17(7):1772-1783.

282. Bunker TD, Esler CN, Leach WJ. Rotator-cuff tear of the hip. *J Bone Joint Surg Br.* 1997;79(4):618-620.

283. Long SS, Surrey DE, Nazarian LN. Sonography of greater trochanteric pain syndrome and the rarity of primary bursitis. *AJR.* 2013;201(5):1083-1086.

284. Blankenbaker DG, Ullrick SR, Davis KW, De Smet AA, Haaland B, Fine JP. Correlation of MRI findings with clinical findings of trochanteric pain syndrome. *Skeletal Radiol.* 2008;37(10):903-909.

285. Silva F, Adams T, Feinstein J, Arroyo RA. Trochanteric bursitis: Refuting the myth of inflammation. *J Clin Rheumatol.* 2008;14(2):82-86.

286. Johnston CA, Lindsay DM, Wiley JP. Treatment of iliopsoas syndrome with a hip rotation strengthening program: A retrospective case series. *J Orthop Sport Phys.* 1999;29(4):218-224.

287. Tormenta S, Sconfienza LM, Iannessi F, et al. Prevalence study of iliopsoas bursitis in a cohort of 860 patients affected by symptomatic hip osteoarthritis. *Ultrasound Med Biol.* 2012;38(8):1352-1356.

288. Ho GW, Howard TM. Greater trochanteric pain syndrome: More than bursitis and iliotibial tract friction. *Curr Sports Med Rep.* 2012;11(5):232-238.

289. Sayegh F, Potoupnis M, Kapetanos G. Greater trochanter bursitis pain syndrome in females with chronic low back pain and sciatica. *Acta Orthop Belg.* 2004;70(5):423-428.

Chapter 25

1. Childs JD, Cleland JA, Elliott JM, et al. Neck pain: Clinical practice guidelines linked to the International Classification of Functioning, Disability, and Health from the Orthopedic Section of the American Physical Therapy Association. *J Orthop Sport Phys.* 2008;38(9):A1-A34.

2. Logerstedt DS, Snyder-Mackler L, Ritter RC, Axe MJ, Godges JJ. Knee stability and movement coordination impairments: Knee ligament sprain. *J Orthop Sport Phys* 2010;40(4):A1-A37.

3. Logerstedt DS, Snyder-Mackler L, Ritter RC, Axe MJ. Knee pain and mobility impairments: Meniscal and articular cartilage lesions. *J Orthop Sport Phys.* 2010;40(6):A1-A35.

4. Bachmann LM, Kolb E, Koller MT, Steurer J, ter Riet G. Accuracy of Ottawa ankle rules to exclude fractures of the ankle and mid-foot: Systematic review. *BMJ.* 2003;326(7386):417.

5. Robertson A, Nutton RW, Keating JF. Dislocation of the knee. *J Bone Joint Surg Br.* 2006;88(6):706-711.

6. Butler DL, Noyes FR, Grood ES. Ligamentous restraints to anterior-posterior drawer in the human knee. A biomechanical study. *J Bone Joint Surg Am.* 1980;62(2):259-270.

7. Duthon VB, Barea C, Abrassart S, Fasel JH, Fritschy D, Menetrey J. Anatomy of the anterior cruciate ligament. *Knee Surg Sport Tr A.* 2006;14(3):204-213.

8. Amis AA, Gupte CM, Bull AM, Edwards A. Anatomy of the posterior cruciate ligament and the meniscofemoral ligaments. *Knee Surg Sport Tr A.* 2006;14(3):257-263.

9. Janousek AT, Jones DG, Clatworthy M, Higgins LD, Fu FH. Posterior cruciate ligament injuries of the knee joint. *Sports Med.* 1999;28(6):429-441.

10. Grood ES, Noyes FR, Butler DL, Suntay WJ. Ligamentous and capsular restraints preventing straight medial and lateral laxity in intact human cadaver knees. *J Bone Joint Surg Am.* 1981;63(8):1257-1269.

11. Brindle T, Nyland J, Johnson DL. The meniscus: Review of basic principles with application to surgery and rehabilitation. *J Athl Train.* 2001;36(2):160-169.

12. Kutzner I, Heinlein B, Graichen F, et al. Loading of the knee joint during activities of daily living measured in vivo in five subjects. *J Biomech.* 2010;43(11):2164-2173.

13. Rothstein JM, Echternach JL. Hypothesis-oriented algorithm for clinicians. A method for evaluation and treatment planning. *Phys Ther.* 1986;66(9):1388-1394.

14. Kolt GS, Snyder-Mackler L. *Physical Therapies in Sport and Exercise.* Edinburgh, Scotland: Churchill Livingstone; 2003.

15. Calmbach WL, Hutchens M. Evaluation of patients presenting with knee pain: Part II. Differential diagnosis. *Am Fam Physician.* 2003;68(5):917-922.

16. Griffin LY, Albohm MJ, Arendt EA, et al. Understanding and preventing noncontact anterior cruciate ligament injuries: A review of the Hunt Valley II meeting, January 2005. *Am J Sports Med.* 2006;34(9):1512-1532.

17. Shimokochi Y, Shultz SJ. Mechanisms of noncontact anterior cruciate ligament injury. *J Athl Train.* 2008;43(4):396-408.

18. Jackson JL, O'Malley PG, Kroenke K. Evaluation of acute knee pain in primary care. *Ann Intern Med.* 2003;139(7):575-588.

19. Madhusudhan T, Kumar T, Bastawrous S, Sinha A. Clinical examination, MRI and arthroscopy in meniscal and ligamentous knee injuries—a prospective study. *J Orthop Surg.* 2008;3:19.

20. Brukner P, Khan K. *Clinical Sports Medicine.* Sydney, Australia: McGraw-Hill; 2006.

21. Bansal P, Deehan DJ, Gregory RJ. Diagnosing the acutely locked knee. *Injury.* 2002;33(6):495-498.

22. Hambly K, Griva K. IKDC or KOOS: Which one captures symptoms and disabilities most important to patients who have undergone initial anterior cruciate ligament reconstruction? *Am J Sports Med.* 2010;38(7):1395-1404.

23. Stratford PW, Kennedy DM. Performance measures were necessary to obtain a complete picture of osteoarthritic patients. *J Clin Epidemiol.* 2006;59(2):160-167.

24. Stratford PW, Kennedy DM, Woodhouse LJ. Performance measures provide assessments of pain and function in people with advanced osteoarthritis of the hip or knee. *Phys Ther.* 2006;86(11):1489-1496.

25. Fitzgerald GK, Lephart SM, Hwang JH, Wainner RS. Hop tests as predictors of dynamic knee stability. *J Orthop Sport Phys.* 2001;31(10):588-597.

26. Dobson F, Hinman RS, Roos EM, et al. OARSI recommended performance-based tests to assess physical function in people diagnosed with hip or knee osteoarthritis. *Osteoarthr Cartilage.* 2013;21(8):1042-1052.

27. Risberg MA, Holm I, Tjomsland O, Ljunggren E, Ekeland A. Prospective study of changes in impairments and disabilities after anterior cruciate ligament reconstruction. *J Orthop Sport Phys.* 1999;29(7):400-412.

28. Mizner RL, Petterson SC, Clements KE, Zeni JA Jr, Irrgang JJ, Snyder-Mackler L. Measuring functional improvement after total knee arthroplasty requires both performance-based and patient-report assessments: A longitudinal analysis of outcomes. *J Arthroplasty.* 2011;26(5):728-737.

29. Logerstedt D, Lynch A, Axe MJ, Snyder-Mackler L. Symmetry restoration and functional recovery before and after anterior cruciate ligament reconstruction. *Knee Surg Sport Tr A.* 2013;21(4):859-868.

30. Lynch AD, Logerstedt DS, Grindem H, et al. Consensus criteria for defining 'successful outcome' after ACL injury and reconstruction: A Delaware-Oslo ACL cohort investigation [published online ahead of print July 23 2013]. *Brit J Sport Med.* 2013.

31. Clayton RA, Court-Brown CM. The epidemiology of musculoskeletal tendinous and ligamentous injuries. *Injury.* 2008;39(12):1338-1344.

32. Beattie KA, Boulos P, Pui M, et al. Abnormalities identified in the knees of asymptomatic volunteers using peripheral magnetic resonance imaging. *Osteoarthr Cartilage.* 2005;13(3):181-186.

33. Kaplan LD, Schurhoff MR, Selesnick H, Thorpe M, Uribe JW. Magnetic resonance imaging of the knee in asymptomatic professional basketball players. *Arthroscopy.* 2005;21(5):557-561.

34. LaPrade RF, Burnett QM, Veenstra MA, Hodgman CG. The prevalence of abnormal magnetic resonance imaging findings in asymptomatic knees. With correlation of magnetic resonance imaging to arthroscopic findings in symptomatic knees. *Am J Sports Med.* 1994;22(6):739-745.

35. Kocabey Y, Tetik O, Isbell WM, Atay OA, Johnson DL. The value of clinical examination versus magnetic resonance imaging in the diagnosis of meniscal tears and anterior cruciate ligament rupture. *Arthroscopy.* 2004;20(7):696-700.

36. Menashe L, Hirko K, Losina E, et al. The diagnostic performance of MRI in osteoarthritis: A systematic review and meta-analysis. *Osteoarthr Cartilage.* 2012;20(1):13-21.

37. Quatman CE, Hettrich CM, Schmitt LC, Spindler KP. The clinical utility and diagnostic performance of magnetic resonance imaging for identification of early and advanced knee osteoarthritis: A systematic review. *Am J Sport Med.* 2011;39(7):1557-1568.

38. Galea A, Giuffre B, Dimmick S, Coolican MR, Parker DA. The accuracy of magnetic resonance imaging scanning and its influence on management decisions in knee surgery. *Arthroscopy.* 2009;25(5):473-480.

39. Crawford R, Walley G, Bridgman S, Maffulli N. Magnetic resonance imaging versus arthroscopy in the diagnosis of knee pathology, concentrating on meniscal lesions and ACL tears: A systematic review. *Brit Med Bull.* 2007;84:5-23.

40. Oei EH, Ginai AZ, Hunink MG. MRI for traumatic knee injury: A review. *Semin Ultrasound CT.* 2007;28(2):141-157.

41. Panisset JC, Ntagiopoulos PG, Saggin PR, Dejour D. A comparison of Telos™ stress radiography versus Rolimeter™ in the diagnosis of different patterns of anterior cruciate ligament tears. *Orthop Traumatol Surg Res.* 2012;98(7):751-758.

42. Navali AM, Bazavar M, Mohseni MA, Safari B, Tabrizi A. Arthroscopic evaluation of the accuracy of clinical examination versus MRI in diagnosing meniscus tears and cruciate ligament ruptures. *Arch Iran Med.* 2013;16(4):229-232.

43. Stiell IG, Greenberg GH, Wells GA, et al. Derivation of a decision rule for the use of radiography in acute knee injuries. *Ann Emerg Med.* 1995;26(4):405-413.

44. Bauer DC, Hunter DJ, Abramson SB, et al. Classification of osteoarthritis biomarkers: A proposed approach. *Osteoarthr Cartilage.* 2006;14(8):723-727.

45. Nicolaas L, Tigchelaar S, Koëter S. Patellofemoral evaluation with magnetic resonance imaging in 51 knees of asymptomatic subjects. *Knee Surg Sport Tr A.* 2011;19(10):1735-1739.

46. Emparanza JI, Aginaga JR. Validation of the Ottawa Knee Rules. *Ann Emerg Med.* 2001;38(4):364-368.

47. Bachmann LM, Haberzeth S, Steurer J, ter Riet G. The accuracy of the Ottawa knee rule to rule out knee fractures: A systematic review. *Ann Intern Med.* 2004;140(2):121-124.

48. Seaberg DC, Jackson R. Clinical decision rule for knee radiographs. *Am J Emerg Med.* 1994;12(5):541-543.

49. Seaberg DC, Yealy DM, Lukens T, Auble T, Mathias S. Multicenter comparison of two clinical decision rules for the use of radiography in acute, high-risk knee injuries. *Ann Emerg Med.* 1998;32(1):8-13.

50. Simon LV, Matteucci MJ, Tanen DA, Roos JA, Riffenburgh RH. The Pittsburgh Decision Rule: Triage nurse versus physician utilization in the emergency department. *J Emerg Med.* 2006;31(3):247-250.

51. Cheung TC, Tank Y, Breederveld RS, Tuinebreijer WE, de Lange-de Klerk ES, Derksen RJ. Diagnostic accuracy and reproducibility of the Ottawa Knee Rule vs the Pittsburgh Decision Rule. *Am J Emerg Med.* 2013;31(4):641-645.

52. Beall DP, Googe JD, Moss JT, et al. Magnetic resonance imaging of the collateral ligaments and the anatomic quadrants of the knee. *Radiol Clin N Am.* 2007;45(6):983-1002, vi.

53. Buckwalter JA, Mankin HJ, Grodzinsky AJ. Articular cartilage and osteoarthritis. *Instr Course Lect.* 2005;54:465-480.

54. Buckwalter JA, Martin JA. Osteoarthritis. *Adv Drug Deliv Rev.* 2006;58(2):150-167.

55. Guermazi A, Hayashi D, Roemer FW, Felson DT. Osteoarthritis: A review of strengths and weaknesses of different imaging options. *Rheum Dis Clin N Am.* 2013;39(3):567-591.

56. Schmid MR, Pfirrmann CW, Hodler J, Vienne P, Zanetti M. Cartilage lesions in the ankle joint: Comparison of MR arthrography and CT arthrography. *Skeletal Radiol.* 2003;32(5):259-265.

57. Omoumi P, Mercier GA, Lecouvet F, Simoni P, Vande Berg BC. CT arthrography, MR arthrography, PET, and scintigraphy in osteoarthritis. *Radiol Clin N Am.* 2009;47(4):595-615.

58. Williams GN, Buchanan TS, Barrance PJ, Axe MJ, Snyder-Mackler L. Quadriceps weakness, atrophy, and activation failure in predicted noncopers after anterior cruciate ligament injury. *Am J Sport Med.* 2005;33(3):402-408.

59. Chmielewski TL, Hurd WJ, Snyder-Mackler L. Elucidation of a potentially destabilizing control strategy in ACL deficient non-copers. *J Electromyogr Kines.* 2005;15(1):83-92.

60. Di Stasi SL, Snyder-Mackler L. The effects of neuromuscular training on the gait patterns of ACL-deficient men and women. *Clin Biomech (Bristol, Avon).* 2012;27(4):360-365.

61. Baliunas AJ, Hurwitz DE, Ryals AB, et al. Increased knee joint loads during walking are present in subjects with knee osteoarthritis. *Osteoarthr Cartilage.* 2002;10(7):573-579.

62. Mündermann A, Dyrby CO, Hurwitz DE, Sharma L, Andriacchi TP. Potential strategies to reduce medial compartment loading in patients with knee osteoarthritis of varying severity: Reduced walking speed. *Arthritis Rheum.* 2004;50(4):1172-1178.

63. Miyazaki T, Wada M, Kawahara H, Sato M, Baba H, Shimada S. Dynamic load at baseline can predict radiographic disease progression in medial compartment knee osteoarthritis. *Ann Rheum Dis.* 2002;61(7):617-622.

64. Laubenthal KN, Smidt GL, Kettelkamp DB. A quantitative analysis of knee motion during activities of daily living. *Phys Ther.* 1972;52(1):34-43.

65. Delitto A, Erhard RE, Bowling RW. A treatment-based classification approach to low back syndrome: Identifying and staging patients for conservative treatment. *Phys Ther.* 1995;75(6):470-485, discussion 485-479.

66. Donelson R, Aprill C, Medcalf R, Grant W. A prospective study of centralization of lumbar and referred pain. A predictor of symptomatic discs and anular competence. *Spine (Phila Pa 1976).* 1997;22(10):1115-1122.

67. Laslett M, Oberg B, Aprill CN, McDonald B. Centralization as a predictor of provocation discography results in chronic low back pain, and the influence of disability and distress on diagnostic power. *Spine J.* 2005;5(4):370-380.

68. Vroomen PC, de Krom MC, Wilmink JT, Kester AD, Knottnerus JA. Diagnostic value of history and physical examination in patients suspected of lumbosacral nerve root compression. *J Neurol Neurosur Ps.* 2002;72(5):630-634.

69. van der Windt DA, Simons E, Riphagen II, et al. Physical examination for lumbar radiculopathy due to disc herniation in patients with low-back pain. *Cochrane Db Syst Rev.* 2010;2:CD007431.

70. Stankovic R, Johnell O, Maly P, Willner S. Use of lumbar extension, slump test, physical and neurological examination in the evaluation of patients with suspected herniated nucleus pulposus. A prospective clinical study. *Man Ther.* 1999;4(1):25-32.

71. Laslett M, McDonald B, Aprill CN, Tropp H, Oberg B. Clinical predictors of screening lumbar zygapophyseal joint blocks: Development of clinical prediction rules. *Spine J.* 2006;6(4):370-379.

72. Laslett M, Young SB, Aprill CN, McDonald B. Diagnosing painful sacroiliac joints: A validity study of a McKenzie evaluation and sacroiliac provocation tests. *Aust J Physiother.* 2003;49(2):89-97.

73. Laslett M, Aprill CN, McDonald B, Young SB. Diagnosis of sacroiliac joint pain: Validity of individual provocation tests and composites of tests. *Man Ther.* 2005;10(3):207-218.

74. Reiman MP, Goode AP, Hegedus EJ, Cook CE, Wright AA. Diagnostic accuracy of clinical tests of the hip: A systematic review with meta-analysis. *Brit J Sport Med.* 2013;47(14):893-902.

75. Piriyaprasarth P, Morris ME. Psychometric properties of measurement tools for quantifying knee joint position and movement: A systematic review. *Knee.* 2007;14(1):2-8.

76. Clapper MP, Wolf SL. Comparison of the reliability of the Orthoranger and the standard goniometer for assessing active lower extremity range of motion. *Phys Ther.* 1988;68(2):214-218.

77. Shelbourne KD, Gray T. Results of anterior cruciate ligament reconstruction based on meniscus and articular cartilage status at the time of surgery. Five- to fifteen-year evaluations. *Am J Sport Med.* 2000;28(4):446-452.

78. Mauro CS, Irrgang JJ, Williams BA, Harner CD. Loss of extension following anterior cruciate ligament reconstruction: Analysis of incidence and etiology using IKDC criteria. *Arthroscopy.* 2008;24(2):146-153.

79. Bezuidenhout B. *The Intra- and Interexaminer Reliability of Motion Palpation of the Patella* [dissertation]. Durban, South Africa: Durban University of Technology; 2002.

80. Vaghmaria J. *An Investigation Into the Inter-Examiner Reliability of Motion Palpation of the Patella in Patellofemoral Pain Syndrome and Osteoarthritis* [dissertation]. Durban, South Africa: Durban Institute of Technology; 2006.

81. Farrimond C. *The Inter-Examiner Reliability and Comparison of Motion Palpation Findings of the Knee Joint in Patellofemoral Pain Syndrome and Asymptomatic Knee Joints* [dissertation]. Durban, South Africa: Durban University of Technology; 2010.

82. Bohannon RW. Manual muscle testing: Does it meet the standards of an adequate screening test? *Clin Rehabil.* 2005;19(6):662-667.

83. Knapik JJ, Bauman CL, Jones BH, Harris JM, Vaughan L. Preseason strength and flexibility imbalances associated with athletic injuries in female collegiate athletes. *Am J Sport Med.* 1991;19(1):76-81.

84. Nadler SF, Malanga GA, Feinberg JH, Prybicien M, Stitik TP, DePrince M. Relationship between hip muscle imbalance and occurrence of low back pain in collegiate athletes: A prospective study. *Am J Phys Med Rehabil.* 2001;80(8):572-577.

85. Fousekis K, Tsepis E, Poulmedis P, Athanasopoulos S, Vagenas G. Intrinsic risk factors of non-contact quadriceps and hamstring strains in soccer: A prospective study of 100 professional players. *Brit J Sport Med.* 2011;45(9):709-714.

86. Baumhauer JF, Alosa DM, Renstrom AF, Trevino S, Beynnon B. A prospective study of ankle injury risk factors. *Am J Sport Med.* 1995;23(5):564-570.

87. Soderman K, Alfredson H, Pietila T, Werner S. Risk factors for leg injuries in female soccer players: A prospective investigation during one outdoor season. *Knee Surg Sport Tr A.* 2001;9(5):313-321.

88. Hewett TE, Di Stasi SL, Myer GD. Current concepts for injury prevention in athletes after anterior cruciate ligament reconstruction. *Am J Sport Med.* 2013;41(1):216-224.

89. Palmieri-Smith RM, Thomas AC, Wojtys EM. Maximizing quadriceps strength after ACL reconstruction. *Clin Sports Med.* 2008;27(3):405-424, vii-ix.

90. Oberlander MA, Shalvoy RM, Hughston JC. The accuracy of the clinical knee examination documented by arthroscopy. A prospective study. *Am J Sport Med.* 1993;21(6):773-778.

91. Yoon YS, Rah JH, Park HJ. A prospective study of the accuracy of clinical examination evaluated by arthroscopy of the knee. *Int Orthop.* 1997;21(4):223-227.

92. Hegedus EJ, Cook C, Hasselblad V, Goode A, McCrory DC. Physical examination tests for assessing a torn meniscus in the knee: A systematic review with meta-analysis. *J Orthop Sport Phys.* 2007;37(9):541-550.

93. Meserve BB, Cleland JA, Boucher TR. A meta-analysis examining clinical test utilities for assessing meniscal injury. *Clin Rehabil.* 2008;22(2):143-161.

94. Konan S, Rayan F, Haddad FS. Do physical diagnostic tests accurately detect meniscal tears? *Knee Surg Sport Tr A.* 2009;17(7):806-811.

95. Pookarnjanamorakot C, Korsantirat T, Woratanarat P. Meniscal lesions in the anterior cruciate insufficient knee: The accuracy of clinical evaluation. *J Med Assoc Thai.* 2004;87(6):618-623.

96. Jaddue D, Tawfiq F, Sayed-Noor A. The utility of clinical examination in the diagnosis of medial meniscus injury in comparison with arthroscopic findings. *Eur J Orthop Surg Tr.* 2010;20:389-392.

97. Mirzatolooei F, Yekta Z, Bayazidchi M, Ershadi S, Afshar A. Validation of the Thessaly test for detecting meniscal tears in anterior cruciate deficient knees. *Knee.* 2010;17(3):221-223.

98. Evans PJ, Bell GD, Frank C. Prospective evaluation of the McMurray test. *Am J Sport Med.* 1993;21(4):604-608.

99. Karachalios T, Hantes M, Zibis AH, Zachos V, Karantanas AH, Malizos KN. Diagnostic accuracy of a new clinical test (the Thessaly test) for early detection of meniscal tears. *J Bone Joint Surg Am.* 2005;87(5):955-962.

100. Akseki D, Ozcan O, Boya H, Pinar H. A new weight-bearing meniscal test and a comparison with McMurray's test and joint line tenderness. *Arthroscopy.* 2004;20(9):951-958.

101. Kurosaka M, Yagi M, Yoshiya S, Muratsu H, Mizuno K. Efficacy of the axially loaded pivot shift test for the diagnosis of a meniscal tear. *Int Orthop.* 1999;23(5):271-274.

102. Fowler PJ, Lubliner JA. The predictive value of five clinical signs in the evaluation of meniscal pathology. *Arthroscopy.* 1989;5(3):184-186.

103. Sae-Jung S, Jirarattanaphochai K, Benjasil T. KKU knee compression-rotation test for detection of meniscal tears: A comparative study of its diagnostic accuracy with McMurray test. *J Med Assoc Thai.* 2007;90(4):718-723.

104. Mariani PP, Adriani E, Maresca G, Mazzola CG. A prospective evaluation of a test for lateral meniscus tears. *Knee Surg Sport Tr A.* 1996;4(1):22-26.

105. Anderson AF, Lipscomb AB. Clinical diagnosis of meniscal tears. Description of a new manipulative test. *Am J Sport Med.* 1986;14(4):291-293.

106. Noble J, Erat K. In defence of the meniscus. A prospective study of 200 meniscectomy patients. *J Bone Joint Surg Br.* 1980;62-B(1):7-11.

107. Wagemakers HP, Heintjes EM, Boks SS, et al. Diagnostic value of history-taking and physical examination for assessing meniscal tears of the knee in general practice. *Clin J Sport Med.* 2008;18(1):24-30.

108. Jerosch J, Riemer S. How good are clinical investigative procedures for diagnosing meniscus lesions? [in German]. *Sportverletz Sportschaden.* 2004;18(2):59-67.

109. Simonsen O, Jensen J, Mouritsen P, Lauritzen J. The accuracy of clinical examination of injury of the knee joint. *Injury.* 1984;16(2):96-101.

110. Rose NE, Gold SM. A comparison of accuracy between clinical examination and magnetic resonance imaging in the diagnosis of meniscal and anterior cruciate ligament tears. *Arthroscopy.* 1996;12(4):398-405.

111. Kocher MS, DiCanzio J, Zurakowski D, Micheli LJ. Diagnostic performance of clinical examination and selective magnetic resonance imaging in the evaluation of intraarticular knee disorders in children and adolescents. *Am J Sport Med.* 2001;29(3):292-296.

112. Wagemakers HP, Luijsterburg PA, Boks SS, et al. Diagnostic accuracy of history taking and physical examination for assessing anterior cruciate ligament lesions of the knee in primary care. *Arch Phys Med Rehab.* 2010;91(9):1452-1459.

113. Benjaminse A, Gokeler A, van der Schans CP. Clinical diagnosis of an anterior cruciate ligament rupture: A meta-analysis. *J Orthop Sport Phys.* 2006;36(5):267-288.

114. Dejour D, Ntagiopoulos PG, Saggin PR, Panisset JC. The diagnostic value of clinical tests, magnetic resonance imaging, and instrumented laxity in the differentiation of complete versus partial anterior cruciate ligament tears. *Arthroscopy.* 2013;29(3):491-499.

115. Rubinstein RA Jr, Shelbourne KD, McCarroll JR, VanMeter CD, Rettig AC. The accuracy of the clinical examination in the setting of posterior cruciate ligament injuries. *Am J Sport Med.* 1994;22(4):550-557.

116. Kastelein M, Wagemakers HP, Luijsterburg PA, Verhaar JA, Koes BW, Bierma-Zeinstra SM. Assessing medial collateral ligament knee lesions in general practice. *Am J Med.* 2008;121(11):982-988.e2.

117. Näslund J, Näslund UB, Odenbring S, Lundeberg T. Comparison of symptoms and clinical findings in subgroups of individuals with patellofemoral pain. *Physiother Theory Pract.* 2006;22(3):105-118.

118. Sweitzer BA, Cook C, Steadman JR, Hawkins RJ, Wyland DJ. The inter-rater reliability and diagnostic accuracy of patellar mobility tests in patients with anterior knee pain. *Phys Sportsmed.* 2010;38(3):90-96.

119. Haim A, Yaniv M, Dekel S, Amir H. Patellofemoral pain syndrome: Validity of clinical and radiological features. *Clin Orthop Relat R.* 2006;451:223-228.

120. Nunes GS, Stapait EL, Kirsten MH, de Noronha M, Santos GM. Clinical test for diagnosis of patellofemoral pain syndrome: Systematic review with meta-analysis. *Phys Ther Sport.* 2013;14(1):54-59.

121. Nijs J, Van Geel C, Van der auwera C, Van de Velde B. Diagnostic value of five clinical tests in patellofemoral pain syndrome. *Man Ther.* 2006;11(1):69-77.

122. Cook C, Hegedus E, Hawkins R, Scovell F, Wyland D. Diagnostic accuracy and association to disability of clinical test findings associated with patellofemoral pain syndrome. *Physiother Can.* 2010;62(1):17-24.

123. Elton K, McDonough K, Savinar-Nogue E, Jensen GM. A preliminary investigation: History, physical, and isokinetic exam results versus arthroscopic diagnosis of chondromalacia patella. *J Orthop Sport Phys.* 1985;7(3):115-123.

124. Cook JL, Khan KM, Kiss ZS, Purdam CR, Griffiths L. Reproducibility and clinical utility of tendon palpation to detect patellar tendinopathy in young basketball players. Victorian Institute of Sport tendon study group. *Brit J Sport Med.* 2001;35(1):65-69.

125. Sijbrandij S. Instability of the proximal tibio-fibular joint. *Acta Orthop Scand.* 1978;49(6):621-626.

126. Baciu CC, Tudor A, Olaru I. Recurrent luxation of the superior tibio-fibular joint in the adult. *Acta Orthop Scand.* 1974;45(5):772-777.

127. Sturgill LP, Snyder-Mackler L, Manal TJ, Axe MJ. Interrater reliability of a clinical scale to assess knee joint effusion. *J Orthop Sport Phys.* 2009;39(12):845-849.

128. Kastelein M, Luijsterburg PA, Wagemakers HP, et al. Diagnostic value of history taking and physical examination to assess effusion of the knee in traumatic knee patients in general practice. *Arch Phys Med Rehab.* 2009;90(1):82-86.

129. Stratford PW, Kennedy DM, Maly MR, Macintyre NJ. Quantifying self-report measures' overestimation of mobility scores postarthroplasty. *Phys Ther.* 2010;90(9):1288-1296.

130. Gage BE, McIlvain NM, Collins CL, Fields SK, Comstock RD. Epidemiology of 6.6 million knee injuries presenting to United States emergency departments from 1999 through 2008. *Acad Emerg Med.* 2012;19(4):378-385.

131. Ingram JG, Fields SK, Yard EE, Comstock RD. Epidemiology of knee injuries among boys and girls in US high school athletics. *Am J Sport Med.* 2008;36(6):1116-1122.

132. Powell JW, Barber-Foss KD. Injury patterns in selected high school sports: A review of the 1995-1997 seasons. *J Athl Train.* 1999;34(3):277-284.

133. O'Keeffe SA, Hogan BA, Eustace SJ, Kavanagh EC. Overuse injuries of the knee. *Magn Reson Imaging Clin N Am.* 2009;17(4):725-739.

134. Buckwalter JA, Saltzman C, Brown T. The impact of osteoarthritis: Implications for research. *Clin Orthop Relat R.* 2004;427(suppl):S6-S15.

135. Griffin LY, Agel J, Albohm MJ, et al. Noncontact anterior cruciate ligament injuries: Risk factors and prevention strategies. *J Am Acad Orthop Surg.* 2000;8(3):141-150.

136. Murphy L, Schwartz TA, Helmick CG, et al. Lifetime risk of symptomatic knee osteoarthritis. *Arthritis Rheum.* 2008;59(9):1207-1213.

137. Daniel DM, Stone ML, Dobson BE, Fithian DC, Rossman DJ, Kaufman KR. Fate of the ACL-injured patient. A prospective outcome study. *Am J Sport Med.* 1994;22(5):632-644.

138. Fitzgerald GK, Axe MJ, Snyder-Mackler L. A decision-making scheme for returning patients to high-level activity with nonoperative treatment after anterior cruciate ligament rupture. *Knee Surg Sport Tr A.* 2000;8(2):76-82.

139. Irrgang JJ, Snyder-Mackler L, Wainner RS, Fu FH, Harner CD. Development of a patient-reported measure of function of the knee. *J Bone Joint Surg Am.* 1998;80(8):1132-1145.

140. Irrgang JJ, Anderson AF, Boland AL, et al. Development and validation of the international knee documentation committee subjective knee form. *Am J Sport Med.* 2001;29(5):600-613.

141. Irrgang JJ, Anderson AF, Boland AL, et al. Responsiveness of the International Knee Documentation Committee Subjective Knee Form. *Am J Sport Med.* 2006;34(10):1567-1573.

142. Roos EM, Roos HP, Lohmander LS, Ekdahl C, Beynnon BD. Knee Injury and Osteoarthritis Outcome Score (KOOS)—Development of a self-administered outcome measure. *J Orthop Sport Phys.* 1998;28(2):88-96.

143. Briggs KK, Lysholm J, Tegner Y, Rodkey WG, Kocher MS, Steadman JR. The reliability, validity, and responsiveness of the Lysholm score and Tegner activity scale for anterior cruciate ligament injuries of the knee: 25 years later. *Am J Sport Med.* 2009;37(5):890-897.

144. Marx RG, Stump TJ, Jones EC, Wickiewicz TL, Warren RF. Development and evaluation of an activity rating scale for disorders of the knee. *Am J Sport Med.* 2001;29(2):213-218.

145. Wright RW. Knee injury outcomes measures. *J Am Acad Orthop Surg.* 2009;17(1):31-39.

146. Chmielewski TL, Jones D, Day T, Tillman SM, Lentz TA, George SZ. The association of pain and fear of movement/reinjury with function during anterior cruciate ligament reconstruction rehabilitation. *J Orthop Sport Phys.* 2008;38(12):746-753.

147. Chmielewski TL, Zeppieri G Jr, Lentz TA, et al. Longitudinal changes in psychosocial factors and their association with knee pain and function after anterior cruciate ligament reconstruction. *Phys Ther.* 2011;91(9):1355-1366.

148. Webster KE, Feller JA, Lambros C. Development and preliminary validation of a scale to measure the psychological impact of returning to sport following anterior cruciate ligament reconstruction surgery. *Phys Ther Sport.* 2008;9(1):9-15.

149. Langford JL, Webster KE, Feller JA. A prospective longitudinal study to assess psychological changes following anterior cruciate ligament reconstruction surgery. *Brit J Sport Med.* 2009;43(5):377-378.

150. Lorentzon R, Elmqvist LG, Sjöström M, Fagerlund M, Fuglmeyer AR. Thigh musculature in relation to chronic anterior cruciate ligament tear: Muscle size, morphology, and mechanical output before reconstruction. *Am J Sport Med.* 1989;17(3):423-429.

151. Rudolph KS, Axe MJ, Buchanan TS, Scholz JP, Snyder-Mackler L. Dynamic stability in the anterior cruciate ligament deficient knee. *Knee Surg Sport Tr A.* 2001;9(2):62-71.

152. Fitzgerald GK, Axe MJ, Snyder-Mackler L. The efficacy of perturbation training in nonoperative anterior cruciate ligament rehabilitation programs for physical active individuals. *Phys Ther.* 2000;80(2):128-140.

153. Mayr HO, Weig TG, Plitz W. Arthrofibrosis following ACL reconstruction—Reasons and outcome. *Arch Orthop Trauma Surg.* 2004;124(8):518-522.

154. Harner CD, Irrgang JJ, Paul J, Dearwater S, Fu FH. Loss of motion after anterior cruciate ligament reconstruction. *Am J Sport Med.* 1992;20(5):499-506.

155. McHugh MP, Tyler TF, Gleim GW, Nicholas SJ. Preoperative indicators of motion loss and weakness following anterior cruciate ligament reconstruction. *J Orthop Sport Phys.* 1998;27(6):407-411.

156. Shelbourne KD, Patel DV, Martini DJ. Classification and management of arthrofibrosis of the knee after anterior cruciate ligament reconstruction. *Am J Sport Med.* 1996;24(6):857-862.

157. Chmielewski TL, Stackhouse S, Axe MJ, Snyder-Mackler L. A prospective analysis of incidence and severity of quadriceps inhibition in a consecutive sample of 100 patients with complete acute anterior cruciate ligament rupture. *J Orthop Res.* 2004;22(5):925-930.

158. de Jong SN, van Caspel DR, van Haeff MJ, Saris DB. Functional assessment and muscle strength before and after reconstruction of chronic anterior cruciate ligament lesions. *Arthroscopy.* 2007;23(1):21-28.

159. Eitzen I, Moksnes H, Snyder-Mackler L, Risberg MA. A progressive 5-week exercise therapy program leads to significant improvement in knee function early after anterior cruciate ligament injury. *J Orthop Sport Phys*. 2010;40(11):705-721.

160. Hartigan E, Axe MJ, Snyder-Mackler L. Perturbation training prior to ACL reconstruction improves gait asymmetries in non-copers. *J Orthop Res*. 2009;27(6):724-729.

161. Keays SL, Bullock-Saxton J, Keays AC, Newcombe P. Muscle strength and function before and after anterior cruciate ligament reconstruction using semitendonosus and gracilis. *Knee*. 2001;8(3):229-234.

162. Tsepis E, Vagenas G, Ristanis S, Georgoulis AD. Thigh muscle weakness in ACL-deficient knees persists without structured rehabilitation. *Clin Orthop Relat R*. 2006;450:211-218.

163. Eitzen I, Holm I, Risberg MA. Preoperative quadriceps strength is a significant predictor of knee function two years after anterior cruciate ligament reconstruction. *Brit J Sport Med*. 2009;43(5):371-376.

164. Logerstedt D, Lynch A, Axe MJ, Snyder-Mackler L. Pre-operative quadriceps strength predicts IKDC2000 scores 6 months after anterior cruciate ligament reconstruction. *Knee*. 2012.

165. Keays SL, Bullock-Saxton JE, Newcombe P, Keays AC. The relationship between knee strength and functional stability before and after anterior cruciate ligament reconstruction. *J Orthop Res*. 2003;21(2):231-237.

166. Cooperman JM, Riddle DL, Rothstein JM. Reliability and validity of judgments of the integrity of the anterior cruciate ligament of the knee using the Lachman's test. *Phys Ther*. 1990;70(4):225-233.

167. Grindem H, Logerstedt D, Eitzen I, et al. Single-legged hop tests as predictors of self-reported knee function in nonoperatively treated individuals with anterior cruciate ligament injury. *Am J Sport Med*. 2011;39(11):2347-2354.

168. Logerstedt D, Grindem H, Lynch A, et al. Single-legged hop tests as predictors of self-reported knee function after anterior cruciate ligament reconstruction: The Delaware-Oslo ACL cohort study. *Am J Sport Med*. 2012;40(10):2348-2356.

169. Kopkow C, Freiberg A, Kirschner S, Seidler A, Schmitt J. Physical examination tests for the diagnosis of posterior cruciate ligament rupture: A systematic review. *J Orthop Sport Phys*. 2013;43(11):804-813.

170. Shelbourne KD, Davis TJ, Patel DV. The natural history of acute, isolated, nonoperatively treated posterior cruciate ligament injuries. A prospective study. *Am J Sport Med*. 1999;27(3):276-283.

171. Grassmayr MJ, Parker DA, Coolican MR, Vanwanseele B. Posterior cruciate ligament deficiency: Biomechanical and biological consequences and the outcomes of conservative treatment. A systematic review. *J Sci Med Sport*. 2008;11(5):433-443.

172. MacLean CL, Taunton JE, Clement DB, Regan WD, Stanish WD. Eccentric kinetic chain exercise as a conservative means of functionally rehabilitating chronic isolated insufficiency of the posterior cruciate ligament. *Clin J Sport Med*. 1999;9(3):142-150.

173. Post WR. Clinical evaluation of patients with patellofemoral disorders. *Arthroscopy*. 1999;15(8):841-851.

174. Binkley JM, Stratford PW, Lott SA, Riddle DL. The Lower Extremity Functional Scale (LEFS): Scale development, measurement properties, and clinical application. North American Orthopaedic Rehabilitation Research Network. *Phys Ther*. 1999;79(4):371-383.

175. Laprade JA, Culham EG. A self-administered pain severity scale for patellofemoral pain syndrome. *Clin Rehabil*. 2002;16(7):780-788.

176. Loudon JK, Wiesner D, Goist-Foley HL, Asjes C, Loudon KL. Intrarater reliability of functional performance tests for subjects with patellofemoral pain syndrome. *J Athl Train*. 2002;37(3):256-261.

177. Lowery DJ, Farley TD, Wing DW, Sterett WI, Steadman JR. A clinical composite score accurately detects meniscal pathology. *Arthroscopy*. 2006;22(11):1174-1179.

178. Tanner SM, Dainty KN, Marx RG, Kirkley A. Knee-specific quality-of-life instruments: Which ones measure symptoms and disabilities most important to patients? *Am J Sports Med*. 2007;35(9):1450-1458.

179. Briggs KK, Kocher MS, Rodkey WG, Steadman JR. Reliability, validity, and responsiveness of the Lysholm knee score and Tegner activity scale for patients with meniscal injury of the knee. *J Bone Joint Surg Am*. 2006;88(4):698-705.

180. McLeod MM, Gribble P, Pfile KR, Pietrosimone BG. Effects of arthroscopic partial meniscectomy on quadriceps strength: A systematic review. *J Sport Rehabil*. 2012;21(3):285-295.

181. LaPrade RF, Terry GC. Injuries to the posterolateral aspect of the knee. Association of anatomic injury patterns with clinical instability. *Am J Sport Med*. 1997;25(4):433-438.

182. Indelicato PA. Isolated medial collateral ligament injuries in the knee. *J Am Acad Orthop Surg*. 1995;3(1):9-14.

183. Reider B. Medial collateral ligament injuries in athletes. *Sports Med*. 1996;21(2):147-156.

184. Pressman A, Johnson DH. A review of ski injuries resulting in combined injury to the anterior cruciate ligament and medial collateral ligaments. *Arthroscopy*. 2003;19(2):194-202.

185. Hughston JC, Andrews JR, Cross MJ, Moschi A. Classification of knee ligament instabilities. Part I. The medial compartment and cruciate ligaments. *J Bone Joint Surg Am*. 1976;58(2):159-172.

186. Kannus P. Long-term results of conservatively treated medial collateral ligament injuries of the knee joint. *Clin Orthop Relat R*. 1988;226:103-112.

187. Malanga GA, Andrus S, Nadler SF, McLean J. Physical examination of the knee: A review of the original test description and scientific validity of common orthopedic tests. *Arch Phys Med Rehab*. 2003;84(4):592-603.

188. Marchant MH, Tibor LM, Sekiya JK, Hardaker WT, Garrett WE, Taylor DC. Management of medial-sided knee injuries, part 1: medial collateral ligament. *Am J Sport Med.* 2011;39(5):1102-1113.

189. Peers KH, Lysens RJ. Patellar tendinopathy in athletes: Current diagnostic and therapeutic recommendations. *Sports Med.* 2005;35(1):71-87.

190. Cook JL, Khan KM. What is the most appropriate treatment for patellar tendinopathy? *Brit J Sport Med.* 2001;35(5):291-294.

191. Khan KM, Cook JL, Bonar F, Harcourt P, Astrom M. Histopathology of common tendinopathies. Update and implications for clinical management. *Sports Med.* 1999;27(6):393-408.

192. Maffulli N, Khan KM, Puddu G. Overuse tendon conditions: Time to change a confusing terminology. *Arthroscopy.* 1998;14(8):840-843.

193. Visentini PJ, Khan KM, Cook JL, Kiss ZS, Harcourt PR, Wark JD. The VISA score: An index of severity of symptoms in patients with jumper's knee (patellar tendinosis). Victorian Institute of Sport Tendon Study Group. *J Sci Med Sport.* 1998;1(1):22-28.

194. Hernandez-Sanchez S, Hidalgo MD, Gomez A. Responsiveness of the VISA-P scale for patellar tendinopathy in athletes [published online ahead of print September 25 2012]. *Brit J Sport Med.* 2012.

195. van der Worp H, van Ark M, Zwerver J, van den Akker-Scheek I. Risk factors for patellar tendinopathy in basketball and volleyball players: A cross-sectional study. *Scand J Med Sci Sports.* 2012;22(6):783-790.

196. Backman LJ, Danielson P. Low range of ankle dorsiflexion predisposes for patellar tendinopathy in junior elite basketball players: A 1-year prospective study. *Am J Sport Med.* 2011;39(12):2626-2633.

197. Cook J, Khan K, Maffuli N, Purdam C. Overuse tendinosis, not tendinitis: Applying the new approach to patellar tendinopathy. *Physician Sportsmed.* 2000;28(6):31-46.

198. Wilson JJ, Best TM. Common overuse tendon problems: A review and recommendations for treatment. *Am Fam Physician.* 2005;72(5):811-818.

199. Felson DT, Lawrence RC, Dieppe PA, et al. Osteoarthritis: New insights. Part 1: The disease and its risk factors. *Ann Intern Med.* 2000;133(8):635-646.

200. Fitzgerald GK, Piva SR, Irrgang JJ, Bouzubar F, Starz TW. Quadriceps activation failure as a moderator of the relationship between quadriceps strength and physical function in individuals with knee osteoarthritis. *Arthritis Rheum.* 2004;51(1):40-48.

201. Messier SP, Loeser RF, Hoover JL, Semble EL, Wise CM. Osteoarthritis of the knee: Effects on gait, strength, and flexibility. *Arch Phys Med Rehab.* 1992;73(1):29-36.

202. Guccione AA, Felson DT, Anderson JJ, et al. The effects of specific medical conditions on the functional limitations of elders in the Framingham Study. *Am J Public Health.* 1994;84(3):351-358.

203. Altman R, Asch E, Bloch D, et al. Development of criteria for the classification and reporting of osteoarthritis. Classification of osteoarthritis of the knee. Diagnostic and Therapeutic Criteria Committee of the American Rheumatism Association. *Arthritis Rheum.* 1986;29(8):1039-1049.

204. Parmet S, Lynm C, Glass RM. JAMA patient page. Osteoarthritis of the knee. *JAMA.* 2003;289(8):1068.

205. Foy CG, Penninx BW, Shumaker SA, Messier SP, Pahor M. Long-term exercise therapy resolves ethnic differences in baseline health status in older adults with knee osteoarthritis. *J Am Geriatr Soc.* 2005;53(9):1469-1475.

206. Jiang L, Tian W, Wang Y, et al. Body mass index and susceptibility to knee osteoarthritis: A systematic review and meta-analysis. *Joint Bone Spine.* 2012;79(3):291-297.

207. Blagojevic M, Jinks C, Jeffery A, Jordan KP. Risk factors for onset of osteoarthritis of the knee in older adults: A systematic review and meta-analysis. *Osteoarthr Cartilage.* 2010;18(1):24-33.

208. Oatis CA, Wolff EF, Lennon SK. Knee joint stiffness in individuals with and without knee osteoarthritis: A preliminary study. *J Orthop Sport Phys.* 2006;36(12):935-941.

209. Terwee CB, van der Slikke RM, van Lummel RC, Benink RJ, Meijers WG, de Vet HC. Self-reported physical functioning was more influenced by pain than performance-based physical functioning in knee-osteoarthritis patients. *J Clin Epidemiol.* 2006;59(7):724-731.

210. van Dijk GM, Veenhof C, Schellevis F, et al. Comorbidity, limitations in activities and pain in patients with osteoarthritis of the hip or knee. *BMC Musculoskel Dis.* 2008;9:95.

211. Lin E. Magnetic resonance imaging of the knee: Clinical significance of common findings. *Curr Probl Diagn Radiol.* 2010;39(4):152-159.

212. Kellgren JH, Lawrence JS. Radiological assessment of osteo-arthrosis. *Ann Rheum Dis.* 1957;16(4):494-502.

213. Deyle GD, Allison SC, Matekel RL, et al. Physical therapy treatment effectiveness for osteoarthritis of the knee: A randomized comparison of supervised clinical exercise and manual therapy procedures versus a home exercise program. *Phys Ther.* 2005;85(12):1301-1317.

214. Dekker J, van Dijk GM, Veenhof C. Risk factors for functional decline in osteoarthritis of the hip or knee. *Curr Opin Rheumatol.* 2009;21(5):520-524.

215. van Dijk GM, Dekker J, Veenhof C, van den Ende CH. Course of functional status and pain in osteoarthritis of the hip or knee: A systematic review of the literature. *Arthritis Rheum.* 2006;55(5):779-785.

216. Terwee CB, Mokkink LB, Steultjens MP, Dekker J. Performance-based methods for measuring the physical function of patients with osteoarthritis of the hip or knee: A systematic review of measurement properties. *Rheumatology (Oxford).* 2006;45(7):890-902.

Chapter 26

1. Rao S, Riskowski JL, Hannan MT. Musculoskeletal conditions of the foot and ankle: Assessments and treatment options. *Best Pract Res Cl Rh.* 2012;26(3):345-368.

2. Stanley CJ, Creighton RA, Gross MT, Garrett WE, Yu B. Effects of a knee extension constraint brace on lower extremity movements after ACL reconstruction. *Clin Orthop Relat R.* 2011;469(6):1774-1780.

3. Close JR. Some applications of the functional anatomy of the ankle joint. *J Bone Joint Surg Am.* 1956;38-a(4):761-781.

4. Attarian DE, McCrackin HJ, Devito DP, McElhaney JH, Garrett WE Jr. A biomechanical study of human lateral ankle ligaments and autogenous reconstructive grafts. *Am J Sport Med.* 1985;13(6):377-381.

5. Sartoris DJ. Diagnosis of ankle injuries: The essentials. *J Foot Ankle Surg.* 1994;33(1):102-107.

6. Dutton M. *Orthopaedic Examination, Evaluation and Intervention.* New York, NY: McGraw Hill; 2004.

7. Menz HB, Lord SR. Gait instability in older people with hallux valgus. *Foot Ankle Int.* 2005;26(6):483-489.

8. Riskowski J, Dufour AB, Hannan MT. Arthritis, foot pain and shoe wear: Current musculoskeletal research on feet. *Curr Opin Rheumatol.* 2011;23(2):148-155.

9. Dufour AB, Broe KE, Nguyen US, et al. Foot pain: Is current or past shoewear a factor? *Arthritis Rheum.* 2009;61(10):1352-1358.

10. Barton CJ, Bonanno D, Menz HB. Development and evaluation of a tool for the assessment of footwear characteristics. *J Foot Ankle Res.* 2009;2:10.

11. Martin RL, Irrgang JJ, Burdett RG, Conti SF, Van Swearingen JM. Evidence of validity for the Foot and Ankle Ability Measure (FAAM). *Foot Ankle Int.* 2005;26(11):968-983.

12. Hale SA, Hertel J. Reliability and sensitivity of the Foot and Ankle Disability Index in subjects with chronic ankle instability. *J Athl Train.* 2005;40(1):35-40.

13. Budiman-Mak E, Conrad KJ, Roach KE. The Foot Function Index: A measure of foot pain and disability. *J Clin Epidemiol.* 1991;44(6):561-570.

14. Saag KG, Saltzman CL, Brown CK, Budiman-Mak E. The Foot Function Index for measuring rheumatoid arthritis pain: Evaluating side-to-side reliability. *Foot Ankle Int.* 1996;17(8):506-510.

15. SooHoo NF, Vyas R, Samimi D. Responsiveness of the Foot Function Index, AOFAS clinical rating systems, and SF-36 after foot and ankle surgery. *Foot Ankle Int.* 2006;27(11):930-934.

16. Landorf KB, Radford JA. Minimal important difference: Values for the Foot Health Status Questionnaire, Foot Function Index and Visual Analogue Scale. *The Foot.* 2008;18(1):15-19.

17. Domsic RT, Saltzman CL. Ankle osteoarthritis scale. *Foot Ankle Int.* 1998;19(7):466-471.

18. Binkley JM, Stratford PW, Lott SA, Riddle DL. The Lower Extremity Functional Scale (LEFS): Scale development, measurement properties, and clinical application. North American Orthopaedic Rehabilitation Research Network. *Phys Ther.* 1999;79(4):371-383.

19. Cleland JA, Abbott JH, Kidd MO, et al. Manual physical therapy and exercise versus electrophysical agents and exercise in the management of plantar heel pain: A multicenter randomized clinical trial. *J Orthop Sport Phys.* 2009;39(8):573-585.

20. Mei-Dan O, Kots E, Barchilon V, Massarwe S, Nyska M, Mann G. A dynamic ultrasound examination for the diagnosis of ankle syndesmotic injury in professional athletes: A preliminary study. *Am J Sport Med.* 2009;37(5):1009-1016.

21. Kuwada GT. Surgical correlation of preoperative MRI findings of trauma to tendons and ligaments of the foot and ankle. *J Am Podiatr Med Assn.* 2008;98(5):370-373.

22. Kapoor A, Page S, Lavalley M, Gale DR, Felson DT. Magnetic resonance imaging for diagnosing foot osteomyelitis: A meta-analysis. *Arch Intern Med.* 2007;167(2):125-132.

23. Guggenberger R, Gnannt R, Hodler J, et al. Diagnostic performance of dual-energy CT for the detection of traumatic bone marrow lesions in the ankle: Comparison with MR imaging. *Radiology.* 2012;264(1):164-173.

24. Garras DN, Raikin SM, Bhat SB, Taweel N, Karanjia H. MRI is unnecessary for diagnosing acute Achilles tendon ruptures: Clinical diagnostic criteria. *Clin Orthop Relat R.* 2012;470(8):2268-2273.

25. Kalebo P, Allenmark C, Peterson L, Sward L. Diagnostic value of ultrasonography in partial ruptures of the Achilles tendon. *Am J Sport Med.* 1992;20(4):378-381.

26. Lamm BM, Myers DT, Dombek M, Mendicino RW, Catanzariti AR, Saltrick K. Magnetic resonance imaging and surgical correlation of peroneus brevis tears. *J Foot Ankle Surg.* 2004;43(1):30-36.

27. Park HJ, Cha SD, Kim HS, et al. Reliability of MRI findings of peroneal tendinopathy in patients with lateral chronic ankle instability. *Clin Orthop Surg.* 2010;2(4):237-243.

28. Haverstock BD. Foot and ankle imaging in the athlete. *Clin Podiatr Med Surg.* 2008;25(2):249-262, vi-vii.

29. Stiell IG, Greenberg GH, McKnight RD, Nair RC, McDowell I, Worthington JR. A study to develop clinical decision rules for the use of radiography in acute ankle injuries. *Ann Emerg Med.* 1992;21(4):384-390.

30. Stiell IG, McKnight RD, Greenberg GH, et al. Implementation of the Ottawa ankle rules. *JAMA.* 1994;271(11):827-832.

31. Bachmann LM, Kolb E, Koller MT, Steurer J, ter Riet G. Accuracy of Ottawa ankle rules to exclude fractures of the ankle and mid-foot: Systemic review. *BMJ.* 2003;326(7386):417.

32. Dowling S, Spooner CH, Liang Y, et al. Accuracy of Ottawa Ankle Rules to exclude fractures of the ankle and midfoot in children: A meta-analysis. *Acad Emerg Med.* 2009;16(4):277-287.

33. Martin RL, Davenport TE, Paulseth S, Wukich DK, Godges JJ. Ankle stability and movement coordination impairments: Ankle ligament sprains. *J Orthop Sport Phys.* 2013;43(9):A1-A40.

34. Eggli S, Sclabas GM, Zimmermann H, Exadaktylos AK. The Bernese ankle rules: A fast, reliable test after low-energy, supination-type malleolar and midfoot trauma. *J Trauma.* 2005;59(5):1268-1271.

35. Margetic P, Pavic R. Comparative assessment of the acute ankle injury by ultrasound and magnetic resonance. *Coll Antropol.* 2012;36(2):605-610.

36. McNally EG, Shetty S. Plantar fascia: Imaging diagnosis and guided treatment. *Semin Musculoskelet R.* 2010;14(3):334-343.

37. Campbell SE, Warner M. MR imaging of ankle inversion injuries. *Magn Reson Imaging C.* 2008;16(1):1-18, v.

38. Yu GM, Zhang LH, Lu DL, Zhu Y, Li HM, Huang QL. MSCT diagnosis of foot and ankle tendon injury [in Chinese]. *Zhongguo Gu Shang.* 2013;26(1):73-77.

39. Singh VK, Javed S, Parthipun A, Sott AH. The diagnostic value of single photon-emission computed tomography bone scans combined with CT (SPECT-CT) in diseases of the foot and ankle. *Foot Ankle Surg.* 2013;19(2):80-83.

40. Cornwall MW, McPoil TG. Relationship between static foot posture and foot mobility. *J Foot Ankle Res.* 2011;4:4.

41. Giallonardo LM. Clinical evaluation of foot and ankle dysfunction. *Phys Ther.* 1988;68(12):1850-1856.

42. Gross MT. Lower quarter screening for skeletal malalignment—suggestions for orthotics and shoewear. *J Orthop Sport Phys.* 1995;21(6):389-405.

43. Rozzi SL, Lephart SM, Sterner R, Kuligowski L. Balance training for persons with functionally unstable ankles. *J Orthop Sport Phys.* 1999;29(8):478-486.

44. Eils E, Rosenbaum D. A multi-station proprioceptive exercise program in patients with ankle instability. *Med Sci Sport Exer.* 2001;33(12):1991-1998.

45. Michels F, Guillo S. Tailor's bunionectomy. In: Saxena A, ed. *International Advances in Foot and Ankle Surgery.* London, England: Springer; 2012: 99-106.

46. Mann RA. Pain in the foot. 1. Evaluation of foot pain and identification of associated problems. *Postgrad Med.* 1987;82(1):154-157, 160-152.

47. Hunt G, Brocato R. Gait and foot pathomechanics. In Hunt GC, ed. *Physical Therapy of the Foot and Ankle.* New York, NY: Churchill Livingstone; 1988: 39-57.

48. Root ML, Orien WP, Weed JH. *Normal and Abnormal Function of the Foot. Vol II.* Los Angeles, CA: Clinical Biomechanics; 1977.

49. Garbalosa JC, McClure MH, Catlin PA, Wooden M. The frontal plane relationship of the forefoot to the rearfoot in an asymptomatic population. *J Orthop Sport Phys.* 1994;20(4):200-206.

50. Jain S, Mannan K. The diagnosis and management of Morton's neuroma: A literature review. *Foot Ankle Spec.* 2013;6(4):307-317.

51. Hockenbury RT. Forefoot problems in athletes. *Med Sci Sport Exer.* 1999;31(7)(suppl):S448-S458.

52. O'Neill DB, Micheli LJ. Tarsal coalition. A follow-up of adolescent athletes. *Am J Sport Med.* 1989;17(4):544-549.

53. Brown GP, Feehery RV Jr, Grant SM. Case study: The painful os trigonum syndrome. *J Orthop Sport Phys.* 1995;22(1):22-25.

54. Moore MB. The use of a tuning fork and stethoscope to identify fractures. *J Athl Train.* 2009;44(3):272-274.

55. Lesho EP. Can tuning forks replace bone scans for identification of tibial stress fractures? *Mil Med.* 1997;162(12):802-803.

56. Owens R, Gougoulias N, Guthrie H, Sakellariou A. Morton's neuroma: Clinical testing and imaging in 76 feet, compared to a control group. *Foot Ankle Surg.* 2011;17(3):197-200.

57. Donelson R, Aprill C, Medcalf R, Grant W. A prospective study of centralization of lumbar and referred pain. A predictor of symptomatic discs and anular competence. *Spine (Phila Pa 1976).* 1997;22(10):1115-1122.

58. Laslett M, Oberg B, Aprill CN, McDonald B. Centralization as a predictor of provocation discography results in chronic low back pain, and the influence of disability and distress on diagnostic power. *Spine J.* 2005;5(4):370-380.

59. Vroomen PC, de Krom MC, Wilmink JT, Kester AD, Knottnerus JA. Diagnostic value of history and physical examination in patients suspected of lumbosacral nerve root compression. *J Neurol Neurosur Ps.* 2002;72(5):630-634.

60. van der Windt DA, Simons E, Riphagen II, et al. Physical examination for lumbar radiculopathy due to disc herniation in patients with low-back pain. *Cochrane Db Syst Rev.* 2010;2:CD007431.

61. Stankovic R, Johnell O, Maly P, Willner S. Use of lumbar extension, slump test, physical and neurological examination in the evaluation of patients with suspected herniated nucleus pulposus. A prospective clinical study. *Man Ther.* 1999;4(1):25-32.

62. Laslett M, McDonald B, Aprill CN, Tropp H, Oberg B. Clinical predictors of screening lumbar zygapophyseal joint blocks: Development of clinical prediction rules. *Spine J.* 2006;6(4):370-379.

63. Laslett M, Young SB, Aprill CN, McDonald B. Diagnosing painful sacroiliac joints: A validity study of a McKenzie evaluation and sacroiliac provocation tests. *Aust J Physiother.* 2003;49(2):89-97.

64. Laslett M, Aprill CN, McDonald B, Young SB. Diagnosis of sacroiliac joint pain: Validity of individual provocation tests and composites of tests. *Man Ther.* 2005;10(3):207-218.

65. Reiman MP, Goode AP, Hegedus EJ, Cook CE, Wright AA. Diagnostic accuracy of clinical tests of the hip: A systematic review with meta-analysis. *Brit J Sport Med.* 2013;47(14):893-902.

66. Bachmann LM, Haberzeth S, Steurer J, ter Riet G. The accuracy of the Ottawa knee rule to rule out knee fractures: A systematic review. *Ann Intern Med.* 2004;140(2):121-124.

67. Emparanza JI, Aginaga JR. Validation of the Ottawa Knee Rules. *Ann Emerg Med.* 2001;38(4):364-368.

68. Martin RL, McPoil TG. Reliability of ankle goniometric measurements: A literature review. *J Am Podiatr Med Assn.* 2005;95(6):564-572.

69. Reese NB, Bandy WD. *Joint Range of Motion and Muscle Length Testing.* Philadelphia, PA: Saunders; 2002.

70. Piva SR, Fitzgerald K, Irrgang JJ, et al. Reliability of measures of impairments associated with patellofemoral pain syndrome. *BMC Musculoskel Dis.* 2006;7:33.

71. Wang SS, Whitney SL, Burdett RG, Janosky JE. Lower extremity muscular flexibility in long distance runners. *J Orthop Sport Phys.* 1993;17(2):102-107.

72. David P, Halimi M, Mora I, Doutrellot PL, Petitjean M. Isokinetic testing of evertor and invertor muscles in patients with chronic ankle instability. *J Appl Biomech.* 2013;29(6):696-704.

73. Hebert-Losier K, Newsham-West RJ, Schneiders AG, Sullivan SJ. Raising the standards of the calf-raise test: A systematic review. *J Sci Med Sport.* 2009;12(6):594-602.

74. Rohner-Spengler M, Mannion AF, Babst R. Reliability and minimal detectable change for the figure-of-eight-20 method of measurement of ankle edema. *J Orthop Sport Phys.* 2007;37(4):199-205.

75. Friends J, Augustine E, Danoff J. A comparison of different assessment techniques for measuring foot and ankle volume in healthy adults. *J Am Podiatr Med Assn.* 2008;98(2):85-94.

76. Pugia ML, Middel CJ, Seward SW, et al. Comparison of acute swelling and function in subjects with lateral ankle injury. *J Orthop Sport Phys.* 2001;31(7):384-388.

77. Sell KE, Verity TM, Worrell TW, Pease BJ, Wigglesworth J. Two measurement techniques for assessing subtalar joint position: A reliability study. *J Orthop Sport Phys.* 1994;19(3):162-167.

78. Astrom M, Arvidson T. Alignment and joint motion in the normal foot. *J Orthop Sport Phys.* 1995;22(5):216-222.

79. Nguyen AD, Shultz SJ. Identifying relationships among lower extremity alignment characteristics. *J Athl Train.* 2009;44(5):511-518.

80. Drexler M, Dwyer T, Marmor M, Reischl N, Attar F, Cameron J. Total knee arthroplasty in patients with excessive external tibial torsion >45 degrees and patella instability—surgical technique and follow up. *J Arthroplasty.* 2013;28(4):614-619.

81. Brody DM. Techniques in the evaluation and treatment of the injured runner. *Orthop Clin N Am.* 1982;13(3):541-558.

82. Mueller MJ, Host JV, Norton BJ. Navicular drop as a composite measure of excessive pronation. *J Am Podiatr Med Assn.* 1993;83(4):198-202.

83. Menz HB, Munteanu SE. Validity of 3 clinical techniques for the measurement of static foot posture in older people. *J Orthop Sport Phys.* 2005;35(8):479-486.

84. Williams DS, McClay IS. Measurements used to characterize the foot and the medial longitudinal arch: Reliability and validity. *Phys Ther.* 2000;80(9):864-871.

85. Spörndly-Nees S, Dåsberg B, Nielsen RO, Boesen MI, Langberg H. The navicular position test—a reliable measure of the navicular bone position during rest and loading. *Int J Sports Phys Ther.* 2011;6(3):199-205.

86. Williams DS III, McClay IS, Hamill J. Arch structure and injury patterns in runners. *Clin Biomech (Bristol, Avon).* 2001;16(4):341-347.

87. Glasoe WM, Grebing BR, Beck S, Coughlin MJ, Saltzman CL. A comparison of device measures of dorsal first ray mobility. *Foot Ankle Int.* 2005;26(11):957-961.

88. Glasoe WM, Getsoian S, Myers M, et al. Criterion-related validity of a clinical measure of dorsal first ray mobility. *J Orthop Sport Phys.* 2005;35(9):589-593.

89. Payne C, Chuter V, Miller K. Sensitivity and specificity of the functional hallux limitus test to predict foot function. *J Am Podiatr Med Assn.* 2002;92(5):269-271.

90. DeOrio JK, Shapiro SA, McNeil RB, Stansel J. Validity of the posterior tibial edema sign in posterior tibial tendon dysfunction. *Foot Ankle Int.* 2011;32(2):189-192.

91. Newman P, Adams R, Waddington G. Two simple clinical tests for predicting onset of medial tibial stress syndrome: Shin palpation test and shin oedema test. *Brit J Sport Med.* 2012;46(12):861-864.

92. Reiman M, Burgi C, Strube E, et al. The utility of clinical measures for the diagnosis of Achilles tendon pathology: A systematic review with meta-analysis. *J Athl Training.* 2014;49(6):820-829.

93. Maffulli N, Kenward MG, Testa V, Capasso G, Regine R, King JB. Clinical diagnosis of Achilles tendinopathy with tendinosis. *Clin J Sport Med.* 2003;13(1):11-15.

94. Hutchison AM, Evans R, Bodger O, et al. What is the best clinical test for Achilles tendinopathy? *Foot Ankle Surg.* 2013;19(2):112-117.

95. Maffulli N. The clinical diagnosis of subcutaneous tear of the Achilles tendon. A prospective study in 174 patients. *Am J Sport Med.* 1998;26(2):266-270.

96. Thompson TC, Doherty JH. Spontaneous rupture of tendon of Achilles: A new clinical diagnostic test. *J Trauma.* 1962;2:126-129.

97. De Garceau D, Dean D, Requejo SM, Thordarson DB. The association between diagnosis of plantar fasciitis and Windlass test results. *Foot Ankle Int.* 2003;24(3):251-255.

98. Alshami AM, Babri AS, Souvlis T, Coppieters MW. Biomechanical evaluation of two clinical tests for plantar heel pain: The dorsiflexion-eversion test for tarsal tunnel syndrome and the windlass test for plantar fasciitis. *Foot Ankle Int.* 2007;28(4):499-505.

99. Hertel J, Denegar CR, Monroe MM, Stokes WL. Talocrural and subtalar joint instability after lateral ankle sprain. *Med Sci Sport Exer.* 1999;31(11):1501-1508.

100. Croy T, Koppenhaver S, Saliba S, Hertel J. Anterior talocrural joint laxity: Diagnostic accuracy of the anterior drawer test of the ankle. *J Orthop Sport Phys.* 2013;43(12):911-919.

101. Rosen AB, Ko J, Brown CN. Diagnostic accuracy of instrumented and manual talar tilt tests in chronic ankle instability populations. *Scand J Med Sci Spor.* 2014.

102. Schwieterman B, Haas D, Columber K, Knupp D, Cook C. Diagnostic accuracy of physical examination tests of the ankle/foot complex: A systematic review. *Int J Sports Phys Ther.* 2013;8(4):416-426.

103. van Dijk CN, Mol BW, Lim LS, Marti RK, Bossuyt PM. Diagnosis of ligament rupture of the ankle joint. Physical examination, arthrography, stress radiography and sonography compared in 160 patients after inversion trauma. *Acta Orthop Scand.* 1996;67(6):566-570.

104. DeAngelis NA, Eskander MS, French BG. Does medial tenderness predict deep deltoid ligament incompetence in supination-external rotation type ankle fractures? *J Orthop Trauma.* 2007;21(4):244-247.

105. Beumer A, Swierstra BA, Mulder PG. Clinical diagnosis of syndesmotic ankle instability: Evaluation of stress tests behind the curtains. *Acta Orthop Scand.* 2002;73(6):667-669.

106. de Cesar PC, Avila EM, de Abreu MR. Comparison of magnetic resonance imaging to physical examination for syndesmotic injury after lateral ankle sprain. *Foot Ankle Int.* 2011;32(12):1110-1114.

107. Sman AD, Hiller CE, Rae K, et al. Diagnostic accuracy of clinical tests for ankle syndesmosis injury [published online ahead of print November 19 2013]. *Brit J Sport Med.* 2013.

108. Sman AD, Hiller CE, Refshauge KM. Diagnostic accuracy of clinical tests for diagnosis of ankle syndesmosis injury: A systematic review. *Brit J Sport Med.* 2013;47(10):620-628.

109. Molloy S, Solan MC, Bendall SP. Synovial impingement in the ankle. A new physical sign. *J Bone Joint Surg Br.* 2003;85(3):330-333.

110. Liu SH, Nuccion SL, Finerman G. Diagnosis of anterolateral ankle impingement. Comparison between magnetic resonance imaging and clinical examination. *Am J Sport Med.* 1997;25(3):389-393.

111. Cook C, Hegedus E. *Orthopedic Physical Examination Tests: An Evidence-Based Approach.* 2nd ed. Upper Saddle River, NJ: Prentice Hall; 2012.

112. Oloff LM, Schulhofer SD. Flexor hallucis longus dysfunction. *J Foot Ankle Surg.* 1998;37(2):101-109.

113. Abouelela AA, Zohiery AK. The triple compression stress test for diagnosis of tarsal tunnel syndrome. *Foot (Edinb).* 2012;22(3):146-149.

114. Kinoshita M, Okuda R, Morikawa J, Jotoku T, Abe M. The dorsiflexion-eversion test for diagnosis of tarsal tunnel syndrome. *J Bone Joint Surg Am.* 2001;83-A(12):1835-1839.

115. Garrick JG. The frequency of injury, mechanism of injury, and epidemiology of ankle sprains. *Am J Sport Med.* 1977;5(6):241-242.

116. Yeung MS, Chan KM, So CH, Yuan WY. An epidemiological survey on ankle sprain. *Brit J Sport Med.* 1994;28(2):112-116.

117. Waterman BR, Owens BD, Davey S, Zacchilli MA, Belmont PJ. The epidemiology of ankle sprains in the United States. *J Bone Joint Surg Am.* 2010;92(13):2279-2284.

118. Liu K, Gustavsen G, Kaminski TW. Increased frequency of ankle sprain does not lead to an increase in ligament laxity. *Clin J Sport Med.* 2013;23(6):483-487.

119. Fong DT, Hong Y, Chan LK, Yung PS, Chan KM. A systematic review on ankle injury and ankle sprain in sports. *Sports Med.* 2007;37(1):73-94.

120. Ivins D. Acute ankle sprain: An update. *Am Fam Physician.* 2006;74(10):1714-1720.

121. Tiemstra JD. Update on acute ankle sprains. *Am Fam Physician.* 2012;85(12):1170-1176.

122. Seah R, Mani-Babu S. Managing ankle sprains in primary care: What is best practice? A systematic review of the last 10 years of evidence. *Brit Med Bull.* 2011;97:105-135.

123. Hiller CE, Refshauge KM, Bundy AC, Herbert RD, Kilbreath SL. The Cumberland ankle instability tool: A report of validity and reliability testing. *Arch Phys Med Rehab.* 2006;87(9):1235-1241.

124. Alcock G, Stratford, PW. Validation of the Lower Extremity Functional Scale on athletic subjects with ankle sprains. *Physiother Can.* 2002;54:233-240.

125. Breitenseher MJ, Trattnig S, Kukla C, et al. MRI versus lateral stress radiography in acute lateral ankle ligament injuries. *J Comput Assist Tomogr.* 1997;21(2):280-285.

126. Verhaven EF, Shahabpour M, Handelberg FW, Vaes PH, Opdecam PJ. The accuracy of three-dimensional magnetic resonance imaging in the diagnosis of ruptures of the lateral ligaments of the ankle. *Am J Sport Med.* 1991;19(6):583-587.

127. Oae K, Takao M, Uchio Y, Ochi M. Evaluation of anterior talofibular ligament injury with stress radiography, ultrasonography and MR imaging. *Skeletal Radiol.* 2010;39(1):41-47.

128. Verhagen RA, Maas M, Dijkgraaf MG, Tol JL, Krips R, van Dijk CN. Prospective study on diagnostic strategies in osteochondral lesions of the talus. Is MRI superior to helical CT? *J Bone Joint Surg Br.* 2005;87(1):41-46.

129. Kobayashi T, Suzuki E, Yamazaki N, et al. Fibular malalignment in individuals with chronic ankle instability. *J Orthop Sport Phys.* 2014;44(11):872-878.

130. Kerkhoffs GM, van den Bekerom M, Elders LA, et al. Diagnosis, treatment and prevention of ankle sprains: An evidence-based clinical guideline. *Brit J Sport Med.* 2012;46(12):854-860.

131. Vijayasankar D, Boyle AA, Atkinson P. Can the Ottawa knee rule be applied to children? A systematic review and meta-analysis of observational studies. *Emerg Med J.* 2009;26(4):250-253.

132. Moreira V, Antunes F. Ankle sprains: From diagnosis to management. The physiatric view [in Portuguese]. *Acta Med Port.* 2008;21(3):285-292.

133. van Dijk CN, Lim LS, Bossuyt PM, Marti RK. Physical examination is sufficient for the diagnosis of sprained ankles. *J Bone Joint Surg Br.* 1996;78(6):958-962.

134. Bastien M, Moffet H, Bouyer L, Perron M, Hebert LJ, Leblond J. Concurrent and discriminant validity of the Star Excursion Balance Test for military personnel with lateral ankle sprain. *J Sport Rehabil.* 2014;23(1):44-55.

135. Kerkhoffs GM, Rowe BH, Assendelft WJ, Kelly KD, Struijs PA, van Dijk CN. Immobilisation for acute ankle sprain. A systematic review. *Arch Orthop Traum Su.* 2001;121(8):462-471.

136. Kemler E, van de Port I, Backx F, van Dijk CN. A systematic review on the treatment of acute ankle sprain: Brace versus other functional treatment types. *Sports Med.* 2011;41(3):185-197.

137. Loudon JK, Reiman MP, Sylvain J. The efficacy of manual joint mobilisation/manipulation in treatment of lateral ankle sprains: A systematic review. *Brit J Sport Med.* 2014;48(5):365-370.

138. McKeon PO, Ingersoll CD, Kerrigan DC, Saliba E, Bennett BC, Hertel J. Balance training improves function and postural control in those with chronic ankle instability. *Med Sci Sport Exer.* 2008;40(10):1810-1819.

139. Konradsen L, Voigt M, Højsgaard C. Ankle inversion injuries. The role of the dynamic defense mechanism. *Am J Sport Med.* 1997;25(1):54-58.

140. Wilkerson GB, Pinerola JJ, Caturano RW. Invertor vs. evertor peak torque and power deficiencies associated with lateral ankle ligament injury. *J Orthop Sport Phys.* 1997;26(2):78-86.

141. Kaminski TW, Hartsell HD. Factors contributing to chronic ankle instability: A strength perspective. *J Athl Train.* 2002;37(4):394-405.

142. Youdas JW, McLean TJ, Krause DA, Hollman JH. Changes in active ankle dorsiflexion range of motion after acute inversion ankle sprain. *J Sport Rehabil.* 2009;18(3):358-374.

143. Boytim MJ, Fischer DA, Neumann L. Syndesmotic ankle sprains. *Am J Sport Med.* 1991;19(3):294-298.

144. Norwig J. Injury management update: Recognizing and rehabilitating the high ankle sprain. *IJATT.* 1998;3(4):12-13.

145. Lin CF, Gross ML, Weinhold P. Ankle syndesmosis injuries: Anatomy, biomechanics, mechanism of injury, and clinical guidelines for diagnosis and intervention. *J Orthop Sport Phys.* 2006;36(6):372-384.

146. Fritschy D. An unusual ankle injury in top skiers. *Am J Sport Med.* 1989;17(2):282-285, discussion 285-286.

147. Clanton TO, Paul P. Syndesmosis injuries in athletes. *Foot Ankle Clin.* 2002;7(3):529-549.

148. Takao M, Ochi M, Oae K, Naito K, Uchio Y. Diagnosis of a tear of the tibiofibular syndesmosis. The role of arthroscopy of the ankle. *J Bone Joint Surg Br.* 2003;85(3):324-329.

149. Han SH, Lee JW, Kim S, Suh JS, Choi YR. Chronic tibiofibular syndesmosis injury: The diagnostic efficiency of magnetic resonance imaging and comparative analysis of operative treatment. *Foot Ankle Int.* 2007;28(3):336-342.

150. Vogl TJ, Hochmuth K, Diebold T, et al. Magnetic resonance imaging in the diagnosis of acute injured distal tibiofibular syndesmosis. *Invest Radiol.* 1997;32(7):401-409.

151. Bassewitz HL, Shapiro M. Persistent pain after ankle sprain: Targeting the causes. *Phys Sportsmed.* 1997;25(12):58-68.

152. Amendola A. Controversies in diagnosis and management of syndesmosis injuries of the ankle. *Foot Ankle.* 1992;13(1):44-50.

153. Fincher AL. Early recognition of syndesmotic ankle sprains. *Athl Ther Today.* 1999;4:42-43.

154. Zwipp H, Rammelt S, Grass R. Ligamentous injuries about the ankle and subtalar joints. *Clin Podiatr Med Surg.* 2002;19(2):195-229, v.

155. Mazzone MF, McCue T. Common conditions of the Achilles tendon. *Am Fam Physician.* 2002;65(9):1805-1810.

156. Khan RJ, Fick D, Keogh A, Crawford J, Brammar T, Parker M. Treatment of acute Achilles tendon ruptures. A meta-analysis of randomized, controlled trials. *J Bone Joint Surg Am.* 2005;87(10):2202-2210.

157. Khan NA, Rahim SA, Anand SS, Simel DL, Panju A. Does the clinical examination predict lower extremity peripheral arterial disease? *JAMA.* 2006;295(5):536-546.

158. Nilsson-Helander K, Thomee R, Silbernagel KG, et al. The Achilles tendon Total Rupture Score (ATRS): Development and validation. *Am J Sport Med.* 2007;35(3):421-426.

159. Chiodo CP, Glazebrook M, Bluman EM, et al. American Academy of Orthopaedic Surgeons clinical practice guideline on treatment of Achilles tendon rupture. *J Bone Joint Surg Am.* 2010;92(14):2466-2468.

160. Kujala UM, Sarna S, Kaprio J. Cumulative incidence of Achilles tendon rupture and tendinopathy in male former elite athletes. *Clin J Sport Med.* 2005;15(3):133-135.

161. Carcia CR, Martin RL, Houck J, Wukich DK. Achilles pain, stiffness, and muscle power deficits: Achilles tendinitis. *J Orthop Sport Phys.* 2010;40(9):A1-A26.

162. Jonsson P, Alfredson H, Sunding K, Fahlstrom M, Cook J. New regimen for eccentric calf-muscle training in patients with chronic insertional Achilles tendinopathy: Results of a pilot study. *Brit J Sport Med.* 2008;42(9):746-749.

163. Alfredson H, Cook J. A treatment algorithm for managing Achilles tendinopathy: New treatment options. *Brit J Sport Med.* 2007;41(4):211-216.

164. Alfredson H, Pietila T, Jonsson P, Lorentzon R. Heavy-load eccentric calf muscle training for the treatment of chronic Achilles tendinosis. *Am J Sport Med.* 1998;26(3):360-366.

165. Haims AH, Schweitzer ME, Patel RS, Hecht P, Wapner KL. MR imaging of the Achilles tendon: Overlap of findings in symptomatic and asymptomatic individuals. *Skeletal Radiol.* 2000;29(11):640-645.

166. Wilson JJ, Best TM. Common overuse tendon problems: A review and recommendations for treatment. *Am Fam Physician.* 2005;72(5):811-818.

167. Rome K, Webb P, Unsworth A, Haslock I. Heel pad stiffness in runners with plantar heel pain. *Clin Biomech (Bristol, Avon).* 2001;16(10):901-905.

168. McPoil TG, Martin RL, Cornwall MW, Wukich DK, Irrgang JJ, Godges JJ. Heel pain—plantar fasciitis: Clinical practice guidelines linked to the international classification of function, disability, and health from the orthopaedic section of the American Physical Therapy Association. *J Orthop Sports Phys Ther.* 2008;38(4):A1-A18.

169. Alshami AM, Souvlis T, Coppieters MW. A review of plantar heel pain of neural origin: Differential diagnosis and management. *Man Ther.* 2008;13(2):103-111.

170. Baxter DE, Pfeffer GB. Treatment of chronic heel pain by surgical release of the first branch of the lateral plantar nerve. *Clin Orthop Relat Res.* 1992;(279):229-36.

171. Patel A, DiGiovanni B. Association between plantar fasciitis and isolated contracture of the gastrocnemius. *Foot Ankle Int.* 2011;32(1):5-8.

172. Riddle DL, Pulisic M, Pidcoe P, Johnson RE. Risk factors for plantar fasciitis: A matched case-control study. *J Bone Joint Surg Am.* 2003;85-A(5):872-877.

173. Thordarson DB, Schmotzer H, Chon J, Peters J. Dynamic support of the human longitudinal arch. A biomechanical evaluation. *Clin Orthop Relat R.* 1995(316):165-172.

174. Bolgla LA, Malone TR. Plantar fasciitis and the windlass mechanism: A biomechanical link to clinical practice. *J Athl Train.* 2004;39(1):77-82.

175. Martin RL, Davenport TE, Reischl SF, et al. Heel pain-plantar fasciitis: Revision 2014. *J Orthop Sport Phys.* 2014;44(11):A1-A33.

176. Radford JA, Landorf KB, Buchbinder R, Cook C. Effectiveness of low-dye taping for the short-term treatment of plantar heel pain: A randomised trial. *BMC Musculoskel Dis.* 2006;7:64.

177. Cotchett MP, Munteanu SE, Landorf KB. Effectiveness of trigger point dry needling for plantar heel pain: A randomized controlled trial. *Phys Ther.* 2014;94(8):1083-1094.

178. Neville CG, Houck JR. Choosing among 3 ankle-foot orthoses for a patient with stage II posterior tibial tendon dysfunction. *J Orthop Sport Phys.* 2009;39(11):816-824.

179. Renan-Ordine R, Alburquerque-Sendín F, de Souza DP, Cleland JA, Fernández-de-Las-Peñas C. Effectiveness of myofascial trigger point manual therapy combined with a self-stretching protocol for the management of plantar heel pain: A randomized controlled trial. *J Orthop Sport Phys.* 2011;41(2):43-50.

180. Franklyn M, Oakes B, Field B, Wells P, Morgan D. Section modulus is the optimum geometric predictor for stress fractures and medial tibial stress syndrome in both male and female athletes. *Am J Sport Med.* 2008;36(6):1179-1189.

181. Gaeta M, Minutoli F, Vinci S, et al. High-resolution CT grading of tibial stress reactions in distance runners. *AJR.* 2006;187(3):789-793.

182. Magnusson HI, Ahlborg HG, Karlsson C, Nyquist F, Karlsson MK. Low regional tibial bone density in athletes with medial tibial stress syndrome normalizes after recovery from symptoms. *Am J Sport Med.* 2003;31(4):596-600.

183. Moen MH, Tol JL, Weir A, Steunebrink M, De Winter TC. Medial tibial stress syndrome: A critical review. *Sports Med.* 2009;39(7):523-546.

184. Frost HM. From Wolff's law to the Utah paradigm: Insights about bone physiology and its clinical applications. *Anat Rec.* 2001;262(4):398-419.

185. Aweid O, Del Buono A, Malliaras P, et al. Systematic review and recommendations for intracompartmental pressure monitoring in diagnosing chronic exertional compartment syndrome of the leg. *Clin J Sport Med.* 2012;22(4):356-370.

186. Roberts A, Franklyn-Miller A. The validity of the diagnostic criteria used in chronic exertional compartment syndrome: A systematic review. *Scand J Med Sci Sports.* 2012;22(5):585-595.

187. Arendt EA, Griffiths HJ. The use of MR imaging in the assessment and clinical management of stress reactions of bone in high-performance athletes. *Clin Sport Med.* 1997;16(2):291-306.

188. Lassus J, Tulikoura I, Konttinen YT, Salo J, Santavirta S. Bone stress injuries of the lower extremity: A review. *Acta Orthop Scand.* 2002;73(3):359-368.

189. Plisky MS, Rauh MJ, Heiderscheit B, Underwood FB, Tank RT. Medial tibial stress syndrome in high school cross-country runners: Incidence and risk factors. *J Orthop Sport Phys.* 2007;37(2):40-47.

190. Kortebein PM, Kaufman KR, Basford JR, Stuart MJ. Medial tibial stress syndrome. *Med Sci Sport Exer.* 2000;32(3)(suppl):S27-S33.

191. Spitz DJ, Newberg AH. Imaging of stress fractures in the athlete. *Radiol Clin N Am.* 2002;40(2):313-331.

192. Batt ME, Ugalde V, Anderson MW, Shelton DK. A prospective controlled study of diagnostic imaging for acute shin splints. *Med Sci Sport Exer.* 1998;30(11):1564-1571.

193. Gaeta M, Minutoli F, Scribano E, et al. CT and MR imaging findings in athletes with early tibial stress injuries: Comparison with bone scintigraphy findings and emphasis on cortical abnormalities. *Radiology.* 2005;235(2):553-561.

194. Boden BP, Osbahr DC, Jimenez C. Low-risk stress fractures. *Am J Sport Med.* 2001;29(1):100-111.

195. Edwards PH Jr, Wright ML, Hartman JF. A practical approach for the differential diagnosis of chronic leg pain in the athlete. *Am J Sport Med.* 2005;33(8):1241-1249.

196. Rorabeck CH, Bourne RB, Fowler PJ, Finlay JB, Nott L. The role of tissue pressure measurement in diagnosing chronic anterior compartment syndrome. *Am J Sport Med.* 1988;16(2):143-146.

197. Loudon JK, Dolphino MR. Use foot orthoses and calf stretching for individuals with medial tibial stress syndrome. *Foot Ankle Spec.* 2010;3(1):15-20.

198. Yates B, White S. The incidence and risk factors in the development of medial tibial stress syndrome among naval recruits. *Am J Sport Med.* 2004;32(3):772-780.

199. Winters M, Eskes M, Weir A, Moen MH, Backx FJ, Bakker EW. Treatment of medial tibial stress syndrome: A systematic review. *Sports Medicine.* 2013;43(12):1315-1333.

200. Mendicino SS. Posterior tibial tendon dysfunction. Diagnosis, evaluation, and treatment. *Clin Podiatr Med Surg.* 2000;17(1):33-54, vi.

201. Richie D. Pathomechanics of the adult acquired flatfoot. *Foot Ankle Quart.* 2005;17(4):109-123.

202. Imhauser CW, Siegler S, Abidi NA, Frankel DZ. The effect of posterior tibialis tendon dysfunction on the plantar pressure characteristics and the kinematics of the arch and the hindfoot. *Clin Biomech (Bristol, Avon).* 2004;19(2):161-169.

203. Basmajian JV, Stecko G. The role of muscles in arch support of the foot. *J Bone Joint Surg Am.* 1963;45:1184-1190.

204. Mosier SM, Lucas DR, Pomeroy G, Manoli A II. Pathology of the posterior tibial tendon in posterior tibial tendon insufficiency. *Foot Ankle Int.* 1998;19(8):520-524.

205. Laughlin T. Evaluation and management of posterior tibial tendon dysfunction. *Foot Ankle Quart.* 2000;13(1):1-9.

206. Rosenberg ZS. Chronic rupture of the posterior tibial tendon. *Clin Pod Med Surg.* 1999;16(3):423-438.

207. Kohls-Gatzoulis J, Angel JC, Singh D, Haddad F, Livingstone J, Berry G. Tibialis posterior dysfunction: A common and treatable cause of adult acquired flatfoot. *BMJ.* 2004;329(7478):1328-1333.

208. Johnson KA, Strom DE. Tibialis posterior tendon dysfunction. *Clin Orthop Relat R.* 1989;239:196-206.

209. Myerson MS. Adult acquired flatfoot deformity: Treatment of dysfunction of the posterior tibial tendon. *Instr Course Lect.* 1997;46:393-405.

210. Chao W, Wapner KL, Lee TH, Adams J, Hecht PJ. Nonoperative management of posterior tibial tendon dysfunction. *Foot Ankle Int.* 1996;17(12):736-741.

211. Wapner KL, Chao W. Nonoperative treatment of posterior tibial tendon dysfunction. *Clin Orthop Relat R.* 1999;365:39-45.

212. Squires NA, Jeng CL. Posterior tibial tendon dysfunction. *Oper Techn Orthop.* 2006;16(1):44-52.

213. Taunton J, Ryan M, Clement D, McKenzie D, Lloyd-Smith D, Zumbo B. A retrospective case-control analysis of 2002 running injuries. *Brit J Sport Med.* 2002;36(2):95-101.

214. Perry MB, Premkumar A, Venzon DJ, Shawker TH, Gerber LH. Ultrasound, magnetic resonance imaging, and posterior tibialis dysfunction. *Clin Orthop Relat R.* 2003;408:225-231.

215. Bowring B, Chockalingam N. Conservative treatment of tibialis posterior tendon dysfunction—a review. *Foot (Edinb).* 2010;20(1):18-26.

216. Rabbito M, Pohl MB, Humble N, Ferber R. Biomechanical and clinical factors related to stage I posterior tibial tendon dysfunction. *J Orthop Sport Phys.* 2011;41(10):776-784.

217. Sobel M, Stern SH, Manoni A, et al. The association posterior tibialis tendon insufficiency with valgus osteoarthritis of the knee. *Am J Knee Surg.* 1992;5:59-64.

218. Alvarez RG, Marini A, Schmitt C, Saltzman CL. Stage I and II posterior tibial tendon dysfunction treated by a structured nonoperative management protocol: An orthosis and exercise program. *Foot Ankle Int.* 2006;27(1):2-8.

219. Lin JL, Balbas J, Richardson EG. Results of non-surgical treatment of stage II posterior tibial tendon dysfunction: A 7- to 10-year followup. *Foot Ankle Int.* 2008;29(8):781-786.

220. Nunley JA, Vertullo CJ. Classification, investigation, and management of midfoot sprains: Lisfranc injuries in the athlete. *Am J Sport Med.* 2002;30(6):871-878.

221. Trevino SG, Wade A. Lisfranc fracture dislocation. *Emedicence.* 2009; http://ptcoop.org/wp-content/uploads/2012/08/TTS-CMG.pdf.

222. Reischl SF, Noceti-DeWit LM. . *Current Concepts of Orthopaedic Physical Therapy.* 2nd ed. APTA: Alexandria, VA; 2006.

223. Burroughs KE, Reimer CD, Fields KB. Lisfranc injury of the foot: A commonly missed diagnosis. *Am Fam Physician.* 1998;58(1):118-124.

224. Wadsworth DJ, Eadie NT. Conservative management of subtle Lisfranc joint injury: A case report. *J Orthop Sport Phys.* 2005;35(3):154-164.

225. Brown DD, Gumbs RV. Lisfranc fracture-dislocations: Report of two cases. *J Natl Med Assoc.* 1991;83(4):366-369.

226. Pearse EO, Klass B, Bendall SP. The 'ABC' of examining foot radiographs. *Ann R Coll Surg Engl.* 2005;87(6):449-451.

227. Davies MS, Saxby TS. Intercuneiform instability and the "gap" sign. *Foot Ankle Int.* 1999;20(9):606-609.

228. Curtis MJ, Myerson M, Szura B. Tarsometatarsal joint injuries in the athlete. *Am J Sport Med.* 1993;21(4):497-502.

229. Leeuw M, Goossens ME, Linton SJ, Crombez G, Boersma K, Vlaeyen JW. The fear-avoidance model of musculoskeletal pain: Current state of scientific evidence. *J Behav Med.* 2007;30(1):77-94.

230. Goossens M, De Stoop N. Lisfranc's fracture-dislocations: Etiology, radiology, and results of treatment. A review of 20 cases. *Clin Orthop Relat R.* 1983;176:154-162.

231. Coetzee JC. Making sense of Lisfranc injuries. *Foot Ankle Clin.* 2008;13(4):695-704, ix.

232. Myerson MS. The diagnosis and treatment of injury to the tarsometatarsal joint complex. *J Bone Joint Surg Br.* 1999;81(5):756-763.

233. Thompson MC, Mormino MA. Injury to the tarsometatarsal joint complex. *J Am Acad Orthop Surg.* 2003;11(4):260-267.

234. Diebal AR, Westrick RB, Alitz C, Gerber JP. Lisfranc injury in a West Point cadet. *Sports Health.* 2013;5(3):281-285.

235. Ford LA, Collins KB, Christensen JC. Stabilization of the subluxed second metatarsophalangeal joint: Flexor tendon transfer versus primary repair of the plantar plate. *J Foot Ankle Surg.* 1998;37(3):217-222.

236. Bouché RT, Heit EJ. Combined plantar plate and hammertoe repair with flexor digitorum longus tendon transfer for chronic, severe sagittal plane instability of the lesser metatarsophalangeal joints: Preliminary observations. *J Foot Ankle Surg.* 2008;47(2):125-137.

237. Gregg J, Silberstein M, Schneider T, Marks P. Sonographic and MRI evaluation of the plantar plate: A prospective study. *Eur Radiol.* 2006;16(12):2661-2669.

238. Fortin PT, Myerson MS. Second metatarsophalangeal joint instability. *Foot Ankle Int.* 1995;16(5):306-313.

239. Coughlin MJ. Subluxation and dislocation of the second metatarsophalangeal joint. *Orthop Clin N Am.* 1989;20(4):535-551.

240. Sung W, Weil L, Weil LS, Rolfes RJ. Diagnosis of plantar plate injury by magnetic resonance imaging with reference to intraoperative findings. *J Foot Ankle Surg.* 2012;51(5):570-574.

241. Ford KR, Hoogenboom BJ, Myer GD. Understanding and preventing ACL injuries: Current biomechanical and epidemiologic considerations—update 2010. *N Am J Sports Phys Ther.* 2010;5(4):234-251.

242. Oliver TB, Beggs I. Ultrasound in the assessment of metatarsalgia: A surgical and histological correlation. *Clin Radiol.* 1998;53(4):287-289.

243. Klein EE, Weil L Jr, Weil LS Sr, Coughlin MJ, Knight J. Clinical examination of plantar plate abnormality: A diagnostic perspective. *Foot Ankle Int.* 2013;34(6):800-804.

244. Institute WFaA. Plantar Plate Tears. Available at: www.weil4feet.com/patients/education/plantar-plate-tears/. Accessed January 10, 2014.

245. Coker TP, Arnold JA, Weber DL. Traumatic lesions of the metatarsophalangeal joint of the great toe in athletes. *Am J Sport Med.* 1978;6(6):326-334.

246. McCormick JJ, Anderson RB. Turf toe: Anatomy, diagnosis, and treatment. *Sports Health.* 2010;2(6):487-494.

247. Douglas DP, Davidson DM, Robinson JE, Bedi DG. Rupture of the medial collateral ligament of the first metatarsophalangeal joint in a professional soccer player. *J Foot Ankle Surg.* 1997;36(5):388-390.

248. Fabeck LG, Zekhnini C, Farrokh D, Descamps PY, Delince PE. Traumatic hallux valgus following rupture of the medial collateral ligament of the first metatarsophalangeal joint: A case report. *J Foot Ankle Surg.* 2002;41(2):125-128.

249. Watson TS, Anderson RB, Davis WH. Periarticular injuries to the hallux metatarsophalangeal joint in athletes. *Foot Ankle Clin.* 2000;5(3):687-713.

250. McCormick JJ, Anderson RB. The great toe: Failed turf toe, chronic turf toe, and complicated sesamoid injuries. *Foot Ankle Clin.* 2009;14(2):135-150.

251. Stephens MM. Pathogenesis of hallux valgus. *Eur J Foot Ankle Surg.* 1994;1:7-10.

252. Robinson AH, Limbers JP. Modern concepts in the treatment of hallux valgus. *J Bone Joint Surg Br.* 2005;87(8):1038-1045.

253. Nguyen US, Hillstrom HJ, Li W, et al. Factors associated with hallux valgus in a population-based study of older women and men: The MOBILIZE Boston Study. *Osteoarthr Cartilage.* 2009;18:41-46.

254. Nix S, Smith M, Vicenzino B. Prevalence of hallux valgus in the general population: A systematic review and meta-analysis. *J Foot Ankle Res.* 2010;3:21.

255. Klaue K, Hansen ST, Masquelet AC. Clinical, quantitative assessment of first tarsometatarsal mobility in the sagittal plane and its relation to hallux valgus deformity. *Foot Ankle Int.* 1994;15(1):9-13.

256. Torkki M, Malmivaara A, Seitsalo S, Hoikka V, Laippala P, Paavolainen P. Surgery vs orthosis vs watchful waiting for hallux valgus: A randomized controlled trial. *JAMA.* 2001;285(19):2474-2480.

257. Hudes K. Conservative management of a case of tarsal tunnel syndrome. *J Can Chiropr Assoc.* 2010;54(2):100-106.

258. Plyler B, Martinez M, Melde C, Gieringer M. PT7549. Tarsal tunnel syndrome: A clinical management guideline. 2012;2014. http://ptcoop.org/wp-content/uploads/2012/08/TTS-CMG.pdf.

259. Williams TH, Ah R. Entrapment neuropathies of the foot and ankle. *Orthop Traum.* 2009;23:404-411.

260. Antoniadis G, Scheglmann K. Posterior tarsal tunnel syndrome: Diagnosis and treatment. *Dtsch Arztebl Int.* 2008;105(45):776-781.

261. Dellon AL. Deep peroneal nerve entrapment on the dorsum of the foot. *Foot Ankle.* 1990;11:73-80.

262. DiDomenico LA, Masternick EB. Anterior tarsal tunnel syndrome. *Clin Podiatr Med Surg.* 2006;23(3):611-620.

263. Fabre T, Montero C, Gaujard E, Gervais-Dellion F, Durandeau A. Chronic calf pain in athletes due to sural nerve entrapment. A report of 18 cases. *Am J Sport Med.* 2000;28(5):679-682.

264. Pringle RM, Protheroe K, Mukherjee SK. Entrapment neuropathy of the sural nerve. *J Bone Joint Surg Br.* 1974;56B:465-468.

265. Uritani D, Fukumoto T, Matsumoto D, Shima M. Associations between toe grip strength and hallux valgus, toe curl ability, and foot arch height in Japanese adults aged 20 to 79 years: a cross-sectional study. *J Foot Ankle Res.* 2015;8:18.

266. Hislop, HJ., Montgomery J, Connolly BH, and Daniels L. *Daniels and Worthingham's muscle testing: Techniques of manual examination.* Philadelphia, PA: W.B. Saunders, 1995.

267. Smith TO, Clark A, Neda S, Arendt EA, Post WR, Grelsamer RP, Dejour D, Almqvist KF, Donell ST. The intra- and inter-observer reliability of the physical examination methods used to assess patients with patellofemoral joint instability. *Knee.* 2012;19(4):404-410.

268. Picciano AM, Rowlands MS, Worrell T: Reliability of open and closed kinetic chain subtalar joint neutral positions and navicular drop test. *J Orthop Sports Phys Ther.* 1993;18(4):553-558.

269. Maffulli N, Waterston SW, Squair J, Reaper J, Douglas AS. Changing incidence of Achilles tendon rupture in Scotland: a 15-year study. *Clin J Sport Med.* 1999;9:157-160.

270. Gulati V, Jaggard M, Al-Nammari SS, Uzoigwe C, Gulati P, Ismail N, Gibbons C, Gupte C. Management of Achilles tendon injury: A current concepts systematic review. *World J Orthop.* 2015;6(4):380-386.

271. Maffulli N, Ewen SW, Waterston SW, Reaper J, Barrass V. Tenocytes from ruptured and tendinopathic Achilles tendons produce greater quantities of type III collagen than tenocytes from normal Achilles tendons. An in vitro model of human tendon healing. *Am J Sports Med.* 2000;28:499–505.

272. Järvinen M, Józsa L, Kannus P, Järvinen TL, Kvist M, Leadbetter W. Histopathological findings in chronic tendon disorders. *Scand J Med Sci Sports.* 1997;7:86–95.

273. Sode J, Obel N, Hallas J, Lassen A. Use of fluroquinolone and risk of Achilles tendon rupture: a population-based cohort study. *Eur J Clin Pharmacol.* 2007;63:499-503.

Chapter 27

1. Jonasson P, Halldin K, Karlsson J, et al. Prevalence of joint-related pain in the extremities and spine in five groups of top athletes. *Knee Surg Sport Tra A.* 2011;19(9):1540-1546.

2. Sahler CS, Greenwald BD. Traumatic brain injury in sports: A review. *Rehabil Res Pract.* 2012;2012:659-652.

3. McCrory P, Meeuwisse WH, Aubry M, et al. Consensus statement on concussion in sport: The 4th International Conference on Concussion in Sport held in Zurich, November 2012. *Brit J Sport Med.* 2013;47:250-258.

4. Gilchrist J, Thomas KE, Xu L, McGuire LC, Coronado VG. Nonfatal sports and recreation related traumatic brain injuries among children and adolescents treated in emergency departments in the United States, 2001-2009. *MMWR.* 2011;60(39):1337-1342.

5. Gessel LM, Fields SK, Collins CL, Dick RW, Comstock RD. Concussions among United States high school and collegiate athletes. *J Athl Train.* 2007;42(4):495-503.

6. Kristman VL, Tator CH, Kreiger N, et al. Does the apolipoprotein epsilon 4 allele predispose varsity athletes to concussion? A prospective cohort study. *Clin J Sport Med.* 2008;18:322-328.

7. Delaney JS, Al-Kashmiri A. Neck injuries presenting to emergency departments in the United States from 1990 to 1999 for ice hockey, soccer, and American football. *Brit J Sport Med.* 2005;39(4):1-5.

8. Chen JK, Johnston KM, Collie A, McCrory P, Ptito A. A validation of the post concussion symptom scale in the assessment of complex concussion using cognitive testing and functional MRI. *J Neurol Neurosurg Ps.* 2007;78(11):1231-1238.

9. Maddocks D, Dicker G. An objective measure of recovery from concussion in Australian rules footballers. *Sport Health.* 1989;7(suppl):6-7.

10. Maddocks DL, Dicker GD, Saling MM. The assessment of orientation following concussion in athletes. *Clin J Sport Med.* 1995;5(1):32-35.

11. Dicker G, Maddocks D. Clinical management of concussion. *Aust Fam Physician.* 1993;22(5):750-753.

12. McCrea M, Kelly JP, Randolph C, et al. Standardized assessment of concussion (SAC): On-site mental status evaluation of the athlete. *J Head Trauma Rehab.* 1998;13(2):27-35.

13. Barr WB, McCrea M. Sensitivity and specificity of standardized neurocognitive testing immediately following sports concussion. *J Int Neuropsychol Soc.* 2001;7(6):693-702.

14. Giza C, Kutcher J, Ashwal S, et al. Summary of evidence-based guideline update: Evaluation and management of concussion in sports: Report of the Guideline Development Subcommittee of the American Academy of Neurology. *Neurology.* 2013;80(24):2250-2257.

15. Bell DR, Guskiewicz KM, Clark MA, Padua DA. Systematic review of the Balance Error Scoring System. *Sports Health.* 2011;3(3):287-295.

16. Guskiewicz KM. Assessment of postural stability following sport-related concussion. *Curr Sports Med Rep.* 2003;2:24-30.

17. Schatz PS, Pardini JE, Lovell MR, Collins MW, Podell K. Sensitivity and specificity of the ImPACT Test Battery for concussion in athletes. *Arch Clin Neuropsychol.* 2006;21(1):91-99.

18. Van Kampen DA, Lovell MR, Pardini JE, Collins MW, Fu FH. The "value added" of neurocognitive testing after sports-related concussion. *Am J Sport Med.* 2006;34(10):1630-1635.

19. Fazio V, Lovell MR, Pardini J, Collins MW. The relationship between postconcussion symptoms and neurocognitive performance in concussed athletes. *Neurorehabilitation.* 2007;22:207-216.

20. Lau BC, Colins MW, Lovell MR. Sensitivity and specificity of subacute computerized neurocognitive testing and symptom evaluation in predicting outcome after sports-related concussion. *Am J Sport Med.* 2011;39(6):1209-1216.

21. National Spinal Cord Injury Statistical Center (NSCISC). Spinal cord injury facts and figures at a glance. Available at: www.nscisc.uab.edu/PublicDocuments/fact_figures_docs/Facts%202012%20Feb%20Final.pdf.

22. NSCISC National Spinal Cord Injury Statistical Center: Facts and Figures at a Glance. www.nscisc.uab.edu/PublicDocuments/fact_figures_docs/Facts%202012%20Feb%20Final.pdf.

23. Ghiselli G, Schaadt G, McAllister DR. On-the-field evaluation of an athlete with a head or neck injury. *Clin Sport Med.* 2003;22(3):445-465.

24. Boden BP, Tacchetti RL, Cantu RC, Knowles SB, Mueller FO. Catastrophic cervical spine injuries in high school and college football players. *Am J Sport Med.* 2006;34(8):1223-1232.

25. Banerjee R, Palumbo MA, Fadale PD. Catastrophic cervical spine injuries in the collision sport athlete. Part 1. Epidemiology, functional anatomy, and diagnosis. *Am J Sport Med.* 2004;32:1077-1087.

26. Bailes JE, Petschauer M, Guskiewicz KM, Marano G. Management of cervical spine injuries in athletes. *J Athl Train.* 2007;42(1):126-134.

27. Torg JS, Pavlov H, Genuario SE, et al. Neurapraxia of the cervical spinal cord with transient quadriplegia. *J Bone Joint Surg Am.* 1986;68:1354-1370.

28. Castro FP. Stingers, the Torg ratio, and the cervical spine. *Am J Sport Med.* 1997;25: 603-608.

29. Levitz CL, Reilly PJ, Torg JS. The pathomechanics of chronic, recurrent cervical nerve root neuropraxia. The chronic burner syndrome. *Am J Sport Med.* 1997;25:73-76.

30. Meyer SA, Schulte KR, Callaghan JJ, et al. Cervical spinal stenosis and stingers in collegiate football players. *Am J Sport Med.* 1994;22:158-166.

31. Standaert CJ, Herring SA. Expert opinion and controversies in musculoskeletal and sports medicine: Stingers. *Arch Phys Med Rehab.* 2009;90(3):402-406.

32. Maron BJ, Doerer JJ, Haas TS, Terney DM, Mueller FO. Sudden deaths in young competitive athletes. *Circulation.* 2009;119;1085-1092.

33. Maron BJ. Hypertrophic cardiomyopathy. In: Zipes DP, Libby P, Bonow RO, Braunwald E, eds. *Braunwald's Heart Disease: A Textbook of Cardiovascular Medicine.* 8th ed. St. Louis, MO: WB Saunders; 2007.

34. Maron BJ, Thompson PD, Ackerman MJ, et al. Recommendation and considerations related to preparticipation screening for cardiovascular abnormalities in competitive athletes: 2007 update. A scientific statement from the American Heart Association Council on Nutrition, Physical Activity, and Metabolism: Endorsed by the American College of Cardiology Foundation. *Circulation.* 2007;115(12):1643-1655.

35. Davis JA, Cecchin F, Jones TK, Portman MA. Major coronary artery anomalies in pediatric population: Incidence and clinical importance. *J Am Coll Cardio.* 2001;37(2);593-597.

36. Pelliccia A, Maron BJ. Preparticipation cardiovascular evaluation of the competitive athlete: Perspectives from the 30-year Italian experience. *Am J Cardiol.* 1995;75:827- 829.

37. Maron BJ, Haas TS, Doerer JJ, Thompson PD, Hodges JS. Comparison of U.S. and Italian experiences with sudden cardiac deaths in young competitive athletes and implications for preparticipation screening strategies. *Am J Cardiol.* 2009;104(2):276-280.

38. Lawless CE, Best TM. Electrocardiograms in athletes: Interpretation and diagnostic accuracy. *Med Sci Sport Exer.* 2008;40(5):787-798.

39. Reneman RS, Jageneau AH. The influence of weighted exercise on tissue (intramuscular) pressure in normal subjects and patients with intermittent claudication. *Scand J Clin Lab Inv.* 1973;128(suppl):37-42.

40. George CA, Hutchinson MR. Chronic exertional compartment syndrome. *Clin Sport Med.* 2012;31(2):307-319.

41. Edmundsson D, Toolanen G, Sojka P. Chronic compartment syndrome also affects nonathletic subjects: A prospective study of 63 cases with exercise-induced lower leg pain. *Acta Orthop.* 2007;78:136-142.

42. Lecocq J, Isner-Horobeti ME, Dupeyron A, Helmlinger JL, Vautravers P. Exertional compartment syndrome [in French]. *Ann Readapt Med Phys.* 2004;47(6):334-345.

43. Shubert A. Exertional compartment syndrome: Review of the literature and proposed rehabilitation guidelines following surgical release. *N Am J Sports Phys Ther.* 2007;2(3):170-180.

44. Styf J. *Compartment Syndromes: Diagnosis, Treatment, and Complications.* Boca Raton, FL: CRC Press; 2004.

45. Roberts A, Franklyn-Miller A. The validity of the diagnostic criteria used in chronic exertional compartment syndrome: A systematic review. *Scand J Med Sci Spor.* 2012;22:585-595.

46. Helenius I, Lumme A, Haahtela T. Asthma, airway inflammation and treatment in elite athletes. *Sports Med.* 2005;35(7):565-574.

47. Larsson K, Ohlsen P, Larsson L, et al. High prevalence of asthma in cross-country skiers. *BMJ.* 1993;307:1326-1329.

48. Sue-Chu M, Larsson L, Bjermer L. Prevalence of asthma in young cross-country skiers in central Scandinavia: Differences between Norway and Sweden. *Resp Med.* 1996;90:99-105.

49. Helenius I, Rytila P, Sarna S, et al. Effect of continuing or finishing high-level sports on airway inflammation, bronchial hyperresponsiveness, and asthma: A prospective follow-up study of 42 elite swimmers. *J Allergy Clin Immun.* 2002;109:962-968.

50. Langdeau JB, Turcotte H, Bowie DM, et al. Airway hyperresponsiveness in elite athletes. *Am J Resp Crit Care.* 2000;161:1479-1484.

51. Helenius IJ, Rytila P, Metso T, et al. Respiratory symptoms bronchial responsiveness and cellular characteristics of induced sputum in elite swimmers. *Allergy.* 1998;53:346-352.

52. Helenius IJ, Tikkanen HO, Sarna S, et al. Asthma and increased bronchial responsiveness in elite athletes: Atopy and sport bievent as risk factors. *J Allergy Clin Immun.* 1998;101:646-652.

53. Dosman JA, Hodgson WC, Cockcroft DW. Effect of cold air on the bronchial response to inhaled histamine in patients with asthma. *Am Rev Respir Dis.* 1991;144:45-50.

54. Leuppi JD, Kuhn M, Comminot C, et al. High prevalence of bronchial hyperresponsiveness and asthma in ice hockey players. *Eur Resp J.* 1998;12:13-16.

55. Wilber RL, Rundell KW, Szmedra L, et al. Incidence of exercise-induced bronchospasm in Olympic Winter sport athletes. *Med Sci Sport Exer.* 2000;32:732-737.

56. Helenius IJ, Tikkanen HO, Haahtela T. Association between type of training and risk of asthma in elite athletes. *Thorax.* 1997;52:157-160.

57. Papiris SA, Manali ED, Kolilekas L, Triantafillidou C, Tsangaris I. Acute severe asthma. New approaches to assessment and treatment. *Drugs.* 2009;69(17):2363-2391.

58. Couto M, Silva D, Delgado L, Moreira A. Exercise and airway injury in athletes. *Acta Med Port.* 2013;26(1):56-60.

59. Casa DJ, Guskiewicz KM, Anderson SA, et al. National Athletic Trainers' Association position statement: Preventing sudden death in sports. *J Athl Train.* 2012;47(1):96-118.

60. Lougheed MD, Leniere C, Ducharme FM, et al. Thoracic Society 2012 guideline update: Diagnosis and management of asthma in preschoolers, children and adults: Executive summary. *Can Respir J.* 2012;19(6):e81-e88.

61. Putukian M, Thompson C. Traumatic injuries. In: Casa DJ, ed. *Preventing Sudden Death in Sport and Physical Activity.* Sudbury, MA: Jones and Bartlett Learning; 2012: 143-145.

62. Putukian M. Pneumothorax and pneumomediastinum. *Clin Sport Med.* 2004;23(3):443-454.

63. McGown AT. Blunt abdominal and chest trauma. *Athlet Ther Today.* 2004;9(1):40-41.

64. Price S, Wilson L. *Pathophysiology—Clinical Concepts of Disease Processes.* 4th ed. St. Louis, MO: Mosby-Year Book; 1992: 518-519, 561-562.

65. Smith D. Chest injuries. What the sports physical therapist should know. *Int J Sports Phys Ther.* 2011;6(4):357-360.

66. Howe AS, Boden BP. Heat-related illness in athletes. *Am J Sport Med.* 2007;35(8):1384-1395.

67. Casa DJ, Armstrong LE, Kenny GP, O'Connor FG, Huggins RA. Exertional heat stroke: New concepts regarding cause and care. *Curr Sports Med Rep.* 2012;11(3):115-123.

68. Kerr ZY, Casa DJ, Marshall SW, Comstock RD. Epidemiology of exertional heat illness among U.S. high school athletes. *Am J Prev Med.* 2013;44(1):8-14.

69. Glazer JL. Management of heatstroke and heat exhaustion. *Am Fam Physician.* 2005;71:2133-2140.

70. Casa DJ, Becker SM, Ganio MAS, et al. Validity of devices that assess body temperature during outdoor exercise in the heat. *J Athl Train.* 2007;42(3):333-342.

71. Becker JA, Stewart LK. Heat-related illness. *Am Fam Physician.* 2011;83(11):1325-1330.

72. American Red Cross. *Emergency Response Manual.* Boston, MA: Author; 2001.

73. Cockshott WP, Jenkin JK, Pui M. Limiting the use of routine radiography for acute ankle injuries. *Can Med Assoc J.* 1983;129:129-131.

74. Heyworth J. Ottawa ankle rules for the injured ankle. *Brit J Sport Med.* 2003;37:194.

75. Stiell IG, Greenberg GH, McKnight RD, et al. A study to develop clinical decision rules for the use of radiography in acute ankle injuries. *Ann Emerg Med.* 1996;21:384-390.

76. Stiell IG, Wells G, Laupacis A, et al. Multicentre trial to introduce the Ottawa ankle rules for use of radiography in acute ankle injuries. *Brit Med J.*1995;311:594-597.

77. McBride, Kim L. Validation of the Ottawa ankle rules. Experience at a community hospital. *Can Fam Physician.*1997;43:459.

78. Stiell IG, Wells G, McDowell I, et al. Use of radiography in acute knee injuries: Need for clinical decision rules. *Acad Emerg Med.* 1995;2:966-973.

79. Stiell IG, Greenberg GH, Wells GA, et al. Prospective validation of a decision rule for the use of radiography in acute knee injuries. *JAMA.*1996;275(8):611-615.

80. Bachmann LM, et al. The accuracy of the Ottawa knee rule to rule out knee fractures. A systematic review. *Ann Intern Med.* 2004;140(2):121-124.

81. Stiell IG, Wells GA, Vandemheen KL, et al. The Canadian C-Spine rule for radiography in alert and stable trauma patients. *JAMA.* 2001;286(15):1841-1848.

82. Reid DC, Henderson R, Saboe L, Miller JD. Etiology and clinical course of missed spine fractures. *J Traum.*1987;27:980-986.

83. Diliberti T, Lindsey RW. Evaluation of the cervical spine in the emergency setting: Who does not need an x-ray? *Orthopedics.*1992;15:179-183.

84. Bachulis BL, Long WB, Hynes GD, Johnson MC. Clinical indications for cervical spine radiographs in the traumatized patient. *Am J Surg.*1987;153:473-478.

85. Gbaanador GBM, Fruin AH, Taylon C. Role of routine emergency cervical radiography in head trauma. *Am J Surg.*1986;152:643-648.

86. Bayless P, Ray VG. Incidence of cervical spine injuries in association with blunt head trauma. *Am J Emerg Med.*1989;7:139-142.

87. Vandemark RM. Radiology of the cervical spine in trauma patients: Practice pitfalls and recommendations for improving efficiency and communication. *Am J Roentgenol.*1990;155:465-472.

88. Michaleff ZA. Accuracy of the Canadian C-spine rule and NEXUS to screen for clinically important cervical spine injury in patients following blunt trauma: A systematic review. *Can Med Assoc J.* 2012;184(16):E867-E876.

89. American Diabetes Association. All about Diabetes. Retrieved from: www.diabetes.org/.

90. Jiminez CC, Corcoran, MH, Crawley JT, et al. National Athletic Trainers Association position statement: Management of the athlete with Type 1 diabetes mellitus. *J Athl Train.* 2007;42(4):536-545.

Chapter 28

1. U.S. Department of Health and Human Services. Administration on Aging. *A profile of older Americans: 2013.* Washington DC: Author; 2012:1-17.

2. American Academy of Orthopaedic Surgeons. *Burden of Musculoskeletal Diseases in the United States: Prevalence, Societal, and Economic Cost.* 2008. Available from: www.spinalkinetics.info/Bone_and_Joint_Executive_Summary.pdf.

3. American Academy of Orthopaedic Surgeons. *Burden of Musculoskeletal Disease in the United States: Prevalence, Societal, and Economic Cost.* 2011. Available from: www.spinalkinetics.info/Bone_and_Joint_Executive_Summary.pdf.

4. Haralson RH, Zuckerman JD. Prevalence, health care expenditures, and orthopedic surgery workforce for musculoskeletal conditions. *JAMA.* 2009;302(14):1586-1587.

5. Deyo RA, Rainville J, Kent DL. What can the history and physical examination tell us about low back pain? *JAMA.* 1992;268(6):760-765.

6. Cook C, Brown C, Isaacs R, Roman M, Davis S, Richardson W. Clustered clinical findings for diagnosis of cervical spine myelopathy. *J Man Manip Ther.* 2010;18(4):175-180.

7. Stiell IG, Greenberg GH, Wells GA, et al. Derivation of a decision rule for the use of radiography in acute knee injuries. *Ann Emerg Med.* 1995;26(4):405-413.

8. Seaberg DC, Jackson R. Clinical decision rule for knee radiographs. *Am J Emerg Med.* 1994;12(5):541-543.

9. Stiell IG, Wells GA, Vandemheen KL, et al. The Canadian C-spine rule for radiography in alert and stable trauma patients. *JAMA.* 2001;286(15):1841-1848.

10. Roman M, Brown C, Richardson W, Isaacs R, Howes C, Cook C. The development of a clinical decision making algorithm for detection of osteoporotic vertebral compression fracture or wedge deformity. *J Man Manip Ther.* 2010;18(1):44-49.

11. Cadarette SM, Jaglal SB, Kreiger N, McIsaac WJ, Darlington GA, Tu JV. Development and validation of the Osteoporosis Risk Assessment Instrument to facilitate selection of women for bone densitometry. *Can Med Assoc J.* 2000;162(9):1289-1294.

12. Lydick E, Cook K, Turpin J, Melton M, Stine R, Byrnes C. Development and validation of a simple questionnaire to facilitate identification of women likely to have low bone density. *Am J Manag C.* 1998;4(1):37-48.

13. Koh LK, Sedrine WB, Torralba TP, et al. A simple tool to identify Asian women at increased risk of osteoporosis. *Osteoporosis Int.* 2001;12(8):699-705.

14. Shepherd AJ, Cass AR, Carlson CA, Ray L. Development and internal validation of the male osteoporosis risk estimation score. *Ann Fam Med.* 2007;5(6):540-546.

15. Le Gal G, Righini M, Roy PM, et al. Prediction of pulmonary embolism in the emergency department: The revised Geneva score. *Ann Intern Med.* 2006;144(3):165-171.

16. Litaker D, Pioro M, El Bilbeisi H, Brems J. Returning to the bedside: Using the history and physical examination to identify rotator cuff tears. *J Am Geriatr.* 2000;48(12):1633-1637.

17. Wainner RS, Fritz JM, Irrgang JJ, Delitto A, Allison S, Boninger ML. Development of a clinical prediction rule for the diagnosis of carpal tunnel syndrome. *Arch Phys Med Rehab.* 2005;86(4):609-618.

18. Sugioka T, Hayashino Y, Konno S, Kikuchi S, Fukuhara S. Predictive value of self-reported patient information for the identification of lumbar spinal stenosis. *Fam Pract.* 2008;25(4):237-244.

19. Altman R, Alarcon G, Appelrouth D, et al. The American College of Rheumatology criteria for the classification and reporting of osteoarthritis of the hip. *Arthritis Rheum.* 1991;34(5):505-514.

20. Altman R, Asch E, Bloch D, et al. Development of criteria for the classification and reporting of osteoarthritis. Classification of osteoarthritis of the knee. Diagnostic and Therapeutic Criteria Committee of the American Rheumatism Association. *Arthritis Rheum.* 1986;29(8):1039-1049.

21. Fernandez-de-las-Penas C, Cleland JA, Palomeque-del-Cerro L, Caminero AB, Guillem-Mesado A, Jimenez-Garcia R. Development of a clinical prediction rule for identifying women with tension-type headache who are likely to achieve short-term success with joint mobilization and muscle trigger point therapy. *Headache.* 2011;51(2):246-261.

22. Vicenzino B, Smith D, Cleland J, Bisset L. Development of a clinical prediction rule to identify initial responders to mobilisation with movement and exercise for lateral epicondylalgia. *Man Ther.* 2009;14(5):550-554.

23. Kennedy CA, Haines T, Beaton DE. Eight predictive factors associated with response patterns during physiotherapy for soft tissue shoulder disorders were identified. *J Clin Epidemiol.* 2006;59(5):485-496.

24. Vicenzino B, Collins N, Cleland J, McPoil T. A clinical prediction rule for identifying patients with patellofemoral pain who are likely to benefit from foot orthoses: A preliminary determination. *Brit J Sport Med.* 2010;44(12):862-866.

25. Raney NH, Petersen EJ, Smith TA, et al. Development of a clinical prediction rule to identify patients with neck pain likely to benefit from cervical traction and exercise. *Eur Spine J.* 2009;18(3):382-391.

26. Schellingerhout JM, Verhagen AP, Heymans MW, et al. Which subgroups of patients with non-specific neck pain are more likely to benefit from spinal manipulation therapy, physiotherapy, or usual care? *Pain.* 2008;139(3):670-680.

27. Cai C, Pua YH, Lim KC. A clinical prediction rule for classifying patients with low back pain who demonstrate short-term improvement with mechanical lumbar traction. *Eur Spine J.* 2009;18(4):554-561.

28. Stanton TR, Hancock MJ, Maher CG, Koes BW. Critical appraisal of clinical prediction rules that aim to optimize treatment selection for musculoskeletal conditions. *Phys Ther.* 2010;90(6):843-854.

29. Crowell MS, Wofford NH. Lumbopelvic manipulation in patients with patellofemoral pain syndrome. *J Man Manip Ther.* 2012;20(3):113-120.

30. Rabin A, Shashua A, Pizem K, Dickstein R, Dar G. A clinical prediction rule to identify patients with low back pain who are likely to experience short-term success following lumbar stabilization exercises: A randomized controlled validation study [published online ahead of print November 21 2013]. *J Orthop Sport Phys.* 2013.

31. Cleland JA, Mintken PE, Carpenter K, et al. Examination of a clinical prediction rule to identify patients with neck pain likely to benefit from thoracic spine thrust manipulation and a general cervical range of motion exercise: Multi-center randomized clinical trial. *Phys Ther.* 2010;90(9):1239-1250.

32. Bassey EJ, Harries UJ. Normal values for handgrip strength in 920 men and women aged over 65 years, and longitudinal changes over 4 years in 620 survivors. *Clin Sci.* 1993;84(3):331-337.

33. Boissonnault WG. *Primary Care for the Physical Therapist.* 2nd ed. Philadelphia, PA: Saunders; 2010.

34. American Heart Association. *Older Americans & Cardiovascular Diseases 2014 Fact Sheet.* Dallas, TX: Author; 2014.

35. Lakatta EG. Age-associated cardiovascular changes in health: Impact on cardiovascular disease in older persons. *Heart Fail Rev.* 2002;7:29-49.

36. Monahan KD. Effect of aging on baroreflex function in humans. *Am J Physiol Reg I.* 2007;293:R3-R12.

37. Ferrari AU, Radaelli A, Centola M. Physiology of aging invited review: Aging and the cardiovascular system. *J Appl Physiol.* 2003;95:2591-2597.

38. Wei JY. Age and the cardiovascular system. *New Engl J Med.* 1992;327(24):1735-1739.

39. Wei JY, Gersh BJ. Heart disease in the elderly. *Curr Prob Cardiology.* 1987;12:1-65.

40. United States Census Bureau. The 2012 statistical abstract age-adjusted death rates by major causes. Available at: www.census.gov/compendia/statab/cats/births_deaths_marriages_divorces/deaths.html. Accessed on December 1, 2013.

41. Janssens JP, Pache JC, Nicod LP. Physiological changes in respiratory function associated with ageing. *Eur Respir J.* 1999;13:197-205.

42. Lewis CB, Bottomley JM. *Geriatric Rehabilitation: A Clinical Approach.* 3rd ed. Upper Saddle River, NJ: Prentice Hall; 2008.

43. Murphy SL, Xu J, Kochanek KD. Deaths: Preliminary data for 2010. *National Vital Statistics Reports.* 2012;60(4):1-52.

44. American Lung Association. What are the symptoms of pneumonia? Available at: www.lung.org/lung-disease/pneumonia/symptoms-diagnosis-and.html. Accessed on December 1, 2013.

45. Laurentani F, Russo SR, Bandinelli S, et al. Age-associated changes in skeletal muscles and their effect on mobility: An operational diagnosis of sarcopenia. *J Appl Physiol.* 2003;95:1851-1860.

46. Frontera WR, Hughes VA, Fielding RA, Fiatarone MA, Evans WJ, Roubenoff R. Aging of skeletal muscle: A 12-year longitudinal study. *J Appl Physiol.* 2000;88:1321-1326.

47. Booth FW, Weeden SH, Tseng BS. Effect of aging on human skeletal muscle and motor function. *Med Sci Sport Exer.* 1994;26(5):556-560.

48. Tseng BS, Marsh DR, Hamilton MT, Booth FW. Strength and aerobic training attenuate muscle wasting and improve resistance to the development of disability with aging. *J Gerontol.* 1995;50A:113-119.

49. Loeser RF. Age-related changes in the musculoskeletal system and the development of osteoarthritis. *Clin Geriatr Med.* 2010;26(3):371-386.

50. Visser M, Goodpaster BH, Kritchevsky SB, et al. Muscle mass, muscle strength, and muscle fat infiltration as predictors of incident mobility limitations in well-functioning older persons. *J Gerontol.* 2005;60A(3):324-333.

51. Evans W. Functional and metabolic consequences of sarcopenia. *J Nutr.* 1997;127:998S-1003S.

52. Guralnik JM, Ferrucci L, Balfour JL, Volpato S, Iorio AD. Progressive versus catastrophic loss of the ability to walk: Implications for the prevention of mobility loss. *J Am Geriatr Soc.* 2001;49:1463-1470.

53. Buckwalter JA, Woo SL, Goldberg VM, et al. Soft-tissue aging and musculoskeletal function. *J Bone Joint Surg.* 1993;75(10):1533-1548.

54. Morris CE, Bullock MI, Basmajian JV. Vladimir Janda, MD, DSc: Tribute to a master of rehabilitation. *Spine.* 2006;31:1060-1064.

55. Bollet AJ, Nance JL. Biochemical findings in normal and osteoarthritic articular cartilage. II. Chondroitin sulfate concentration and chain length, water, and ash content. *J Clin Invest.* 1966;45(7):1170-1177.

56. Maldonado DC, Pereira da Silva CP, Neto SE, Rodrigues de Souza M, Rosrigues de Souza R. The effects of joint immobilization on articular cartilage of the knee in previously exercised rats. *J Anat.* 2013;222:518-525.

57. Roughly PJ, White RJ. Age-related changes in the structure of the proteoglycan subunits from human articular cartilage. *J Biol Chem.* 1980;255(1):217-224.

58. Aagaard P, Suetta C, Caserotti P, Magnusson SP, Kjer M. Role of the nervous system in sarcopenia and muscle atrophy with aging: Strength training as a countermeasure. *Scand J Med Sci Spor.* 2010;20:49-64.

59. Jang YC, Van Remmen H. Age-associated alterations of neuromuscular junction. *Exp Gerontol.* 2011;46:193-198.

60. Sabbahi MA, Sedgwick EM. Age-related changes in monosynaptic reflex excitability. *J Gerontol.* 1982;37(1):24-32.

61. Centers for Disease Control and Prevention. Prevalence and characteristics of persons with hearing trouble: United States, 1990-91. Hyattsville, MD: Author; 1994. Available at: http://www.cdc.gov/nchs/data/series/sr_10/sr10_188.pdf.

62. National Eye Institute. Age-related eye diseases. Available at: www.nei.nih.gov/healthyeyes/aging_eye.asp. Accessed on January 2, 2014.

63. Centers for Disease Control and Prevention. Falls among older adults: An overview. Available at: www.cdc.gov/homeandrecreationalsafety/falls/adultfalls.html. Accessed on January 2, 2014.

64. Kenney WL, Munce TA. Physiology of aging invited review: Aging and human temperature regulation. *J Appl Physiol.* 2003;96:2598-2603.

65. Clarkston W, Pantano M, Morley JE, Horowitz M, Littlefield J, Burton F. Evidence for the anorexia of aging: Gastrointestinal transit and hunger in healthy elderly vs. young adults. *Am J Physiol-Reg I.* 1997;272(1):R243-R248.

66. Weinstein JR, Anderson S. The aging kidney: Physiological changes. *Adv Chronic Kidney D.* 2010;17(4):302-307.

67. Jhamb M, Weisbord SD, Steel JL, Unruh M. Fatigue in patients receiving maintenance dialysis: A review of definitions, measures, and contributing factors. *Am J Kidney Dis.* 2008;52(2):353-365.

68. Ginsberg G, Hattis D, Russ A, Sonawane B. Pharmacokinetic and pharmacodynamic factors that can affect sensitivity to neurotoxic sequelae in elderly individuals. *Environ Health Persp.* 2005;113(9):1243.

69. Foxman B. Epidemiology of urinary tract infections: Incidence, morbidity, and economic costs. *Am J Med.* 2002;113(1):5-13.

70. Beveridge LA, Davey PG, Phillips G, McMurdo ME. Optimal management of urinary tract infections in older people. *Clin Interv Aging.* 2011;6:173.

71. Ingham SL, Zhang W, Doherty SA, McWilliams DF, Muir KR, Doherty M. Incident knee pain in the Nottingham community: A 12-year retrospective cohort study. *Osteoarthr Cartilage.* 2011;19(7):847-852.

72. Felson DT, Zhang Y, Hannan MT, et al. Risk factors for incident radiographic knee osteoarthritis in the elderly: The Framingham Study. *Arthritis Rheum.* 1997;40(4):728-733.

73. Dawson J, Juszczak E, Thorogood M, Marks SA, Dodd C, Fitzpatrick R. An investigation of risk factors for symptomatic osteoarthritis of the knee in women using a life course approach. *J Epidemiol Commun H.* 2003;57(10):823-830.

74. Riddle DL, Stratford PW. Body weight changes and corresponding changes in pain and function in persons with symptomatic knee osteoarthritis: A cohort study. *Arthritis Care Res.* 2013;65(1):15-22.

75. Shrier I. Muscle dysfunction versus wear and tear as a cause of exercise related osteoarthritis: An epidemiological update. *Brit J Sport Med.* 2004;38(5):526-535.

76. Davis MA, Ettinger WH, Neuhaus JM, Cho SA, Hauck WW. The association of knee injury and obesity with unilateral and bilateral osteoarthritis of the knee. *Am J Epidemiol.* 1989;130(2):278-288.

77. Tjoumakaris FP, Van Kleunen J, Weidner Z, Huffman GR. Knee sports injury is associated with an increased prevalence of unilateral knee replacement: A case-controlled study. *J Knee Surg.* 2012;25(5):403-406.

78. Uthman OA, van der Windt DA, Jordan JL, et al. Exercise for lower limb osteoarthritis: Systematic review incorporating trial sequential analysis and network meta-analysis. *BMJ.* 2013;347:f5555.

79. Hoy D, Brooks P, Blyth F, Buchbinder R. The epidemiology of low back pain. *Best Pract Res Cl Rh.* 2010;24(6):769-781.

80. Fejer R, Leboeuf-Yde C. Does back and neck pain become more common as you get older? A systematic literature review. *Chiropr Man Ther.* 2012;20(1):24.

81. Andrews AW, Thomas MW, Bohannon RW. Normative values for isometric muscle force measurements obtained with hand-held dynamometers. *Phys Ther.* 1996;76(3):248-259.

82. Norkin C, White D. *Measurement of Joint Motion: A Guide to Goniometry.* 4th ed. Philadelphia, PA: F.A. Davis; 2009.

83. American College of Sports Medicine. *ACSM's Guidelines for Exercise Testing and Prescription.* 8th ed. Baltimore, MD: Lippincott Williams & Wilkins; 2009.

84. Knaggs JD, Larkin KA, Manini TM. Metabolic cost of daily activities and effect of mobility impairment in older adults. *J Am Geriatr.* 2011;59(11):2118-2123.

85. National Osteoporosis Foundation. *Clinician's guide to prevention and treatment of osteoporosis* [revised 2013]. Washington, DC: Author; 2013.

86. Surgeon General. *Bone health and osteoporosis: A report of the Surgeon General.* Rockville, MD: Author; 2004.

87. Kemmis K. *Focus: Physical therapist practice in geriatrics 2011. The aging musculoskeletal system.* La Crosse, WI: American Physical Therapy Association; 2011.

88. Siminoski K, Warshawski R, Jen H, Lee K. Accuracy of physical examination using the rib-pelvis distance for detection of lumbar vertebral fractures. *Am J Med.* 2003;115(3):233-236.

89. Centers for Disease Control and Prevention. Falls are a major threat for your patients. Available at: www.cdc.gov/HomeandRecreationalSafety/pdf/steadi/falls_are_a_major_threat.pdf. Accessed on January 10, 2014.

90. Whitney SL, Hudak MT, Marchetti GF. The dynamic gait index relates to self-reported fall history in individuals with vestibular dysfunction. *J Vestibul Res-Equil.* 2000;10(2):99-105.

91. Cattaneo D, Regola A, Meotti M. Validity of six balance disorders scales in persons with multiple sclerosis. *Disabil Rehabil.* 2006;28(12):789-795.

92. Cakit BD, Saracoglu M, Genc H, Erdem HR, Inan L. The effects of incremental speed-dependent treadmill training on postural instability and fear of falling in Parkinson's disease. *Clin Rehabil.* 2007;21(8):698-705.

93. Centers for Disease Control and Prevention. Algorithm for fall risk assessment and interventions. Available at: www.cdc.gov/HomeandRecreationalSafety/pdf/steadi/algorithm_fall_risk_assessment.pdf. Accessed on December 23, 2013.

94. Centers For Disease Control and Prevention. STEADI (Stopping Elderly Accidents, Deaths and Injuries) tool kit for health care providers. Available at: www.cdc.gov/homeandrecreationalsafety/Falls/steadi/index.html. Accessed on December 23, 2013.

95. Dite W, Temple VA. A clinical test of stepping and change of direction to identify multiple falling older adults. *Arch Phys Med Rehab.* 2002;83(11):1566-1571.

96. Shumway-Cook A, Baldwin M, Polissar NL, Gruber W. Predicting the probability for falls in community-dwelling older adults. *Phys Ther.* 1997;77(8):812-819.

97. Karthikeyan G, Sheikh SG, Chippala P. Test-retest reliability of short form of Berg balance scale in elderly people. *GARJMMS.* 2012;1(6):139-144.

98. Wrisley DM, Kumar NA. Functional gait assessment: Concurrent, discriminative, and predictive validity in community-dwelling older adults. *Phys Ther.* 2010;90(5):761-773.

99. Bowden MG, Balasubramanian CK, Behrman AL, Kautz SA. Validation of a speed-based classification system using quantitative measures of walking performance poststroke. *Neurorehab Neural Re.* 2008;22(6):672-675.

100. Shumway-Cook A, Brauer S, Woollacott M. Predicting the probability for falls in community-dwelling older adults using the Timed Up & Go Test. *Phys Ther.* 2000;80(9):896-903.

101. Di Fabio R, Anacker S. Identifying fallers in community living elders using a clinical test of sensory interaction for balance. *Eur J Phys Rehab Med.* 1996;6(2):61-66.

102. Weiner D, Duncan P, Chandler J, Studenski S. Functional reach: A marker of physical frailty. *J Am Geriatr.* 1992;40(3):203-207.

103. Liu-Ambrose T, Khan KM, Donaldson MG, Eng JJ, Lord SR, McKay HA. Falls-related self-efficacy is independently associated with balance and mobility in older women with low bone mass. *J Gerontol.* 2006;61(8):832-838.

104. Tiedemann A, Shimada H, Sherrington C, Murray S, Lord S. The comparative ability of eight functional mobility tests for predicting falls in community-dwelling older people. *Age Ageing.* 2008;37(4):430-435.

105. Faber MJ, Bosscher RJ, van Wieringen PC. Clinimetric properties of the performance-oriented mobility assessment. *Phys Ther.* 2006;86(7):944-954.

106. Hernandez D, Rose DJ. Predicting which older adults will or will not fall using the Fullerton Advanced Balance scale. *Arch Phys Med Rehab.* 2008;89(12):2309-2315.

107. Verghese J, Buschke H, Viola L, et al. Validity of divided attention tasks in predicting falls in older individuals: A preliminary study. *J Am Geriatrics Society.* 2002;50(9):1572-1576.

108. Lusardi MM, Pellecchia GL, Schulman M. Functional performance in community living older adults. *J Geriatr Phys Ther.* 2003;26(3):14-22.

109. Tinetti ME, Richman D, Powell L. Falls efficacy as a measure of fear of falling. *J Gerontol.* 1990;45(6):P239-P243.

110. Lajoie Y, Gallagher SP. Predicting falls within the elderly community: Comparison of postural sway, reaction time, the Berg balance scale and the Activities-specific Balance Confidence (ABC) scale for comparing fallers and non-fallers. *Arch Gerontol Geriat.* 2004;38(1):11-26.

Chapter 29

1. De Inocencio J. Epidemiology of musculoskeletal pain in primary care. *Arch Dis Child.* 2004;89:431-434.

2. Hansman, CF. Appearance and fusion of ossification centers in the human skeleton. *Am J Roentgenol Ra.* 1962;88:476-482.

3. Roche, A. National Health Survey. Skeletal Maturity of Youths 12-17 Years: Racial, Geographic Area, and Socioeconomic Differentials United States, 1966-1970: Series 11 (No. 160); HRA 77-1642.

4. Ravelli A, Martini A. Juvenile idiopathic arthritis. *Lancet.* 2007;369: 767-778.

5. Colbert, RA. Classification of juvenile spondyloarthritis: Enthesitis-related arthritis and beyond. *Nat Rev Rheumatol.* 2010;6:477-485.

6. Emery AEH. Population frequencies of inherited neuromuscular diseases: A world survey. *Neuromuscular Disord.* 1991;1:19-29.

7. Eagle M, Baudouinb S, Chandlerc C, et al. Survival in Duchenne muscular dystrophy: Improvements in life expectancy since 1967 and the impact of home nocturnal ventilation. *Neuromuscular Disord.* 2002;12:926-929.

8. Passamano L, Talia A, Palladino A, et al. Improvement of survival in Duchenne muscular dystrophy: Retrospective analysis of 835 patients. *Acta Myologica.* 2012;31:121-125.

9. Emery A, Skinner R. Clinical studies in benign (Becker type) X-linked muscular dystrophy. *Clin Genet.* 1976;10(4):189-201.

10. Gregoretti C, Ottonello G, Testa M, et al. Survival of patients with spinal muscular atrophy type 1. *Pediatrics.* 2013;131:e1509-e1514.

11. Angelini C, Tasca E. Fatigue in muscular dystrophies. *Neuromuscular Disord.* 2012;22:S214-S220.

12. Centers for Disease Control. Available from: www.cdc.gov/obesity/data/childhood.html. Accessed on March 12, 2014.

13. Wearing SC, Henning EM, Byrne NM, et al. The impact of childhood obesity on musculoskeletal form. *Obes Rev.* 2006;7:209-218.

14. Restrepo R, Reed M. Impact of obesity in the diagnosis of SCFE and knee problems in obese children. *Pediatr Radiol.* 2009;39(suppl 2):S220-S225.

15. Lazar-Antman M, Leet A. Effects of obesity on pediatric fracture care and management. *J Bone Joint Surg Am.* 2012;94:855-861.

16. Smith SM, Sumar B, Dixon KA. Musculoskeletal pain in overweight and obese children. *Int J Obesity.* 2014;38:11-15.

17. Callewaert B, Malfait F, Loeys B, et al. Ehlers-Danlos syndromes and Marfan syndrome. *Best Pract Res Cl Rh.* 2008;22(1):165-189.

18. Hamod A, Moodie D, Clark B, Traboulsi E. Presenting signs and clinical diagnosis in individuals referred to rule out Marfan syndrome. *Ophthalmic Genet.* 2003;24(1):35-39.

19. Martin E, Shapiro J. Osteogenesis imperfecta: Epidemiology and pathophysiology. *Curr Osteoporos Rep.* 2007;5:91-97.

20. McMaster M, Singh H. Natural history of congenital kyphosis and kyphoscoliosis. *J Bone Joint Surg.* 1999;81(10):1367-1383.

21. Lowe T, Line B. Evidence-based medicine analysis of Scheuermann kyphosis. *Spine.* 2007;32(19)(suppl):S115-S119.

22. Konieczny M, Senyurt H, Krauspe R. Epidemiology of adolescent idiopathic scoliosis. *J Child Orthop.* 2013;7:3-9.

23. Langensiepen S, Semler O, Sobottke R, et al. Measuring procedures to determine the Cobb angle in idiopathic scoliosis: A systematic review. *Eur Spine J.* 2013;22:2360-2371.

24. Cote P, Kreitz B, Cassidy J, et al. A study of the diagnostic accuracy and reliability of the scoliometer and the Adam's forward bend test. *Spine.* 1998;23(7):796-803.

25. Kotwicki T, Chowanska J, Kinel E, et al. Optimal management of idiopathic scoliosis in adolescence. *Adolescent Health, Medicine and Therapeutics.* 2013;4:59-73.

26. Diab M. Physical examination in adolescent idiopathic scoliosis. *Neurosurg Clin N Am.* 2007;18:229-236.

27. Cheng J, Tang D, Chen T, et al. The clinical presentation and outcome of treatment of congenital muscular torticollis in infants: A study of 1,086 cases. *J Pediatr Surg.* 2000;35:1091-1096.

28. Stellwagen L, Hubbard E, Chambers C, Lyons Jones K. Torticollis, facial asymmetry and plagiocephaly in normal newborns. *Arch Dis Child.* 2008;93(10):827-831.

29. de Chalain T, Park S. Torticollis associated with positional plagiocephaly: A growing epidemic. *J Craniofac Surg.* 2005;16(3):411-418.

30. Tatli B, Aydinli N, Cahskan M, et al. Congenital muscular torticollis: Evaluation and classification. *Pediatr Neurol.* 2006;34:41-44.

31. Kaplan S, Coulter C, Fetters L. Physical therapy management of congenital muscular torticollis: An evidence-based clinical practice guideline. *Pediatr Phys Ther.* 2013;25(4):348-394.

32. Ohman A, Nilsson S, Beckung E. Validity and reliability of the muscle function scale, aimed to assess the lateral flexors of the neck in infants. *Physiother Theory Pract.* 2009;25(2):129-137.

33. Ohman A, Nillson S, Lagerkvist A-L. Are infants with torticollis at risk of a delay in early motor milestones compared to a control group of healthy infants? *Dev Med Child Neur.* 2009;51(7):545-550.

34. Abzug J, Kozin S. Evaluation and management of brachial plexus birth palsy. *Orth Clin N Am.* 2014;25:225-232.

35. Eng GD, Koch B, Smokvina MD. Brachial plexus palsy in neonates and children. *Arch Phys Med Rehab.* 1978;59(10):458-464.

36. Curtis C, Stephens D, Clark H, Andrews D. The active movement scale: An evaluative tool for infants with obstetrical brachial plexus palsy. *J Hand Surg.* 2002;27A(3):470-478.

37. Bae D, Waters P, Zurakowski D. Reliability of three classification systems measuring active motion in brachial plexus birth palsy. *J Bone Joint Surg.* 2003;85A(9):1733-1738.

38. Shanley E, Thigpen C. Throwing injuries in the adolescent athlete. *Int J Sports Phys Ther.* 2013;8(5):630-640.

39. Krul M, van der Wouden JC, van Suijlekom-Smit LWA, Koes BW. Manipulative interventions for reducing pulled elbow in young children. *Cochrane Db Syst Rev.* 2012;1:CD007759.

40. Cooper C, Dennison EM, Leufkens HG, Bishop N, van Staa TP. Epidemiology of childhood fractures in Britain: A study using the general practice research database. *Am Soc Bone Mineral Res.* 2004;19(12):1976-1981.

41. Storvold G, Aarethun K, Bratberg G. Age for onset of walking and prewalking strategies. *Early Hum Dev.* 2013;89:655-659.

42. Sutherland D. The development of mature gait. *Gait Posture.* 1997;6:163-170.

43. Bly L. *Motor Skills Acquisition in the First Year.* San Antonio, TX: Therapy Skill Builders; 1994.

44. Nemeth B, Narotam V. Developmental dysplasia of the hip. *Pediatr Rev.* 2012;33:553-561.

45. Choudry Q, Goyal R, Paton R. Is limitation of hip abduction a useful clinical sign in the diagnosis of developmental dysplasia of the hip? *Arch Dis Child.* 2013;98:862-866.

46. Shah H. Perthes disease evaluation and management. *Orthop Clin N Am.* 2014;45:87-97.

47. Sawyer J, Kapoor M. The limping child. A systematic approach to diagnosis. *Am Fam Physician.* 2009;79(3):215-224.

48. Novais E, Millis M. Slipped capital femoral epiphysis: Prevalence, pathogenesis, and natural history. *Clin Orthop Relat Res.* 2012;470:3432-3438.

49. Kocher M, Mandinga R, Zurakowski D, et al. Validation of a clinical prediction rule for the differentiation between septic arthritis and transient synovitis of the hip in children. *J Bone Joint Surg.* 2004;86A(8):1629-1635.

50. Gholve P, Scher D, Khakharia S, et al. Osgood Schlatter syndrome. *Curr Opin Pediatr*. 2007;18:44-50.

51. Wynne-Davies R. Genetic and environmental factors in the etiology of talipes equinovarus. *Clin Orthop*. 1972;84:29-38.

52. Roye D, Roye B. Idiopathic congenital talipes equinovarus. *J Am Acad Orthop Surg*. 2002;10:239-248.

53. Wainwright A, Auld T, Benson M, Thelogis T. The classification of congenital talipes equinovarus. *J Bone Joint Surg Br*. 2002;84B:1020-1024.

54. Dimeglio A, Bensahel H, Souchet PH, et al. Classification of clubfoot. *J Pediatr Orthop*.1995;4(2):129-136.

55. Barry RJ, Scranton PE. Flat feet in children. *Clin Orthop Rel Res*. 1983;181:68.

56. Pfeiffer M, Kotz R, Ledl T, et al. Prevalence of flat foot in preschool-aged children. *Pediatrics*. 2006;118(2):634-639.

57. Mckie J, Radomisli T. Congenital vertical talus: A review. *Clin Podiatr Med Surg*. 2010:27;145-156.

Index

Page numbers ending in an *f* or a *t* indicate a figure or table, respectively.

Cozen's test 615
CPRs (clinical prediction rules) 104-105, 241, 964
Craig's test 763-764
cramps 41
cranial nerve examination 114, 115*t*
craniocervical flexion test (CCFT) 342
craniomandibular complex. *See* temporomandibular joint
crank test 547-548
crepitation test 272
crepitus 174, 261
CRH (cortiocotropin-releasing hormone) 35
cross-body adduction test 537-538, 558
crossed syndrome 220-221, 221*f*
C-sign pattern 742
CT. *See* computed tomography
CTQ (Brigham and Women's carpal tunnel questionnaire) 653
CTS. *See* carpal tunnel syndrome
cubital tunnel syndrome 626-627, 637-638
cuboid dorsal glide 892
cuboid plantar glide 892
CVT (congenital vertical talus) 996
cystic fibrosis 956

D

DASH (Disabilities of the Arm, Shoulder, and Hand) 507, 591, 653
DDH (developmental dysplasia of the hip) 993
decorin 23
deep peroneal nerve palpation 137
deep tendon reflex testing 121, 123*t*
deep venous thrombosis (DVT) 44, 102-103, 879
Deerfield's test 487
deformity, open injury, tenderness, swelling (DOTS) 958
degenerative disc disease
    cervical spine 343-345
    lumbar spine 447-450
deltoid extension lag sign test 563
dendrites 26
De Quervain's tenosynovitis 712-713
dermatomes 26
Description of Specialty Practice for Orthopedic Physical Therapy 175
developmental dysplasia of the hip (DDH) 993
dexterity 706, 707-708*t*
diabetes mellitus (DM) 959-960
diagnostic imaging
    basic competencies 92
    cervical spine 292-297, 293*t*
    computed tomography 96
    considerations for using 96
    elbow and forearm 591-596, 592*t*
    face and head 232-234, 233*t*
    hip joint 736-741, 737*t*, 738-739*f*
    knee joint 807-810, 807*t*, 808*f*, 809*f*
    LLA 871*t*, 871-874, 872*f*, 873*f*
    lumbar spine 407-410, 408*t*, 409*t*
    magnetic resonance imaging 95-96, 95*t*
    for medically related conditions 93-94*t*
    nuclear medicine studies 96
    radiography 92, 94-95
    sacroiliac joint 469-470, 469*t*
    shoulder 508-511, 509*t*, 510*f*
    thoracic spine 370-371, 370*t*
    ultrasound 96-97
    wrist and hand 654-656, 654*t*
dial test 770
differential diagnosis. *See* medical screening examination; triage and screening

Diméglio classification 996
DIP (distal interphalangeal). *See* wrist and hand motion tests
Disabilities of the Arm, Shoulder, and Hand (DASH) 507, 591, 653
dislocations
    causes in the elbow 590
    defined 45
    diagnostic imaging of the elbow 593
    diagnostic imaging of the foot 872*f*, 873
    diagnostic imaging of the hip 738, 740
    elbow pathology assessment 636-637, 642-644, 992
    foot pathology assessment 938
    shoulder pathology assessment 575
    tests for shoulder 513, 554-556, 563
distal biceps rupture assessment 633-634
distal biceps tear/rupture tests
    biceps crease interval 618-619
    biceps squeeze 616
    bicipital aponeurosis flexion 619
    cluster testing 619
    hook 617
    passive forearm pronation 617-618
distal humeral fractures assessment 638-640
distal interphalangeal (DIP). *See* wrist and hand motion tests
distal radius fracture test 701
distraction test 482
Dix-Hallpike test 238, 309
dizziness, cervicogenic (CGD) 363
dizziness, vestibular system 252-254
DM (diabetes mellitus) 959-960
DMD (Duchenne muscular dystrophy) 985
dorsal capitate displacement test 700
dorsiflexion-eversion test 923
dorsiflexion lunge with compression test 919
DOTS (deformity, open injury, tenderness, swelling) 958
drop arm test 540-541
drop foot gait 203
drop sign test 543
drop vertical jump test 183-184
Duchenne muscular dystrophy (DMD) 985
Dupuytren's contracture 728
Durkan's test 689
DVT (deep venous thrombosis) 44, 102-103
Dynamic Gait index 974, 978
dynamic knee test 828
dynamometry, handheld 158
dysarthria 232
dysphasia 232
dysphonia 232

E

ear examination 241-242
EBP. *See* evidence-based practice
eccentric step-down test 843
ectomorph body type 215-216, 216*f*
ECU synergy test 693
edema
    defined 172-173
    tests for 903, 907, 908
effusion test 830
Ege's test 825
Ehler-Danlos syndrome (EDS) 986
EIB (exercise-induced bronchoconstriction) 955
EIP (evidence-informed practice) 52
elastic cartilage 7

About the Author

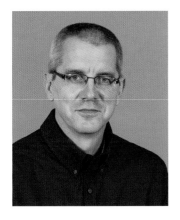

Michael P. Reiman, PT, DPT, OCS, SCS, ATC, FAAOMPT, CSCS, is an assistant professor of physical therapy and the codirector of the orthopaedic manual therapy fellowship program at Duke University Medical Center. As a clinician, Reiman has more than 20 years of experience assessing, rehabilitating, and training athletes and clients. He has presented on orthopedic assessment and treatment methods at national and international conferences and actively participates in research regarding various testing methods for orthopedic examination and intervention and human performance. Reiman coauthored *Functional Testing in Human Performance* and has written 12 book chapters and more than 40 peer-reviewed articles. He currently serves on the editorial boards for multiple sport- and orthopedic-related journals.

Reiman received his doctoral degree in physical therapy from MGH Institute of Health Professions and is currently pursuing his PhD. In addition to his certifications as an athletic trainer and strength and conditioning specialist, Reiman is a manual therapy fellow through the American Academy of Orthopaedic and Manual Physical Therapists, a USA Weightlifting level 1 coach, and a USA Track and Field level 1 coach. He is also the chair of the Sports Section Hip Special Interest Group of the American Physical Therapy Association.

Contributor List

Gary P. Austin, PT, PhD, OCS, FAFS, FAAOMPT

    Associate professor
    Doctor of physical therapy program
    Lynchburg College
    Lynchburg, VA

Robert J. Butler, PT, DPT, PhD

    Assistant professor
    Division of physical therapy
    Michael W. Krzyzewski human performance laboratory
    Duke University
    Durham, NC

Shefali Christopher, PT, DPT, SCS, LAT, ATC

    Clinician educator
    Doctor of physical therapy division
    Duke University
    Durham, NC

John DeWitt, PT, DPT, SCS, ATC

    Clinical assistant professor
    Division of physical therapy
    Rehab manager, OSU sports medicine
    Ohio State University
    Columbus, OH

Christopher Fiander, PT, DPT, OCS, CSCS

    Clinical care coordinator
    Department of physical and occupational therapy
    Duke University
    Durham, NC

Dora J. Gosselin, PT, DPT, PCS, C/NDT

    Senior pediatric physical therapist
    Adjunct associate
    Doctor of physical therapy program
    Duke University
    Durham, NC
    Adjunct faculty
    Doctor of physical therapy program
    Winston Salem State University
    Winston-Salem, NC

Dawn Driesner Kennedy, PT, DPT, OCS, COMT, FAAOMPT

    Senior level physical therapist
    SSM Select Medical Physical Therapy
    Hazelwood, MO

David Logerstedt, PT, PhD, MPT, SCS

    Research assistant professor
    Department of physical therapy and interdisciplinary program in biomechanics and movement science
    University of Delaware
    Newark, DE

Janice K. Loudon, PT, PhD, SCS, ATC

    Associate professor
    Department of physical therapy education
    Rockhurst University
    Kansas City, MO

Adriaan Louw, PT, PhD, CSMT

    CEO, International Spine and Pain Institute
    Story City, IA

B. James Massey, PT, DPT, OCS, FAAOMPT

    Assistant professor of physical therapy
    Doctor of physical therapy program
    Wingate University
    Wingate, NC

Mark F. Reinking, PT, PhD, SCS, ATC

    Associate professor
    Board-certified specialist in sports physical therapy
    Chairman, department of physical therapy and athletic training
    Program director, program in physical therapy
    Doisy College of Health Sciences, Saint Louis University
    St. Louis, MO

Tasala Rufai, PT, DPT, GCS

    Staff physical therapist
    Physical medicine and rehabilitation services
    Durham Veterans Affairs Medical Center
    Durham, NC

Mitch Salsbery, PT, DPT, SCS, CSCS

    Physical therapist
    OSU sports medicine
    Ohio State University
    Columbus, OH

Michael Schmidt, PT, DPT, OCS, FAAOMPT

Codirector orthopaedic manual physical therapy program
Senior level physical therapist
Department of physical and occupational therapy
Duke University Hospital
Durham, NC

Charles Sheets, PT, OCS, SCS, Dip MDT

Codirector orthopaedic physical therapist residency
Department of physical and occupational therapy
Duke University Hospital
Durham, NC
Adjunct associate
Department of orthopaedic surgery
Duke University Medical Center
Durham, NC

Jonathan Sylvain, PT, DPT, OCS, FAAOMPT

Rehabilitation services supervisor
Spine rehabilitation
UConn Health
Farmington, CT

Gilbert M. Willett, PT, PhD, OCS, CSCS

Associate professor
Division of physical therapy education
University of Nebraska medical center
Omaha, NE

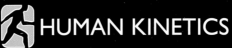
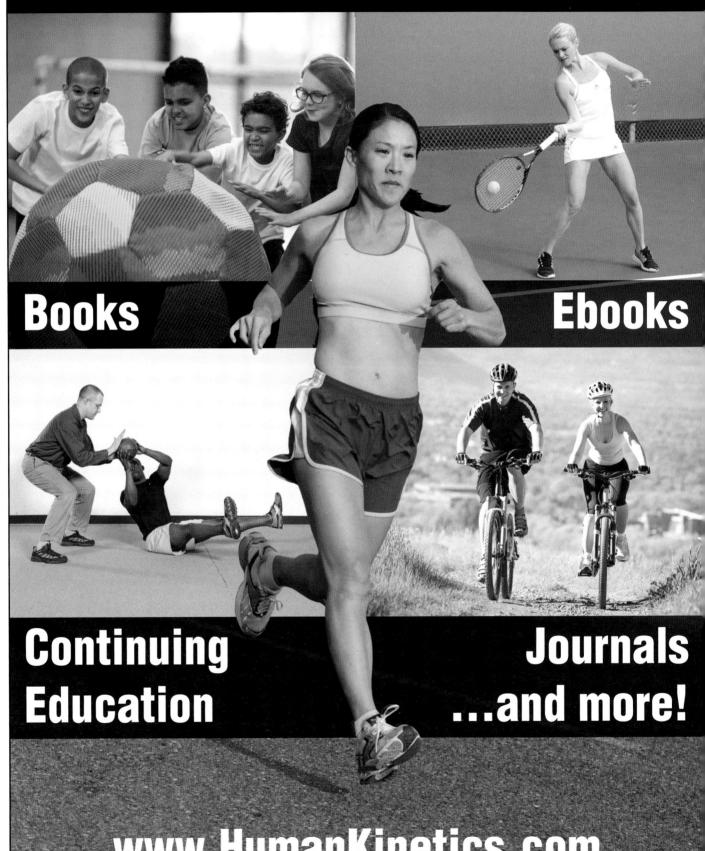